PATHOPHYSIOLOGY
CLINICAL CONCEPTS OF DISEASE PROCESSES

PATHOPHYSIOLOGY
CLINICAL CONCEPTS OF DISEASE PROCESSES

THIRD EDITION

SYLVIA ANDERSON PRICE, Ph.D., R.N.
LORRAINE McCARTY WILSON, Ph.D., R.N.

McGRAW-HILL BOOK COMPANY

New York   St. Louis   San Francisco   Auckland   Bogotá   Hamburg   Johannesburg   London
Madrid   Mexico   Montreal   New Delhi   Panama   Paris
São Paulo   Singapore   Sydney   Tokyo   Toronto

NOTICE

As new medical and nursing research and clinical experience broaden our knowledge, changes in treatment and drug therapy are required. The editors and the publisher of this work have made every effort to ensure that the drug dosage schedules herein are accurate and in accord with the standards accepted at the time of publication. Readers are advised, however, to check the product information sheet included in the package of each drug they plan to administer to be certain that changes have not been made in the recommended dose or in the contraindications for administration. This recommendation is of particular importance in regard to new or infrequently used drugs.

PATHOPHYSIOLOGY:
CLINICAL CONCEPTS OF DISEASE PROCESSES

1 2 3 4 5 6 7 8 9 0   DOWDOW   8 9 8 7 6

ISBN 0-07-050864-X

This book was set in Electra by University Graphics, Inc.
The editors were Sally J. Barhydt and James W. Bradley;
the designer was Anne Canevari Green;
the production supervisor was Phil Galea.
Medical illustrations were done by Margaret Croup Brudon.
R. R. Donnelley & Sons Company was printer and binder.

Library of Congress-in-Publication Data
Main entry under title:

Pathophysiology: clinical concepts of disease processes.

  Includes bibliographies and index.
  1. Physiology, Pathological.   2. Nursing.   I. Price,
Sylvia Anderson.   II. Wilson, Lorraine McCarty.   [DNLM:
1. Pathology—nurses' instruction.   QZ 4 P302]
RB113.P363   1986   616.07   85–18010
ISBN O-07-050864-X

CONTENTS

PART I

INTRODUCTION TO GENERAL PATHOLOGY: MECHANISMS OF DISEASE
Gerald D. Abrams

PART II

DISTURBANCES OF IMMUNE MECHANISMS
William R. Solomon

PART VI

RESPIRATORY PATHOPHYSIOLOGY
Lorraine M. Wilson and Sylvia A. Price

PART VII

RENAL PATHOPHYSIOLOGY
Lorraine M. Wilson

PART VIII

NEUROLOGIC DISORDERS
Mary Carter Lombardo

PART IX

ENDOCRINE AND METABOLIC DISORDERS
David E. Schteingart

PART X

ORTHOPEDICS
Larry S. Matthews

PART XI

RHEUMATIC DISORDERS
Michael A. Carter

PART XII

DERMATOLOGY
Marek A. Stawiski and Jeffrey P. Callen

LIST OF CONTRIBUTORS

Gerald D. Abrams, M.D.
Professor of Pathology
Department of Pathology
The University of Michigan
Medical School
Ann Arbor, Michigan

Catherine M. Baldy, R.N., M.S.
Clinical Nurse Specialist in Hematology
Henry Ford Hospital
Detroit, Michigan

Jeffrey P. Callen, M.D.
Assistant Clinical Professor of Medicine
(Dermatology)
University of Louisville
School of Medicine
Louisville, Kentucky

Michael A. Carter, D.N.Sc., R. N., F.A.A.N.
Professor and Dean
College of Nursing
The University of Tennessee
Center for the Health Sciences
Memphis, Tennessee

Daniel J. Fall, M.D.
Clinical Associate Professor of Internal Medicine
The University of Michigan
Ann Arbor, Michigan

Penny J. Ford, R.N., M.S.
Cardiovascular Clinical Nurse Specialist
Massachusetts General Hospital
Boston, Massachusetts

Ellen Kinnealy, R.N., M.S.
Inservice Educator
Intensive Care Nursing Service
Massachusetts General Hospital
Boston, Massachusetts

Mary Carter Lombardo, R.N., B.S.N., M.S.N.
Assistant Professor of Nursing
Howard Community College
Columbia, Maryland

Nancy Reidy MacDonald, R.N., B.S.
Technical Director, Vascular Laboratory
Massachusetts General Hospital
Boston, Massachusetts

Larry S. Matthews, M.D.
Professor of Surgery
Section of Orthopaedic Surgery
The University of Michigan
Medical School
Ann Arbor, Michigan

Madeline M. O'Donnell, R.N., M.S.
Inservice Educator
Cardiac Surgery Intensive Care
Massachusetts General Hospital
Boston, Massachusetts

Sylvia Anderson Price, Ph.D., R.N.
Research Associate
Former coordinator of pathophysiology course
The University of Michigan
School of Nursing
Ann Arbor, Michigan

David E. Schteingart, M.D.
 Professor of Internal Medicine
 The University of Michigan
 Medical School
 Ann Arbor, Michigan

William R. Solomon, M.D.
 Professor of Internal Medicine
 The University of Michigan
 Medical School
 Ann Arbor, Michigan

Marek A. Stawiski, M.D.
 Clinical Assistant Professor of Dermatology and
 Postgraduate Medicine
 The University of Michigan
 Ann Arbor, Michigan
 Clinical Assistant Professor of Internal Medicine
 Michigan State University
 East Lansing, Michigan

F. Michael Vislosky, R.N., B.S.
 Head Nurse, Coronary Care
 Massachusetts General Hospital
 Boston, Massachusetts

Lorraine McCarty Wilson, Ph.D., R.N.
 Associate Professor of Nursing
 Oakland University
 Rochester, Michigan
 Former coordinator of pathophysiology course
 The University of Michigan
 Ann Arbor, Michigan

PREFACE

The third edition of *Pathophysiology: Clinical Concepts of Disease Processes* retains the same philosophy and organization as the two previous editions, which have been used extensively as major textbooks in nursing and other professions in the health care field. Our focus is on alterations in biological processes which affect the body's dynamic equilibrium or homeostasis, a conceptual approach that is designed to integrate knowledge from the basic and clinical sciences.

Pathophysiology emphasizes the *dynamic* aspects of disease. It is concerned with the disruption of normal physiology: the alterations, derangements, and mechanisms involved and their manifestations as signs, symptoms, and physical and laboratory findings. Pathophysiology provides the common bond linking anatomy, physiology, and biochemistry to clinical practice. The study of pathophysiology is essential to understanding the rationale for medical and surgical therapy.

This edition incorporates significant changes suggested by faculty, students, and others who have used the book. Major revisions and additions appear in Part V, "Cardiovascular Pathophysiology," which now includes an extensive discussion of cardiogenic shock and congestive heart failure, an updating of cardiovascular techniques with the many advances in noninvasive techniques, the latest advances and hemodynamic monitoring techniques, and a complete revision of the chapter on vascular disease. In Part VI, "Respiratory Pathophysiology," the chapter on respiratory failure has been rewritten to include more extensive treatment of respiratory acid-base disturbances and blood gas interpretations, and the discussion of respiratory distress syndrome has been expanded. In Part VII, "Renal Pathophysiology," the chapter on acute renal failure has been completely rewritten and expanded and contains new material on neurogenic bladder. The discussion of transplant immunology includes advances in the field. Part VIII, "Neurologic Disorders," contains new material on Alzheimer's disease, Reyes's syndrome, and nutritional degenerative diseases. Part IX, "Endocrine and Metabolic Disorders," has been extensively revised to incorporate the most recent advances in diagnostic procedures relative to endocrine disorders and new material on disorders of the female reproductive cycle. Part XI, "Rheumatic Disorders," has been completely rewritten to include an extensive discussion of pathophysiological mechanisms that underlie rheumatic disorders. Finally, Part XII, "Dermatology," has been extensively revised with new material on acquired immune deficiency syndrome (AIDS) and cutaneous infections.

Throughout this edition, the authors have incorporated recent research findings, new diagnostic procedures, and current treatment principles. Many illustrations have been replaced and over 100 new ones added. There are over 200 new end-of-chapter questions.

This textbook is designed to meet the sophisticated needs of health care professionals. Because of the numerous advances in the biomedical sciences, changes in patterns of health care delivery, and consumer influence to decrease health care expenditures, nurses and other health care professionals must be accountable for the implementation of quality client-centered care. The role of the practitioner in the health care delivery system continues to change. Nurses are functioning as independent practitioners in a variety of health care settings, such as primary health care. Nurses assume major responsibility for managing the holistic health care of clients. They work cooperatively with professionals from other health disciplines to ensure that quality client-centered care is administered. It is essential that health care professionals synthesize pathophysiological concepts in order to understand the rationale for therapeutic regimens.

The unique feature of this book is that the subject is presented in a self-instructional format. Objectives are included for each part and chapter. These objectives focus the learner's attention on the important concepts presented. The conceptual material is then followed by questions and answers on the content. This self-instructional method enables the student to actively participate in the learning process through reading, reasoning, and demonstrating in writing his or her mastery of the concepts as opposed to merely memorizing factual material. The authors believe that this method enables one to achieve maximum understanding of the subject material. In addition, the pace may be one that the student finds most comfortable.

The conceptual model is presented in the following fashion. First, the general concepts of disease processes are discussed; then the various disorders of an organ or organ system are reviewed. Emphasis is on understanding the roots of a given disorder, which is an essential factor in the development of insight. For example, consider disorders of the kidney. The student who thoroughly understands the nephron, which is the fundamental work unit of the kidney, is better able to predict what diseases will occur when certain pathophysiological processes involve the kidney. That student will understand the basis for such diseases as pyelonephritis, glomerulonephritis, and the nephroses. Moreover, the student will understand the rationale for the treatment.

This textbook provides the reader with an in-depth presentation of pathophysiological mechanisms that are essential to the understanding of disease processes. In order to reduce the subject matter to manageable dimensions, the authors have focused on relevant concepts that are applicable to optimum practices of modern health care delivery.

ACKNOWLEDGMENTS

Our sincere appreciation:

To Karol Carstensen, former Nursing Editor at McGraw-Hill Book Company, for her contributions during the initial phase of revision.

To Sally J. Barhydt, Nursing Editor, and Eileen Dowd, former Editorial Assistant at McGraw-Hill Book Company, for their support and enthusiasm.

To James W. Bradley, Senior Editing Supervisor at McGraw-Hill Book Company, for the excellent quality of his editorial assistance.

To Susan Zenow for the excellent quality of her work in typing the manuscript.

We also appreciate the review and suggestions on selected portions of the manuscript offered by the following: Francile C. Clevenger, Colleen C. Miller, Phyllis Coindreau Patterson, and Paula Wilson Saari.

Sylvia Anderson Price
Lorraine McCarty Wilson

PART I

GERALD D. ABRAMS

INTRODUCTION TO GENERAL PATHOLOGY: MECHANISMS OF DISEASE

The intent of Part I of this book is to provide the reader with the background necessary for the understanding of the many different diseases to which human beings fall victim. The number of specific human diseases is immense and the variety is great, given the fact that no organ or organ system within the body is exempt from disease. However, the basic ways in which an organ can become diseased are quite limited, and the large and bewildering array of diseases actually represents different combinations and permutations of a smaller number of basic biological processes leading to the alterations of structure and function that are recognized clinically. It is on these basic biological processes that this first section will be focused.

The study of such basic disease processes is usually called *general pathology*. Pathology is the science or study of disease. In its broadest sense, pathology is literally abnormal biology, the study of sick or disordered life. As a basic biological science, the study of pathology includes such fields as plant pathology, insect pathology, and veterinary and comparative pathology, as well as human pathology, which is the major focus of this text.

Pathology, in the context of human medicine, is not only a basic or theoretical science but also a clinical medical specialty. Pathologists are specialists in laboratory medicine; they provide a consultative service to other physicians, thereby assisting in the diagnosis and treatment of disease. The scope of laboratory medicine is such as to include all of the many types of studies performed on samples derived from patients, including samples of tissue and of blood and other body fluids. Some laboratory studies which fall under the general heading of *anatomic pathology* involve the study and assessment of morphologic alterations in cells and tissues. Surgical pathology, exfoliative cytology, and autopsy pathology are included in this division. Many types of studies are done by other than morphologic means, and these areas of *clinical pathology* include such things as clinical chemistry, microbiology, hematology, immunology, and immunohematology.

In this part the specifics of individual diseases will not be discussed. However, fundamental disease processes, such as inflammation, neoplasia, and immunologic injury, will be described. Following the elucidation of these fundamental processes, the details of specific illnesses will be addressed in later parts of the text.

OBJECTIVES

At the completion of this part you should be able to:

1. Describe the essential features of basic disease processes including the body's reactions to injury and infection, the immune response, disturbances of circulation, and abnormalities of cellular growth.
2. Interpret the natural history and clinical manifestations of specific illnesses in terms of their etiology and pathogenesis.

GENERAL CONCEPTS OF DISEASE—HEALTH VERSUS DISEASE

OBJECTIVES

At the completion of this chapter you should be able to:

1. Define *pathology*.
2. Formulate a definition of pathophysiology.
3. Explain the complexities associated with the concept of normalcy.
4. Differentiate between etiology and pathogenesis in relation to disease.
5. Critically assess the essential elements involved in the disease process.
6. Identify and use the following terms when describing the manifestations of a disease: symptom, sign, lesion, sequel, complication.

CONCEPT OF NORMALCY

In terms of their personal experiences, most people have some notion of what it is to be "normal" and would define disease or illness in terms of deviation from or absence of that normal state. However, on closer scrutiny, the concept of normalcy turns out to be a complex one which cannot be defined succinctly; correspondingly, the concept of disease is far from simple.

Selecting any parameter of measurement which might be applied to an individual or group of individuals, we define *normal* as some sort of average value for that parameter. Thus, average values for parameters such as height, weight, and blood pressure are derived from observations on many individuals. Implicitly, a certain amount of variation from the average is ac-

cepted as being permissible or normal. Thus, the usual concept of normalcy involves both an average value and some range of variation either above or below that value.

Variation in normal values actually stems from several different sources. First, it is recognized that individuals differ from one another because of differences in their genetic makeup. Thus, no two individuals in the world, except for those derived from the same fertilized ovum, have exactly the same genes. Second, there is variation related to the fact that individuals differ in their life experiences and in their interaction with the environment. Third, even in a single individual, many physiologic parameters vary because of the way in which the control mechanisms of the body function. For instance, measurement of blood glucose concentrations in a healthy person would reveal significant variations at different times during the day, depending upon food intake, activities of the individual, and so forth. These variations would generally occur within a certain range. The situation is somewhat analogous to a room with thermostatically controlled temperature which may dip slightly below the desired or ideal level before such a drop is sensed by the thermostat. The corrective action then triggered by the thermostat may, in turn, overshoot the ideal slightly before the heat input is halted. Indeed such variations in body temperature, even in the normal state, do occur in all individuals. Finally, for those physiologic parameters that must be measured by fairly intricate means, a significant amount of variation in observed values may be derived from error or imprecision inherent in the measurement process itself.

Because of the above considerations, establishing limits on this "normal" range of variation from an average value is a matter of some complexity. This complexity relates to such things as knowing the degree of physiologic oscillation of a particular measurement, accounting for the degree of variation among normal individuals even under baseline conditions, and figuring the precision of the measurement method. Then, finally, the biological significance of the measurement must be estimated. It is thus evident that single measurements, observations, or laboratory results which seem to be indicative of abnormality must always be judged in the context of the entire individual. A single reading of elevated blood pressure does not make an individual hypertensive; a single slightly elevated blood glucose level does not relegate an individual to the category of diabetics; and a single hemoglobin value lower than average does not necessarily indicate anemia.

Finally, to place all of the above considerations in perspective, it should be noted that concepts of normalcy and even of disease are, to an extent, arbitrary and are influenced by cultural values as well as by biological realities. For example, in our culture, a defect of central nervous system function manifesting itself as a significant reading disability would be labeled as an abnormality, whereas the same defect might never be noted in a primitive culture. Furthermore, a trait which might be average and thus normal in one population might be considered distinctly abnormal in another. Consider, for instance, how a "normal" person from our population would be viewed by a group of central African pygmies; or conversely, how an infant from a primitive culture, with the "normal" chronic diarrhea and poor weight gain, might be viewed in one of our well-baby clinics!

Bearing in mind the many nuances in the concept of normalcy, *disease* can be defined as a form of life beyond the limits of normal. The most useful biological yardstick for these limits of normalcy relates to the ability of the individual to meet the demands placed on the body and to adapt to these demands or changes in the external environment in such a way as to maintain reasonable constancy of the internal environment. All cells in the body need a certain amount of oxygen and nutrients for their continuing survival and function and also require an environment which affords such things as narrow ranges of temperature, water content, acidity, and salt concentration. Thus, the maintenance of internal conditions within fairly narrow limits is an essential feature of the normal body. When some of the structures and functions of the body deviate from the norm to the point where the ability to maintain homeostasis is destroyed or threatened or where the individual can no longer meet environmental challenges, disease is said to exist. A person's subjective perception of disease is related to impairment of the ability to carry on daily activities comfortably as those limits of normalcy are passed.

Another important element in the concept of disease is the recognition that disease does not involve the development of a completely new form of life but rather is an extension or distortion of the normal life processes that are present in the individual. Even in the case of an obviously infectious disease, where the body is literally invaded, the infectious agent itself does not constitute the disease but only serves to evoke the changes in the subject that ultimately are manifested as disease. Thus, disease is actually the sum of the physiologic processes which have been distorted. In order to understand and adequately treat the disease one must take into account the identity of the normal processes interfered with, the character of the disturbances, and the secondary effects of such disturbances on other vital processes.

An alternative view of disease, certainly not unknown in history, has held that disease is actually a new form of life, a sort of possession of the body by an outside agent. From this notion it would follow that some form of exorcism, which is directed at driving out that agent, is proper therapy of disease. However, even in the instance of an invasive infectious agent, attempted treatment with antibiotics alone may not be sufficient to cure the patient if proper attention is not directed toward the intrinsic body processes which have become deranged.

A theme that will recur, with variations, throughout this volume is that disease above all is part and parcel of the patient. *Normal and abnormal processes represent different points on the same continuous spectrum.* In fact, very often the seeds of disease actually lie within the adaptive machinery of the body itself, machinery which constitutes a potential two-edged sword. For instance, the very same machinery which allows us to become immune to certain infections evokes reactions such as hay fever and asthma when some of us are challenged by particular environmental agents. Similarly, the machinery of cellular proliferation that allows us to repair wounds and constantly to renew cell populations in various tissues may run amok, giving rise to cancer.

DEVELOPMENT OF DISEASE

Etiology

Etiology, in its most general definition, is the assignment of causes or reasons for phenomena. A description of the etiology of a disease includes the identification of those causal factors that, acting in concert, provoke the particular disease. Thus, the tubercle bacillus is designated as the etiologic agent of tuberculosis. Other etiologic factors in the development of tuberculosis which influence the course of the infection include the age, nutritional status, and even the occupation of the individual. It is sufficiently important to mention again that even in the case of an infectious disease such as tuberculosis the agent itself does not constitute the disease. Rather, the resultant of all the responses to that agent, all the perversions of biological processes taken together, constitute the disease. In the etiology of a particular disease, then, a range of extrinsic or exogenous factors in the environment must be considered along with a variety of intrinsic or endogenous characteristics of the host.

Pathogenesis

Pathogenesis of a disease refers to the development or evolution of the disease. To continue with the above example, a description of the pathogenesis of tuberculosis would indicate the mechanisms whereby the invasion of the body by the tubercle bacillus ultimately leads to the observed abnormalities.

Such an analysis of pathogenesis would relate the proliferation and spread of tubercle bacilli to the evolving inflammatory responses, to the immunologic defenses of the host, and to the actual destruction of cells and tissues. The pattern and extent of the tissue damage would ultimately be related to the overt manifestations of clinical disease. The study of pathogenesis also takes into account the sequential occurrence of certain phenomena and the temporal aspects of the evolving disease. Implicit in this approach is the notion that a given disease is not a static affair but rather a dynamic phenomenon with a rhythm and natural history of its own.

In the diagnostic evaluation of patients and the assessment of therapy, it is essential to keep in mind this concept of natural history and the range of variation among different diseases with respect to their natural history. Some diseases, for example, are characteristically of rapid onset, while others have a long prodrome. Some diseases are self-limited; i.e., they clear up spontaneously in a brief time. Others most often become chronic, while yet others are subject to frequent remissions and exacerbations.

When considering the totality of human disease, the number of etiologic factors and the number of separately named diseases seem to be endless. However, even though there are many different diseases with unique natural histories, the situation is not as difficult as indicated by sheer numbers. The response mechanisms of the body are finite. Therefore, disease A differs from disease B because it varies somewhat in terms of this or that pathogenetic mechanism being exaggerated. Thus, the understanding of a manageable number of pathogenetic mechanisms and their evolution permits understanding of a very large number of seemingly different diseases.

Manifestations

Early in the development of a disease, the etiologic agent or agents may provoke a number of changes in biological processes which can be detected by laboratory analysis even though there is no recognition by the patient that these changes have occurred. Thus, many diseases have a *subclinical stage* during which the patient functions normally even though the disease processes are well established. It is important to understand that the structure and function of many organs provides a large reserve or safety margin, so that functional impairment may become evident only when disease has become quite advanced anatomically. For example, chronic renal disease could completely destroy one kidney and partly destroy the other before any symptoms related to decreased renal function would be perceived. Conversely, it is important to recognize that some diseases seem to begin as functional derangements and actually reach the clinical horizon although no anatomic abnormalities can be detected at the time. Such functional illnesses may lead ultimately to secondary structural abnormalities.

As certain biological processes are encroached upon, the patient begins to feel subjectively that something is wrong. These subjective feelings are termed *symptoms* of disease. By definition, symptoms are subjective and can be reported only by the patient to an observer. When, however, the manifestations of the disease involve objectively identifiable aberrations, these are termed *signs* of the disease. Nausea, malaise, and pain are symptoms, while fever, reddening of the skin, and a palpable mass are signs of disease. A demonstrable structural change produced in the course of a disease is referred to as a *lesion*. Lesions may be evident at a gross and/or a microscopic level. The outcome of a disease is sometimes referred to as a *sequel* (plural, *sequelae*). For example, the sequel to an inflammatory process in a given tissue might be a scar in that tissue. The sequel to acute rheumatic inflammation of the heart might be scarred, deformed cardiac valves. A *complication* of disease is a new or separate process that may arise secondarily because of some change produced by the original entity. For example, bacterial pneumonia may be a complication of viral infection of the respiratory tract. Fortunately, many diseases can also undergo what is termed *resolution,* and the host returns to a completely normal state, without sequelae or complications. Resolution can occur spontaneously, i.e., owing to body defenses, or can be a result of successful therapy.

Finally, it is essential to reemphasize that disease is dynamic rather than static. The manifestations of disease in a given patient may change from day to day as biological equilibriums shift and as compensatory mechanisms are brought into play. Environmental influences that are brought to bear upon the patient will also affect the disease. Therefore, every disease has a *range* of manifestations and a *spectrum* of expressions which may vary from patient to patient.

QUESTIONS

General concepts of disease—Health versus disease

Directions: Answer the following questions on a separate sheet of paper.

1. Formulate a definition of pathology and pathophysiology.
2. What is the difference between anatomic and clinical pathology? List at least three examples of types of studies included under each of these divisions.
3. What is the difference between etiology and pathogenesis?
4. Explain the complex factors associated with the concept of normalcy.

Directions: Circle the letter preceding each item below that correctly answers the question. More than one answer may be correct.

5. The study and evaluation of morphologic alterations in cells and tissues is referred to as:
   a. Pathophysiology   *b.* Anatomic pathology
   c. Clinical pathology   *d.* Comparative pathology
6. The outcome of a disease is termed a:
   a. Sequel   *b.* Complication   *c.* Resolution
   d. Lesion
7. In the course of a disease process, a demonstrable structural change which is produced is termed a:
   a. Symptom   *b.* Sign   *c.* Lesion
   d. Sequel   *e.* Complication
8. Which of the following would be considered symptoms?
   a. Edema   *b.* Pallor   *c.* Cyanosis
   d. Headache

CHAPTER 2

HEREDITY, ENVIRONMENT, AND DISEASE; INTERACTION OF HEREDITY AND ENVIRONMENT

OBJECTIVES

At the completion of this chapter you should be able to:

1. Differentiate between extrinsic and intrinsic factors in relation to the disease process.
2. Describe the importance of hereditary factors in disease.
3. Explain the way in which deoxyribonucleic acid (DNA) carries genetic information.
4. Contrast transcription and translation during the process of protein synthesis.
5. Describe how DNA is involved in programming the function of cells.
6. Explain what occurs with regard to DNA and chromosomes during the process of cell division, distinguishing between mitosis and meiosis.
7. Describe the process of differentiation.
8. Explain the process by which genes control the development of a particular trait.
9. Define and discuss the significance of a mutation.
10. Differentiate between dominant and recessive genes.
11. Explain the ways in which chromosomal abnormalities can develop.
12. Define karyotype.
13. Describe the importance of karyotypic anomalies.
14. Identify the way in which genetic abnormalities may be expressed as disease.
15. Identify for Down's syndrome the chromosomal abnormality, physical traits, and risk factors.
16. Explain the rationale for the amniocentesis procedure.
17. Assess the consequences of abnormalities of a single gene.
18. Critically analyze the purpose of genetic counseling.

EXTRINSIC FACTORS IN DISEASE

If one were asked to list some of the important causes of human disease, such things as infectious agents, mechanical trauma, toxic chemicals, radiation, extremes of temperature, nutritional problems, and even psychological stress would likely be mentioned. All of these, along with many others usually placed on such a list, actually represent variations in the environment which can produce disease when brought to bear upon the subject. Certainly it is true that such *extrinsic factors* are exceedingly important causes of human misery, and attention is directed to them in an attempt to prevent and alleviate disease. However, since disease is actually part of the life of the afflicted individual—the sum of the physiologic processes which have been distorted—a view of disease causation that takes into account only extrinsic factors is necessarily incomplete. The intrinsic biological processes must also be taken into consideration.

INTRINSIC FACTORS IN DISEASE

Many characteristics of the individual host must be considered as *intrinsic factors* in disease, inasmuch as they will have significant impact on the evolution of various conditions. Age, sex, and even abnormalities acquired in the course of previous illnesses are factors that need to be considered in the pathogenesis of a disease. Above all, the genetic constitution or *genome* of the individual is an essential part of the "equation." This is true because the anatomic characteristics of the host, the myriad of physiologic mechanisms of everyday life, and the modes of responding to injury are all determined by the genetic information assembled at the moment of conception of the individual. A more familiar way of stating this principle is that in studying the biology of disease one must always take into account both heredity and environment.

Interaction of extrinsic and intrinsic factors— A spectrum

We often hear the question, "Is this disease hereditary?" In a sense, that question is improper. With recognition of the fact that heredity is almost always vitally important, the question should be phrased, "To what extent is heredity important in this disease?" The exceptions to this principle are relatively few and quite extreme. Admittedly, heredity plays no real role in determining the outcome when one is involved in an ex-

plosion or struck by a speeding truck; but, such instances aside, it is always a factor. Even in an exogenous infectious disease, it is clear that genetic factors can influence susceptibility to the infectious agent and also the pattern of disease produced by that agent.

With regard to the relative balance of heredity and environment in the causation of disease, there exists a broad spectrum. At one end of the spectrum are those diseases which are largely determined by some environmental agent irrespective of the individual's hereditary background, while at the other end are those diseases which represent faulty heredity, that is, faulty genetic programming of the body's machinery. These latter diseases include those usually identified as *hereditary diseases*, diseases which are expressed in almost any bearer of the faulty genetic information regardless of extrinsic influences. Between these two ends of the spectrum most human diseases occur and involve a significant interplay between genetic and extrinsic factors. A brief commentary on heredity and an exploration of some of the ways that an inherited abnormality can be expressed would be instructive at this point.

THE NATURE OF THE GENOME

The "stuff" of heredity

Nucleic acids are the chemical materials which are responsible for storing, duplicating, and transmitting all of the information needed for programming the functions of a single cell and thereby those of an entire individual. Nucleic acids are composed of nitrogen-containing bases (purines and pyrimidines), sugar (ribose or deoxyribose), and phosphoric acid. A nucleic acid which contains deoxyribose is called *deoxyribonucleic acid* or DNA, while one which contains ribose is called *ribonucleic acid* or RNA. Nucleic acids are long-chain molecules composed of many mononucleotides, each of which contains a base, a sugar, and phosphoric acid. DNA actually is the carrier of genetic information (i.e., the instructions for the synthesis of proteins), while RNA acts to execute the instructions contained in DNA by serving an intermediary role in protein synthesis.

DNA carries genetic information in a coded form using purine and pyrimidine bases to construct the code. DNA contains four of these nucleotide bases (adenine, guanine, cytosine, and thymine); any three *in a particular order* within the DNA molecule code for a particular amino acid ultimately to be inserted into a given protein. Such three-base sequences are called *codons*. Proteins of the body are made up of some 20 different amino acids and their derivatives, so that the 64 possible three-base sequences that can be derived from various permutations of the four bases in DNA are more than enough codons to control protein biosynthesis. A gene is actually only a portion of a DNA molecule—that portion containing enough information (i.e., enough codons) to determine the sequence of amino acids making up a single polypeptide. A given DNA molecule is large enough to contain many genes. In addition to carrying the genetic code necessary to control protein biosynthesis, DNA has the property of being able to replicate itself during cell division, thus assuring the transmission of genetic information to daughter cells.

These functional properties of DNA depend upon the chemical affinity of certain purine and pyrimidine bases for one another. Adenine pairs with thymine; guanine, with cytosine. Cellular DNA is arranged in twin strands linked in the form of a double helix, and the base sequence in one strand complements that of the other. In fact, as DNA replicates, the sequence of bases in one strand "automatically" determines that in the other. In the course of preparation for cell division, the base-paired strands of the double helix separate, and each one serves as a sort of template for the synthesis of a new complementary strand. In this fashion, just before a cell divides, its DNA content is doubled with great precision, so that identical genetic information is passed to each daughter cell.

Base pairing is also of fundamental importance during the process of protein biosynthesis, but the pairing involves RNA as well as DNA. Virtually all of the DNA in a cell resides in the nucleus, while actual synthesis of protein from individual amino acids occurs in the cytoplasm. RNA plays an intermediary role, transmitting the coded information from nucleus to cytoplasm and then aiding in the assembly of the peptide chains. The transfer of information from nucleus to cytoplasm is accomplished by so-called messenger RNA. Early in the process of protein synthesis, messenger RNA is synthesized in the nucleus by a process involving base pairing. In this process, free nucleotides are paired with the sequences of nucleotides in the DNA, yielding complementary RNA. The fourth base in RNA is uracil rather than thymine, but the process is as described above. Once formed, this messenger RNA enters the cytoplasm and attaches to structures termed *ribosomes*. Free amino acids do not attach directly to messenger RNA but are assembled after first being bound to so-called transfer RNA. There is transfer RNA for each of the 20 amino acids. This latter form of RNA "finds" the proper place to deliver a given amino acid by base pairing with messenger RNA on the ribosomes. This complex pairing system ultimately allows the amino acids to be linked in a sequence originally determined by DNA in the nucleus. The transfer of genetic information from DNA to messenger RNA is known as *transcription*, while the final use of the information to assemble amino acids into peptides is called *translation*.

There is a very large variety of ways that the nucleotides of DNA can be assembled, so that there is an

enormous number of different kinds of DNA, and hence, of complementary RNA. A given portion of DNA may "instruct" a cell to produce a particular chemical product by controlling the biosynthesis of the requisite enzyme systems within the cell. Similarly, other kinds of DNA can instruct cells to develop certain kinds of structures. Ultimately it is the DNA that determines exactly how the billions of cells which make up the body are assembled, and, in fact, whether the individual will be a dog, a cat, or a human being. Portions of the DNA also determine the limits of the individual's stature, the racial features, and a multitude of traits and processes that characterize the individual. Some DNA is even used to control other DNA, by instructing the cell when to "switch on" and use some portion of the DNA information stored in it (see Fig. 2-1).

In the nondividing cell, the DNA is found almost entirely within the nucleus. Even with the microscope, individual DNA molecules cannot be seen as distinct structures but only as part of ill-defined, deeply staining material within the nucleus (Fig. 2-2). As the cell begins to divide, the material in the nucleus arranges itself into strands called *chromosomes* (Fig. 2-3). The cells of the human body generally contain 46 chromosomes, or 23 pairs each (22 pairs of autosomes plus 1 pair of sex chromosomes). Prior to this point in cell division the DNA has been duplicated, so that with splitting of each chromosome and separation of the newly formed structures, identically endowed daughter cells are formed. By means of this form of cell division, termed *mitosis*, which begins with the fertilized ovum, identical genetic information is passed to every somatic or nongerm cell of the developing body. As a result of this process in a given individual, a cell of the epidermis will have exactly the same genetic information as does a cell within the liver. The reason that a skin cell differs from a liver cell is that in the course of development different portions of the "program" encoded in the DNA have actually been *expressed*. That is to say, "switching-on" of genes which code for the characteristics of skin cells leads to the phenotypic development of skin cells, while much additional genetic information remains unused in those cells. The process by which cells begin to diverge in their structure and function is referred to as *differentiation*.

There occurs a special kind of cell division termed *meiosis* which does not involve an even distribution of genetic material to the two daughter cells. Meiosis is involved in the formation of sperm and ova. In the course of meiosis, the distribution of chromosomes to daughter cells is such that each receives only 23 chromosomes, i.e., *one* member of each pair. This occurs during a *reduction division* in meiosis. By virtue of this, each sperm or ovum has only half the number of chromosomes present in somatic cells. Then, at the moment of conception, the union of the two half-sets of chromosomes produces a fertilized ovum having the proper number of chromosomes, one of each pair from each parent.

The genetic shuffle

The unit of heredity is the *gene*, a portion of DNA that controls the development of a particular trait, ultimately by specifying the production of some particular polypeptide within the cells of the body. Any given chromosome contains a tremendous number of genes. Genes controlling a particular trait are located at a specific position (locus) on a definite chromosome pair. Of a given pair of chromosomes in the somatic cells of an individual, one is derived from each parent; correspondingly, at a specific locus is a pair of genes, one gene from each parent. Tremendous genetic variability from individual to individual is due to the fact that there is a random sorting of chromosomes in each germ cell during reduction division. Furthermore, there is random union of sperm and ovum. Thus, although relatives are more likely to share portions of their DNA than are nonrelated individuals, the only individuals possessing identical genomes are twins derived from the same fertilized ovum, i.e., identical twins. Another source of genetic variation is a change occurring in some portion of the DNA of a germ cell. Such a chemical change in the DNA is termed a *mutation;* the result is that the trait

FIGURE 2-1
Functions of DNA. (Adapted from Luciano, Vander, and Sherman, *Human Anatomy and Physiology: Structure and Function,* 2d ed., McGraw-Hill, New York, 1983, p. 45.)

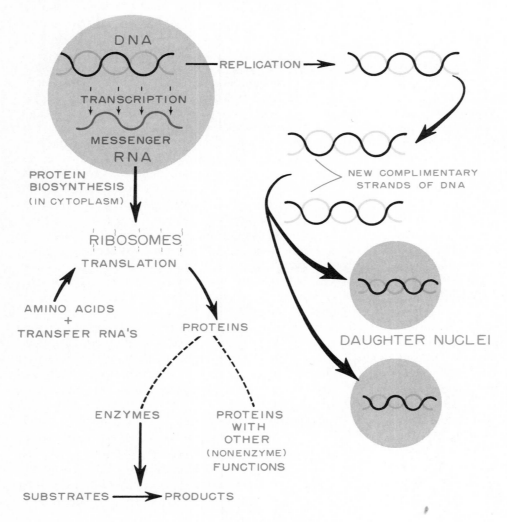

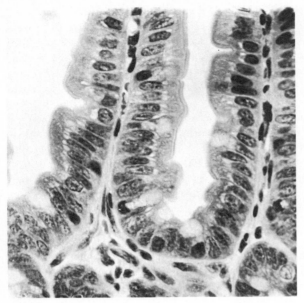

FIGURE 2-2
Nuclei of nondividing cells. The ovoid nuclei of these intestinal lining cells are arranged in regular rows. The DNA that controls the cells is within these nuclei, forming part of the deeply stained material called chromatin. (Photomicrograph, ×800.)

programmed by that particular gene may be altered in the individual receiving it.

The presence of individual genes cannot be detected with a microscope, but their presence can be inferred merely from the appearance of a demonstrable trait, a *phenotypic* trait, in the bearer. At a given genetic locus, if the paternal and maternal genes differ, one of the traits produced may be *dominant* and thus

FIGURE 2-3
Nuclei of dividing cells. As a cell divides, the nuclear material is arranged in strands called chromosomes. The starlike figure to the right of center is a cluster of chromosomes in a dividing cell. Just below this is a pair of horizontally oriented dark masses which actually represent masses of chromosomes dividing into two daughter cells. (Photomicrograph, ×800.)

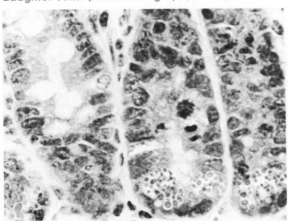

will appear in the phenotype. The effect of the second gene is thus not expressed (or is expressed to a minor degree), and the trait determined by that gene is termed *recessive*. A recessive gene will not express itself fully in the phenotype unless it is matched by a similar recessive gene from the other parent. Thus a particular trait, seemingly absent in both parents, may appear in the child if one recessive gene of the pair is supplied by each parent. Inheritance of a particular trait governed by a single gene pair as described is sometimes called *Mendelian* inheritance. However, many phenotypic traits are not so simply determined but are the result of the additive effect of multiple genes.

Abnormality of the hereditary material in an individual may thus arise and be expressed in a variety of ways. A particular abnormality may appear in a child without being a total surprise if the phenotypic expression of that trait is evident in the parents or immediate family. On the other hand, an abnormality may appear without previous evidence of the trait in a family by the combination of two preexisting recessive genes, by the process of mutation in the germ cell of one of the parents, or by a complex polygenic combination not present in either parent. In addition, abnormalities of entire chromosomes, or major portions of a chromosome, may arise during the development of germ cells and then be transmitted to the individual created by that germ cell.

PHENOTYPIC EXPRESSION OF GENETIC ABNORMALITY

Chromosomal anomalies

The coarsest sort of abnormality of genetic material is that which is associated with a visible morphologic peculiarity of chromosomes. Chromosomal abnormalities can develop in a variety of ways as cells divide. If such accidents occur during the production of germ cells, the individual formed from such an abnormal ovum or sperm will carry the chromosomal abnormality in all cells of the body, because as the original fertilized egg (with its abnormal chromosome) divides, subsequent generations of daughter cells receive the chromosomal abnormality in the process of cell division. One common way for a chromosomal abnormality to develop is for one or more chromosomes to break and the broken ends to "stick" inappropriately to other chromosomes, with the formation of a fused, abnormal chromosome. Another type of abnormality involves faulty separation of the two chromosomes of a given pair during the meiotic reduction division, which normally leads to a chromosome number of 23 in sperm or ovum. If such faulty separation occurs, a germ cell would be formed with a *pair* of chromosomes in a particular location instead of a single chromosome, which results in 24 chromosomes instead of 23. Fertilization of such a cell, for instance, an ovum, by a normal sperm with 23 chromosomes would yield a cell with 47 chromosomes—with a *triplet* instead of a *pair* of chromosomes in a given location.

The presence of a chromosomal abnormality in an individual patient can be detected by sampling some living cells, usually white blood cells, encouraging them to divide in an artificial culture, and then studying the details of microscopic anatomy of the chromosomes formed during cell division. The array of chromosomes observed in this fashion is referred to as a *karyotype*. Conventionally, the pairs of chromosomes are given a number designation based on the length and shape of the particular chromosomes. A given karyotype might be deemed abnormal because of an extra chromsome in a particular numerical location (trisomy) or even a deletion of one chromosome of a pair. Individual chromosomes might also be morphologically abnormal even though present in normal numbers. In contemporary practice, even the substructure of chromosomes can be analyzed by the use of staining techniques which reveal various banding patterns on particular chromosomes.

The results of karyotypic anomalies can be extremely serious, presumably because of the large quantity of DNA and the many genes involved on even a single chromosome. There is also the fact that genes on other chromosomes will be operating in a situation of abnormal imbalance if a particular chromosome is faulty in structure. It has been found that many spontaneously aborted embryos or fetuses have abnormal chromosomes, which indicates that the abortion occurred because the chromosomal abnormality present at the moment of conception was lethal to the developing individual. However, some chromosomal abnormalities do permit birth of a live baby, though they may produce severe defects in that individual. Because of the grossness of the genetic defect in such instances, multiple organ systems are often involved.

An example of a chromosomal abnormality, which unfortunately is not rare, is the common form of Down's syndrome, formerly termed mongolism, in which there is an extra chromosome in one pair, yielding a total chromosome number of 47. As shown in Fig. 2-4, the typical karyotype of an affected person shows three chromosomes in the so-called 21 position, and the condition is therefore referred to as *trisomy 21*. Affected individuals have a number of familiar and distinctive physical traits. They are generally mentally retarded and have a variety of internal anatomic abnormalities. The basic problem in this form of Down's syndrome often stems from a failure of separation of one chromosome pair that occurs in the development of the maternal germ cell, the ovum. Advanced maternal age in particular carries an increased risk of this sort of accident. Recent studies also implicate accidents of spermatogenesis, i.e., a *paternal* abnormality, in some instances.

Given the high risk of such pregnancies, it may be desirable to make or to rule out the diagnosis of Down's syndrome before the fetus becomes independently viable. This is accomplished by studying the chromosomes of fetal cells obtained by puncturing the amniotic sac around the fetus and aspirating a bit of amniotic fluid which contains some of the cells of the fetus. This procedure, which is called *amniocentesis*, generally does not harm the developing fetus. The amniotic fluid itself can be analyzed for certain substances whose concentration may indicate one or another abnormality in the fetus. Fetal cells suspended in the amniotic fluid can be cultured and subjected not only to karyotyping for detection of Down's syndrome but also to enzyme assays to detect some of the hereditary metabolic diseases discussed below.

Many other chromosomal anomalies have been described in individuals who have multiple defects. It is

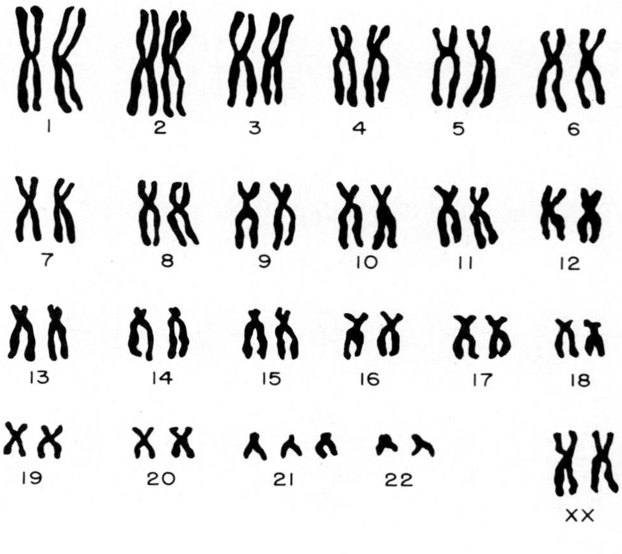

FIGURE 2-4

Karyotype of a female with Down's syndrome (formerly called mongolism). In the position conventionally designed as 21 are three chromosomes instead of two. This trisomy 21 is present in all of the cells of the affected individual and is expressed in terms of abnormalities in several organ systems.

estimated that 10 to 15 percent of infants born with multiple malformations and mental retardation have abnormal karyotypes. Approximately 5 percent of stillborns have abnormal chromosomes, as do approximately one-half of spontaneous abortuses. Fortunately, however, genetic abnormalities so gross as to involve karyotypic abnormality constitute but a small fraction of hereditary abnormality.

Single gene abnormalities

Abnormalities of a single gene are more prevalent than the defects described above. These genetic abnormalities cannot be identified by microscopic examination of cells since the karyotype of the affected individual is normal. The presence of the abnormal gene is inferred by the detection of an abnormal phenotypic trait in the individual and in the family tree. Single gene abnormalities, both dominant and recessive, can be expressed in a variety of ways, ranging from simple localized anatomic defects to subtle and complex disturbances of body chemistry.

Localized malformations are perhaps the most readily observed effects of single gene abnormalities. When, for instance, a dozen individuals in three generations of a family have identically deformed hands and the pattern of incidence follows the laws of Mendelian inheritance, there is no difficulty in recognizing what is involved. However, it should be noted that the bulk of birth defects do not fit into this single gene category but are more often the result of several separate gene abnormalities, possibly along with some environmental effects, or are the result of an intrauterine accident such as drug exposure or rubella. *Congenital* and *hereditary*

are not synonymous terms. An abnormality may be congenital, i.e., present at birth, and not be genetically determined. Conversely, a genetically determined abnormality may manifest itself for the first time in some instances only when the patient is middle-aged.

Single gene abnormalities may be expressed as *inborn errors of metabolism*. This designation refers to a situation in which an abnormal gene leads to the production of a faulty product or to an absence of production of a product. If the product is an enzyme, the result of the genetic abnormality is the loss of services of that enzyme, a situation sometimes referred to as *enzymopathy*. Enzymopathies have three general sorts of consequences. First, if the lack of enzyme prevents some metabolic reaction from occurring, the subject may exhibit the lack of the result of that reaction. The albino illustrates this in the lack of melanin, the brown pigment of the body, because of a genetically determined deficiency of an enzyme essential to its production.

A second sort of consequence of enzymopathy involves the accumulation of some substance in the body when, with an essential enzyme missing, the substance cannot be properly eliminated from the body. The precise results of such a *storage disease* depend on where in the body the substance accumulates. For example, in the adult type of Gaucher's disease a complex lipid accumulates within cells scattered in the liver, spleen, lymph nodes, and bone marrow of affected individuals (Fig. 2-5). Signs and symptoms of this storage disease

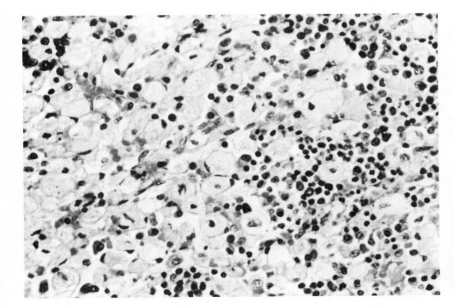

FIGURE 2-5
Gaucher cells in the bone marrow. Much of this field, especially on the left, is occupied by large, pale cells stuffed with stored lipid. These Gaucher cells crowd out the normal blood-forming elements, seen relatively concentrated at the right. Similar changes occur in many other organs. (Photomicrograph, ×500.)

may be quite mild and may not appear until adult life, when normal cells of the bone marrow begin to be crowded out by the Gaucher cells or when the spleen becomes enlarged and results in the formation of an abdominal mass. Tay-Sachs disease is an even more serious example. In this condition, because of a missing enzyme, the affected subject progressively accumulates a certain lipid within the neurons of the brain. Resulting degeneration of these cells leads to blindness, paralysis, and death, usually before 4 years of age.

The third type of consequence of enzymopathy is typified by the disease phenylketonuria, or PKU, in which the genetic defect leads to accumulation of improperly metabolized substances which have a toxic effect on certain bodily functions, especially those of the growing, developing brain. The result in the untreated case is severe mental retardation. Fortunately, in this disease early diagnosis, with dietary restriction of the substances which are not properly metabolized, can circumvent the disastrous effects on the growing infant.

In yet another category of single gene abnormality, aberrant DNA may lead to the production of an abnormal protein molecule, for example, the hemoglobin molecule. A slight deviation in the structure of hemoglobin may give it unusual physical properties which can be magnified into a serious disease. For example, in sickle cell anemia the abnormal recessive gene "instructs" the red blood cells to produce hemoglobin molecules which are prone to deform when the oxygen concentration in the blood is reduced. These sickled red cells form tangled masses and are rapidly destroyed, producing a variety of severe signs and symptoms characteristic of anemia in an individual homozygous for the gene.

Other single gene abnormalities cover a broad spectrum of phenotypic expression. Thus, there are genetically determined defects in the growth of bones or in the chemistry of connective tissue and genetically determined diseases such as cystic fibrosis. In cystic fibrosis there is an abnormality of many exocrine secretions, such as sweat and pancreatic and bronchial secretions. Because of the last abnormality, affected individuals frequently die prematurely of pulmonary infection. There have also been recognized a number of genetically determined conditions in which the individual is normal in all respects except for an unusual response to some environmental agent such as a drug. This latter sort of phenomenon has resulted in the recent development of the field of *pharmacogenetics*, the study of hereditary variations in response to drugs. The list of abnormal phenotypes determined by Mendelian inheritance includes many hundreds of diverse conditions.

Polygenic conditions

Even more prevalent than any of the situations outlined above are the many things that "run in families" but do not follow the usual patterns of Mendelian or single gene inheritance. Analysis of many of these diseases suggests that the interaction of several separate genes and several environmental factors determines the outcome. An excellent example of this type of pattern is observed in atherosclerotic coronary artery disease (refer to Chap. 27). Evidence indicates that the incidence of coronary artery disease is more prevalent in members of the immediate family of patients with the disease than in the general population. However, it is equally clear that environmental factors such as cigarette smoking, diet, and perhaps psychological stress make a significant contribution to the incidence and severity of the disease, along with associated conditions such as diabetes and high blood pressure. In such polygenic or *multifactorial* disease, the approach to prevention can clearly proceed along nongenetic lines with the expectation that environmental manipulation such as dietary limitations or alternatives in life-style and smoking habits will be beneficial regardless of genetic constitution.

Congenital anomalies or malformations constitute another category of conditions generally resulting from the interaction of multiple genes with certain environmental agents. Most congenital anomalies occur in a setting where there is no clear pattern of inheritance. Studies of twins have shown, however, that the likelihood of both members of a pair having a particular anomaly is higher in identical than in fraternal (dizygotic and, therefore, genetically different) twins. Furthermore, many family studies have shown that the relatives of a patient with a particular anomaly manifest a much higher incidence of the condition than do the general population. The role of environmental factors is evident, conversely, in the fact that even in identical twins the frequency of concordance for a particular anomaly is never 100 percent. At the other end of the spectrum are diverse environmental factors, such as chemical toxins, drugs, physical agents, and viruses, which can produce congenital anomalies. However, even for an obvious and powerful environmental teratogen such as thalidomide, other factors (genetic and/or environmental) must be involved, since not all fetuses exposed at the critical time have shown anomalies. Needless to say, the complex interactions between multiple genes and environmental factors in producing anomalies are not completely understood.

To recapitulate, some human diseases arise as a direct result of abnormality of DNA, the "stuff" of heredity. The basic problem may be one involving a single gene, multiple genes, or even an entire chromosome; the expression of the abnormality may range from a localized anatomic malformation, to a complex chemical and metabolic problem, to an increased susceptibility to something in the environment.

PREVENTIVE MEDICINE AND GENETIC COUNSELING

Very often the pronouncement to a patient that some condition is "hereditary" is met with feelings of hopelessness and despair and a sense of the irreversibility of what one has been dealt by nature. These feelings are, to an extent, a realistic expression of the fact that the era of genetic engineering has not yet arrived, that it is not yet possible to reverse such things as Tay-Sachs disease in a dying infant. Nonetheless, the total perspective of genetics and disease is far different from what is initially suggested by the permanence of DNA.

Many conditions that are inherited are not inevitably *expressed* in the bearer of the abnormal DNA despite the presence of a single or even several abnormal genes. As previously discussed, the ravages of phenylketonuria can be prevented, even in an infant with a hereditary lack of critical enzymes, by careful dietary manipulation. The progression of coronary artery disease can be influenced by manipulations ranging from drug treatment to changes in personal habits. The task of human genetics in such instances is not simply one of noting and cataloging the inevitable but is one of identifying subjects at unusual risk on a genetic basis and minimizing that risk by some environmental manipulation. Modifying the expression of genetic abnormality is an advancing frontier of biomedicine.

In those conditions that have not yielded even partly to such an approach, the outlook is necessarily somewhat different and is based ultimately on prevention of the disease—that is, through prevention of the birth of individuals afflicted with the disorder in question. This process, in turn, has two operational levels, both of which involve decisions on the part of the concerned individuals.

At the first level, a pregnancy likely to yield an abnormal individual can be electively avoided by the couple. At the second level, a pregnancy can be terminated by elective abortion prior to independent viability of a fetus determined to be affected with the condition in question. In the first example it is essential that the parents are accurately informed of the risk of conceiving an individual with an abnormality. The subject of risk often arises when an earlier pregnancy has already yielded an affected infant or when there is a strong family history of some particular condition. Also, there is a general risk in belonging to a population group where there is an increased incidence of some conditions. One example of such a population is the group of eastern European Jews who display an increased incidence of Tay-Sachs disease.

For some conditions it is now possible by means of specific tests applied to normal parents to detect the presence of a recessive gene which *in a double dose* would yield an afflicted infant. This is the case, for instance, with both Tay-Sachs disease and sickle cell disease. In these situations if both parents are found to be carriers of the gene, then the couple can be informed that the likelihood of producing an affected infant would be one pregnancy in four. Based on this knowledge the parents could decide, in keeping with their own particular religious or ethical systems, whether to avoid pregnancy entirely, whether to take the calculated risk, or whether to proceed with the pregnancy and seek prenatal diagnosis of the anticipated condition with possible termination of the pregnancy. For example, in Tay-Sachs disease it is now possible to secure fetal cells by amniocentesis and determine their content of the particular enzyme involved in the disease. This type of approach has allowed couples to produce families when the risk of abnormality is such that pregnancy would previously not have been considered by them.

Extremely difficult and sensitive decisions in this area must ultimately be made by the prospective parents. This requires that accurate and understandable information related to the nature and prognosis of the particular disease, the mode of its inheritance, and the probability of the disease appearing in the offspring be made available. In many instances this is the task of a person who has special skills in genetic counseling.

Identifying a condition as hereditary is not without pitfalls for the inexperienced. As emphasized above, many congenital conditions may be essentially nonhereditary, while nearly identical conditions may in fact be hereditary. Even conditions that are definitely *familial*, in terms of their greater frequency in a given family, may be nonhereditary but due to some environmental influence to which the entire family is exposed. Even more important, a given individual may appear to be afflicted with disease A associated with a gene but actually may have disease B which closely mimics disease A but is associated with a different gene and with a different pattern of inheritance. The subject might even be afflicted with disease C, which could be a nonhereditary look-alike. The counselor must be aware of such mimicry and be able to interpret appropriate studies which range from chromosomal and chemical analyses of cells secured from patient and/or family to careful evaluation of the family tree for evidence of disease.

In summary, the medical counselor must have the skill and perception to render as accurate a diagnosis as currently possible. The counselor must possess the ability to explain to the parents humanely but understandably the nature and prognosis of the disease and its impact on affected individuals, the mode of available treatment, and the means of preventing the occurrence of the disease. The ultimate decision as to any action is made by the parents or patients in the light of available options, and therapeutic measures are administered by the members of the health team in accordance with that decision. While the issues are perhaps more obvious in the case of so-called hereditary disease, the sequence just outlined is not unique. It describes the essence of medical practice.

QUESTIONS

Heredity, environment, and disease; interaction of heredity and environment

Directions: Answer the following questions on a separate sheet of paper.

1. Explain the ways in which DNA is responsible for storing, duplicating, and transmitting all of the information necessary for programming the functions of a cell.

2. Illustrate the role of DNA in the mechanism of transmitting genetic information.

3. Describe the ways in which chromosomal abnormalities can develop.

4. State the purposes of genetic counseling.

Directions: Circle the letter preceding each item below that correctly answers the question. More than one answer may be correct.

5. The functional properties of DNA are dependent upon the chemical affinity of which of the following bases to one another:
   a. Thymine with adenine   *b.* Thymine with cytosine   *c.* Cytosine with adenine   *d.* Guanine with cytosine

6. DNA functions include:
   a. Carrying genetic information   *b.* Executing the instructions of the given cell   *c.* Ability to replicate itself during cell division   *d.* Playing intermediate role in protein synthesis

7. Characteristics of Down's syndrome include:
   a. Affected individuals most often have a trisomy 21 karyotype pattern.   *b.* It is associated with an inborn error of metabolism.   *c.* Advanced maternal age is an increased risk factor.   *d.* It has high association with mental retardation.

8. Which of the following are extrinsic factors in relationship to the disease process?
   a. Microorganisms   *b.* Race   *c.* Sex   *d.* Nutrition

9. Which of the following best describes a *hereditary* disease?
   a. It is largely determined by an environmental agent.   *b.* Faulty genetic "programming" of the body's machinery results only from external influences.   *c.* It is expressed in nearly every bearer of faulty genetic information regardless of external influences.   *d.* An infectious agent is the usual causal agent.

10. Differentiation refers to the process by which:
    a. There is a decrease in the number of cells in a given population   *b.* Cells containing identical genetic information begin to diverge in their structure and function   *c.* There is a chemical change in the DNA   *d.* The nucleus arranges itself into strands

11. Meiosis is a type of cell division which:
    a. Involves DNA molecules making exact duplicates of themselves when the cell divides
    b. Does *not* involve an even distribution of genetic material to the two daughter cells   *c.* Involves a chemical change in DNA   *d.* Is involved in the formation of sperm and ova

12. Characteristic features of autosomal *dominant* disorders include:
    a. They are not expressed as disease if dominant gene is present   *b.* They manifest as disease even when only one abnormal gene is present and the partner on the homologous chromosome is normal   *c.* The trait will be altered when an individual has a mutation of a single dominant gene   *d.* Individuals who are homozygous for dominant genes are usually less severely affected than those who are heterozygous for recessive genes

13. The portion of DNA that is responsible for the development of a particular trait is which of the following:
    a. Chromosome   *b.* Purine   *c.* Gene   *d.* Pyrimidine

14. Which of the following genetic diseases are inherited as autosomal *recessive* disorders?

a. Sickle cell anemia   b. Down's syndrome
c. Phenylketonuria (PKU)   d. Tay-Sachs
disease

15. Which of the following diseases is an example of a genetic disease due to an abnormal karyotype?
    a. Phenylketonuria (PKU)   b. Albinism
    c. Down's syndrome   d. Sickle cell anemia

Directions: Circle T if the statement is true and F if it is false. Correct the false statements.

16. T   F   The presence of individual abnormal genes can be detected with a microscopic examination.

17. T   F   The term *genetic trait* means that the trait is inherited because of the DNA which is passed from generation to generation.

18. T   F   An arrangement of the chromosomes present in a cell is called a karyotype.

19. T   F   An inborn error of metabolism results from a genetically determined enzymatic defect that may involve the body's handling of protein, carbohydrates, lipids, etc.

20. T   F   The decoding process of protein biosynthesis is termed transcription.

CELLULAR INJURY AND DEATH

OBJECTIVES

At the completion of this chapter you should be able to:

1. Describe the organization of a hypothetical "typical" cell.
2. List the modalities by which cells may be injured or killed.
3. Describe the sequential stages of cell damage.
4. Describe the relationship of these stages to functional abnormalities of a cell.
5. Distinguish between the several forms of degenerative changes that occur in injured cells.
6. State at least one example of each of these degenerative cell changes.
7. Differentiate between atrophy and hypertrophy.
8. Explain the concept "point of no return" in relation to cell injury.
9. Explain the concept of necrosis.
10. Identify the types and causes of necrosis.
11. State at least one example of each type of necrosis.
12. Describe the effects of necrosis.
13. Explain what happens to necrotic tissue in the body.
14. Identify and distinguish the various types of pathologic calcification.
15. Define *somatic death*.
16. Describe the typical postmortem changes.

CELLULAR ORGANIZATION

Although within the body there are many different kinds of cells with highly specialized functions, all cells, to a large extent, have similar life-styles and similar structural elements. They have parallel requirements for such things as oxygen and nutrient supplies, for constancy of temperature, for water supply, and for means of waste disposal. The cell is literally the unit of life, the smallest entity that manifests the various phenomena which are associated with living. Therefore, the cell is also the basic unit of disease.

The organization of a hypothetical "typical" cell is diagramed in Fig. 3-1. The cell is bounded by a *cell membrane*, which not only gives the cell its shape but also attaches it to other cells. Even more importantly, the cell membrane serves as the gateway to and from the cell, allowing only certain things to pass in either direction and even actively transporting some things in a selective fashion. It is also the cell membrane that must receive many of the control signals from around the body and transmit these signals to the interior of the cell.

Within the cell is the *nucleus*, which serves as the control center by virtue of the fact that the DNA is concentrated within it. The instructions coded within the nuclear DNA are actually executed within the *cytoplasm*, the portion of the cell outside the nucleus. The cytoplasm is a watery medium containing many structures so small that they can be seen only with the electron microscope. These ultramicroscopic organs are termed *organelles*, and they are highly specialized as to function even within the confines of a single cell.

The *mitochondria* are organelles devoted to energy production within the cell. They are the power plant of the cell, for within them various foodstuffs are oxidized to produce the driving force for other cellular activities. The *endoplasmic reticulum* and *Golgi apparatus* constitute a sort of manufacturing, processing, and plumb-

ing system within the cytoplasm. The endoplasmic reticulum is a network of interconnecting tubules and cisterns, while the Golgi complex is a closely related array of flattened cisterns and associated vesicles. Protein synthesis is carried out along the endoplasmic reticulum under control of RNA (ribonucleic acid) in the *ribosomes*. The cytoplasmic RNA is actually produced and directed by nuclear DNA to act as a sort of assembly team in relation to the executive role of DNA. The ribosomes carry out protein synthesis by assembling amino acids into complex molecules according to the directions supplied by DNA. The Golgi apparatus is a packaging device which wraps the cell products for export (secretion) or for storage within the cell. Certain glycoprotein complexes are also elaborated within the Golgi apparatus. The *lysosomes* are membrane-bound packages of digestive enzymes prepared by the cell and held inactive until needed. Yet other organelles not shown in Fig. 3-1 account for additional special functions within the cell, such as providing rigidity and/or movement in the manner of a musculoskeletal system. The various organelles represent a total organism in mi-

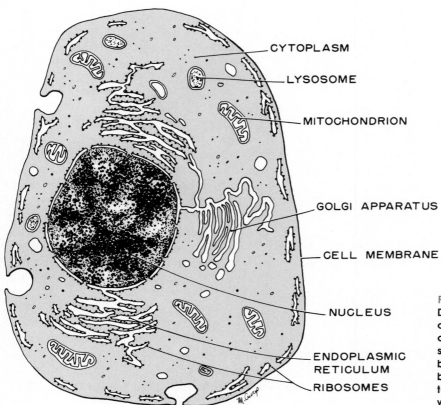

CYTOPLASM

LYSOSOME

MITOCHONDRION

GOLGI APPARATUS

CELL MEMBRANE

NUCLEUS

ENDOPLASMIC RETICULUM

RIBOSOMES

FIGURE 3-1

Diagram of a hypothetical typical cell. The structural basis for division of labor within the cell is shown. It should be noted that in the living body, the cell membrane not only bounds the cell and controls access to the interior but also joins the cell with others to form tissues.

crocosm, and their activity must be closely coordinated and controlled to preserve cellular integrity.

It should be emphasized that individual cells relate to one another in a variety of ways as they assemble into tissues and organs. Some tissues, such as lining or covering epithelia, consist of densely packed cells directly and tightly adherent to one another with little intervening space. Groups of cells of this type are soft and pliable and could not maintain the form of various organs or the strength of the entire body. It is actually *connective tissue* which holds the body together by virtue of its *intercellular substance*—literally, material between the cells. This substance includes collagen, which is a protein produced in the form of extremely tough fibers (like those in tendons and ligaments) and elastin, which is also a protein assembled into fibers but which also has elastic properties. Between these fibers is a jellylike matrix or ground substance. The combination of tough and elastic fibers and matrix gives the body its strength, form, and resiliency. In the skeleton, the intercellular substance is impregnated with calcium salts, producing the rigid bony support of the body.

MODALITIES OF CELLULAR INJURY

There are many ways in which cells can be injured or killed, but important modalities of injury tend to fall into just a few categories. One of the most common factors in cellular injury is a *deficiency of oxygen or other critical nutrient material.* Cells are particularly dependent upon a continuous supply of oxygen, because it is the energy of oxidative chemical reactions which drives the machinery of the cell and maintains the integrity of the various components of the cell. Therefore, without oxygen the various maintenance and synthetic activities of cells quickly come to a halt.

A second important type of injury is *physical,* which involves actual disruption of cells or at least disturbance of the usual spatial relationships between the various organelles or of the structural integrity of one or more types of organelles. Thus, mechanical and thermal means of injury are significant in the causation of human disease.

Living infectious agents constitute a third category of injurious modalities, and there are a wide variety of means by which particular organisms injure cells.

Chemical agents constitute a final common means of cellular injury. Not only do toxic substances find their way into cells from the environment, but accumulation of endogenous substances (as with genetically determined metabolic "errors") may likewise injure cells.

When an injurious stimulus is applied to a cell, the first important effect is what has been called a *biochemical lesion.* This involves a change in the chemistry of one or more metabolic reactions within the cell. It is interesting to note that very few types of injury are actually understood at this level. Although biochemical changes can be noted in injured cells, very often the abnormalities noted are second- or third-order effects rather than evidence of the primary biochemical lesion. When a biochemical lesion is established, the cell may or may not manifest a functional abnormality. In the case of many injuries, the cell possesses sufficient reserve to perform without significant functional impairment; in other instances there can be a failure of contraction, secretion, or other activities of the cell.

Finally, accompanying these biochemical and functional abnormalities there may *or may not* be a detectable morphologic change in the affected cell. The limitation here is one of technique. Changes that are evident upon routine microscopic examination are generally late changes, since many biochemical and functional abnormalities may have occurred before the anatomic abnormality becomes evident. With the advent of electron microscopy it is becoming possible to detect earlier and earlier microscopic lesions of the various organelles, but with presently available techniques it is still true that many functionally impaired cells may not yield evidence of their impairment in morphologic terms.

The result of an attack upon a cell is not always impairment of function. In fact, there are cellular mechanisms of *adaptation* to various kinds of adversity. For example, a common reaction of a muscle cell placed under abnormal stress is to gain strength by enlargement, a process called *hypertrophy.* Thus, the heart muscle cells of an individual with high blood pressure will enlarge in order to cope with the strain of pumping against increased resistance. A similar type of adaptation occurs in regard to certain chemical challenges. Barbiturates and certain other substances are ordinarily metabolized in liver cells, under the influence of enzyme systems found within these cells in association with the endoplasmic reticulum. In an individual taking barbiturates, there is often a striking increase in the amount of endoplasmic reticulum within liver cells, and this is associated with an increased enzyme content in these cells and an increased ability to metabolize the drug.

MORPHOLOGIC CHANGES IN SUBLETHALLY INJURED CELLS

Often when cells are injured but not killed, they manifest easily identifiable morphologic changes. These sublethal changes are at least potentially reversible. That is, if the injurious stimulus can be withdrawn, the cells return to their previous state of health. On the other hand, these changes may be a step toward cell death if the noxious influence cannot be corrected. Sublethal changes in cells are traditionally called *degenerations* or *degenerative changes*. Although any cells of the body may manifest such changes, metabolically active cells such as those in liver, kidney, and heart are commonly involved. Degenerative changes tend to involve the cytoplasm of cells, while nuclei maintain their integrity as long as the cell is not lethally injured. Although there is an extremely large number of injurious agents or specific ways of attacking cells, the repertory of morphologic expression of injury is actually quite limited.

The commonest form of cellular degenerative change involves the accumulation of water within the affected cells. The injury in effect causes loss of volume control on the part of the cells. Ordinarily, in order to maintain constancy of its internal environment, a cell must expend metabolic energy to pump sodium ion out of the cell. This occurs at the level of the cell membrane. Anything which disturbs energy metabolism in the cell or slightly injures the cell membrane may render the cell unable to pump out sufficient sodium ion. The natural osmotic result of increased intracellular concentration of sodium is an influx of water into the cell. The result is a morphologic change termed *cellular swelling*. An older name for this change was *cloudy swelling*, which reflected the fact that an organ whose cells suffered this change acquired a peculiar parboiled appearance grossly and the affected cells acquired an unusual granular appearance of the cytoplasm microscopically. These changes reflect the fact that when water accumulates within the cytoplasm, the cytoplasm organelles also absorb it, causing mitochrondrial swell-

ing, dilatation of the endoplasmic reticulum, and so forth.

Microscopically the changes of cellular swelling are quite subtle and involve simply an enlargement of the cell and a slight change in its texture. The gross counterpart of this is the enlargement of the affected tissue or organ usually detectable by a moderate increase in weight. If the noxious influence which has produced cellular swelling can be removed, after a period of time the cells usually begin to extrude sodium, and along with it water, and the volume returns to normal. This change is but a slight perturbation of the normal state of affairs.

If there is a severe influx of water, some of the cytoplasmic organelles such as the endoplasmic reticulum may be converted into water-filled sacs. Upon microscopic examination, the cytoplasm of the cell is seen to be vacuolated (Fig. 3-2). This is termed *hydropic change* or sometimes *vacuolar change*. The gross appearance of affected organs and the significance of the change are identical to those of cellular swelling.

A more striking and significant change than simple cellular swelling involves the intracellular *accumulation of lipid* within affected cells. This type of change commonly involves the kidneys, heart muscle, and liver, particularly the latter. Microscopically, the cytoplasm of the affected cells appears vacuolated in a fashion quite similar to that seen in hydropic change, but the content of the vacuoles is lipid instead of water. In the case of the liver, the amount of lipid accumulating within a cell is often relatively large, so that the nucleus of the cell is pushed to one side and the cytoplasm of the cell is oc-

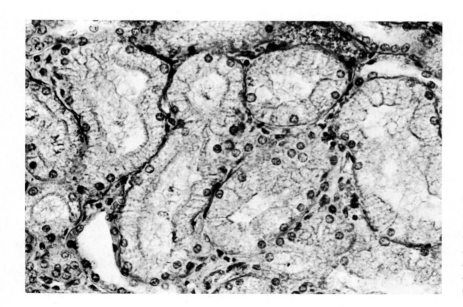

FIGURE 3-2
Hydropic change in renal tubular epithelium. The epithelial cells lining these convoluted tubules are enlarged and have vacuolated, lacy-appearing cytoplasm due to intracellular accumulation of water. (Photomicrograph, ×500.)

cupied by one lipid-containing vacuole (Fig. 3-3). The counterpart of such changes with respect to the gross appearance of affected tissues involves swelling of the tissues, increase in weight of the affected organ, and very often a distinct yellowish cast to the tissue due to contained lipid. Severely affected livers are in fact often bright yellow and greasy to touch. This type of change is termed *fatty change* or sometimes *fatty degeneration*, or *fatty infiltration*.

Fatty change occurs commonly because it can be produced by so many different mechanisms, particularly in the liver. Hepatocytes (and other types of cells) normally are involved in an active metabolic exchange of lipids. These substances are constantly mobilized from adipose tissue into the bloodstream from which they are extracted by the liver cells. Some of the lipid which is absorbed by the cell is oxidized, while some of it is combined with protein synthesized by the cell and then exported from the cell (i.e., into the bloodstream) in the form of lipoprotein.

Accumulation of fat within the cell can be produced by interfering with the usual exchange processes at any of several points. For example, if an excess of lipid is presented to the liver cell, the metabolic and synthetic capabilities of the cell may be exceeded, whereupon the lipid will accumulate intracellularly. If, on the other hand, normal amounts of lipid reach the cell but oxidation is impaired by some cellular injury, lipid will accumulate. Finally, if the process of lipoprotein synthesis and export is interfered with at any of several points, lipid will also accumulate. For these reasons one may encounter a fatty liver in diverse situa-

tions ranging from malnutrition, which will impair protein synthesis, to overfeeding, which will in effect swamp the liver with lipids. Hypoxia will sufficiently impair cellular metabolism to produce fatty accumulation, and numerous toxic substances from the environment will affect the cells in such a manner as to promote lipid accumulation. One of the most potent and widespread toxins in our environment that produces fatty livers is alcohol. This substance is directly toxic to the liver cell as well as indirectly injurious to individuals whose alcohol intake is extreme, because this often leads to malnutrition. Fatty change is potentially reversible but frequently reflects a severe injury to the cell and thus constitutes a step on the way to cell death.

Another response of cells under attack is to undergo a reduction in mass, quite literally a shrinkage. Such an acquired reduction in the size of a cell, a tissue, or an organ is referred to as *atrophy*. Seemingly, the atrophic cell or tissue is able to achieve an equilibrium under the adverse conditions imposed upon it by virtue of reducing the total demand it must meet. Grossly, of course, atrophic tissues or organs are smaller than normal.

In the course of becoming atrophic the cell must absorb some of its constitutents. This involves what is sometimes called *autophagocytosis* or *autophagy*, literally a self-eating process. This involves the enzymatic digestion of portions of the cell contained within cytoplasmic vacuoles. This same process occurs not only in the cell undergoing atrophy but also in the wear and tear of everyday cellular existence. That is to say, cytoplasmic organelles are damaged from time to time and are sequestered within the cytoplasmic vacuole and digested enzymatically. The digestion process tends to leave traces of residual indigestible material which gradually accumulate within the cells. This material is derived for the most part from membranous structures within the cells and generally has a dark-brown color.

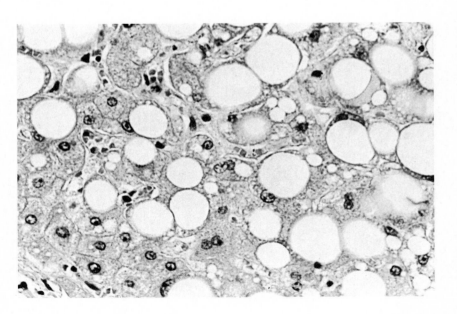

FIGURE 3-3
Fatty change in liver. Many liver cells have several small "holes" in their cytoplasm or a single huge vacuole which distorts the entire cell. These apparently empty spaces once contained abundant lipid which was dissolved during histologic preparation. The liver cells at the lower left are virtually normal. (Photomicrograph, ×500.)

Insoluble residual material may also accumulate as the result of *heterophagocytosis* or *heterophagy*, which is the cellular uptake of materials from outside the cell. As cells age, they accumulate more and more of this intracytoplasmic pigment, which is referred to as *lipofuscin, aging pigment,* or *wear-and-tear pigment.* As cells become atrophic, lipofuscin may become even more concentrated because of increased autophagocytic activity. Sometimes the atrophic tissue is pigmented even grossly; the process responsible is referred to as *brown atrophy.*

A discussion of degenerative changes must inevitably touch upon the topic of aging. Clearly the process of aging or senescence of an individual is an exceedingly complex one involving many genetic, endocrine, immunologic, and environmental factors. The process is poorly understood at all levels, i.e., from the level of the whole individual down to the level of single cells. It has been postulated that aging may result from an actual genetic limitation on the replicative ability of cells, coupled with the progressive accumulation of structural abnormalities in cells which no longer proliferate. However, it has not yet been possible to identify any cellular features specific to the process of aging, and the true functional implications of even the nonspecific changes are not known.

CELLULAR DEATH

If the noxious influence on a cell is severe enough or continued long enough, the cell will reach a point at which it can no longer compensate and cannot carry on metabolically. At some hypothetical point of no return, the processes become irreversible, and the cell is in effect dead. At this hypothetical instant of death, when the cell just reaches the *point of no return*, it may not be possible to recognize morphologically that the cell is irreversibly dead. However, if a group of cells that has reached this state remains in the living host for even a few hours, additional things occur which permit the recognition of the cells or the tissue as being dead. All cells have within them a variety of enzymes, many of them lytic. While the cell is alive, these enzymes do no damage to the cell, but they are released upon cell death and begin to dissolve various cellular constituents. In addition, as the dead cells change chemically, the living tissues immediately adjacent respond to the changes and mount an acute inflammatory reaction (see Chap. 4). Part of this latter reaction is the delivery of many leukocytes or white blood cells to the area, and these assist in the digestion of the dead cells. Thus, from their own digestive enzymes or as a result of the inflammatory process, the cells that have reached the point of no return begin to undergo discernible morphologic changes.

When a cell or group of cells or tissue in a living host are recognizably dead, they are referred to as *necrotic. Necrosis,* then, represents local cell death.

In general, although the lytic changes which occur in necrotic tissue may involve the cytoplasm of cells, it is the nuclei which manifest the changes most clearly indicative of cell death. Commonly, the nucleus of the dead cell shrinks, develops an irregular outline, and stains densely with the usual dyes used by pathologists. This process is referred to as *pyknosis,* and the nuclei are termed *pyknotic.* Alternatively, nuclei may crumble, leaving scattered fragments of chromatin material within the cell. This process is referred to as *karyorrhexis.* Finally, in some instances, the nuclei of dead cells lose their staining ability and simply disappear, the process being referred to as *karyolysis* (see Fig. 3-4).

The morphologic appearance of necrotic tissue varies depending upon the results of lytic activities within the dead tissue. If the activity of lytic enzymes is inhibited somewhat by local conditions, the necrotic cells will maintain their outline and the tissue will maintain its architectural features for some period of time. This type of necrosis is called *coagulative necrosis* and is particularly common when necrosis has been caused by deprivation of blood supply (Fig. 3-5). In general, coagulative necrosis is the most commonly encountered type of necrosis. In some instances the necrotic tissue gradually liquefies by enzymatic action, the process being

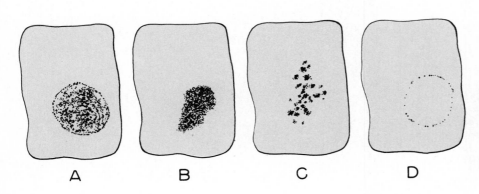

A   B   C   D

FIGURE 3-4

Nuclear changes in cell death. The morphologic changes most clearly indicative of cell death involve the nucleus. Diagramed are a normal nucleus (A), a pyknotic nucleus (B), a karyorrhectic nucleus (C), and one which has undergone karyolysis (D).

called *liquefactive necrosis*. This is particularly likely to occur in an area of necrotic brain, and the result is literally a hole in the brain filled with fluid (Fig. 3-6). In yet other instances the necrotic cells disintegrate, but the finely divided cellular fragments remain in the area for months or even years, virtually undigested. This type of necrosis is referred to as *caseous necrosis* because the area so affected has the appearance of crumbly cheese when viewed grossly (see Fig. 3-7). The prototype situation giving rise to caseous necrosis is tuberculosis, although this type of necrosis can arise in many other situations.

Certain special local conditions can give rise to yet other variants of necrosis. *Gangrene* is defined as coagulative necrosis, usually due to deprivation of blood supply, with superimposed growth of saprophytic bacteria. Gangrene thus occurs in necrotic tissues that are exposed to living bacteria. This is especially common in the extremities (Fig. 3-8) or in a segment of bowel which becomes necrotic (Fig. 3-9). Sometimes the shriveled, blackened tissue of a gangrenous area on an extremity is described as being the seat of *dry gangrene*, while an internal area which cannot become desiccated is designated as *moist gangrene*. In either situation the process involves the growth of saprophytic bacteria superimposed upon necrotic tissue.

Necrotic adipose tissue constitutes another special case. If the duct system of the pancreas is ruptured, either by trauma or in the course of spontaneous disease

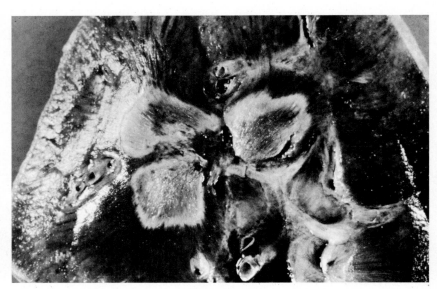

FIGURE 3-5
Coagulative necrosis. In this close-up of the cut surface of a kidney, three pale areas of necrosis can be seen approximately in the center of the field. The architectural outlines are obviously maintained in the dead tissue, hence the designation of coagulative necrosis. (Since the renal papillae are involved, this condition is specifically termed *renal papillary necrosis.***)**

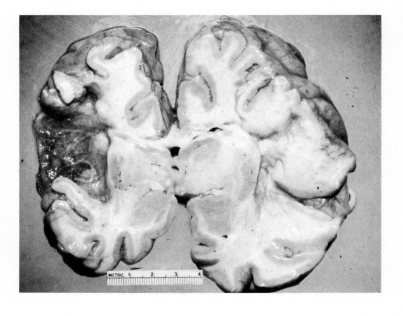

FIGURE 3-6
Liquefactive necrosis. A large defect is seen at the left in this section of brain. The brain substance in this area became necrotic owing to deprivation of blood supply. As is generally true in this organ, the necrotic tissue gradually softened, then liquefied, leaving a permanent defect.

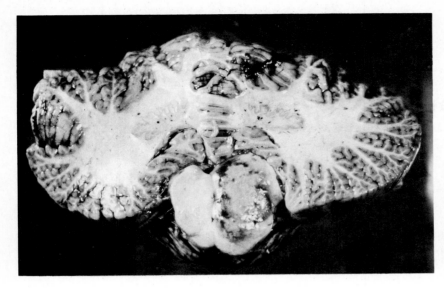

FIGURE 3-7
Caseous necrosis. A large necrotic area is evident in the brainstem at the right of center. In this instance, the dead tissue crumbled but did not liquefy. Because of a fancied gross resemblance to cheese, this type of necrosis is termed caseous. (This particular lesion was the result of tuberculosis, one of many causes of caseation.)

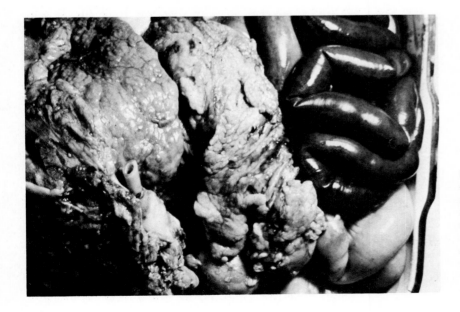

FIGURE 3-8
Gangrene. The toes of this foot have become necrotic because of poor blood supply. Saprophytic microorganisms are growing in the blackened dead tissue. On the extremities gangrene of this sort is frequently termed "dry."

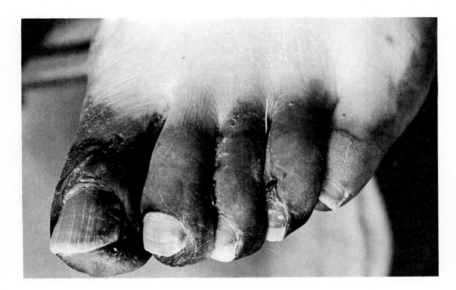

FIGURE 3-9
Gangrene. In this instance, a major portion of small intestine has been deprived of its blood supply. The gangrenous loops of intestine at the upper right contrast with the viable ones at the lower right. Saprophytes flourish in the necrotic tissue. Internal gangrene of this sort is inevitably "moist" as contrasted to that on the extremities.

of the pancreas, the pancreatic enzymes ordinarily carried within the duct may be spilled into the surroundings. The secretions of the pancreas contain many powerful hydrolytic enzymes, including lipases which cleave the lipids of adipose tissue. When this cleavage occurs, free fatty acids are formed by enzymatic action, and these are rapidly combined with metallic ions (such as calcium ions) in the area, producing deposits of soaps. This *enzymatic* (or *pancreatic*) *fat necrosis* is largely restricted to the abdominal cavity since that is the area exposed to leaking pancreatic enzymes. If adipose tissue elsewhere becomes necrotic, spillage of lipid from the dead cells may evoke an inflammatory response, but there is no formation of the yellow, chalky deposits characteristic of enzymatic fat necrosis.

Effects of necrosis

The most obvious effect of necrosis, of course, is *loss of function* of the dead area. If the necrotic tissue represents a small fraction of an organ with a large reserve (e.g., the kidney), there may be no functional impact on the host. On the other hand, if the area of necrosis is in a portion of brain, severe neurologic deficit or even death might be the result. In addition, the necrotic area in some instances can become a *focus of infection,* representing an excellent culture medium for the growth of certain organisms which might then spread elsewhere in the body. Even without becoming infected, the presence of necrotic tissue within the body may evoke certain *systemic changes,* such as fever, increased numbers of leukocytes within the circulating blood, and a variety of subjective symptoms. Finally, the necrotic tissue often *leaks its constituent enzymes* into the bloodstream as the cells die and the permeability of cell membranes increases. It is possible to analyze a specimen of blood and determine the level of various enzymes such as creatine phosphokinase (CPK), lactic dehydrogenase (LDH), or glutamic-oxaloacetic transaminase (GOT). Then an increased level of one or another enzyme may indicate that the patient does in fact have an area of necrosis hidden deep in some tissue. This principle has given rise to an important diagnostic field, clinical enzymology.

FATE OF NECROTIC TISSUE

Most often when an area of tissue becomes necrotic, the event evokes an inflammatory response on the part of the adjacent tissues (see Chap. 4). As a result of this inflammatory response, the dead tissue is ultimately demolished and removed, making way for the reparative process which replaces the necrotic area with regenerating cells of the sort lost or, in many instances, with scar tissue. If the necrotic tissue is located on a body surface, e.g., along the lining of the gastrointestinal tract, it may simply slough off, leaving a gap in the continuity of the surface which is referred to as an *ulcer.* Finally if the necrotic area is neither demolished nor cast off, it commonly will be encapsulated by fibrous connective tissue and will ultimately be impregnated with calcium salts precipitated from the circulating blood in the area of necrosis. This process of calcification may lead to the necrotic area becoming stony hard and remaining so for the life of the individual.

PATHOLOGIC CALCIFICATION

The deposition of insoluble calcium salts from the bloodstream which renders tissues rigid and hard is of course perfectly normal in the formation of bones and teeth. Elsewhere when such a phenomenon occurs, it is abnormal and is referred to as *pathologic calcification* or *heterotopic calcification.* This may occur in several situations. Most commonly, as described above, injured tissue or necrotic tissue which is not quickly demolished may become a site of calcification. This particular form of calcification is referred to as *dystrophic.* Since an area of caseous necrosis by its very nature remains undigested for long periods of time, it commonly becomes calcified. Thus, because tiny foci of tuberculosis or other infections occur in lung and in the lymph nodes draining the lung, small foci of dystrophic calcification commonly appear in these areas. They are not particularly important biologically but often appear on x-rays because of the opacity of the dense deposits of calcium salts. Another common site of dystrophic calcification is in the wall of arteries which have become atherosclerotic (see Chap. 7). In fact, the texture of this "hardening of the arteries" is due to the calcium deposition. Calcium salts also tend to deposit, with advancing age, in previously cartilaginous areas such as the rib cartilages. Ultimately dystrophic calcific deposits in any location may undergo actual conversion to bone, the process being termed *heterotopic ossification.*

In certain other circumstances calcium salts may be deposited in the soft tissues of the body in the absence of prior tissue damage or necrosis. This type of calcification is referred to as *metastatic calcification.* This process occurs not because of an abnormality of tissues but because there is an abnormal concentration of calcium and phosphorus salts within the circulating blood. Specifically, if the concentration of these substances rises beyond a certain critical level, their solubility product is exceeded, and precipitation occurs in a variety of tissues, especially lung, kidney, stomach, and the walls of blood vessels. The concentrations of calcium and phosphates in the blood are affected by activity of the parathyroid glands, renal function, intake of calcium and vitamin D in the diet, and the integrity of the skeleton. Thus, metastatic calcification may be seen with hyperparathyroidism, decreased renal function, abnormal diet, and destructive lesions of the skeletal system which liberate large quantities of calcium salts from the bones.

Calcium salts may also be deposited in the form of stones, or *calculi*, within the duct systems of a variety of organs. Calculi are formed from a variety of locally available materials, i.e., materials within the secretions of the particular organ. Thus, although they frequently contain calcium as one constituent, many calculi are not primarily calcific. Some calculi form as a result of encrustation of necrotic debris within a duct, while others form because of an imbalance in the constituents of a particular secretion such that there is precipitation from what is ordinarily a dissolved state. For a variety of reasons, then, calculi are commonly encountered in the biliary tract (Fig. 3-10), the pancreas, the salivary glands, the prostate, and the urinary system.

While calculi are often silent and discovered incidentally if at all, many move along the duct system of the particular organ and cause pain and bleeding. Frequently calculi will move until they lodge in the narrow part of the duct system and produce obstruction of the outflow of the particular secretion. When this occurs, there is often infection of the obstructed organ and atrophy of the parenchyma (Fig. 3-11).

SOMATIC DEATH

Death of the entire individual, as contrasted to localized death or necrosis, is referred to as *somatic death*. In past years the definition of somatic death was a relatively simple matter. An individual was decleared dead when "vital functions" ceased beyond any chance of reversal. Thus, if an individual stopped breathing and could not be resuscitated, the heart rather quickly stopped beating as a result of anoxia, and the individual was indisputably dead. Today, with technological advances, a patient can be attached to a mechanical respirator if breathing stops. If the patient's heart begins to falter, an electrical pacemaker may be put in place. With such "life-sustaining" machinery available, the definition of death becomes an exceedingly difficult one. In fact, it should be pointed out that not all cells of the body die at once. Living tissue cultures have been established from tissues removed from corpses. In hospitals today a common definition of somatic death concerns the activity of the central nervous system, specifically the brain. When the brain is dead, electrical activity ceases and the electroencephalogram becomes isoelectric or "flat." When the absence of electrical activity has been demonstrated for a predetermined period of time under rigidly defined circumstances, medical authorities will consider the patient dead despite the fact that heart and lungs could be kept going artificially for some time.

Following death certain so-called postmortem changes ensue. Because of a chemical reaction in the muscles of the dead subject, a stiffness called *rigor mortis* develops. The phrase *algor mortis* refers to the inevitable cooling of a dead subject as the body temperature approaches environmental temperature. Another set of changes is referred to as *livor mortis* or postmortem lividity. Generally, such lividity is due to the fact that when the circulation stops, the blood within the vessels settles according to the pull of gravity, and the

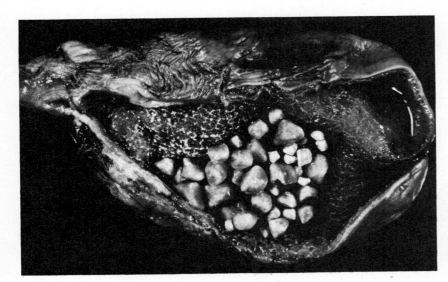

FIGURE 3-10
Gallstones within the gallbladder. Calculi of this sort are composed largely of bile pigments and cholesterol. It is apparent that stones of this size may be propelled into the common bile duct, where they can obstruct the flow of bile.

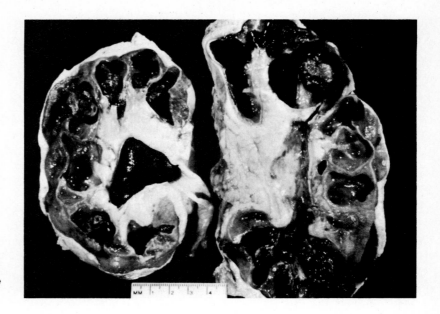

FIGURE 3-11

Renal calculi. Numerous large stones are present within the calyces and pelvis of these hemisected kidneys. The associated obstruction of urine flow and infection have led to marked loss of renal parenchyma.

tissues lowermost in the body develop a purple discoloration due to their increased content of blood. At a microscopic level, as the individual tissues within the corpse die, their enzymes are released locally, and lytic reactions begin. These reactions, termed *postmortem autolysis* (literally self-dissolution), are very similar to the changes seen in necrotic tissue but, of course, are not accompanied by an inflammatory reaction. The speed of onset of various postmortem changes is extremely variable, depending on individual as well as on associated environmental characteristics. Thus the amazingly accurate pinpointing of the time of death by medical authorities in detective fiction is largely just that, fiction.

QUESTIONS

Cellular injury and death

Directions: Circle the letter preceding each item below that correctly answers the question. More than one answer may be correct.

1. The part of the cell which serves as the control center because DNA is concentrated within it is the:
   a. Cell membrane   b. Cytoplasm
   c. Mitochondria   d. Nucleus

2. Within the cytoplasm of the cell, protein synthesis is carried out in association with:
   a. Lysosomes   b. Endoplasmic reticulum
   c. Mitochondria   d. Lipofuscin granules

3. Structural alterations in cells which are *reversible* include all of the following *except*:
   a. Cloudy swelling or cellular swelling.
   b. Hydropic change   c. Fatty infiltration
   d. Karyolysis

4. Accumulation of lipid within liver cells may be related to:

a. Starvation of the patient   b. Excessive alcohol intake by the patient   c. Obesity   d. Toxic injury to liver cells   e. All of the above

5. An increase in the size of a tissue or an organ due to an increase in the size of the individual cells without an increase in the number of component cells would be termed:
   a. Atrophy   b. Hypertrophy   c. Autophagocytosis
   d. Karyolysis

6. The death of cells or tissue within a living host is:
   a. Somatic death   b. Putrefaction   c. Necrosis
   d. Inflammation

7. Necrosis that results in a cheeselike appearance of affected tissue due to disintegration of the dead cells and that is frequently caused by tuberculosis is termed:
   a. Liquefactive necrosis   b. Caseous necrosis   c. Coagulative necrosis   d. Enzymatic fat necrosis

8. A common type of necrosis that is caused by deprivation of blood supply is termed:

a. Coagulative necrosis   b. Caseous necrosis   c. Enzymatic fat necrosis   d. Liquefactive necrosis

9. Gangrene is most likely to develop in a large area of ischemic necrosis in the:
a. Heart   b. Pancreas   c. Brain   d. Intestine

10. A type of calcification which occurs when damaged or dead cells cannot be eliminated from the body is:
a. Dystrophic   b. Metastatic   c. Calcinosis   d. Hypertrophic

11. Which of the following would probably *not* be associated with the presence of a calculus (stone) in the excretory duct of an organ?
a. Colic   b. Bleeding into the duct system of the organ   c. Infection   d. Proliferation of the secretory cells of the organ   e. Obstruction to the flow of the particular secretion

Directions: Fill in the blanks with the correct words.

12. The sequence of events involved in cellular degeneration includes _____, _____, and finally _____ alterations.

13. Three major categories of pathologic calcification are _____, _____, and _____ .

14. Following death, a chemical reaction in the muscles causing them to stiffen produces _____.

Directions: Match the type of necrosis in col. A with its characteristic manifestation or description in col. B.

Column A

15. ____ Coagulative necrosis

16. ____ Liquefactive necrosis

17. ____ Caseation

18. ____ Enzymatic fat necrosis

19. ____ Gangrene

Column B

a. Massive necrosis with superimposed bacterial growth

b. Characteristic of tuberculosis or fungal infections

c. Characteristic of brain

d. Characteristic necrosis of heart and kidney due to ischemia

e. Related to rupture of the pancreatic duct system

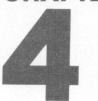
RESPONSE OF THE BODY TO INJURY—INFLAMMATION AND REPAIR

OBJECTIVES

At the completion of this chapter you should be able to:

1. Define *inflammation* and identify some possible causes.
2. Explain why inflammation is considered a major defense mechanism of the body.
3. Explain why inflammation can originate only within viable tissue and in a living host.
4. Distinguish inflammation from infection.
5. Identify the cardinal signs of acute inflammation and the mechanism responsible for each.
6. Identify the forces which normally govern the transport of fluid between the intravascular and interstitial spaces.
7. Describe the major events (vascular and cellular response) of acute inflammation and their order of occurrence.
8. Cite the evidence which indicates that mediators elicit the phenomena of inflammation.
9. Identify the four recognized types of hypersensitivity reactions.
10. Describe the role of histamine, components of the complement system, arachidonic acid metabolites, and cell-derived substances in the inflammatory response.
11. Describe the margination, adhesion, and emigration of blood leukocytes.
12. Define and contrast *exudate* and *transudate*.
13. Define *lymphadenitis* and describe the mechanism causing it in inflammation.
14. Define *chemotaxis* and *chemotactic substances*.
15. Describe the defensive or adaptive role of phagocytosis.
16. Define *opsonin* and *lysosome*.
17. Describe the morphologic and functional characteristics of the five types of blood leukocytes.

18. Differentiate between monocytes, macrophages, and histiocytes.

19. Describe the role of mast cells in acute inflammation.

20. Contrast the characteristics of neutrophils and macrophages.

21. Identify the major locations, components, and function of the *monocyte-macrophage system*, which was originally described as the *reticuloendothelial system (RES)*.

22. Differentiate between acute, subacute, and chronic inflammation on the basis of duration and predominant cell types.

23. Describe the characteristics of a granuloma, the mechanism responsible for its formation, and the causative agents involved.

24. Differentiate between these patterns of inflammation on the basis of variations in their exudate and give examples of each: serous, fibrinous, catarrhal, purulent, pseudomembranous, phlegmonous (cellulitis).

25. Identify the components of pus.

26. Define *suppuration, abscess, empyema, sinus, fistula, ulcer*.

27. Describe the possible fate of inflamed areas.

28. Define and differentiate between *healing by first intention* and *healing by second intention* in terms of time, sequence of events, outcome, and factors determing which course will be followed.

29. Identify the local and systemic factors affecting healing.

30. List several complications of wound healing.

31. Describe the systemic effects of inflammation.

AN OVERVIEW OF THE INFLAMMATORY REACTION

Whenever cells or tissues of the body are injured or killed, so long as the host survives, there is a striking response on the part of the surviving adjacent tissues. This response to injury is called *inflammation*. More specifically, inflammation is a vascular reaction whose net result is the delivery of fluid, dissolved substances, and cells from the circulating blood into the interstitial tissues in an area of injury or necrosis.

There is a natural tendency to view inflammation as something undesirable since, under ordinary circumstances, one would rather not have an inflamed throat, skin, soft tissue, or the like. However, it cannot be emphasized too strongly that inflammation is actually a beneficial and defensive phenomenon, the net result of which is the neutralization and elimination of an offending agent, the demolition of necrotic tissue, and the establishment of conditions necessary for repair and restitution. The beneficial character of the inflammatory reaction is dramatically demonstrated in our hospitals by what happens when patients cannot produce a needed inflammatory reaction, e.g., when it has become

necessary to administer high doses of drugs which have the side effect of suppressing such reactions. Under these conditions there is a high incidence of extremely severe, rapidly spreading, or even lethal infections caused by ordinarily harmless microorganisms.

The inflammatory reaction is actually a dynamic and continuous succession of well-coordinated events. In order to manifest an inflammatory reaction a tissue must be alive and in particular must possess a functional microcirculation. One corollary to this requirement is that if an area of tissue necrosis is extensive, the inflammatory reaction will be found not in its midst but rather at its edges, i.e., at the interface between the dead tissue and living tissue with an intact circulation. Another corollary is that if a particular injury kills the host instantly, there will be no evidence of an associated inflammatory reaction, since this would take time to develop.

The causes of inflammation are numerous and varied. There is no profit in attempting to list these causes, but it is essential to understand that *inflammation and infection are not synonymous*. Thus, *infection* (the presence of living microorganisms within the tissue) is but one cause of inflammation. In many instances inflammation occurs under conditions of perfect sterility, as happens when a portion of tissue dies because of deprivation of blood supply. Because of the broad range of situations which result in inflammation, an understanding of the process is basic to much of biology and medicine. Without an understanding of the process one cannot begin to comprehend the principles of infectious disease; the principles of surgery, wound healing, and the response to a variety of kinds of trauma; or the principles of how the body copes with catastrophes of tissue death such as strokes, "heart attacks," and the like.

Despite the large number of causes of inflammation and the variety of situations in which it appears, the train of events set in motion tends to be the same in general outline, with various types of inflammation differing largely in quantitative detail. Happily, therefore, one can study the inflammatory reaction as a general phenomenon and deal with the quantitative variations secondarily.

GROSS FEATURES OF ACUTE INFLAMMATION

Acute inflammation is the *immediate* response of the body to injury or cell death. The gross features are familiar to all of us, as a moment's reflection on past scrapes, cuts, and minor infections will recall. In fact, these obvious features of inflammation were described some 2000 years ago and are still known as *cardinal signs of inflammation*. These include redness, warmth, pain, and swelling, or in the classical Latin, *rubor*, *calor*, *dolor*, and *tumor*. A fifth cardinal sign, altered function, or *functio laesa*, was added in the last century.

Redness

Redness, or rubor, is usually the first thing to be noted in an area that is in the process of becoming inflamed. As the inflammatory reaction begins, the arterioles supplying the area become dilatated, thus allowing more blood into the local microcirculation. Capillaries previously empty or perhaps only partly distended quickly become packed with blood (Fig. 4-1). This condition, termed *hyperemia* or *congestion*, accounts for the local blush of acute inflammation. The production of hyperemia at the start of an inflammatory reaction is controlled by the body both neurogenically and chemically, via the release of substances like histamine.

Heat

Heat, or calor, parallels the redness of an acute inflammatory reaction. Actually, heat is a characteristic only of the inflammatory reactions at the body surface, which is normally cooler than the 37°C temperature of the interior of the body. An area of cutaneous inflammation becomes warmer than the surroundings because there is more blood (at 37°C) being conducted from the inside of the body to the surface in the affected area than there is in a normal area. This phenomenon of local warmth is not observed in inflamed areas deep within the body, since such tissues will already be at the core temperature of 37°C and local hyperemia would make no difference.

Pain

The pain, or dolor, of an inflammatory reaction is probably produced in a variety of ways. Change in local pH or in the local concentration of certain ions can stimulate nerve endings. Similarly, the release of certain chemicals such as histamine or other bioactive chemicals can stimulate the nerves. In addition, swelling of the inflamed tissues leading to increased local pressure can undoubtedly produce pain.

Swelling

Perhaps the most striking aspect of acute inflammation is the local swelling (tumor). This is produced by the transfer of fluid and cells from the bloodstream to the interstitial tissues. This mixture of fluid and cells that accumulates in an area of inflammation is termed an *exudate*. Early in the course of inflammatory reactions most of the exudate is fluid. A classic example of such exudate fluid is that which appears quickly within a blister following a minor burn of the skin. Somewhat later, white blood cells, or leukocytes, leave the bloodstream and accumulate as part of the exudate.

Altered function

The fact of altered function, *functio laesa*, is a familiar one. In a superficial way, it is easy to understand why a swollen, painful part with an abnormal circulation and abnormal local chemical environment should function abnormally. In truth, however, we do not understand in detail the means whereby function of an inflamed tissue is impaired.

FLUID ASPECTS OF INFLAMMATION

Exudation

In order to understand the very rapid flux of fluid across vessel walls into the tissue in an area of inflammation it is necessary to recall the principles governing fluid transport under more normal conditions. Ordinarily, the walls of the smallest vascular channels (such as capillaries and venules) will allow small molecules to pass

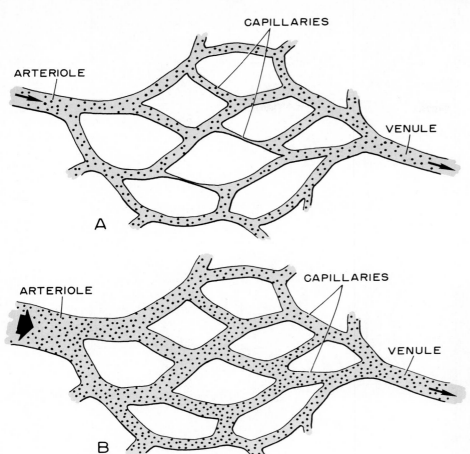

CAPILLARIES

ARTERIOLE

VENULE

A

CAPILLARIES

ARTERIOLE

VENULE

B

FIGURE 4-1

Mechanism of hyperemia in acute inflammation. The caliber of the arteriole controls the volume flow of blood into a capillary bed. In the normal state (A), the flow is such that some capillaries appear collapsed and others extremely narrow. With arteriolar dilatation (B), the increased volume of blood flowing into the capillaries distends them and produces the gross red-purple discoloration of tissue due to increased blood content.

but will retain large molecules such as plasma proteins within the vascular lumen. The result of this semipermeable character of the vessels is that there is an osmotic force tending to keep fluid within the vasculature. This is counterbalanced by the outward thrust of hydrostatic pressure within the vessels. A simplified diagram of the balance of forces is shown in Fig. 4-2. It can be seen that the lymphatics function to siphon off fluid which has reached the interstices of the tissue, and an equilibrium is thus normally maintained.

Shifts of fluid in the evolving inflammatory reaction are exceedingly rapid, as illustrated by the previously cited example of a blister following thermal injury. When such inflammatory exudates are analyzed, it is found that they contain significant amounts of plasma protein. Thus, a key event in acute inflammation is the alteration of permeability of the tiny vessels in the area, which leads to protein leakage. This is followed by a shift in osmotic balance and, in effect, water follows the protein, producing swelling of the tissues. The arteriolar dilatation which produces local hyperemia and redness also results in an increase in intravascular pressure locally as vessels become engorged. This, too, augments the fluid shift (Fig. 4-2). The major factor, however, is the increase in vascular premeability to protein.

It is the endothelial cells which line the small vessels that are responsible for the usual semipermeable character of the vessels, and it is these same cells which change their relationship to one another in acute inflammation, producing the leakage of protein and fluid. Figure 4-3 shows the situation diagrammatically. In the normal small vessel at the left, the endothelial lining cells are joined tightly to one another. The dots in the lumen represent large molecules such as those of serum proteins or of large marker particles injected experimentally to simulate protein molecules. Ordinarily these large molecules or particles cannot penetrate the intercellular junctions. However, if one induces an inflammatory reaction locally, there develops an actual separation between contiguous endothelial cells in the area, and the marker particles (and presumably the protein molecules) exit from the lumen as shown at the right of Fig. 4-3. If one uses a pigmented marker particle for such an experiment, entire vessels become discolored, and it becomes possible to see which part of the microcirculation is actually leaking in the course of inflammation. In most instances studied in this fashion, the leak seems to occur chiefly at the venular end of the microcirculation rather than within the true capillaries (Fig. 4-3).

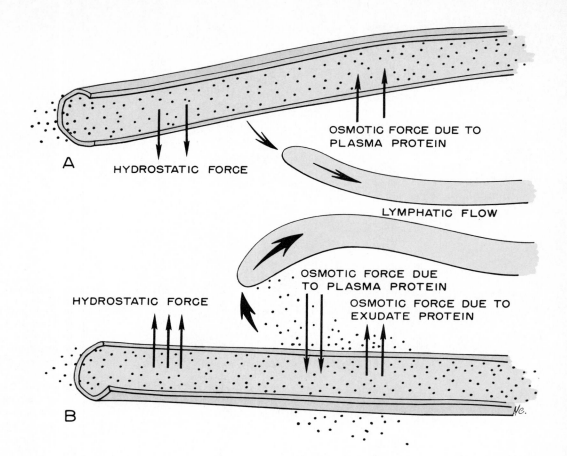

OSMOTIC FORCE DUE TO
PLASMA PROTEIN

A HYDROSTATIC FORCE

LYMPHATIC FLOW

HYDROSTATIC FORCE

OSMOTIC FORCE DUE
TO PLASMA PROTEIN

OSMOTIC FORCE DUE TO
EXUDATE PROTEIN

B

FIGURE 4-2

Factors involved in fluid exchange between blood vessels and tissues. In the normal or resting state (A), hydrostatic forces tend to push fluid into the interstitial spaces. This is largely balanced by the osmotic force exerted by plasma proteins (dots) which ordinarily do not pass through vessel walls. The fluid which does pass into the interstices drains via the lymphatics. In acute inflammation (B), protein escapes from the vessels as permeability increases. This, along with a smaller contribution from the increased hydrostatic pressure related to hyperemia, accounts for a significant fluid flux. Lymphatic flow is correspondingly increased.

Lymphatics and flow of lymph

The lymphatic system participates in the acute inflammatory reaction in parallel with the blood vascular system. Ordinarily there is a slow percolation of interstitial fluid into lymphatic channels in the tissue, and the lymph thus formed is carried centrally in the body ultimately to rejoin venous blood. As an area becomes inflamed, there is usually a striking increase in the flow of lymph draining from the area. It is known that in the course of acute inflammation, the contiguous lining cells of the smallest lymphatics separate somewhat, just as they do within the venules, thus allowing more ready access to material from the interstices of tissues into the lymphatics. There is even evidence that lymphatic channels are maintained in an open position as a tissue swells by a system of connective tissue fibers anchored to the walls of the lymphatics. In any event, not only does the flow of lymph increase but the protein and cell content of the lymph likewise increases during acute inflammation.

On the one hand, this increased flow of material through lymphatics is beneficial since it tends to minimize the swelling of the inflamed tissue by draining off a portion of the exudate. On the other hand, the price we pay is that potentially injurious agents can be carried by the lymphatics from a primary site of inflammation to a distant point in the body. By such means, for instance, infectious agents may spread. The spread is often limited by the filtering action of regional lymph nodes through which the lymph flows as it moves centrad in the body, but agents or materials carried within the lymph may pass through the nodes and reach the bloodstream.

For these reasons one must always be aware of the possible involvement of the lymphatic system in inflammation of any cause. When a lymphatic vessel itself becomes inflamed, this is termed *lymphangitis*. If a lymph node becomes inflamed, the phenomenon is termed *lymphadenitis*. Regional lymphadenitis is an exceedingly common accompaniment of inflammation. One familiar example is the enlarged, tender cervical lymph nodes seen with tonsillitis. The more general term

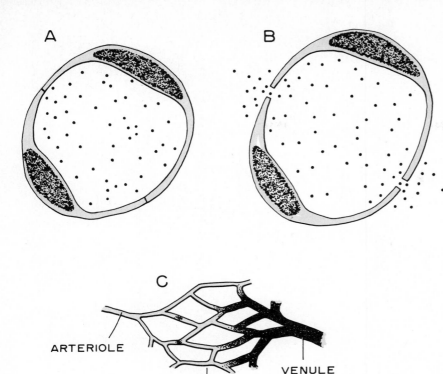

FIGURE 4-3

Mechanism of increased vascular permeability in acute inflammation. In normal vessels (A), the junctions between endothelial lining cells are sufficiently tight to keep large molecules (dots) within the lumen. In acute inflammation (B), contraction of endothelial cells creates gaps allowing leakage of macromolecules. As shown in (C), the permeability change is at the venular side of the microcirculatory bed.

lymphadenopathy is used to describe virtually any abnormality of lymph nodes. In practice the term refers not only to lymphadenitis but to any *enlargement* of lymph nodes, most nodal reactions being accompanied by enlargement.

CELLULAR ASPECTS OF INFLAMMATION

Margination and emigration

Early in acute inflammation as arterioles dilate, the flow of blood into the inflamed area increases. Soon, however, the character of the blood flow changes. As fluid leaks out of the microcirculation with its increased permeability, large numbers of the so-called formed elements (red blood cells, platelets, and white blood cells) are left behind, and the viscosity of the blood increases. The circulation within the affected area then slows, leading to some important consequences. In a normal situation (Fig. 4-4A), the flow of blood is more or less streamlined, and the formed elements do not bump up against the sides of the vessel appreciably. As the viscosity of the blood increases and the flow slows, the leukocytes begin to *marginate*; that is, they move to the periphery of the stream, along the lining of the vessel (Fig. 4-4B). With progression of the phenomenon, the marginated leukocytes begin to adhere to the endothelium. The result is an appearance reminiscent of a cobblestone street, leading to the designation of this event

as *pavementing*. Actually margination and pavementing are but preludes to emigration of the leukocytes from the blood vessels to the surrounding tissue.

Figure 4-4C is a diagrammatic representation of leukocytic emigration. Leukocytes move in an ameboid fashion. They seem able to extend a pseudopod into the potential space between two endothelial cells and then push gradually through to appear on the other side, a process requiring a matter of minutes. The net result, given the fact that this event is repeated in innumerable venules and that more and more leukocytes are delivered into the area via the circulating blood, is that tremendous numbers of cells are delivered into the area of inflammation in a relatively short time. Literally millions of cells emigrate into even a small area of inflammation within a period of several hours.

Chemotaxis

The active motility of the leukocytes in the interstices of inflamed tissues once they emigrate is apparently not random but is directionally oriented. This is accomplished by a variety of chemical "signals." The phenomenon of attraction to a substance by directional orientation of movement is referred to as *chemotaxis*. Many different things may provide a chemotactic signal to attract leukocytes, ranging from infectious agents, to damaged tissues, to substances activated within the protein fraction of plasma leaking from the bloodstream. Thus,

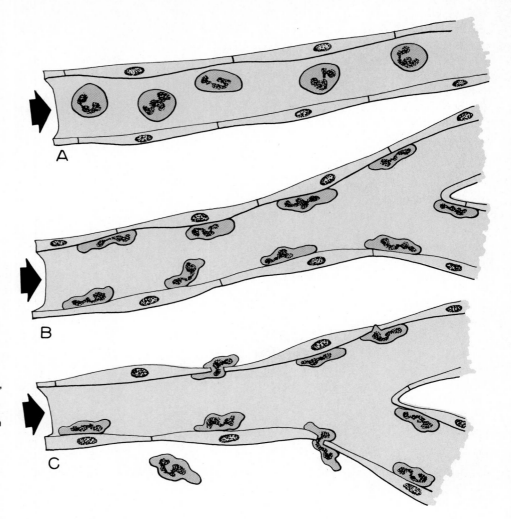

FIGURE 4-4
Blood flow and cellular phenomena in acute inflammation. Normally (A), formed elements of the blood, especially the leukocytes shown, are carried in the mainstream. As the circulation slows (B), margination of leukocytes occurs. This is a prelude to emigration of leukocytes between endothelial cells (C).

a smooth combination of increased delivery of leukocytes to the area (as a result of hyperemia), changes in blood flow resulting in margination and pavementing, and chemotactic orientation of leukocyte motion results in the rapid accumulation of a significant leukocytic component in the exudate.

Mediation of inflammation

The dramatic vascular, fluid, and cellular phenomena of inflammation, which make up a carefully focused reponse to injury, are obviously under meticulous control. While some injurious modalities directly damage vascular endothelium and thus by themselves lead to leakage of protein and fluid in the zone of injury, many bits of convergent evidence suggest that injury generally triggers the formation and/or release of chemical substances within the body, and that these so-called mediators elicit the phenomena of inflammation. The ability of many kinds of injuries to trigger the activation of the same endogenous mediators would explain the stereotyped character of the inflammatory response to diverse stimuli. The presence of a latent period between application of an injurious stimulus and the development of inflammatory response also points to the role of mediators; the ability to frustrate certain aspects of the reaction with pharmacologic blocking agents emphasizes the importance of mediators.

In recent years many endogenously released substances have been identified as mediators of the inflammatory response. This sort of knowledge has, on the one hand, led to a better understanding of deficiencies and perturbations of the inflammatory response and, on the other hand, suggested the means of squelching unwanted inflammation when dictated by the clinical setting. Although the list of proposed mediators is long and complex, the better recognized mediators fall into several classes: (1) vasoactive amines, (2) substances produced by plasma enzyme systems, (3) arachidonic acid metabolites, and (4) miscellaneous cell products.

The most important vasoactive amine is histamine, which is capable of producing vasodilatation and increased vascular permeability. Large amounts of histamine are stored within the granules of connective tissue cells known as *mast cells*, which are widely distributed in the body (histamine is also present in blood basophils and platelets). The stored histamine is inactive and exerts its vascular effects only when released. Many physical injuries lead directly to mast cell degranulation and histamine release. Some injuries first trigger activation of the serum complement system (described below and in Chap. 5), certain components of which then lead to histamine release. Some immunologic reactions (detailed in Chap. 5) also trigger release of this mediator from mast cells. Histamine seems particularly important early in inflammation and is a prime mediator in some common allergic reactions. Antihistamines are drugs designed to block the mediator effects of histamine.

The blood plasma is a rich source of a number of important mediators. These are formed through the action of certain proteolytic enzymes which make up a sort of interconnected defensive system. The key agent coordinating these systems is the so-called Hageman factor (factor XII), which is present in the plasma in an inactive form and which can be activated by a variety of injuries. Activated Hageman factor triggers the clotting cascade, leading to the formation of fibrin (see Chap. 18). Clotting, per se, is an important defensive reaction to injury, but certain products derived from fibrin also act as vasoactive mediators in inflammation. Hageman factor also activates the plasminogen system, liberating plasmin or fibrinolysin. This protease is capable not only of splitting fibrin but also of activating the complement system. Several components of the complement system function as important inflammatory mediators. For example, derivatives of the third and fifth components, so-called anaphylatoxins, release histamine and affect vascular permeability. A derivative of the fifth component and a complex of the fifth, sixth, and seventh components are potent chemotactic agents when activated in tissues. These effects are important in many examples of inflammation, not just in immunologically provoked reactions (although, as described in Chap. 5, union of antigen and certain antibodies is a potent activator of the complement system). Activated Hageman factor also converts prekallikrein (an inactive substance in plasma) to kallikrein (a proteolytic enzyme). This, in turn, acts on plasma kininogen to liberate bradykinin, a peptide which dilates blood vessels and increases permeability.

In recent years attention has been directed to arachidonic acid metabolites as important inflammatory mediators. Arachidonic acid is derived from the phospholipid of many cell membranes when phospholipases are activated by injury (or, in fact, by other mediators). Subsequently, arachidonic acid can be metabolized by two different pathways, the cyclooxygenase pathway and the lipoxygenase pathway, yielding a variety of so-called prostaglandins, thromboxanes, and leukotrienes as shown in Fig. 4-5. These substances show a broad range of vascular and chemotactic effects in inflammation, and are important in hemostasis as well. It is now recognized that aspirin and many nonsteroidal anti-inflammatory drugs act by inhibiting the cyclooxygenase pathway.

In addition to the above mediators a variety of cell-derived substances have been shown to have properties suggesting that they may also be important in inflammation. A partial list would include such things as oxygen metabolites produced by neutrophils and macrophages, lysosomal contents of these cells (see below), and so-called lymphokines released by activated lymphocytes (see Chap. 5).

Thus, the total list of proposed mediators of inflammation is a truly extensive one, and our knowledge of which substances are significantly involved in a given reaction is still quite limited. There appears to be considerable overlap and redundancy of mediators, which perhaps explains the difficulty involved in effectively blocking inflammatory reactions.

Types of leukocytes and their functions

The leukocytes which circulate in the bloodstream and emigrate into inflammatory exudates originate in the bone marrow, where not only leukocytes but also red blood cells and platelets are continuously produced (see Chap. 15). Normally, within the bone marrow there can be found large numbers of immature leukocytes of various kinds and a "pool" of mature leukocytes being held in reserve for release into the circulating blood. The numbers of each type of leukocyte circulating in the peripheral blood are closely controlled within certain limits (see Chap. 17) but are altered "on demand" when an inflammatory process arises. That is to say, with the instigation of an inflammatory response, feedback signals to the bone morrow alter the rate of production and release of one or more kinds of leukocytes into the bloodstream.

Granulocytes constitute a class of leukocytes which includes neutrophils, eosinophils, and basophils. These three types of cells are named by virtue of the granules within their cytoplasm visible after the application of certain dyes. Two additional types of leukocytes, monocytes and lymphocytes, do not contain the numerous cytoplasmic granules that characterize the above-named cells. Although each of the types of cells listed is available in the circulating blood, the appearance of leukocytes within exudates is not a random affair but probably represents the result of specific chemotactic signals arising in the evolution of the inflammatory process.

The first cells to appear in large numbers within exudates in the early hours of inflammation are neutrophils. The nuclei of these cells are irregularly lobed or polymorphous (Fig. 4-6). These cells are therefore

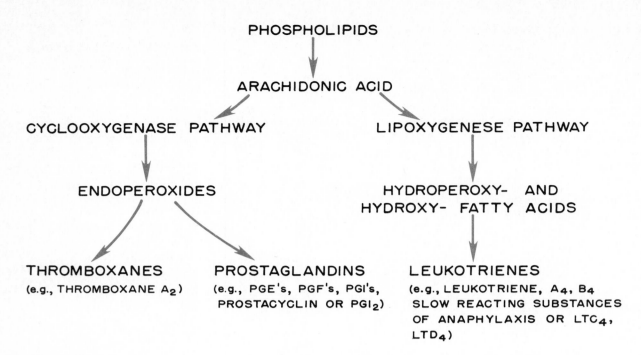

PHOSPHOLIPIDS

ARACHIDONIC ACID

CYCLOOXYGENASE PATHWAY

LIPOXYGENESE PATHWAY

ENDOPEROXIDES

HYDROPEROXY- AND HYDROXY- FATTY ACIDS

THROMBOXANES
(e.g., THROMBOXANE A_2)

PROSTAGLANDINS
(e.g., PGE's, PGF's, PGI's, PROSTACYCLIN OR PGI_2)

LEUKOTRIENES
(e.g., LEUKOTRIENE, A_4, B_4 SLOW REACTING SUBSTANCES OF ANAPHYLAXIS OR LTC_4, LTD_4)

FIGURE 4-5
Arachidonic acid metabolism and inflammatory mediators.

called *polymorphonuclear neutrophils, PMN's,* or *"polys."* These cells have a developmental sequence within the bone marrow which requires approximately 2 weeks for completion. When they are released into the circulating blood, their circulatory half-life is 6 hours or so. There are approximately 5000 neutrophils per cubic millimeter of blood in circulation at any given time, with approximately 100 times this number being held in reserve as mature cells within the bone marrow ready to be released on signal. Amazingly, although literally billions of neutrophils per day are replaced by the bone marrow, their production and release is quite rigidly controlled.

When released into the bloodstream, polymorphonuclear neutrophils are ordinarily incapable of further cell division or significant synthesis of cellular products. The numerous granules visible within the cytoplasm of the neutrophils, however, actually represent membrane-bound packets of enzymes, i.e., *lysosomes,* produced during maturation of the cells. These enzymes include a wide variety of hydrolases, including proteases, lipases, phosphatases, etc. In addition, associated

FIGURE 4-6
Macrophages and neutrophils in connective tissue. These cells are part of a voluminous exudate which has formed, in this instance, in response to bacterial infection. Most of the cells shown are neutrophils. Their cytoplasmic granules cannot be seen at this magnification, but their irregularly lobed *(polymorphous)* nuclei are evident. The macrophages are severalfold larger and, in this particular exudate, have a bubbly-appearing cytoplasm. They are scattered, but are prominent in the lower center and lower left of the field. (Photomicrograph, ×500)

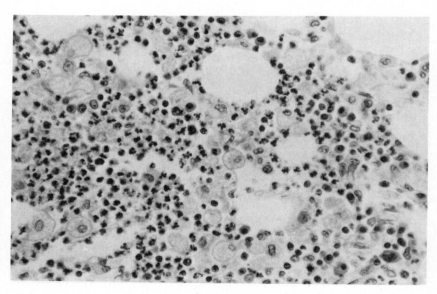

with the granules are a variety of antimicrobial substances. Thus, in effect, the mature polymorphonuclear neutrophil is a traveling bag of enzyme-loaded and antimicrobial particles.

Polymorphonuclear neutrophils are capable of active ameboid motion and are able to engulf a variety of materials by a process termed *phagocytosis*. As illustrated in Fig. 4-7, the neutrophil approaches the particle (for instance, a bacterium) to be phagocytosed, flows its cytoplasm around the particle, and eventually takes the particle into the cytoplasm enveloped in a membrane-bound vesicle which pinches off from the cell membrane of the neutrophil. This phagocytic process is aided by certain substances which coat the object to be ingested and render it more easily internalized by the leukocyte. These kinds of leukocytosis-promoting substances, called *opsonins*, include immunoglobulins (antibodies) and components of the so-called complement system (see Chap. 5). Having ingested a particle and incorporated it into the cytoplasm of a *phagocytic vacuole* or *phagosome*, the leukocyte's next task is to kill the particle, if it is a living microbial agent, and to digest it. Killing of living agents is accomplished in a variety of ways, including alteration in intracellular pH following phagocytosis, release of antibacterial substances into the phagocytic vacuole, and production of antibacterial substances such as hydrogen peroxide (and other highly reactive oxygen metabolites) as a result of cellular metabolic processes initiated following the phagocytic event. The digestion of phagocytosed particles is generally accomplished within the vacuoles formed by fusion of lysosomes with phagosomes. The previously inactive digestive enzymes are now activated within the so-called *phagolysosomes*, resulting in the enzymatic digestion of the objects.

Under certain other circumstances, these same potent digestive enzymes of the neutrophils may be released into the host tissues rather than into intracellular phagolysosomes. When this occurs, the neutrophilic enzymes become potent agents of tissue injury. This extracellular release occurs with death and disintegration of neutrophils; it occurs following phagocytosis of certain crystals such as urates by neutrophils (because phagocytosis of these crystals is followed by rupture of phagolysosomes); it also occurs when neutrophils attempt to ingest immune complexes under certain circumstances. These kinds of situations will be described more fully below.

The *eosinophil* is another type of granulocyte which may appear in inflammatory exudates, although usually in relatively small numbers. Eosinophils have irregular nuclei much like neutrophils, but the cytoplasmic granules stain a bright red with the dye eosin and are much more prominent than the lavender-colored granules of neutrophils. The granules of eosinophils are actually packets of enzymes quite similar to those of neutrophils. In fact, functionally eosinophils do

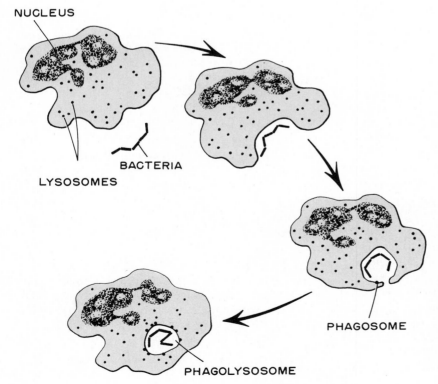

NUCLEUS

BACTERIA

LYSOSOMES

PHAGOSOME

PHAGOLYSOSOME

FIGURE 4-7
Diagram of phagocytosis. Neutrophils and monocytes ingest particles by flowing their cytoplasm around the objects and internalizing them in an envelope of cell membrane, the phagosome. The digestive enzymes of the lysosomes are then released into the phagolysosome.

many of the same things: they respond to chemotactic stimuli, they phagocytose various kinds of particles, and they even kill certain microorganisms. What appears to be distinctive about eosinophils, however, is that they respond to certain unique chemotactic stimuli generated in the course of allergic reactions and that they contain enzymes which are capable of counteracting the effects of certain inflammatory mediators released in such reactions. Apparently correlated with these features is the fact that eosinophils tend to accumulate in significant concentrations at the site of allergic reactions, where they may be acting as "firemen." Eosinophils also appear to be active in the body's defense against certain parasites.

The third type of granulocyte is the basophil, whose cytoplasm is crowded with large granules which stain a deep blue with basic dyes. Although these cells come from the bone marrow like other granulocytes, they have many features in common with certain cells of the connective tissues called *mast cells* or *tissue basophils*. The granules of both of these kinds of cells contain a variety of enzymes, heparin, and histamine. Blood basophils seem to respond to chemotactic signals released in the course of certain immunologic reactions. Ordinarily they are present in very small numbers in exudates. Blood basophils and tissue mast cells are stimulated to release the contents of their granules into the surroundings in a variety of injurious circumstances, including both immunologic and nonspecific reactions. In fact, the mast cells are a major source of histamine early in any acute inflammatory reaction. The immunologic means of stimulating granule release by mast cells or basophils will be discussed in Chap. 5.

The *monocyte* is an important form of leukocyte which differs from the granulocytes by virtue of its nuclear morphology and the relative agranular character of its cytoplasm (Fig. 4-6). The monocyte originates within the bone marrow just as do the granulocytes, but its circulatory life is 3 to 4 times longer than that of granulocytes. In the course of acute inflammatory reactions monocytes begin to emigrate at approximately the same time as do neutrophils, but they do so in much smaller numbers and at a slower rate. Consequently in the early hours of inflammation there are relatively few such cells within exudate. However, as exudates age, the percentage of these cells frequently increases. The same cell which is called a monocyte in the circulating blood is called a *macrophage* when it appears within exudates. In fact, the same type of cell is found wandering in small numbers through the connective tissues of the body even in the absence of overt inflammation. These wandering macrophages in the connective tissues are frequently referred to as *histiocytes*.

In many ways the functions of macrophages most closely parallel those of polymorphonuclear neutrophils in that macrophages are actively motile cells which respond to chemotactic stimuli, are actively phagocytic, and are able to kill and digest a variety of agents. A number of important differences between macrophages and neutrophils exists. For one thing, the life cycle of macrophages is very different in that these cells may survive weeks or even possibly months within the tissues, in contrast to the short-lived neutrophils. In addition, when the monocyte enters the bloodstream from the bone marrow and when it enters the tissues from the bloodstream, it is not a fully mature cell in the sense that the neutrophil is. This latter cell is incapable of further division and is also incapable of active synthesis of digestive enzymes. Monocytes, on the other hand, can be stimulated under some circumstances to divide within the tissues, and they are capable of responding to local conditions by synthesizing a variety of intracellular enzymes. This ability to undergo "on-the-job-training" is a vital property of macrophages, particularly in certain immunologic reactions where they are trained by lymphocytes. In such circumstances macrophages are known to increase their metabolic activities, become more effective in phagocytosis, and become more efficient in killing and digesting certain microbes. In addition, macrophages may alter their form as they undergo such changes, giving rise to cells which have been traditionally referred to as *epithelioid cells*. Macrophages are also able to fuse together to form *multinucleated giant cells*. These forms will be illustrated below.

Although macrophages are significant components of various exudates, they are widely distributed in the body under normal baseline conditions. This was recognized many years ago, and the term *reticuloendothelial system* (RES) was coined in recognition of the existence of a population of mononuclear cells sharing the same property, namely, phagocytosis. The name of *monocyte-macrophage system* is now being applied to the RES, because this name is actually more descriptive. As ordinarily conceived, the RES, or monocyte-macrophage system, includes not only the blood monocytes and tissue histiocytes, or wandering macrophages, but a large population of more or less fixed mononuclear phagocytic cells closely related to the more mobile members of the system. This population of less mobile cells includes lining cells along blood channels within the spleen, the liver (where the cells are known as Kupffer cells), and the bone marrow. Similar fixed macrophages are present along many of the lymphatic channels within the lymph nodes of the body. There are, in addition, many macrophages within the serosal cavities of the body, within the lungs, and even within the central nervous system.

The important functions of this system involve, of course, the vigorous phagocytic activities of the component cells. These cells are responsible for cleaning the blood, the lymph, and the interstitial spaces of foreign material, thus performing a vital defensive function. Experimentally if one injects even millions of microorganisms into the circulating blood, they are removed within a matter of a few hours by the many millions of macrophages located strategically around the body. This is exceedingly important in everyday life inasmuch as the release of at least a few microorganisms into the circulating fluids of the body is a fairly frequent event. It is known, for instance, that with vigorous brushing of the teeth, with defecation, or, in fact, with certain medical or dental manipulations organisms frequently enter the bloodstream. Because of the phagocytic activities of the macrophage system such episodes of *bacteremia* are transient and trivial. The macrophages in the body cavities and connective tissues perform a similar police function. In addition, the uptake of foreign material by macrophages is an essential first step in the chain of events which leads to the induction of an immune response (see Chap. 5).

An important everyday function of the monocyte-macrophage system involves the processing of the hemoglobin of red blood cells which have reached the end of their life span. It is the function of macrophages to trap and recycle the components of this essential substance. These cells are capable of splitting hemoglobin into an iron-containing moiety and a non-iron-containing moiety. The iron is recycled in the body for the building of other red blood cells in the bone marrow; the non-iron-containing moiety is further processed liberating a substance known as *bilirubin*, which is carried in the bloodstream to the liver, where the hepatocytes extract it and secrete it as part of the bile.

One type of leukocyte, the *lymphocyte*, has not yet been mentioned. Lymphocytes generally are present in exudates only in very small numbers until the exudates are quite old—that is, until the inflammatory reactions have become chronic. Since the known functions of lymphocytes are all within the immunologic realm, these cells will be more fully described in Chap. 5.

The essential features of the acute inflammatory response having been described, it might be well to reflect at this point on the beneficial or adaptive nature of the response, each component of which has a unique importance. The function of the vasodilatation early in acute inflammation is to bring to the area the "raw materials" for the reaction. It is known that if the arteriolar dilatation and increased blood flow are frustrated by local conditions or by the administration of certain drugs, later aspects of the inflammatory reaction are significantly frustrated. The increased vascular permeability accomplishes not only the outpouring of fluid which may act to dilute noxious agents but also accomplishes the transfer of some important protein substances such as opsonins or other antibodies to the "battleground." Furthermore, one of the proteins which leaks into the area of inflammation is *fibrinogen*, which is quickly converted to form *fibrin*, which may act as kind of a sealer or "glue" in wounds. Because of its fibrillar character,

fibrin may act as a scaffold for migration of phagocytic leukocytes and ultimately for the cells which form scar tissue in the reparative phase. The mobilization of leukocytes is of obvious defensive value not only in terms of the apprehension of invading microbes but also because leukocytes are responsible for demolition of tissue debris so that repair processes can begin.

PATTERNS OF INFLAMMATION

Although the inflammatory reaction tends to evolve by the mechanisms described above, a number of different patterns of inflammation can emerge based on the type of exudate that is formed, the particular organ or tissue involved, and the duration of the inflammatory process. The nomenclature of inflammatory processes takes into account each of these variables. Different sorts of exudates are given descriptive names. The duration of the inflammatory response is designated as *acute* during the phase of active exudation, as *chronic* when there is evidence of advanced repair along with the exudation, and as *subacute* when there is but early evidence of repair along with the exudation. The location of the inflammatory reaction is designated by the organ name to which is appended the suffix *-itis* (e.g., appendicitis, tonsillitis, arthritis).

Noncellular exudates

In some instances of inflammation, the exudate consists almost entirely of fluid and dissolved substances with very few leukocytes. The simplest sort of noncellular exudate is a *serous* exudate, which consists basically of the protein which leaks from permeable blood vessels in an area of inflammation along with the accompanying fluid. The most familiar example of serous exudate is blister fluid. Similar accumulations of serous exudate are frequent within body cavities such as the pleural cavity or the peritoneal cavity and, although not as striking, serous exudates frequently spread through connective tissues.

Sometimes collections of fluid occur in body cavities for reasons other than inflammation—usually increased hydrostatic pressure or depletion of plasma protein. Such noninflammatory collections are termed *transudates*, and are protein-poor and cell-poor as compared to exudates.

A second type of noncellular exudate is *fibrinous* exudate. Such an exudate forms when the protein which is extravasated in an area of inflammation contains abundant fibrinogen. This fibrinogen is converted to fibrin, which is a sort of sticky, elastic meshwork (perhaps more familiar as the backbone of blood clot). Fibrinous exudates are frequently encountered on inflamed serosal surfaces such as the pleura and the pericardium, where the precipitated fibrin is compacted into a shaggy layer on the involved membrane (Fig. 4-8). When such a shaggy layer of fibrin has accumulated on serosal surfaces, it is frequently accompanied by the symptom of pain when one surface rubs on another. Thus, for instance, the patient with pleuritis feels pain upon respiration when the roughened surfaces rub together during inspiration. This rubbing of shaggy surfaces also produces a sign called *friction rub*, which is audible through the stethoscope over the affected area, be it pleura, pericardium, or the like.

Yet another noncellular exudate is the *mucinous* or *catarrhal* exudate. This type of exudate can form only on the surface of a mucous membrane, where there are cells capable of secreting mucin. This type of exudate differs from others in that it represents a cellular secretion rather than something which escapes from the bloodstream. Mucin secretion is obviously a normal property of mucous membranes, and mucinous exudate represents nothing more than an acceleration of a basic physiologic process. The most familiar and homely example of a mucinous exudate is the runny nose which accompanies many upper respiratory infections.

Cellular exudates

Probably the most common exudates are those which consist predominantly of polymorphonuclear neutrophils, in such numbers as to overshadow the fluid and proteinaceous parts of exudate. Such neutrophilic exudates are referred to as *purulent*. Purulent exudates (Fig. 4-9) are very commonly formed in response to bacterial infection. They are also seen in response to many aseptic injuries and are prominent in situations where tissues have become necrotic almost anywhere in the body.

Not infrequently (most often with bacterial infection) extremely high concentrations of neutrophils accumulate in a tissue, and many of these cells die and liberate their powerful hydrolytic enzymes into the surroundings. Under such circumstances the enzymes of

the neutrophils literally digest the underlying tissue and liquefy it. This combination of neutrophil aggregation and liquefaction of underlying tissues is referred to as *suppuration*, and the exudate thus formed is referred to as *suppurative exudate*, or, more commonly, *pus*. Thus, pus consists of polymorphonuclear neutrophils, living, dying, and disintegrated; liquefied digestion products of underlying tissue; fluid exudate of the inflammatory process; and, very often, the inciting bacteria. The significant difference between suppurative and purulent inflammation is that with suppuration, there is liquefactive necrosis of underlying tissue. Figure 4-10 illustrates the significant difference between purulent and suppurative inflammation. (Although there exists a significant difference between purulent and suppurative inflammation, many authors unfortunately use the terms interchangeably.)

When localized suppuration occurs within a solid tissue, the resulting lesion is termed an *abscess*. As seen in Fig. 4-10, an abscess is quite literally a hole in the involved tissue filled with pus. Abscesses are difficult lesions for the body to handle because of their tendency to expand with the liquefaction of more tissue, their tendency to burrow, and their resistance to healing. In fact when an abscess has formed, it is difficult to deliver therapeutic agents such as antibiotics into the abscess via the bloodstream. In general the handling of abscesses by the body is greatly aided by draining them

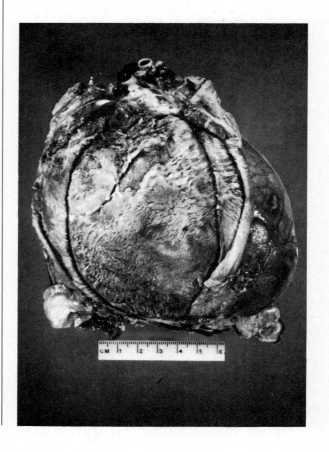

FIGURE 4-8

Fibrinous exudate on the surface of the heart. The pericardium has been opened and, instead of the normally smooth epicardial surface, a shaggy layer of fibrin is evident. This has formed from fibrinogen that has exuded from underlying vessels. Classically this condition has been termed "bread-and-butter heart."

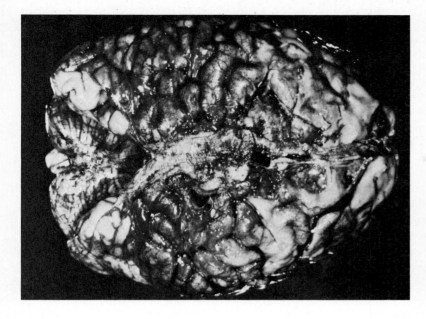

FIGURE 4-9
Purulent exudate within the cerebral meninges. The membranes covering the brain contain literally millions of neutrophils forming a purulent exudate. The creamy patches of exudate are especially prominent at the right. The gyri in the center of the photograph are dark because of intense vascular congestion, part of the inflammatory response. (This is pneumococcal meningitis.)

surgically, thus allowing the closed space previously filled with pus to collapse and heal. If abscesses are not surgically drained by pathways chosen by the surgeon, they tend to expand, destroying additional structures in their path. An abscess in a lung might burrow until it communicates with the pleural cavity, and if the contents are discharged into the pleural cavity and infection spreads, the result might be *empyema*, which is a purulent inflammatory process involving the entire pleural cavity. Occasionally an abscess will rupture onto a surface and produce a draining tract which ends blindly in the space of the abscess. Any such blind tract communicating with a surface is referred to as a *sinus*. If, on the other hand, an abscess extended to two separate surfaces, it might result in an abnormal tract communicating between two organs or between the lumen of a hollow organ and the body surface. Such an abnormal communication is referred to as a *fistula*. (Fistulas are named according to their communications, e.g., gastrocolic, bronchopleural, colocutaneous.)

When purulent inflammation extends diffusely through a tissue, the process is referred to as *phlegmonous*. Perhaps more commonly the term *cellulitis* is used clinically to describe an area of phelgmonous inflammation. Such a spreading purulent process is seen usually as a result of bacterial infection when the particular agent is capable of spreading rapidly through the loose connective tissue of the body.

As one would expect, there are frequently mixtures of noncellular and cellular exudates, and these are

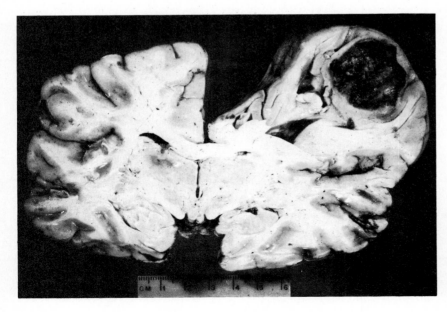

FIGURE 4-10
Brain abscess. As a result of bacterial infection in the cerebral hemisphere on the right, large numbers of neutrophils emigrated into the region. Liquefaction of the regional tissue by lysosomal enzymes of the neutrophils produced the defect illustrated.

named accordingly. Thus there are *fibrinopurulent* exudates, which consist of fibrin and polymorphonuclear neutrophils, *mucopurulent* exudates consisting of mucin and neutrophils, *serofibrinous* exudates, etc. Certain of these exudates such as mucinous and mucopurulent are, of course, unique to mucous membranes.

Frequently, in association with damage to mucous membranes, a necrotic area may actually slough off, leaving a gap in the continuity of the mucosal surface. Such a defect is termed an *ulcer*. Most often the bed of an ulcer will be surfaced by fibrinopurulent exudate emanating from the underlying blood vessels (Fig. 4-11). Sometimes broad areas of mucous membrane will become necrotic, and the dead cells may become enmeshed in a web of fibrinopurulent exudate, which coats the mucosal surface. Such an area grossly resembles a ragged mucous membrane and hence this type of process is referred to as *pseudomembranous* or simply *membranous* inflammation (Fig. 4-12). The classic example of pseudomembranous inflammation in bygone days was the pseudomembrane of diphtheria within the respiratory tract. Thus such membranes are occasionally referred to as *diphtheritic*. Pseudomembranous inflammation is now more commonly observed within the gastrointestinal tract, particularly the colon, as the result of an upset in the microbial ecology of the tract usually brought about by the administration of antibiotics.

A unique and distinctive pattern of inflammation which can occur virtually anywhere is *granulomatous* inflammation. This type of inflammation is characterized by the massing of large numbers of macrophages and their aggregation into nodular clumps referred to as *granulomas*. Although many inflammatory exudates contain appreciable numbers of macrophages, in granulomatous inflammation the field is dominated by sheets of these cells or their derivatives such as epithelioid cells or multinucleated giant cells. Granulomas take time to evolve and generally pass through rather nondescript acute stages where there is exudation of fluid, neutrophils, and protein. It is the continued emigration of monocytes and also the local proliferation of these cells which leads to their massing as a granuloma. Granulomas usually form because of the persistence within the tissues of some offensive agent resistant to the efforts of the body to dispose of it. Such agents can include insoluble but sterile materials or particularly resistant microorganisms. The prototypical microorganism which evokes the formation of granulomas is the *Mycobacterium tuberculosis*, or tubercle bacillus. The response to this organism is characteristically granulomatous, and usually the macrophages mass in nodular aggregates of epithelioid cells and giant cells. This sort of a nodular mass of epithelioid cells is referred to as a *tubercle* (Fig. 4-13). Granulomas also form in response to foreign bodies such as suture materials (Fig. 4-14). In general the presence of a granuloma is the hallmark of "tissue indigestion." As the granuloma evolves in some instances, the macrophages acquire increasing ability to handle the offensive agent, in which case it is eliminated. In other instances the agent remains refractory, and the net effect of the granuloma formation is to wall off that agent from the remainder of the body.

FATE OF THE INFLAMMATORY REACTION

Given the presence of an inflammatory reaction, the happiest result that can be obtained occurs when there actually has been little or no destruction of underlying

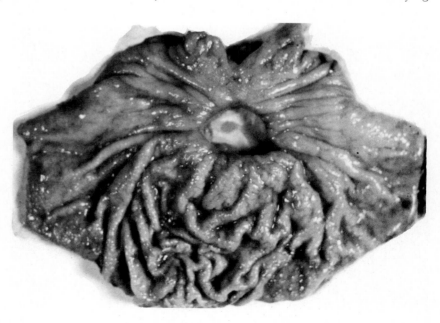

FIGURE 4-11
Gastric ulcer. A gap such as this in the continuity of a surface is termed an ulcer. An inflammatory reaction is invariably present in the base. Blood vessels may be eroded, giving rise to hemorrhage, or the full thickness of wall may be perforated.

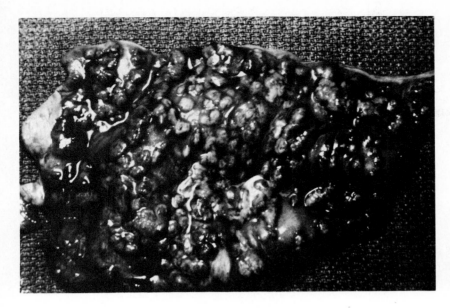

FIGURE 4-12
Pseudomembranous colitis. The many plaquelike lesions on the colonic mucosal surface represent patches of *pseudomembrane* consisting of fibrinopurulent exudate and necrotic epithelial debris.

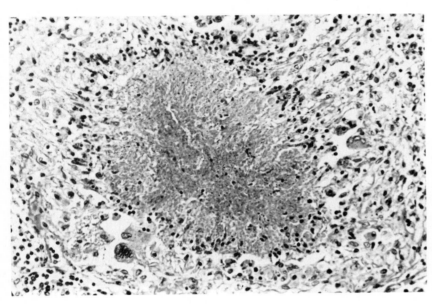

FIGURE 4-13
Epithelioid tubercle. A tubercle is a mass of macrophages which have acquired an *epithelioid* appearance. The zone of ill-defined light-staining cells at the periphery of the field (outer one-third) consists of epithelioid macrophages and multinucleated giant cells (three o'clock and seven o'clock). The center of the tubercle has undergone caseous necrosis. The small dark cells are lymphocytes. (Photomicrograph, ×315.)

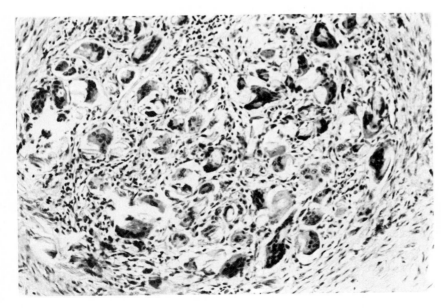

FIGURE 4-14
Foreign body granuloma. In this instance the granuloma is a mass of macrophages which have fused to form many giant cells. Many of these have engulfed fibrils, which represent fragments of suture material. (Photomicrograph, ×200.)

45

tissue. In such instances when the offending agent has been neutralized and removed, the stimulus for continuing exudation of fluid and cells gradually disappears. The small blood vessels in the area regain their usual semipermeability, fluid flux ceases, and emigration of leukocytes likewise stops. The fluid which has been previously exuded is gradually absorbed by the lymphatics, and the cells of the exudate disintegrate, wander off via the lymphatics, or are actually eliminated from the body (as, for instance, by being coughed up in the case of exudates within the lung). The net result of this process is that the previously inflamed tissue is left precisely as it was before the reaction started. This phenomenon is referred to as *resolution*.

In contrast, when significant amounts of tissue have been destroyed, resolution cannot occur. There must be *repair* of the destroyed tissue by proliferation of adjacent surviving host cells. Repair actually involves two separate but coordinated components. One, referred to as *regeneration*, actually involves proliferation of parenchymal elements identical to those lost, the net result being replacement of those lost elements by the same kind of cells. The second component of repair involves the proliferation of connective tissue elements leading to the formation of *scar*. In most tissues there is a combination of these two activities.

The abilities of different kinds of cells and tissues to regenerate differ widely. Most epithelial tissues, such as the covering of the skin and the lining of the mouth, pharynx, and gastrointestinal tract, regenerate beautifully following loss of a portion of the tissue. Other epithelial cells, such as those of the liver parenchyma,

renal tubules, or the secretory elements of certain glands, regenerate well providing that the outlines of the tissue are maintained without extensive collapse during the inflammatory process. Unfortunately some tissues regenerate very poorly or not at all. Useful regeneration is extremely limited in involuntary and voluntary muscle if it is present at all, and there is absolutely no regeneration in heart muscle, which is unfortunate given the frequency of necrosis of portions of myocardium in our population. Finally it should be pointed out that there is no regeneration of neurons or nerve cells within the central nervous system. When such cells are lost, the loss is permanent.

Repair by formation of scar is an efficient process in virtually any tissue of the body. Formation of scar involves proliferating connective tissue from areas adjoining the necrotic tissue extending into the area as the tissue is demolished by the inflammatory reaction. Such ingrowth of a proliferating young connective tissue into an area of inflammation is referred to as *organization*, and the connective tissue itself is referred to as *granulation tissue*. The components of granulation tissue actually include proliferating fibroblasts, proliferating capillary sprouts (the endothelial cells are sometimes referred to as *angioblasts*), various leukocytes of the inflammatory process, fluid portions of the exudate, and a loose semifluid connective tissue ground substance. Organization occurs in situations where abundant tissue has become necrotic, it occurs when inflammatory exudates persist and do not resolve, and it occurs where masses of blood (hematomas) or blood clots do not resolve quickly. The fibroblasts and angioblasts of granulation tissue originate from preexisting fibroblasts and capillaries in the surroundings, and their migration is somehow oriented so there is gradual extension of this tissue into the appropriate area (Fig. 4-15).

The earliest evidence of organization usually oc-

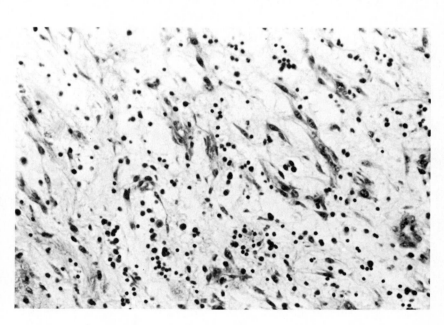

FIGURE 4-15
Early organization. The field depicts granulation tissue growing into an area of repair. The elongated, spindle-shaped cells are fibroblasts. Capillary sprouts are recognized as tubular structures, round in cross section (as at the lower right). The small dark cells are leukocytes, and the interstitial spaces contain exudate fluid and connective tissue ground substance. Compare with Fig. 4-16. (Photomicrograph, ×315.)

curs several days after the start of the inflammatory re-action. By the end of a week or so, the granulation tissue is still very loose and cellular. At this point the fibro-blasts of the granulation tissue gradually begin to se-crete the soluble precursors of the protein *collagen,* which gradually precipitates as fibrils in the interstices of the granulation tissue. With the passage of time, more and more collagen is deposited in the granulation tissue, which is now gradually maturing to a rather dense collagenous connective tissue or scar (Fig. 4-16). While the scar achieves much of its strength by the end of 2 weeks or so, there is a continuing remodeling pro-cess and a continuing increase in the density and strength of the scar over the ensuing weeks. The gran-ulation tissue, which at first was quite cellular and vas-cular, gradually becomes less cellular and less vascular and more densely collagenous. The gross counterpart of this evolution is familiar in the appearance of healing incisions, where the resulting scar is at first somewhat loose and quite pink because of the vascularity, ulti-mately becoming denser and paler as the blood vessels regress.

The coordination of scar formation and regenera-tion is perhaps most easily illustrated in the case of the healing of cutaneous wounds. The simplest type of heal-ing is that seen in the body's handling of wounds such as surgical incisions, where the wound edges can be brought together for the healing process to begin. Such healing is referred to as *primary healing* or *healing by first intention.* As seen in Fig. 4-17, immediately after wounding the wound edges are bound together by a bit of blood clot, the fibrin of which acts somewhat like a glue. Immediately thereafter an acute inflammatory re-action develops at the edges of the wound, and the in-flammatory cells, particularly macrophages, enter the blood clot and begin to demolish it. On the heels of this exudative inflammatory reaction, the ingrowth of gran-

ulation tissue into the area formerly occupied by the clot begins. Thus in a period of several days the wound is bridged by granulation tissue which is destined to ma-ture to a scar. While this is going on (Fig. 4-17), the surface epithelium at the edges begins to regenerate, and within a period of a few days a thin layer of epithe-lium migrates across the wound surface. As the scar be-neath matures, this epithelium also thickens and ma-tures so that it comes to resemble the adjacent skin. The net result (Fig. 4-17) is a reconstituted skin surface and an underlying scar which may be virtually invisible or barely visible as a thickened line. Many skin wounds heal in just this fashion with no medical attention. In others, sutures are placed to hold the wound edges in apposition until healing can occur. Sutures can be re-moved when organization and epithelial regeneration have progressed to the point where the edges will not gape when the sutures are removed. Thus, in an area of skin where there is relatively little tension, sutures can be removed in several days, long before maximal strength of the scar has been achieved, and in fact be-fore appreciable amounts of collagen have been laid down. In areas under stress, sutures must be left in place longer to hold the tissue together until a tough scar can form.

A second pattern of healing occurs when the wounding of skin is such that the edges cannot be brought together during the healing process. This is re-ferred to as *healing by second intention* or sometimes *healing by granulation* (Fig. 4-18). This type of healing is qualitatively identical to that described above. The difference lies only in the fact that much more granu-

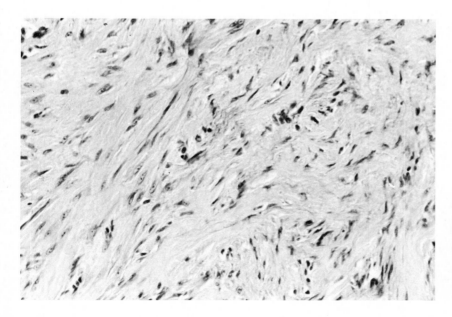

FIGURE 4-16

Maturing scar. As granulation tissue matures, the fibroblasts synthesize collagen which forms the tough scar. In this field, the interstitial material has a "stringy" appearance due to abundant collagen in fibrillar form. As scar ages, it becomes less cellular, more densely collagenous. (Photomicrograph, ×315.)

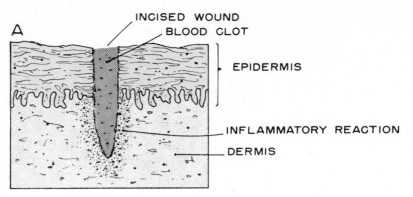

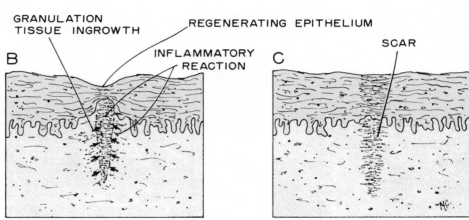

FIGURE 4-17
Healing of an incised, primarily closed wound. The wound edges are initially held together by blood clot (A) and perhaps also by sutures. An acute inflammatory response is mounted in the adjacent tissue, and it leads to ingrowth of granulation tissue after several days (B). At this stage epidermal regeneration is under way. The usual result is complete epidermal regeneration and a compact dermal scar, which forms as the granulation tissue matures (C).

lation tissue is formed, much more epithelial regeneration is necessary, and usually a larger scar is formed. The entire process, of course, takes longer than healing by primary intention. Very often in such large open wounds, granulation tissue can be observed covering the floor of the wound as a delicate nappy carpet which bleeds easily on touch. In other situations the granulation tissue actually grows beneath a scab, and epithelial regeneration likewise occurs beneath the scab. Ultimately in such circumstances the scab is cast off when healing is complete. Most of us can recall having impatiently removed a scab approximately in the stage shown in Fig. 4-18B to reveal a central pinpoint of bleeding granulation tissue where epithelial regeneration was not yet total. Although identical in many ways to healing by primary intention, secondary healing is less desirable (not that there is often a choice!) because of the time involved and the termination in a much larger and potentially disfiguring scar.

Healing in virtually any tissue of the body occurs by a process paralleling that described for the skin, with local variations depending upon the ability of the tissues to regenerate, etc.

The designation of an inflammatory process as acute, subacute, or chronic reflects the duration in terms of the extent of repair. Acute inflammation by definition has no reparative aspects; it consists only of the exudative phenomena of inflammation. In subacute inflam-

mation there is beginning granulation tissue ingrowth and perhaps beginning regeneration. In chronic inflammation there is evidence of advanced repair side by side with continuing exudation. Evidence of advanced repair includes extensive regenerative proliferation and extensive formation of scar with abundant collagen.

FACTORS AFFECTING INFLAMMATION AND HEALING

In some situations the inflammatory process may be impaired from the beginning, i.e., in its exudative stages. The entire inflammatory process is dependent upon an intact circulation to the affected area. Thus, when there is a deficiency of blood supply to an area, the result may be very sluggish inflammatory processes, persistent infections, and poor healing. Another requisite for efficient exudative inflammation is a liberal supply of leukocytes in the circulating blood. Patients whose marrow is destroyed or depressed, as, for instance, by malignant disease or as the result of adverse reaction to drugs, are unable to produce cellular exudates with normal function and as a result are liable to severe infections. More rarely the functions of leukocytes, even when they are present in normal numbers, may be imparied (e.g., abnormal chemotaxis, abnormal phagocytosis, or abnor-

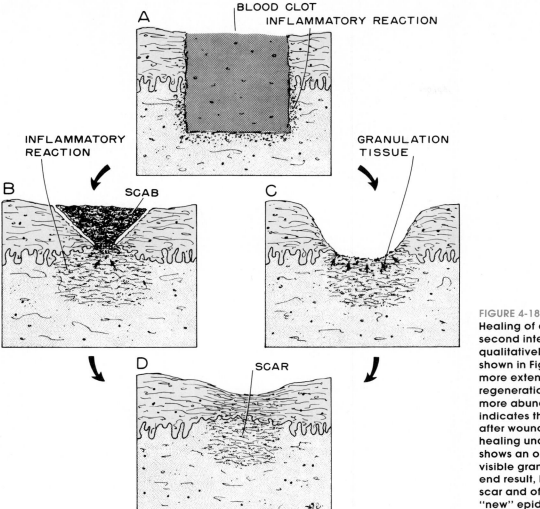

A
BLOOD CLOT
INFLAMMATORY REACTION

INFLAMMATORY REACTION

GRANULATION TISSUE

B
SCAB

C

D
SCAR

FIGURE 4-18
Healing of an open wound by second intention. The process is qualitatively similar to that shown in Fig. 4-17 but involves more extensive epithelial regeneration and formation of more abundant scar. Diagram A indicates the situation shortly after wounding, B represents healing under a scab, while C shows an open wound with visible granulation tissue. The end result, D, involves a large scar and often a thin area of "new" epidermis devoid of hair and other appendages.

mal intracellular killing and digestion), and the patient is rendered similarly liable to aggressive infections. Since leukocyte function is assisted by certain antibodies (see Chap. 5), the inflammatory reaction is also less than normally effective in immunodeficient patients. Finally, certain drugs are capable, in sufficiently high doses, of inhibiting essential aspects of the inflammatory response.

Many factors can affect the healing of wounds or other areas of tissue injury and inflammation. The healing process, dependent as it is on cellular proliferation and synthetic activity, is particularly sensitive to local deficiencies of blood supply (with attendant impairment of raw material delivery) and is also sensitive to the nutritional state of the host. Patients who are markedly malnourished do not heal wounds optimally. The healing of wounds is also adversely affected by the presence of foreign material or necrotic tissue in the wound, by the presence of wound infection, and by incomplete immobilization and apposition of wound edges.

Even if healing proceeds adequately on a cellular level, there are occasionally complications as an end result. It is in the nature of scar tissue to shorten and to become more dense and compact with the passage of time. The result of this is sometimes *contracture*, which may disfigure an area, limit motion at a joint, etc. If the scar tissue encircles a tubular structure, e.g., the urethra, the result may be a *stricture*, which narrows the structure in question and may produce serious difficulty. When serosal surfaces are inflamed and the exudate does not resolve, granulation tissue and eventually scar may come to bind serosal surfaces together forming what are called *adhesions*. In many areas, such as the pleura or the pericardium, adhesions are generally trivial as far as organ function is concerned. Within the peritoneal cavity, however, adhesions, whether between loops of bowel or between abdominal viscera and the body wall, may produce webs which can constrict portions of the gastrointestinal tract or can actually entrap them, forming internal hernias which may strangulate and become gangrenous. Another complication seen occasionally in healing wounds of the body wall is the so-called *incisional hernia*. In this situation the granulation tissue and scar which bridge the surgical defect in the body wall gradually yield to intraperitoneal pressure, and a bulging sac in the incision is formed. Another minor local complication of healing is the protrusion of a bit of granulation tissue above the surface of the healing wound, forming what is sometimes called "proud flesh" or a *pyogenic granuloma*. Healing generally proceeds well when such excrescences are cauterized or nipped off. A complication of healing occasionally encountered is the so-called *amputation* or *traumatic neuroma* which simply represents regenerative proliferation of nerve fibers into the area of healing where they become entrapped in dense scar. Such a neuroma may constitute an unsightly or even painful lump within a scar. Finally some individuals, apparently on a genetic basis, handle the production and/or remodeling of collagen in a healing wound abnormally, so that an excess of collagen is formed, leading to a protrusion called a *keloid*. These are somewhat commoner in blacks and Asians and in younger patients. Keloids are biologically trivial but cosmetically may assume great importance.

SYSTEMIC ASPECTS OF INFLAMMATION

The emphasis of all of the foregoing description has been on strictly local aspects of the response to injury. It must be pointed out that systemic accompaniments of the local reaction are frequently present. *Fever* is a familiar phenomenon occurring in parallel with many local inflammatory processes, noninfectious as well as infectious. While many causes of fever exist, a final pathway of mediation seems to be the release of so-called *endogenous pyrogens* from neutrophils and macrophages. These substances affect the temperature-regulating centers in the hypothalamus, in effect resetting the body's "thermostat" and producing fever. Another striking accompaniment of local inflammation is the set of hematologic changes commonly observed. Stimuli emanating from the locus of inflammation influence the process of maturation and the release of leukocytes from the bone marrow leading to an increase in the circulating numbers of one or another type of leukocyte, the increase being referred to as *leukocytosis*. Changes in certain blood proteins also occur, along with alterations in the so-called sedimentation rate of the blood. With severe injuries, striking metabolic and endocrinologic changes occur. Finally, local inflammatory reactions are often accompanied by a variety of ill-defined "constitutional" symptoms including malaise, anorexia or loss of appetite, and varying degrees of disability or even prostration. The causes and mediation of most of these systemic changes are poorly understood or unknown.

QUESTIONS

Response of the body to injury—Inflammation and repair

Directions: Circle the letter preceding each item below that correctly answers the question. More than one answer may be correct.

1. The best definition of inflammation is:
   a. Accumulation of water in the cells due to failure of the sodium pump   *b.* Invasion of tissue by living pathogenic organisms   *c.* Margination of leukocytes along the vascular lining   *d.* Local reaction of the tissues to an injury

2. The *ultimate* purpose of the inflammatory response is to:
   a. Increase fatty infiltration in the affected tissue in preparation for the process of healing   *b.* Release lysosomes which promote the synthesis of cellular proteins to promote healing   *c.* Localize, destroy, neutralize, and remove injurious agents in preparation for the process of healing   *d.* Restore function by promoting hydropic changes in cells

3. An acute inflammatory reaction in the host can be expected:
   a. Following cell injury by pathogenic bacteria   *b.* Following introduction of a *sterile* but irritating foreign material   *c.* Around an area of necrosis in a sterile area   *d.* In the center of a necrotic area   *e.* Shortly following death

4. Which of the following are cardinal signs of acute inflammation?
   a. Calor   *b.* Rigor   *c.* *Functio laesa*   *d.* Algor   *e.* Rubor

5. Which of the cardinal signs of inflammation result from increased blood flow in the affected area?
   a. Swelling   *b.* Heat   *c.* Pain   *d.* Redness

6. Manifestations of inflammation resulting from increased vascular permeability include:
   a. Swelling   *b.* Heat   *c.* Pain   *d.* Redness

7. Which of the following are believed to be causes of pain in an inflamed area?
   a. Pressure of the exudate   *b.* Changes in the pH due to acidic breakdown products   *c.* Release of chemical mediators which stimulate nerve endings   *d.* Increased flow of lymph

8. The two *major* forces which normally govern the transport of fluid between the intravascular and interstitial spaces are:
   a. The hydrostatic pressure of the blood   *b.* The contractility of endothelial cells   *c.* The osmotic pressure of the plasma proteins   *d.* The permeability of connective tissue

9. Which one of the following reactions occurs in an acute inflammatory response?
   a. Lymph flow decreases, producing edema. *b.* Arterioles in the area dilate to produce active congestion.   *c.* Protein follows water into the interstitial spaces.   *d.* The permeability of the venules decreases owing to the release of local chemical mediators.

10. An exudate differs from a transudate in that:
    a. Exudates contain more cells derived from the blood.   *b.* Transudates are much smaller in quantity.   *c.* A transudate is a result of a noninflammatory situation.   *d.* Exudates have a higher protein content than do transudates.

11. The rapid shift of fluid into the interstitial tissue during inflammation is a result of:
    a. Increased hydrostatic pressure within the vessel *b.* Increased osmotic pressure within the vessel *c.* Increase in the lymphatic flow   *d.* Increase in the permeability of the vessel walls to protein

12. Which of the following best describes histamine?
    a. It produces vasoconstriction.   *b.* It increases vascular permeability.   *c.* It is released from mast cells early in inflammation.   *d.* It has an important role in chronic inflammation.

13. Hageman factor is known to:
    a. Increase vascular permeability   *b.* Be present in plasma in an active form   *c.* Trigger the clotting cascade system   *d.* Be an important inflammatory mediator

14. The cyclooxygenase pathway is responsible for generating which of the following mediators of inflammation?
    a. Histamine   *b.* Hageman factor   *c.* Prostaglandins   *d.* Leukotrienes

15. In an acute inflammatory reaction, the first cells to appear at the site of injury are generally the:
    a. Monocytes   *b.* Lymphocytes   *c.* Plasma cells *d.* Polymorphonuclear neutrophils (PMNs)

16. The cells least likely to be found in large numbers (dominant in the exudate) in chronic inflammation are:
    a. Lymphocytes   *b.* Plasma cells   *c.* Macrophages   *d.* Fibroblasts   *e.* Neutrophils (PMNs)

17. Opsonization refers to:
    a. Removal of extracellular debris by specific digestive enzymes   *b.* Enzymatic destruction of large particles of foreign material over a long period of time   *c.* Destruction of the fibrin barrier formed around some bacterial infection sites *d.* A process by which bacteria are rendered more susceptible to phagocytosis

18. The polymorphonuclear neutrophil is associated with:
    a. Phagocytosis of bacteria in acute inflammation *b.* Cytoplasmic granules (lysosomes) which stain bright red with eosin dye   *c.* Heparin production *d.* Synthesis of antibody in allergic reactions

19. Basophils:
    a. Have many features in common with mast cells in connective tissue   *b.* Have cytoplasmic granules which stain deep blue with basic dyes *c.* Are generally present in large numbers in exudates   *d.* Are granulocytes which contain histamine and heparin in their cytoplasmic granules

20. The mechanisms of leukocytosis in the course of an inflammatory reaction include:
    a. Increased production of leukocytes by the bone marrow   *b.* Increased life span of leukocytes during inflammation   *c.* Increased release of leukocytes from the bone marrow reserves into the blood   *d.* Stimulation of the vascular endothelium by pyrogens

21. The monocyte-macrophage system:
    a. Was originally called the reticuloendothelial system   *b.* Provides a major defense against the spread of infection in the body   *c.* Removes foreign material from circulating blood, lymph, and tissue spaces.   *d.* Includes as components blood monocytes, wandering macrophages, and fixed mononuclear phagocytic cells   *e.* Is present in the bone marrow, spleen, lymph nodes, and liver

22. Epithelioid cells:
    a. Are altered epithelial cells   *b.* Are common components of granulomatous inflammation *c.* Serve to wall off an agent which cannot be destroyed or eliminated from the body   *d.* Are altered macrophages

23. Pus contains:
    a. Dead and dying neutrophils   b. Micro-organisms   c. Tissue debris   d. Water and solutes

24. Which of the following cells are capable of regeneration following necrosis?
    a. Myocardial cells   b. Epithelial cells of the gastrointestinal tract   c. Neurons   d. Hepatocytes   e. Lymphoid cells

25. What *two* cell types play the primary role in organization?
    a. Fibroblasts producing collagen   b. Osteoblasts producing mature scar tissue   c. Endothelial cells producing new blood vessels   d. Parenchymal cells producing new connective tissue

26. Which of the following may organize?
    a. Unresolved exudate   b. Necrotic tissue   c. Persistent blood clots   d. Collagen fibers

27. In comparison to healing by first intention, one would expect healing by secondary intention to involve:
    a. Good apposition of wound edges   b. A longer time for the process to be completed   c. Less scarring   d. Formation of more granulation tissue   e. A greater amount of exudate

28. The outcome of inflammation is affected by:
    a. Vascularity of the tissue   b. Nutritional status of the host   c. Presence of debris   d. Immunologic capability

29. Systemic manifestations associated with inflammation include:
    a. Leukocytosis   b. Malaise (vague feeling of discomfort)   c. Fever   d. Agranulocytosis

Directions: Circle T if the statement is true and F if it is false. Correct false statements.

30. T   F   When a specific area of the body is infected, the regional lymph nodes may act as filters preventing further spread of the bacteria in the body.

31. T   F   A chemotactic effect can be exerted only by the injurious agent.

32. T   F   Monocytes and neutrophils both respond to chemotactic signals.

33. T   F   Mast cells are the primary source of histamine.

34. T   F   Lysosomes are packets of digestive enzymes within the cytoplasm of neutrophils and other cells.

35. T   F   Monocytes differ from neutrophils in that they are capable of synthesizing intracellular enzymes and dividing after migration to the tissues while neutrophils are not.

36. T   F   When a circulating monocyte appears in an exudate, it is called a mast cell.

37. T   F   Granulation tissue consists primarily of proliferating young connective tissue.

38. T   F   Healing by secondary intention requires a longer time period and leaves a larger scar than healing by primary intention.

39. T   F   Granulomas may result from a foreign material such as a nonabsorbable suture left in the body or from certain bacteria, such as the tubercle bacillus, which are resistant to phagocytosis or enzymatic digestion.

40. T   F   Granuloma formation indicates that the body cannot easily overcome or eliminate the agent responsible.

41. T   F   Giant cells are formed by the fusion of neutrophils in chronic granulomatous inflammation.

42. T   F   Subacute inflammations show evidence of advanced repair along with exudation.

43. T   F   A keloid represents disordered wound healing and is caused by the proliferation of nerve fibers and their entrapment in dense scar tissue.

44. T   F   Arachidonic acid is derived from cell membrane phospholipids when phospholipases are activated by injury.

45. T   F   Prostaglandins are important vascular and chemotactic mediators of inflammation.

Directions: Match the following types of exudates in col. A to the statements in col. B.

Column A

46. ____ Catarrhal
47. ____ Suppurative
48. ____ Phlegmonous (cellulitis)
49. ____ Serous
50. ____ Pseudomembranous

Column B

a. Poorly limited spreading or diffuse inflammation

b. Occurs only on mucous membranes and contains mucin

c. Includes a web of fibrinopurulent exudate coating the necrotic mucosal surface

d. Contains very few cells (e.g., blister fluid)

e. Contains many living and
dead neutrophils and debris
liquefied by enzymes released
from the dead neutorphils

Directions: Fill in the blanks with the correct words.

51. A(n) _____ is a lesion within solid tissue containing dead cells, liquefied tissue, neutrophils, and often bacteria.

52. A(n) _____ is a local gap in the continuity of the mucosal surface.

53. The accumulation of pus in the pleural cavity is called _____.

54. A blind tract opening to the body surface is called a(n) _____.

55. An abnormal communication tract between two organs or the lumen of a hollow organ and the body surface is called a(n) _____.

56. The suffix for inflammation is _____.

57. _____ is the term describing the movement of leukocytes from the axial stream to the periphery of the blood vessel lumen.

58. _____ is the term used to describe leukocytes inserting pseudopodia in intercellular junctions and sliding and wriggling through to the extravascular spaces.

59. The resorption of exudate with return of the area to normal is called _____.

60. _____ is the replacement of dead or injured tissues by new cells of parenchymal or stromal origin.

61. Inflammation of the lymph nodes is termed _____.

62. The correct sequence of the following events as they occur in an inflammatory reaction is _____.
a. Tissue injury   b. Increased local blood flow leading to heat and redness   c. Emigration of leukocytes   d. Slowing of blood flow; margination of leukocytes   e. Increased vascular permeability

RESPONSE OF THE BODY TO IMMUNOLOGIC CHALLENGE

OBJECTIVES

At the completion of this chapter you should be able to:

1. Describe in general terms the biological significance of immune responses.
2. Describe the nature of antigens.
3. Describe the two basic modes of immunologic response which may be elicited when lymphoid tissue is exposed to antigens.
4. State the general properties associated with immunologic reactions.
5. Identify three sorts of phenomena manifested by antigen-stimulated lymphocytes.
6. Describe the components of the lymphoid system including their location, structure, interconnections, and functions.
7. Trace the development of lymphocytes.
8. Compare and contrast T and B lymphocytes, "null cells," and natural killer (NK) cells as to their function.
9. Describe the steps in the process of immunoglobulin synthesis.
10. Contrast the sequence of events that occurs when an antigen is first introduced into the body with the sequence when that material is re-introduced into the same individual.
11. Compare active and passive immunization.
12. Characterize the several different classes of immunoglobulins as to occurrence and function.
13. Identify characteristics that are common to the several different types of immunoglobulins.
14. Describe the means of histamine release in the course of immunologic reactions.
15. Explain how the interaction of antigen and antibody results in the activation of the complement system and describe the consequences of such activation.
16. Describe the cellular phenomena which may occur when lymphocytes interact with antigen in the effector phase of a cellular immune response.

17. Differentiate between the mechanisms of antibody-mediated (immediate) and cell-mediated (delayed) hypersensitivity according to the type of response, cell changes, and reactions.
18. Describe the four basic types of immunologic injuries as classified by Gell and Coombs.
19. List three types of allergic reactions due to humoral immunity and three types due to cellular immunity.
20. Describe the events which may trigger autoimmunity.
21. Define immunodeficiency syndromes.
22. Cite examples and discuss the etiology of primary and secondary immunologic deficiencies.

THE NATURE OF IMMUNOLOGIC REACTIONS

Antigens

When a foreign material is introduced into the tissues of a living host, there is generally a response mounted to the presence of that material. That response has the general characteristics of the inflammatory reaction described in Chap. 4. Many foreign materials, if introduced into the host body on multiple occasions, elicit precisely the same response on each occasion. Certain foreign materials, however, are capable of inducing a change in the host such that reactions to subsequent exposures are different from the reaction to the first introduction of the material. Such altered responses on the part of the host are referred to as immunologic responses, and the materials eliciting them are termed *antigens* or *immunogens*. *The essence of an immune response is that the offending material is neutralized, destroyed, or eliminated from the host body more rapidly than would otherwise be the case.*

As indicated above, not all foreign materials are antigenic. Those materials which do function as antigens are generally of relatively high molecular weight, usually in excess of 10,000. Most antigens are proteins, but certain polysaccharides, polypeptides, and nucleic acids of large size may also function antigenically. Antigens may be chemically pure substances, or, as is often the case, might be incorporated in complex form as part of the structure of a bacterium, a virus, or even of a living tissue. In provoking a response the entire molecule of antigen does not necessarily play a vital role. In fact it appears that only certain active portions of the molecule, called *determinant groups*, are specifically essential to the reactions. From the standpoint of general biology as well as of human medicine it is important to note that certain small molecules which are unable in and of themselves to act as antigens are able to join chemically with larger molecules, such as proteins within the host body, creating a sort of complex which may then behave as an antigen. In such an instance, the specificity of the reactions provoked is related in large part to determinant groups of the small molecule. Such molecules are called *haptens*, and the larger molecules are referred to as *carriers*.

Properties of the immune response

The "business" of the immune response, i.e., the expeditious elimination of antigenic materials, is accomplished by the host body in two sorts of ways. The first type of response, the *humoral immune response*, is effected by *immunoglobulins*, the gamma globulins of the blood, which are synthesized by the host in response to introduction of the antigenic material. These immunoglobulins are capable of reacting specifically with the antigens which provoke their production, and in so reacting, sometimes with the aid of one or another "amplification system," they lead to elimination of the antigen.

The second sort of immunologic reaction, the *cell-mediated reaction*, is carried out directly by lymphocytes which have proliferated in response to introduction of the antigen and which react specifically with the antigen (without the intervention of ordinary immunoglobulins).

Immunologic reactions, whether mediated by immunoglobulin antibodies or directly by cells, display the property of *self-recognition*. That is to say, these reactions will be mounted only against materials which are sensed as being foreign and will not ordinarily be mounted against constituents of the host's own body. A second property of immunologic response is *memory*, by virtue of which the production of immunoglobulin antibodies or the expansion of a clone of specifically re-

active cells proceeds more rapidly with repeated introduction of the antigen. The cellular mechanisms of the
body, in effect, remember the antigen. Last but not
least, *specificity* is an extremely important property of
immunologic reactions. That is to say, the antibodies
whose formation is elicited by a particular antigen react
uniquely with that antigen (or with molecules bearing
virtually identical determinant groups).

Immunoreactive tissues

The part of the immune response which leads to the
production of immunoglobulin antibodies or to the proliferation of antigen-reactive cells is sometimes referred
to as the *afferent limb* or *induction phase* of the immune response. Lymphocytes and macrophages are the
cells chiefly responsible for this portion of the response.
More specifically, it is the so-called lymphoid tissues of
the body which are involved. Once antibody has been
synthesized or antigen-reactive cells have proliferated,
they become widely disseminated in various tissues of
the body so that when antigens are reintroduced in almost any location, an efficient immunologic reaction
may ensue. In other words, the effector cells or immunoglobulin molecules, although produced in the lymphoid tissues, may participate in the *efferent limb* or *effector phase* of the immunologic response virtually
anywhere in the body.

BIOLOGY OF LYMPHOCYTES AND LYMPHOID TISSUES

Properties of lymphocytes

Lymphocytes are, morphologically speaking, among the
most nondescript cells of the body. Lymphocytes, in
general, have large, roughly spherical, rather deeply
staining nuclei and relatively little cytoplasm. Even
under scrutiny with the electron microscope lymphocytes tend to be rather uninspiring in appearance, with
relatively little in the way of intracytoplasmic organelles. As seen with the ordinary microscope, lymphocytes tend to differ from one another largely in respect
to their size and amount of cytoplasm.

Although lymphocytes certainly give no such hint
from their drab morphology, they are in point of fact
extremely dynamic cells and are remarkably heterogeneous in a variety of respects. Probably the variation in
size is the most trivial aspect of lymphocyte heterogeneity. Lymphocytes actually differ in terms of how they
(1) differentiate in the course of development, (2) differ
in their life cycles, (3) stream along different pathways
in the body, (4) have different surface characteristics,
and most importantly, (5) serve different functions.
Some lymphocytes, when properly stimulated, are capable of secreting soluble substances termed *lymphokines*, which have exceedingly important effects on
other cells within the body. Other types of lymphocytes, when properly stimulated, actually change their
structure, acquire the cytoplasmic "machinery" of protein synthesis, and become producers of immunoglobulin antibody. When lymphocytes have undergone this
type of modulation, they are referred to as *plasma cells*

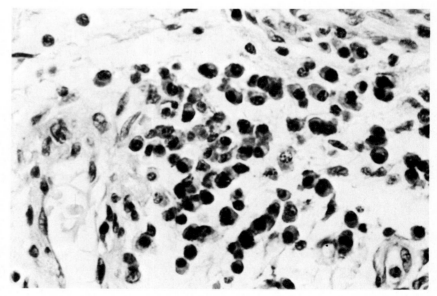

FIGURE 5-1

**Plasma cells in tissue. These cells
represent lymphocytes which have
modulated into immunoglobulin-
synthesizing cells. They differ from
"ordinary" lymphocytes by virtue of their
relatively abundant, deeply staining
cytoplasm. (Photomicrograph, ×800.)**

(Fig. 5-1). Viewed with the electron microscope, the abundant basophilic cytoplasm that develops when a lymphocyte becomes a plasma cell is seen to contain an extensive rough endoplasmic reticulum, which is the locus of immunoglobulin synthesis. Some lymphocytes are also capable, when properly stimulated, of undergoing what is termed *blast transformation*. That is, they become dividing lymphoblasts and give rise to expanding numbers of cells having the same properties. These various reactions of different kinds of lymphocytes are triggered by reactions which occur at the level of the cell membrane.

Components of the lymphoid system

Lymphocytes are almost everywhere in the body but tend to be concentrated in certain tissues (the lymphoid tissues) which together constitute a coordinated system. The components of this system include lymph nodes, spleen, thymus, lymphoid tissues associated with mucosal surfaces, and bone marrow.

Lymph nodes (Fig. 5-2) are the most numerous components of this system. These encapsulated masses of lymphoid tissues are present in virtually every area of the body, perhaps the most familiar being the nodes palpable in the neck or groin. They are like filters placed at intervals in lymphatic channels. The entering or afferent lymphatics pierce the capsule of the node, and the lymph immediately enters an anastomosing system of sinusoids lined by macrophages. The node is, in effect, a meshwork of sinusoids with nodules of lymphoid tissue called *follicles* arranged in the meshwork at the periphery of the node (the cortex). In the inner part, or medulla of the node, there are cords of lymphoid tissue between the sinusoids. In both cortex and medulla of lymph nodes are quantities of lymphocytes; these are able to interact with one another and with macrophages, often in the presence of antigenic materials percolating through the node after having entered by the afferent lymphatics. Efferent lymphatics exit from the node from the region of the medulla. An important detail of lymph node structure is the fact that lymph nodes also have a rich blood supply, which is important to the traffic of lymphocytes within the body.

The *spleen* is, in effect, a large mass of lymphoid and reticuloendothelial cells, or macrophages, interposed in the course of the bloodstream. Instead of being filled with lymph, the sinusoids of the spleen are filled with blood. Interspersed in this meshwork of blood sinusoids with their reticuloendothelial cell, or macrophage, lining are nodules of lymphoid tissue similar to those in the cortex of lymph nodes (Fig. 5-3). As in the case of the lymph nodes, the structure of the spleen allows close interaction between lymphocytes, macrophages, and materials carried in the bloodstream.

The *thymus* is a somewhat less familiar lymphoid tissue which is located in the thorax anterior to the upper part of the heart and great vessels. This organ consists of a reticular framework densely infiltrated with lymphocytes arranged in the pattern of cortex and medulla (Fig. 5-4). The lymphoid tissue of the thymus has a rich blood supply.

An extremely important component of the lymphoid system is the lymphoid tissue associated with *mucosal surfaces* in the body such as those in the gastrointestinal tract and the respiratory tract. Although in any one area this type of lymphoid tissue does not form par-

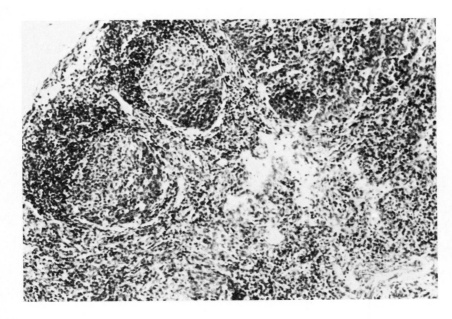

FIGURE 5-2
Lymph node. The capsule and the underlying sinusoid are seen at the upper left. Two prominent lymphoid follicles are evident in the subjacent cortex. The open spaces (center and right) are sinusoids, while the intervening clusters of cells are cords of lymphocytes composing the medulla. (Photomicrograph, ×200.)

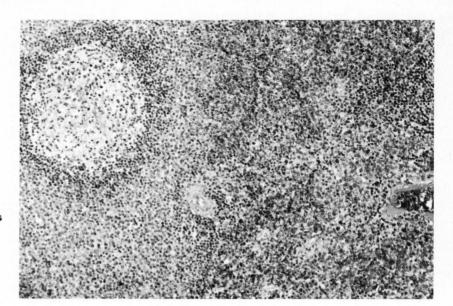

FIGURE 5-3
Spleen. At the upper left is a lymphoid follicle in the so-called white pulp. This is similar to the cortical follicles of lymph nodes. The right half of the field is occupied by so-called red pulp, a meshwork of blood sinusoids and intervening cells. (Photomicrograph, ×200.)

ticularly large nodules, the diffuseness of its distribution renders this tissue highly important. It is also strategically placed in terms of antigen reactivity and defensive function by virtue of being at the interface between the host and the environment. This type of lymphoid tissue is particularly prominent within the gastrointestinal tract, distributed diffusely in the so-called lamina propria of the mucosa (see Fig. 5-5) and in nodular aggregates referred to as Peyer's patches.

Finally, the *bone marrow* should be designated as an important part of the lymphoid system. Although attention is usually focused on hematopoietic elements in the marrow which are responsible for producing granulocytes, platelets, and red blood cells, many millions of lymphocytes are scattered within the bone marrow.

Lymphocytic traffic within the body

The various components of the lymphoid system are joined together by a sort of double plumbing system, the blood vascular system and the lymphatic system. At any given time millions of lymphocytes are moving within both the blood and the lymph. The various lymphatic channels in the body drain fluid from the interstices of organs and tissues and conduct it centrad, where ultimately the various channels join together and enter the bloodstream via a large vein in the thorax. Thus, there is a constant flow of lymph back into the blood and a constant formation of lymph by movement of fluid from the blood out into the tissues. In a similar fashion there is a constant recirculation of lymphocytes

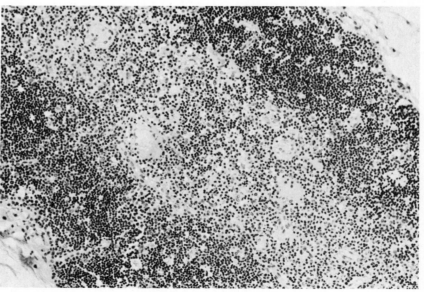

FIGURE 5-4
Thymus. The framework of this organ is infiltrated by myriads of lymphocytes, more densely in the cortex (periphery), less so in the medulla. The thymic tissue tends to atrophy with age. (Photomicrograph, ×200.)

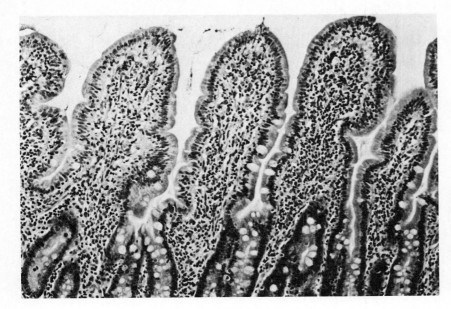

FIGURE 5-5

Mucosal lymphoid tissue. In this section of small intestine, large numbers of lymphocytes are present in the connective tissue beneath the epithelium. This is of obvious importance, given the antigen load impinging on a mucosal surface. (Photomicrograph, ×200.)

themselves. If one were to sample the lymph within the large central lymphatic channel (the thoracic duct) many lymphocytes would be found. In fact sufficient numbers of lymphocytes flow through the thoracic duct to replace the total number in circulation in the bloodstream several times per day.

Most of the lymphocytes flowing in the thoracic duct are actually being "recycled." In recent years it has been recognized that lymphocytes leave the bloodstream by specialized venules within lymphoid tissues; they spend variable lengths of time within the lymphoid tissues and then circulate via the stream of lymph to rejoin the lymphocytes in circulating blood. Lymphocytes differ quite strikingly from one another with respect to their movements around the body. Some lymphocytes are remarkably long-lived (many months or even years) and travel and recycle extensively. Other lymphocytes are relatively short-lived and do not move around quite as freely. It also appears that certain groups of lymphocytes may have preferential "homing" patterns with respect to various parts of the lymphoid system. The key point here is that there exists within the lymphoid system provision for moving lymphocytes from one area to another. The biological importance of this lies in the fact that members of a particular clone of lymphocytes which initially proliferate in one given location may circulate around the body and be available for interaction with antigen at many locations.

Ontogeny of lymphocytes

The body's supply of lymphocytes begins embryologically in the yolk sac and liver, and the supply function is ultimately taken over by the lymphocyte population of the bone marrow. Lymphocytes are continually ex-

ported from the bone marrow, and some of them migrate to the thymus, where their development is conditioned. That is to say, by virtue of their exposure to certain substances within the thymus, these lymphocytes acquire certain reactive properties. Such cells are known as *thymus-dependent* lymphocytes or *T lymphocytes*. These lymphocytes are subsequently exported from the thymus, and they populate the various other lymphoid tissues of the body. Other lymphocytes are apparently independent of the thymic influence and thus have properties which differ from the T lymphocytes. The thymus-independent cells are referred to as *B lymphocytes*. It is these latter lymphocytes which, under appropriate conditions, change into plasma cells. The populating of so-called peripheral lymphoid tissues by B and T lymphocytes is not a random affair, and these tissues have actually been mapped in terms of preferential concentration of one or another type of cell. Although these specific localizations are not important for purposes of the present discussion, it is vital to reemphasize that the design of lymphoid tissue is such as to allow the interaction of T lymphocytes, B lymphocytes, macrophages, and antigenic materials carried in blood or lymph or entering via a mucosal surface.

There is even greater heterogeneity of lymphocytes than the simple division into the T and B classes outlined above. A number of subsets of T lymphocytes have been described. Some of these act as "helper" cells, augmenting the activities of other lymphocytes. Conversely, some act as suppressor cells. Yet others act as directly cytotoxic or killer cells, bringing about the lysis of target cells with whose surface antigens these lymphocytes are specifically reactive.

The various subsets of T lymphocytes have distinctive surface "markers" distinguishing one subset from another and from B lymphocytes. Other lymphocytes, called "null cells," lack surface markers of either the T or B series. Certain of these cells have receptors for portions of the immunoglobulin G (IgG) molecule and function in so-called antibody-dependent cell-mediated cytotoxic reactions described below. Finally, another subset of lymphocytes, which morphologically are large and granular, are known as *natural killer* or NK cells. These cells can destroy certain tumor cells and virus-infected cells without prior sensitization, and thus appear to play an important role as a sort of first line of defense.

ANTIBODY–MEDIATED IMMUNITY

Induction of immunoglobulin synthesis

The requisites for synthesis of immunoglobulins or antibodies are such that no one organ has a monopoly on antibody production. Generally speaking, when antigen can be brought into the presence of macrophages, B lymphocytes, and T lymphocytes, immunoglobulin production may result. Conditions are right within the lymph nodes, the spleen, and certain of the nodular lymphoid tissues along mucosal surfaces. Thus if antigen enters the subcutaneous tissues, as commonly is the case with injections, the material drains via the lymphatics to the regional lymph nodes, where antibody production subsequently takes place. If antigen enters the bloodstream directly, the spleen is a major locus of antibody production. In either situation there may be "spillover." For instance, following subcutaneous injection, antigen may actually pass through the regional lymph nodes to get into the blood circulation to the spleen. In a similar fashion, antigenic material entering by mucosal surfaces may stimulate the associated lymphoid tissues and may drain to regional lymph nodes.

When an antigen enters a lymphoid tissue, the initial step involves uptake of the antigenic material by macrophages. These cells are responsible either for presenting the antigen in the proper form to the lymphocytes or possibly for processing the antigen to produce a highly immunogenic molecule of some sort. The antigen then functions to "select" certain lymphocytes and react with them. That is to say, there are within the lymphoid tissues at least a small number of lymphocytes whose surface receptors are such as to react with the determinant groups of the antigen. The net result of such interaction is an increase in the number of lymphocytes of that particular type and a modulation of the B lymphocytes into antibody-producing plasma cells. In the case of most antigens, a population of T lympho-

cytes functions as "helper cells," somehow influencing B lymphocyte activities. The net results of this interaction that are appreciated both grossly and microscopically are an enlargement of the reacting lymph node, a marked increase in the number of lymphocytes within it, and an expansion of the follicles within the cortex and the cords of cells within the medulla. As the plasma cells synthesize immunoglobulin antibody, it is secreted into the lymph and thence circulates widely in the body. Part of the result of the induction in an immune reaction is the production of "memory lymphocytes." Presumably such cells circulate widely in the body so that cellular memory of the antigen does not remain a localized affair.

When an antigen is first introduced into the body, there is a latent period usually amounting to several days before significant amounts of antibody appear in the circulating fluids. This time is required for the various cellular interactions, proliferation, and modulation to occur. In this so-called *primary response* the level of antibody rises somewhat slowly and then gradually diminishes as the immunoglobulin is catabolized. The nature of immunologic memory is such that when antigen is introduced the second time, even in another location and even after immunoglobulin levels have dwindled, the machinery of antibody production is put into motion much more rapidly, so that immunoglobulin appears after a shorter latent period and usually reaches higher levels in the circulating fluids.

These principles provide the rationale for immunization against many diseases. Immunization is referred to as *active* when the antigen is introduced into the host, who subsequently activates the machinery of immunoglobulin synthesis. *Passive immunization* is accomplished by injecting preformed immunoglobulin directly into a host, i.e., with another individual or animal having done the immunologic "work." With passive immunization, once the immunoglobulin has been catabolized by the recipient there is no memory, so the host is protected only during the circulatory life of the administered antibody. With active immunization, however, memory is induced (stimulated by an occasional "booster" injection), so that if the host is challenged by the agent of the corresponding disease, antibody production will be prompt and efficient, thus protecting the individual.

The nature of immunoglobulin molecules

Immunoglobulins, or antibodies, are protein molecules which possess as part of their structure unique sequences of amino acids permitting highly specific interactions with the corresponding antigens. Each molecule of immunoglobulin (Ig) consists of four peptide chains, two heavy (H) chains and two light (L) chains, chemically bonded together. Immunoglobulins belong to several different classes, each one of which is characterized by a certain constancy of structure (in the H chains) in addition to the variable, antigen-reactive portion of the molecule. These classes are named with the letters G, M, A, E, and D and are usually designated as IgG, IgM, IgA, IgE, and IgD. The constant portions of these various immunoglobulin molecules determine the general biological effects of the particular kind of antibody, while the variable regions determine specifically which antigens will be reacted with. The antibodies most commonly found in circulating fluids and in many tissues belong to the IgG group. These antibodies are important in resistance to infection and are able to cross the placenta from mother to child, passively immunizing the latter. IgM antibodies are found largely within circulating fluids and are generally the first sort to be synthesized early in the antibody response. IgA antibodies are produced in the lymphoid tissues along mucosal surfaces, and these molecules are actually combined with a protein in the mucosa and secreted onto the mucosal surfaces as so-called secretory antibody. This type of antibody protects the exposed surface against certain agents in the lumen. IgE antibodies are produced within lymphoid tissues (usually near boundary surfaces in the body) and secreted into the circulating fluids, but they rapidly attach to the myriads of mast cells or tissue basophils around the body. These cells have specific receptors on their surfaces for a portion of the IgE molecule. Via their effects on the release of chemical mediator substances from the mast cells, IgE molecules are involved in the regulation of vascular permeability and mucosal secretion. Relatively little is known of the function of IgD.

Functions of immunoglobulin molecules

The basic function of any immunoglobulin molecule is, of course, to react with the corresponding antigen. This particular interaction involves the variable portion of the immunoglobulin molecule. The biological effects of the interaction, i.e., those which lead to antigen neutralization or elimination, are mediated by other portions of the immunoglobulin molecule. The results of these latter kinds of reactions take a number of forms. If the antigen is a soluble protein molecule, for instance, one result of the interaction with antibody (usually of the IgG or IgM class) is the linking together of numerous antigen and antibody molecules to form a large latticework, which results in the formation of a precipitate. Such precipitation reactions can be demonstrated in vitro and presumably may be important in vivo, where insoluble precipitates would be more rapidly cleared by phagocytic cells than soluble molecules would be. If the antigen is on the surface of a large structure such as a bacterial cell, the interaction with immunoglobulin may again form a complexly linked structure. This time, the result will be agglutination of numerous bacteria bearing the antigen on their surfaces. Another function of

immunoglobulin may be to coat an antigenic particle and by interacting with receptors on the surface of phagocytic cells, such as neutrophils or macrophages, render that particle more easily phagocytosed (opsonization). Immunoglobulin may also interact with the pharmacologically important part of toxin molecules, thus neutralizing the toxin. Secretory immunoglobulin of the IgA class appears to function by preventing adherence of antigen (e.g., antigen on the surface of a microorganism) to the mucosa. These sorts of direct effects of antigen-antibody interaction can be visualized as having the net effect of eliminating the offensive material with dispatch. Certain kinds of immunoglobulin molecules, in addition, serve as effectors of immune responses in conjunction with certain "amplification systems."

Antibodies of the IgE class act in conjunction with mast cells when responding to antigen. These particular immunoglobulin molecules have such a high affinity for receptors on the surface of mast cells that they are rapidly fixed to a variety of tissues in the body and do not circulate in body fluids in high concentrations. The fixation of IgE antibodies to the surface of mast cells does not alter the function of these cells or injure them. It does, however, prepare them for action. In this attachment of IgE molecules their antigen-reactive portions remain free. When antigen molecules contact the corresponding IgE, the antigen-antibody interaction triggers release of the contents of the mast cells. One of the released substances is histamine, a potent vasodilator which is also capable of altering vascular permeability, causing contraction of certain smooth-muscle cells, and increasing the rate of secretion of certain mucosal cells. A second substance released from mast cells under these circumstances is ECF-A, the eosinophil chemotactic factor of anaphylaxis. As the name suggests, this substance is responsible for the accumulation of eosinophils where this type of antigen-antibody interaction occurs. Yet another important mediator, called SRS-A (slow reacting substance of anaphylaxis) is generated as mast cells are activated. This material, an arachidonic acid metabolite from the cell membrane, is capable of increasing vascular permeability, causing contraction of certain smooth-muscle cells, and altering pulmonary physiology. The net effect of antigen-antibody interaction, then, is the explosive release of substances which alter the physiology of the microcirculation locally. Some evidence indicates that this sort of reaction may be important in the defense of mucosal surfaces against certain agents in the environment. Unfortunately, as will be described below, the same sort of reaction is responsible for certain allergic responses.

Another means whereby the interaction of immunoglobulin and antigen is biologically amplified is via the *complement system,* in which there are nine interacting components. These components are proteins which circulate in the blood in an inactive form. So-called complement-fixing antibodies, IgG and IgM, are capable of activating the various complement proteins.

As shown in Table 5-1, the interaction of antigen and antibody results in the activation of the first component of the system. This activated product, C1, in turn interacts with the second and fourth components of the system, yielding several cleavage products. From these a complex, C4b2a, is formed. This complex is able to interact with C3 and is therefore also called C3 convertase. One of the cleavage products of C3 forms a complex, C4b2a3b, which functions as C5 convertase. A cleavage product of C5 then interacts with the later

components of the system. The activation of the entire system through C8 and C9, when it occurs on a cell surface, radically alters the cell membrane, leading to lysis. If the original antigen-antibody interaction occurred on the surface of a bacterial cell, the activation of this system would lead to lysis of that bacterium, clearly an event of some significance.

Table 5-1 also discloses that the fragments of various components activated earlier in the sequence have exceedingly important biological activities. Thus portions of C3 and C5 are capable of releasing histamine from mast cells, leading to contraction of smooth muscle and alteration of vascular permeability. These fragments are sometimes referred to as *anaphylatoxins.* Portions of the third component are also important in opsonization. Finally, a fragment of the fifth component and a complex of the fifth, sixth, and seventh components are strongly chemotactic for leukocytes. Clearly, activation of the various parts of the complement system provides an immense biological leverage to the original antigen-antibody interaction.

It should be noted here that although the comple-

TABLE 5-1

The complement system

ACTIVATING AGENTS	ACTIVATION SEQUENCE	PRODUCT BIOACTIVITY
ANTIGEN + ANTIBODY (IgG, IgM) PLASMIN] ----> $C1qrs$		
	$C\bar{1}$	$C\bar{1}$: ESTERASE ACTIVITY
	$C2$ $C4$	
	$C2b$ $C2a$ $C4b$ $C4a$	C_{2a4b}: C_3 CONVERTASE
ALTERNATE (PROPERDIN) PATHWAY AGGREGATED GLOBULINS ENDOTOXINS TISSUE PROTEASES LYSOSOMAL ENZYMES PLASMIN] ----> $C3$		C_{3a}: ANAPHYLATOXIN MAST CELL DEGRANULATION HISTAMINE RELEASE SMOOTH MUSCLE CONTRACTION INCREASED VASCULAR PERMEABILITY
	$C3a$ $C4b2a3b$ $C3b$	C_{3b}: IMMUNE ADHERENCE ENHANCED PHAGOCYTOSIS
LYSOSOMAL ENZYMES TISSUE PROTEASES] --------> $C5$		C_{4b2a3b}: C_5 CONVERTASE
	$C5a$ $C5b$	C_{5a}: ANAPHYLATOXIN LEUKOCYTE CHEMOTAXIS
	$C\overline{567}$	$C\overline{567}$: LEUKOCYTE CHEMOTAXIS
	$C8, C9$	C_8, C_9: CYTOLYSIS

ment system is an important amplifier of immunologic reactions, it also serves importantly in nonimmunologic settings. There are ways of activating the third component and subsequent components in the system directly without the intervention of antigen-antibody interactions. Various tissue proteases, lysosomal contents, and plasmin (fibrinolysin) can directly cleave and activate complement components. There also exists a so-called alternate pathway which, when activated nonimmunologically, can bypass C1, C2, and C4 to activate C3 directly. Thus it appears on the basis of current evidence that a number of components of the complement system are important mediators of many nonspecific inflammatory responses.

Although this discussion has emphasized the adaptive or beneficial aspects of the complement system, it should be pointed out once again that we usually pay a price for having various response mechanisms within the body. The complement system is, in fact, involved in a number of potentially harmful reactions, as described later in this chapter.

CELL–MEDIATED IMMUNITY

The nature of the response

This second of the two modes of immunologic response of the body does not involve circulating immunoglobulin molecules as effectors of the response. Instead, the various interactions with antigens are directly mediated by T lymphocytes which are specifically reactive with a particular antigen. The reason why some antigens stimulate immunoglobulin production and others induce the development of cell-mediated immunity is not entirely clear. The difference seems to lie in the mode of presentation of the antigen to the host. Simple proteins when injected almost always evoke humoral responses, i.e., those mediated by immunoglobulin. It seems that when the antigen is complex, especially when it is part of something like a bacterial body or part of some other living cell, cellular immunity is effectively evoked. The two types of immunity are not necessarily mutually exclusive; in the course of an infectious disease, elements of both kinds of immunologic reactions may be demonstrable.

Induction of the cell-mediated response

The afferent or inductive limb of the cellular immune response takes place within the lymphoid tissues of the body just as it does in the case of humoral immunity. The end point of the process, however, is proliferation of clones of T lymphocytes that are specifically reactive with a particular antigen, with no synthesis of immunoglobulin. The specifically reactive lymphocytes enter the circulating fluids of the body, migrate widely, and are available virtually anywhere to react with the antigen when it is reintroduced.

Cellular immune functions

Appropriately sensitized lymphocytes appear capable of killing target cells by some mechanism involving direct contact. T lymphocytes so occupied are known as "killer" lymphocytes.

Biological amplification of cell-mediated reactions is provided by various *lymphokines*, the soluble substances released by T lymphocytes when they are stimulated by the appropriate antigen. A number of different lymphokine activities have been described, and these have different cellular targets. Some lymphokines such as interleukin 2 or T-cell growth factor are able to induce blast transformation and proliferation of other lymphocytes, in effect recruiting the services of such cells. Another lymphokine is *transfer factor*, which is capable of transferring the specific reactivity from one set of lymphocytes to another. *Lymphotoxins* seem able to cause necrosis of the living cells which bear the corresponding antigens on their surfaces.

Still other lymphokines exert their major effects on macrophages. One such lymphokine, migration inhibiting factor (MIF), is able to suppress the migration of macrophages in vitro. Such an effect in vivo might well serve to keep macrophages in an area where lymphocytes had come into contact with the antigens with which they were reactive. Lymphocytes are also capable of secreting substances which are chemotactic for macrophages. The in vivo counterpart of this activity would be the efficient formation of macrophage-rich exudates in areas of challenge. Finally, certain lymphokines have the effect of activating or "arming" macrophages, rendering them more effective as phagocytic and microbicidal cells. Gamma interferon is one such substance, which also has antiviral activity. Thus the net effect of lymphokine release is that it will accelerate the handling and disposal of foreign antigenic material.

The classic example of cellular immune function is encountered in the development and evolution of tuberculosis. It has long been known that previous experience with tuberculous infection results in some measure of resistance to the disease upon later challenge. It has been known for many years that this protection is not mediated by any demonstrable immunoglobulin antibody but seems to reside within host cells. More specifically, it is possible to demonstrate by appropriate experiments that macrophages derived from individuals who have had a tuberculous infection at some time in the past are better able to deal with tubercle bacilli than are macrophages derived from naive hosts. In the latter, intracellular killing of phagocytized living organisms proceeds very slowly if at all, whereas in the macrophages from the experienced individual, the rate of intracellular killing is enhanced. Furthermore, it can be shown that when tubercle bacilli are introduced into experienced hosts, the inflammatory reaction in response to the bacilli evolves much more rapidly and efficiently than it does in inexperienced hosts. Although in the expression of protection against tubercle bacilli the macrophages are the essential cells, it is now known that the accumulation and function of these cells is actually enhanced by T lymphocytes which are specifically reactive with antigens of the tubercle bacilli. In short, what happens is that the initial exposure to tubercle bacilli leads to proliferation of specifically reactive lymphocytes (usually 2 weeks or so after the infection) and dissemination of these cells around the body. The result of subsequent contact between these lymphocytes and additional tubercle bacilli is the release of lymphokines leading to the critical effects on macrophages. Interestingly, the interaction between lymphocytes and antigens of tubercle bacilli is highly specific, but once these cells activate the macrophages, the superior properties of the macrophages seem to function equally well against a variety of agents regardless of antigenic specificity. It should be emphasized that a state of cellular immunity evolves even during the first infection with the tubercle bacilli and is, in fact, responsible for assisting the host in arresting that infection. During the first 2 weeks or so following introduction of tubercle bacilli, bacillary multiplication proceeds relatively unhindered by the host's inflammatory response. During this time the macrophages that appear within the exudate around

the organisms seem incapable of coping with them. When specifically reactive lymphocytes appear on the scene at the end of the induction phase, the interaction of these cells with antigen leads to the progressive increase in the microbicidal efficiency of macrophages, and the host eventually (in most instances) arrests the spread of the infection.

These same sorts of cellular reactions form the basis for skin testing to detect the cellular immune state. If a bit of protein derived from tubercle bacilli is injected into the skin of an individual who has never been infected with the tubercle bacillus, there ensues a very mild, nonspecific acute inflammatory reaction, as would occur in response to any minimally irritating foreign material. This inflammatory response is transient, and by 24 hours after the injection the site usually appears completely normal. This is considered a negative test. On the other hand, if antigen is injected into the skin of an individual who has been infected with the tubercle bacillus at some time in the past, a pronounced local inflammatory response evolves slowly, so that by 24 hours after injection the local area is indurated (that is, thickened and swollen). Microscopic examination (Fig. 5-6) reveals that the induration is due to dense infiltration of the area by mixture of lymphocytes and macrophages. This constitutes a positive reaction. Actually, only a few of the many lymphocytes at the site of the reaction are specifically antigen-reactive cells. The remaining lymphocytes and macrophages have been "recruited" into the area as a result of substances released by the antigen-reactive cells. It should be noted that a positive test does *not* mean that the subject has the clinical disease of tuberculosis. A positive reaction indicates that the subject has contacted the organism at some time, with the resulting development of a clone of reactive T lymphocytes. A person with a positive skin test

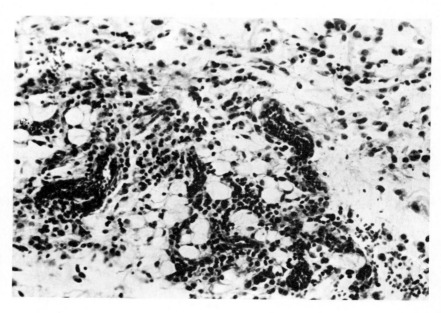

FIGURE 5-6
Positive tuberculin skin test. The area of antigen injection becomes densely packed with lymphocytes and macrophages, especially perivascularly. This produces the gross induration which constitutes the positive reaction. (Photomicrograph, ×315.)

could have the disease but most often does not. The test is clinically useful in differential diagnosis and in screening. In the former instance, if the subject has evidence of a disease which could be tuberculosis but might not be, a negative skin test (i.e., evidence of the subject not having previous contact with the tubercle bacillus) would be evidence in favor of some other etiologic diagnosis. In the latter instance, skin testing is useful in screening populations such as medical and nursing personnel who are exposed occupationally to tuberculosis. Continuing negativity on tests repeated at regular intervals affords reasonable assurance that no infection has been acquired. If a previously negative individual converts to positive, this indicates infection since the previous test. With such a finding, appropriate tests can be undertaken to make certain that clinically significant disease does not exist, and a program of prophylactic administration of antituberculous drugs might be undertaken to eliminate the very slight possibility that infection might progress. Once an individual has been found to be positive on skin test there is usually no point in repeating the test at later intervals since such positivity is most often permanent.

A measure of protection against tuberculosis can be afforded skin test–negative individuals by means of vaccination designed to induce a cellular immune state. The material generally used is referred to as BCG (bacillus of Calmette and Guérin), which is a live but attenuated strain of tubercle bacillus. These organisms are incapable of producing a progressive infection in normal individuals, but they will result in the development of a clone of T lymphocytes specifically reactive against tuberculoproteins. The protection afforded by such a procedure is not total and is usually not deemed desirable in relatively low-risk situations. Persons in such situations are more efficiently handled by serial skin testing and chemoprophylaxis as indicated.* More recently, BCG vaccination has been employed in the attempted immunotherapy of malignant disease. The rationale for this approach is that once activated by the BCG, the cellular immune defenses of the host may also operate against the cancer cells.

As for transfer of immunity, because cellular immune functions reside in the lymphocytes, immunity cannot be transferred passively by means of serum the way humoral immunity can be.

IMMUNITY AND HYPERSENSITIVITY

Relationship between the two

The several humoral and cell-mediated reactions outlined above are clearly of adaptive value to the host.

---

*This is more efficient since tuberculin-negative subjects do not require frequent chest x-rays to rule out acute tuberculosis, while tuberculin-positive subjects (including those positive because of BCG) do.

When one speaks of immunity, one generally refers to such beneficial phenomena mediated by the immunologic apparatus of the body. However, the price we pay for having this adaptive machinery is that occasionally the interaction of antibodies or T lymphocytes with antigen may result in injury to the host. These injurious reactions are frequently referred to as *hypersensitivity* reactions. The term *allergy* is also used to describe certain clinically observed hypersensitivity reactions in humans.

According to terminology evolved many years ago, hypersensitivity reactions mediated by immunoglobulins are sometimes referred to as *immediate-type hypersensitivity* reactions while those mediated by cellular immune mechanisms are called *delayed hypersensitivity* reactions. (Sometimes the latter reactions are also referred to as tuberculin-type hypersensitivity reactions or bacterial hypersensitivity reactions, because of prototypical examples.) While this terminology is occasionally employed currently, it is less than completely precise because of considerable overlapping in the velocity of the various kinds of reactions. A more useful classification of immunologic injuries is that proposed by Gell and Coombs. This scheme recognizes four types of mechanisms: Type I reactions are mediated by IgE antibodies fixed to the surface of mast cells. Type II reactions are mediated by IgG- or IgM-type antibodies reacting with antigens on the surface of the target cell. Type III reactions are mediated through the formation of antigen-antibody complexes, largely with IgG antibodies. Type IV reactions are mediated by sensitized T lymphocytes.

Modes of tissue injury

In Type I reactions, also referred to as *anaphylactic-type* reactions, the subject must be sensitized by prior exposure to a particular antigen. During the inductive phase of the response IgE antibodies are made, circulated, and fixed to the surface of mast cells widely scattered about the body. When antigen is then reintroduced into the subject, interaction of antigen with mast-cell-fixed antibody results in explosive release of substances contained within the cells. If the amount of antigen introduced is small and of local extent, mediator release is local, and the result is nothing more than an area of vasodilatation and increased permeability leading to a bit of local swelling. (This mechanism of reaction forms the basis for skin testing by the allergist.) If, however, a larger amount of antigen is introduced intravenously into the sensitized subject, release of mediators may be massive and widespread. A classic example of this type of *generalized anaphylactic reaction* can be relatively easily produced experimentally in the guinea pig. The animal is initially sensitized by injection of some foreign antigen by one of a variety of routes. When that same antigen is subsequently introduced by intravenous injection, signs of distress appear within a few moments, and the animal may die quickly after a period of agitation or even of convulsions. Autopsy of such an animal reveals that the lungs are markedly hyperinflated. This phenomenon is due to bronchiolar obstruction which leads to trapping of inspired air within the lungs, ventilatory failure, and rapid suffocation. This chain of events is due to the release of mediator substances from mast cells, the chief target then being the bronchiolar smooth muscle, which is thrown into a state of continuous spastic contraction. The precise pattern of response to widespread mediator release from mast cells varies from species to species but can be equally dramatic in humans in a number of different situations (see Part II).

Type II reactions are basically *cytotoxic*. In these sorts of reactions, the circulating IgG or IgM antibody unites with the corresponding antigen on the surface of a cell (i.e., the antigen is either attached to or a part of the cell's surface). The net result of the interaction might be accelerated phagocytosis of the target cell or might be actual lysis of the target cell following activation of the eighth and ninth components of the complement sequence. If the target cell is a foreign one such as a bacterium, the outcome of this type of reaction is beneficial. However, as is sometimes the case, the target cell may be a host erythrocyte, in which case the result may be a form of hemolytic anemia. Another sort of Type II reaction is termed *antibody-dependent cell-mediated cytotoxicity* (ADCC). In this type of reaction, antibody directed against surface antigens of a cell bind to that cell, and then leukocytes (neutrophils, macrophages, and null cells) having receptors for a particular portion (the Fc portion) of the immunoglobulin molecules bind to the cell and bring about its destruction. This sort of reaction is known in vitro and may be operative in vivo as well.

Type III reactions take a number of forms, but they are mediated ultimately by immune complexes, that is, complexes of antigen with antibody, usually of the IgG type. The prototype of this sort of reaction is the *Arthus reaction*. Classically, this type of reaction is elicited by first sensitizing an experimental animal to some foreign protein and subsequently challenging the subject by an intracutaneous injection of the same antigen. The reaction typically evolves over a period of several hours, passing through a phase of swelling and redness; the area ultimately becomes necrotic and hemorrhagic in severe examples. The microscopic appearance of a typical Arthus reaction is shown in Fig. 5-7. The essence of the lesion is severe vascular damage brought about by large numbers of neutrophils which infiltrate vessel walls in the region of the challenge. In this phenomenon, the basic mechanism involves the formation of antigen-antibody complexes in vascular walls as injected antigen diffuses into the walls and combines with antibody diffusing out of the circulation. A key element in the reaction is activation of the complement cascade by the immune complexes within vascular walls. This activation results in the formation of chemotactic factor ($C\overline{567}$), which attracts neutrophils from the circulation. The final effectors of vascular damage are the powerful lytic enzymes released from lysosomes of the leukocytes

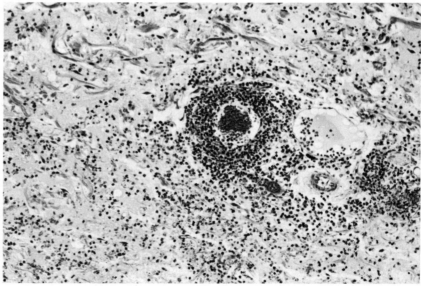

FIGURE 5-7
The Arthus reaction. In the center of the field is a blood vessel densely infiltrated by neutrophils which are attracted to the site by the Type III reaction. Severe damage is inflicted on the vessel by the leukocytic enzymes. (Photomicrograph, ×200.)

which are attracted. It is important to note that the reaction triggered by the immune complexes bears no immunologic relationship to the vascular walls. The presence of the immune complexes within vascular walls and the subsequent damage to those walls represent a sort of mechanical outcome of the circumstances of challenge. Other immune complexes of a similar sort, formed in other situations, could produce parallel reactions.

This, in fact, is what occurs in so-called *serum sickness*, which is another classic sort of immune complex disease. The basic mechanism of production of serum sickness involves the formation of immune complexes within the circulatory system, with subsequent deposition of these complexes in a number of locations. The entire chain of events can be initiated by a *single* injection of foreign protein provided that the amount injected is relatively massive. If the amount of the foreign material is sufficient, abundant antigen will still be in circulation when immunoglobulin production and release begin several days after the original injection. As antibody is formed, it enters the circulation and combines with the still-circulating antigen, forming circulating immune complexes. These complexes are deposited in many points of the vascular system, and at each of those points complement is activated, leukocytes are attracted, and a vasculitis similar to that of the Arthus phenomenon is produced (Fig. 5-8). Another important component of serum sickness is the characteristic renal lesion. The circulating immune complexes are filtered out as the blood passes through renal glomeruli, and the glomeruli are injured by the complexes, producing the characteristic *glomerulonephritis* of serum sickness. Again it should be noted that tissue damage is initiated by the deposition of immune complexes which in themselves are not immunologically related to the tissues injured. Thus, in a real sense, the numerous vessels and glomeruli involved in serum sickness are "innocent bystanders."

Immune complex, or Type III, reactions precisely analogous to those described above can be elicited in human beings, as will be described in Part II. Thus, serum sickness is a potential clinical problem, and immune complex glomerulonephritis develops in a number of settings, including certain infections.

Type IV reactions mediated by the contact of sensitized T lymphocytes with the corresponding antigen can be seen in a number of settings. Tuberculosis affords a classic example. The protective or beneficial effects of T-lymphocyte-mediated reactions in tuberculosis have been described above. Accompanying these sorts of reactions there is often extensive necrosis of tissue, which, in fact, is quite characteristic of the disease. Such necrosis is now recognized to be a result of cell-mediated immunity rather than being directly caused by any toxic moiety of the tubercle bacillus. It appears that necrosis is the result of lymphocytotoxicity, i.e., the effect of lymphocytes activated by the tuberculoprotein of the bacilli.

Type IV reactions are also exemplified by so-called *allergic contact dermatitis*, which can be induced experimentally and also has a spontaneous human counterpart. In this type of situation a simple chemical material is applied to the skin of the subject, and the material acts as a *hapten*, combining with proteins in the skin. The complex molecules thus formed induce the proliferation of a clone of sensitized lymphocytes

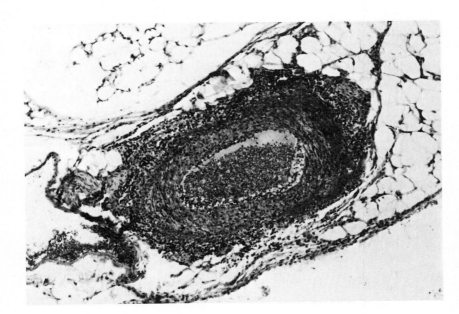

FIGURE 5-8
Serum sickness. The mesenteric artery is being damaged by leukocytes in a mechanism analogous to that depicted in Fig. 5-7. The circumstances of immune complex formation differ. (Photomicrograph, ×125.)

which subsequently interact with the antigen in the skin. The cells of the skin then bear the brunt of lymphocytotoxicity and of the secondary effects triggered by lymphokines released in the reaction. The clinical counterparts of this are described in Part II.

This type of reaction is also mounted in the rejection of foreign grafts. When a living tissue from one individual is grafted into another, whether it is a patch of skin or an entire organ such as a kidney, unless the donor and recipient are genetically identical, the graft tissue is sensed by the recipient's immune system as being foreign and antigenic. After a brief induction phase, lymphocytes specifically sensitized to so-called *histocompatibility* or *transplant antigens* of the graft invade the graft and lead to its destruction or rejection by a number of mechanisms involving either direct lymphocytotoxicity or the involvement of macrophages. While T lymphocytes play a major role in graft rejection, under some circumstances immunoglobulins play a significant parallel role. It is these sorts of rejection reactions which limit our ability to replace defective organs in one individual with organs taken from another.

AUTOIMMUNITY

Generally speaking, immunologic phenomena involve self-recognition such that the lymphoid system of the host does not react against antigens of the host body. However, it is now recognized that in a number of diseases, antibody-mediated or cell-mediated reactions against self antigens can be demonstrated. While some of these reactions are of only secondary importance, in other instances autoimmunity is thought to be a key factor in the pathogenesis of disease. Most often the triggering event in autoimmunity is not recognized, but several theoretical possibilities exist which might explain the loss of tolerance to self antigens. In some instances, it appears that an infectious agent may have antigenic determinant groups similar to those of certain host tissues. Then, in reaction to that agent, host tissues may be injured by cross-reaction. A second set of circumstances involves changes in the antigenic structure of host proteins brought about by injury, infection, or complexing with a haptene from outside of the host. With altered antigenic structure, a given tissue may then evoke an immunologic reaction as if foreign. Another explanation is the sudden "exposure" of previously isolated or sequestered self antigens to the lymphoid tissues. This sort of phenomenon is seen in autoimmune reactions to sperm constituents or to ocu-

lar constituents following physical injury which disrupts normal anatomy. Finally, it appears that some autoimmune reactions may be precipitated by the loss of T-cell function, involving suppressor T cells which ordinarily hold autoimmune reactions in check.

IMMUNODEFICIENCY SYNDROMES

At the opposite extreme, so to speak, an individual may develop disease because of a deficiency in the immunologic machinery itself, i.e., an inability of the lymphoid tissue to react normally to various antigens. These sorts of diseases are manifested clinically as an unusual susceptibility to infection, which may be so severe as to be lethal. The pattern of infection will be determined by the precise sort of immunodeficiency.

Immunologic deficiencies may be primary, i.e., may have a genetic basis, and various parts of the immune system may be involved. For instance, in X-linked agammaglobulinemia, the deficiency is of B cells, with almost total absence of immunoglobulin production. The deficiency can be of one particular type of immunoglobulin, e.g., IgA. There are also primary deficiencies of the T-cell system, and even so-called severe combined immunodeficiency wherein the affected individual has virtual absence of all immunologic reactivity.

Immunologic deficiency may also be secondary, i.e., acquired in the course of other disease. Certain malignant states, for instance, may involve lymphoid tissues extensively enough to impair their function. Cytotoxic drug therapy may also destroy these tissues. The result will be greatly increased susceptibility to infection.

Within the past few years, a devastating form of acquired immunologic deficiency has been recognized. This so-called acquired immunologic deficiency syndrome (AIDS) has been seen primarily in homosexual or bisexual males with multiple sexual contacts, intravenous (IV) drug abusers, and recipients of blood products, especially hemophiliacs who receive material from numerous donors. The epidemiology of AIDS suggests an infectious etiology; recently, a form of HTLV (human T-cell leukemia virus) has been implicated. It appears that infection by this virus leads to obliteration of helper T-cell function, with consequent profound depression of cell-mediated defenses (and other more subtle deficiencies as well). Affected individuals fall victim to "opportunistic" infection with agents ordinarily harmless to immunocompetent individuals, e.g., cytomegalovirus, a protozoan named *Pneumocystis carinii*, and various other protozoa, bacteria, and fungi. Some patients with AIDS also develop unusual forms of cancer. The mortality of the full-blown syndrome, with its exquisite sensitivity to infection, appears to approach 100 percent (see Chaps. 14 and 77).

Response of the body to immunologic challenge

Directions: Answer the following questions on a separate sheet of paper.

1. What is the essential biological significance of an immune response?

2. Describe the nature of antigens in terms of their structure and their effects on the host.

3. Describe two different modes of immunologic responses which may be evoked when lymphoid tissue is exposed to antigens.

4. List three properties generally associated with immunologic reactions.

5. What are the possible reactions of lymphocytes stimulated by antigen?

6. Describe the mechanism by which antibodies appear to be formed.

7. Illustrate how the complement system is activated and the consequences of such activation.

Directions: Circle T if the statement is true and F if it is false. Correct any false statements.

8. T F The sinusoids of the spleen are filled with lymph.

9. T F Lymphocytes are widely distributed within the bone marrow.

10. T F If antigen enters the bloodstream directly, the regional lymph nodes are a major locus of antibody production.

11. T F Passive immunization refers to the situation wherein an antigen is introduced into the host and the process of immunoglobulin synthesis is activated.

12. T F People normally have only minute amounts of IgE present in their blood serum.

13. T F Immediate hypersensitivity is a cell-mediated response.

14. T F Mediators of cellular immunity are sensitized T lymphocytes working either directly or via substances which are elaborated when the cell encounters its antigen.

Directions: Circle the letter preceding each item below that correctly answers the question. More than one answer may be correct.

15. All of the following are components of the lymphoid system *except*:
a. Lymph nodes b. Spleen c. Liver
d. Thymus e. Bone marrow

16. The thymus converts stem cells from the bone marrow to:
a. T lymphocytes b. B lymphocytes c. Both a and b d. Neither a nor b

17. When an antibody reacts with its corresponding antigen:
a. A precipitate may be produced from a previously soluble antigen b. A biologically "toxic" complex may be formed c. The elimination of the antigen (in the intact host) may be accelerated d. A particulate antigen may be caused to agglutinate e. All of the above

18. An antibody which can coat the surface of bacteria so that phagocytosis by PMNs and macrophages is enhanced is called a(n):
a. Hapten b. Agglutinin c. Opsonin
d. Precipitin

19. When stimulated by antigen, sensitive T lymphocytes release:
a. SRS-A b. ECF-A c. Secretory IgA
d. Macrophage-inhibiting factor

20. IgE antibody has a special affinity for:
a. Mast cells b. Eosinophils c. Basophils
d. Histiocytes

21. The principal role of IgE in allergic reactions is to:
a. Form a precipitating complex with allergens
b. Fix the complement with tissue-damaging effects c. Generate eosinophilic chemotactic factor d. Combine with allergen on the mast cell surface and induce secretion of contained materials

22. Which of the following is an important function of IgG?
a. Protection of mucosal surfaces b. Mediation of the tuberculin skin test c. Defense against pyogenic infections d. Participation in anaphylactic reactions

23. Complement activation would be anticipated with:
a. Reactions of antigens with cell-bound IgE
b. Reactions of antigens with sensitized T lymphocytes c. Reactions of antigens with IgG
d. Addition of antigens alone to complement-rich serum

24. Biological effects of activation of complement components include all of the following *except:*
a. Production of lesions in target cell membranes
b. Release of histamine with resulting vascular permeability changes   c. Attraction of white blood cells   d. Development of "transfer factor" in sensitized lymphocytes   e. Facilitation of phagocytosis by white blood cells

25. Mast cell granules contain substances that are involved in hypersensitivity reactions. Which of the following statements is/are true regarding these substances?
a. Histamine effects are never evident before 1 hour.   b. SRS-A causes increased vessel permeability.   c. ECF-A causes constriction of bronchial smooth muscle.   d. Histamine causes lymphokine generation.

26. Reactions due to delayed hypersensitivity may have all of the following features *except:*
a. Involvement of nonsensitive macrophages recruited by specifically sensitive lymphoid cells
b. Mediation by circulating IgM antibody
c. Passive transfer by means of specifically sensitized lymphocytes   d. Responsibility for immunity to some bacterial and fungal infections.

27. All of the following statements about anaphylaxis are true *except:*
a. It is a condition caused by an immunologic reaction.   b. It is a potentially fatal condition.
c. It may occur in minutes or even seconds after exposure to causative agent.   d. Patient need not have been previously exposed to the causative agent or a closely related one.   e. It is thought to be mediated by IgE.

28. Which of the following are characteristic of serum sickness?
a. It is a delayed hypersensitivity reaction.   b. It requires many periods of exposure to a particular antigen.   c. It is IgE-mediated.   d. Circulating antibody-antigen complexes are present as the disease evolves.   e. It may occur following administration of animal serums to an individual not previously sensitized to the antigen.

29. Delayed hypersensitivity reactions, such as the positive tuberculin response, reflect a recruitment of cells by factors released by:

a. IgE   b. Neutrophils   c. Lymphocytes
d. The complement system   e. Macrophages

30. The function or properties of subsets of T lymphocytes include:
a. Involvement in antibody-dependent cell-mediated cytotoxic reactions   b. Destruction of certain tumor cells which augment activities of the lymphocytes   c. Augmentation of the activities of other lymphocytes   d. Presence of portions of IgG molecules

31. Examples of a Type II hypersensitivity reaction include:
a. Anaphylactic reaction   b. Hemolytic anemia
c. Antibody-dependent cell-mediated cytotoxicity (ADCC)   d. Arthus reaction

32. Which of the following phenomena are implicated in the pathogenesis of autoimmune disease?
a. Changes in the antigenic structures of host proteins   b. Loss of function of suppressor T cells   c. Inability of lymphoid tissue to react normally to various antigens   d. Deficiency of B lymphocytes

Directions: Match the characteristics in col. A with the type of immune mechanism generally involved in col. B.

Column A

33. ____ Antibody-mediated

34. ____ Mediated by sensitized T lymphocytes

35. ____ B lymphocytes involved

36. ____ Can be induced by simple protein molecules

37. ____ Response more likely to be immediate

38. ____ Anaphylactic shock following penicillin injection

39. ____ Positive tuberculin skin test

Column B

a. Humoral immunity
b. Cellular immunity

CHAPTER

6

RESPONSE OF THE BODY TO INFECTIOUS AGENTS

OBJECTIVES

At the completion of this chapter you should able to:

1. State the general requirements for the estabishment of an infection.
2. Distinguish an infection from an infectious disease.
3. Identify the modes of entry of an infectious agent into the host.
4. Describe the local and systemic means of dissemination in the host body once an infectious agent is established.
5. Describe the normal body defenses against penetration and spread of infectious agents in the following and give examples of each:

    a Skin and mucosal surface
    b Inflammatory reaction
    c Monocyte-macrophage system
6. Define *bacteremia, septicemia, septicopyemia.*
7. List the direct and indirect means of transmission of organisms from the source to a susceptible host.
8. Describe the characteristics of an organism which affect its transmissibility, invasiveness, and pathogenicity.
9. Identify several mechanisms by which microorganisms cause injury.
10. Define *commensalism, mutualism.*
11. Describe the concept of an opportunistic infection.
12. Identify the host and environmental factors which determine resistance, susceptibility, and outcome of an infection.
13. Explain why the normal microbial flora of the body is essential for the health of the human host.

Infection is a universal aspect of life. Plants and animals of all sizes and descriptions are infested with a variety of living microbes, and human beings are certainly no exception. The purpose of the following discussion is not to catalog the many specific infections to which human beings fall victim but rather to discuss in a most general way the biological principles which govern the interaction between host and infectious agents. In particular, a goal of this chapter is to provide a proper perspective of the universe of infection, i.e., to establish firmly the view that *infectious disease* is but an occasional outcome of the interaction between host and microbe.

HOST DETERMINANTS OF INFECTION

A requirement for the production of any infection is that the infectious organism must be able to *adhere to, colonize,* or *invade* the host and proliferate at least to some extent. It is not surprising, therefore, that in the course of evolution, animal species, including human beings, have evolved certain elaborate defense mechanisms at the various interfaces with the environment.

Skin and oropharyngeal mucosa

A major interface between the environment and the human body is, of course, the skin. Figure 6-1 shows the structure of a typical area of human skin. Clearly the intact skin with its keratinized or horny layer at the outer surface and multilayered epithelium beneath con-

stitutes an excellent *mechanical* barrier to infection. Ordinarily it is exceedingly difficult for any microorganism to breach this mechanical barrier. However, cuts, abrasions, or areas of maceration (such as those folds of the body which are kept constantly moist) may allow infectious agents to enter. In addition to being a simple mechanical barrier, the skin also has a certain ability to *decontaminate* itself. Thus, organisms which adhere to the outer layers of skin (assuming they do not simply die as they dry out) will be shed as the outer flakes of skin fall off. In addition to this physical sort of decontamination there is a chemical decontamination attributable to the properties of sweat and sebaceous secretions which bathe the surface of the skin. Finally, associated with the skin is a so-called *normal flora* (described more fully later in this chapter), which may exert a sort of *biological* decontaminative effect by inhibiting the multiplication of organisms which land on the cutaneous surface.

The lining of the mouth and much of the pharynx is similar to the skin in that it is surfaced by a multilayered epithelium which constitutes a formidable mechanical barrier to microbial invasion. This mechanical barrier, however, may actually be breached along gingival margins and in the region of the tonsils. The oropharyngeal mucosa is also decontaminated by the flow of saliva, which simply washes many particles away mechanically. In addition, there are substances in the saliva that are inhibitory to certain microorganisms. Finally, there is a rich microbial flora within the mouth and pharynx that may also act to impair the growth of some potential invaders.

Gastrointestinal tract

The gastric mucosa is of a glandular sort and is not a particularly impressive mechanical barrier. Frequently

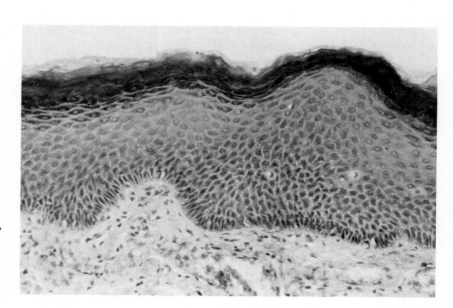

FIGURE 6-1

Skin. The epidermis (upper two-thirds of field) consists of multiple layers of cells, the most superficial of which are flattened, keratinized, and without nuclei. In toto, these layers constitute a formidable mechanical barrier. (Photomicrograph, ×300).

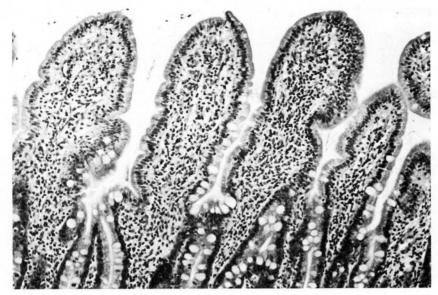

FIGURE 6-2
Small intestine. The epithelium separating bowel contents from underlying tissue is actually quite delicate and is not a particularly good mechanical barrier. The surface is protected by mucus secreted by the light-staining "goblet cells," by antibody produced by the underlying lymphoid tissues, and by peristaltic emptying. (Photomicrograph, ×200.)

there are small defects or erosions of the gastric lining, but these are of no consequence in relation to infection, because the gastric environment is extremely hostile to many microorganisms. This is due largely to the pronounced acidity of gastric secretions. Also, the stomach tends to empty its contents relatively rapidly into the small intestine. The lining of the small intestine (Fig. 6-2) is likewise not particularly tough mechanically, and it is potentially easily penetrated by many bacteria. However, peristaltic propulsion of the intestinal contents is extremely rapid in the small intestine, and bacterial populations are thereby kept quite sparse within the lumen. When intestinal motility is impaired, microbial counts are sharply elevated within the small intestine, and invasion of the mucosa may then occur. Several

other features of the small intestine assist in the rapid propulsion of organisms through the tract. Abundant mucus is constantly secreted by intestinal lining cells, forming a viscous blanket over the intestinal surface, trapping bacteria, and propelling them distally by peristalsis. In addition, adhesion of bacteria to the mucosal surface is inhibited by the presence of antibodies within the intestinal secretions. In the large intestine (Fig. 6-3) the lining is likewise not particularly tough mechanically. In this location propulsion is not especially rapid, and in fact there is relative stagnation of intestinal contents. Here, the major defense against establishment of invading microbes is the presence of astronomic numbers of "normal" microbial inhabitants which coexist peacefully with the host. This mass of normal bacteria

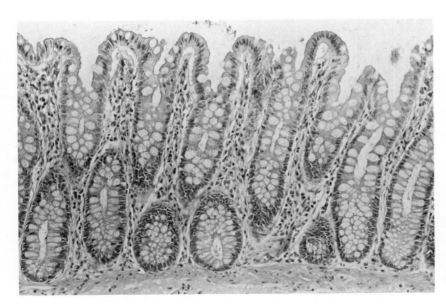

FIGURE 6-3
Colon. This epithelium contains many mucus-secreting cells. During life, the surface is bathed in a layer of mucus, but after tissue processing, only wisps remain (upper right). The rich microbial flora which "defends" the colon is not visible in this preparation. (Photomicrograph, ×200).

has many ecologic ways of discouraging invaders either by competition for foodstuffs or by actually secreting antibacterial (antibiotic) substances.

Respiratory tract

Represented in Fig. 6-4 is a microscopic view of the mucosal surface typical of conducting portions of the respiratory tract (e.g., the lining of the nose, the nasopharynx, the trachea, and the bronchi). The epithelium consists of tall cells, some of which are mucus-secreting, but most of which are equipped with cilia at their lumenal surfaces. These tiny projections beat like whips with the action stroke directed upward toward the mouth, nose, and exterior of the body. The mucus-secreting cells produce a sticky blanket which rides on top of the cilia and glides continuously upward. If microbes are inhaled, they tend to impinge on the mucous blanket, to be moved outward and either expectorated or swallowed. This protective action is enhanced by the presence of antibodies within the secretions. If some agents elude these defenses and reach the air spaces in the lung itself, the macrophages always present there provide another line of defense.

OTHER DEFENSIVE BARRIERS

Other surfaces in the body are similarly equipped with defensive mechanisms. Within the urinary tract the lining is a multilayered epithelium which provides a mechanical barrier, but one of the main antimicrobial defenses is the flushing action of urine flow. Anything which interferes with the normal flow of urine, whether it be obstruction of a ureter or simply bad habits of long-delayed micturition, will promote infection. The ocular conjunctiva is likewise defended in part mechanically and in part by the flow of tears. The vaginal mucosa is a tough, multilayered epithelium whose mechanical properties are augmented by a rich resident flora and by mucous secretions.

Inflammation as a defense

If an infectious agent manages to penetrate one or another of the barriers of the body and enter the tissues, the *next line of defense* is the *acute inflammatory reaction*. From the discussion in Chap. 4, the value of the inflammatory reaction in this regard should be evident. It might be reemphasized at this point that the inflammatory reaction is an arena in which humoral (antibody) and cellular aspects of bodily defense converge. The antimicrobial activities of the phagocytes, for instance, are augmented by the opsonizing effects of antibodies and complement components. The defensive properties of macrophages, as another example, may be enhanced by so-called *cellular immune mechanisms* (see Chap. 5).

In the event that the acute inflammatory reaction is not sufficient to handle the invader, the infection may spread elsewhere in the body. The usual means of spread is largely passive as regards microbial action, and usually involves currents of body fluid carrying the organisms. Locally, even the outpouring of exudate fluid may move the organisms about, and a phagocyte may actually be an agent of spread if it does not kill the ingested organism but wanders to another location. Spread tends to occur across natural spaces. For instance, if something perforates part of the gastrointestinal tract and the contained microorganisms enter the peritoneal cavity, they can spread along the entire peritoneal surface. If some agent reaches a connective tissue

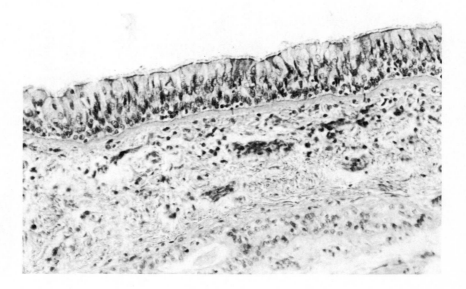

FIGURE 6-4
Trachea. This type of epithelium is equipped with cilia, visible as a fringe along the upper surface. These are responsible for propelling a protective mucous blanket over the exposed surface of the air passages. (Photomicrograph, ×315.)

plane, such as that along a muscle, it may spread rapidly along that plane. When infectious organisms gain access to the meninges (the coverings around the central nervous system), there is frequently rapid spread along the entire cerebrospinal axis.

Lymphatics in infection

For reasons outlined in Chap. 4, the flow of lymph is accelerated in acute inflammation. This means, unfortunately, that infectious agents on occasion may also spread quite rapidly along the course of lymphatics with the flowing lymph. Sometimes lymphangitis is the result, but more often the infectious agents are carried directly to the lymph nodes, where they are rapidly phagocytosed by macrophages. In such instances the effluent lymph moving centrally beyond a lymph node may be free of living organisms.

The final defenses

If spreading infectious agents are not arrested within lymph nodes or if such agents directly invade venous channels at the primary site, there may be actual infection of the bloodstream. Bursts of bacteria in the bloodstream are actually not uncommon, and the episodes of so-called *bacteremia* are usually handled quickly and effectively by the macrophages of the monocyte-macrophage system. If large numbers of organisms are fed into the bloodstream, however, and if these organisms are sufficiently resistant, the macrophage system may be overwhelmed. This will result in persistence of organisms in circulation, with associated symptoms of malaise, prostration, and signs of fever, chills, etc. This condition is called *septicemia*, often referred to by the laity as "blood poisoning." Finally in some instances organisms reach such high numbers that they are circulating in clumps, lodging in many organs, and producing myriads of microabscesses (Fig. 6-5). This overwhelming situation is called *septicopyemia*, or simply *pyemia.*

MICROBIAL DETERMINANTS OF INFECTION

Transmissibility

An obviously essential feature in the production of infection is the transport of the living infectious agent to the host. Perhaps the most obvious means of transmission of infection is *directly* from person to person, e.g., by coughing, sneezing, and kissing.

Organisms are transmitted *indirectly* in a variety of ways. Infected individuals shed organisms into the environment, and these are deposited on various surfaces and can be resuspended in air at a later time, thus spreading indirectly to other hosts. Similarly, organisms can get into the soil, the water, the food, or other chains of indirect transmission. Around hospitals, infection can also be spread via exudates and excreta. Blood transfusions may also be a means of spreading infection, as in the case of viral hepatitis. More complex types of indirect transmission involve vectors such as insects. These may act in a strictly mechanical fashion, carrying the microbial agents from one place to another, or may act in a biological fashion, i.e., by serving as intermediate hosts in some essential part of a life cycle of the infectious agent.

Certain intrinsic characteristics of microorganisms sharply influence their transmissibility or communicability. Organisms which are very resistant to drying, e.g., spore-forming organisms, are readily transmissible through the environment. On the other hand, some organisms, e.g., the spirochetes of syphilis, are extremely sensitive to drying and temperature change, factors which sharply limit the mode of this transmission. In hospitals a sort of natural selective factor which influences the communicability of microbial agents is their resistance to antibiotics. It is distressingly common to

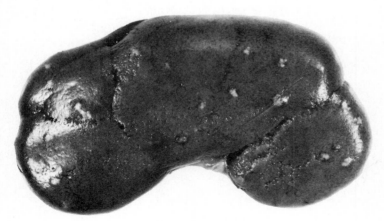

FIGURE 6-5
Kidney in septicopyemia. The light-colored lesions scattered over the cortical surface are actually small abscesses formed as a result of lodgement of blood-borne bacteria.

find antibiotic-resistant strains of microorganisms emerging and then being communicated relatively freely in the hospital environment.

Invasiveness

Once comunicated to a new host, the microbial agent must establish itself on or in the host in order to produce infection. There is great variability in the means adopted by various infectious agents for becoming established on or in the host individual. *Cholera*, for instance, is caused by an organism that never invades the tissues but only colonizes the lining of the intestine, apparently by being able to adhere to some component of the surface and thus avoid being washed away. There are some other organisms, e.g., those which produce bacillary dysentery, which invade only the superficial lining of the bowel but never go any farther into the body. Then there are organisms such as the causative agent of typhoid, which not only invades the superficial lining of the bowel but eventually reaches the bloodstream and disseminates around the body. Another efficient spreader is the spirochete of syphilis, which penetrates mucous membrane or skin at the portal of entry and is disseminated via the bloodstream with great rapidity.

Some organisms, even after gaining access to the tissues and becoming established, never spread to any extent. The organisms which produces tetanus, for instance, do not actually spread around the body. When they grow locally, they secrete a toxin which is carried via the bloodstream to produce the widespread effects that characterize the disease. The reasons for these differences in invasiveness of various organisms are not clearly understood but undoubtedly are related to specific chemical requirements of the organism and the extent to which these requirements can be met in various locales.

Microorganisms have evolved certain ways of breaching host barriers or eluding defense mechanisms. For example, some organisms develop a slimy capsule such that the phagocytic cells of the host cannot ingest them efficiently. In the course of evolution other organisms have developed the enzymatic means of spreading through the ground substance of connective tissue by a sort of chemical digestive process. Yet other organisms are able to secrete toxins which kill leukocytes, thus eluding capture. Some organisms have even evolved a resistance to the intracellular environment within phagocytes, and these organisms (for instance, the tubercle bacillus) tend to persist as intracellular parasites.

Ability to produce disease

At the level of explaining in a chemical or molecular way the mechanism whereby the presence of an infectious agent produces disease, our knowledge has been relatively meager and is only now growing. Best understood are those situations in which the infectious agent actually secretes a soluble *exotoxin* which then circulates and produces well-defined physiologic changes by acting on specific cells. Thus the chemical mechanisms of disease production in tetanus and in diphtheria, for instance, are relatively well understood.

Many other microorganisms, such as the gram-negative bacteria, contain as part of their structure a complex *endotoxin* which is released with lysis of the microorganism. Although the biological role of such endotoxins is far from completely understood, it is known that the release of endotoxin can be associated with the production of fever and, under more extreme circumstances such as gram-negative septicemias, with the production of a shock syndrome.

Some organisms actually injure the host, largely by immunologic means. The tubercle bacillus, for instance, appears to have no direct toxin of its own. Rather, the patient becomes allergic to the tubercle bacillus (cell-mediated immune mechanism), and the caseous necrosis typical of the disease is produced on an immunologic basis. In a similar vein, some organisms affect the host by contributing to the formation of antigen-antibody complexes which may subsequently be injurious, e.g., via the development of immune complex glomerulonephritis.

At the far end of the spectrum are viruses which are obligate intracellular parasites. In effect, viruses are simply chunks of genetic material (DNA, RNA) equipped to insert themselves into host cells. The cells are subsequently injured (if at all) by the new genetic information being expressed in altered cell function. One expression of such added genetic information is the replication of additional infectious virus, which may be accompanied by lysis of the affected cell. The cell may also be altered without actually becoming necrotic. In fact, the cell may even be stimulated to proliferate, as in the case of virally induced tumors. Viruses may also injure the host by evoking a variety of immunologic reactions in which some moiety of the virus behaves as an antigen.

MODES OF INTERACTION OF HOST AND MICROBE

It is common to view the interaction between a host and an infectious agent in terms of all-out war or a "fight to the death." There is a great tendency to view infectious agents as intrinsically "bad" things, designed to produce disease. However, the real business, biologically speaking, of any living agent is not to produce disease but to produce more of the same kind of agent. In effect, a given microbial agent "could not care less" about producing disease in the host individual. In fact an ideal infectious agent would simply reproduce within a given host (who constitutes a food supply) and not harm the host or otherwise "rock the boat."

Thinking in evolutionary terms, if a particular infectious agent were to be so effective in producing disease that it would be lethal to each host it entered, the organism would rapidly run out of a food supply and quickly become extinct. The other side of the coin is that if a particular host species is to survive in the course of evolution, one of the things that it must face successfully is infectious agents within the environment. Natural selection obviously would favor the hardier hosts. So, in the course of evolution, more resistant hosts and less lethal infectious agents tend to be developed. Thus, the dictates of evolution are such that most interactions between host and infectious agent should turn out eventually to be rather happy ones, producing significant harm to neither party. When a relationship between host and infectious agent is inoffensive to either species, that type of interaction is referred to as *commensalism*. When the interaction affords both parties some benefit, the interaction is referred to as *mutualism*. Commensalism and mutualism are the most frequent outcomes of infectious interactions in nature, and the production of *infectious disease* is in an evolutionary sense (and in fact numerically) an aberrant circumstance.

By this line of reasoning one would predict that most infectious diseases should be mild, or even that most infections should be unaccompanied by disease. As a matter of fact, it does turn out, even for most microbial "pathogens," that the presence of the organism on or in the host is most commonly trivial or inapparent and only as the exception is significant disease produced. Thus, for every individual suffering from an infectious disease of a particular sort there are probably several individuals in the population who are *infected* with the same organism and are *not at all sick*. Pneumococcus, staphylococcus, meningococcus, and many other pathogens can be recovered easily from perfectly healthy individuals in the population.

There are certainly exceptions to the principle that infection is most often mild or even inapparent. Interestingly these exceptions can usually be explained on evolutionary grounds. Rabies, for instance, is almost 100 percent fatal to human beings. Our species has not evolved with the virus but is only accidentally inserted into the chain of infection, which usually involves other mammalian species better adapted to the infection. The same is true of many other animal diseases in which human beings "get in the way;" they become much

more ill than the particular animal species adapted to that infection. Another sort of evolutionary exception is seen when "new" organisms are introduced into previously isolated human populations. Thus, when primitive tribes are suddenly invaded by individuals from the outside world or when island populations are exposed to agents that are commonplace in our experience (e.g., measles), the attack and fatality rates may be striking. This same evolutionary principle is involved in the spread of certain strains of influenza virus around the world. In this latter instance the virus behaves as if it were "new" because of the development of antigenic traits which are unknown to the population at risk.

For these reasons it has become obvious that simply knowing the line of transmission of an infectious agent from host to host does not explain fully the incidence of an *infectious disease*. To understand the epidemiology of such a disease completely, we must understand those aspects of the interaction between host and microbe which convert an ordinarily innocuous or inapparent infection into a clinically significant infectious disease.

OPPORTUNISTIC INFECTION

The concept of *opportunistic infection* reflects our recognition of the fact that there are many organisms which we do not think of as doing much to a healthy individual but which, given the wrong circumstances, will take over and produce an infectious disease. Such organisms are referred to as opportunists because they seemingly take advantage of the special circumstances of the host. Many opportunists are organisms which reside constantly within the host, and these are sometimes referred to as *endogenous* infectious agents. Some *exogenous* agents are likewise opportunistic in their behavior.

Opportunistic infections emerge when some factor or set of factors has compromised intrinsic defense mechanisms of the host or has in some way altered the ecology of the normal resident microbes (see later). Many opportunistic infections are seen in our hospitals in patients who have been significantly debilitated by diseases which impair their nutrition, their immunologic reactions, or their ability to produce effectively functioning leukocytes. Leukemias and other forms of cancer are high on the list of such diseases associated with opportunistic infections. Similarly, pharmacologic agents which must be administered in the treatment of certain diseases may have as an undesirable side effect the suppression of immunologic or inflammatory reactions, thus paving the way for opportunistic infections. Adrenal corticosteroids, which behave in many ways as anti-inflammatory agents, are high on this list, as are cytotoxic agents given in the course of cancer chemotherapy or immunosuppressive therapy. Antimicrobial therapy sometimes also leads to opportunistic infection apparently via suppression of part of the normal microbial flora. It may alter the critical ecologic balance such that another member of the flora may emerge and grow out of all proportion, thus producing disease. Antimicrobial therapy may also render a host more susceptible to some agent which ordinarily could not get a foothold because of the normal microbial flora.

Many other things happen to hospitalized patients that tend to tip the scales in favor of an infectious organism rather than of the patient. These include certain phenomena associated with anesthesia, shock, and burns, to mention but a few instances. Finally there are many examples of diseases that predispose individuals to the occurrence of infectious diseases. For example, certain cancers which involve the lymphoid tissues of the body result in *defective cellular immune reactions*. Individuals with these deficiencies develop infectious diseases due to agents ordinarily controlled by the lymphocyte-macrophage system. Finally, one infectious disease may predispose to another. For example, an individual may develop a viral "cold" and thereby become likely to develop bacterial pneumonia as a complication.

There are numerous environmental factors in the community at large that tip the scales in favor of a particular organism rather than of the host. An example of such an environmental factor involving a single individual would be occupational exposure, such as exposure to silica dust predisposing to tuberculosis. Entire populations of individuals may be involved at one time, as in famine conditions where depression of host response results in virtual epidemics of diseases such as tuberculosis. Finally, in deference to our grandmothers who seemed to know about such things, it should be pointed out that meteorologic changes may also influence the incidence of *infectious disease* as compared to infection. A variety of studies have indicated in this regard that certain infectious agents can be found within human populations the year round, but *symptomatic* infections with those agents have a seasonal incidence, perhaps related to the weather.

None of the above discussion is intended to belittle the importance of germs in disease or to discourage attempts at interrupting the cycle of transmission of infectious agents between individuals. What should be emphasized, though, is that a given organism may be a necessary condition for the production of a particular disease without in itself being a sufficient condition. It is the complex interaction of many host and environmental factors that ultimately determines the precise outcome in a given instance of infection. For these reasons when one considers the "virulence" or the "pathogenicity" of a particular microorganism, it must be done in relation to the status of the given host at that time.

NORMAL MICROBIAL FLORA

In the above discussion, in several places, the *normal or indigenous microbial flora* was mentioned. It should be emphasized that the host together with this microbial flora constitutes a sort of ecosystem whose equilibriums are an essential part of what we consider to be health.

Quantitatively, the normal microbial flora of animal hosts (including the human species) represents a staggering sort of load. For example, a significant fraction of the dry weight of feces actually consists of bacterial carcasses. We all excrete trillions of organisms each day from the gastrointestinal tract. The skin likewise has a large resident flora, estimated to be in concentration of greater than 10,000 organisms per square centimeter of skin. It should be pointed out that these are not simply organisms adhering to dirty skin but organisms which live deep within the various epithelial structures of the skin (and in fact are shed in larger numbers with scrubbing). Astronomic numbers of organisms also live within the mouth. Scrapings taken from the surfaces of teeth or gums may contain millions of organisms per milligram of material, and saliva may contain as many as 100 million organisms per milliliter.

Another point to be emphasized is that this impressive microbial flora is not a random population. Of the many species of microbes encountered within the environment as we move about each day, only relatively few have become adapted in the course of their own evolution to the particular environments that we afford in various tissues. Therefore, within certain limits the flora of a given animal species is predictable, and within a given species, such as our own, the flora of particular tissues is quite predictable. An interesting point about the flora is that in most tissues that have been studied carefully the anaerobic bacteria seem to outnumber the aerobic bacteria. This is especially true in the bowel, where the ratio is as high as 1000:1.

Biologists have known of the existence of the normal microbial flora for many decades, but opinions concerning the significance of the flora have varied tremendously through the years. In the early years of this century some authorities had a very dim view of the flora, judging it at best to be a neutral mass, and at worst to be a cause of the degenerative diseases of aging.

Gradually this view has been replaced, with the increasing recognition that no animal species would evolve with a particular flora in a disadvantageous relationship. To the contrary, one would predict that a mutually advantageous relationship should evolve.

Clearly, indigenous microbes do many good things for us. Many chemical reactions within the lumen of the bowel, for instance, are actually carried out by the resident microbes. The ecologic functions of such microbes in repelling potential invaders has already been alluded to. In fact, however, carrying this argument on evolutionary grounds even further, one would predict that many traits of our species have evolved as they did partly as a result of the presence of the microbial associates. In everyday terms this means that a number of anatomic and physiologic traits of the host that we consider normal and innate actually develop as a response to the presence of the flora. Putting this in another way, the host depends for normalcy to a significant extent upon the microbial flora. It is known, for instance, that the structure and function of the lining of the gastrointestinal tract are influenced by the presence of the flora, that the motility of the tract is influenced by the flora,

and that many of the reactions of the tract to challenge are similarly conditioned by the flora.

Although such considerations are perhaps more obvious within the gastrointestinal tract, the direct and indirect effects of the indigenous flora are not limited to that area. There is reason to believe that even immunologic function and leukocyte function are influenced by the flora.

The actual means by which the microbial flora acts upon the host are not well understood. In fact, even the identity of some components of the flora in human beings is far from clear. We are only now beginning to learn what it is that controls the usual ecologic balance of the flora itself: a combination of factors involving microbe-to-microbe and host-to-microbe interactions. What is evident at this point, however, is that when one disrupts the normal ecology of the microbal flora, it is done at significant risk to the host.

QUESTIONS

Response of the body to infectious agents

Directions: Answer the following questions on a separate sheet of paper.

1. What are the criteria used to determine that a host is infected? Does a host who is infected necessarily have an infectious disease?

2. Name at least five portals of entry of infectious agents into the host. Describe the characteristics of the defenses at each of these portals.

3. Briefly describe what can occur if an acute inflammatory reaction is unable to contain an invading microorganism locally.

4. What is the final line of defense against widespread dissemination of an infectious agent throughout the body?

5. What is meant by an opportunistic infection?

6. What are some situations which can change an inapparent infection into an infectious disease?

7. Briefly discuss the interaction of the human host and the bacteria forming the normal flora on body surfaces. What value does this relationship provide for the host?

8. List several known mechanisms causing tissue injury by infectious agents.

Directions: Circle the letter preceding each item below that correctly answers each question. More than one answer may be correct.

9. All of the following may directly deter or prevent the invasion and spread of infectious agents *except:*
   a. Inflammatory response   *b.* Intact skin
   c. Alveolar macrophages   *d.* Fibroblasts
   e. Monocyte-macrophage system

10. When microorganisms reach such a high number in the circulation that they lodge in tissues and form abcesses, the condition is termed:
    a. Septicemia   *b.* Bacteremia   *c.* Septicopyemia
    d. Polycythemia

11. In relationships between hosts and infectious agents evolution has favored:
    a. Weak, nonresistant hosts   *b.* Hardier, resistant hosts   *c.* Very lethal infectious agents
    d. Less lethal infectious agents

Match the organisms listed in col. A with their specific invasive characteristic in col. B.

Column A	Column B
12. ___ Cholera vibrio	*a.* Penetrates the mucous membrane or skin and enters the

13. ____ Typhoid bacillus

14. ____ Syphilis spirochete

15. ____ Tetanus bacillus

bloodstream; disseminated widely in body

b. Invades the lining of the bowel and enters the bloodstream

c. Colonizes bowel lumen, never invades

d. Remains local but secretes a toxin which is carried in the bloodstream

Match the terms in col. A, which indicate the type of relationship between two dissimilar organisms living in close association (e.g., human being and microorganism), to their correct interpretation in col. B.

Column A

16. ____ Commensalism

17. ____ Parasitism

18. ____ Mutualism

Column B

a. The association is beneficial to one but detrimental to the other.

b. The association is beneficial to one without injury to the other.

c. The association is beneficial to both.

DISTURBANCES OF CIRCULATION

OBJECTIVES

At the completion of this chapter you should be able to:

1. Describe the two mechanisms by which congestion (hyperemia) may be produced.
2. State at least one example of each type of congestion.
3. Identify the systemic causes of passive congestion.
4. Describe the effects of chronic passive congestion in areas such as the lungs, liver, and veins.
5. Differentiate between acute passive congestion and chronic passive congestion in terms of their effects on the involved tissue.
6. Define *edema.*
7. Discuss the pathogenesis of edema in terms of factors governing fluid flux across vascular membranes.
8. Compare an exudate to a transudate as to pathogenesis and give an example of each type.
9. Describe the significance of generalized edema.
10. Define the following terms associated with hemorrhage: *hematoma, petechiae, ecchymoses.*
11. Describe the various causes of hemorrhage.
12. Describe the body's mechanisms for stopping hemorrhage.
13. Describe the local and systemic effects of hemorrhage.
14. Discuss the etiology, pathogenesis, and morphology of thrombi.
15. Distinguish between factors predisposing to the development of thrombi in arteries and veins.
16. Contrast the consequences of arterial and venous thrombi.
17. Describe the process of embolism.
18. Trace the route taken when fragments of venous thrombi from deep veins of the leg or pelvis break off and are dislodged into the circulation.
19. Describe the potential consequences of pulmonary arterial emboli, caisson disease, air emboli, and traumatic fat emboli.
20. Define *arteriosclerosis.*

21. Differentiate between Mönckeberg's sclerosis, arteriolosclerosis, and atherosclerosis in terms of morphology and clinical significance.
22. Identify for atherosclerosis the area(s) of involvement, unit lesion, etiology, incidence, and consequences.
23. Discuss the possible causes of ischemia and the effects of affected tissue.
24. Describe the possible outcome of occlusion of major blood vessels.
25. Define an *infarct*.
26. Discuss the factors which determine whether an ischemic area actually undergoes infarction.
27. Describe the morphologic features of an infarct.
28. Cite examples of infarcts commonly encountered clinically.

CONGESTION

Simply stated, *congestion* is an overabundance of blood *within* the vessels in a given region. Another word for congestion is *hyperemia*. When observed grossly, an area of tissue or an organ which is congested has a deeper red (or purplish) color than usual because of the increase in blood within the tissue. Microscopically the capillaries in a hyperemic tissue are dilated and engorged with blood. Basically there are two mechanisms by which congestion may be produced: (1) by an actual increase in the amount of blood flowing into an area and (2) by a decrease in the amount of blood draining from an area.

Active congestion

When the flow of blood into an area is increased and produces congestion, the phenomenon is referred to as *active congestion,* in the sense that more blood than usual is actively flowing into the area. This increase in local blood flow is accomplished by dilatation of arterioles which behave as valves governing the flow into the local microcirculation. One common example of active congestion is the hyperemia accompanying acute inflammation which accounts for the redness described in Chap. 4 (see Fig. 4-1). Another example of active congestion is a blush, which is basically a matter of vasodilatation produced in response to a neurogenic stimulus. A physiologic example of active congestion is the delivery of more blood upon "demand" of a working tissue such as an actively contracting muscle. This is also termed *functional hyperemia*. By its very nature, active congestion is often short-lived. As the stimulus to arteriolar dilatation is withdrawn, the flow of blood to the affected area is decreased, and the situation returns to normal.

Passive congestion

As the name suggests, *passive congestion* does not involve an increase in the amount of blood flowing into an area but rather some impairment in drainage of blood from the area. Anything which compresses the venules and veins draining a tissue may produce passive congestion. When one places an elastic tourniquet about the arm prior to drawing blood from a vein, one is actually inducing an artificial form of passive congestion. A similar and more significant change could be produced, for instance, by a tumor compressing the local venous drainage from an area. In addition to such local causes of passive congestion there are central or systemic reasons for impaired venous drainage. Not infrequently the heart fails in its pumping action (see Part V), and this leads to impaired venous drainage. For instance, if the left side of the heart fails in its pumping action, the flow of blood returning to the heart from the lung will be somewhat impaired. Under such circumstances blood will be dammed back into the lung, producing passive congestion of the pulmonary vasculature. Similarly if the right side of the heart fails, the damming-up of blood affects systemic venous return, and many tissues throughout the body become passively congested. In point of fact, very often patients suffer simultaneously from right- and left-sided cardiac failure.

Passive congestion may be relatively short-lived, in which case it is termed *acute passive congestion,* or it may be of long standing, in which case it is termed *chronic passive congestion*. If the passive congestion is short-lived, there are no effects on the involved tissue.

In chronic passive congestion, however, there may be permanent changes in the tissues. These changes are due in large part to the fact that in a passively congested area, if the change in blood flow is marked enough, there is an element of tissue hypoxia which may lead to shrinkage or even loss of cells of the involved tissue. In certain organs this also leads to an increase in the amount of fibrous connective tissue. In many areas there is also evidence of local breakdown of red blood cells, which results in the deposition of hemoglobin-derived pigments within the tissues.

The effects of chronic passive congestion are particularly notable in lungs and liver. In the case of the lungs (Fig. 7-1), the walls of air spaces tend to become thickened, and numerous macrophages are found to contain *hemosiderin* pigment, a product of the breakdown of hemoglobin from red blood cells which escape the congested vessels into the air spaces. Such hemosiderin-containing macrophages are sometimes termed *heart failure cells* and can be found in the sputum of patients in chronic left-sided cardiac failure. In the case of the liver, chronic passive congestion leads to marked dilatation of the blood channels in the center of each hepatic lobule, with shrinkage of liver cells in this area. The result of this is a striking gross appearance of the liver (Fig. 7-2) produced by the hyperemic centrilobular zone alternating with the less affected peripheral areas of each lobule. This gross appearance is sometimes referred to as "nutmeg liver" because of the fancied resemblance of the cut surface of such a liver to the cut surface of a nutmeg.

Another effect of chronic passive congestion is dilatation of the veins in the affected area. As the walls of affected veins are chronically stretched, they become somewhat fibrotic, and the veins also tend to lengthen. Because veins are fixed at various points along their length they necessarily become tortuous as they lengthen; i.e., they twist back and forth between points of fixation. Dilated, somewhat tortuous, thick-walled veins are referred to as *varicose veins* or *varices*. Varicose veins in the legs are a familiar sight. Also common are *hemorrhoids*, which are actually varicose veins of the anus (in the hemorrhoidal plexus of veins). More importantly, venous varices sometimes form in the lower esophagus in cases of chronic liver disease (see Chap. 19), and rupture of such congested varices may lead to fatal hemorrhage.

EDEMA

Edema is an accumulation of excess fluid between the cells of the body or within the various body cavities. (Some authors also include in the definition the accumulation of excess fluids intracellularly.) When edema accumulates in a cavity, it is usually called an *effusion*, e.g., pericardial effusion, pleural effusion. An accumulation of fluid in the peritoneal cavity is usually termed *ascites*. Massive generalized edema is frequently referred to as *anasarca*. *Hydrops* and *dropsy* are older terms also referring to edema.

Etiology and pathogenesis of edema

The development of edema can be explained by considering the various forces normally controlling fluid exchange across vessel walls (see Fig. 4-2 and Chap. 4).

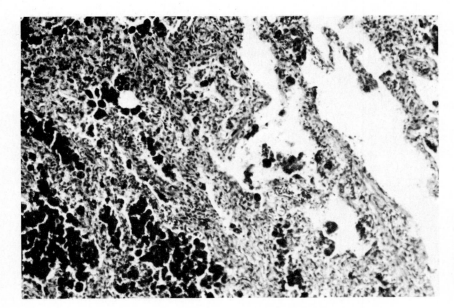

FIGURE 7-1
Chronic-passive congestion of lung. Alveolar septa are thickened (evident at the right), and many air spaces contain deeply pigmented macrophages containing hemosiderin. (Photomicrograph, ×200.)

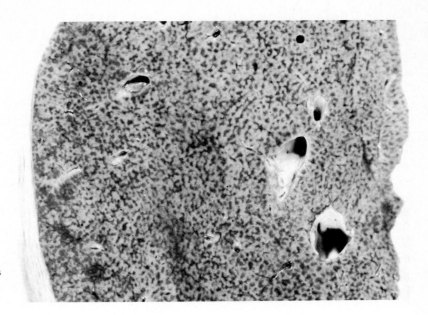

FIGURE 7-2
Chronic passive congestion of liver. Dark areas on this cut surface are hyperemic centrilobular zones, while light areas are less affected peripheral zones. The result is this typical "nutmeg" pattern.

Local factors include the hydrostatic pressure within the microcirculation and the permeability of vessel walls. Increases in hydrostatic pressure will tend to force fluid into the interstitial spaces of the body. For this simple reason, congestion and edema tend to go together. As was explained in the discussion of inflammation, a local increase in the permeability of vessel walls to protein will allow these large molecules to escape the vessels, and fluid will follow osmotically. Therefore, edema is a prominent part of the acute inflammatory reaction. Another local cause of edema formation is obstruction of lymphatic channels, which are normally responsible for drainage of the interstitial fluid. When these channels become obstructed for any reason, an important pathway of egress of fluid is lost, leading to accumulation of fluid, which is referred to as *lymphedema*. Lymphedema is seen in a variety of inflammatory conditions affecting the lymphatics but is perhaps most commonly encountered in hospitals following either excision or irradiation of local lymphatics as part of cancer therapy. A specific example of this type of edema is swelling of the upper extremity sometimes seen following radical mastectomy.

Systemic factors may also favor edema formation. Since fluid balance is dependent on osmotic properties of serum protein, conditions accompanied by a lower concentration of this protein may lead to edema. In the so-called *nephrotic syndrome*, massive amounts of protein are lost in the urine, and the patient becomes hypoproteinemic and edematous. The hypoproteinemia of advanced liver disease may also favor the formation of edema. In famine situations massive edema may likewise accompany the nutritional hypoproteinemia.

Transudates versus exudates

When fluid accumulates in a tissue or space because of increased vascular permeability to protein, this accumulation is referred to as an *exudate*. Thus, inflammatory edema represents an exudate. When fluid accumulates in the tissues or spaces because of reasons other than changes in vascular permeability, the accumulation is referred to as a *transudate*. In hospital situations probably cardiac failure is the leading cause of transudate formation. Sometimes it becomes important clinically to determine whether a particular fluid accumulation represents a transudate or an exudate. Exudates by their very nature tend to contain more protein than transudates and tend, therefore, to have higher specific gravities. In addition, the protein of exudates often includes fibrinogen, which will precipitate as fibrin, causing clotting of the exudate fluid. Transudates do not clot generally. Finally, exudates will frequently contain leukocytes as part of the inflammatory process, while transudates tend to be cell-poor.

Morphology of edema

The morphology of edema involves simply a swelling of the affected part because of too much fluid contained within the interstices. The swelling is generally of a soft sort, and, unless it is largely intracellular, the fluid actually can be moved about. This latter feature is utilized clinically in diagnosing subtle degrees of edema. While a massively swollen ankle is easily diagnosed on sight, a slight degree of edema may be present without being particularly visible. In this instance gentle pressure of a thumb against the side of the ankle will tend to displace some of the edema fluid temporarily, and when the thumb is removed after a few moments, a depression is left in the tissues. This is referred to as *pitting edema*. This same mobility of edema fluid within the interstices of tissues accounts for certain postural effects. Sometimes, when first admitted to the hospital, a patient will have demonstrably edematous ankles, because in the ambulatory situation the edema moves with gravity toward the lower extremities. However, when the patient has been in bed for a time with the lower extremities not in a dependent position, the ankles may become slimmer, and edema may become demonstrable over the sacrum instead.

Effects of edema

Edema is important primarily as an indicator of something being amiss. In other words, the swollen ankles per se do not harm the patient other than, perhaps, in a cosmetic sense but do serve as an indicator of protein loss, congestive heart failure, etc. In certain locations edema in and of itself is extremely important. Edema of the lungs, as, for instance, in left-sided heart failure, is an acute medical emergency if extensive. If a sufficient number of air spaces in the lungs fill with edema fluid, the patient may literally drown. Massive pulmonary edema can be lethal within a matter of minutes. Lesser degrees of pulmonary edema which can be tolerated in a ventilatory sense may be dangerous to bedridden patients. In such instances the fluid may collect posteriorly at the lung bases and serve as a focus for the development of bacterial pneumonia, sometimes referred to as *hypostatic pneumonia*. Edema is also life-threatening when it affects the brain. This is so because the skull represents a closed space with no room to spare. As the brain becomes edematous, it swells and is compressed against the bony confines of the skull. At some point, in severe cases, increased intracranial pressure will compromise blood flow within the brain, leading to death.

HEMORRHAGE

Hemorrhage is the escape of blood from the confines of the cardiovascular system, with accumulation in tissues or spaces of the body or with actual escape from the body. Special descriptive terms are used to designate various circumstances of hemorrhage. An accumulation of blood within tissues is referred to as a *hematoma*. When the blood escapes into various spaces in the body, it is named according to the space, e.g., *hemopericardium*, *hemothorax* (hemorrhage into the pleural space), *hemoperitoneum*, *hematosalpinx* (hemorrhage into the fallopian tube). Pinpoint hemorrhages visible on cutaneous or mucosal surfaces or on cut surfaces of organs are referred to as *petechiae*. Larger, blotchy areas of hemorrhage are referred to as *ecchymoses*, and a condition characterized by widespread blotchy hemorrhages is sometimes referred to as *purpura*.

Etiology of hemorrhage

The commonest cause of hemorrhage is loss of integrity of vascular walls, which permits the escape of blood. This is most often due to external trauma such as we all experience from time to time with injuries accompanied by bruising. The discoloration of a bruise is due to the blood accumulated in the interstices of the traumatized tissue. Vascular walls may be disrupted as a result of disease as well as of trauma.

A number of mechanisms exist within the body to counteract hemorrhage (see Part III). One mechanism of hemostasis involves the *blood platelets*, which are made in the bone marrow and circulate in the blood in large numbers. Platelets act directly to plug small leaks in vessels by aggregating in the area and blocking the flow. Platelets also lead to hemostasis by triggering the *clotting mechanism* of the blood. The "backbone" of a blood clot is fibrin, which is precipitated from its circulating precursor, fibrinogen. The precipitation of fibrin is controlled by a number of clotting factors which are activated under certain circumstances (see Chap. 18).

Hemorrhage may be caused by an abnormality of these hemostatic mechanisms. For instance, hemorrhage accompanies a state of *thrombocytopenia*, a deficiency in the number of circulating platelets. Thrombocytopenia can arise because of destruction or suppression of the bone marrow, e.g., by malignancy or by some drug, with consequent failure of platelet production. Thrombocytopenia may also occur if circulating platelets are rapidly destroyed, as occurs in certain diseases. When the platelet count in the peripheral blood drops beyond a certain point, the patient begins to bleed "spontaneously," meaning that the trauma of normal motion leads to widespread hemorrhages. A deficiency of any of the various clotting factors may likewise lead to hemorrhage. Such deficiency may be hereditary (e.g., hemophilia), but may also be acquired. Certain of the blood clotting factors are synthesized in the liver, and with advanced hepatic disease the level of such factors available in the blood may drop precipitously. Paradoxically, in certain situations excessive clotting of the blood may lead to an acquired deficiency of platelets and/or clotting factors. Usually this involves the formation of myriads of tiny clots around the body, so-called *disseminated intravascular coagulation* (DIC), and the acquired deficiency state is sometimes referred to under the general heading of *consumptive coagulopathy*.

Effects of hemorrhage

The *local effects* of hemorrhage are related to the presence of extravasated blood in the tissues and can range from trivial to lethal. Perhaps the most trivial local effect is a bruise, which may be of only cosmetic importance. The initial bluish discoloration of the bruise is related directly to the presence of spilled red blood cells accumulated in the tissue. These extravasated erythrocytes break down fairly rapidly and are phagocytized by macrophages arriving as part of the associated inflammatory response. These macrophages process the hemoglobin in the same manner as that used in the normal recycling of old red cells but in a much more accelerated, concentrated fashion. As the hemoglobin is metabolized within these cells, an iron-containing complex called *hemosiderin* is formed, along with a non-iron-containing moiety which in tissues is termed *hematoidin* (although it is chemically identical with *bilirubin*). Hemosiderin has a rusty-brown color, and hematoidin a light-yellow color. It is the play of these pigments in a resolving bruise that produces the familiar range of colors as the "black-and-blue mark" fades through varying shades of brown and yellow, ultimately to disappear as the macrophages wander off, and restitution of the tissue is complete. Sometimes, when a hematoma is of considerable volume, it may actually organize rather than resolve completely, leaving some degree of local scarring.

At the other extreme, strictly local hemorrhage may be fatal, even if of small volume, if it is in the wrong place. Thus, as seen in Fig. 7-3, a relatively small volume of hemorrhage in a vital area of the brain can produce death. Similarly if a few hundred milliliters of blood are aspirated into the tracheobronchial tree, the patient may be suffocated. Another area wherein a relatively small volume of hemorrhage may produce death is the pericardial sac. If hemopericardium develops quickly and the tough, fibrous pericardial sac does not have the opportunity to stretch, pressure within the sac builds up rapidly as blood accumulates. Sometimes, with accumulation of only a few hundred milliliters, the pressure is sufficient to impair diastolic filling of the heart, leading to death by *cardiac tamponade*.

The systemic effects of blood loss are related directly to the volume of blood extravasated. Obviously, if a major portion of the circulatory volume is lost, as with massive trauma, the patient may die of *exsanguination* very quickly. It should be noted that a patient may exsanguinate with absolutely no external evidence of hemorrhage. This occurs when the extravasated blood accumulates within a large body cavity such as the pleural cavity or peritoneal cavity. This type of lethal internal hemorrhage is seen all too often in crushing injuries associated with motor vehicle accidents, when broken ribs lacerate a lung or abdominal trauma results in rupture of the spleen or liver. (In emergency room practice such internal hemorrhage is identified by needle aspiration of the cavity in question.) The effects of a given volume of hemorrhage are also related to the rate at which the loss occurs, a larger volume loss being better tolerated if it occurs gradually rather than instantaneously.

Short of death, the rapid loss of a sufficient volume

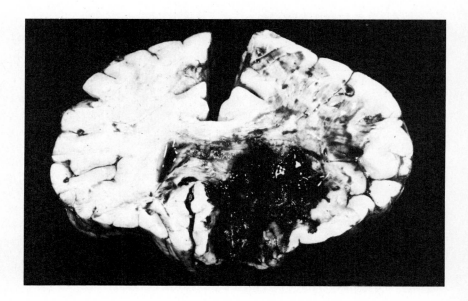

FIGURE 7-3
Cerebral hemorrhage. In an instance such as this, a relatively small volume of hemorrhage may lead to death because of local destructive effects.

of blood may lead to a condition of *shock*. A detailed consideration of the various shock syndromes is beyond the scope of this discussion, but it should be pointed out that shock can be produced not only by the loss of blood volume but also by neurogenic causes, cardiac causes, or even accompanying systemic sepsis. Although the various shock syndromes differ in detail, they are all basically accompanied by a decrease in blood pressure and by an element of loss of control over the regulation of blood flow, leading ultimately to inadequate perfusion and oxygenation of the vital tissues of the body.

If a patient survives the acute loss of a given volume of blood, the circulatory volume is quickly regained by an influx of fluid into the cardiovascular system. This leads to a relative dilution of the red blood cell mass remaining, and the patient at that point would be found to be somewhat anemic. Under such conditions the marrow is stimulated to produce red blood cells in an accelerated fashion, and the anemia would gradually be corrected. Under conditions of chronic loss of even relatively small volumes of blood, the compensatory abilities of the marrow may be exceeded, and the patient may become progressively more anemic. Not infrequently, patients with chronic loss of blood present themselves with signs and symptoms of the anemia rather than of the blood loss itself. Thus, many a patient with a cancer of the colon, which oozes blood for many months unnoticed into the feces, may ultimately seek medical attention because of fatigue, pallor, lack of energy, etc. Thus, occult loss of blood is a consideration in the investigation of many anemias.

THROMBOSIS

The process of formation of a blood clot or coagulum within the vascular system (i.e., the blood vessels or the heart) during life is referred to as *thrombosis*. The coagulum of blood is called a *thrombus*. The accumulation of blood which clots outside of the vascular system, e.g., a hematoma, is *not* referred to as a thrombus. Furthermore, the clots that form within the cardiovascular system after death are not called thrombi. They are called *postmortem clots*.

Thrombosis is obviously of great adaptive value in case of hemorrhage. That is to say, a thrombus acts as a very effective hemostatic plug. However, thrombosis may also occur inappropriately when the normal control mechanisms are defective and, under these circumstances, prove to be harmful to the host.

Etiology and pathogenesis of thrombosis

Three sets of factors ordinarily guard against inappropriate thrombus formation. First of all, the normal vascular system has a smooth, slick lining of endothelial cells to which platelets and fibrin do not readily adhere.

Secondly, the normal flow of blood within the vascular system is a fairly streamlined one so that platelets are not hurled against lining surfaces. Finally, the clotting mechanism (see Chap. 18) has built into it a number of chemical checks and balances to control clot formation. Correspondingly, there are three basic kinds of situations in which clots form inappropriately: those in which there is abnormality of the vessel wall and lining, those in which blood flow is abnormal, and those in which the coagulability of the blood itself is increased.

The flow of blood on the arterial side of the circulation is a high-pressure flow of rapid velocity, and the arteries themselves are rather thick-walled and not easily deformed. For these reasons the usual cause of arterial thrombosis is disease in the lining and wall of the artery, particularly atherosclerosis (see discussion later). On the venous side of the circulation the blood flow is one of low pressure and relatively lower velocity, and the veins are sufficiently thin-walled that they can be deformed readily by external pressures. For these reasons, the usual causes of thrombosis on the venous side of the circulation relate to diminished flow of blood. Finally, chemical changes occur in the blood of patients with a variety of diseases, leading to a hypercoagulable state which may further complicate any of the above situations.

Morphology and fate of thrombi

Thrombi consist of varying combinations of aggregated platelets, precipitated fibrin, and enmeshed red blood cells and leukocytes. The precise configuration of a thrombus depends on the conditions under which it was formed. If the thrombus begins to form in flowing blood, very often the first element is a clump of platelets adhering to the endothelium. This may occur because of abnormal flow allowing platelets to settle against or to be hurled against the endothelium; it may occur because of a roughening of the endothelial lining, which would produce a nidus for platelet aggregation. As platelets aggregate, they release substances which encourage the precipitation of fibrin, so that soon the platelet aggregates come to be surrounded by fibrin and trapped blood cells. Successive waves of events of this sort can lead to a complex, ribbed structure of a thrombus. On the other hand, if a thrombus forms in a vessel in which the flow has virtually stopped, the clot may simply consist of a diffuse meshwork of fibrin trapping the formed elements of the blood more or less homogeneously. It should be noted here that, in contrast to the processes just described, postmortem clotting occurs quite slowly so that the formed elements of the blood

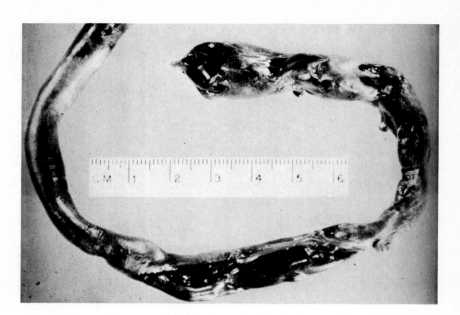

FIGURE 7-4

Venous thrombus. This thrombus was extracted from a leg vein at autopsy. Such a finding is unfortunately quite common and is associated with many dire consequences. Reference to the scale emphasizes the magnitude of the clot.

layer out before the clot solidifies, giving rise to a stratified structure in which red blood cells, white blood cells, and fibrin may be quite separate. Such postmortem clots tend to be more elastic than true thrombi and are much less likely to be adherent to vascular walls.

Thrombi may occur literally in any part of the cardiovascular system for a variety of causes. Figure 7-4 illustrates a thrombus from a large deep vein of the leg. Such thrombi are all too common in hospitalized, bedridden patients. Their occurrence is generally related to the decreased rate of flow through these veins, in turn secondary to the loss of pumping action of muscular activity. The situation is aggravated in many instances by sluggish peripheral circulation related to chronic cardiac failure. It cannot be emphasized too strongly that *phlebothrombosis*, the formation of thrombi in veins, is an ever-present danger stalking hospitalized patients. Such thrombi may develop relatively silently or may be accompanied by signs and symptoms of inflammation of the vein wall, which are presumably secondary to the presence of the thrombus. (When inflammatory signs dominate, the condition is sometimes referred to as *thrombophlebitis*.) The most feared consequence of such venous thrombi is the breaking off of a portion, which is then transported in the bloodstream to lodge at a distant site.

Figure 7-5 illustrates a thrombus within the left atrium of the heart. In this instance the thrombus formed because of an abnormal flow and pattern of circulation through the atrium related to stenosis of the

FIGURE 7-5

Atrial thrombus. A huge thrombus has formed in the left atrium because of malfunction of the scarred mitral valve. The position of this clot renders it of great potential danger.

mitral valve. Occasionally such atrial thrombi may behave as "ball valves," suddenly occluding the atrioventricular orifice and producing instant death. More often such thrombi act as the source of fragments which are propelled distally in the bloodstream.

Figure 7-6 illustrates a thrombus on a cardiac valve. In this instance the cause is bacterial infection of the

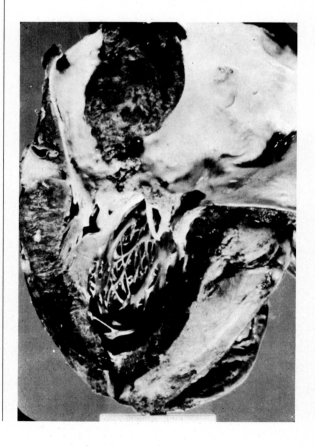

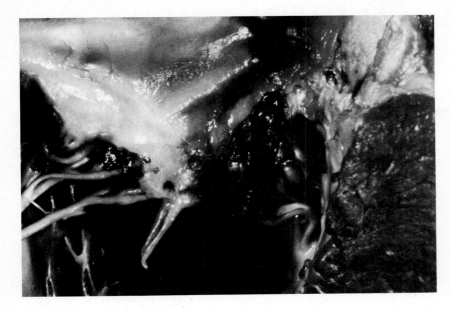

FIGURE 7-6
Infective endocarditis. The dark vegetations on this mitral valve are actually thrombotic masses formed around foci of bacterial infection of the valve. The valve was previously scarred (note thickening of leaflets and chordae) and therefore was susceptible to infection during a burst of bacteremia.

valve, and the thrombus is frequently referred to as a *vegetation*. Vegetations of infective endocarditis are exceedingly dangerous because of local damage to the valve and because fragments may be propelled to other sites in the body where additional vessels may become occluded and infected.

Figure 7-7 illustrates a thrombus within the left ventricle of the heart. When a thrombus such as this one is adherent to the wall of the cardiovascular system but does not totally occlude the area, it is referred to as a *mural thrombus*. The usual reason for the formation of a ventricular mural thrombus is death of the underlying myocardium with an associated inflammatory reaction reaching the lining of the heart. The tendency to thrombosis is also aggravated by decreased local motion of the necrotic heart wall.

Figure 7-8 illustrates a thrombus within an artery. Clearly evident in the picture is the thickening of the wall of the artery which has given rise to the thrombus. The roughening in this instance is due to a disease (atherosclerosis) and is a precipitating cause of thrombosis.

Very often, when the subject survives the formation of a thrombus, the fate of the thrombus is to undergo resolution. The body possesses fibrinolytic mechanisms which, along with the action of leukocytes, may lead to the dissolution of clots. Probably all of us form tiny thrombi now and then, and these are resolved without ever reaching the clinical horizon. On the other hand, the fate of some large thrombi is to undergo organization, with granulation tissue growing in from an adjacent vascular lining. In such instances, the involved vessel may become permanently plugged by scar. Some-

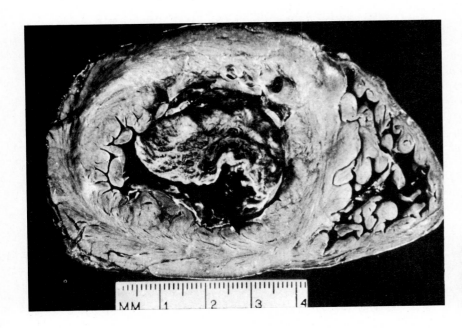

FIGURE 7-7
Mural thrombus in heart. In this transverse section a large mural thrombus overlies an area of previous myocardial necrosis in the wall of the left ventricle.

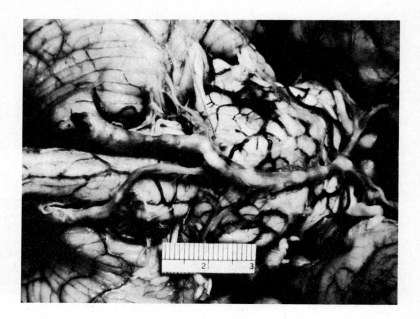

FIGURE 7-8
Thrombus in a sclerotic artery. The artery above the brainstem (left of center) is atherosclerotic and gnarled. The lumen is occluded by a thrombus which protrudes from the cut end at the left.

times the vascular channels within the young granulation tissue organizing a thrombus may anastomose in such a manner as to provide new channels through the area occupied by thrombus. This phenomenon is referred to as *recanalization*. Unfortunately, in many instances, before the thrombus either organizes or resolves, portions of it break off and are propelled in the bloodstream, ultimately lodging elsewhere and occluding additional vessels.

Effects of thrombi

The consequences of thrombosis are perhaps most obvious in the case of arterial thrombi. If an artery is occluded by a thrombus, the tissues served by that artery will suffer loss of their blood supply. The results of this may range from functional abnormality of tissue to death of the tissue or death of the subject. The consequences of venous thrombi are somewhat different. The anatomy of the venous system is such that if one vein is plugged, chances are that the blood will find its way back to the heart via some anastomosing channel. It is only when a very large vein is occluded by thrombus that local problems with passive congestion become evident. The most ominous problem associated with venous thrombi is their fragmentation and transport to distant points in the body. Similarly, the effects of cardiac thrombi are largely related to their moving elsewhere within the cardiovascular system.

EMBOLISM

Definition and types

The carriage of a physical mass in the bloodstream from one place to another with lodgement in the new loca-

tion is termed *embolism*. The physical mass itself is called an *embolus*. The commonest emboli in human subjects are derived from thrombi and are termed *thromboemboli*. Many other things, however, can become embolic. Bits of tissue can embolize if they enter the vascular system, usually with trauma. Cancer cells may embolize, constituting a devastating means of spread of the disease (see Chap. 8). Foreign materials injected into the cardiovascular system may embolize. Droplets of liquid which form in the circulation under a variety of circumstances or are injected into the circulation may embolize, and even gas bubbles may become embolic.

Pathogenesis, routes, and effects of embolism

The commonest sources of emboli within the body are venous thrombi, most often in the deep veins of the legs or the pelvis. When fragments of such venous thrombi break off and float with the flow of blood, they enter the vena cava and then the right side of the heart. Such fragments do not lodge along this path because of the large size of the vessels and cardiac chambers involved. The blood leaving the right ventricle, however, flows into the main pulmonary artery, which branches into right and left pulmonary arteries, which in turn branch to smaller vessels. For these reasons of anatomy, emboli originating in venous thrombi usually terminate as *pulmonary arterial emboli*. When a very large fragment of thrombus becomes an embolus, a major portion of the pulmonary arterial supply may suddenly be occluded (Fig. 7-9). This can produce virtually instantaneous death of the subject. On the other hand, smaller pulmonary arterial emboli may be silent, may lead to pulmonary hemorrhage secondary to the vascular damage, or may actually result in necrosis of a portion of lung.

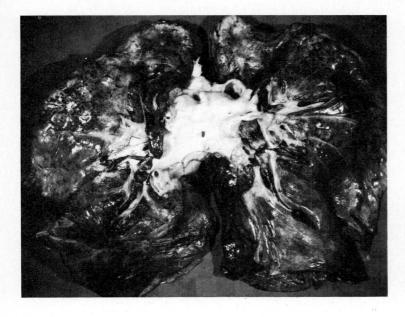

FIGURE 7-9
Massive pulmonary emboli. The opened pulmonary arteries supplying these lungs are seen in the center of the photograph. The several dark cylindrical masses are emboli which originated from venous thrombus in a leg, similar to that shown in Fig. 7-4. The patient died within moments of lodgement of the emboli.

Pulmonary emboli of various sizes can be found in a significant fraction of patients dying within hospitals, sometimes contributing to the death of the subject, sometimes being only of incidental importance. Showers of tiny pulmonary emboli over a long period of time may produce sufficient occlusion of the pulmonary vascular bed as to cause the right side of the heart to become overloaded and to fail.

Emboli which lodge on the arterial side of the circulation take their origin on the "left side" of the circulatory system either in the left cardiac chambers or in the large arteries. The only way that an embolus originating on the venous side of the circulation could lodge on the arterial side is to bypass the lungs via a defect in the interatrial or interventricular septum of the heart. This situation, termed *paradoxical embolism*, is exceedingly rare. Most often an arterial embolus is found to have originated from an intracardiac thrombus or, more rarely, from a mural thrombus in the aorta or one of its large branches.

Gas bubbles may become embolic in a variety of circumstances. One such circumstance has been termed *caisson disease*, more popularly known as "the bends." This situation arises when a subject has been living under markedly increased atmospheric pressure such as that within a pressurized caisson or in underwater diving gear. In such circumstances increased amounts of atmospheric gases are dissolved within the bloodstream. If decompression is sufficiently abrupt, the result is analogous to what is seen when a warm bottle of soda pop is suddenly opened. The myriads of tiny gas bubbles appearing within the circulation are carried to a variety of places in the body where they lodge in the microcirculation and occlude the blood flow to those tissues. In hospitals an analogous circumstance sometimes arises when atmospheric air enters venous channels due to

faulty handling of an intravenous infusion or indwelling vascular catheter, or sometimes in the course of a surgical procedure when large vascular channels must be traversed. With massive air embolism a large "bolus" of air may enter the right side of the heart, and at autopsy a large foamy mass of air and blood is seen distending the heart and pulmonary vessels.

An example of embolism of liquid droplets is so-called *traumatic fat embolism*. As the name suggests, these emboli, composed of fat globules, tend to form within the circulation following trauma. The usual point of lodgement is the microcirculation of the lung. Minor degrees of fat embolism probably follow most surgical procedures where fatty tissue is incised and lipidic material is allowed to enter vascular channels. In such circumstances the few scattered emboli which lodge in the lung are completely silent and trivial. A similar circumstance arises when bones are fractured, apparently with liberation of lipid into the sinusoids of the bone marrow. Again, such scattered pulmonary fat emboli as result in this circumstance are trivial and clinically inapparent. Occasionally, however, following traumatic injury, fat embolism may be massive. It is not clear whether all the fat droplets in such a circumstance originate from trauma to adipose cells. Some evidence suggests that in this type of circumstance there is actually coalescence of lipid normally carried within the bloodstream. In any event, with sufficiently massive fat embolism, symptoms of respiratory distress may appear, usually in the first day or two after trauma. In severe instances the emboli lodge in a variety of places in the body beyond the lungs, including the skin and, more importantly, the central nervous system. In both of these latter areas each microscopic fat embolus is associated with a petechial hemorrhage. In the case of the brain, a tiny focus of necrosis surrounds each occluded vessel. In these rare instances, fat embolism can be fatal, usually because of cerebral damage.

ATHEROSCLEROSIS

Arteriosclerosis, or "hardening of the arteries," is an exceedingly important disease phenomenon in most developed countries. The term arteriosclerosis actually encompasses any condition of arterial vessels that results in a thickening and/or hardening of the walls. Three conditions are generally included under this heading: *Mönckeberg's sclerosis*, *arteriolosclerosis*, and *atherosclerosis*. Mönckeberg's sclerosis involves deposition of calcium salts in the muscular wall of medium-sized arteries. Although this can be detected grossly and even seen on x-rays, this form of arteriosclerosis is not clinically significant since the lining of the involved vessel is not roughened and the lumen is not narrowed. Arteriolosclerosis refers to a thickening of arterioles, seen frequently in patients with elevated blood pressure and to some extent in association with aging. The most important type of arteriosclerosis is atherosclerosis, and generally when the term arteriosclerosis is used, it is used synonymously with atherosclerosis.

Atherosclerosis is a disease which involves the aorta, its large branches, and medium-sized arteries such as those supplying portions of the extremities, the brain, the heart, and the major internal viscera. Atherosclerosis does not involve arterioles, and it does not involve the venous side of the circulation. The disease is a multifocal one, and the unit lesion, or *atheroma* (also termed *atherosclerotic plaque*), consists of an elevated mass of fatty material associated with fibrous connective tissue, very often with secondary deposits of calcium salts and blood products. The plaques of atherosclerosis begin in the intima or inner layer of the vessel wall but with growth may extend to encroach upon the media or musculoelastic portion of the vessel wall.

Morphology of atherosclerosis

The typical gross appearance of moderately severe atherosclerosis is shown in Fig. 7-10. When it is recalled that a smooth endothelial lining of vessels is an important protection against thrombus formation, it is not at all difficult to realize why atherosclerosis should involve considerable liability to arterial thrombosis. The microscopic appearance of an atheroma is illustrated in Fig. 7-11. The dominance of both fibrous and fatty material in the lesion is evident (the term *athero* refers to the *mushy* and *sclerosis* to the *hard* character of the lesions). In large vessels such as the aorta even numerous and severe atheromas do not generally lead to occlusion of the lumen but only to roughening of the lining surface. In smaller vessels, the atheromas may actually become circumferential, leading to marked narrowing of the lumen (Fig. 7-12).

Etiology and incidence of atherosclerosis

Atherosclerosis is truly a multifactorial disease, and it is therefore not possible to cite a single or dominant etiologic factor. The various factors which contribute to the development of atherosclerosis are so widespread in the populations of more affluent countries that none but the youngest individuals in the population are spared by the disease. In fact, autopsies performed on young adults dying "in their prime" as a result of trauma always reveal lesions of atherosclerosis, sometimes surprisingly severe. In general, the earliest fatty deposits can be seen in young children, and these tend to increase with age (speaking of the population as a whole). The rate at which atheromas increase in size and number is influenced by a wide variety of factors. Certainly genetic factors are important here, and atherosclerosis and its complications often tend to run in families. Subjects with

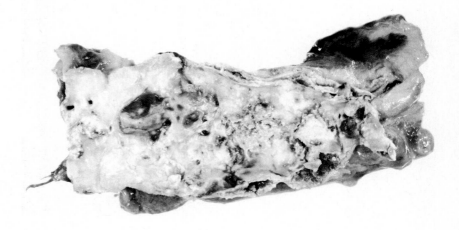

FIGURE 7-10

Atherosclerosis of aorta. This photograph depicts the intimal (lining) surface of the opened abdominal aorta. Instead of being pearly and smooth, the surface is a roughened mass of atherosclerotic plaques.

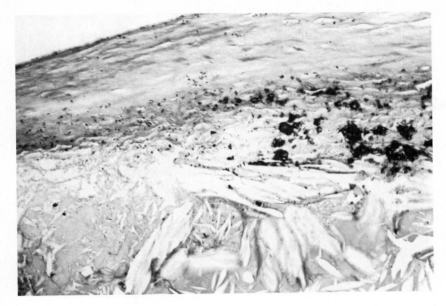

FIGURE 7-11
Atherosclerotic plaque. The clefts in the depths of the plaque represent large deposits of cholesterol. The dark material at the right is a dystrophic calcific deposit, and the horizontal band across the top is a fibrous "cap" of the lesion. The elevated rough lesions in Fig. 7-10 have this microscopic appearance.

abnormalities of their blood lipids are often susceptible to accelerated atherosclerosis, as are individuals with diabetes mellitus. Blood pressure is an important factor in the incidence and severity of atherosclerosis. Patients with hypertension are much likelier to have earlier and more severe atherosclerosis; the severity of the disease is correlated with the blood pressure even in the so-called normal range. In this regard it is interesting to note that atherosclerosis is not seen within the pulmonary arteries (usually a low-pressure circuit) unless the pressure is abnormally elevated, a state termed *pulmonary hypertension*. Without an undue lengthening of the list of "risk factors" in the development of atherosclerosis, it should be emphasized that *cigarette smoking* is a major environmental factor leading to increased

severity of atherosclerosis. The precise way in which these various factors contribute to the pathogenesis of the lesions of atherosclerosis has not been completely elucidated.

Consequences of atherosclerosis

The consequences of atherosclerosis depend in part on the size of the artery involved. If the artery is a medium-sized one such as a major branch of the coronary artery, with a lumen perhaps a few millimeters in diameter, atherosclerosis may lead gradually to narrowing or even total obstruction of the lumen. In contrast to this slowly developing occlusion, complications of atherosclerosis may lead to an abruptly developing occlusion. One such

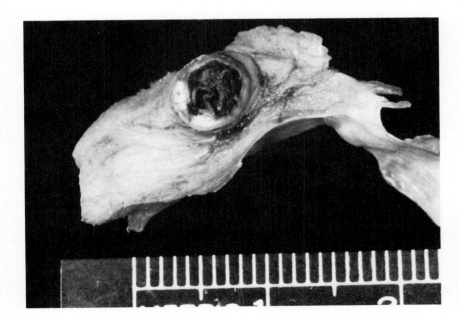

FIGURE 7-12
Atherosclerotic coronary artery seen in cross section. The circumferential atheroma has left only a tiny lumen (at eight o'clock) in this cross section of coronary artery. Consequences in terms of blood flow are obvious.

93

circumstance is thrombus formation superimposed upon the intimal roughening produced by atherosclerotic plaques. Thrombosis tends to be occlusive in a small or medium-sized artery but may be in the form of a relatively thin mural deposit in a large vessel like the aorta. Another complication of atherosclerosis is hemorrhage into the soft center of the plaque. In a vessel the size of the coronary artery this may result in swelling of the plaque with sudden occlusion of the lumen. Another complication which may lead to acute arterial occlusion is a rupture of the plaque with welling-up of the soft lipidic contents into the lumen and lodgement in a narrower "downstream" segment of the vessel. Finally, if extensive and severe enough, lesions of atherosclerosis may encroach upon the muscular and elastic wall (the media) of an artery, thus weakening it. In the abdominal aorta, a frequent site of severe arthrosclerosis, the result of such medial damage may be the formation of an atherosclerotic *aneurysm*, which is a ballooning of the weakened arterial wall (Fig. 7-13). Although a thrombus may form within such an aneurysm because of the abnormal swirling of the blood and because of the roughened intima, the feared complication of an aneurysm is rupture with exsanguination.

ISCHEMIA AND INFARCTION

Ischemia is simply inadequacy of blood supply in an area. When tissues are rendered ischemic, they suffer by virtue of being deprived of necessary oxygen and nutrients. It is possible that the accumulation of metabolic wastes within the poorly perfused tissue may also contribute to tissue damage. Literally anything which affects the flow of blood may produce tissue ischemia. One tends to think first of local arterial obstruction related to atherosclerosis, thrombosis, or embolism. In less usual circumstances, venous obstruction may lead to ischemia when the flow of blood through the tissue virtually reaches a standstill. There are even systemic causes of tissue ischemia. For instance, if heart failure is sufficiently severe, a tissue might become ischemic simply because of the low level of perfusion. Similarly, prolonged shock may lead to significant tissue ischemia.

The effects of ischemia are conditioned by a number of variables such as the intensity of the ischemia, the rate of onset, and the metabolic demands of the particular tissue. In some instances of ischemia, usually involving muscular tissues, pain may be a symptom of diminished blood supply. For example, an elderly person with atherosclerosis of the leg arteries and consequent decrease in blood flow may have sufficient blood supply when at rest but not during activity. When such an individual walks briskly, increasing the metabolic demand of the leg muscles, the onset of relative ischemia may cause pain and limping. The same type of thing happens in the heart muscle with narrowing of the coronary arterial circulation. In such an instance, a patient may, with activity, develop a feeling of oppression or squeezing pain within the chest, this phenomenon being referred to as *angina pectoris*. By definition, anginal pain recedes with rest, when the metabolic demand of the heart muscle diminishes to the point where the narrowed coronary arterial circulation is adequate.

Another effect of ischemia, if it is of gradual onset

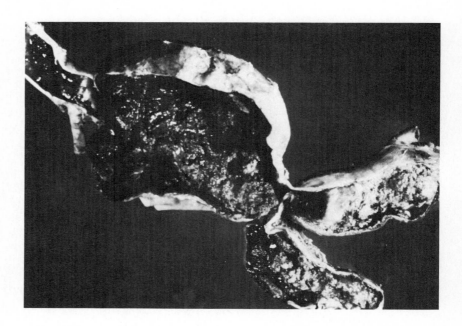

FIGURE 7-13
Atherosclerotic aneurysms. A large aneurysm distorts the distal aorta and each iliac artery. The walls of such aneurysms are prone to rupture.

and prolonged duration, is that the involved tissue may atrophy, that is, shrink. A common example of this is readily observed in a patient who has atherosclerosis which diminishes the circulation to the lower extremities. Often the legs exhibit loss of muscle mass, and the skin becomes smooth, thin, and hairless, all the result of chronic ischemia.

The most extreme effect of ischemia is the death of the ischemic tissue. An area of ischemic necrosis is termed an *infarct,* and the process of forming an infarct is termed *infarction.* Whether or not an ischemic area actually undergoes infarction is conditioned by a variety of local and systemic factors. For instance, a degree of arterial occlusion will be better tolerated if it occurs slowly, if the metabolic demand of the tissue is low and if there is development of collateral circulation (that is, auxiliary supply of the involved area by branches of neighboring arteries). In addition, the effects of a given degree of ischemia will be worsened if the oxygen carriage within the blood is diminished for any reason.

The morphologic features of infarcts vary from organ to organ, but in general the tissue necrosis produced by ischemia is accompanied by an element of hemorrhage from damaged vessels at the edges of the infarcted area. In loose tissues such as the lung, this hemorrhage is extensive, and the infarcted area literally becomes stuffed with blood producing a *hemorrhagic* or *red infarct.* In other organs, e.g., the kidney or the heart, the hemorrhage accompanying infarction is minimal, and the infarct tends to be *pale.* It should be borne in mind that in hemorrhagic as well as in pale infarcts the basic cause of the damage is ischemia of the tissues. In most infarcts the necrosis produced by ischemia is of coagulative type, and the outlines of the tissue are maintained (Fig. 7-14). In the lung, hemorrhage dominates the picture, while in the brain an area of infarction grad-

ually softens and undergoes liquefactive change so that the result is a hole in the tissue.

The presence of infarcted tissue excites an inflammatory reaction at the margins interfacing with viable tissue. Soon neutrophils and macrophages invade the dead area to begin the job of demolition. Subsequently, the area is gradually organized as demolition proceeds, and the usual outcome is scarring of the infarcted area. In many organs an infarct is not particularly important in and of itself, given the amount of reserve of that organ. Thus even a moderately large renal infarct will not endanger the life of the subject because of the ability of one kidney or even part of one kidney to maintain homeostasis. The presence of a pulmonary infarct likewise is not particularly threatening in terms of ventilatory function. In this latter instance, however, the occurrence of pulmonary infarction is somewhat ominous, because it is usually the result of pulmonary embolism. Therefore, there is always concern that larger and more threatening emboli may originate from the source of the first embolus. In the case of the brain and of the myocardium, the results of infarction are much more significant because there is less reserve in these organs, each area being important, and in particular because in these two areas there is no possibility of regeneration of infarcted elements. Finally, in some areas exposed to bacterial populations, the infarcted tissue will serve as a focus of growth of saprophytic microorganisms. Thus, infarcts of bowel quickly become gangrenous, and infarcts of portions of the extremity are initially recognized as areas of gangrene.

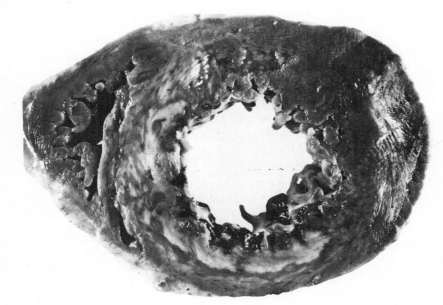

FIGURE 7-14
Myocardial infarct. Myocardial ischemia has resulted in coagulative necrosis (light area) of much of the septum and ventricular wall.

Disturbances of circulation

Directions: Answer the following questions on a separate sheet of paper.

1. Describe how the mechanisms involved in active congestion differ from those in passive congestion.

2. Explain how congestion could be produced by a cardiac problem.

3. What are the effects on the involved tissue of acute passive congestion and chronic passive congestion?

4. Define *edema*.

Directions: Circle the letter preceding each item below that correctly answers the question. More than one answer may be correct.

5. Which of the following is the best example of *active* congestion?
   a. The lung in acute left ventricular failure
   b. The tissues of the leg in femoral vein thrombosis   *c.* The red "halo" around an area of cutaneous inflammation

6. The individual with chronic right-sided heart failure who develops persistent hyperemia of the liver has which type of congestion?
   a. Active   *b.* Chronic active   *c.* Chronic passive   *d.* Acute passive

7. Chronic passive congestion may lead to which of the following changes in the liver?
   a. Dilatation of the blood channels in the centrilobular zone of each hepatic lobule   *b.* Enlargement of liver cells of each hepatic lobule
   c. Constriction of blood channels in the peripheral zone of each hepatic lobule   *d.* Shrinkage of liver cells in the centrilobular zone of each hepatic lobule

8. The accumulation of fluid in the peritoneal cavity is called:
   a. Pericardial effusion   *b.* Peritonitis   *c.* Ascites   *d.* Pleural effusion

9. Which of the following would likely contribute to the formation of edema?
   a. Elevation of venous pressure in a tissue
   b. Dehydration   *c.* Marked decrease in serum protein   *d.* Arterial obstruction in a tissue
   e. Increased phagocytosis in lymph nodes draining the area

10. In acute inflammatory states, which of the following statements apply:
    a. Protein molecules move from inside the vessels of the area to the interstitial spaces   *b.* Arterioles in the area dilate to produce active congestion
    c. Water "follows" protein into the interstitial spaces   *d.* Edema develops because of diminution of lymphatic drainage

11. Which of the following edematous conditions is potentionally the *most* serious?
    a. Pleural effusion   *b.* Ascites   *c.* Cerebral edema   *d.* Facial edema

12. Exudates differ from transudates in that:
    a. Exudates tend to contain more leukocytes
    b. Transudates have a higher specific gravity than do exudates   *c.* Exudates have a higher protein content than transudates   *d.* Exudates contain large numbers of basophils

13. Pinpoint hemorrhages visible on cutaneous or mucosal surfaces are referred to as:
    a. Ecchymoses   *b.* Petechiae   *c.* Hematomas   *d.* Purpura

Directions: Answer the following questions on a separate sheet of paper.

14. What is the commonest cause of a hemorrhage?

15. What are two basic mechanisms for stopping hemorrhage?

16. Describe the local and systemic effects of hemorrhage.

17. Describe two clinical implications of thrombosis.

18. List some local causes of ischemia.

19. Describe possible effects of ischemia.

Directions: Circle the letter preceding the item below that correctly answers each question. More than one answer may be correct.

20. Thrombi consist of all of the following *except*:
    a. Aggregated platelets   *b.* Precipitated fibrin
    c. Basophils   *d.* Enmeshed erythrocytes and leukocytes

21. In the formation of a thrombus which event usually occurs first?
    a. Platelet aggregation   *b.* Precipitation of fibrin   *c.* Vascular dilatation   *d.* Hemolysis

22. Thrombosis is favored by all of the following *except*:
    a. Decreased viscosity of the blood   *b.* Venous stasis   *c.* Increase in blood platelets   *d.* Rough vessel lining

23. The carriage of a physical mass in the bloodstream from one place to another with lodgement in the new location is:
    a. Ischemia   *b.* Infarction   *c.* Embolism   *d.* Thrombosis

24. Emboli which lodge on the arterial side of the circulation generally originate from a(n):
    a. Mural thrombus in the aorta   *b.* Right atrium
    c. Intracardiac thrombus   *d.* Femoral vein

25. If decompression is sufficiently abrupt or when atmospheric air enters venous channels, gas bubbles may appear within the circulation, where they lodge in the microcirculation and occlude the blood flow to the area. Examples of this condition would include:
    a. A diver who has been living under increased atmospheric pressure   *b.* A surgical procedure in which large vascular channels were traversed
    c. A patient with a fractured femur   *d.* Generalized traumatic injury involving adipose tissue

26. All of the following conditions contribute to atherosclerosis *except:*
    a. Certain genetic factors   *b.* Increased serum cholesterol levels   *c.* Diabetes mellitus
    d. Hypotension   *e.* Cigarette smoking

27. The atherosclerotic plaque usually initially involves the:
    a. Arterioles   *b.* Intima of an artery   *c.* Media of an artery   *d.* Intima of a vein

28. All of the following generally cause ischemia except:
    a. Diminished clotting factors   *b.* Local arterial obstruction   *c.* Thrombosis   *d.* Atherosclerosis

29. Which of the following describes an infarcted area located in the lung?
    a. The hemorrhage accompanying infarction is minimal, and the infarction tends to be pale.
    b. The hemorrhage is extensive, and the infarcted area tends to be red.   *c.* The infarction gradually softens and undergoes liquefactive change.

Directions: Circle T if the statement is true and F if it is false. Correct any false statements.

30. T   F   Mönckeberg's sclerosis is a clinically significant form of arteriosclerosis since the lining of the involved vessel is roughened and the lumen is narrowed.

31. T   F   Atherosclerosis is the most important form of arteriosclerosis.

32. T   F   An atheroma is an elevated mass of fatty material and associated fibrous connective tissue.

33. T   F   Atherosclerosis can usually be ascribed to a single etiologic factor.

34. T   F   Complications of atherosclerosis may lead to an abruptly developing occlusion.

35. T   F   The results of infarction in the brain and myocardium are very significant particularly because there is no possibility of regeneration of infarcted elements.

36. T   F   Infarct is a term used to denote a type of circulatory abnormality.

DISTURBANCES OF GROWTH, CELLULAR PROLIFERATION, AND DIFFERENTIATION

OBJECTIVES

At the completion of this chapter you should be able to:

1. Distinguish between agenesis, hypoplasia, and atrophy as to etiology and possible consequences.
2. List at least two common causes of atrophy.
3. Contrast hypertrophy and hyperplasia.
4. Identify an example of physiologic and of nonphysiologic hyperplasia.
5. Describe the phenomenon referred to as metaplasia.
6. Explain the significance of dysplasia.
7. Define a neoplasm.
8. Differentiate between benign and malignant neoplasms according to architecture, rate of growth, and pattern of enlargement and spread.
9. State two dangerous properties of malignant neoplasms which distinguish them from benign neoplasms.
10. Trace the pathways by which malignant neoplasms disseminate through the body.
11. Describe the effects of benign and malignant neoplasms on the host.
12. Explain the pattern of organization of tumor cells and stroma.
13. Identify the terms used to describe the microscopic resemblance of tumor cells to their normal ancestors.
14. Explain the basis of exfoliative cytology.
15. State the criteria used in the classification of neoplasms.
16. Identify with an example the following terms used to describe neoplasms: adeno-, -oma, polyp, papilloma, carcinoma, fibroma, osteoma, chondroma, sarcoma, lymphoma.
17. Describe the possible cellular basis of malignant behavior.
18. Describe the environmental and genetic factors that seem to be involved in the causation of neoplasia.
19. Describe the rationale used in establishing the diagnosis and determining the treatment modalities for neoplasia.

This chapter focuses on a number of extremely diverse conditions having very different etiologies and consequences for the host. The unifying concept throughout the chapter is that each of the conditions discussed is characterized by an abnormality in (1) the size and/or number of cells in a tissue, (2) the mode of cellular proliferation, or (3) the character of cellular differentiation. These abnormalities may lead to tissues that are smaller or larger than normal and to tissues that have abnormal functional specialization. In the extreme, the abnormal cells may form masses, the behavior of which is generally beyond the influence of normal homeostatic controls.

ORGANS AND TISSUES SMALLER THAN NORMAL

Not infrequently one encounters a tissue, organ, or part of the body that is smaller than normal. This situation can arise in two ways: as a result of a developmental defect or as an acquired abnormality. Stated in a slightly different way, the organ or tissue may never have grown to a definitive size, or, alternatively, it may have reached definitive size and then secondarily have shrunk.

In the course of development it may come to pass that the embryonic rudiment of an organ never forms. This phenomenon is referred to as *agenesis*, and the result is the absence of the particular organ. Thus, for instance, as a result of agenesis some individuals are born with but a single kidney. A related situation is *aplasia*, which involves the embryonic rudiment of an organ failing to grow at all once it has formed (some use the terms agenesis and aplasia interchangeably and, indeed, there is little practical difference). Yet another abnormal developmental situation is that in which the embryonic rudiment forms and grows but never quite reaches definitive or adult size, yielding a dwarfed organ. This phenomenon is called *hypoplasia*. Hypoplasia might, like agenesis and aplasia, involve any portion of the body, might involve one of a pair of organs, or might even involve both organs of a pair. Minor degrees of hypoplasia of some organ might be well tolerated for long periods of time, the net effect being some encroachment on the usual degree of reserve of that organ.

Organs which reach definitive size in the course of development and then secondarily shrink are referred to as *atrophic*. Atrophy has a variety of causes, and some instances of atrophy are actually normal or physiologic, as, for instance, the atrophy of certain parts of the embryo or fetus in the course of development. Some forms of atrophy are inevitable with advancing age, such as the endocrine atrophy which occurs when hormonal support is withdrawn from a tissue like the mammary gland. An extremely common cause of atrophy is chronic ischemia. Another common type of atrophy, primarily involving skeletal muscle, is so-called disuse atrophy. When, for instance, a broken leg is placed in an immobilizing cast for a period of weeks or months, the mass of the extremity is significantly reduced owing to atrophy of the unused muscle. In this situation the individual muscle cells are of reduced size, but the state is a reversible one. In other instances of atrophy there is actually a loss of cellular elements.

ORGANS AND TISSUES LARGER THAN NORMAL

Hypertrophy

Hypertrophy is defined as an enlargement of a tissue or organ because of enlargement of individual cells. Hypertrophy can be seen in a variety of tissues but is particularly prominent in various types of muscle. An increased workload on a muscle is a very strong stimulus to hypertrophy. The bulging biceps of the weight lifter are an obvious example of muscular hypertrophy. The same type of thing happens as an important adaptive response in the case of the myocardium. If a subject has an abnormal cardiac valve which imposes an unusual mechanical load, say, on the left ventricle, or if the ventricle is pumping against an elevated systemic blood pressure, the result is hypertrophy of the myocardium with thickening of the ventricular wall. A similar phenomenon can occur in smooth muscle which is forced to work against an increased load. Thus the wall of the urinary bladder may become hypertrophic when there is obstruction to the free outflow of urine. In each of these instances hypertrophic enlargement of cells is actually accompanied by an increase in the contractile elements of the tissue and thus the response is an adaptive one. Hypertrophy is stimulus-related so that it tends to regress at least to some extent if the abnormal workload is withdrawn.

Hyperplasia

Hyperplasia is an increase in the absolute number of cells within a tissue leading to an increase in the size of that tissue or organ. This obviously can occur only in a tissue capable of cell division. (In such tissues hyperplasia may also be accompanied by hypertrophy of individual cells.) Hyperplasia occurs in a wide variety of tissues under many different circumstances, some of them completely physiologic. For instance, with the hormonal stimulus of pregnancy and lactation there is extensive proliferation of epithelial elements within the breast with an increase in the size of breast tissue due to this hyperplasia. An example of nonphysiologic hyperplasia is a callus, which is a thickening of skin, developing in response to a mechanical stimulus. Microscopic examination of a callus reveals a marked increase in the number of epidermal cells and in the number of layers of cells in the epidermis, clearly an adaptive response.

Although certainly an abnormal stimulus (e.g., one associated with endocrine imbalance) may give rise to hyperplasia which is nonadaptive, many examples of hyperplasia represent "rational" responses on the part of the body to some imposed demand. As with hypertrophy, if the abnormal circumstance is reversed, the signal to cellular proliferation is withdrawn, and there is regression of the hyperplasia and return to more normal conditions. In the above examples, the enlarged breast shrinks to a more normal size following lactation, and the callus gradually disappears when the mechanical stimulus to the skin is no longer applied.

ABNORMAL DIFFERENTIATION—DEFINITIONS

Metaplasia

The character of cellular *differentiation* in a given tissue may also change under abnormal circumstances. Differentiation is the process by which the progeny of dividing *stem cells* become specialized to perform a particular task. For instance, dividing cells in the deepest layer of the epidermis gradually migrate upward, and as they do so, they acquire the specialized protective characteristics of outer epidermal cells and produce a proteinaceous substance known as *keratin*. Similarly,

within the lining of the respiratory tract some of the dividing cells in the epithelium develop into tall columnar cells with cilia on their luminal surfaces.

When differentiating cell systems of this type are placed under adverse circumstances, the pattern of differentiation may change so that the dividing cells begin to differentiate into types of cells not ordinarily found in the area but that would be perfectly reasonable elsewhere in the body. This phenomenon is referred to as *metaplasia*. For instance, when the lining of the uterine cervix is chronically irritated, portions of the columnar epithelium are replaced by an epidermislike squamous epithelium (Fig. 8-1). Presumably, this "squamous metaplasia" is adaptive; i.e., the squamous epithelium is more resistant to irritation than is the original epithelium. The process of metaplasia seems to be under tight control; that is, the "new" type of differentiation is perfectly regular as well as being adapative. Metaplasia is potentially reversible, so that if the cause of the original change can be eliminated, the stem cells in the population once again differentiate to form the specialized types of cells usually found in that locale.

Dysplasia

Dysplasia is an abnormality in the differentiation of proliferating cells such that there occurs an abnormal degree of variation in the size, shape, and appearance of the cells with a disturbance in the usual arrangement of those cells (Fig. 8-2). In essence, dysplasia represents a degree of loss of control over the affected cell population. Minor degrees of dysplasia are frequently encountered in association with areas of inflammation, and these are potentially reversible if the irritant stimulus can be reversed. However, in some instances the stimulus leading to dysplasia cannot be identified, and the

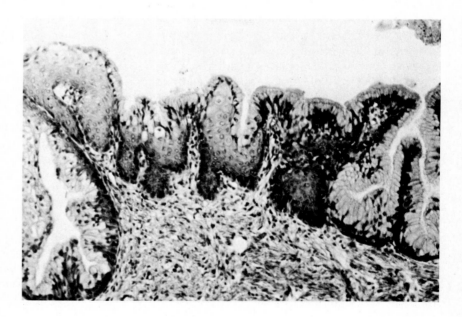

FIGURE 8-1
Squamous metaplasia. In this lining epithelium of uterine cervix, the usual cell type is columnar, as at the right. Most of the epithelium has altered its differentiation to form an epidermislike squamous epithelium. (Photomicrograph, ×200.)

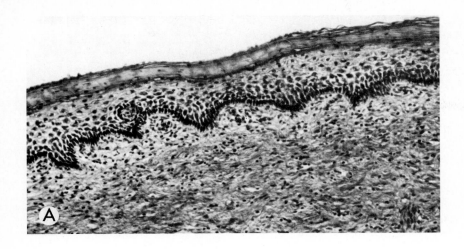

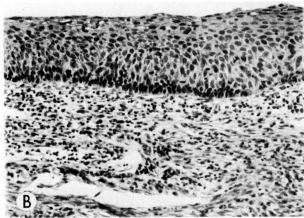

FIGURE 8-2
Dysplasia versus normal cells. In the normal epithelium (A) the cells are very regular in a given zone and the layering is orderly. In dysplasia (B) there is marked morphologic variation in the cells and layering is disordered. (Photomicrograph, ×200.)

changes may become progressively more severe, terminating eventually in the development of malignant disease.

Neoplasia

A *neoplasm*, literally a "new growth," is an abnormal mass of proliferating cells. The cells of a neoplasm are derived from previously normal cells, but in undergoing neoplastic change they acquire a certain degree of autonomy. Neoplastic cells are autonomous in the sense of growing at a rate which is uncoordinated with the needs of the host and functioning quite independently of the usual homeostatic controls over most other cells of the body. The growth of neoplastic cells is usually progressive; i.e., it does not reach equilibrium but results rather in an ever-increasing mass of cells having the same properties. A neoplasm serves no adaptive purpose as far as benefiting the host is concerned and, in fact, is frequently harmful. Finally, in keeping with the autonomous character of neoplastic cells, even if the stimulus that caused the neoplasm is withdrawn, the neoplasm continues to grow progressively.

The word *tumor* is used more or less synonymously with the word neoplasm. Originally the word tumor meant simply swelling or lump, so that occasionally the phrase "true tumor" is used to denote a neoplasm as contrasted with some other sort of lump. Two basic types of neoplasms are distinguished on the basis of their behavior. Some are referred to as *benign,* while others are termed *malignant. Cancer* is a general term referring to any malignant neoplasm. Thus, there are many tumors or neoplasms which are noncancerous.

CHARACTERISTICS OF NEOPLASMS

Characteristics of benign neoplasms

A benign (i.e., noncancerous) neoplasm is a strictly local affair. The proliferating cells which constitute the neoplasm tend to be quite cohesive, so that as the mass of neoplastic cells grows, there is centrifugal expansion of the mass with a fairly well-defined border. Since the proliferating cells do not fall away from each other, the edges of the neoplasm tend to move outward more or less smoothly, pushing adjacent tissue away in the process. In so doing, benign neoplasms may acquire a capsule of compressed connective tissue separating them from their surroundings. Above all, as indicated in Fig. 8-3A, the benign neoplasm remains a strictly local affair

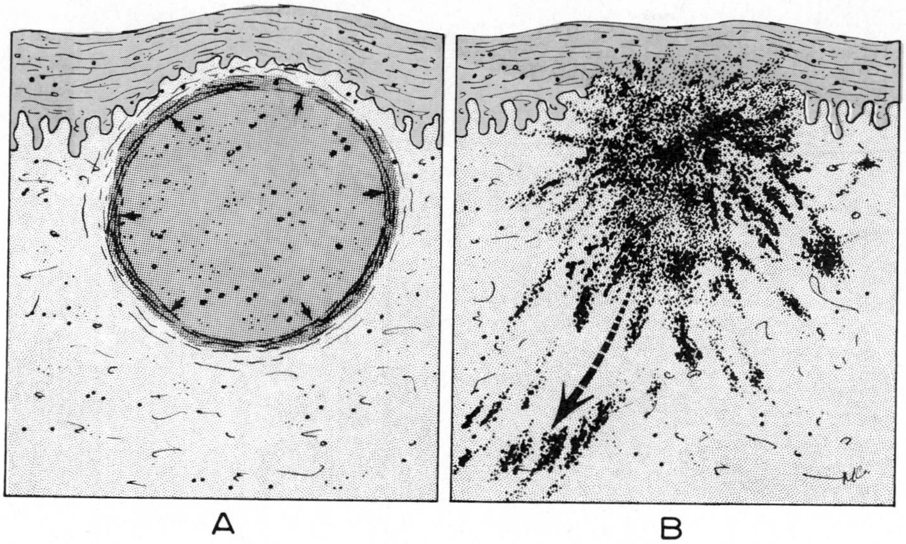

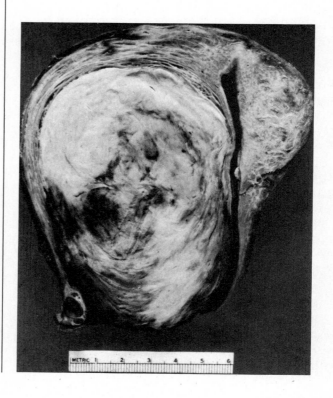

FIGURE 8-3

Diagram of benign versus malignant growth. A "typical" benign neoplasm (A) is cohesive, centrifugally expanding, smooth-bordered, and often encapsulated. Adjacent tissue is compressed. A malignant neoplasm (B) is less cohesive, has an irregular border, and invades adjacent tissue. Malignant cells are also capable of metastasis (dotted arrow).

A   B

and does not spread to a distant site. The rate of growth of benign neoplasms is often rather leisurely, and some seem to plateau and remain at a more or less stable size for many months or years.

Characteristics of malignant neoplasms

Many of the characteristics of malignant neoplasms contrast sharply with those of their benign counterparts. Malignant neoplasms generally grow more rapidly than benign ones and almost always grow in a relentlessly progressive manner if not removed. The cells of a malignant neoplasm are not as cohesive as are benign cells, and consequently the pattern of expansion of a malignant neoplasm is often quite irregular (Fig. 8-3B). Malignant neoplasms tend not to be encapsulated, and they are usually not easily separable from their surroundings in the way that benign neoplasms are. In fact malignant neoplasms characteristically *invade* their surroundings rather than simply push them aside. Malignant cells, whether in clusters, cords, or singly, seem to cut their way through adjacent tissue in a destructive fashion. The gross features of benign and malignant neoplasms are contrasted in Figs. 8-4 and 8-5.

An additional property of malignant neoplasms, the most devastating of all, is related to the ability of proliferating cancer cells to break away from the parent tumor (the so-called *primary* tumor) and enter the circulation to float elsewhere. When such embolic cancer cells lodge, they are able to extravasate, continue their proliferation, and form a *secondary* focus of tumor. Ac-

tually a single primary focus of cancer can give rise to numerous embolic fragments which, in turn, may form dozens or even hundreds of secondary nodules at considerable distance from the primary. The process of discontinuous spread of malignant neoplasms is referred to as *metastasis*, and the daughter foci or areas of secondary growth are referred to as *metastases* (singular, *metastasis*). Thus, the two dangerous properties of malignant neoplasms which distinguish them from noncancerous neoplasms are the ability to invade normal tissue and the ability to form metastases. A benign neoplasm has neither of these abilities.

FIGURE 8-4

Benign neoplasm. In this section of uterus, the right half is normal. On the left is a large benign neoplasm (leiomyoma).

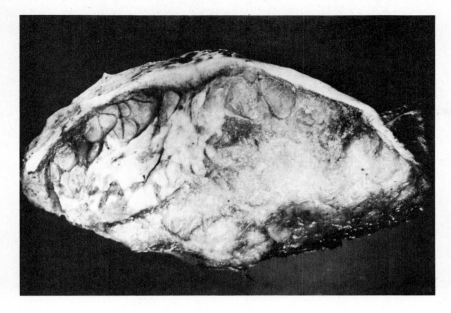

FIGURE 8-5
Malignant neoplasm. In this section of breast, a whitish tissue infiltrates the breast to the left of center. This is a malignant neoplasm, specifically, a carcinoma. Contrast the gross features of this with the benign neoplasm in Fig. 8-4.

Metastasis can occur by a variety of routes. Invasion of blood vascular channels gives rise to hematogenous metastasis in a pattern which at first may be quite predictable. That is to say, for instance, if cancer cells originating from a primary location in the wall of the gastrointestinal tract enter the venous drainage of the tract, they very likely will lodge in the liver, since portal venous blood must flow through that organ before returning to the heart. On the other hand, hematogenously borne cells originating from, say, a malignant neoplasm in the leg will flow via the vena cava to the right side of the heart and then to the lungs, where the secondary foci may grow. In an analogous fashion malignant cells may invade lymphatic channels and float centrad with the streaming of lymph. In such instances metastases would be expected to appear in the regional lymph node group filtering the lymph emanating from a particular organ. Thus, for instance, lymphogenous metastases from a primary cancer of the breast may be anticipated in the axillary lymph nodes, and lymphogenous metastases from a primary cancer in the oral cavity would be sought in cervical lymph node groups. In addition to metastasizing via blood vessels and lymphatics, cancer cells may metastasize directly by being transported across a body cavity (e.g., the peritoneal cavity) and implanting on a distant surface of that cavity. In this fashion a malignant neoplasm which invades through the entire thickness of the wall of an abdominal organ may "seed" the entire peritoneal cavity, producing literally hundreds of metastases by the direct route. Similarly, if malignant cells are picked up on surgical instru-

ments in the course of an operation they may be implanted elsewhere in the incision, ultimately to grow into metastatic foci. Figures 8-6 to 8-8 illustrate metastases encountered at autopsy.

In all likelihood, most cancer cells which enter the blood or lymphatic circulation or various body cavities fail to form progressively growing metastases. This is due in part to the fact that the growth of such cells is

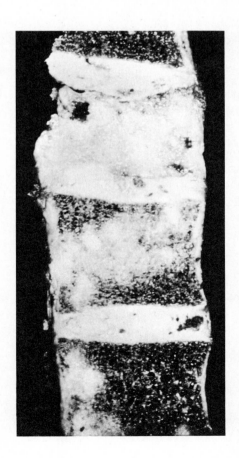

FIGURE 8-6
Vertebral metastases. The whitish nodules of metastatic carcinoma within the bone grew from cells originating in the lung and spreading hematogenously.

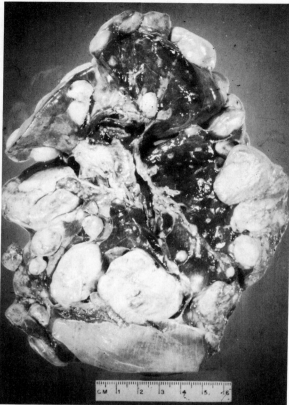

FIGURE 8-7
**Pulmonary metastases. This lung is extensively replaced
(as was the contralateral lung) by malignant neoplasm
originating in the kidney.**

inhibited by various bodily defenses (e.g., immunologic
defenses) and is also related to the fact that growth conditions in an organ of secondary lodgement may not be
adequate for the particular cells. Presumably on this
basis many cancers have characteristic patterns of me-

tastases which become important in diagnosis and
treatment.

NEOPLASM–HOST INTERACTION

Effects of neoplasms on the host

Neoplasms affect the host in a variety of ways. Since
benign neoplasms do not invade or metastasize, the
problems they cause are generally local. These can
range from trivial to lethal. For example, a small, strictly
benign tumor in the loose subcutaneous tissue of the
arm might constitute a cosmetic problem but little else.
At the opposite end of the spectrum, a perfectly benign
tumor (in the sense defined above) growing in a vital
area such as the cranial cavity might actually kill the
patient by virtue of exerting pressure on some vital part
of the brain as the neoplasm expands locally. For such
reasons "benign" does not necessarily mean incon-
sequential.

Local problems caused by benign neoplasms might
involve plugging of various body passages. A vein or a
part of the gastrointestinal tract might become obstructed by a perfectly benign neoplasm impinging
upon it. Benign neoplasms can also become ulcerated
and infected, and they may give rise to significant hemorrhage. Finally, benign tumors are capable of producing striking effects which are not mechanical but are related rather to the metabolic properties of the tumor
cells. For instance, the cells of the islets of Langerhans
of the pancreas may give rise to a benign neoplasm only
a few millimeters in diameter that would never produce
mechanical problems. Sometimes, however, such neoplastic cells retain the function of the parent cells and
produce insulin. Because neoplasms do not respond appropriately to homeostatic signals, such a neoplasm of
islet cells might produce insulin inappropriately and in
great excess, causing abnormally low blood sugar levels.
Patients with such neoplasms might thus suffer a variety
of systemic signs and symptoms of hypoglycemia.

Malignant neoplasms are capable of doing everything that benign tumors do but usually do so in a much

FIGURE 8-8
**Hepatic metastases. Many neoplasms spread
to the liver, particularly, as in this case, those
arising in the gastrointestinal tract. The whitish
tissue is metastatic carcinoma.**

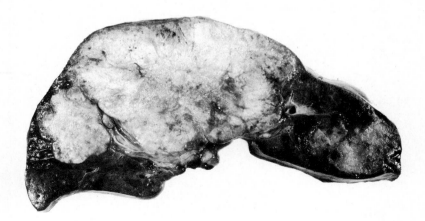

more aggressive, destructive fashion related to the generally faster growth rate of malignant neoplasms and to their ability to invade, destroy local tissues, and spread to form distant metastases. Many advanced malignant neoplasms even appear to compete nutritionally with the patient, literally trapping nutrient materials to the detriment of the host. Thus, all too frequently patients with advanced cancers have the appearance of severe malnutrition, a state referred to as *tumor cachexia*. Commonly the life of such a debilitated patient with an advanced cancer is finally terminated by an episode of pneumonia or systemic sepsis.

Host impact on neoplasms

Although a key event in the life history of any neoplasm is the development of a "runaway" clone of proliferating cells which are unresponsive to homeostatic signals within the body, even highly malignant neoplasms are not completely autonomous. Obviously, neoplasms are in need of a supply of oxygen and nutrients for the proliferating neoplastic cells, and these must be supplied by the host. In fact, neoplastic cells are able to evoke from the neighboring nonneoplastic tissues the formation of a vascular supply to nourish the tumor cells. Thus, the supporting framework or *stroma* of neoplasms includes not only a fibrous connective tissue but also numerous finely branching, thin-walled blood vessels (Fig. 8-9). The connective tissue cells and blood vessels are actually not part of the neoplastic clone of cells but represent nonneoplastic host cells whose proliferation has been stimulated by substances released from the tumor cells.

It has become evident that various processes within the host body may modulate the growth of neoplastic cells and in effect constitute antineoplastic defenses. It has been demonstrated that many neoplastic cells are sufficiently different antigenically from the corresponding normal host cells that the body may mount an immunologic reaction against the neoplasm. Although there is no doubt of the existence of such immunologic defenses, the current state of knowledge about them does not permit the routine widespread use of immunotherapeutic measures at present. There have been promising demonstrations of beneficial immunologic effects in the treatment of certain neoplasms, and efforts are now made to consider the immunologic status of the host in the planning and conduct of various modes of antineoplastic therapy.

STRUCTURE OF NEOPLASMS

As indicated above, neoplasms consist of the proliferating neoplastic cells associated with a logistical support system referred to as a *stroma*. The pattern of organization of tumor cells and stroma varies widely between neoplasms, and, in fact, the relative balance of stromal elements may lend the neoplasm distinctive characteristics. A tumor which contains an extremely dense fibrous stroma is very hard grossly and is sometimes referred to as *scirrhous*. A tumor which consists predominantly of neoplastic cells with relatively little stroma is much softer and is sometimes referred to as *medullary*.

Since neoplastic cells are derived from previously normal cell populations, they may have many of the

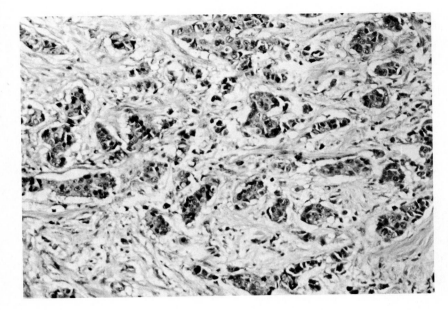

FIGURE 8-9

Microscopic structure of a neoplasm. The dark clumps of cells are the actual carcinoma cells (i.e., cells of the malignant clone), while the remaining tissue is a fibrovascular stroma supplied by the host tissue.

characteristics of normal cell populations metabolically and microscopically. However, tumors vary in their degree of resemblance to normal tissues. If the microscopic resemblance of tumor cells to their normal ancestors is close, the neoplasm is frequently referred to as *well-differentiated* (Fig. 8-10). If the resemblance of neoplastic cells to their forebears is very slight, so that the tumor consists largely of unspecialized proliferating elements, the neoplasm is frequently termed *poorly differentiated, undifferentiated,* or *anaplastic.* The neoplasm in Fig. 8-9 is rather poorly differentiated. The level of differentiation may be expressed in terms of the structure of individual cells, in terms of the production of some cell products such as mucin or keratin, or in the arrangement of neoplastic cells in relation to one another. Thus, for instance, a well-differentiated neoplasm arising from a mucin-producing glandular epithelium may be composed of tumor cells which individually resemble the nonneoplastic glandular tissue, are arranged in a pattern of tubules or glands like the parent tissue, and may manifest mucin secretion. An anaplastic tumor arising from such a tissue might lack individual cellular resemblance, might lack glandular arrangement, and might manifest no evidence of mucin secretion. In general, benign neoplasms are very well differentiated; i.e., they resemble parent tissues very closely. Malignant neoplasms occupy a rather broad spectrum with regard to differentiation. Many highly aggressive destructive cancers are poorly differentiated or anaplastic microscopically, but in some instances even well-differentiated neoplasms may behave in a malignant fashion.

In the case of many malignant neoplasms, individual cells manifest morphologic abnormalities which seem to mirror the malignant behavioral potential of the cells. Many cancer cells have an altered ratio of nuclear volume to cytoplasmic volume, irregular contour of nuclei, and irregular chromatin patterns. These individual cytologic manifestations of malignancy form the basis of exfoliative cytology, that is, the examination of individual cells which have exfoliated or dropped from the surface of tissues into the secretion bathing those tissues. The familiar Pap smear, named after the originator of the method, George Papanicolaou, is a smear of this sort made of any of a variety of body fluids including such things as pleural fluid, gastric aspirate, sputum specimens, bronchial washings, and uterine cervical scrapings. Specimens for cytologic examination can frequently be obtained with minimal inconvenience to the patient and provide exceedingly valuable diagnostic information should morphologically malignant cells be found on the smear. Figure 8-11 illustrates benign and malignant cells seen in a cytologic smear.

CLASSIFICATION AND NOMENCLATURE OF NEOPLASMS

A classification of neoplasms is important in terms of predicting the possible or probable course of disease in a particular patient and thereby planning rational modes of therapy. The usual contemporary scheme of classification of neoplasms utilizes several different sets of criteria. The most important of these is the distinction between benign and malignant biological behavior. If a particular neoplasm has already invaded neighboring nonneoplastic tissue or has produced metastases, it is obviously malignant. However, it is important to rec-

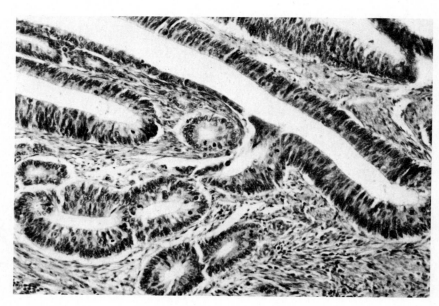

FIGURE 8-10
Well-differentiated adenocarcinoma.
This carcinoma of colon resembles the
parent tissue to the extent of forming
glands that are easily recognizable (see
Fig. 6-3); thus it is "well-differentiated."
(Photomicrograph, ×200.)

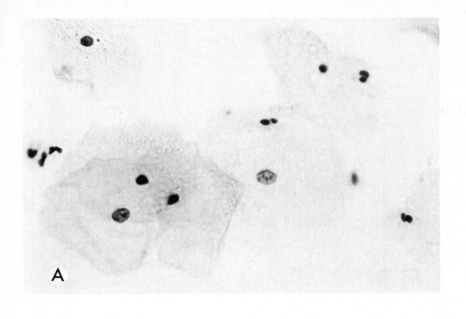

A

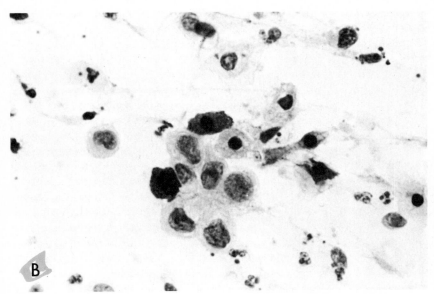

B

FIGURE 8-11
Benign and malignant cells in vaginal cytologic smears. In A the cells are benign. The ratio of nucleus to cytoplasm is small, and nuclei are regular. In B, taken from a patient with carcinoma of the uterine cervix, the ratio of the nucleus to cytoplasm is increased, and the nuclei are irregular. These features allow the diagnosis of malignancy. (Photomicrograph, ×800.)

ognize that even in the absence of such established invasion or metastasis, the pathologist can classify a neoplasm as malignant if its *potential* for malignant behavior can be predicted. That is to say, a particular neoplasm will be called malignant on the basis of its microscopic appearance alone if experience has shown that neoplasms of that type will invade and metastasize if not treated. Other parts of the classification scheme take into account the cell type of origin of the neoplasm and the organ of origin of the neoplasm. Classification of neoplasms on the basis of these several kinds of criteria is useful in that years of accumulated experience have shown that a tumor with a particular appearance of cells, of a certain level of differentiation, arranged in a certain way, and originating in a certain organ will behave with a degree of predictability. This allows the

health care team to plan therapy based on the knowledge of what has happened to many patients with similar neoplasms in the past.

This kind of classification of neoplasms is expressed in a system of naming that serves as a sort of shorthand, condensing abundant information into a relatively few terms. An attempt to display the entire system of tumor nomenclature at this point would prove tedious. Abundant specific information is contained in subsequent chapters. However, a few generalizations here might be in order. Many neoplasms encountered in our species arise from epithelium, which includes cells covering surfaces, lining organs, and forming glands of various kinds. The root *adeno-* is used to denote something of glandular origin. The suffix *-oma* refers to a neoplasm (with some exceptions). Thus in the usual system of nomenclature an *adenoma* is a benign neoplasm of glandular epithelial origin. Examples of such neoplasms would include adenomas of thyroid gland, adrenal gland, or the lining glandular epithelium within the gastrointestinal tract. In the instance of neoplasms arising and projecting from lining epithelia, topographic terms are sometimes used. Thus an adenoma of the colonic lining epithelium which projects into the lumen either as a broad-based mass or hangs into the lumen on a "stem" is frequently referred to as a *polyp*. Such a growth projecting into the lumen of an organ in finger-like projections is often referred to as a *papilloma*. These topographic terms are not restricted in their usage, however, so that the usual nasal polyp, for instance, is not a neoplasm at all but a polypoid fold of swollen nasal mucosa. A malignant neoplasm arising from epithelium is referred to as *carcinoma*. Various qualifying prefixes and adjectives can then be added to the name. A malignancy of glandular epithelium would be referred to as an *adenocarcinoma*, while a malignant neoplasm arising from a squamous epithelium would be referred to as a *squamous cell carcinoma*. The designation of a neoplasm might also include some comment about the level of differentiation, so that one encounters such phrases as "well-differentiated, mucin-forming adenocarcinoma" or "well-differentiated, keratinizing squamous cell carcinoma." In addition, topographic descriptors may be used such as "papillary adenocarcinoma" or "fungating (literally, mushrooming) carcinoma" for a projecting lesion.

Neoplasms derived from the supporting tissues of the body are named according to the specific tissue of origin. Thus a benign neoplasm on a fibrous tissue would be termed a *fibroma*, a benign neoplasm of bone would be referred to as an *osteoma*, a benign neoplasm of cartilage would be referred to as a *chondroma*, etc. A malignant neoplasm derived from supporting tissue is referred to as a *sarcoma*. The specific tissue of origin is prefixed to this term. Thus a malignant neoplasm arising from fibrous tissue is a *fibrosarcoma*, one arising from bone is an *osteosarcoma*, and one arising from cartilage is a *chondrosarcoma*.

Neoplasms arising from lymphoid tissue are referred to as *lymphomas*. Such neoplasms generally behave in a malignant fashion, so that the term lymphoma generally is used synonymously with *malignant lymphoma*. Lymphomas may arise from lymphoid tissue anywhere in the body, i.e., not only from lymph nodes and spleen but from lymphoid cells in virtually any organ. Lymphomas may come to involve the bone marrow extensively, and in many patients the lymphoma cells circulate in the blood in large numbers, giving rise

to *leukemia*. The term leukemia literally means "white blood" and pertains not only to lymphoid malignancy but also to malignancy of bone marrow cells with circulating malignant elements. The nomenclature of leukemias and lymphomas is quite complicated and will be discussed more fully in Part III.

Many special names are used for neoplasms arising in specific sites and from particular specialized tissues. Thus, *gliomas* arise from the glial supportive cells in the central nervous system, *mesotheliomas* arise from the lining cells of body cavities, *retinoblastoma* arises within the eye, etc. A simplified summary of the classification of neoplasms is presented in Table 8-1.

BIOLOGY OF CANCER

As indicated above, cancer cells are derived from previously normal cell populations within the body. What is not yet understood completely is what is actually happening at a cellular level during the "transformation" or cancerigenic event, i.e., what is actually happening to a cell when it becomes a cancer cell. In the last analysis, the behavior of cancer cells is "antisocial" with regard to normal cells of the body. Malignant cells disobey the usual territorial rules and grow in inappropriate locations. They do not respond to the usual restraints on the size of cell populations or on the rate of growth of those populations. Evidence is beginning to accumulate which seems to indicate that the important abnormalities of cancer cells lie within the membranes of the cell. It is obviously on the cell membrane that homeostatic signals are received from other cells and from other points in the body and transmitted to the interior of the cell. Abnormalities in this important membrane may thus result in abnormal reception of control signals or abnormal responses to them. There is also evidence that events at the cell membrane are important in controlling cellular proliferation. The antigenic structure of cell membranes is certainly important with regard to the immunologic interactions of the cell with its surroundings.

Several explanations in terms of cellular genetics and control mechanisms can be invoked to explain the "phenotypic" expression of malignancy in cells. A classical notion is that of *somatic mutation*, which suggests that the basic cancerigenic event involves a chemical change in the DNA of a cell—that is, a mutation. This type of event would be similar to a mutation occurring in a germ cell but would instead involve a nongerm cell or somatic cell. This notion of mutation would explain the fact that once a cell is transformed into a neoplastic cell, its characteristics breed true, and it gives rise to an expanding clone of cells with similar properties. Another explanation of a change in cells is through the addition of genetic information to the genome of the cells. This, of course, is precisely what happens when a cell

TABLE 8-1

109

BIOLOGY OF CANCER

Classification of neoplasms

Cell or tissue of origin	Benign	Malignant
Epithelium		
Stratified, squamous	Squamous papilloma	Squamous cell carcinoma (epidermoid carcinoma)
Glandular (lining fluid-filled spaces)	Adenoma (cystadenoma)	Adenocarcinoma (cystadenocarcinoma)
Melanocytes	Nevus	Melanoma
Connective tissue		
Fibrous	Fibroma	Fibrosarcoma
Adipose	Lipoma	Liposarcoma
Cartilage	Chondroma	Chondrosarcoma
Bone	Osteoma	Osteosarcoma
Muscle		
Smooth	Leiomyoma	Leiomyosarcoma
Striated	Rhabdomyoma	Rhabdomyosarcoma
Endothelium		
Blood vessel	Hemangioma	Hemangiosarcoma
Lymphatic	Lymphangioma	Lymphangiosarcoma
Nervous tissue		
Nerve sheath	Neurofibroma	Neurofibrosarcoma
Glial cells		Glioma, glioblastoma
Meninges	Meningioma	
Hematopoietic-lymphoid tissue		
Lymphoid tissue		Lymphoma, Hodgkins's disease Lymphocytic leukemia Plasmacytoma (multiple myeloma)
Bone marrow		Granulocytic (myelogenous, monocytic, erythroleukemia, polycythemia rubra vera)
Germinal tissue	Teratoma	Malignant teratoma, teratocarcinoma, seminoma, embryonal carcinoma

is infected by a virus. More recently, evidence has been found that the transformational or cancerigenic event may involve neither mutation nor addition to the total genetic information of the cell but may instead involve a change in the *expression* of genetic information present normally. According to this notion, there is within the total genome of any somatic cell the information necessary for the expression of malignant behavior, but this information is normally not expressed during adult life. Accordingly, the transformation of the normal cell

to a tumor cell may involve inappropriate derepression of genes normally present. By this mechanism, cancer may be a disease of abnormal differentiation.

It is not possible to speak of a single etiology of cancer. There are obviously many different types of cancer with different epidemiologic patterns of occurrence and different etiologic factors. In most instances of human neoplasia the causes are yet unknown. The weight of circumstantial and experimental evidence, however, seems to indicate that the environment is the source of most tumorigenic agents. There is certainly no doubt that many chemical substances within the environment are carcinogenic. This is evident from animal experimentation, from the incidence of certain tumors in industrial workers, and above all from the devastating incidence of lung cancer in cigarette smokers. The role of viruses in tumorigenesis has been elucidated in many species of animals; while total proof is yet lacking in our species, there is little reason to believe we differ from other animals in this regard. Physical agents within the environment are also known to be potentially tumorigenic. Such agents would include ionizing radiations such as x-radiation and even ultraviolet radiation such as encountered in exposure to the sun.

Needless to say, genetic factors are also important in the causation of neoplasms. Again, animal experimentation has shown that it is possible to develop strains of individuals that are highly susceptible to one or another type of neoplasm on a genetic basis. It should be pointed out, however, that even in a strain of mice with a very high incidence of breast cancer, not all individuals are affected; this indicates the operation of certain environmental factors in addition to the genetic factors. The breeding habits of our species being what they are, there tends to be a dilution of this sort of genetic effect, and certainly in human beings there is nothing approaching the situation of inbred strains of rodents. Nonetheless, genetic factors do seem to be important in human neoplasia. Generally there is not inheritance of an *overall susceptibility* to cancer of various kinds, but rather an increased likelihood of developing one particular type of tumor or another is inherited. Thus, females in a family where several related women have developed breast cancer, particularly at an early age, are more likely than the general population to develop a breast cancer but probably no more likely to develop a bladder cancer. In most instances we do not know what is actually being inherited in those individuals who are genetically more susceptible to the development of a particular neoplasm. Even in such individuals there must be a significant interaction between genetic and environmental factors, and an exciting avenue of research is the attempt to identify individuals at genetic risk and separate them somehow from the precipitating environmental factors. Finally, it must be emphasized that neoplasms are sufficiently common in our species that several persons within a family group may develop a neoplasm for other than genetic reasons. That is to say, the occurrence of multiple neoplasms within a family may be totally unrelated to significant hereditary factors. Even when there appears to be a geniune *familial* incidence of a particular neoplasm, this may be related to some environmental factor within the family and may not be a strictly genetic affair.

CLINICAL ASPECTS OF NEOPLASIA

From the previous discussion it should be evident that the variety of signs and symptoms which can be produced by neoplasms is virtually endless. Therefore, the astute clinician considers the possibility of neoplasm with many different modes of patient presentation. Given the nonreversibility of neoplasms, however, a clue of particular value is the persistence (if not progression) of a given manifestation, e.g., a sore that does not heal, chronic hoarseness. In each case, clinical judgment must be guided by knowledge of the incidence of various kinds of neoplasms in different organs, in the two sexes, and at various ages, as shown in Table 8-2. Thus, hoarseness in a young child will suggest a much different list of possibilities (and approaches) than the same sign would in a 60-year-old adult smoker, who may have a carcinoma of the larynx. A collection of fluid behind the eardrum of a 3-year-old with repeated sore throats is more likely to be related to a benign, reversible condition than is a similar collection in an adult who feels well but may harbor a pharyngeal cancer blocking a eustachian tube. The finding of an iron-deficiency anemia in an elderly patient is likely to be associated with a chronically bleeding colonic cancer, whereas the same finding in a teen-age girl may be explained by a nutritionally inadequate diet combined with the onset of menstrual blood loss.

In any case, whether the index of suspicion is based on circumstances or on physical findings, the presence of the neoplasm must be definitively confirmed, since nonneoplastic conditions can produce identical manifestations in almost any situation. In a few instances certain blood tests may provide additional circumstantial evidence of a particular neoplasm. Ultimately, a space-occupying mass must be identified and delineated, whether by simple palpation during physical examina-

tion, x-ray, ultrasonography, radionuclide scanning, or any of several endoscopic procedures for direct visualization of internal organs. A final step in making the diagnosis of neoplasm involves morphologic confirmation by the pathologist, based on microscopic examination of the tissue in question. The diagnostic biopsy procedure may be curative, e.g., when the questionable lump is totally excised as a primary procedure with little risk or morbidity to the patient and is found to be benign. In other instances, however, only a wedge biopsy can be obtained from a larger mass, a tiny core of tissue is removed from the mass with a special biopsy needle, or a small amount of fluid containing neoplastic cells is aspirated by needle from the mass.

Cytologic examination of a Pap smear made from some fluid or secretion bathing the area in question may also yield valuable diagnostic information. A positive cytologic examination, i.e., one indicating the presence of cancer cells, is usually confirmed by biopsy before treatment is undertaken. One value of the Pap smear is that the fluid sampled may contain cancer cells from an area that is not visible by ordinary examination (e.g., the upper endocervical canal) and thereby may direct attention to that precise area. Another value of the Pap smear is in screening, that is, sampling large numbers of individuals from a population on a routine basis even when signs and symptoms of abnormality may not have been noted. Obviously, routine biopsy of asymptomatic people is not feasible; however, sampling cervicovaginal mucus is an innocuous procedure which may yield some "positives" leading to the diagnosis of cancer, possibly in a very early stage.

Microscopic examination of the tissue, while constituting the essential step in distinguishing neoplastic from nonneoplastic and malignant from benign conditions, has additional value in planning therapy. Identifying the precise type and classification of a cancer will allow some important *general* predictions of its likely behavior. Thus, accumulated experience with a particular neoplasm might suggest an extremely high probability of metastases in regional lymph nodes, lungs, or other sites, even in the absence of clinical evidence. In this situation, simple excision of the primary lesion with no additional therapy would generally not be successful. With certain malignant neoplasms the predictions may be more accurate if they take into account the histologic *grade* of the neoplasm. This is a classification based on the microscopic appearance, arrangement, and degree of differentiation of the cancer cells, features which may correlate with the behavioral aggressiveness of the tumor.

These predictions are very general and provide correspondingly broad guidelines for therapy. However, decisions regarding treatment can be refined by determining the *clinical stage* of the cancer in the patient. The concept of staging is based on the fact that a certain type of cancer is likely to manifest a sequence of progression. A small primary tumor with limited local invasion may be less likely than a larger, more invasive tumor of the same type to have metastasized to the local lymph nodes. Thus, a patient with a limited primary tumor would be at an earlier clinical stage. A patient with established lymph nodal metastases may be more likely than the patient without lymph nodal metastases to harbor occult distant metastases and thus would be at a more advanced stage. A patient with overtly evident distant metastases would, of course, be in an extremely advanced stage of the disease.

The purpose of clinical staging is not only to determine prognosis but also to plan rational therapy, preferably a step ahead of the neoplasm. The patient in a late stage of disease may well require an entirely differ-

ent treatment regimen from a patient in an early stage, and the particular therapeutic regimen may be associated with sufficient risk and/or morbidity that the clinician would not desire to institute it unless it is clearly indicated. Since different types of neoplasms have strikingly different natural histories, the staging schemes and methods will vary accordingly. For example, a patient with biopsy-proven carcinoma of the uterine cervix will be staged by a different procedure than that used for a patient found to have lymphoma in a lymph node in the

TABLE 8-2

CANCER INCIDENCE BY SITE AND SEX, 1984*

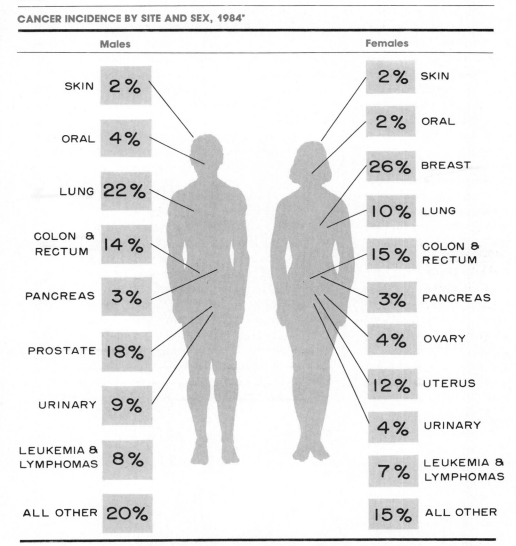

*The figures shown are drawn from overall statistics and do not include carcinoma in situ or nonmelanoma skin cancer. For children under 15, the figures differ strikingly: Leukemias, cancers of the nervous system, and lymphomas account for approximately 30, 26, and 14 percent respectively.
Source: American Cancer Society, 1984. Reproduced with permission from the American Cancer Society, Michigan Division.

neck. Staging may involve physical examination, various radiologic techniques, or even surgical biopsy of certain tissues distant from the primary.

Several different modalities of cancer treatment exist, and each might be employed simultaneously or serially in a given patient. Each of these modalities is based on a differential effect such that the cancerous tissue is eradicated with an acceptable degree of loss or damage to normal tissues.

The oldest and best known of these treatment modalities involves the attempt to extirpate the cancerous tissue surgically. This approach is extremely efficacious if excision of the primary tumor, along with a margin of normal tissues and perhaps the regional lymph nodes, eliminates all cancer cells from the body (or, some would claim, reduces the total body load of cancer cells to the point where host defenses can eliminate the remainder). Many tumors are not amenable to this type of therapy when discovered; i.e., they are "inoperable." In some cases this is because the primary cannot be totally excised without sacrificing essential local structures. In other cases, distant metastases may be evident at the time of diagnosis, indicating that extirpation of the primary tumor would not eradicate all the neoplasm. Also, the natural history of some diseases (e.g., leukemia) renders surgery inappropriate at any stage.

Another mode of therapy is radiotherapy, which refers to the application of ionizing radiation to the neoplasm. This approach is based on the fact that the lethal effect of radiation is greater on proliferating, poorly differentiated cancer cells than on adjacent normal cells. Thus, if the field of a cancer is irradiated, the normal tissues may by injured to a tolerable, reparable degree, while the cancer cells infiltrating the tissues are eliminated. In a favorable situation, a cure can be effected without a need to sacrifice some vital structure. This mode of therapy also has limitations. Some tumors by their nature are *radioresistant*, being no more sensitive to the effects of irradiation than are the surrounding normal cells which would be exposed. Other tumors, widespread at the time of diagnosis, cannot be treated by radiotherapy, since irradiation of broad areas of the body would risk unacceptable morbidity or could be lethal.

A more recent and rapidly evolving treatment modality is that of *chemotherapy*, which is based on the differential sensitivity of proliferating cancer cells and normal cells to a variety of cytotoxic chemical agents. The exciting potential of chemotherapy is that widely disseminated cancer cells beyond the confines of surgical or radiation therapy might be eliminated by a systemically adminstered drug where the toxic effects on normal cells are low enough to be acceptable. This potential has been realized in a number of cancer cases. However, different kinds of cancers are sensitive to different drugs or combinations of drugs, and no one regimen is applicable to all tumors. Unfortunately, in many instances chemotherapy is limited by the toxicity of the agents for rapidly proliferating normal cells such as the hematopoietic cells of the bone marrow or the lining epithelial cells of the bone marrow or the lining epithelial cells of the gastrointestinal tract. In this rapidly developing field, however, reports are emerging of previously uncontrollable neoplasms proving to be sensitive to a new chemotherapeutic approach.

Mention should also be made of immunotherapy of cancers. As noted above, cancer cells often differ antigenically from normal host cells to a degree that immunologic reactions may be mounted against them. Such reactions are demonstrable in laboratory situations but are not yet controllable at a practical clinical level. However, evidence is accumulating which suggests that therapeutic measures aimed at immunologic stimulation of the cancer patient may be helpful.

In contemporary practice, the approach to the cancer patient is not limited to the use of a single treatment modality but instead involves a team approach tailored to the unique needs of the individual patient with a particular neoplasm at a given clinical stage. It should be emphasized in conclusion that even if a neoplasm is deemed "incurable," several modes of therapy may provide dramatic palliation, significantly prolonging the span of comfortable, useful life for the cancer patient.

QUESTIONS

Disturbances of growth, cellular proliferation, and differentiation

Directions: Match the term in col. A related to disturbances of cellular growth and proliferation to its proper description in col. B.

Column A	Column B
1. ____ Aplasia	a. Abnormal degree of variation
2. ____ Hyperplasia	in size, shape, and appearance of the cells with an abnormal arrangement of cells
3. ____ Hypertrophy	b. Lack of differentiation or specialization in a group of neo-

4. ____ Meta-
   plasia
5. ____ Dysplasia
6. ____ Neoplasia
7. ____ Anaplasia

plastic cells; representation as a mass of pleomorphic primitive cells

c. Failure of structure to grow in the course of organogenesis

d. Increase in the absolute number of cells leading to an increase in the size of that tissue or organ

e. Differentiation of dividing cells into types of cells not ordinarily found in the area, but types of cells that would be perfectly reasonable elsewhere

f. Increase in size of existing cells without an increase in their number

g. Formation of an abnormal mass of proliferating cells, possessing a significant degree of autonomy

Directions: Circle the letter preceding each item below that correctly answers the question. More than one answer may be correct.

8. Which of the following are types of abnormal development?
   a. Hyperplasia b. Agenesis c. Aplasia
   d. Atrophy

9. Failure to reach definitive or adult size is:
   a. Atrophy b. Hypoplasia c. Both a and b
   d. Neither a nor b

10. The pressure of an enlarged prostate causes urethral obstruction. The resultant thickening of the bladder wall muscle is referred to as:
    a. Hypertrophy b. Hypoplasia c. Atrophy
    d. Neoplasia

11. A callus formed on the hand of a gardener from handling a hoe is an example of:
    a. Dysplasia b. Hyperplasia c. Metaplasia
    d. Neoplasia

12. Neoplasia differs from all other pathologic processes in that it:
    a. Involves proliferation of the cells of affected tissues b. Is relatively autonomous of the body's controls c. Is detrimental to the host d. May affect the host's nutritional state adversely

13. Malignant neoplasms differ from benign neoplasms in that malignant neoplasms:
    a. Have an infiltrative pattern of growth b. Are

encapsulated c. Give rise to metastases
d. Compress adjacent tissue

14. A carcinoma of the stomach would be most likely to produce its earliest metastases in:
    a Bone b. Lung c. Liver d. Kidney

15. An osteosarcoma of the femur would be most likely to produce its earliest metastases in the:
    a. Kidney b. Liver c. Brain d. Lung

16. A benign neoplasm of glandular epithelial origin would be termed a(n):
    a. Carcinoma b. Myoma c. Adenoma
    d. Chondroma

17. A malignant neoplasm arising in fibrous tissue (mesenchymal origin) would be termed a:
    a. Fibroma b. Carcinoma c. Fibrocarcinoma
    d. Fibrosarcoma

18. A malignant neoplasm arising from the glial supportive cells in the central nervous system would be termed a:
    a. Neurofibrosarcoma b. Glioma c. Neurofibroma d. Glioblastoma

Directions: Circle T if the statement is true and F if it is false. Correct the false statements.

19. T F Neoplastic cells are sufficiently different antigenically from the normal host cells that the body may mount an immunologic reaction against the neoplasm.

20. T F At present, there is widespread routine use of immunotherapeutic measures in the treatment of neoplasms.

21. T F A tumor which contains dense fibrous stroma and very hard growth is referred to as a medullary tumor.

22. T F Benign neoplasms tend to be very well differentiated; i.e., they resemble parent tissues very closely.

23. T F A malignant neoplasm of smooth muscle is classified as a rhabdomyosarcoma.

24. T F A Papanicolaou smear is a cytologic diagnostic examination used only for uterine cervical scrapings or secretions.

Directions: Complete the following statements by filling in the blanks.

25. Some causes of atrophy are _____
    and _____.

26. Two dangerous properties of malignant neoplasms
    which distinguish them from benign neoplasms are
    _____and _____.

*Directions: Answer the following questions on a
separate sheet of paper.*

27. List at least three pathways by which malignant
    neoplasms disseminate through the body.

28. How do neoplasms (benign and malignant) affect
    the host?

29. What are the criteria used in the classification of
    neoplasms?

30. What is actually happening at a cellular level dur-
    ing the "transformation" or cancerigenic event?

31. In terms of cellular control mechanisms explain the
    "phenotypic" expression of malignancy in cells.

32. What are the environmental and genetic factors
    that seem to be related to the causation of neopla-
    sia?

33. What are the means and the criteria used to estab-
    lish the diagnosis and to determine the therapeutic
    modalities for treatment of neoplasia?

REFERENCES FOR PART I

AMERICAN CANCER SOCIETY, *CAA Cancer Journal for
Clinicians,* **34**(1)F: , January/February 1984.

BECKER, F. F. (ed.): *Cancer, A Comprehensive Treatise,*
Plenum, New York, 1982.

BELLANTI, J. A.: *Immunology II,* Saunders, Philadephia,
1978.

COCKBURN, A.: *The Evolution and Eradication of Infectious Diseases,* Johns Hopkins, Baltimore, 1963.

COPENHAVER, W. M., D. E. KELLY, and R. L. WOOD:
Bailey's Textbook of Histology, 17th ed., Williams
& Wilkins, Baltimore, 1978.

FROHLICH, E. E. (ed.): *Pathophysiology. Altered Regulatory Mechanisms in Disease,* Lippincott, 1984.

HARVEY, A. M., R. J. JOHNS, A. H. OWENS, and R. S.
ROSS: *The Principles and Practice of Medicine,* 20th
ed., Appleton Century Crofts, New York, 1980.

HENRY, J. D.: *Clinical Diagnosis and Management by
Laboratory Methods,* 17th ed., Saunders, Philadelphia, 1984.

HILL, R. B. and M. F. LaVIA: *Principles of Pathobiology,* 3d ed., Oxford University Press, New York,
1980.

JAWETZ, E., J. MELNICK, and E. ADELBERG: *Review of
Medical Microbiology,* 16th ed., Lange, Palo Alto,
Cal., 1984.

KING, D. W., C. M. FENOGLIO, and J. H. LEFKOWITCH:
General Pathology. Principles and Dynamics, Lea &
Febiger, Philadelphia, 1983.

LUCIANO, D., A. VANDER, and J. SHERMAN: *Human
Anatomy and Physiology: Structure and Function,*
2d ed., McGraw-Hill, New York, 1983.

MARTIN, G. M. and H. HOEHN: "Genetics and Human

Diseases," *Human Pathology,* **5**(4): 387–405, July
1974.

MOVAT, H. A.: *Inflammation, Immunity and Hypersensitivity. Cellular and Molecular Mechanisms,* 2d ed.,
Harper & Row, Hagerstown, Md., 1979.

NORA, J. J. and F. C. FRASER: *Medical Genetics: Principles and Practice,* Lea & Febiger, Philadelphia,
1974.

PEACOCK, E. E. and W. VAN WINKLE: *Surgery and Biology of Wound Repair,* Saunders, Philadelphia,
1970.

POMERANCE: A. and M. J. DAVIES: *The Pathology of the
Heart,* Blackwell, Oxford, 1975.

PREHN, R. T. and L. M. PREHN: "Pathobiology of Neoplasia," *American Journal of Pathology,* **80**: (3):529–
550, September 1975.

ROBBINS, S. L., R. S. COTRAN, and V. KUMAR: *Pathologic Basis of Disease,* 3d ed., Saunders, Philadelphia,
1984.

ROSS, R. and J. A. GLOMSET: "Pathogenesis of Atherosclerosis" (part 1), *New England Journal of Medicine,* **295**(6): 369–377, August 5, 1976.

———: "Pathogenesis of Atherosclerosis" (part 2),
New England Journal of Medicine **295**(8): 420–425,
August 19, 1976.

SIMON, H. J.: *Attenuated Infection,* Lippincott, Philadelphia, 1960.

YUNIS, J. J. and M. E. CHANDLER: "The Chromosomes
of Man—Clinical and Biologic Significance," *American Journal of Pathology,* **88**(10): 466–495, August
1977.

PART II

WILLIAM R. SOLOMON

DISTURBANCES OF IMMUNE MECHANISMS

Unfavorable effects of immune processes underlie much human disease and may impair the function of any major organ system. In addition, characteristic changes in immune reactants that provide essential diagnostic clues *accompany* many conditions as effects or parallel events. It is now clear that normal antibody and cell-mediated responses involve serial steps, each of which is modulated by groups of specific cells. Defects in these control processes may be the source of excessive or inappropriate immune reactions. Less commonly, disease results when normally protective immediate and delayed hypersensitivity mechanisms become impaired or fail to develop normally. The figure below depicts various immunologic states in terms of a *balance* between the pathogenic effects of

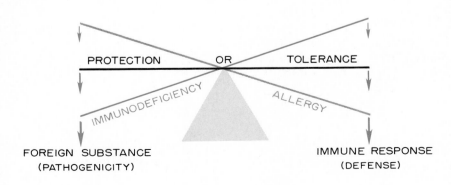

PROTECTION   OR   TOLERANCE

IMMUNODEFICIENCY   ALLERGY

FOREIGN SUBSTANCE
(PATHOGENICITY)

IMMUNE RESPONSE
(DEFENSE)

Immunologic states depicted as a *balance* between the dangers posed by a foreign substance (left) and by the tissue effects resulting from a defensive reaction (right). When the pathogen threat and the immune response are alike in intensity, a state of effective protection is recognized. The impact of *tolerance* may be similar when no immune response is developed to a substance that has no pathogenic potential. When the protective response to a pathogen is relatively inadequate, *immunodeficiency* exists. By contrast, we recognize *allergy* whenever the defensive response is excessive— especially when the foreign substance has little potential for harming the host.

two groups of factors: potentially harmful foreign agents of disease (e.g., microorganisms) and incidental tissue damage due to the body's defensive responses.

It is often difficult to confront the fact that protective immunity and allergic diseases share common processes of tissue response to substances recognized as "foreign" by the host. Immune mechanisms provide essential defense against invasion by injurious organisms and the emergence of malignant tumors, functions which have ensured their retention throughout vertebrate evolution. However, these same processes may be called forth by relatively innocuous extrinsic agents and occasionally may focus the reaction on host tissue components. In these circumstances the *net* effects of exposure and specific host response are unfavorable; patterns of overt illness that result are recognized as immunologic diseases. The resulting conditions are diverse in type and range in severity from trivial, chronic disorders of the skin or mucous membranes to catastrophic events that may be fatal within seconds. The tissue processes responsible and their relationship to a practical classification of human immunologic disorders have been described in Chap. 5. Since these diseases are determined by host reactivity as well as by the type and strength of antigenic exposure, regional differences in their prevalence are prominent. Overall, however, these disorders are remarkably common, and their impact on human comfort and productivity is evident universally.

OBJECTIVES

At the completion of this part you should be able to:

1. Describe the relationship between the immune processes and immediate and delayed hypersensitivity mechanisms.
2. Identify the etiology, pathogenesis, diagnosis, and treatment of selected immunologic diseases.

FAMILIAR ALLERGIC DISORDERS: ANAPHYLAXIS AND THE ATOPIC DISEASES

OBJECTIVES

At the completion of this chapter you should be able to:

1. Identify the immunologic processes which are most clearly recognized as immunologic disease.
2. Define *hypersensitivity* and *sensitization*.
3. Explain the immunologic effects which may result following exposure to a *single* antigen.
4. Identify the characteristics of allergy as an immunologic response.
5. Describe the tissue changes elicited by the reaction of immunoglobulin E (IgE) with antigen.
6. Describe immunoglobulin E–mediated (Type I) allergic problems as to type of cells involved, location, and reactions that occur.
7. Identify the characteristics of an acute systemic (anaphylactic) reaction in terms of etiology, onset, signs and symptoms, and tissue response.
8. Describe the unique properties of angioedema in relation to acute systemic reactions.
9. Explain the treatment modalities for anaphylaxis.
10. Cite the usual requirements necessary to elicit anaphylaxis sensitization in human beings.
11. Describe the characteristics of the atopic state in terms of familial predisposition, tissues most often affected, allergens involved, type of antibody necessary to mediate the reaction, and circumstances in which immune responses occur.
12. Identify for seasonal and perennial allergic rhinitis the common etiologies, signs and symptoms, distinctive features, complications, diagnostic procedures, and treatment.
13. Explain, for skin tests that elicit a wheal-and-flare reaction, the techniques utilized and significance of a positive reaction in evaluating respiratory allergy.
14. Explain for the radioallergosorbent test (RAST) the purpose of the procedure, and compare its clinical value to direct testing.

15. List three principal considerations which dominate the management of respiratory allergy as exemplified by allergic rhinitis.

16. State at least two examples of the treatment modalities used in the management of respiratory allergy.

17. Identify the classes, actions, side effects, and mode of administration of medications used in treating respiratory allergy as exemplified by allergic rhinitis.

18. Appreciate, for hyposensitization, the indications, practical characteristics, and efficacy of the procedure as well as its possible modes of action.

Immunologic processes are most evident as clinically perceived reactions of immediate or delayed hypersensitivity. In this context, *hypersensitivity* denotes the capacity, acquired through prior contact with a specific, chemically characterizable agent, to hyperreact to that agent. The cellular events that follow exposure and establish a capacity for responses of hypersensitivity are termed *sensitization*. Reexposure to defined antigens may reveal that sensitized cells, as well as one or more types of immunoglobulins, have been produced in the course of this specific "defensive" response. Not surprisingly, clinical hypersensitivity reactions in human beings often show evidence of more than one immunologic process, each with its specific amplification system(s). Such complexity is easy to accept where the "invader" is itself antigenically complex, (e.g., a microorganism) but can be elicited also by *single, defined* proteins.

A remarkable variety of immunologic effects may be recognized following exposure to a *single* antigen, with both humoral (antibody-dependent) and cell-mediated immunity often developing. In addition, depending on the size and form of the antigen and the route of exposure, and depending on the respondent's age, health, and prior exposure to that sensitizer, the antibody response may embrace *one or more* immunoglobulin classes. For example, first exposure to an injected agent often will elicit an IgM response which, in days, changes to IgG synthesis; reexposure typically elicits only IgG production. Very low antigen doses often have favored IgE synthesis, while mucosal exposure promotes an IgA response which may be "local" in the challenged organ. A *single* antigen-antibody interaction also can provoke different effects depending on the circumstances (or test system) in which it is observed. This implies, for example, that human IgG molecules specific for an antigen may precipitate the antigen from solution, agglutinate insoluble particles coated with the antigen, or activate complement proteins after interacting

with the antigen in either form. The effects observed depend largely on antigen-antibody concentrations, the relative proportions of these reactants, and the presence of additional components which often serve as "indicators" in laboratory test systems. When such interactions occur in vivo, their effects depend upon similar factors as well as local tissue responses to the primary antigen-antibody reaction and to activation of secondary amplification mechanisms (see also Chap. 5).

Studies of antibody structure and function have shown that antigen *specificity* is directed by the two combining sites present on the antibody fragment (Fab) portions of immunoglobulin molecules. These antigen-reactive sequences of amino acids specifically determine with which molecules a given antibody will interact. The biological consequences of the reaction generally are identified with activities of the crystallizable fragment (Fc fragment) of antibodies. The Fc portion determines the tissue localization of certain immunoglobulins, and receptors on phagocytic cells may recognize this region, facilitating the uptake of antigen-antibody complexes and of particles bearing surface-bound immunoglobulins. Activation of the "classical" complement pathway (as depicted in Table 5-1) also appears to involve the Fc region; as a result, activities including target cell lysis, leukocyte attraction, and release of permeability-enhancing factors may be generated. In addition, the class-specific properties of immunoglobulins which determine their tissue localization and function as *antibodies* are expressed on the Fc region.

Although it is the least plentiful of the five recognized antibody classes, immunoglobulin E (IgE) plays a disproportionately major role in human allergic* re-

---

*The term *allergy* was proposed by von Pirquet in 1906 to denote all instances of acquired altered reactivity that promote "supersensitivity." Current usage equates allergy with clinically evident responses of immediate or delayed hypersensitivity.

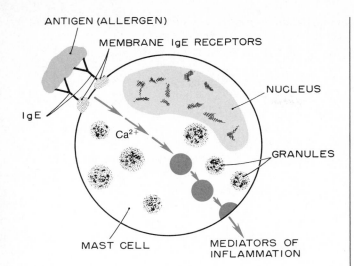

FIGURE 9-1

Mast cell secretion provoked by bridging of adjacent IgE molecules by a multivalent antigen or allergen. The process is calcium-dependent and, if manifestations of allergy are produced, proceeds in steps after membrane IgE receptors are brought together. As developed further later (see Fig. 10-6), the secretion process is affected by levels of cyclic nucleotides (cyclic AMP and GMP) within the mast cell. Many drugs can affect mast cell activity by their effects on cyclic nucleotides, although separate membrane receptors occur for these and other substances.

sponses. IgE molecules bind readily to surface receptors of tissue mast cells and blood basophils. As a result, *bound* IgE is *concentrated* in the respiratory and gastrointestinal tracts as well as in the intravascular compartment (i.e., circulating blood) although it is readily demonstrated at other sites, including skin. When adjacent IgE molecules combine with groupings of a multiple reactive antigen, a series of events, shown in Fig. 9-1 can occur, with liberation from the cell of tissue-reactive "mediator" substances including histamine, leukotrienes (formerly termed SRS-A) and eosinophil chemotactic factor(s) of anaphylaxis (ECF-A); substances that attract neutrophils and lead to the formation of kinins also have been described. Additional

products may include an anticoagulant (heparin), a proteolytic enzyme (chymotrypsin), and a highly reactive oxygen radical (superoxide) as well as prostaglandins. Individual characteristics of some of these agents are summarized in Table 9-1; however, their combined effects promote dilatation and hyperpermeability of small blood vessels (principally venules), spasm of the walls of hollow viscera, and increased secretion by mucous membranes. Heightened venule permeability should promote diminished circulating blood volume and arterial pressure as well as collections of fluid outside of vessels. In fact, these effects are all more or less easily observed in clinically significant human responses involving IgE.

TABLE 9-1

SOME MEDIATORS OF INFLAMMATION RELEASED BY HUMAN MAST CELLS* AND BASOPHILS

Mediator	Chemical characteristics	Biological activity
Histamine	Simple amine, mol wt 111	Contracts visceral smooth muscle; increases permeability of capillaries; increases respiratory mucous gland activity; produces sensation of itching
Leukotrienes (C_4, D_4, E_4)†	Acid lipids, mol wt 400–600	Cause *prolonged* visceral smooth-muscle spasm; dilate and increase permeability of venules
Prostaglandin D_2	mol wt $\sim$ 350	Contracts smooth muscle; increases mediator release by basophils
Eosinphil chemotactic factor of anaphylaxis (ECF-A)	Pair of acidic tetrapeptides	Attracts eosinophils selectively
Platelet-activating factor (PAF)	Phospholipid(s?), mol wt < 500	Aggregates and degranulates platelets; contracts some smooth muscle; produces wheal-and-flare skin responses
Neutrophil chemotactic factor (NCF-A)	Not defined, mol wt > 10,000	Causes directed migration of neutrophils
Basophil kallikrein‡	Not defined	Causes formation of bradykinin

*Serotonin is present in human *platelets* and in the mast cells of other species. Additional materials released by human mast cells probably remain to be confirmed but seem to include heparin and activators of additional proinflammatory systems.
†Formerly called SRS-A.
‡Released from basophils but not as yet described from mast cells.

As Fig. 9-1 suggests, the release of mediator substances from mast cell granules is modulated by cellular levels of agents—especially cyclic nucleotides—with cyclic AMP depressing and GMP facilitating release. Both cholinergic and alpha-adrenergic stimuli seem to increase GMP (guanosine monophosphate), while beta-adrenergic agents promote adenylate cyclase activity and augmented AMP (adenosine monophosphate). Both histamine and certain prostaglandins depress mediator release by receptors either unique to these agents or shared with beta-adrenergic agonists.

ANAPHYLAXIS—A TYPE I DISORDER

Acute systemic reactions—often resulting in death—first were recognized in several species almost 100 years ago during immunization experiments with foreign toxins. In many animals, sensitization did not confer protection; rather, on readministration of the toxin, there was prompt development of shock, airway obstruction, and/or visceral congestion in species-specific patterns. The term *anaphylaxis* (*ana* = back or reverse; *phylaxis* = protection) was derived from this paradoxical outcome. Similar human reactions were noted early in this century and remain the most rapidly developing and dangerous form of allergic response. Acute systemic reactions generally follow the *injection* of a potent antigen *(allergen)* into a highly sensitive subject, although, rarely, exposure occurs by ingesting the offending agent. In the past, antiserums derived from other species (especially equine antiserums) were most often responsible for these reactions; more recently, injected penicillins have become the principal offenders, with serums, adrenocorticotropic hormone (ACTH), insulin, and other drugs less often implicated. Comparable reactions also may follow insect stings and the less frequent attacks of other venomous creatures upon *previously sensitized* subjects.

Acute systemic reactions generally begin within minutes after introduction of an allergen; a delay longer than 1 hour is distinctly rare. In extreme sensitivity, injection of an allergen may cause death or a sublethal reaction almost instantly, with maximally severe responses often appearing the most promptly. Affected persons report a sense of uneasiness, rapidly followed by light-headedness, which may lead to syncope (loss of consciousness). Itching of the palms and scalp is often felt and may herald hives (urticaria) that cover much of the skin surface. Localized tissue swellings (angioedema) may appear within minutes and distort especially the eyelids, lips, tongue, hands, feet, and genitalia. *Angioedema* denotes a discrete swelling, involving tissues deep to skin or mucous membranes, produced by a localized increase in vascular *permeability* without frank injury to the small veins and capillaries involved. Angioedema is, by nature, reversible within a short time. It differs from other forms of edema in which abnormal pressure or blood vessel injury promotes passage of fluid into tissues. Swelling (edema) of the uvula and larynx are less evident to casual inspection but are especially prominent in human anaphylaxis, and may cause death by respiratory obstruction. Laryngeal edema induces prominent air hunger, impaired phonation, noisy breathing, and a "barking" or high-pitched cough. Respiratory difficulty also may arise owing to bronchial narrowing, with audible wheezes mimicking spontaneous asthma (see Chap. 10). Less often, spasm of the gut, bladder, or uterus is prominent, with cramping pain, loss of visceral contents, or vaginal spotting. Figure 9-2 summarizes the most prominent manifestations of human anaphylaxis.

All current evidence suggests that clinical anaphylaxis in both animals and humans involves a sudden multifocal reaction of allergen with mast cell–bound, specific IgE, followed by widespread tissue response to the mediator substances [e.g., histamine and leukotrienes (SRS-A)] released. Many features of these responses—including urticaria—can be induced by injection of agents that directly release mediators from mast cells in vivo, although *not* by injection of histamine alone. Systemic reactions to certain injected agents (e.g., x-ray contrast media) may exemplify such nonimmunologic release of mediators, since rises in their plasma levels and in levels of activated complement components have been shown to occur. Differences among species in patterns of anaphylactic response seem to reflect differences both in the distribution of mast cells and in relative responsiveness of tissues to mediator substances.

Effective treatment of anaphylaxis requires, first, assurance of a patent airway. Careful and continuous observation is essential since oropharyngeal intubation or tracheostomy may become necessary to prevent asphyxia from laryngeal edema. Hypotension, which, if severe and/or prolonged, may lead to brain, kidney, or heart damage, poses a threat only slightly less grim. Since this problem reflects, primarily, loss of intravascular fluid due to leaky vessels, it may be corrected most directly by replacing plasma volume with normal saline solution, half-normal saline solution, or plasma. Several thousand milliliters of fluid often are required to restore normal blood pressure. Vasoconstrictor drugs (e.g., norepinephrine) can be of further value but offer limited benefit without adequate volume replacement. Epinephrine remains the preferred drug to limit or reverse the anaphylactic process and should be the first agent administered. A dose of 0.3 ml of 1:1000 epinephrine may be injected subcutaneously (see Chap. 10) and repeated several times, if needed, at intervals of 15 minutes; small children may receive 0.022 ml/kg to a maximum of 0.3 ml per dose. The absorption of epinephrine from subcutaneous depots is slow with severe hypotension; when shock is present, the drug may be diluted to 1:10,000 and infused slowly intravenously to provide comparable total doses. Injected antihistaminics (e.g., diphenhydramine or chlorpheniramine) may speed the resolution of urticaria and relieve cramps originating in hollow viscera. Adrenocortical steroids are often given for their favorable effects on inflammation and abnormal vascular permeability; however, benefit derived from such agents is *not* realized immediately. While the steroids rarely may be lifesaving in *prolonged* shock, they should be considered only after the airway is secure, volume repletion has been begun, and epinephrine administered.

Systemic reactions, comparable to those induced by drugs and serums, follow insect stings (e.g., bee, wasp, hornet, and yellow jacket) and, rarely, insect bites (e.g., deerfly) in some persons. These responses, too, appear to be IgE-mediated and, without treatment mentioned above, may terminate fatally. Besides avoiding situations favored by stinging insects, susceptible persons are urged to carry commercially prepared, preloaded syringes of epinephrine whenever feasible. Such persons must be *prepared* to self-administer the drug in 0.3-ml subcutaneous doses and to apply a tourniquet if an extremity has been attacked. *Immunotherapy* or *hyposensitization* with incremental injected doses of sterile, aqueous dilutions of purified venoms is now available and is extremely effective in reducing risks of anaphylaxis if adequate doses can be aministered over many months. This approach has entirely replaced the former practice of injecting "whole-body" extracts of incriminated insects.

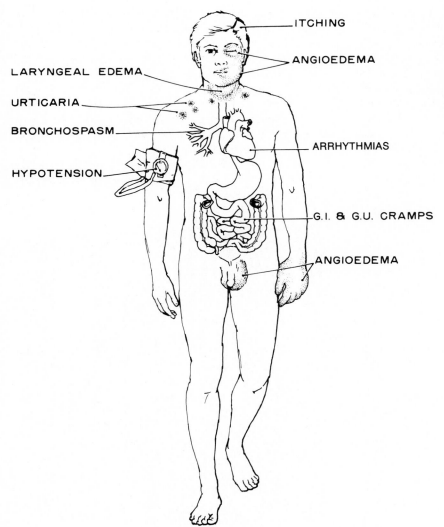

ITCHING

ANGIOEDEMA

LARYNGEAL EDEMA

URTICARIA

BRONCHOSPASM

HYPOTENSION

ARRHYTHMIAS

G.I. & G.U. CRAMPS

ANGIOEDEMA

FIGURE 9-2

Prominent manifestations of anaphylaxis in the human being. Laryngeal edema and profound hypotension usually pose the greatest dangers for affected persons. Cardiac effects may be primary or secondary to lowering of blood pressure.

THE ATOPIC DISEASES

Anaphylactic sensitization in human beings generally requires the *injection* of potent allergens, although certain gastrointestinal and respiratory parasites also elicit prominent IgE responses in a majority of those exposed. In addition, a substantial fraction of persons make specific IgE in response to *mucosal* contact (viz., by inhalation or ingestion) with quite innocuous materials including foods, pollens, and animal emanations (danders). The presence of allergen-specific IgE fixed to tissue may be demonstrated conveniently by performing skin tests and observing the development in 5 to 15 minutes of local redness (erythema)—often with a central hive (wheal). A *proportion* of persons, easily sensitized for such Type I (IgE-mediated) responses by mucosal exposure, also manifest one or more related illnesses, of which the most common types—allergic rhinitis, allergic (extrinsic) asthma, and atopic dermatitis—will be described subsequently. In addition, gastrointestinal allergy, allergic conjunctivitis, and instances of acute urticaria and angioedema may coexist. Those with gastrointestinal allergy may show, in response to specific foods, perioral pruritus (itching), tongue and mucous-membrane swelling, difficulty in swallowing (dysphagia), nausea, vomiting, abdominal cramps, diarrhea, and perianal itching—singly or in combination. *Food allergy* may also affect distant organs including the skin and bronchi and rarely may underlie generalized reactions. These familiar conditions often are grouped as *atopic diseases,* and the predisposition that favors their occurrence is termed *atopy.** The pathophysiological basis of atopy still is not entirely clear; however, prominent IgE production from mucosal exposure to (benign) allergens appears to be a principal marker and one fundamental characteristic. The tissue-fixing IgE antibodies formed in this manner are often termed *atopic reagins.* In addition, health histories of affected subjects commonly include *more than one* of the atopic conditions (e.g., eczema in infancy, then allergic rhinitis and/or asthma). Furthermore, familial clustering of these

---

*Atopy is derived from the Greek ατοπια, which means strange or out of place. The term probably was chosen to express the inappropriateness of an immune response to entirely innocuous environment agents.

FIGURE 9-3
Upward deflection of the nasal tip is a common mannerism among children with allergic rhinitis. This "allergic salute" serves briefly to allay pruritus and open the nasal airway.

conditions is very prominent, although it seems to be the atopic constitution, rather than any specific form of illness, that is hereditable. In most North American reports, more than one-half of overtly affected subjects have close relatives with atopic conditions, while in subjects free of atopic disease, a positive family history is definable only in about 10 percent.

Allergic rhinitis

Nasal allergy is the most commonly encountered atopic condition, affecting as many as 20 percent of certain pediatric and young-adult populations in North America and western Europe. Elsewhere, rates of this and other atopic illnesses appear to be lower, although prevalence data often are incomplete. Persons with allergic rhinitis experience prominent nasal stuffiness and may report excessive nasal secretion (rhinorrhea) and sneezes occurring in rapid succession. Pruritus (Fig. 9-3) of the nasal mucosa, throat, and ears often is distressing and is accompanied by conjunctival redness, ocular pruritus, and lacrimation. The involved mucous membranes show dilatation of blood vessels (especially venules) and extensive edema with prominent accumulation of eosinophils in both tissue and secretions. Many of these features, including the pruritus, can be duplicated by applying histamine alone to the normal mucosa, and allergic rhinitis may reflect the straightforward tissue effects of recognized mast cell–derived mediator substances (see earlier in this chapter). A release of histamine, leukotrienes, prostaglandin D, etc., from the mucosa has been shown after direct nasal challenge of sensitive subjects with pollen allergens.

Although no *absolute* distinction is implied, allergic rhinitis is often divided into "seasonal" and "perennial"

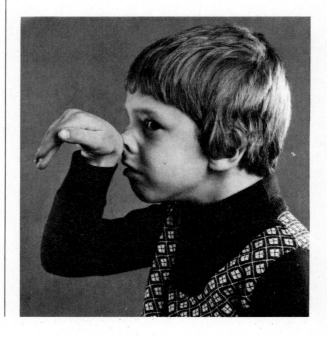

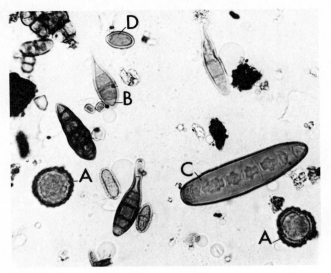

FIGURE 9-4
Particles recovered during atmospheric sampling in late summer. Prominent sources of hay fever including ragweed pollen grain (A), and fungus spores of *Alternaria* (B) and *Helminthosporium* (C) species are evident. Many spores, such as those of mushrooms (D), remain to be evaluated as allergens.

forms. Seasonal allergic rhinitis, or "hay fever," usually involves a specific period of symptoms in successive years, reflecting sensitivity principally to airborne pollens and/or fungus spores (Fig. 9-4) with defined schedules of prevalence. Seasonal rhinitis is mild in many persons who do not seek medical care but can be an exhausting illness for some because of continual sneezing, copious rhinorrhea, and unremitting pruritus. Intense pallor and swelling of mucous membranes usually accompany these dramatic symptoms, and eosinophils abound in nasal secretions (Fig. 9-5). By contrast, perennial rhinitis seldom shows major annual variations in severity, and symptoms are often dominated by unremitting nasal obstruction; prominent offenders include foods, house dust, and animal emanations to which daily exposure is commonplace. Not surprisingly, persons with multiple clinical sensitivities often experience perennial rhinitis as well as one or more predictable seasonal flares annually.

Although perennial allergic rhinitis rarely is a source of dramatic symptoms, persistent partial nasal obstruction can promote distressing complications. In most instances, the affected person resorts to mouth breathing with resulting complaints of snoring and oropharyngeal dryness. Dark circles and redundant tissue

often develop beneath the eyes; while popularly termed "allergic shiners," these changes may reflect long-standing nasal obstruction of any cause. The swollen mucosa readily sustains bacterial infection, and obstruction of paranasal sinus openings is common; these lead to recurrent or chronic sinusitis. Drainage from foci of nasal infection promotes sore throat and can foster bronchial soiling and infection. Especially with recurrent infection, the swollen nasal mucosa is prone to form local projections, or *polyps*, that further obstruct the airway. In addition, especially in children, the pharyngeal openings of the eustachian tubes may become blocked by swollen mucosa, enlarged lymphoid tissue, or exudate. Without normal access to air, the middle ears develop negative pressure and fill with fluid, creating a *chronic serous otitis* marked by at least transient hearing loss and, often, recurrent middle ear infection.

Although it is acknowledged that allergic rhinitis sufferers tend to develop bronchial asthma with above normal frequency, the extent of this increased risk remains unclear. In one population of rhinitic persons, *unselected for symptom severity*, less than 10 percent were observed to develop asthma as a new manifestation. However, this sequence has been recorded far more often in persons whose problems eventually prompted evaluation by an allergist. In general, the risk of subsequent asthma appears to rise with increasing severity of rhinitis, with prominent sinobronchial infection, and when asthma has been present in the past.

Although the pruritus, repetitive sneezing, and watery, profuse rhinorrhea of hay fever are distinctive, they are not unique to this disorder, and the symptoms of perennial rhinitis readily mimic those of other conditions. The *distinctive* feature of allergic rhinitis is that *compatible symptoms* appear or worsen predictably in

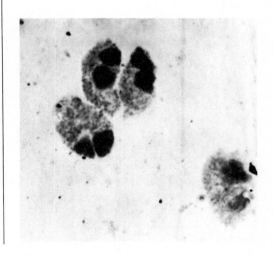

FIGURE 9-5
Eosinophils from nasal secretions of a child with florid ragweed hay fever. Bilobed nuclei and discrete, round granules are familiar features of these cells, when suitably stained.

response to *specific allergen exposures*. Therefore, in diagnosis, careful analysis of the factors precipitating rhinitis is of overriding importance. Many persons with *nonallergic vasomotor rhinitis* experience similar nasal stuffiness and marked rhinorrhea, some also showing intense nasal eosinophilia. However, this group is, by definition, without response to identifiable allergens. Instead, their complaints relate largely to airborne irritants, extremes of temperature and humidity, pregnancy, stages of the menstrual cycle, and emotional factors. Long-standing nasal complaints due to recurrent or chronic infection, nasal polyps, marked deviation of the nasal septum, hypothyroidism, and antihypertensive or ovulatory suppressant drugs also must be distinguished from perennial allergic and nonallergic forms of rhinitis.

A clinical history of symptoms on exposure provides the clearest indication of offenders in respiratory allergy. Symptom variations during and after travel deserve special attention, and the effects of overt exposure to agents including house dust, animals and fur products, feathers, seed derivatives, silk, and kapok fibers may be sought directly. Where casual observations are insufficient, history may be "created" by markedly increasing and/or reducing specific exposures, such as exposures to foods or house pets, for brief periods to observe the results. In addition, the time or place of symptom occurrence may furnish etiological clues not readily evident to the sufferer. Specific pollen sensitivities, for example, may be deduced if the resulting symptoms can be dated precisely and "seasons" of prevalence for local airborne pollens are known (Fig. 9-6). Similarly, recognition of the heavy fungus exposures associated with leaf collection, lawn care, and gardening as well as with hiking in tall vegetation helps to explain associated symptoms.

Skin tests eliciting a wheal-and-flare reaction provide useful *correlates* for a detailed clinical evaluation and are widely performed. However, even strongly positive reactions indicate only the immunologic "apparatus" for response and provide no assurance that symptoms arise from exposure to the allergens in question. The ultimate value of skin tests is to support or contradict impressions formed during clinical fact-finding. For wheal-and flare tests, in common clinical practice, aqueous extracts are used and testing is performed initially by pricking the skin through applied drops of these materials to produce epidermal or "prick" tests or by injecting small quantities (usually 0.02 ml) intracutaneously (Figs. 9-7 and 9-8, respectively). Since even this volume of extract may be hazardous in exquisitely sensitive persons, prick tests are usually done first and persons with negative reactions are considered for intracutaneous (IC) testing; where IC tests are done exclusively, very dilute materials must be used. Since occasional persons manifest whealing with any skin trauma (i.e., *dermographism*), all reactions must be compared with those at control sites tested with the sterile diluent alone. Wheal and erythema reactions may be reduced factitiously by oral antihistaminic drugs (see later in this section); of these, hydroxyzine (Atarax, Vistaril) may cause suppression lasting 2 to 3 days. Cortisonelike drugs, by contrast, have little effect on immediate skin reactivity, while suppression due to theophylline and sympathomimetic amines is minor, at best.

Few additional test procedures furnish help in evaluating respiratory allergy. Initial hopes that levels of total serum IgE could distinguish clearly between symptomatic atopic patients and others have not been sustained. Recently, however, measurement of allergen-specific IgE has become possible in vitro using venous blood. This procedure, the radioallergosorbent test

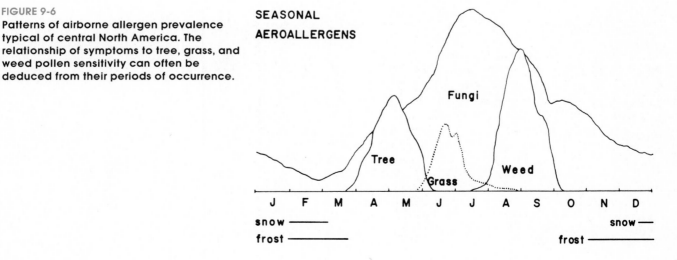

FIGURE 9-6

Patterns of airborne allergen prevalence typical of central North America. The relationship of symptoms to tree, grass, and weed pollen sensitivity can often be deduced from their periods of occurrence.

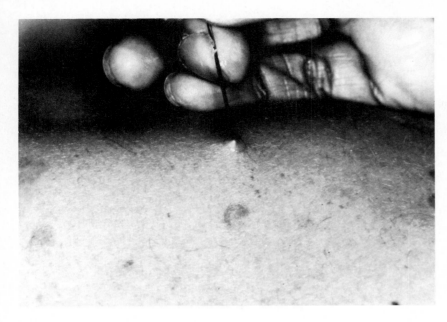

FIGURE 9-7
Technique of epidermal (prick) testing using a sterile, straight needle. Since only the epidermis is penetrated, bleeding should not occur.

(RAST), diagramed in Fig. 9-9, offers certain logistic advantages over direct testing and eliminates rare adverse reactions that accompany that procedure; however, neither the sensitivity nor the specificity of RAST exceeds that of conventional skin tests.

The demonstration of eosinophils as the predominating cell in nasal or lacrimal secretions suggests an associated Type I allergic inflammatory process but may be found in nonallergic conditions. In suitably stained material, the bilobed nuclei and abundant, discrete, red, refractile granules of eosinophils are evident by oil-immersion microscopy (Fig. 9-5).

Three principal considerations dominate the management of respiratory allergy as exemplified by allergic rhinitis: (1) efforts to reduce allergen (and irritant) ex-

posure, (2) suppressive medications to mitigate symptom severity *nonspecifically,* and (3) *specific* hyposensitization to reduce responsiveness to *unavoidable* allergen challenge. Avoidance measures are most feasible for allergens associated with home and work situations, such as house dust, animal emanations, and agricultural products. However, even pollen exposure can be reduced significantly by the patient remaining indoors with windows closed—a strategy that often requires air conditioning for success. House dust avoidance is fostered by provision of smooth, simple surfaces that facilitate cleaning (e.g., bare floors and uncluttered table and dresser tops) as well as by elimination or plastic-encasing of bedding and upholstered furnishings (Fig. 9-10). Filters or electrostatic particle precipitators

FIGURE 9-8
Technique of intradermal (intracutaneous) skin testing.

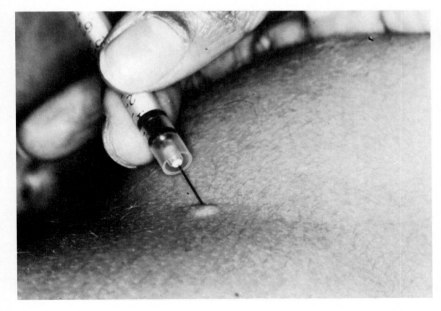

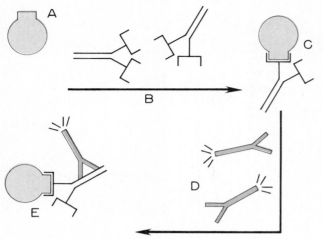

FIGURE 9-9

The radioallergosorbent test (RAST), a technique for quanititating allergen-specific immunoglobulin E. In this procedure allergens are linked chemically to carrier particles (A), and the resulting conjugate reacted (B) with serum presumably containing specific IgE. If IgE is bound (C), it will react with and bind radiolabeled antihuman IgE (D) to form a radioactive complex (E). By counting bound radioactivity, the original specific IgE present may be estimated.

FIGURE 9-10

Measures designed to minimize exposure to house dust (and other inhalant allergens) as applied to a bedroom. Objectives include covering pillows (A) and mattresses and box springs (B) with plastic encasings; maintaining a bare floor (C) and uncluttered surfaces (D); applying final filters to warm-air ducts (E); keeping closet doors closed (F); and minimizing window coverings (G), upholstered furnishings (H), and wall decorations (I).

are helpful where central forced air heating is used but do not replace a careful antidust program at room level. Recent recognition that mites in house dust often contribute to its allergenic potency provides a new rationale for these traditional measures, which are known to reduce mite populations also.

Where sensitivity to animal emanations (dander) is confirmed, total avoidance of the source usually is justified. Although danders are popularly equated with hair, far more potent allergen sources include epidermal scales, saliva, lacrimal secretions, and even urine. House pets are the most persistently troublesome dander sources. However, occupational exposures also may plague laboratory workers, veterinarians, and livestock handlers. In addition, products derived from animal sources may retain sensitizing properties for prolonged periods; these include feather- and down-filled materials, fur-trimmed clothing and toys, furniture and rug pads (cattle and horse hair), and raw silk. Mohair and camel hair fabrics are occasionally implicated as allergen sources, although commercially processed sheep's wool appears not to be an offender.

Tobacco smoke is an acknowledged respiratory irritant, containing a remarkable assortment of toxic agents, but without confirmed activity as an allergen. By contrast, plant products such as cottonseed, flaxseed, and castor bean meals are among the most potent sensitizers and are major symptom sources in industry.

For several decades, antihistaminic drugs have been the most useful agents in the symptomatic (i.e., nonspecific) treatment of allergic nasal disease. While many antihistaminics share anticholinergic, antiserotonin, and/or tranquilizing properties, their capacity to compete with histamine for tissue receptors seems to underlie their effectiveness in hay fever, etc. These drugs are generally effective orally and may be admin-

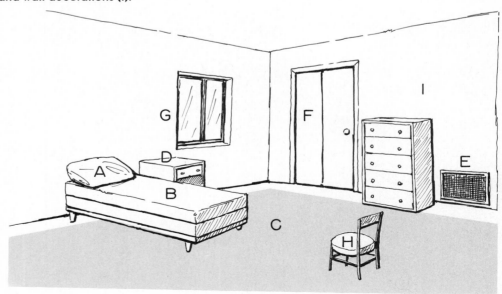

istered in several doses daily for prolonged periods, if necessary. Side effects are common though seldom severe in normal persons and generally may include drowsiness, lethargy, mucous membrane dryness, and occasionally, nausea, cramps, or light-headedness. However, because of these symptoms and a frequent impairment of depth perception, activities involving moving vehicles, dangerous machinery, or fine hand-eye coordination in general must be undertaken with care by those receiving antihistaminics. Recently, several effective newer agents that do not cross the blood-brain barrier have been shown to produce little or no sedation. In practice, several antihistaminic agents often must be tried in turn before an optimal (or even a satisfactory) one is identified, and the results of such trials defy prediction at the outset. In choosing drugs for comparison by individuals, it must be recalled that many marketed preparations are merely different *forms* of a few agents (e.g., chlorpheniramine) and that efficacy trials should compare *different* chemical species. Patients often report a waning of previous antihistaminic effectiveness, requiring substitution (or addition) of different agents.

Sympathomimetic amines offer additional benefit in allergic rhinitis and are often marketed in combinations with antihistaminic agents. Drugs including ephedrine, isoephedrine, and phenylpropanolamine act as mucosal decongestants and, by causing more or less psychomotor stimulation, can offset the sedative effects of antihistaminic agents. Whether orally administered sympathomimetic drugs *significantly* affect the release of mediator substances from tissue mast cells is unclear, although (opposing) beta- and alpha-adrenergic effects (see Chap. 10) both are possible. In addition, these agents produce side effects that may impair ocular, cardiac, gastrointestinal, and genitourinary function (see Chap. 10). The *topical* use of sympathomimetic agents as drops, sprays, and vapors is widespread and provides prompt mucosal shrinkage which is helpful in acute illness (e.g., bacterial sinusitis). Unfortunately, these preparations are easily obtained and frequently abused. With prolonged overuse, an irritant effect often supervenes so that each dose gives transient decongestion followed by a prolonged obstructive response, prompting further self-medication. In habituated persons, the resulting mucosal inflammation, or *rhinitis medicamentosa*, produces obdurate nasal stuffiness and a congested, or edematous, appearance. In approaching this problem, complete withdrawal of topical nasal medication is mandatory and, where possible, oral agents are substituted. In some cases, several weeks of topical nasal corticosteroid spray must be given to make this change tolerable. Choosing recently introduced agents such as beclomethasone and flunisolide, which are both locally effective and rapidly metabolized by the liver, offers considerable advantages over older dexamethasone sprays.

Intranasal steroids are useful also in suppressing the primary symptoms of allergic rhinitis but are preferred mainly for brief, seasonal periods of exquisite severity. In addition, systemic corticosteroids will suppress hay fever manifestations when other remedies have failed. However, the widespread side effects of these systemically active agents make their *chronic* administration for nasal allergy unacceptable.

Except for antibiotics, when indicated, very few additional drugs offer benefit to rhinitis sufferers. Aspirin in conventional oral doses may have limited value for occasional persons with allergic and nonallergic vasomotor rhinitis. Evidence is accumulating that cromolyn sodium (see Chap. 10) can attenuate manifestations of allergic rhinitis and conjunctivitis by appropriate topical application. However, the place of this drug and certain of its oral congeners in managing upper airway disease remains to be defined.

Immunotherapy (hyposensitization) continues to provide an important *allergen-specific* approach to the treatment of respiratory allergy. This procedure typically entails the subcutaneous injection of incremental doses of extracts of a recognized allergen over prolonged periods in an attempt to somehow modify clinical reactivity. After reaching an empirically indicated "maximum" level, this dose is maintained pending evaluation of symptoms, and adjustments in the program are carried out accordingly. Valid indications for immunotherapy may include allergic asthma, as well as allergic rhinitis or conjunctivitis that is inadequately controlled despite optimal avoidance measures and antihistaminic treatment. In each instance, sensitivity to *specific, inhalant* allergens must be confirmed, since any nonspecific benefits of injection treatment are unpredictable; food factors are approached by diet modification exclusively. A typical treatment schedule is illustrated in Fig. 9-11. Properly controlled clinical trials have confirmed the value of hyposensitization for grass and ragweed pollen and have suggested that tree pollen, animal dander, and house dust immunotherapy *may* be beneficial. Hyposensitization for other materials either has been shown to be valueless (e.g., for respiratory bacterial vaccines) or remains unstudied (e.g., for fungus extracts). Trials of pollen extracts have indicated also that (1) optimal symptom suppression is seen when the largest well-tolerated extract doses are given, (2) symptom suppression due to treatment may carry over to a subsequent year in which injections are withheld, and (3) a placebo, or inert material, given by injection may decrease symptoms in one-third to one-half of subjects in control groups, which reemphasizes the need for proper controls in evaluating treatment results.

The basis of the efficacy of immunotherapy remains unclear although several tissue effects that might promote benefit are known. It was initially assumed that the procedure induced active immunization against a pollen toxin, but this rationale has been entirely discredited. Subsequently, it has been postulated that immunotherapy might "turn off" specific IgE production. However, RAST values and skin test positivity often do not substantially decrease during extended successful treatment, and specific IgE values usually rise early in the injection sequence. The appearance in serum of IgG antibodies specific for the injected allergen is well documented, and these factors can compete with IgE for allergen, thus showing "blocking" capabilities. Although a general correlation between blocking antibody titer and clinical improvement is seen, the relationship is far from perfect, and exceptions (e.g., persons with

high titers and unabated rhinitis) imply that other factors must also contribute. Recently described elevations, with immunotherapy, of IgG and IgA (blocking) antibodies in respiratory tract secretions suggest an alternative mechanism of tissue effect. In addition, blood basophils from persons receiving high-dose immunotherapy have been noted to release progressively less histamine on allergen challenge in vitro and, in some cases, to become wholly unresponsive. The significance of this effect is not clear, and some workers have alleged that its allergen-specificity is questionable. At present, therefore, although the clinical value of hyposensitization for selected allergens is established, the responsible mechanisms are not; current evidence justifies major interest in the role of blocking factors, however.

Although serious, *long-term* adverse effects of immunotherapy are nowhere evident, significant transient local or systemic reactions can occur. Locally, redness, whealing, and tender swelling lasting up to 36 hours may develop if dosage is excessive. These reactions usu-

FIGURE 9-11

Dosage schedule form used at the Allergy Clinic of the University Hospital, Ann Arbor, for patients whose injection treatment will be administered by their personal physicians. The steps shown form a commonly useful sequence, although additional dilutions or dosage volumes may be desirable for specific persons.

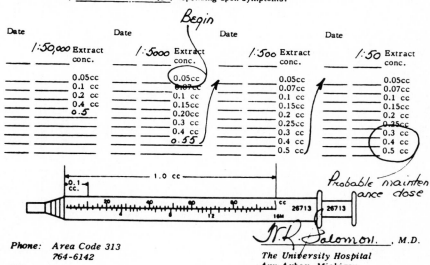

ally mandate a reduction in the amount of allergen next injected. However, their severity also may be decreased by care in wiping the needle with a sterile swab before injection to remove adhering extract and application of firm pressure to the site following injection to prevent retrograde dissection of fluid along the needle track. Acute systemic reactions often are preceded by increasingly prominent local swellings but may occur in their absence. Generalized reactions exemplify human anaphylaxis, but the reaction also may be accompanied by or confined to rhinitis and/or asthma symptoms; management has been described previously. Since extract should be given into a site sufficiently distal to allow placement of a proximal tourniquet, this opportunity also should be exploited. In addition, 0.1 to 0.2 ml of epinephrine is commonly introduced at the point of previous injection to slow allergen absorption. Although adverse reactions may occur capriciously, their risk increases with conditions that elevate cutaneous blood flow, including high environmental temperature, fever, physical exertion, hyperthyroidism, and pregnancy. Human error also is a factor. Such error may occur owing to misreading of previously recorded doses or of vial labels; confusion of persons with similar names commonly is implicated. In general, reactions that will require treatment have onset within 20 minutes following injection; therefore most clinics require their patients to remain quietly seated in a well-ventilated room for 15 to 20 minutes after they receive injections. The low but inescapable risk of systemic reactions and a corresponding need for rapid, complex treatment measures leave little justification for self-administration of extract by any patient.

At present, skin testing and most injection treatment are carried out with sterile, aqueous extracts containing, usually, an antimicrobial agent [e.g., phenol or thimerosal (Merthiolate)] and occasionally a protein stabilizer such as human serum albumin. Attempts to establish standards of biological activity for these materials have had limited success, although assays of defined allergens in ragweed and grass pollen extracts are now feasible as indicators of potency; other materials commonly are rated on a "weight-by-volume" basis. In this system, a 1:500 ragweed pollen extract is the solution resulting when one gram of defatted ragweed pollen is extracted under defined conditions in five hundred milliliters of fluid. Alternative approaches based on assays of total protein or total nitrogen are no more instructive. Comparisons of extract potency based upon ability to inhibit RAST carried out with standard reaginic serums appear feasible in the future. In addition, interest has become increasingly focused on therapeutic materials suitable for infrequent administration and combining low skin reactivity with prominent immunizing potency. Currently, alum-precipitated aqueous extracts are available with modestly long-acting properties, although local and systemic adverse reactions can occur. Directions of future work will emphasize the use of allergens aggregated by or absorbed to carriers as well as those chemically modified by agents such as formalin or glutaraldehyde.

QUESTIONS

Familiar allergic disorders: anaphylaxis and the atopic diseases

Directions: Answer the following questions on a separate sheet of paper.

1. Differentiate between hypersensitivity and sensitization in the context of immunologic events.
2. Contrast angioedema with lymphedema.
3. Describe the pathogenesis of an acute systemic (anaphylactic) reaction.
4. What accounts for differences among species in patterns of an anaphylactic response?
5. What are the necessary conditions for anaphylactic sensitization in human beings?
6. List three principal considerations which dominate the management of respiratory allergy as exemplified by allergic rhinitis.

Directions: Circle the letter preceding each item below that correctly answers the question. More than one answer may be correct.

7. Immunologic processes which are most clearly recognized as immunologic disease are reactions of:
   a. Delayed hypersensitivity *b.* Immediate hypersensitivity *c.* Both *a* and *b*. *d.* Neither *a* nor *b*
8. All of the following are important characteristics of clinical hypersensitivity (allergy) as an immunologic response *except:*
   a. Specificity—reaction is to a specific, exogenous antigen *b.* Response usually involves immunologic mechanisms *c.* Reaction is abnormal (inappropriate or damaging) *d.* Prior contact with a

specific substance (allergen) is not necessary to elicit a response

9. IgE antibody has specific affinity for:
   a. Mast cells   b. Neutrophils   c. Basophils
   d. Red blood cells

10. Which of the following characteristics may be associated with IgE?
    a. It is a tissue-fixing antibody associated with allergic rhinitis.   b. It participates in reactions leading to release of histamine.   c. It is involved in immunologically induced wheal-and-flare reactions   d. All of the above are associated with IgE.

11. The Fc fragment (crystallizable fragment) of antibodies is the portion of the immunoglobulin which involves the following activities:
    a. Activation of the complement pathway   b. Facilitation of the uptake by phagocytes of antigen-bound immunoglobulins   c. Combination with specific antigenic components   d. Determination of the tissue location of certain immunoglobulins

12. Which of the following immunoglobulin types is most important in the body's defense against pyogenic infections?
    a. IgA   b. IgE   c. IgG   d. IgM

13. Tissue effects of the classical complement pathway include all of the following except:
    a. Production of direct lesions in cell membranes   b. Lysis of target cells   c Release of transfer factor from sensitized lymphocytes   d. Attraction of leukocytes   e. Release of permeability-enhancing factors

14. Manifestations of acute systemic (anaphylactic) reaction include all of the following except:
    a. Pruritus of the scalp and palms of the hands   b. Eczema   c. Severe laryngeal edema and bronchial obstruction   d. Hypovolemic shock caused by exudation of fluid from the vascular compartment

15. All of the following statements about anaphylaxis are true except:
    a. It is a condition caused by an immunologic reaction   b. It is a potentially fatal condition   c. It is thought to be mediated mainly by IgG   d. Acute systemic reactions generally begin within minutes after introduction of an allergen

16. Important considerations to be observed in treating acute systemic (anaphylactic) reactions include which of the following?
    a. Maintaining a patent airway   b. Improving vascular or blood vessel integrity or intactness   c. Supporting the blood pressure   d. Promoting rapid absorption of the allergen   e. Administering antipruritic lotions to the skin

17. A 25-year-old male has collapsed following an intramuscular (IM) penicillin injection; he is unconscious, has generalized hives, and his blood pressure is 60/20. Initial treatment should be:
    a. IM, penicillinase   b. Intravenous (IV) adrenalin and IM diphenhydramine (Benadryl)   c. IV corticosteroids in normal saline solution   d. Subcutaneous adrenalin and IV saline solution e. IV corticosteroids and IM diphenhydramine

18. Common characteristics of the atopic state include:
    a. A strong family history of chronic bronchitis and emphysema   b. The occurrence of typical infantile eczema without evident precipitating allergens   c. The genetically inherited predisposition to become hypersensitive   d. Presence of numerous wheal-and-flare reactions on testing the skin with food and pollen extracts

19. The most prevalent atopic condition in North America among young adult populations is:
    a. Allergic asthma   b. Nasal allergy   c. Eczema   d. Gastrointestinal allergy

20. Jane, a 15-year-old female, presents with pruritus, repetitive sneezing, and watery profuse rhinorrhea. Her diagnosis is allergic rhinitis. Which of the following data would be most significant in diagnosing the allergen responsible for this allergic rhinitis?
    a. Positive reaction to an intradermal skin test   b. Clinical history of symptoms on exposure to a specific allergen in her home   c. Levels of total serum IgE   d. Predominance of basophils in nasal or lacrymal secretions

21. A 20-year-old male has a large wheal-and-flare reaction on skin testing with ragweed pollen extract; a comparable test with the diluent is nonreactive. He may be told, with confidence, that:
    a. He has large amounts of IgG-blocking antibody specific for ragweed pollen allergens in his blood   b. He has ragweed hay fever   c. He is immune to ragweed pollen and will never have difficulty related to it in the future   d. He has IgE antibodies specific for ragweed pollen allergens fixed at skin sites

22. Antihistaminic drugs:
    a. Prevent the release of histamine from mast cells   b. Prevent the release of histamine from macrophages   c. Are highly beneficial in treatment of severe asthma   d. At least partially control symptoms in a majority of patients with hay fever

23. Which of the following drugs should be immediately available when intracutaneous skin tests are being performed with atopic allergens?
    a. Epinephrine   *b.* Cortisone tablets   *c.* Horse serum   *d.* Antihistamine tablets

24. All of the following describe recognized effects of hyposensitization (immunotherapy) *except:*
    a. This causes an immediate decrease in IgE in the blood   *b.* This often causes an increase in IgG which may compete with IgE for antigens   *c.* Decreased histamine release from sensitized mast cells occurs with specific amounts of added allergen   *d.* Treated persons are able to tolerate progressively larger amounts of *injected* allergen

25. Injection treatment (hyposensitization) would be most appropriate for:
    a. A 30-year-old mother of three with severe wheezing due to a guinea pig present in the home for 3 months   *b.* A 60-year-old vice-president of IBM with angioedema following ingestion of abalone (and other snails)   *c.* A 30-year-old veterinarian with well-identified asthma due to dog dander   *d.* A 9-month-old infant with severe eczema known to be worsened by egg   *e.* A 20-year-old nursing student with grass and ragweed pollen hay fever, readily controlled with an antihistamine-decongestant drug preparation

26. Persons with seasonal allergic rhinitis or hay fever:
    a. Are less likely than normal to have had asthma or atopic dermatitis   *b.* Usually have other members in their family with atopic conditions   *c.* Develop sensitivity to penicillin in over 70 percent of cases   *d.* Typically wheeze with exposure to offending allergens in normal seasonal concentrations

27. John, a 19-year-old male, has had severe allergic reactions to insect stings (bee, wasp, hornet, and yellow jacket). Which of the following precautions *must* be followed to avoid a likely systemic reaction?
    a. He must avoid situations favored by stinging insects.   *b.* He must always have available and be able to self-administer preloaded syringes of epinephrine.   *c.* He must undergo hyposensitization therapy which includes injecting "whole-body" extracts of incriminated insects.   *d.* He should undergo incremental injections of dilutions of purified venoms.

Directions: Circle T if the statement is true and F if it is false. Correct the false statements.

28. T   F   Individuals normally have minute amounts of IgE present in their blood serum.

29. T   F   The distinctive feature of allergic rhinitis is that compatible symptoms appear or worsen predictably in response to specific exposures.

30. T   F   Strongly positive skin tests eliciting wheal-and-flare reactions provide assurance that symptoms of allergic respiratory conditions do arise from exposure to the allergens in question.

31. T   F   The preferred method of skin testing for clinical evaluation of respiratory allergy is to inject highly concentrated aqueous extracts of allergenic material intracutaneously.

32. T   F   The radioallergosorbent test (RAST) is used to measure allergen-specific IgE using venous blood in vitro.

CHAPTER 1

BRONCHIAL ASTHMA— ALLERGIC AND OTHERWISE

OBJECTIVES

At the completion of this chapter you should be able to:

1. Formulate a definition of bronchial asthma.
2. Explain the pattern of ventilatory dysfunction observed in asthma.
3. Describe the relationship of atopy to bronchial asthma and distinguish other *clinical* forms.
4. Relate autonomic innervation to the abnormal bronchial lability that is characteristic of asthmatic persons.
5. Describe the relationship of viral and respiratory infection with asthma in both children and adults.
6. Describe the tissue changes associated with *uncomplicated* asthma.
7. Identify for distressed asthmatic patients the signs and symptoms related to their condition.
8. Assess the significance of exercise in provoking an asthma attack.
9. Discuss the relationship of the signs and symptoms that simulate bronchial asthma.
10. Explain the measures used to differentiate asthma from other obstructive airway problems.
11. Identify for allergic aspergillosis the pathogenesis, signs and symptoms, treatment, and prognosis.
12. Compare chronic bronchitis, pulmonary emphysema, and bronchial asthma (unassociated with atopic factors) in terms of pathologic anatomy, symptoms, and diagnosis.
13. Explain the rationale for long-term treatment considerations in bronchial asthma.
14. Identify the drugs, mode of administration, dosages, side effects, and range of serum levels used in both acute and long-term management of asthma.
15. State the problems related to self-administration of adrenergic agents.
16. Describe the appropriate urgent treatment of asthma.
17. Identify for severe asthma or status asthmaticus the signs and symptoms, complications, treatment, and prognosis.

Asthma is a clinically defined condition marked by recurrent, discrete episodes of *reversible* bronchial narrowing, separated by periods in which ventilation approaches normality. These transient events are readily provoked in asthma-prone subjects by a variety of stimuli; this denotes a state of *bronchial hyperreactivity*.

Tissue changes in uncomplicated asthma (Fig. 10-1) are confined to bronchial airways and consist of smooth-muscle spasm, mucosal edema, and hypersecretion of viscid mucus. Mobilization of luminal secretions is compromised by airway narrowing and by the shedding of ciliated bronchial epithelial cells that normally subserve the clearance of mucus.

VENTILATORY DYSFUNCTION

In asthma a fundamental inability to achieve normal rates of air flow during respiration (especially expiration) results in flattening of the curve relating total expired volume and time (Fig. 10-2). Since many narrowed airways cannot fill and empty quickly enough, there is uneven lung aeration and a loss of the normal spatial matching of ventilation and pulmonary blood flow (Fig. 10-3). Depending on their severity, these defects may produce no symptoms or merely a sense of tracheal ir-

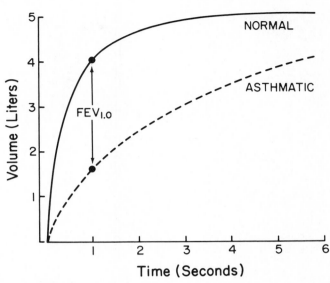

FIGURE 10-2
Forced expiratory curves produced by two 20-year-old males—one normal and one with moderately severe asthma. The slope of these curves at any point is equivalent to flow rate. An inability to move air quickly is the major ventilatory defect in asthma.

FIGURE 10-1
Bronchial changes in chronic asthma. This small bronchus shows increased width of the epithelial basement membrane (arrow) and partial loss of mucosal cells. The lumen (A) is filled with mucus and cellular debris, while the submucosa (B) is densely infiltrated with inflammatory cells including many eosinophils. (From J. M. Sheldon, R. G. Lovell, and K. P. Mathews, *A Manual of Clinical Allergy*, 2d ed., Saunders, Philadelphia, 1967.)

ritation; in other cases respiratory distress may be intolerable. Airstream turbulence and the vibrations of bronchial mucus lead to audible wheezing during asthmatic attacks; however, this physical sign also is prominent in other obstructive airway problems. Distressed asth-

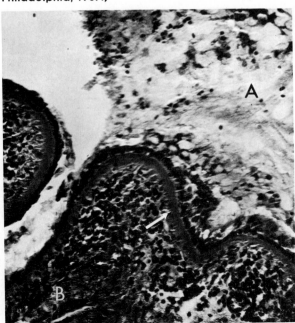

FIGURE 10-3
Mismatching of ventilation and perfusion in asthma. Owing to narrowing of its bronchus, alveolus A does not properly oxygenate its share of pulmonary artery blood; B functions normally. As a result of these contributions, average O_2 saturation of pulmonary venous blood is abnormally low. In asthma, a shift of blood flow from A- to B-type alveoli occurs secondarily but is usually quite incomplete. Furthermore, hyperventilation of B with room air cannot compensate for the "shunting" at A.

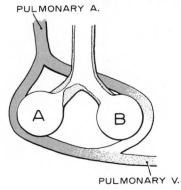

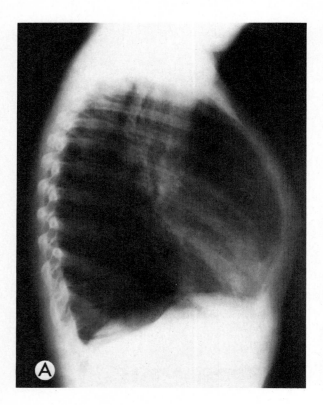

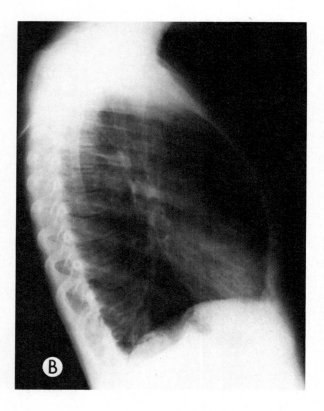

matic people commonly breathe more rapidly than normal (even though this tends to increase resistance to airflow) and avoid unnecessary activity. In addition, the chest assumes a position of maximum inspiration, which is voluntarily achieved at first and serves to dilate the airways. Later this appearance is sustained owing to incomplete emptying of alveoli, which results in progressive hyperinflation of the thorax (Fig. 10-4). In *uncomplicated* asthma, cough is prominent only as attacks resolve, when it serves to clear accumulated secretions. Between bouts of asthma the patient is typically free of wheezes and symptoms, although heightened bronchial reactivity and defects in ventilation remain demonstrable by special techniques. However, with chronicity, symptomless interludes may disappear, which leads to a state of continuous asthma—often with secondary infection.

Asthmatic people as a group, both those with and those without allergic mechanisms, share an abnormal bronchial lability which promotes airway narrowing by many factors which have no effect on normal persons. The basis of this tendency remains unclear; however, asthmatic airways behave as though their beta-adrenergic innervation (which helps preserve airway patency) is incompetent, and much evidence suggests that, at least functionally, partial blockage of beta-adrenergic receptors exists in typical asthma. Without adequate bronchodilator tone, bronchoconstrictor influences, known to be mediated normally by parasympathetic (cholinergic) and alpha-adrenergic pathways, would tend to predominate. In clinical practice, the bronchial lability of asthmatic patients may be confirmed by demonstrating their brisk airway obstructive responses to extremely low concentrations of inhaled histamine and methacholine. (The latter is a substance with activity resembling that of acetylcholine.) Related mechanisms probably contribute to the bouts of asthma that often follow inhalation of cold air as well as exposure to myriad mists, dusts, and volatile irritants. Poorly understood nervous pathways are available also to mediate airway closure in response to psychic stimuli, which commonly worsen symptoms in both adults and children. (Asthma due *solely* to emotional factors is exceptionally rare, however.) Reflex pathways promoting bronchospasm with forced chest deflation are also especially effective in asthmatic persons and are activated by maneuvers such as laughing, blowing up a balloon, or providing a full expiration for ventilatory testing.

FIGURE 10-4

Hyperinflation of the chest shown by an 8-year-old boy with asthma. One X-ray (A) was taken during severe status asthmaticus which later required mechanical ventilation. (Note especially the broad space between the heart and sternum.) The other film (B) was taken during a symptom-free interlude 4 months later and shows far less severe changes.

Asthma must be distinguished from two conditions described in detail in Chap. 34. These are *chronic* bronchitis, marked by continuous bronchial hypersection, and *emphysema*, in which loss of supporting lung tissues allows severe airway narrowing to occur with expiration. Although atopy is readily implicated in many instances of bronchial asthma, a substantial number of asthmatics lack demonstrable allergic factors even after exhaustive study. Such persons, including many infants as well as middle-aged and older adults, are often said to have "intrinsic" asthma, although their problem is more properly "idiopathic" (i.e., unexplained).

A subset of adults with idiopathic asthma also manifest nasal polyps, recurrent sinusitis, and severe airway obstructive responses to *aspirin* in various combinations. Less frequently, other nonsteroidal anti-inflammatory drugs (e.g., ibuprofen and indomethacin) or the FDA-approved food coloring tartrazine (Yellow No. 5) also precipitate severe attacks in these patients. Moderate asthma is often persistent in these patients even when recognized offenders are avoided, however, and prominent vasomotor rhinitis frequently ushers in the disease. A willingness to accept the patient's report of respiratory distress after aspirin is essential, since *no* safe confirmatory test is available.

Flares of asthma commonly accompany viral or bacterial respiratory infections and may progress in severity, ultimately requiring inpatient care. Where responsible pathogens have been sought in childhood asthmatic patients, rhinovirus and parainfluenza virus infections have been especially implicated. The presence of significant secondary infection may be manifested by fever, purulent expectoration, elevated white blood cell count, or recovery of pathogens from sputum; however, often persistent asthma provides the *only* signal. Many children with infection-triggered asthma in preschool years go on to develop classic nasal allergy or allergic (atopic) asthma in later life. However, there are few indications that microbial sensitivity is responsible for asthma accompanying infection. Rather, since invading organisms frequently destroy already compromised ciliated epithelium and localize agents of inflammation in labile bronchi, their adverse effect on asthma is predictable. In addition, animal studies have suggested that microbial substances may further weaken already inadequate beta-adrenergic activity.

Many severely asthmatic patients experience increased wheezing and dyspnea (abnormal shortness of breath) promptly with exertion of any intensity. In addition, a specific form of exercise-induced asthma (EIA) often is noted in which, following several minutes of brisk activity and, often, well after its termination, significant bronchospasm occurs. EIA is most commonly evident in children and characteristically appears in subjects symptomless before beginning exertion. Although a *minimum* total energy expenditure is necessary, above this critical level the risk of symptoms varies with the type of activity; generally, at comparable work levels, sprint running is most and swimming least conducive to EIA. Current evidence suggests airway cooling due to evaporation of moisture from the mucosa as an important determinant of EIA.

DIFFERENTIAL DIAGNOSIS

Since bronchial asthma is an abnormal *pattern* of response rather than a discrete disease, differential diagnosis requires attention to the clinical form and major determinants of this syndrome,* as well as to its distinction from other obstructive airway problems. Rarely, persons who overbreathe with psychic stress or children with noisy respiration due to large adenoids, a short neck, or a "floppy" epiglottis are suspected of having asthma. In adults, at least, this possibility often may be excluded by demonstrating a normal test response to inhalation of methacholine, while the childhood problems usually are clarified by careful examination and resolve, in time, with developmental changes. However, at any age, the impaction of a foreign body or growth of a localized tumor in the bronchi (or larynx) may lead to *diffuse* wheezing, simulating asthma. More typical recurrent symptoms may be encountered in certain forms of diffuse vascular inflammation (vasculitis) and with secreting carcinoid tumors when these are metastatic to the liver (see also Chap. 38).

Severe airway obstruction, capable of producing respiratory failure and associated with fever, is characteristic of the bronchiolitis of small children. This illness is often recurrent and appears frequently owing to infection with respiratory syncytial virus. Severe local inflammation promotes closure of the small, distal airways involved, although humoral immune mechanisms also may contribute to this process.

A striking picture occurs in occasional allergic asthmatic people owing to carriage of the fungus *Aspergillus fumigatus* in their bronchial lumina. Although there is little or no tissue invasion, this organism excites an intense, apparently immunologically directed, inflammatory response with fever, pulmonary infiltrates on chest x-ray, and prominent tissue and peripheral blood eosinophilia. Affected persons experience fatigue, weight loss, severe asthma, and expectoration of bronchial

---

*A syndrome is a set of signs and symptoms that occur together and characterize a specific illness.

mucus plugs that may show the fungus as minute, dark growth points. Immediate wheal-and-flare skin reactivity to the fungus organism is striking, and *total* serum IgE levels are extremely high. IgG-precipitating antibodies with specificity for this organism also are demonstrable in over 70 percent of this *allergic bronchopulmonary aspergillosis* group. Suppression of the disease with adequate doses of adrenal cortical steroids (see later in this chapter) is feasible and also essential if irreversible bronchial damage (bronchiectasis) is to be averted (Fig. 10-5).

Especially in older adults, chronic bronchitis and pulmonary emphysema often require distinction from bronchial asthma when the latter is unassociated with atopic factors. *Chronic bronchitis* denotes a prolonged and often slowly progressive condition of bronchial inflammation and hypersecretion manifested by cough and sputum production extending over months and years. In addition, a proportion of chronic bronchitic people also experience episodic bouts of airway obstruction—in effect, a form of idiopathic asthma—late in the disease. *Pulmonary emphysema*, by contrast, presents prominent, *irreversible* anatomic changes with diffuse loss of the alveolar walls that normally exert outward traction on the bronchi that they surround. Deprived of this source of support, the airways tend to close in expiration wherever pressure outside their walls exceeds that within. Affected persons develop predictable periods of dyspnea and wheezing with any increase (usually exertional) in respiratory effort rather than experiencing *spontaneous attacks*, typical of asthma, which

readily begin at rest or, often, during sleep. Because the prognosis of emphysema is quite unfavorable, with variably increasing disability the rule, this diagnosis cannot be proposed lightly. However, since, with recurrent infection, asthmatic individuals also may acquire chronic bronchitis, and severely bronchitic patients ultimately may show emphysema as well, a sharp distinction between these disorders may be impossible at times. On the other hand, when chest hyperinflation, evident on x-ray or physical evaluation, is casually (and erroneously) designated "emphysema," a grave stigma may be implied without basis. In fact, the hyperinflation and resulting thoracic deformity of young asthmatics may be totally reversed with successful treatment, leaving them anatomically and functionally normal.

LONG-TERM TREATMENT CONSIDERATIONS IN BRONCHIAL ASTHMA

The protracted course typical of asthma and its associated state of bronchial hyperreactivity determine a chronic need for treatment measures. Where atopic factors are evident, efforts to reduce exposure to and institution of immunotherapy for selected inhalant allergens (see Chap. 9) have established value and, again, deserve attention. Avoidance of irritants—especially tobacco smoke—and prompt treatment of unresolved bacterial respiratory infections are frequently overlooked, although of major benefit to asthmatic people generally.

Perfumes, aerosol cleaners and cosmetics, strong cooking odors, solvents, and paint fumes also pose potentially avoidable risks that must be appreciated. Cold air is an additional bronchoconstrictor influence that may be mitigated by wearing a scarf or gauze mask over the nose and mouth as a heat exchanger. Adding moisture to dry indoor air (to maintain a relative humidity of at least 30 percent) is desirable, although poorly maintained humidifiers can become sources of microbial aerosols. In addition, programs of regular medication can effectively reduce bronchial lability and thereby raise the threshold for obstructive airway responses.

At present, the maintenance of adequate blood levels of theophylline is a first objective in the drug treatment of bronchial asthma (Fig. 10-6). The desired effect of theophylline seems to be exerted by its inhibition of intracellular enzymes (viz., phosphodiesterases) which otherwise would degrade the nucleotide 3'5'-cyclic adenosine monophosphate (cyclic AMP). This substance mediates beta-adrenergic effects in many tissues,

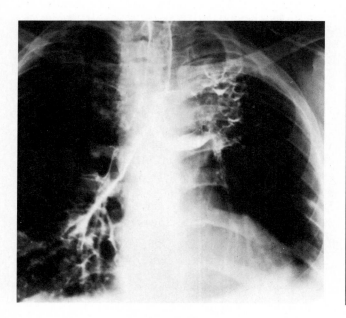

FIGURE 10-5
Saccular (saclike) bronchiectasis of the left upper lobe demonstrated by bronchography in an adult with long-standing allergic bronchopulmonary asperigillosis. Bronchi in lower lung fields are essentially uninvolved. (Film courtesy of Dr. Terry Silver.)

and, as intracellular levels of cyclic AMP rise in bronchial smooth muscle, relaxation (a beta effect) is notably increased. Cyclic AMP levels also strongly modify the allergen-induced release of inflammatory mediators [e.g., histamine, leukotrienes (SRS-A), and ECF-A] from IgE-sensitized mast cells or blood basophils (Figs. 9-1 and 10-6). In these systems, *increasing* cyclic AMP levels serve to *reduce* mediator liberation and thereby provide an additional mode of effectiveness for both theophylline and direct beta-adrenergic agonists in bronchial asthma.

Serum levels of theophylline correlate closely with the occurrence of favorable or of toxic effects. Toxicity is uncommon below a concentration of 20 μg/ml, but its risk rises progressively above this point; similarly, favorable effects generally are suboptimal at levels below 10 μg/ml. Serum levels in the desired range of 10 to 20 μg/ml are usually achieved by administering doses of 5 to 6 mg of anhydrous theophylline per kilogram of body weight every 6 hours to adults receiving rapidly absorbed preparations; children require proportionately *larger* doses. However, individuals may differ as much as fivefold in their rates of hepatic metabolism of this drug. As a result, regular doses well above or below 5 to 6 mg/kg may be essential for a *safe* therapeutic effect. Many slowly released oral theophylline preparations have been introduced; they allow successful dosing twice (or even just once) daily. In general, these also require lower 24-hour drug totals to maintain stable serum levels than do more rapidly absorbed formulations. "Long acting" theophylline preparations promote improved patient compliance and promise to become a standard form of therapy.

Theophylline administration must be approached cautiously—especially where liver function is im-

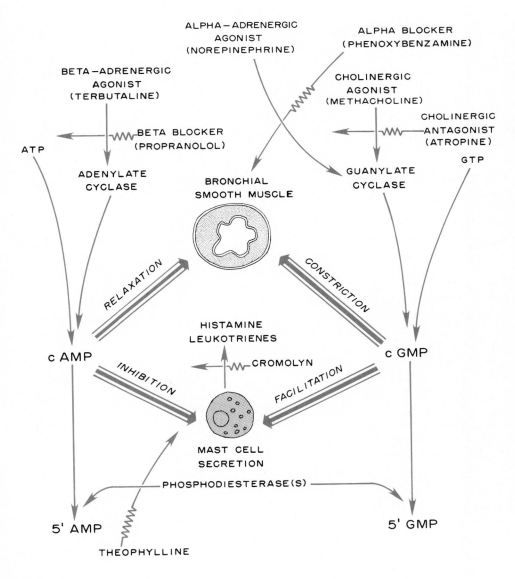

FIGURE 10-6

Actions of drugs that affect bronchial patency either directly (upper portion) or by modifying mediator substance release from mast cells (below). Smooth lines indicate potentiation of an effect; wavy lines signify inhibitory influences. The central importance and opposing effects of cyclic AMP and GMP deserve special attention. Cyclic AMP levels are increased by beta agonists acting on adenylate cyclase and by inhibition of phosphodiesterase effect (e.g., by theophylline). Cyclic GMP levels are increased by cholinergic agents (e.g., methacholine) and possibly by alpha-adrenergic agents. Effects of theophylline and other drugs on cyclic GMP–active phosphodiesterases are not clear. Bronchoconstrictive effects of alpha agents may reflect inhibition of cyclic AMP or promotion of GMP synthesis. The mechanism(s) of corticosteroid effect is uncertain but is associated with increased responsiveness to beta-adrenergic agents, among other effects.

paired—since convulsions, cardiac rhythm disturbance, and/or hypotension may be the first sign(s) of serious overdosage. More commonly, headache, nausea, vomiting, diarrhea (which is rarely bloody), or muscle tremor are the principal manifestations of toxicity. In addition, occasional patients (especially children) may show hyperactivity, mental depression, or misperception of their surroundings at relatively modest doses.

Direct assay of the serum theophylline level has become increasingly available recently as a rational guide for dosage determination. Elixirs of theophylline offer more rapid absorption, facilitating the acute treatment of asthmatic attacks, although adequate blood levels are maintained *only briefly*. Theophylline salts such as aminophylline (theophylline ethylenediamine) also may be given rectally as aqueous solutions or in cocoa butter suppositories; however, absorption is erratic, and this route is rarely preferred. In addition, sterile solutions of aminophylline are widely used for intravenous treatment of serious asthma (see later) but cause intense pain and tissue injury if injected by other routes.

Drugs with intrinsic beta-adrenergic effects continue to be useful for both acute and long-term management of asthma (although most also manifest a measure of alpha activity). The effectiveness of these agents is thought to reflect *direct* stimulation of an enzyme, adenylate cyclase, which promotes the synthesis of 3′5′ cyclic AMP (Fig. 10-6). Cyclic AMP-induced effects (i.e., relaxation of bronchial smooth muscle and inhibition of mediator release from mast cells and basophils) are, therefore, shared by beta-adrenergic agents with theophylline, and additive effects of these two groups of drugs often result when they are administered together. Epinephrine, by subcutaneous injection, remains the most widely useful agent for relief of brief, acute asthmatic attacks. A dose of 0.3 ml of a 1:1000 solution is appropriate for most adults, while 0.022 ml/kg may be used (up to 0.3 ml) for small children. The therapeutic effect of aqueous epinephrine is maximum 10 to 15 minutes after injection and essentially gone after 1 hour. Therefore successive injections at 20-minute intervals are often employed to obtain a gradual, incremental effect.*

Beta-adrenergic drugs are available for inhalation as well as for oral administration. Unlike epinephrine, these agents are commonly self-administered by pa-

tients, which creates a potential for voluntary overdosage. Unwanted side effects *do* vary among these drugs; however, all tend to produce sleeplessness, psychomotor stimulation, and muscle tremor as dosage levels rise. In addition, loss of appetite, constipation, and difficulty in urination can result—especially in the elderly—although patients rarely associate these difficulties with their medications. Since beta agonists (e.g., isoproterenol) have both desired (beta-2) effects on airways and undesired (beta-1) side effects, especially cardiac effects, interest in agents with only beta-2 activity has been keen. Beta-1 effects tend to raise the force of cardiac contraction, elevate heart rate, and increase the activity of abnormal foci of electrical activity in the myocardium and conducting system. These effects are potentially harmful in many types of cardiovascular disease and may increase blood flow to poorly ventilated areas of lung, resulting in a *lowering* of arterial oxygen tension. Recently introduced agents [metaproterenol, terbutaline, and albuterol (Salbutamol)] appear to impose lower cardiovascular side effects than do longer-established remedies such as ephedrine and isoproterenol.

Problems related to self-administration of adrenergic agents have arisen, especially with aerosol preparations administered either from pressurized cannisters or hand bulb-driven nebulizers. Several agents are available by this route for rapid relief of transient asthma attacks, and at times aerosol use virtually becomes a conditioned reflex. Such behavior rapidly leads to overdosage—especially when asthma is severe and only barely responsive to adrenergic agents. Aerosol users are prone to side effects as described above and may experience dangerous disturbances of cardiac rhythm associated with hypoxia and toxicity of fluorinated hydrocarbons (viz., Freons) used as gaseous propellants. In addition (Fig. 10-7) protracted *overuse* of nebulizers often leads to temporarily altered bronchial reactivity in which inhalation of the drug induces brief (about 5 to 10 minutes) improvement followed by a sustained obstructive response. In persons who respond in this way, severe, sustained asthma may improve promptly when aerosols are *stopped*. These concerns mandate careful patient selection and close professional control of nebulizers. Instruction of all patients in the correct use especially of pressurized units will also promote more favorable results. The delivery port should be positioned about two finger breadths from the open lips and the unit activated early in inspiration. Connectors that slow aerosol velocity may be used to improve airway penetration.

Especially in controlling *allergic* (extrinsic, atopic) asthma, regular use of disodium cromoglycate (cromolyn sodium) may provide a valuable supplement, or rarely, an alternative to conventional bronchodilator drugs. Both the structure and tissue effects of cromolyn are unique among antiasthmatic agents; indeed, inhibition of mediator release from allergen-challenged, sen-

---

*Efforts to obtain an epinephrine product with prolonged activity have been only partially successful. Sus-Phrine is widely used for this purpose and has superseded intramuscular epinephrine in oil. Recently interest has shifted to the sustained effects of newer injected agents such as terbutaline.

sitized mast cells remains its only established effect. In addition, this agent may block phosphodiesterases (in the manner of theophylline) or suppress airway lability by other means. Oral absorption of cromolyn is poor, and its local tissue effects predominate. The drug is administered, in 20-mg doses, by inhalation of the dry powder in a lactose carrier or as a nebulized solution. Cromolyn substantially blocks obstructive airway responses to aerosolized allergen extracts inhaled under test conditions by sensitive subjects and, remarkably, also prevents anticipated exercise-induced asthma in many persons. Regular treatment with cromolyn often reduces the overall asthma burden, especially benefiting young allergic persons; however, improvement has been observed even in some with adult-onset, idiopathic disease. Cromolyn is without value in treating established attacks of asthma and often must be withheld until acute symptom flares have been resolved. As with other inhaled medications, the delivery unit must be directed toward the pharynx, and the patient is instructed to take a deep breath, pausing briefly at peak inspiration before exhaling slowly.

Adrenal cortical steroids have proved to be extremely effective antiasthmatic drugs. However, in view of their potential side effects, these agents are reserved for symptoms not otherwise controllable by a combination of safer measures. The anti-inflammatory properties of steroids and their ability to increase the tissue effects of beta-adrenergic agents are well documented; however, additional effects may contribute to their antiasthmatic potency. These drugs are especially helpful when given in high-dose "bursts" for brief periods to terminate sustained, epinephrine-resistant asthma but

also may be required in long-term, outpatient programs. When used chronically, the *minimum* steroid dose required to maintain tolerable function and comfort is the one appropriate. In many persons, corticosteroid control of asthma may be maintained at a lower cost in side effects by administering medication on alternate days (qod). For this purpose, relatively short-acting agents (e.g., prednisone) are especially appropriate in single, early morning doses. Although *several times* the daily drug requirement may be necessary on alternate days there usually is a lessening of somatic side effects, including growth retardation in children. In addition, comparable control of symptoms is potentially possible using steroids on alternate days, with *less* suppression of the patient's adrenal cortical function as reflected by levels of serum cortisol measured 48 hours after medication. However, in a small number of steroid-dependent asthmatic people, drugs on alternate days, in any reasonable dose, will not suffice.

Corticosteroids also may be given by inhalation to achieve a predominantly local bronchial effect; currently, beclomethasone dipropionate is the preferred preparation in doses of up to 100 mg, 4 times a day. The addition of beclomethasone may confer success on an otherwise inadequate program lacking oral corticosteroids, or it may reduce the steroid dose required daily or on alternate days for control of asthma. Overly aggressive treatment with beclomethasone by aerosol has led to pharyngeal irritation and a predisposition to oropharyngeal *Candida* infections. In addition, excessively rapid withdrawal of systemic steroids when beclomethasone is begun may precipitate adrenal cortical insufficiency and permit a sudden flare of previously suppressed inflammatory problems (e.g., allergic rhinitis and rheumatoid arthritis).

Few additional medications have proven merit in managing long-term asthma. Antihistaminic drugs rarely are beneficial—even in allergic asthma—and, by their drying effect on secretions, may compound the problem of sputum mobilization when airway obstruction is severe. The expectorant properties of iodides and

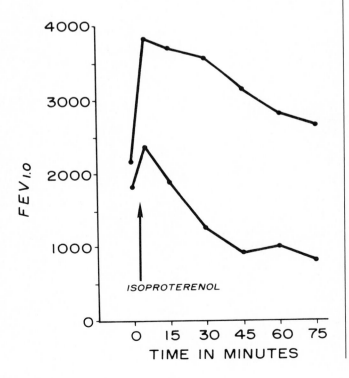

FIGURE 10-7

Responses to nebulized isoproterenol of a 23-year-old person with chronic asthma. The lower curve was obtained after 5 months of isoproterenol overuse with up to 30 inhalations per day; a brief rise in $FEV_{1.0}$ followed by a sustained fall is shown. The upper curve is a response to isoproterenol after 6 months of abstinence from the drug. It shows a normal (therapeutic) $FEV_{1.0}$ rise. The $FEV_{1.0}$ (or volume of air produced in the first second of a forced expiration) is a convenient and widely used test variable.

glyceryl guaiacolate (guaifenesin) remain controversial at doses that do not produce gastrointestinal irritation uniformly. In addition, unpredictable adverse responses to iodides may include painful parotid swelling ("iodide mumps"), prolonged fever, worsening of acne, and the appearance of other skin rashes. Benefits of simple systemic hydration should not be overlooked when sputum mobilization is a problem, and many mild asthma attacks may be curtailed if the patient sits calmly, breathes slowly, and drinks small portions of a warm liquid. Theoretical considerations also have focused interest upon alpha-adrenergic and cholinergic *antagonists* as possible bronchodilators. Several reports also have suggested the safety and efficacy of inhaled atropine; however, the antiasthmatic potential and practical usefulness of these drugs remain to be established.

The treatment approach to severe asthma

Although proper management can assure a good prognosis for most asthmatics, flares of the disease *do* occur, requiring hospitalization and rarely resulting in fatalities. A sustained increase in symptoms often follows re-

spiratory infection or the sudden withdrawal of a necessary suppressive medication; nebulizer abuse is sometimes crucial. However, allergen exposure *alone* rarely precipitates hospitalization.

Medical aid is often sought only after many days of increasing symptoms. During this period, poor fluid and calorie intake coupled with increased respiratory work and fluid loss may produce significant dehydration and metabolic acidosis as well as augmented bronchial mucus plugging. As previously emphasized, the extent of airway obstruction is not uniform and, despite vascular compensation, this leads to an imperfect matching of ventilation and blood flow in local areas of lung. As a result of these disparities, portions of the pulmonary blood flow escape aeration, which produces hypoxia and tends to impede CO_2 clearance. The deficit for CO_2 is overcome readily by the asthmatic person's respiratory effort, which can clear this readily diffusible gas by hyperventilating a *minority* of adequately perfused alveoli. Since hyperventilation typically is present, the partial pressure of CO_2 (P_{CO_2}) in arterial blood is often *below* the normal value (40 mmHg) with asthma of mild or moderate severity. A rise to normal or elevated P_{CO_2} levels, therefore, signifies that an advanced and perilous stage of obstruction (and of ventilation-perfusion mismatching) has been reached. Similar compensation is not possible even transiently for deficient O_2 uptake; as a result, arterial P_{O_2} values fall progressively as asthma worsens. Substantial increases in respiratory work compound these defects by markedly raising the O_2 cost of breathing and its penalty in CO_2 production. Ultimately, ventilation may not suffice even for the metabolic needs of the respiratory system. Figure 10-8 sum-

FIGURE 10-8

Changes in the work of breathing as well as in arterial pH, P_{O_2}, and P_{CO_2} observed in asthmatic patients with increasingly severe airway obstruction (left to right). Hyperventilation is adequate to decrease P_{CO_2} and raise pH until airway narrowing and plugging are severe.

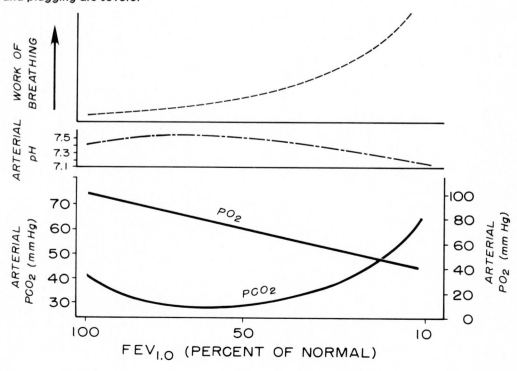

marizes changes observed in several parameters during increasingly severe asthma.

Epinephrine administration remains an appropriate first step in the urgent treatment of asthma, although inhaled beta-agents (e.g., metaproterenol, albuterol) often are equally effective. Standard amounts may be given subcutaneously at 20-minute intervals for a gradual incremental effect; however, if three or, at most, four such sequential doses fail, other measures must be substituted. Epinephrine-fast asthma often yields to intravenous aminophylline, although oral theophyllines (including hydroethanolic preparations) rarely suffice. Since many hours of self-medication with ephedrinelike drugs or with theophylline as tablets, elixirs, and suppositories may have occurred, an estimate of *residual* drug effects is mandatory. Where possible, rapid determination of theophylline serum levels can be used to predict dosage requirements initially. Persons without theophylline "on board" may receive 5 to 6 mg/kg of the drug intravenously by manual injection over at least 10 minutes, or by a "drip" infusion. Care will minimize instances of vomiting, hypotension, and seizures; however, a treatment facility must be prepared to handle these side effects promptly. Severe asthma, persistent for at least 24 hours, which is not substantially benefited by optimal doses of epinephrine and theophylline is often termed *status asthmaticus*. This condition presents a serious threat to life and should prompt intensive *inpatient* care.

Most hospitalized asthmatic patients require supplementary hydration to replace water deficits which may amount to several liters. The oral route rarely is adequate to achieve this, and a significant risk of aspiration must be faced unless fluids and medication are given parenterally to patients with air hunger. Without supplementary oxygen, hypoxemia is present almost uniformly in status asthmaticus and should be corrected to a level of at least 70 mmHg following initial arterial blood gas determinations. Supplementary humidified oxygen is best provided by 24 percent or 28 percent Venti-mask (Fig. 10-9) or, lacking these units, by nasal prongs.

Where bronchial unresponsiveness to epinephrine has been confirmed, this agent is withheld initially, although some patients may benefit from regular doses of inhaled adrenergic agents. However, aminophylline remains the mainstay of bronchodilator therapy, and after an initial "priming" dose of 5 to 6 mg/kg, this amount is given by continuous drip during each succeeding 6- to 8-hour period. Appropriate dosage adjustments are facilitated by determining serum theophylline levels. In addition, the need for antibiotic drugs must be decided after appropriate cultures are obtained.

Adrenal cortical steroids may be lifesaving in status asthmaticus and are usually begun if significant improvement is not evident within several hours of admission. High doses are given promptly also to those who have *required* steroids either to terminate previous bouts of severe asthma or, within the previous 6 to 9 months, as a regular outpatient medication. Preparations of hydrocortisone or methylprednisolone for intravenous infusion are preferred, although even with these, several hours often are required for initial therapeutic effects.

A favorable outcome in status asthmaticus often hinges on the willingness of responsible personnel to monitor the patient's condition closely, to recognize deterioration promptly, and to anticipate problems. Prominent complications can include pneumothorax, pneumomediastinum, aspiration, drug toxicity or idiosyncrasy, and cardiac failure or rhythm disturbance. Widespread plugging of airways may develop rapidly; it is manifested by a *decrease* in wheezing—but also by distant breath sounds over affected areas (an ominous combination). Obvious deterioration often is heralded

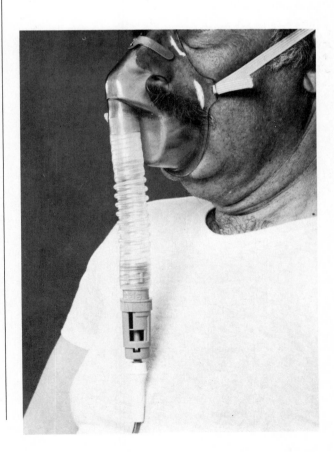

FIGURE 10-9
Variable concentration oxygen mask, utilizing a venturi effect, is a useful device for controlled O$_2$ administration. With this particular device, inspired O$_2$ concentrations of between 30 and 55 percent may be chosen.

by drowsiness, confusion, and decreased muscle tone, as well as by a flagging of respiratory effort signaling general physical exhaustion. This situation readily leads to inadequate alveolar ventilation with mounting hypoxia and rising arterial levels of CO_2. The clinical state and arterial P_{CO_2} correlate closely, and an *upward trend* is disquieting even though the absolute value may be normal (i.e., 40 mmHg) or only minimally elevated. When P_{CO_2} levels exceeding 55 mmHg are encountered, despite a period of optimal treatment, they commonly signify a need for mechanical ventilation to reestablish adequate gas transfer. A volume-cycled respirator is usually chosen for this purpose after placement of a *soft*, cuffed endotracheal tube; tracheostomy rarely is required. Details of respirator care are beyond the scope of this discussion. Ventilatory assistance in status asthmaticus usually is needed for only 24 to 60 hours, when improvement engendered by bronchodilators, steroids, antibiotics, etc., usually has become evident.

For gravely ill asthmatic children, prolonged, carefully controlled, intravenous (IV) infusion of isoproterenol (Isuprel) has been proposed as an alternative to conventional measures, and, in skilled hands, this approach often can obviate mechanical ventilation. However, IV isoproterenol carries a prohibitive risk of cardiovascular complications, including arrhythmias, in those beyond adolescence, and its place, if any, in treating children remains to be defined.

For many inpatients with severe asthma, attaining an audibly clear chest is a realistic and useful predischarge goal, even though ventilatory test results (expiratory time, 1-second forced expiratory volume, maximum midexpiratory flow rate, etc.) may remain somewhat abnormal; in others, irreversible bronchopulmonary changes may preclude a wheeze-free state. In either case, intensive treatment is continued until the anticipated maximum benefit is manifest, and then preparations are made for an outpatient program. During recovery bronchial responsiveness to epinephrine generally reappears, and adrenergic agents (e.g., injected Sus-Phrine or terbutaline every 8 hours) may be reutilized. Sputum production often increases during recovery; however, clearance of secretions may remain difficult despite optimal hydration and use of iodides or glyceryl guaiacolate (which have equivocal expectorant properties). Chest physiotherapy (viz., repetitive manual percussion of the chest with postural drainage) is available now in most hospitals. This approach appears to promote sputum mobilization and can, at times, dislodge obstinate bronchial plugs, permitting reexpansion of atelectatic areas.

QUESTIONS

Bronchial asthma—allergic and otherwise

Directions: Answer the following questions on a separate sheet of paper.

1. Formulate a definition of bronchial asthma.

2. What is the pattern of ventilatory dysfunction in asthma?

3. What is the relationship of atopy to bronchial asthma?

4. Describe a postulated basis for the abnormal bronchial lability that is characteristic of asthmatic people. In clinical practice, how is this bronchial lability confirmed?

5. Why do flares of asthma commonly accompany viral or bacterial respiratory infections?

6. What is the advantage of prescribing slowly released oral theophylline preparations as a therapeutic regimen in asthma?

7. Explain why drugs with intrinsic beta-adrenergic effects continue to be useful for acute and long-term management of asthma.

8. What are the measures used in the long-term treatment of bronchial asthma?

Directions: Circle the letter preceding each item below that correctly answers the question. More than one answer may be correct.

9. Which of the following tissue changes are associated with uncomplicated asthma?
a. Gradual loss of supporting lung tissues
b. Irreversible anatomic changes with diffuse loss of the alveolar walls   *c.* Atrophy of bronchial smooth muscle   *d.* Smooth-muscle spasm, mucosal edema   *e.* Hypersecretion of viscid mucus

10. Evidence suggests that an important determinant of exercise-induced asthma (EIA) is:
a. High serum IgG levels in bronchial tree mucus
b. Airway cooling due to evaporation of moisture from the mucosa   *c.* Decrease in viscid mucus secretion   *d.* Dilation of smooth bronchial muscle

11. Which of the following manifestations are typical of distressed asthmatic people?
a. "Allergic salute" due to pruritus of nasal mucosa   *b.* Hyperinflation of the thorax

c. Rhinorrhea   d. Dyspnea   e. Prolonged expiration and wheezing

12. All of the following substances may be responsible for severe airway obstructive responses in a subset of adults with idiopathic asthma *except*:
a. Aspirin   b. Corticosteroids   c. Ibuprofen and other nonsteroidal anti-inflammatory agents
d. Tartrazine (Yellow No. 5) food coloring

13. Which of the following may precipitate individual attacks of asthma?
a. Volatile irritants from organic solvents   b. Exposure to mists and dusts in industrial plants
c. Inhalation of cold air   d. Psychic stimuli
e. All of the above

14. In what range (μg/ml) should theophylline blood serum levels be maintained for optimal therapeutic effect in asthma?
a. 5 to 10   b. 10 to 15   c. 10 to 20   d. 20 to 30

15. Serum levels of theophylline in the desired range are usually achieved by the administration of doses of how many mg per kilogram of body weight every 6 hours to adults receiving rapidly absorbed preparations?
a. 1 to 4   b. 5 to 6   c. 7 to 10   d. 10 to 15

16. Which of the following are recognized effects of excessive dosing with theophylline?
a. Headache   b. Nausea   c. Bloody diarrhea
d. Vomiting   e. Hair loss

17. Aminophylline may be given appropriately to treat asthma:
a. Orally as a liquid or tablets   b. Intravenously
c. Rectally as a suppository   d. By inhalation

18. Jane S. was six when she suffered her first asthmatic attack. She was admitted to the hospital emergency room in acute respiratory distress. Jane was very anxious and had shortness of breath. Her temperature was 99.2°F rectally, her pulse was 100 per minute, and her respirations were 30 per minute. Chest examination revealed expiratory wheezing and normal resonance. She was felt to be experiencing an acute attack of asthma. The most appropriate initial treatment would have been:
a. Phenobarbital 25 mg orally   b. 0.2 ml of 1:1000 epinephrine subcutaneously   c. Aminophylline 50 mg rectally   d. Potassium iodide 2 g orally

19. Prominent manifestations of status asthmaticus include all of the following *except*:
a. Wheezing evident only on exertion   b. Widespread plugging of airways   c. Hypoxemia
d. Increasing respiratory fatigue

20. In status asthmaticus, when arterial P_{CO_2} levels exceeding 55 mmHg are encountered despite a prolonged period of optimal treatment, there is usually need for:

a. Mechanical ventilation using a soft, cuffed endotracheal tube   b. A tracheostomy   c. Both a and b   d. Neither a nor b

Directions: Circle T if the statement is true and F if it is false. Correct the false statements.

21. T   F   Exercise-induced asthma (EIA) is most commonly evident in older adults with idiopathic asthma and does not occur unless mild wheezing is present before exertion.

22. T   F   Diffuse wheezing is a manifestation characteristic only of asthma.

23. T   F   In over 70 percent of asthmatic people with allergic aspergillosis, serum precipitins are demonstrable, and almost all patients have elevated IgE levels.

24. T   F   In early uncomplicated asthma the patient is usually symptom-free between attacks.

Directions: Match the disease condition in col. A with the appropriate description in col. B. More than one letter may be used in col. A.

Column A
25. ____ Chronic bronchitis
26. ____ Pulmonary emphysema
27. ____ Bronchial asthma

Column B
a. Irreversible anatomic changes with loss of supporting lung tissue associated with severe airway narrowing with exertion

b. A prolonged and slowly progressive condition of bronchial inflammation and hypersecretion with or without airway obstruction

c. Predictable periods of dyspnea and wheezing with any increase in respiratory effort

d. Daily cough and increased sputum production extending over months and years

e. Spontaneous attacks of wheezing and dyspnea often occurring at rest; between attacks the patient is typically free of symptoms

ATOPIC DERMATITIS— URTICARIA

OBJECTIVES

At the completion of this chapter you should be able to:

1. Characterize atopic dermatitis by identifying the susceptible population and the typical skin test reactions.
2. Describe the established skin lesions of atopic dermatitis.
3. Identify for infantile eczema the age group affected, type of skin lesion, areas involved, and complications.
4. Explain the rationale of treatment measures used for atopic dermatitis.
5. Identify typical manifestations and treatment for acute flares of atopic dermatitis.
6. Identify the prevalence and type of hypersensitivity reaction(s) associated with urticaria (hives).
7. Describe the lesions of urticaria, their appearance and duration, and the symptoms produced.
8. Assess the significance of environmental influences for chronic urticaria.
9. Describe the objectives for evaluating persons with unexplained hives that persist for months or years.
10. Compare anaphylactic reactions and acute urticaria with regard to the possible mechanisms and the implicated agents.
11. Contrast heat-, light-, and cold-induced urticaria and cholinergic urticaria as to clinical patterns and complications.
12. Explain the significance of dermographism in normal persons.
13. Identify the characteristics of hereditary angioedema (HANE) in terms of etiology, areas involved, signs and symptoms, complications, and treatment.
14. Explain the treatment measures used for acute urticaria and angioedema.

Atopic dermatitis is a common, chronic skin disorder (or group of related disorders) found with particular frequency among persons manifesting allergic rhinitis and asthma as well as among their family members. In addition, high total serum IgE levels and multiple positive immediate skin test reactions are commonly noted with this condition. These associations appear to justify regarding atopic dermatitis as a de facto "atopic disease." However, the lesions of atopic dermatitis are not readily explained in terms of the transient wheal-and-flare response typical of IgE-mediated reactions. Rather, established skin lesions of atopic dermatitis show edema and variable infiltration with mononuclear cells and eosinophils as well as fluid collections within the skin (forming clinically evident vesicles). Rupture of numerous tiny blisters leads to crusting and scaling. These changes and severe pruritus, which precedes and accompanies the eruption, are associated with an excessively dry skin. Sweating also is impaired in this condition, and sweat retention often leads to prominent heat-induced itching. In addition, sebaceous secretions are deficient, and the skin shows both a low threshold for pruritus-inducing stimuli and an abnormal tendency to lichenification (viz., thickening of the skin with accentuation of normal markings).

Atopic dermatitis most commonly appears in response to scratching in the first year of life (as "infantile eczema") with red, raised, pruritic, scaling areas involving the cheeks, scalp, and diaper area. In a majority of children, the condition remits by age 5 but often only after the neck, antecubital and popliteal fossae, wrists, ankles, and waist also have become affected. The latter areas are prominently involved when this problem still is present in late childhood or when, following onset in infancy or adolescence, it persists into adult life (Fig. 11-1).

Intractable itching and painful cracks in the skin are major sources of discomfort for eczematous persons. In addition, the abraded, fissured epidermis is readily infected by bacteria—especially staphylococci—and by viruses which localize in skin. As a result, contact with herpes simplex virus, the "cold sore" agent, may produce a generalized eruption (Fig. 11-2), fever, and toxicity. An even more severe illness, *eczema vaccinatum*, may follow exposure to vaccinia virus,* and eczematous persons must scrupulously avoid receiving smallpox vaccination as well as exposure to unhealed vaccinated sites.

As many as one-half of eczematous children may manifest overt respiratory allergy prior to puberty. Despite this strong association, it is rare to identify one or more allergens that substantially determine the activity of any case of atopic dermatitis. In persons with strong skin reactivity, factors such as house dust, animals, etc., may worsen the rash but appear to act by direct contact with an abraded epidermis rather than through dissemination after inhalant exposure. Foods—especially egg white—can be shown to cause skin lesions to flare in a minority of children and deserve careful attention. Although the importance of ingestant allergens appears to

*Recently the high mortality rate associated with eczema vaccinatum has been substantially reduced by administration of vaccinia immune globulin and by improved supportive care.

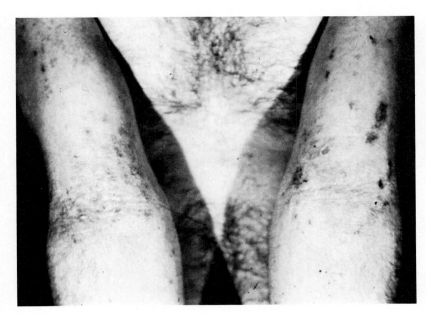

FIGURE 11-1

Chronic lesions of atopic dermatitis (atopic eczema) on the flexor surfaces of the arms of a young man; erosions, pigmentary changes, and a deepening of skin creases (lichenification) are evident. Additional typical lesions in a child and an adult are shown in Figs. 73-1 and 73-2, respectively. (From J. M. Sheldon, R. G. Lovell, and K. P. Mathews, *A Manual of Clinical Allergy*, 2d ed., Saunders, Philadelphia, 1967.)

decline sharply with increasing age, prolonged avoidance of food offenders which have been identified by test challenge clearly is justified.

Since there is no basis for allergen-specific measures in most cases, the approach to treatment of atopic dermatitis remains largely symptomatic (i.e., by nonspecific symptom suppression). Care to avoid potential irritants and topical sensitizers is essential. Prolonged use of bland, inexpensive lubricants is the foundation of most treatment programs and often suffices to keep the disorder quiescent. Oil-in-water emulsions (e.g., water washable base USP) may be adequate and act as minimally greasy vanishing creams. More effective lubrication can be obtained with water-in-oil emulsions (ointments), including hydrophilic ointment USP, Eucerine®, and Aquaphor®. Inert oils such as yellow and white petrolatum provide maximum greasiness and protection from dry air, etc., but their occlusive properties often promote retention of debris and evoke troublesome pruritus.

Topical corticosteroids are widely useful in atopic dermatitis, but these costly preparations should be employed for their anti-inflammatory properties alone

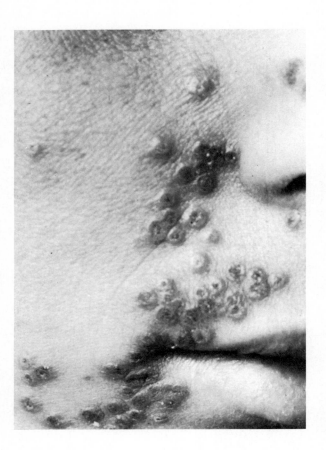

rather than for general lubrication. Where indicated, topically applied steroids may be covered with an occluding layer of polyethylene to promote absorption of the drug, a strategy especially feasible at night. Steroids have largely replaced the once-popular coal tar preparations as anti-inflammatory agents. Tars are still used rarely to reduce lichenification and cracking, although urea-containing ointments are more cosmetically acceptable agents to promote healing and restoration of skin texture.

In managing atopic dermatitis, reduction of pruritus is both an end in itself and a means of interrupting the harmful "scratch-itch" cycle. Oral antipruritic agents such as diphenhydramine (Benadryl) and hydroxyzine (Atarax, Vistaril) are especially useful at night when subconscious scratch responses can do serious damage. Fingernails and toenails should be kept as short as possible (consistent with comfort) to minimize trauma, and, for young children, soft, padded mittens or frank restraint of the extremities may be essential to sustain improvement. Well-washed cotton clothing is generally preferred, and, as a rule, fibers such as wool and synthetics that "snag" the skin must be avoided because of palpable irritant effects. Chapping due to cold dry air is quite harmful to eczematous persons, and well-maintained sources of humidification can offset the tendency of the rash to worsen in winter; organic solvents that defat even normal skin also must be scrupulously avoided. A more subtle drying effect is inflicted by the regular use of soap and water or by contact with water alone. This problem may be approached, in part, by using skin cleaners with low emulsifying activity. In addition, application of topical lubricants after washing or use of emulsified oils in bath water is often helpful. However, frequent bathing by eczematous persons is rarely desirable, and water temperature should be maintained in a tepid range since body heating commonly will increase pruritus.

Acute flares of atopic dermatitis are especially frequent in children and present prominent redness, vesicle formation, and oozing, which may require in-patient care. Brief periods of high-dose systemic corticosteroids will usually speed resolution, and antimicrobial agents may be required. In addition, cool soaks will reduce itching and remove cutaneous debris. Where involvement is general, cool tap-water baths, with or without agents such as colloidal oatmeal, may provide an antipruritic effect more efficiently. As acute lesions begin to resolve, "shake" lotions are employed, followed by the progressively greasier applications emphasized in chronic care programs.

FIGURE 11-2

Facial lesions of eczema herpeticum in a young adult with lifelong atopic dermatitis.

Hives (urticaria) are familiar skin lesions which, at some time, probably affect at least 25 percent of the population. Many clinical forms of urticaria exist, which suggests that a variety of determinants ultimately will be recognized. At present, it seems clear that *some* types of urticaria reflect immunologic processes (especially those involving IgE) while others remain totally unexplained. This practical reality must be faced, since the resemblance of urticarial wheals to IgE-mediated skin reactions often has prompted the false inference that hives per se indicate allergy. Microscopically, most urticarial lesions present only edema, variable dilatation of vessels, and occasional neutrophils and eosinophils; in some patients, however, *grossly identical* lesions can show a definite vasculitis with disruption of blood vessel walls and infiltrating phagocytes. The discrete, raised, pruritic, nontender lesions of urticaria appear most often on the trunk and proximal extremities, individual wheals rarely lasting over 36 hours; angioedema (see Chap. 9) manifested by painless and minimally pruritic swelling of subcutaneous and submucosal tissues is occasionally associated.

Most episodes of urticaria are brief and self-limited, especially in childhood when hives commonly are related to preceding respiratory infections. However, in a minority of adults (and rarely children) unexplained hives may persist for many months or years. The evaluation of such persons requires, first, exclusion of a serious underlying disease as the factor promoting urticaria; prominent among these are lymphomas, systemic lupus erythematosus, hyperthyroidism, and nonlymphoid neoplasms. While chronic foci of bacterial infection and intestinal parasites are often sought in these patients, they are rarely shown to cause the chronic hives.

Like anaphylactic reactions, urticaria can result from IgE-mediated responses to protein allergens. In both situations, the implicated agents usually are ingestants—especially such foods as egg, fish, diverse shellfish, and nuts, including the peanut. In addition, drugs and drug metabolites which are complete antigens or are capable of stable bonding to proteins (e.g., penicillin derivatives) are prominent factors in systemic or urticarial Type I reactions (see Chap. 9). However, many drugs also appear to cause urticaria by mechanisms exclusive of IgE. Aspirin is probably the most frequent offender in this group and has been said to worsen *nonspecifically* 25 percent of chronic urticaria cases.

Physical factors are the major determinants in a proportion of patients with chronic urticaria, and of these environmental influences, cold is probably most frequently implicated. Cold urticaria especially affects young adults and may appear with the most minor degrees of chilling. Hives develop in some as skin temperature falls but generally require rewarming for their ap-

pearance. Cold urticaria has been associated with elevated plasma histamine levels (e.g., in venous blood from a chilled extremity), and both headache and hypotension may result. This effect has led to disaster occasionally when affected persons have developed syncope while swimming and have drowned as a result. Urticaria also may be elicited specifically by local heating, the lesions being immediate in some subjects and delayed as long as several hours in others. Total body heating (e.g., in a warm bath) also can worsen pruritus and whealing of diverse additional causes. In addition, *cholinergic urticaria* is a clinically distinct syndrome in which physical exertion, emotional stress, and environmental warmth elicit crops of tiny wheals, each surrounded by a broad border of redness. Affected persons commonly show abnormally large whealing or erythematous responses to intradermal methacholine, although the pathogenetic significance of this reactivity remains unclear. A period of sustained running usually elicits typical wheals which permit confirmation of the diagnosis. Local urtication (hive formation) or angioedema also may follow exposure to sustained pressure, various wavelengths of light, or vibratory stimuli. Some of these rare conditions appear to be familial. Furthermore, in certain examples of heat-, light-, or cold-induced urticaria, local specific reactivity can be conferred on normal subjects by transfer of IgE in serum of affected persons. At present, it is not clear whether these "passive transfer" phenomena involve classic antigen-antibody reactions or alternative mechanisms.

Urticaria due to pressure most commonly occurs in those with dermographism (Fig. 11-3), in whom firm stroking will produce definite whealing responses. Dermographism is long-standing in a small proportion of normal persons but also may be acquired, appearing after adverse drug reactions or in disease states promoting infiltration of skin by mast cells. Dermographic persons typically develop wheals at pressure points including the buttocks and soles of the feet as well as beneath watch straps, belts, and tight underclothing.

Instances of angioedema accompanying acute urticaria are occasionally confused with hereditary angioedema (HANE), a familial defect in the control of inflammation. HANE manifests as recurrent bouts of edema involving peripheral structures as well as the larynx and bowel, the last producing intense abdominal pain and often leading to exploratory laparotomies. These episodes rarely appear before age 10 and may recur indefinitely, although their frequency often decreases after the sixth decade. Emotional stress or physical trauma (often quite subtle) may precede the edema, but many bouts are unexplained. Laryngeal edema poses a serious threat to life in these patients, and pedigree analysis usually reveals one or more instances in each family where this complication has caused death by asphyxiation. Swelling in this condition usually develops over many hours, regresses equally slowly, and is *not* accompanied by urticaria. HANE patients are known to share low activity levels of the factor that normally inhibits the activated first component of the complement system (C1) as well as additional components concerned with clotting, inflammation, and fibrinolysis. As a result of this deficiency, C1 effects are unopposed, and C1 proceeds to activate and consume the early components of the sequence, C4 and C2, which on assay are demonstrably low in this condition. A kininlike peptide has been described as a by-product of C2 activation, and its excessive generation in HANE may underlie this condition. However, additional permeability-promoting factors, normally checked by the C1 inhibitor, may be responsible for the swellings in this condition. Treatment measures are properly focused on preservation of the airway, avoidance of needless laparotomy when bowel edema occurs, and general support. Currently available drugs contribute little to acute care; however, regular use of either methyltestosterone or other anabolic agents of limited androgenic potency (e.g., danazol and stanozolol) stimulates synthesis of the deficient factor and can greatly reduce attack frequency.

Few additional conditions lend confusion to the evaluation of ordinary urticaria and angioedema. Occasionally, penetrants such as stinging plant hairs or insects produce troublesome whealing reactions, and the possibility of dermographism should not be overlooked. Chronic, pruritic, raised papules, termed *papular urticaria*, often follow insect bites, especially on the legs in childhood, but the persistence and induration (viz., firm consistency) of these lesions usually sets them apart. Typical urticaria may accompany serious primary disease or may follow trivial viral syndromes; however, frequently no cause is evident initially. Drugs or chemical additives in foods and beverages are often identified as sources of urticaria and should be evaluated carefully, although confirmatory in vitro tests rarely are available. Similarly, a painstaking review of historical details may provide evidence implicating foods, physical agents, or psychogenic factors.

Since bouts of hives generally are self-limited and vary in duration as well as in severity, the value of treatment measures for affected individuals often is difficult to evaluate. However, epinephrine has demonstrated effectiveness in speeding the resolution of acute urticaria and angioedema. Agents such as diphenhydramine and hydroxyzine also are acknowledged to have value in this condition, although both cause prominent sedation. These drugs are considered to inhibit a type of histamine receptor termed H_1. A second histamine receptor type (H_2) is blocked by drugs including cimetidine and ranitidine; these may provide additional relief for patients with urticaria. Adrenal cortical steroids have been beneficial in severe acute hives but often fail to influence the course of longer established disease. In chronic urticaria, justifiable reassurance and use of optimal antihistaminic-sympathomimetic medications are of paramount importance; of these, hydroxyzine often is the single most valuable agent. Although repeated study of such patients rarely is fruitful, all concerned should remain receptive to clues that may implicate a responsible factor.

FIGURE 11-3
Dermographism evident 2 minutes after the back is lightly stroked with a fingernail. The subject had occasional urticarial wheals at the beltline and on the buttocks.

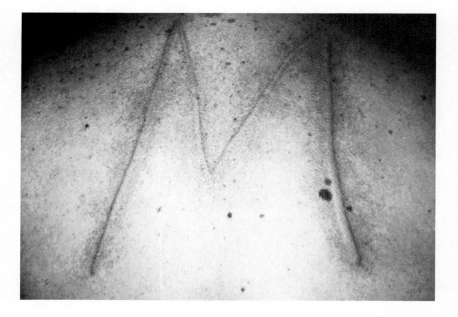

Atopic dermatitis—Urticaria

Directions: Answer the following questions on a separate sheet of paper.

1. Identify the agents usually implicated in both anaphylactic reactions and urticaria.
2. Discuss the treatment measures used for acute urticaria and angioedema.
3. What is the prevalence of urticaria (hives)?
4. Why are treatment modalities for urticaria difficult to evaluate?

Directions: Circle the letter preceding each item below that correctly answers the question. More than one answer may be correct.

5. Patients with atopic dermatitis usually have increased serum levels of:
   a. IgE   *b.* IgM   *c.* IgG   *d.* IgA

6. All of the following descriptions are typical of the skin lesions of atopic dermatitis *except:*
   a. Edema   *b.* Typical wheal-and-flare response
   c. Crusting and scaling   *d.* Infiltration with mononuclear cells and eosinophils

7. Atopic dermatitis occurs with particular frequency among persons manifesting:
   a. Hay fever   *b.* Allergic rhinitis   *c.* Allergic eczematous contact dermatitis   *d.* Bronchial asthma

8. Which of the following are characteristics of infantile eczema?
   a. It usually appears in the first year of life.   *b.* It is associated with a great increase in sebaceous activity producing an excessively oily skin.   *c.* In all cases, it resolves permanently by 3 years of age.
   d. It is associated with red, raised, pruritic, scaling areas involving the cheeks, scalp, and diaper area.

9. All of the following are potential complications of infantile eczema *except:*
   a. Infection with pyogenic (pus-forming) bacteria
   b. Massive hemorrhage into affected skin
   c. Sweat retention and severe itching   *d.* Thickening and lichenification of skin

10. In children acute flares of atopic dermatitis which are characterized by prominent redness, vesicle formation, and oozing may be treated by all of the following *except:*
    a. Systemic corticosteroids   *b.* Antipruritic agents   *c.* Oral coal tar preparations   *d.* Antimicrobial agents

11. Most urticarial lesions show microscopically:
    a. Edema   *b.* Variable dilatation of vessels

c. Neutrophils and eosinophils   *d.* Severe destructive vasculitis

12. Which of the following groups are most often affected by cold urticara:
    a. Infants   *b.* Young children   *c.* Young adults
    d. Elderly persons

13. The occurrence of cold urticara has been associated with elevated levels of:
    a. IgE   *b.* IgG   *c.* IgM   *d.* Plasma histamine

14. Which of the following characteristics are true of urticaria?
    a. There are pruritic, nontender lesions.
    b. There is inflammatory swelling of subcutaneous tissue.   *c.* Lesions appear most often on the face, palms, and soles.   *d.* Angioedema is always present.

15. The evaluation of persons with unexplained hives which persist for months or years requires exclusion of which of the following diseases?
    a. Hay fever   *b.* Lymphomas   *c.* Bronchial asthma   *d.* Systemic lupus erythematosus

16. In the causation of chronic urticaria, which of the following physical factors is probably the most frequently responsible?
    a. Cold   *b.* Light   *c.* Heat   *d.* Vibration

17. All of the following factors may elicit generalized cholinergic urticaria *except:*
    a. Physical exertion   *b.* Emotional stress
    c. Environmental cold   *d.* Intradermal methacholine

18. Hereditary angioedema (HANE):
    a. Involves the same mechanism as angioedema accompanying acute urticaria   *b.* Manifests as recurrent bouts of edema involving peripheral structures as well as the larynx and bowel   *c.* Produces laryngeal edema which usually develops in a matter of minutes and is accompanied by urticaria
    d. Implies low activity levels of the factor that normally inhibits the activated first component of the complement system

Directions: Circle T if the statement is true and F if it is false. Correct the false statements.

19. T   F   In persons with atopic dermatitis, factors such as house dust, animal danders, etc., commonly worsen the rash through inhalant exposure.

20. T   F   The approach to the treatment of

atopic dermatitis remains largely symptomatic.

21. T   F   Topical corticosteroids are used properly in atopic dermatitis for their general lubricating properties.

22. T   F   Oral antipruritic agents such as diphenhydramine and hydroxyzine are especially useful in atopic dermatitis at night when subconscious scratch responses can do serious damage.

23. T   F   Coal tar preparations are, at present, the most widely used preparations for reducing lichenification and cracking.

24. T   F   In order to prevent chapping due to cold dry air in eczematous persons, organic solvents should be used.

25. T   F   Both anaphylactic reactions and urticaria can result from IgE-mediated responses to protein allergens.

26. T   F   Hives per se indicate allergy.

27. T   F   Local urtication (hive formation) may follow exposure to local body heating.

28. T   F   Dermographism in normal persons may appear after adverse drug reactions or in disease states promoting infiltration of the skin by mast cells.

AUTOIMMUNE AND IMMUNE COMPLEX–INDUCED DISEASES

OBJECTIVES

At the completion of this chapter you should be able to:

1. Define *autoantibodies*.
2. Explain what the appearance of autoantibodies denotes.
3. Illustrate with an example the way in which immune responses to autologous (i.e., host-derived) tissue components could arise.
4. Explain the way in which autoaggressive immune reactions may originate.
5. Describe Goodpasture's syndrome as an apparent example of antibody-mediated human autoimmunity.
6. Identify the characteristics of idiopathic thrombocytopenic purpura (ITP), its relationship to antiplatelet antibodies, and its treatment.
7. Illustrate, with examples, immunohemolytic (IH) processes.
8. Explain the purpose of a Coombs' test and the significance of a positive reaction.
9. For hemolytic reactions to transfused blood, describe the signs and symptoms, population at risk, complications, feasibility of prevention, and desirable precautions.
10. In addition to manifestations of hemolysis, list the forms of adverse reactions that may accompany transfusions of blood or blood products.
11. Describe the effects of infusing serums containing potent leukoagglutinins.
12. Describe the nature and origin of adverse reactions to transfusion in persons deficient in IgA.
13. State how the reactions described in objective no. 12 may be averted.
14. Explain for spontaneously developing immunohemolytic phenomena (viz., "warm" and "cold" autoantibodies to red blood cells) the hypersensitivity reaction, age group affected, disease entities, signs and symptoms, and treatment.
15. Describe the clinical manifestations of serum sickness following a *first* exposure to equine antiserum.
16. Describe the pathogenesis of serum sickness.

17. Identify the etiology, onset, signs and symptoms, type of hypersensitivity reaction, laboratory findings, and associated clinical conditions of serum sickness.

18. Describe the reactions that occur with prolonged antigen exposure in individuals making only modest antibody responses.

19. Describe the characteristics of allergic eczematous contact dermatitis by identifying the type of hypersensitivity it connotes, abnormality produced, areas involved, examples of topical irritants and sensitizers, treatment, and characteristics of the diagnostic tests used.

ANTIBODY–MEDIATED, AUTOIMMUNE (TYPE II) DISORDERS

Although injury to the host often is *incidental* to immune processes, host tissues, understandably, are rarely the target of the body's own direct antibody or cell-mediated attack. In many conditions, autoantibodies (i.e., antibodies that react with autologous tissue components) arise, providing valuable diagnostic markers. However, these serum factors appear seldom to be responsible for direct tissue injury.

The appearance of autoantibodies denotes a failure of safeguards which normally prevent immune responses to host tissues (autoimmunity); however, responsible factors are rarely identifiable. In some instances (e.g., ocular pigment and endocrine gland cell components) the inciting antigens are normally sequestered in closed tissue compartments throughout development and maturity; therefore, they may remain "foreign" even to mature lymphoid tissues. If injury releases these heretofore locally confined materials into the general circulation, an immune response may readily occur, with secondary damage to the injured organ and antigenically related structures. This mechanism does, in fact, appear to operate in certain eye conditions (e.g., sympathetic ophthalmia) and in several endocrine deficiency states. Immune responses to host tissue components could arise also following more subtle injury incident to microbial invasion. The possibility that infecting bacteria and viruses may produce *limited* changes in host tissue components that render them "foreign" to immune surveillance has also been proposed. Antibodies (or sensitized lymphocytes) resulting from this process might have specificities broad enough to permit reaction with *native* as well as modified tissue determinants. In addition, autoimmune phenomena could result if an invading organism (or other introduced agent) and host tissues shared an antigen or closely similar antigenic groups as a result of parallel evolution. Although invoked especially with regard to

the pathogenesis of poststreptococcal glomerulonephritis and rheumatic fever, this mechanism remains theoretical. Finally, it is reasonable to speculate that autoaggressive immune reactions may originate with mutant ("forbidden") clones of lymphoid cells programmed to recognize normal host components as "foreign." Such cells might be antigen-specific or nonspecific T_4^+ (helper/promotor) lymphocytes that foster the immune responses of both T and B lymphocytes. Alternatively, disease, including viral invasion, may damage T_8^+ (suppressor) cells that normally repress T- and B-cell responses to "self" components.

Although the disorder is rare, Goodpasture's syndrome has attracted considerable attention as an apparent example of antibody-mediated human autoimmunity causing major damage to internal organs. The typical clinical picture of recurrent pulmonary hemorrhage (Fig. 12-1) and anemia coupled with progressive kidney failure is described in Part VII; however, the relative severity of these features varies among patients. Most Goodpasture's cases present no evident inciting cause, although the disease *has* followed viral and chemical insults to the lungs. Circulating antibodies, reactive with glomerular (kidney) and alveolar (lung) basement membranes, are usually present and, along with complement components, form linear deposits at these sites in vivo. The associated tissue damage is thought to reflect, in part, complement-mediated cytotoxicity and local effects of recruited neutrophils.*

Human antibody-dependent, autoimmune disorders most often affect formed elements of the blood, with platelets and red blood cells attacked predomi-

---

*Many mononuclear cells have membrane receptors which cause them to gather at sites of IgG deposition. Direct contact with these activated cells leads to cytotoxic effects and other tissue damage without a requirement for complement activation. This process, termed *antibody-dependent cell-mediated cytotoxicity* (ADCC), may play a part in Goodpasture's syndrome and many other hypersensitivity disorders.

nantly. Increasing evidence has linked the disease idiopathic thrombocytopenic purpura (ITP) with circulating IgG molecules reactive with host platelets. Even when fixed to platelet surfaces, these antibodies do not cause localization of complement proteins or lysis of platelets in the free circulation. However, platelets bearing IgG molecules are more readily removed and destroyed by macrophages bearing membrane receptors for IgG in the spleen and liver. Evidence supporting this mechanism for thrombocytopenia has come from studies of ITP patients and of experimental subjects who have shown severe but brief platelet deficits after receiving ITP serums; transient thrombocytopenia, noted in infants delivered by mothers with ITP, also is consistent with IgG-dependent damage due to placentally transmitted antibody. ITP may follow infections—especially in childhood—but often appears without prior event and commonly resolves after days or weeks. Persistent ITP usually may be suppressed by corticosteroids which are thought to act largely by reducing platelet removal by spleen and liver. However, when the disease has lasted 6 or more months, the prospect of prolonged high-dose steroid treatment with its inherent side effects generally prompts a splenectomy. Platelet counts usually rise and may become normal after this procedure despite continued sequestration by the liver; in either case, lower steroid requirements result in most patients (see Chap. 18).

Red blood cell membranes carry literally hundreds of described antigens, and immunoglobulins reacting with one or more of these are found in ill as well as in otherwise normal persons. Depending upon the type, specificity, and number of antibody molecules involved, their fixation to membrane sites may have no effect or may shorten cell life by allowing extravascular removal or intravascular lysis. Where decreased survival results,

stigmata of increased turnover of heme pigments (see Part III) usually can be demonstrated, and frank anemia will develop if the host's erythropoietic capacity cannot fully compensate for the losses. Generically, these conditions often are described as immunohemolytic (IH) processes. Hemolytic transfusion reactions are a distinctive form of IH process occurring usually when a recipient already sensitized to "foreign" human red blood cell antigens by pregnancy or prior transfusion receives blood containing these antigens. Far less often, transfused blood contains antibodies reactive with the recipient's erythrocytes. However, most IH processes (spontaneous processes) arise through production by the host of antibodies reactive with his or her own red blood cells.

The Coombs' test provides information central to the description of IH disorders. In this procedure, antibodies derived from other species (e.g., goat) and directed toward human immunoglobulins and/or complement components are mixed with washed human erythrocytes. If these cells have the appropriate human serum components bound to their surfaces, then the foreign antiserum, by reacting with molecules on adjacent cells, will tend to link the cells and cause them to clump visibly (Fig. 12-2). In practice, the foreign (Coombs') serum is usually mixed directly with cells from drawn blood. A positive (clumping) reaction in this "direct Coombs' test" indicates that circulating cells with significant numbers of bound immunoreactive molecules are present. At times, the direct test is negative despite the presence in serum of antibodies reactive with

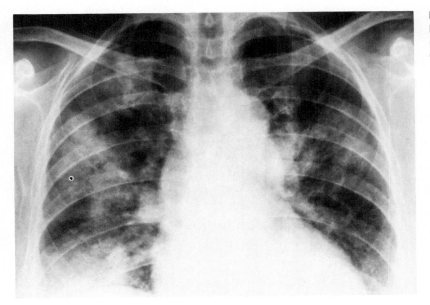

FIGURE 12-1

Frontal chest x-ray during active pulmonary involvement in Goodpasture's syndrome. (Film courtesy of Dr. Terry Silver.)

human erythrocytes other than those of the host. These may be detected by incubating the serums with human red blood cells of compatible ABO and Rh types and then performing a direct Coombs' test. Red blood cell agglutination in this "indirect Coombs' test" serves as an indicator of unsuspected serum antibody and as an important warning of danger prior to an intended blood transfusion. Direct Coombs' reactions are often performed with antiserums specific for human IgG or the third component of serum complement (C3).

Hemolytic reactions to transfused blood provide the most dramatic and dangerous IH phenomena observed clinically. These responses almost always appear *during* infusion of the offending blood and are marked by rapid intravascular lysis of red blood cells because of the circulating antibodies. Those at risk largely comprise persons sensitized to red blood cell antigens by prior pregnancy, transfusion, or unknown factors that may include bacterial or viral infection. Victims of transfusion reactions tend to manifest chills, fever, and low back pain—occasionally preceded by urticaria or flushing and often by uneasiness and mild air hunger. In addition, when cell lysis is massive, the resulting debris may trigger widespread *intravascular* clotting with consumptive depletion of coagulation factors and bleeding from wounds and venipuncture sites. Survivors of severe acute reactions also share a high risk of acute

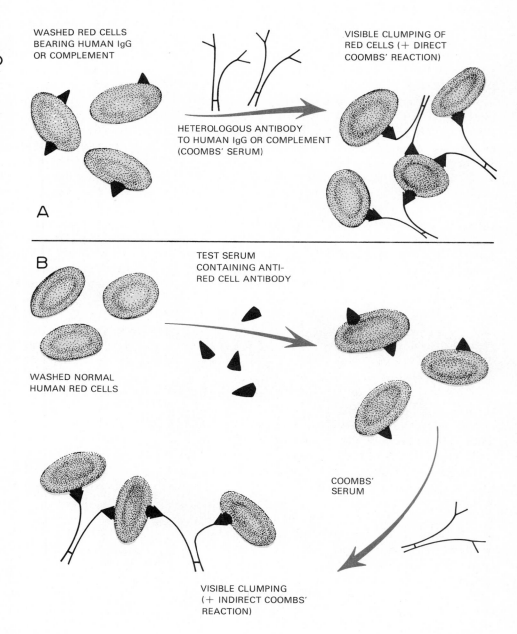

FIGURE 12-2
Reaction sequences in the direct (A) and the indirect (B) Coombs' test.

WASHED RED CELLS BEARING HUMAN IgG OR COMPLEMENT

HETEROLOGOUS ANTIBODY TO HUMAN IgG OR COMPLEMENT (COOMBS' SERUM)

VISIBLE CLUMPING OF RED CELLS (+ DIRECT COOMBS' REACTION)

A

B

TEST SERUM CONTAINING ANTI-RED CELL ANTIBODY

WASHED NORMAL HUMAN RED CELLS

COOMBS' SERUM

VISIBLE CLUMPING (+ INDIRECT COOMBS' REACTION)

kidney failure promoted by shock and massive hemoglobinuria.

Considering these dire consequences, every reasonable measure to prevent or mitigate hemolytic transfusion reactions is justified. Basic to this effort is care in identifying the source and proper recipient of blood products as well as continual surveillance of persons receiving blood—especially of those whose mobility or awareness is impaired. Any serious evidence suggesting an incipient reaction should prompt discontinuance of the questioned infusion, maintenance of intravenous access, and close clinical observation. A carefully drawn venous sample from the recipient should be checked for serum hemoglobin, a sign of intravascular red cell breakdown, and the compatibility of donor and recipient should be reconfirmed. Without exception, *all* materials used for transfusion should be saved to facilitate serological and microbiological testing. Special precautions to monitor urine output are essential, and examination of serial centrifuged specimens for hemoglobin may be instructive since clearance of serum hemoglobin is rapid. Maintenance of adequate hydration and urine flow are important considerations in all survivors, and osmotic diuresis with cautiously administered IV mannitol (beginning with an adult dose of 25 g) may help in achieving this goal. Safe fluid therapy demands precise and regular evaluation of cardiopulmonary and renal function. Measures to combat shock, pulmonary edema, acute renal failure, and/or defibrination with bleeding may be required.

In addition to manifestations of hemolysis, several forms of adverse reaction may accompany transfusion of blood or blood products. Urticaria alone occurs rarely in recipients and, especially in atopic persons, may reflect trace amounts of food or other allergens in transfused serum. In those requiring blood repeatedly or in those who have had multiple pregnancies, antibodies directed to human leukocyte membrane antigens often develop. With subsequent transfusion of "foreign" whole blood, these factors are available to agglutinate leukocytes and, at times, platelets. Such reactions are the most common source of transfusion-associated fever, although vital organs are little affected. Suitable blood for those with leukoagglutinins may be obtained by filtration through nylon fibers or reconstitution from the frozen state, both preparations being essentially leukocyte-free. Where *serums* containing potent leukoagglutinins have been infused, recipients have developed fever, cough, shortness of breath, and lung shadows on chest x-ray; several days have been required for full resolution.

Persons deficient in IgA also may suffer severe reactions from transfused IgA in plasma as a result of antibodies formed to this immunoglobulin or its subgroups. Clinically, these episodes often resemble anaphylaxis with dyspnea, flushing, abdominal cramps, and diarrhea, as well as fever and chills. Reactions may be averted by using IgA-deficient donors or thoroughly washed red blood cells. In addition to these problems, personnel supervising transfusion therapy must be alert for possible air embolism, volume overload, septicemia from microbial contamination, chilling from excessively cold blood, and calcium or platelet deficiency following massive blood replacement.

Spontaneously developing IH phenomena are divisible into three general categories: (1) types associated with medications (see Chap. 13); (2) types with "warm" red blood cell autoantibodies reacting at $37°C$; and (3) a group of conditions with "cold" antibodies that bind at lower temperatures and often only in a range of 4 to $15°C$. Warm autoantibodies are usually of the IgG class and are recognized primarily in middle-aged adults. In more than one-half of these, a serious primary disease such as chronic lymphocytic leukemia, lymphoid (and rarely nonlymphoid) tumors, or systemic lupus erythematosus will become evident, and these conditions substantially determine the prognosis for affected individuals. The IH disorder may be manifested only as a positive Coombs' test (with antihuman IgG); it rarely may lead to symptoms or fulminant, fatal hemolysis. Most commonly, however, shortened red blood cell life leads to chronic morbidity with pallor, fatigue, and weakness as well as recurrent fever and jaundice; dyspnea arising from heart failure, angina pectoris, and vascular thrombosis also are common. Splenic enlargement is a frequent finding, since this organ functions as the main site of red blood cell destruction. Splenic trapping of erythrocytes is most marked when both IgG autoantibody and C3 are present on their surfaces. Where treatment is necessary, adrenocortical steroids are a proper first consideration; they induce remissions in over two-thirds of patients, although relapses are common when these drugs are withdrawn. Splenectomy is undertaken where steroids, in acceptable doses, have proved inadequate alone. In addition, immunosuppressive (cytotoxic) agents (e.g., cyclophosphamide and azathiaprine) may provide additional value in highly selected patients. Since warm hemolysins commonly react with cells of essentially all potential normal donors, transfusions pose extreme difficulties and are avoided if possible. Where no other choice remains, addition of Coombs' serum following incubation of the patient's serum with panels of cells permits the least incompatible ones to be chosen.

Cold autoantibodies to red blood cells generally bind at temperatures well below $32°C$; however, these molecules become dissociated at the warmer levels required for the "fixation" (i.e., cell-surface localization) of complement. Because of this, hemolysis may be absent and red blood cell agglutination minor despite extremely high levels of autoantibody. IgM class cold agglutinins are demonstrable often in infectious mononucleosis and *Mycoplasma pneumoniae* infections, although decreased red blood cell survival rarely results. Chronic cold-dependent hemolysis is evident, however, in certain elderly persons, many of whom have lymphoid neoplasms and IgM autoantibodies. Besides stigmata of chronic hemolysis, these patients display signs of red blood cell agglutination (e.g., pain and cyanosis) in the peripheral circulation on exposure to cold. High titers of cold agglutinins in serum are prominent, and complement components are usually demonstrable on the red blood cells. Treatment considerations usually focus on the associated malignancy (where present), although corticosteroids or immunosuppressive drugs have seemed beneficial in individual cases. A quite different situation involving IgG hemolysins has been seen with syphilis as well as with viral infections and in some apparently normal persons. Termed *paroxysmal cold hemoglobinuria*, this condition presents short bouts of back and extremity pain, fever, chills, and hemoglobinuria precipitated by cold exposure. Sensitization of red blood cells usually occurs below 15°C, and, on rewarming, complement factors are fixed to membrane sites permitting brisk hemolysis.

Antibodies apparently reactive with normal tissue components are associated with diverse additional human disease states. However, in the majority of these conditions, antibody-induced *damage* has not been demonstrated, although in some instances (e.g., systemic lupus erythematosus), pathogenic immune complexes are recognized. Complexes containing antibody to double-stranded DNA in combination with that antigen are important factors in the nephritis of lupus. In addition, antibodies to organ-specific components and to both nuclear and cytoplasmic antigens occur in that disease. Since these various serum factors currently are associated more with diagnostic than pathogenetic considerations, they are discussed briefly in chapters treating diseases of major organ systems.

SERUM SICKNESS AND OTHER CONDITIONS INDUCED BY CIRCULATING IMMUNE COMPLEXES (TYPE III DISORDERS)

Serum sickness was among the earliest recognized hypersensitivity diseases and is considered the prototypic immune complex–induced illness. Originally observed following administration of large volumes of unfractionated equine antiserums for prophylaxis of diphtheria, tetanus, etc., this condition is most prevalent today after administration of drugs (e.g., penicillin and sulfonamides). The development of serum sickness requires administration (usually by injection) of an antigenic material that will remain in the circulation until a specific antibody response occurs, as shown in Fig. 12-3. At that

FIGURE 12-3
Trends in immune reactants during the course of serum sickness.

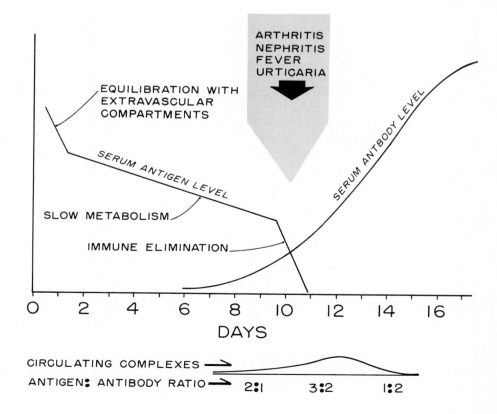

time, the slowly diminishing blood levels of antigen drop sharply, denoting the formation of immune (antigen-antibody) complexes which are cleared from circulation rapidly by macrophage-monocyte scavenging and other mechanisms (viz., "immune elimination"). Complexes are formed initially in considerable antigen excess, with small aggregates comprising one antibody molecule and two antigen molecules (or determinate groups) on a single molecule predominating. As antibody synthesis and immune elimination of the antigen proceed, a state of antibody excess develops progressively. Between these extremes is a period (usually brief) when modest antigen excess occurs and somewhat larger complexes with molecular proportions approaching three antigen to two antibody molecules predominate. Such complexes are capable of activating complement components and probably other amplification systems that mediate inflammation. Furthermore these complexes, because of their physical properties, are readily deposited in the walls of small vessels in many organs including the kidneys; inflammatory changes follow at these sites.

After initial exposure to an appropriate sensitizer, manifestations of serum sickness classically appear in 10 to 14 days; shorter latent periods precede second or subsequent attacks if exposure is repeated. Frequently the most prominent manifestation (Fig. 12-4) is urticaria—often severe and confluent—and angioedema, although skin lesions may resemble bruises or the rash of measles. In addition, many persons develop fever, muscle soreness, and malaise. Lymphadenopathy, with enlarged and tender nodes, is often generalized and may be especially striking in those groups draining the site of introduction of the causative agent. Joint pain (arthralgia) may occur alone, or frank arthritis may affect several large joints together or sequentially. Although genitourinary symptoms are rare, urinalysis may reveal excessive excretion of albumin and, occasionally, of erythrocytes and white blood cells. Gastrointestinal complaints

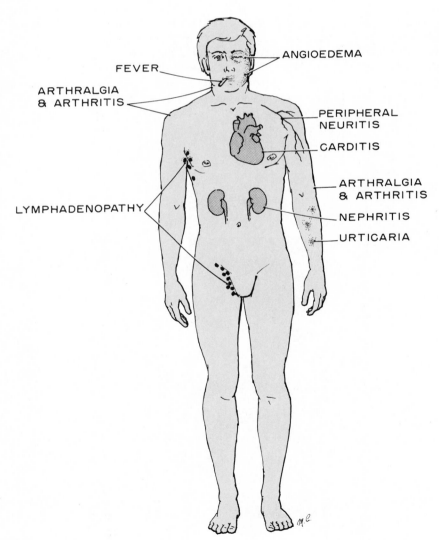

FIGURE 12-4
Manifestations that may occur during serum sickness. Despite these diverse possibilities, many patients experience only fever with skin and/or joint problems.

of nausea, vomiting, and abdominal pain infrequently dominate the picture, and cardiac or peripheral nerve dysfunction is seen rarely. In view of these diverse manifestations it is often difficult to distinguish serum sickness from certain infectious (especially viral) processes as well as from such conditions as rheumatic fever, sickle cell crisis, glomerulonephritis, and bacterial endocarditis. Laboratory findings offer limited guidance in this differential process, although a modest leukocytosis, elevated red blood cell sedimentation rate, and *transient* depression of serum complement activity are characteristic of serum sickness.

As indicated above, complement-fixing immune complexes, presumably containing specific IgG and/or IgM, are implicated strongly in the causation of serum sickness. Among the complement system products formed (see Chap. 5) are *anaphylatoxins* (C5a and C3a) which can release histamine and other proinflammatory agents from mast cells. In addition, a majority of affected persons show tissue-fixing antibodies that mediate wheal-and-flare skin reactivity to the implicated antigen and may contribute additionally to clinical urticaria and angioedema.* There is, furthermore, growing evidence that mast cell–derived mediator substances which increase the permeability of small-vessel walls favor the deposition of complement-fixing complexes. In support of this mechanism are data *suggesting* that prophylactic use of antihistaminic agents may reduce the incidence of clinical serum sickness in high-risk human populations—an effect also clearly shown in animal models.

Serum sickness typically is a brief illness and may require substantially no medication. However, considerable relief of discomfort may be achieved with regular doses of aspirin for fever and rheumatic complaints, as well as antihistaminic drugs and, if needed, epinephrine, to suppress urticaria and angioedema. Where these measures do not suffice, especially if urinary tract or neurological changes are pronounced, a brief course of corticosteroid treatment is justifiable. Careful prospective avoidance of the implicated antigen is essen-

*A majority of these factors probably are IgE; however, in a few cases studied, this activity also seems to reside in other immunoglobulin classes.

tial, since acute systemic reactions as well as a more prompt reappearance of serum sickness may develop if exposure recurs.

Prolonged antigen exposure occurring in individuals making only *modest* antibody responses can promote a chronic condition in which complexes formed in relative antigen excess circulate continuously. This situation may be produced readily in laboratory animals and, in human beings, occurs with systemic lupus erythematosus, bacterial endocarditis, and prolonged infections including malaria, syphilis, and leprosy. Deposition of immune complexes affects especially the kidney, where antigen as well as host antibody and complement (singly or in combination) may be demonstrated along the glomerular basement membrane or between adjacent capillaries (Fig. 12-5). As an apparent result of these deposits, inflammatory cells accumulate, the basement membranes thicken, and glomerular cells swell and proliferate, obliterating normal nephron structure. Changes in other organs also are recognized owing largely to accumulation of complexes in vascular walls.

A syndrome of fever, arthritis, urticaria, and low serum complement levels has been observed early in the course of hepatitis B infection associated with circulating complexes of viral surface antigen (HBsAg) and host antibody. As liver involvement becomes manifest, this syndrome clears; its subsidence correlates, in time, with rising antibody titers and, usually, disappearance of HBsAg from serum. It seems probable that additional examples of immune complex–induced systemic vascular damage will be appreciated in the future. In addition, effects of locally formed complexes have been implicated increasingly in conditions including extrinsic allergic alveolitis (hypersensitivity pneumonitis) and rheumatoid synovitis. While offending antigens remain

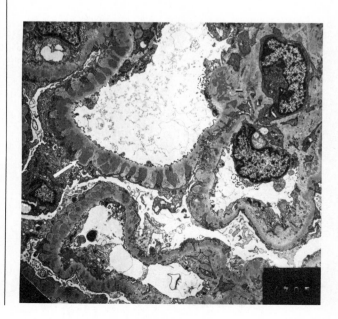

FIGURE 12-5
Antigen-antibody complex depostion (arrow) in the glomerular basement membrane of a nephritic subject. (Electron micrograph courtesy of Dr. Branka Baic.)

speculative in many cases, long-standing viral infections and pollutant chemicals deserve special consideration.

CONTACT DERMATITIS—A TYPE IV RESPONSE

Delayed-type hypersensitivity (DTH), mediated by specifically sensitized lymphocytes, provides a major defensive resource opposing attack by fungi, viruses, and bacteria adapted to intracellular growth and is also a deterrent to growth of malignant cells. Inflammation incident to these necessary responses often injures normal host tissues. However, there are relatively few situations in which DTH underlies a response which is not substantially protective, and of these, the most familiar is allergic eczematous contact dermatitis (AECD). Indeed, in the North American population as a whole, AECD (especially that due to poison ivy and its relatives) is the most frequently encountered *allergic* disorder.

AECD typically presents a pruritic, reddened, thickened area of skin which often shows relatively fragile vesicles (Fig. 12-6). Edema of the involved area often is intense at the outset and, if the face, genitalia, or a distal extremity is involved, may simulate angioedema. With chronicity, although pruritus remains, the rash comes to resemble "eczema" of any cause, with prominent lichenification and scaling. Involved skin shows an influx of mononuclear cells, especially about minute blood vessels, and separation, by edema, of cells in deeper layers of the epidermis (spongiosis) and the adjacent dermis. In many lesions, mast cells are uniquely prominent in the inflammatory infiltrate. AECD reflects application of a sensitizer to the skin, and the rash typically is confined to the area of exposure. Although

any portion of the skin surface may become affected, hairless areas, especially the eyelids, are more commonly involved. Reactions of contact sensitivity occur rarely on the oral, vaginal, and anal mucous membranes.

Contact sensitizers are highly reactive substances which often have quite simple chemical structures. Studies in laboratory animals suggest that these materials, on application to skin, penetrate to the deeper epidermal layers where they complex, as haptens, with cutaneous proteins. The resulting conjugates are presented to cells of draining lymph nodes where lymphocytes specifically able to recognize conjugates of the hapten and adjacent portions of the protein carrier are generated. Hapten-protein conjugation recurs with subsequent contact exposures, and sensitized lymphocytes respond, providing direct cytotoxicity and lymphokine-generated inflammation.

AECD should be suspected in highly pruritic eruptions having patterns of distribution that suggest specific topical exposure. Potential offenders are assessed through a comprehensive environmental review with special attention to topical medications, plant oils, cosmetics and perfumes, cleaning supplies, and work-associated materials. Possible sensitizers may be evaluated by attempting to create the disease in miniature through the use of patch tests. With this approach, extracts or solid fragments of test materials are placed on the unabraided skin, covered with a water-repellent patch, and taped in place. After 48 hours, the sites are uncovered and examined for induration and vesicle formation (Fig. 12-7). Positive reactions may be intense with painful skin erosions as a possible result, and subjects should be prepared to remove patches promptly if itching is severe; offending sites then should be washed thoroughly. In addition, patch testing may worsen ongoing dermatitis and should be deferred until the skin is substantially clear. For many substances, concentrations appropriate for testing may be found by consulting standard references. Tests with other materials must be carried out also on normal (control) subjects, who may be expected to respond comparably to primary irritant agents but not consistently to bland but sensitizing materials. Systemic corticosteroid drugs can partially suppress patch reactivity and are withheld, if possible, for at least 24 hours before as well as during testing; anti-

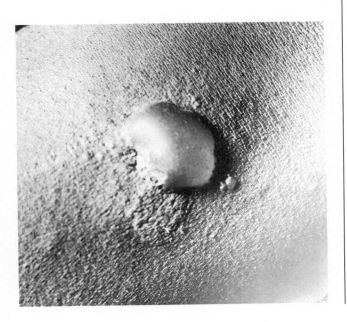

FIGURE 12-6
Large vesicles at the site of application of a crushed leaf of poison ivy 72 hours previously. The subject had had recurrent poison ivy dermatitis for many years.

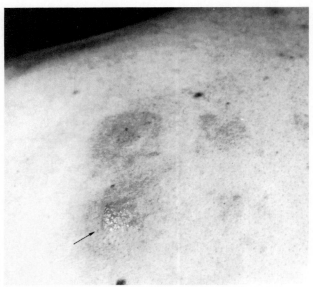

FIGURE 12-7
Patch test reactions to procaine applied in several concentrations to the back of a sensitive dentist. Vesicles (arrow) denote the strongest grade of reaction.

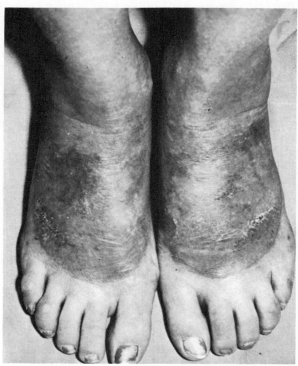

FIGURE 12-8
Phototoxic reaction in a subject taking dimethylchlortetracycline. (From J. M. Sheldon, R. G. Lovell, and K. P. Mathews, *A Manual of Clinical Allergy*, 2d ed., Saunders, Philadelphia, 1967.)

histaminic drugs and sympathetic agonists appear to have negligible effects. As with wheal-and-flare skin reactions, positive patch tests *cannot* be equated with causation of dermatitis, especially since contact sensitivity to some substances (e.g. specific plant oils) may occur in over one-half of exposed persons. However, test results provide essential correlates for use with clinical data in implicating exposure.

Certain substances (i.e., photocontact sensitizers) become allergenic only after skin to which they have been applied is exposed to visible light or adjacent bands. In the recent past, a family of antimicrobial agents (i.e., halogenated salicylanilides) found in commercial soaps caused widespread skin eruptions in this fashion. The resulting rash—restricted to light-exposed areas—must be distinguished from eruptions caused by wind-borne contact sensitizers (e.g., plant *oils*) or direct photosensitizers (e.g., tetracyclines, phenothiazines, psoralens, etc.), which produce *phototoxic* reactions (Fig. 12-8).

AECD often develops after several years of unabated exposure or, through an unexplained "hardening" process, may diminish or resolve completely despite persistent contact with an offending agent. However,

since, in many persons, dermatitis follows exposure indefinitely, avoidance of implicated sensitizers remains essential. A special risk exists in health care personnel who develop contact sensitivity to handled medications (e.g., local anesthetics, penicillins, and aminoglycoside antibiotics) that they themselves may receive systemically. Injection of contact-sensitive persons with these drugs may provoke a severe erythematous or maculopapular rash, with fever and toxicity, progressing occasionally to extensive exfoliation of skin.

Established dermatitis is managed with soaks when open vesicles predominate and, subsequently, with creams for partially healed lesions. Topical corticosteroids provide substantial though limited benefit, although finite courses of systemic steroids often promote rapid resolution of the dermatitis. At present, no available means of reducing sensitivity is sufficiently safe and effective to justify its recommendation. Patch test reactivity may be reduced during *prolonged* periods of ingestion or injection of specific agents (e.g., poison ivy oils). However, the limited results achieved rarely are worth the time, effort, and expense required for such therapy or the substantial risk of inducing local and/or systemic dermatitis.

Autoimmune and immune complex–induced diseases

Directions: Answer the following questions on a separate sheet of paper.

1. What is the significance of the appearance of autoantibodies?

2. Describe the way in which immune responses to tissue components could arise.

3. Describe Goodpasture's syndrome as an apparent example of antibody-mediated human autoimmunity.

4. What are the usual manifestations (signs and symptoms) of transfusion reactions?

5. Evaluate the measures that *must* be employed to prevent or mitigate hemolytic transfusion reactions.

6. What reactions can occur when serums containing potent leukoagglutinins have been infused or when persons deficient in IgA receive whole blood? How can the latter reactions be averted?

Directions: Circle T if the statement is true and F if it is false. Correct the false statements.

7. T F Human antibody-dependent, autoimmune disorders affect formed elements of the blood, with neutrophils and eosinophils attacked predominantly.

8. T F Hemolytic transfusion reactions comprise a distinct form of immunohemolytic process occurring usually when a recipient already sensitized to "foreign" human red blood cell antigens receives blood containing these antigens.

9. T F Autoaggressive immune reactions may originate with mutant clones of lymphoid cells programmed to recognize normal host components as foreign.

10. T F The pathogenesis of serum sickness probably involves complement system–derived products termed *anaphylatoxins* (C5a and C3a).

11. T F Viral infection reactions may foster the immune response to self antigens by damaging T_4^+ helper/promoter lymphocytes.

Directions: Circle the letter preceding each item below that correctly answers the question. More than one answer may be correct.

12. Increasing evidence has linked the disease idiopathic thrombocytopenic purpura (ITP) with:
a. Circulating IgG molecules reactive with platelet surfaces   b. Prominent decrease in complement levels   c. Catastrophic lysis of platelets in the free circulation   d. Platelets with bound IgG molecules that are more readily removed and destroyed by macrophages in spleen and liver

13. Persistent ITP may be suppressed by:
a. Corticosteroid therapy   b. Splenectomy   c. Both a and b   d. Neither a nor b

14. Individuals at risk for hemolytic reactions to transfused blood are those sensitized to red blood cell antigens by prior:
a. Transfusions   b. Pregnancy   c. Both a and b   d. Neither a nor b

15. All of the following spontaneously developing immunohemolytic phenomena are characteristic of "warm" red blood cell autoantibody reactions *except:*
a. Hemolysis may be absent and red cell agglutination minor   b. Autoantibodies are usually of the IgG class and are recognized primarily in middle-aged adults   c. Hemolysis is evident with rewarming after cold exposure   d. The IH disorder may be evident only as a positive Coombs' test (with antihuman IgG)

16. In serum sickness, the pathogenicity of the antigen-antibody complex depends upon the antigen-antibody ratio. Symptoms occur 10 to 14 days after first administration of an antigenic material when this ratio is such that:
a. There is a relative antibody excess—three antibody molecules (Ab) to two antigen molecules (Ag).   b. There is a relative antigen excess—three Ag to two Ab.   c. The antigen-to-antibody ratio is equal to one.

17. Serum sickness:
a. Occurs only after the administration of foreign serums to human beings   b. Occurs within a few minutes following administration of the offending antigen   c. May cause joint pain (arthralgia), lymph node enlargement (lymphadenopathy), and neuritis   d. Requires many previous periods of exposure to an offending antigen before frank disease is seen

18. Mr. J. received an antibiotic injection 12 days prior to his admission to the emergency room. He presents with a fever and angioedema and is complaining of pain in his hip, antecubital fossa, and knee joints. His diagnosis is serum sickness. Which of the following is true regarding the pathogenesis of this condition?
    a. It is an immune complex–induced illness.   *b.* It is only IgE-mediated.   *c.* Circulating antibody-antigen complexes are capable of activating complement components.   *d.* It is a delayed hypersensitivity reaction.

19. The treatment of serum sickness may require:
    a. No medication   *b.* Aspirin for fever and rheumatic complaints   *c.* Epinephrine to relieve urticaria and angioedema   *d.* High doses of corticosteroids for carditis or neurological manifestations   *d.* All of the above

20. The following statement(s) is/are true of allergic eczematous contact dermatitis:
    a. It is exemplified by burns due to caustic detergents.   *b.* It may be appropriately studied by patch tests applied to unbroken skin.   *c.* It is exemplified by poison ivy dermatitis.   *d.* It is a form of atopic eczema.

21. An obstetrical nurse has developed an allergic contact dermatitis to penicillin ointment. She last received intramuscular penicillin as a high school student without ill effect. An injection of penicillin at this time:
    a. Can be given with no fear of adverse reaction
    b. Would almost certainly produce anaphylaxis
    c. Would almost certainly produce serum sickness
    d. Would impose a definite risk of a generalized drug rash

Directions: Match the immunologic mechanisms in col. B to the condition to which it corresponds in col. A. More than one letter from col. B may be used.

Column A	*Column B*
22. ____ Goodpasture's syndrome	a. Immune complex–induced systemic reaction
23. ____ Serum sickness	b. Cellular immune reaction
24. ____ Wheal-and-flare skin response	c. Antibody-mediated human autoimmunity reaction
25. ____ Poison ivy	d. Immediate hypersensitivity reaction
26. ____ Hepatitis B infection with hives and arthritis	

CHAPTER
13

ADVERSE REACTIONS TO DRUGS AND RELATED SUBSTANCES

OBJECTIVES

At the completion of this chapter you should be able to:

1. Describe at least four mechanisms responsible for adverse reactions to drugs.

2. Identify the significance of a wheal-and-flare reaction at the site of an injection of morphine sulfate.

3. Give an example of a Type I reaction that is apparently mediated by IgE antibodies and can occur with systemically administered agents.

4. Explain the relationship between IgE-mediated responses to injected antigens and the atopic population.

5. Relate products of penicillin metabolism to types of adverse reaction following administration of the drug.

6. Appreciate for skin testing with penicilloyl polylysine (PPL) the indictions for, practical approach to, and information forthcoming from the procedure.

7. List three agents for which an immunologic basis usually can be shown for acute systemic and urticarial reactions.

8. Discuss the signs and symptoms and apparent basis of reactions to local anesthetics.

9. List medications that may induce formation of antinuclear antibodies.

10. Describe the drug-induced reactions that are associated with hemolysis.

11. Identify for drug-associated circulating complexes the type of reactions recognized and examples of responsible drugs.

12. List at least two topically applied agents that are known to elicit contact sensitivity readily.

13. Identify for drug-related fever reactions the postulated basis of the reactions and some associated agents.

14. Identify for nitrofurantoin-induced reactions the organs affected, signs and symptoms, useful diagnostic studies, and prognosis.

15. Describe the characteristic liver changes, clinical syndromes, and courses of adverse reactions to the following therapeutic agents: anabolic steroids, some oral contraceptives, chlorpropamide, isoniazid, phenytoin (Dilantin), and halothane.

16. Describe the skin lesions that are typical of a majority of cutaneous adverse drug reactions.
17. Describe the rashes that may be associated with the administration of penicillin.
18. Discuss the considerations which are helpful in the prevention of adverse drug reactions.

ADVERSE REACTIONS TO DRUGS AND RELATED SUBSTANCES

Well over 10 percent of patients who receive indicated drugs experience unforeseen adverse effects from their medication. Taken together, these events constitute a substantial public health problem and cause a serious waste of human and material resources.

Nonimmunologic reactions

Many adverse responses represent unwanted (but recognized) associated effects of drugs or frank toxicity arising from the dose employed or its rate of administration. However, some individuals manifest unique and inappropriate reactions, and this propensity is termed *idiosyncrasy*. Both these personal response patterns and instances of readily induced toxicity may arise from inborn deficiencies in drug-metabolizing capability or related *pharmacogenetic* defects. Reactions that mimic immunologic events are seen with drugs that cause direct histamine release from human mast cells (Fig. 13-1). Agents including morphine alkaloids, thiamine, polymyxin, and *d*-tubocurarine share this property and produce whealing at injection sites or, rarely, generalized hives and flushing following injection. A similar mechanism may be responsible for certain occurrences (e.g., flushing, hypotension, urticaria) following intravenous injection of x-ray contrast media. Local anesthetics commonly precipitate distressing reactions marked by syncope, hypotension, cardiac rhythm disturbances, and, at times, convulsions. Although reminiscent of anaphylaxis, these reactions are more probably a direct toxic effect of the large doses of drug commonly required for local infiltration. High blood levels may result, especially where these agents are injected with some force into restricted tissue compartments, as often occurs for dental procedures. There remain a large number of reactions involving skin and/or internal organs which are not otherwise explained and are often termed *allergic*; however, a causative immunologic process has been established in only a small fraction of these.

Immunologic reactions

Type I reactions, apparently mediated by IgE antibodies, occur with systemically administered agents (e.g., ACTH and insulin) which serve as complete antigens as well as with those of small molecular size that are

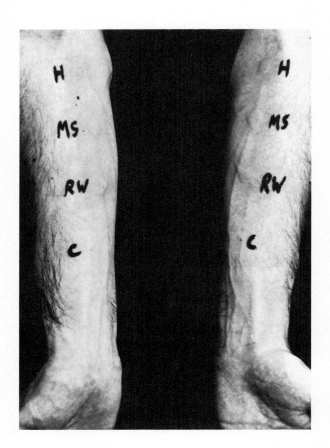

FIGURE 13-1
Skin test sites injected intracutaneously with histamine, morphine sulfate (a histamine releaser), ragweed pollen extract, and a saline solution control. Several mechanisms have produced quite similar wheals in this ragweed-sensitive subject.

capable of stable protein bonding. Adverse reactions to penicillins exemplify the latter mechanism, in which a drug and/or its metabolites serve as haptens. Administration of the sensitizing agent may produce immediately a complete or partial picture of anaphylaxis as well as "late" urticaria with onset after 48 to 72 hours (with penicillins, immunohemolytic reactions, serum sickness, and allergic eczematous contact dermatitis may also occur). Since IgE responses to *injected* antigens are possible in most persons, the risk of immediate systemic and urticarial reactions is not confined to, or even concentrated among, the atopic population. In human subjects, penicillin metabolism can proceed along several potential pathways involving many final and intermediate products, some of which are allergenic. Of the resulting substances, the penicilloyl radical appears to be the predominant sensitizer, and antibodies of this specificity are commonly associated with late urticarial and, at times, acute systemic reactions. By contrast, systemic (anaphylactic) responses with serious or, at times, fatal consequences make up a major proportion of the misadventures referable to native penicillin G or derivatives including penicilloic and penilloic acids. In view of the *frequency* of associated reactions (rather than their relative *severity*) the penicilloyl radical is often designated as the "major determinant" of penicillin allergy and the others as "minor determinants."

Clarification of the antigens responsible for penicillin sensitivity gave direction to efforts to identify reactive subjects. This goal was attained, however, only after development of a skin-reactive but nonsensitizing "major determinant" reagent, through conjugation of numerous penicilloyl groups to the synthetic peptide poly-L-lysine. Skin testing with the product, penicilloyl polylysine (PPL),* is now widely performed and, although minor determinant materials are less readily available, their value is generally acknowledged. Both materials assist in the evaluation of reported previous reactions and of the future risk of untoward events. In practice, epidermal tests are performed initially with PPL, a mixture of minor determinants, and a saline solution control. Penicillin G is applied in a strength of 10,000 units/ml unless extreme sensitivity is suggested, when testing is begun at 10 units/ml. Since higher levels may produce skin irritation, 10,000 units/ml is the highest penicillin G concentration employed for testing. If epidermal sites are negative, intracutaneous tests are performed (see Chap. 9) with 0.02-ml portions of PPL, penicillin G, other minor determinants, and saline solution control. Persons who react negatively to all of these materials have been shown empirically to tolerate therapeutic doses of penicillin with essentially no danger of *acute systemic* reactions. A small portion of *nonreactors* to PPL may show late urticarial responses or,

ultimately, a picture of serum sickness. In addition, there are indications that not *all* persons with positive PPL reactions would have adverse response to administered penicillin. However, the predictive value of these test procedures is strong, and the high risk associated with positive skin reactivity (especially to minor determinants) is especially noteworthy. Unfortunately, patterns of skin and systemic reactivity to semisynthetic penicillins (e.g., methicillin, ampicillin, carbenicillin) do not always parallel those to penicillin G and its derivatives. These disparities are especially distressing since only the unmodified, parenteral forms of the newer penicillins are available for testing (usually performed at 6 mg/ml). Furthermore, even with penicillin G, other minor determinants, and PPL in hand, a single set of negative skin tests cannot predict *lifelong* freedom from adverse reactivity when that drug is administered in repeated courses.

An immunologic basis usually can be shown for acute systemic and urticarial reactions to various immunizing biologicals, penicillins, and cephalosporins but rarely for additional agents, including aspirin.

In rare instances, autoimmune phenomena also are clearly related to the administration of specific medications. Several drugs, for example, including hydralazine, procainamide, diphenylhydantoin, and certain ovulatory suppressants may promote formation of antinuclear antibodies. Furthermore, in some affected persons, manifestations mimicking systemic lupus erythematosus have become evident, receding slowly only after the offending drug has been withdrawn. Additional agents, most notably alpha-methyldopa, in some way induce red blood cell autoantibodies which lead to positive direct Coombs' tests and, in a minority, bring on spherocytosis and frank hemolysis. Drug-associated hemolysis also has occurred in persons receiving large intravenous doses of penicillin owing to acquired sensitivity to a penicillin-conjugated red blood cell substance. Responsible IgG molecules participate in the direct and indirect Coombs' reactions using, respectively, patients' cells and "penicillinized" normal cells. Hemolysis characteristically begins 1 to 2 weeks after initiation of high-dose penicillin treatment but ceases shortly after the drug has been stopped.

Although hemolysis is not a feature of classic serum sickness, drug-associated circulating complexes are known to facilitate red blood cell, leukocyte, and platelet destruction in certain cases. These occurrences have been associated prominently with quinidine, and antituberculous drugs (*para*-aminosalicylic acid and isoniazid), and sulfonamides, although other medications have been implicated. Initially, complexes of host IgG or IgM

*Available as Pre-Pen.

and drug (or drug-protein conjugate) become attached to one or more blood cell types. Complement components then are localized to these surface sites, and their interaction (see Table 5-1) results in discrete membrane lesions or rapid removal of affected cells from the circulation, the formed elements being injured as "'innocent bystanders" rather than as direct participants. Following fixation of complement factors, the immune complexes initially responsible often dissociate from affected membranes. Such cells show Coombs' reactivity using antiserums specific for human complement (i.e., positive "nongamma" Coombs' tests) alone.*

Many *additional* forms of adverse drug reactivity are encountered with some frequency; however, of these, only AECD also has a well-defined immunologic basis, viz., in Type IV (cell-mediated) hypersensitivity (see Chap. 12). A remarkably high proportion of topically applied agents are known to elicit such contact sensitivity; among the foremost offenders are penicillin, aminoglycoside antibiotics, antihistaminic drugs, and local anesthetics.

ADDITIONAL, APPARENTLY IMMUNOLOGIC REACTIONS OF UNCERTAIN MECHANISM

Fever is a feature of many drug reactions and occasionally is the sole manifestation of an adverse response. Since both granulocytes and monocytes release substances that indirectly elevate body temperature, it is not surprising that fever accompanies a variety of health problems. Drug-related fever has been noted particularly with penicillin, sulfonamides, iodide, streptomycin, phenytoin (Dilantin), and additional agents.

Nitrofurantoin, a drug commonly employed to treat urinary tract infections, has been associated with distinctive adverse effects centered in the respiratory tract. Affected persons manifest fever, cough, and variable chest discomfort—often with a marked increase in peripheral blood eosinophil leukocytes. Chest x-rays obtained during these reactions often are abnormal, showing diffuse lung infiltrates and, at times, fluid in the pleural spaces. These rapidly developing changes are thought to resolve completely if nitrofurantoin is promptly discontinued; however, a chronic increase in lung fibrous connective tissue may occur *without* acute manifestations in those receiving the drug over long periods.

Many drugs are directly nephrotoxic (i.e., they cause kidney dysfunction and/or damage). In addition, several of the penicillins—especially methicillin—have been implicated in diffuse renal inflammatory reactions, or "interstitial nephritis." Drug-specific antibody responses often are demonstrable but their significance remains controversial. Kidney damage also has been associated with fever and skin rashes frequently and may result from immune complex deposition.

The liver is a principal site of drug metabolism and commonly bears the brunt of adverse reactions to therapeutic agents. A spectrum of tissue effects is recognized, with certain agents characteristically leading to cholestasis (a failure of bile transport) with little or no inflammation while others mimic florid viral hepatitis in causing necrosis of liver cells and collapse of supporting tissues. Bland cholestasis is an infrequent complication of treatment with certain anabolic steroids as well as some oral contraceptives, erythromycin estolate,* chlorpropamide, etc. Bile stasis and jaundice also occur in reactions to chlorpromazine; however, pathologically, dense infiltration of portal areas with neutrophils, eosinophils, and macrophages is an additional feature, and progression to permanent liver damage is seen rarely. Frank hepatitis has resulted during treatment with isoniazid, alpha-methyldopa, phenytoin, thiazide diuretics, and additional drugs including the anesthetic agents halothane and methoxyflurane. These drugs may be associated with acute fatal reactions or may lead to a picture of chronic liver inflammation and scarring (viz., a form of cirrhosis). In some instances, evidence of liver involvement may be preceded by fever, joint pains, peripheral blood eosinophilia, and/or any of a variety of skin rashes. Although such manifestations have led to increased speculation concerning an "allergic" basis for these reactions, the case for immune causation is preliminary, at best.

By far the largest proportion of familiar adverse drug reactions affect the skin. The resulting lesions generally are transient and not at all distinctive. A majority of "drug rashes" consist of macules (flat red spots) or papules (raised red spots) which are highly pruritic and tend to coalesce into a morbilliform eruption (i.e., like measles). In the case of penicillin, maculopapular rashes may be associated with reactions in tissue of drug-specific IgM antibodies; however, similar correlations have not been suggested for other agents. Failure to withdraw the responsible medication can, at times, lead to an exfoliative dermatitis in which the skin effectively is shed, leading to serious infection as well as heat and fluid losses. Additional common skin manifestations of adverse response to systemic medication include eruptions that are erythematous (diffuse flush), eczematous, vesicular (small blisters), bullous (large blisters), petechial (tiny hemorrhagic spots), purpuric (large hemor-

---

Nongamma Coombs' test reactions are obtained using antiserums to human serum components other than the gamma globulin fraction or specific immunoglobulin classes that it comprises.

*But rarely other salts of erythromycin.

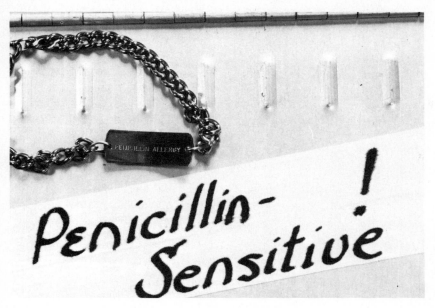

FIGURE 13-2

Adverse drug reactivity may be minimized by clearly stigmatizing those at risk. Well-marked health records and personal indentification, as shown, complement patient education.

rhagic patches), and urticarial. *Firm* hemorrhagic spots often accompany inflammatory lesions of small blood vessels (vasculitis), which can involve diverse organs. Reactions to iodides (and bromides) may consist of pustules or merely a worsening of lesions of acne vulgaris on the face and upper dorsal area. Skin reactions occasionally are confined to discrete patches of rash (viz., "fixed drug eruptions") which become active with each administration of the responsible systemic agent.

The prevention of adverse drug reactions is a serious responsibility which all health care personnel share. An effective approach to this problem requires knowledge of the potential complications of medication and a willingness to consider adverse drug reactivity as a possible cause of *any* unexpected clinical event. Since untoward responses usually are repetitive, no drug should be given without first reviewing the individual's past experience with that agent. Similarly, the clinical data

base requires no less than a comprehensive assessment of past drug reactivity. Health care personnel also must be prepared to accept, on face value, reports of previous problems arising from medication until these have been disproved conclusively.

Close surveillance can reveal the earliest stigmata of drug reactions, facilitating prompt withdrawal of the offender and, often, limiting morbidity. Once recognized, adverse reactivity must be clearly indicated in the clinical record (Fig. 13-2) and, if possible, the sensitivity should be identified for the patient or responsible family members. Documentation is aided, for practical purposes, if the patient can carry a card, bracelet, or medallion indicating medication(s) to be avoided. Careful instruction is necessary also where a risk of reaction from related agents exists or when, like aspirin, the offender has many readily available and poorly identified sources.

QUESTIONS

Adverse reactions to drugs and related substances

Directions: Circle the letter preceding each item below that correctly answers the question. More than one answer may be correct.

1. Which of the following statements are true regarding adverse drug reactions?
   a. Toxicity may arise through inborn deficiencies in drug-metabolizing capability. *b.* A causative immunologic process has been established in the majority of reactions involving the skin and/or internal organs. *c. Idiosyncrasy* is an adverse

drug reaction that is unrelated to the expected pharmacological effect. *d.* Over 10 percent of patients who receive indicated drugs experience adverse reactions from their medication.

2. Wheal-and-flare reactions are readily produced by local:
   a. Injection of histamine into most normal persons *b.* Injection of ragweed pollen extract into most normal persons *c.* Injection of morphine into most normal persons *d.* Application of local anesthetics to the skin of a person with a specific

allergic eczematous contact dermatitis to these agents

3. Type I reactions, apparently mediated by IgE, occur with systemically administered agents that serve as:
   a. Complete antigens   b. Haptens that are capable of stable protein binding   c. Both a and b   d. Neither a nor b

4. Regarding the predictive value of the results of skin testing with penicilloyl polylysine (PPL), which of the following statements is true?
   a. There are indications that not all persons with positive PPL reactions would have adverse responses to subsequently administered penicillin.
   b. Persons with negative reactions to PPL and other penicillin metabolites have been shown to tolerate therapeutic doses of penicillin with no danger of acute systemic reactions.   c. This test accurately predicts skin and systemic reactions to semisynthetic penicillins.   d. A single set of negative skin tests can predict lifelong freedom from adverse reactivity when the drug is administered in repeated doses.

5. An immunologic basis usually can be shown for acute systemic and urticarial reactions to all of the following except:
   a. Certain biologicals   b. Aspirin   c. Penicillin   d. Cephalosporins

6. Autoimmune phenomena are clearly related to the administration of which of the following medications that may induce formation of antinuclear antibodies:
   a. Alpha-methyldopa   b. Aspirin   c. Hydralazine   d Procainamide

7. Adverse drug reactions to nitrofurantoin are manifested by:
   a. Fever   b. Diffuse lung infiltrates and fluid in the pleural spaces   c. Decrease in eosinophil leukocytes   d. Jaundice

Directions: Circle T if the statement is true and F if it is false. Correct the false statements.

8. T   F   The risk of IgE-mediated responses (immediate systemic and urticarial reactions) to injected antigens is usually confined to atopic individuals.

9. T   F   Drug-associated circulating complexes are known to facilitate red blood cell, leukocyte, and platelet destruction in certain cases.

10. T   F   Drug-related fever has been associated with penicillin, sulfonamides, iodide, streptomycin, phenytoin (Dilantin), and additional agents.

Directions: Match the medication in col. A with its characteristic reaction in col. B. More than one item from col. B may be used in col. A.

Column A	Column B
11. ___ Chlorpropamide	a. Bile stasis and jaundice
12. ___ Isoniazid	b. Hepatitis
13. ___ Iodides	c. Maculopapular rashes
14. ___ Halothane	d. Chronic liver inflammation and scarring
15. ___ Penicillin	e. Pustules or a worsening of facial and upper-dorsal lesions of acne vulgaris

Directions: Answer the following questions on a separate sheet of paper.

16. Explain the basis of the adverse reactions observed with drug-associated circulating complexes that affect blood elements.

17. List the reactions commonly associated with the administration of local anesthetics. What is the probable mechanism of these reactions?

18. Discuss the considerations which are helpful in reducing the prevalence of adverse drug reactions.

APPROACHES TO IMMUNE DEFICIENCY STATES

OBJECTIVES

At the completion of this chapter you should be able to:

1. Identify for deficits in humoral immunity the infectious agent(s) involved and host reactions that are impaired most prominently.

2. Describe the methods used to evaluate antigen-specific antibody activity associated with one or more immunoglobulin classes.

3. Identify for IgA immunodeficiency the fraction of the population affected, serum levels encountered, and consequences in affected persons.

4. Compare X-linked hypogammaglobulinemia of infancy and acquired, common variable hypogammaglobulinemia in terms of manifestations, natural history, complications, and treatment.

5. List the disease conditions in which cell-mediated immune function is inadequate.

6. Identify for the Di George syndrome and combined (B- and T-cell) immunodeficiency the etiology and treatment considerations.

7. State the relationship between peripheral blood lymphocyte counts and T-cell defects.

8. Describe the place of delayed-type hypersensitivity (DTH) skin tests as indicators of cellular immune competence.

9. State the purpose of the dinitrochlorobenzene (DNCB) skin sensitization test.

10. Describe three additional tests reflecting T-cell function.

11. Describe an example of an antigen-specific defect in cell-mediated immunity by identifying the responsible infectious agent, organ(s) involved, complications, and treatment.

Current views of immune function emphasize the complex integration of antigen-specific components and effector systems required for normal humoral and cellular hypersensitivity. Both inborn and acquired defects have been recognized at many points in this usually well-coordinated system. The resulting flaws in immune competence may have no clinical consequences or may open the way for catastrophic infection or neoplastic disease. No attempt will be made to describe or catalog the various immunodeficiency disease states. Instead, this section will focus briefly on methods of evaluating immune function, as they relate to deficiency states of several major types.

Deficits in humoral (i.e., antibody-mediated) immunity commonly undermine defenses against virulent bacteria, many of which are encapsulated and stimulate pus formation. Impaired hosts are prone to suffer recurrent infections of the skin, middle ear, and meninges as well as of the paranasal sinuses and bronchopulmonary structures. Repeated attacks by bacteria of a *single* antigenic type are often demonstrable, and, in those with the greatest impairment, naturally acquired viral infections and *live* viral vaccines also may cause grave illness.

Assay of serum immunoglobulins by radial immunodiffusion (Fig. 14-1) provides a widely available, direct measurement of circulating molecules having potential antibody activity. In this procedure, test serums and samples of known immunoglobulin (Ig) content are placed in separate wells cut into agar containing antiserums, derived from other species, to human IgA, IgG, IgM, or IgD. As human serum diffuses outward, a line

of precipitation forms at the forward edge where a favorable ratio of antiserum and specific human Ig is achieved; within this perimeter, an excess of the Ig (i.e., the antigen) suppresses precipitation. The ring diameter around each well is proportional to the Ig content of the serum added, and absolute levels are derived by referring to assayed "known" samples. Determination of IgE content requires alternative techniques employing radioactive markers, because of the lower range in which levels of this Ig fall. Normal total values for specific Ig classes are indicated in Table 14-1.

Several methods are available to evaluate *antigen-specific* antibody activity associated with one or more Ig classes; these include:

1. Determination of naturally occurring (IgM) antibodies to ABO blood group substances which are absent from the subjects' red blood cells. Normal persons consistently demonstrate such *isohemagglutinins* by the age of 1 year.

2. Schick testing of persons previously immunized with diphtheria toxoid. If adequate levels of specific (IgG) antibody have been produced, tissue breakdown at the site of toxin injection is prevented.

3. Determination of antibody titers before and after *nonviable* immunizing materials such as tetanus toxoid and typhoid or influenza vaccines.

In addition, estimates of circulating B-lymphocyte numbers may be made by immunofluorescent staining of the Ig molecules that are prominent on their cell surfaces. In the blood of normal persons, approximately 15 to 20 percent of lymphocytes bear such markers, identifying them as B lymphocytes.

The most frequently encountered form of continuing antibody-dependent immunodeficiency is a selective deficit of IgA, which is observed in 1 in every 500 to 1000 persons. Serum levels of IgA are below 5 mg per 100 ml in this condition and, at mucosal surfaces, the normal preponderance of IgA commonly is replaced by IgG and IgM. Some affected persons remain free of evident illness, but most manifest recurrent paranasal sinus and pulmonary infections. In addition, increased risks of atopic allergic problems as well as certain rheumatic and gastrointestinal diseases seem to exist in this condition. Replacement of deficient serum IgA is not feasible, and systemic reactions due to anti-IgA antibod-

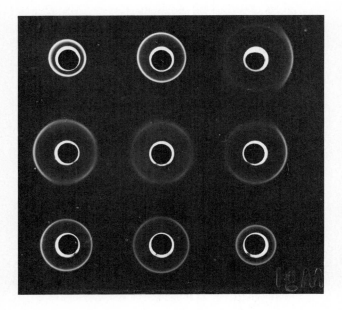

FIGURE 14-1

Determination of immunoglobulin levels by radial immunodiffusion. The agar plate shown contains goat antihuman IgM. The IgM content of samples added to the wells is evidenced by the diameters of the resulting circles of precipitation. The uppermost row of wells contain known serums of increasing IgM content (from left to right).

TABLE 14-1

NORMAL SERUM IMMUNOGLOBULIN LEVELS AT VARIOUS AGES*

Age	IgG, mg/ 100 ml	IgA, mg/ 100 ml	IgM, mg/ 100 ml	IgE, IU/ml†
At birth	650–1250	1–6	5–35	1–3
1–3 yr	250–1320	15–160	15–115	10–500
5–10 yr	550–1450	20–220	30–135	15–600
10–15 yr	620–1450	30–230	35–150	20–750
Adult	720–1800	60–300	45–160	25–900

*Values are approximations of expected ranges derived from several sources.
†IU (international unit) = 2.3 nanograms (ng) IgE.

ies may follow transfusion of human blood products (see Chap. 12).

Males with X-linked hypogammaglobulinemia of infancy exhibit the most severe selective deficiency of humoral immune function, with virtual absence of circulating immunoglobulins and B cells. In addition, these individuals have marked reduction in the size and structural organization of lymph nodes and lymphoid tissues of pharynx and gut (see Chap. 5). Recurrent purulent (viz., pus-forming) infections usually begin after 4 to 6 months of age, when transplacentally acquired levels of maternal IgG have been cleared and are no longer protective. Otitis media, bronchitis, pneumonitis, meningitis, and skin infections are prominent and often lead to permanent organ damage (e.g., bronchiectasis). In addition, viruses, including hepatitis B and attenuated strains present in certain vaccines, may produce severe illnesses, at times with central nervous system damage, if administered to these patients. Rapidly progressive tooth decay and chronic conjunctivitis often add to the patients' discomfort, and an eczematous dermatitis, arthritis resembling rheumatoid disease, and intestinal malabsorption are frequently associated. The administration of commercial gamma globulin by intramuscular injection controls many of these problems and complements appropriate antibiotic treatment; adequate doses usually approximate 0.2 to 0.4 ml/kg every 2 to 4 weeks. These preparations contain no IgA or IgM, and possibly as a result, fail to control infection in some persons despite maximum doses. Better results may follow regular plasma infusions from single donors, free of hepatitis antigen, providing a humoral "buddy system." Recently, the availability of human gamma globulin preparations for intravenous use has allowed high dose replacement for IgG-deficient persons.

Persons of either sex with low Ig levels and infections beginning after infancy are seen with some frequency. This group with acquired, "common, variable hypogammaglobulinemia" often have prominent lymph nodes and intestinal lymphoid aggregates as well as normal numbers of circulating B cells. However, immunoglobulin synthesis and/or secretion tends to be deficient.

As a result, they experience recurrent and sustained sinopulmonary infections as well as intestinal malabsorption, often augmented by infection with the protozoan *Giardia lamblia*. In both affected persons and their relatives, an increased risk of autoantibodies and related diseases (including ITP, immunohemolytic anemia, pernicious anemia, systemic lupus, and rheumatoid arthritis) are noted. Laboratory evidence of impaired T-cell function also has been obtained in some patients. Appropriate antibiotic therapy and Ig replacement using gamma globulin or suitably screened plasma provides substantial benefit in most cases.

Humoral immunodeficiency is especially prominent in certain malignant states such as multiple myeloma and chronic lymphocytic leukemia and contributes to deficits occurring when tumor cells of any source infiltrate lymphoreticular structures. Similar infectious problems (with pyogenic bacteria) may develop in persons deficient in one or more serum complement factors as well as with inadequate leukocyte numbers or function. Serum levels of C3 may be assayed by radial immunodiffusion.* In addition, overall complement activity is commonly estimated from the ability of test serums to facilitate hemolysis of optimally sensitized red blood cells; this capacity is expressed as "CH$_{50}$ activity." Granulocyte deficiencies may be inborn or may accompany conditions such as alcoholism or corticosteroid excess. Defects in leukocyte function may affect random movement, directed movement (chemotaxis), phagocytosis, formation of enzymatically active vacuoles, and intracellular killing by white blood cells. These modalities can be examined *individually* with acceptable precision in a minority of laboratories. More generally available studies include the white blood cell count, leukocyte morphology in peripheral blood smears, and peroxidase stain to confirm the content of myeloperoxidase, a leukocyte enzyme required for intracellular killing of certain ingested organisms. In addition, the quantitative assay of nitroblue tetrazolium (NBT) dye reduction provides a valuable clue to the diagnosis of chronic granulomatous disease (of childhood). Recurrent infection by *Staphylococcus aureus* (*Micrococcus pyogenes*), *Pseudomonas* species, and *Escherichia coli* as well as organisms normally of low virulence (e.g., *Serratia*, *Staphylococcus epidermidis*, and *Candida*) are typical of this X-linked disorder.† Offending organisms are ingested normally but escape death

*This technique may be used for additional complement components although the necessary reagents are not available universally.
†A variant form in females is known to occur rarely.

death and can multiply intracellularly, ultimately destroying the inept phagocytes; a clinical picture of recurrent abscesses, indolent drainage of lymph nodes, osteomyelitis, pneumonia, and persistent diarrhea is the result. Defective killing appears to reflect impaired leukocyte metabolism with decreased generation of hydrogen peroxide and related substances that participate in a microbicidal system. The metabolic defect also precludes the normal reduction of NBT to a readily visible blue-black form, a deficit easily quantitated by colorimetric assay.

Cell-mediated immune function is inadequate in many disease states either as a "primary defect" or secondary to disorders including sarcoidosis, Hodgkin's disease, certain non-Hodgkin's neoplasms, and uremia; therapy with corticosteroids or cytotoxic drugs (e.g., cyclophosphamide) is also a frequent factor. In addition, cellular immunity may be impaired *transiently* by viral infections such as rubeola (measles). Of the steadily growing list of conditions associated with abnormalities of T-cell function, a large majority also display aberrant humoral (i.e., B-cell) immunity. Overall, victims of these disorders are prone to infection by characteristic spectra of organisms which may include bacteria, viruses, protozoa (especially *Pneumocystis carinii*), and fungi. Lymphoreticular malignancies are common terminal complications of many of these disorders.

Relatively complete absence of T-cell function occurs when the thymus fails to develop (viz., the Di George syndrome), and affected infants have been restored immunologically to adequate function with grafts of early fetal thymus tissue. The most compromised individuals are those with severe combined immunodeficiency, who totally lack B-cell as well as T-cell function, often succumbing within the first year of life. Transplantation of bone marrow from optimally matched donors has permitted survival, and partial reconstitution has been achieved with early fetal liver or thymus grafts. Bone marrow recipients often have developed severe *graft vs. host* disease due to cytotoxicity of donor lymphocytes reacting against transplantation antigens of the host. Deficiencies of specific cellular enzymes required for normal nucleoprotein metabolism are demonstrable in certain cases of combined immunodeficiency. A variety of other conditions with combined defects are recognized; most often observed are the Wiskott-Aldrich syndrome (eczema, platelet deficiency, low IgM level) and ataxia telangiectasia (ataxia, spontaneous movements, vascular malformations of skin and conjunctiva, and mental retardation), both of which are familial. In addition an acquired immunodeficiency syndrome (AIDS) transmitted by intimate contact and (apparently) by blood products has received increasing attention (see Chaps. 5 and 77).

Although numerous correlates and functional components of cell-mediated immunity are recognized, only a few are widely tested at present. T-cell defects may be reflected in decreased numbers of peripheral blood lymphocytes, and counts consistently below 1200 per microliter (2000 per microliter in infancy) suggest cellular immunodeficiency. Reactivity to delayed-type hypersensitivity (DTH) skin tests provides a readily available indicator of cellular immune competence. For this purpose, intradermal injections are performed with 0.1-ml portions of substances that elicit DTH and to which a previous sensitizing exposure may be assumed; commonly used materials include purified protein derivative of the tubercle bacillus (PPD), streptokinase and streptodornase, (enzymes of beta-hemolytic streptococci), and antigens from *Candida albicans*, mumps virus, *Histoplasma capsulatum*, and fungi of superficial skin infections. Test sites are observed and palpated after 48 hours, and an indurated area with a diameter of 10 mm or larger generally is regarded as a positive reaction. Using a "battery" of such materials, at least one positive test should be evident in the vast majority of normal individuals (excluding infants). For nonreactors, a more stringent test of cellular competence is provided by attempting contact sensitization with dinitrochlorobenzene (DNCB). This potent material, which is *absent* elsewhere in the environment, is applied (usually as a 30% solution in acetone) to a small skin area; sensitivity testing with a 1% solution at a distant site is performed 14 days later (if a flare is not present at the original point of application at that time).* Over 95 percent of normal persons acquire contact allergy by this procedure, confirming at least partial T-cell function. DNCB in 30% solution is also a strong primary irritant, and patients should recognize that a small scar may develop where it is applied. DNCB sensitization is seldom used, at present. Instead, questions concerning cell-mediated mune function often may be answered by determining subset of T and B cells through appropriate tagging of antigens on their surfaces. Automated approaches to such assays (i.e., by *flow cytometry*) can estimate levels of helper/induced, suppressor/cytotoxic and null cells as well as functional subcomponents within these groups. Additional tests reflecting T-cell function may include:

1. Response of lymphocytes in short-term tissue culture to antigens and nonspecific agents (e.g., phytohemagglutinin) that stimulate cell division and associated nucleic acid synthesis. An increase in the incorporation of added thymidine tagged with tri-

---

*Usually a 1% solution also is applied initially to detect the rare person previously sensitized to DNCB.

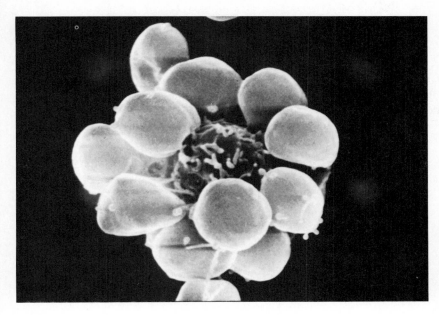

FIGURE 14-2
Human T-cell rosette. A central T lymphocyte is shown surrounded by adherent sheep red blood cells. (Scanning electron micrograph courtesy of Dr. Michael Deegan and Dr. Bertram Schnitzer.)

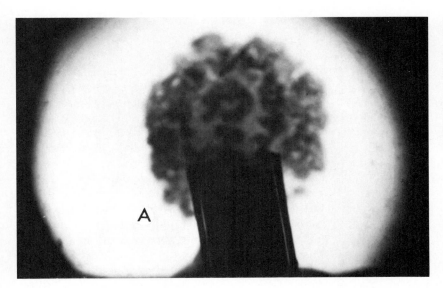

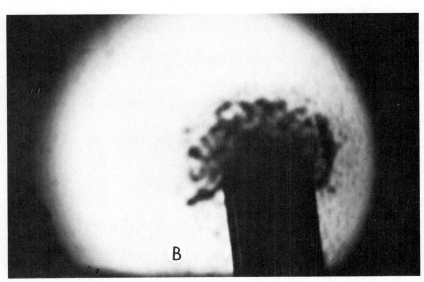

FIGURE 14-3
Macrophage inhibitory factor (MIF) effects as seen in a capillary tube assay. Both tubes contain machophages plus lymphocytes from a tuberculin-sensitive donor. Tuberculin has been added to the tissue culture medium for B, but not for A. The restricted "fan" of migrating cells in B may be measured as an indicator of MIF production by lymphocytes.

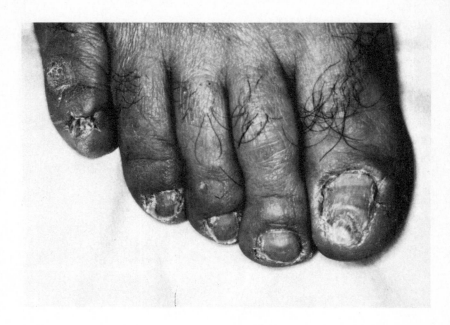

FIGURE 14-4
Skin and nail lesions on the foot of a patient with chronic mucocutaneous candidiasis. (Photograph courtesy of Dr. Jeffrey Callen.)

tium is observed normally in response to these agents.

2. Peripheral aggregation of sheep red blood cells (i.e., "rosette formation") around human peripheral lymphocytes (T lymphocytes) when the two are mixed and incubated (Fig. 14-2). Normally, over 60 percent of lymphocytes demonstrate rosetting, although a teleological basis for the sheep cell receptor is unknown.

3. Assays of lymphokines produced in response to appropriate antigens added to lymphocyte preparations (see Chap. 5). To date, most studies have focused on the macrophage inhibiting factor (MIF), and defects at several stages prior to its release have been described (Fig. 14-3).

Antigen-specific defects in cell-mediated immunity also are recognized; perhaps the best-studied example is chronic mucocutaneous candidiasis (Fig. 14-4). In this condition, indolent *Candida albicans* infection with granuloma formation occurs. Although systemic dissem-

ination is almost unknown, oral candidiasis *(thrush)*, esophageal involvement with dysphagia (difficulty in swallowing), and *Candida* vaginitis may cause severe distress. In addition, affected individuals often show autoantibodies reactive with endocrine tissues and defects in endocrine function—especially adrenal and parathyroid deficiencies—as a possible result. Although cell-mediated immunity to *Candida* is ineffective in this condition, other T-cell functions usually are found to be intact. Defective responses to *Candida* antigens vary among patients, being total in some while others show intact lymphocyte mitogenic responses and/or MIF production despite negative skin tests at 48 hours; in a few, circulating inhibitors of *Candida*-directed cellular immunity occur. Although treatment with amphotericin B can provide temporary improvement, drug toxicity and the expectation of posttreatment relapse limit its usefulness. Repeated injection of transfer factor (see Chap. 5) prepared from lymphocytes of persons with strong DTH to *Candida* has led to prolonged remissions in some cases.

QUESTIONS

Approaches to immune deficiency states

Directions: Circle the letter preceding each item below that correctly answers the question. More than one answer may be correct.

1. Deficits in humoral immunity commonly impair defenses against:
   a. Tubercle bacilli   *b.* Herpes simplex
   c. *Giardia lamblia*   *d.* Virulent pus-forming bacteria

2. Which of the following characteristics are true of acquired, common variable hypogammaglobulinemia?
   a. Virtual absence of circulating B cells   *b.* Only males involved   *c.* Normal number of circulating B cells   *d.* Low Ig levels

3. The usual treatment of X-linked hypogammaglobulinemia includes:
   a. The administration of commercial gamma globulin   *b.* Appropriate antibiotic therapy
   c. Both *a* and *b*   *d.* Neither *a* nor *b*

4. Cell-mediated immune function is inadequate in or may be impaired transiently by:
   a. Cytotoxic drugs   b. Viral infections
   c. Adrenal corticosteroids   d. Streptococcal pharyngitis

Directions: Circle T if the statement is true and F if it is false. Correct the false statements.

5. T   F   Assay of serum immunoglobulins by radial immunodiffusion provides a widely available, direct measurement of circulating molecules having potential antibody activity.

6. T   F   The most frequently encountered form of continuing immunodeficiency is a selective deficit of IgG.

7. T   F   Some persons with a deficit of IgA (level below 5 mg per 100 ml) remain free of evident illness, but most manifest recurrent paranasal sinus and pulmonary infections.

8. T   F   Humoral immunodeficiency is present most commonly as an isolated immunologic deficit in non-Hodgkin's lymphoma and uremia.

9. T   F   Patients with Di George syndrome totally lack B- as well as T-cell function because the thymus fails to develop.

10. T   F   Chronic mucocutaneous candidiasis is an example of an antigen-specific defect in cell-mediated immunity and is characterized by indolent *Candida albicans* infections of the skin, nails, and mucous membranes with granuloma formation.

Directions: Answer the following questions on a separate sheet of paper.

11. List three methods used to evaluate antigen-specific antibody activity associated wtih one or more Ig classes.

12. Explain the significance of delayed-type hypersensitivity (DTH) skin tests as an indicator of cellular immune competence.

13. Describe three additional laboratory tests reflecting lymphocyte function.

REFERENCES FOR PART II

ALTMAN, L. C.: *Clinical Allergy and Immunology*, G.K. Hall, Boston, 1984.

BIERMAN, C. W. and D. S. PEARLMAN: *Allergic Diseases of Infancy, Childhood, and Adolescence*, Saunders, Philadelphia, 1980.

BLAYLOCK, W. K.: "Atopic Dermatitis: Diagnosis and Pathobiology," *Journal of Allergy and Clinical Immunology*, **57**:(1): 62–79, January 1976.

DeSWARTE, R. D.: "Drug Allergy," in R. Paterson (ed.), *Allergic Diseases*, 2d ed., Lippincott, Philadelphia, 1980, pp. 452–583.

FISHER, A. A.: *Contact Dermatitis*, 2d ed., Lea & Febiger, Philadelphia, 1973.

LICHTENSTEIN, L. M. et al.: "Insect Allergy: State of the Art," *Journal of Allergy and Clinical Immunology*, **64**:(1): 5–12, July 1979.

MATHEWS, K. P.: "Urticaria and Angioedema," *Journal of Allergy and Clinical Immunology*, **72**:(1): 1–14, July 1983.

MIDDLETON, E., JR., C. E. REED, and E. F. ELLIS: *Allergy: Principles and Practice*, 2d ed., Mosby, St. Louis, 1983.

PARKER, C. W.: "Drug Allergy," *New England Journal of Medicine*, **292**:(10): part 1, 511–514, March 6, 1975.

———: "Drug Allergy," *New England Journal of Medicine*, **292**(14): part 2, 732–736, April 3, 1975.

———: "Drug Allergy," *New England Journal of Medicine*, **292**(18): part 3, 957–960, May 1, 1975.

SCHLUETER, D. P.: "Response of the Lung to Inhaled Antigens," *American Journal of Medicine*, **57**:(3): 476–492, September 1974.

SELL, S.: *Immunology, Immunopathology, and Immunity*, 3d ed., Harper & Row, Hagerstown, Md., 1980.

SHEFFER, A. L. and K. F. AUSTEN: "Exercise-Induced Anaphylaxis," *Journal of Allergy and Clinical Immunology*, **66**:(2): 106–111, August 1980.

STIEHM, E. R. and V. A. FULGINITI: *Immunological Disorders in Infants and Children*, Saunders, Philadelphia, 1980.

WILLIAMS, R.: *Immune Complexes in Clinical and Experimental Medicine*, Harvard, Cambridge, Mass., 1980.

ZIEGER, R. S. et al.: "Immunotherapy of Atopic Disorders," *Medical Clinics of North America*, **65**:(5): 987–1012, September 1981.

PART III

CATHERINE M. BALDY

HEMATOLOGIC DISORDERS

Hematology is a science which deals with blood and the blood-forming tissues. This hematologic system also includes the monocyte-macrophage (mononuclear phagocyte) system, originally described as the reticuloendothelial system (RES), which is located throughout the body, especially in the spleen, liver, lymph nodes, and bone marrow. It phagocytizes foreign materials ranging from microorganisms to dying red blood cells from the blood and body tissues. Disorders arising from these systems, called *blood dyscrasias*, range from mild and curable to rapidly progressing and lethal diseases. Diagnosis and treatment focus on the accurate interpretation of historical data, careful physical assessment, and laboratory examination.

This section will examine the blood-forming tissues, the blood, and its components, with emphasis on alterations relating to red blood cells, white blood cells, platelets, and the clotting factors.

OBJECTIVES

At the completion of this part you should be able to:

1. Identify the component parts of the blood.
2. Describe how pathologic hematologic conditions are manifested as disease processes.
3. Describe the sequence of events in the mechanism of blood clotting.
4. Develop skill in identifying etiology, pathogenesis, and treatment of hematologic disorders.

CHAPTER
15

THE COMPOSITION OF THE BLOOD AND THE MONOCYTE-MACROPHAGE SYSTEM

OBJECTIVES

At the completion of this chapter you should be able to:

1. Formulate a definition of hematology.

2. List the components of the hematologic system.

3. Differentiate between the aqueous and cellular components of the blood as to composition, function, and percentages of water, protein, and solids.

4. List the major cells found in the particulate matter of blood.

5. Explain the theory of formation and maturation of blood cells (hematopoiesis).

6. Describe the assessment process used in diagnosing hematologic disorders (blood dyscrasias).

7. Identify and differentiate among the methods used to examine blood (blood cell count unit, differential blood cell count) as to process and purpose.

8. Explain for hemoglobin the synthesis process, function, concentration, and method of identification.

9. State the purpose of obtaining red cell indices.

10. Identify for red cell count, hemoglobin concentration, and hematocrit the purpose of each, a description of each test, and the normal values.

11. Differentiate among mean corpuscular volume (MCV), mean corpuscular hemoglobin concentration (MCHC), and mean corpuscular hemoglobin measurement (MCH) as to purpose and normal range.

12. Discuss the purpose and process of the reticulocyte count.

13. Cite for the white blood count, the differential count, and the platelet count a description of the procedure and the normal values.

14. Discuss the purpose of and the procedure for a bone marrow aspiration and biopsy.

179

COMPONENTS OF NORMAL BLOOD

Blood is a suspension of particulate material in an aqueous colloid solution containing electrolytes. It serves as a medium of exchange between the fixed cells of the body and the external environment and possesses properties protective to the organism as a whole and to itself in particular.

The aqueous component of blood, termed *plasma*, consists of 91 to 92 percent water as a transport medium and 7 to 9 percent solids. The solids include such proteins as albumin, globulin, and fibrinogen; inorganic constituents including sodium, calcium, potassium, magnesium, phosphorus, iron, and iodine; and organic constituents such as nonprotein nitrogenous substances, urea, uric acid, xanthine, creatinine, amino acids, neutral fats, phospholipids, cholesterol, glucose, and various enzymes such as amylase, protease, and lipase. A supernatant serum remains after the removal of fibrinogen and the clotting factors from plasma. Even though all the elements play a vital role in homeostasis, the plasma proteins are often involved in blood dyscrasias. Of the three major types, albumin formed in the liver accounts for approximately 53 percent of the serum protein. The major role of albumin is in the maintenance of blood volume by providing colloid osmotic pressure, pH and electrolyte balance, and the transport of metal ions, fatty acids, steroids, hormones, and drugs (Brobeck, 1979). Globulins, accounting for 43 percent of the protein, are formed in the liver and lymphoid tissues. They are responsible for antibody and prothrombin formation. Fibrinogen, accounting for only 4 percent, is essential for blood clotting.

The cellular component of whole blood consists of red blood cells (erythrocytes, red corpuscles, or RBCs), several different types of white blood cells (leukocytes, white corpuscles, or WBCs), and fragments of cells called platelets (or thrombocytes). The function of red blood cells is the transport or exchange of O_2 and CO_2, whereas white blood cells are responsible for infection control, and platelets for hemostasis. Because these cells have a finite life span, a constant optimum production is necessary to maintain levels required to meet tissue needs. In adults this production, which is called *hematopoiesis* (formation and maturation of blood cells), takes place in the bone marrow of the skull, vertebrae, pelvis, sternum, ribs, and the proximal epiphyses of the long bones. During periods of increased demand as in hemorrhage or cell destruction (hemolysis), production may resume in all the long bones, as is the case in children.

On the basis of sophisticated karyotype (chromosomal) studies, all normal blood cells are thought to derive from a single pluripotential *stem cell* with mitotic capability. Stem cells can differentiate into lymphoid and hematopoietic stem cells which become progenitor cells. Progenitor cells differentiate along a single pathway. Through a series of divisions and maturational changes, these cells become specific mature cells in the circulating blood (Fig. 15-1). The marrow stem cells steadily replace normally dying cells and respond to acute changes such as hemorrhage or infection by differentiating into the *specific cell lines* needed.

The monocyte-macrophage system is a part of the hematologic system and includes circulating monocytes and their precursor cells in the bone marrow. The more mature tissue monocyte is called a *macrophage* (a specific WBC responsible for phagocytosis in the inflammatory reaction). This system is described in Chap. 4.

METHODS FOR STUDYING BLOOD

Inherent in an accurate diagnosis of hematologic disorders (blood dyscrasias) is an in-depth assessment of the individual. This assessment includes a thorough history (i.e., past and current illnesses, drug exposure, bleeding tendencies, nutritional habits, and family history), physical examination, and selective diagnostic studies. Specific studies attempt to quantitate the various constituents of blood and bone marrow. This may be accomplished by examining a specified volume of blood. For the most accurate results, a venous blood sample, which is obtained by a venipuncture, is preferred. However, capillary blood specimens may be obtained by pricking the free margin of the earlobe or the palmar surface of the fingertips.

Descriptive terms and methods of measurement

Blood cell count refers to an actual count of the number of formed elements, i.e., red blood cells, white blood cells, and platelets, in a specific volume of blood. Red blood cells must be lysed (destroyed) before the white blood cells can be counted. These counts are usually expressed as a number of cells per cubic millimeter (mm^3) of blood, but may be expressed as the number of cells per liter as recommended by the International Committee for Standardization in Hematology. Abnormal cell counts are a reflection of the body's response or lack of response to certain processes.

Differential blood cell count determines the morphologic characteristics of blood cells. This is done by extracting a drop of capillary blood from the fingertip or the earlobe and carefully spreading a thin film on a glass slide. The slide is stained with Wright's stain which imparts different colors to the various cell structures according to their pH. Colors range from blue to

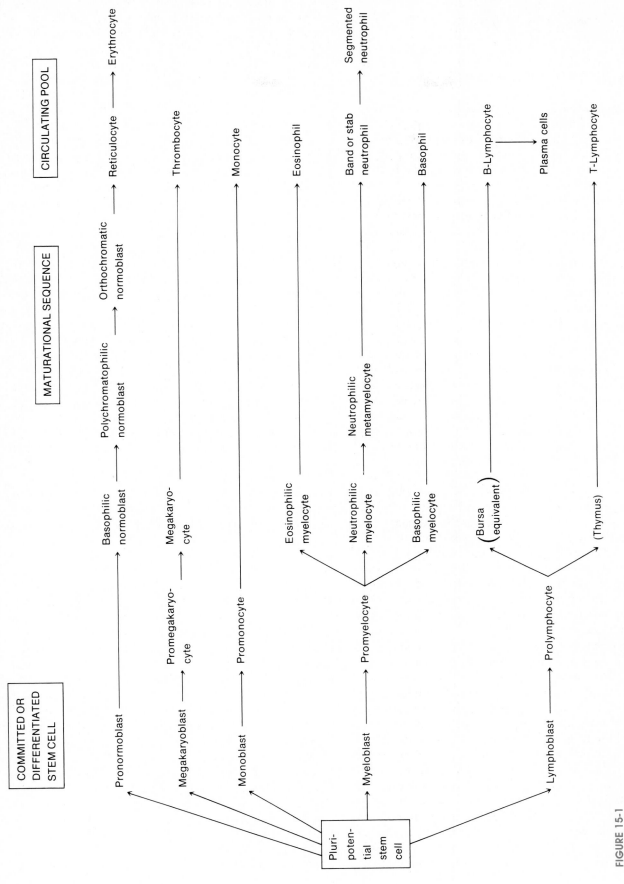

FIGURE 15-1

Theory of formation and maturation of blood cells (hematopoiesis).

pink or red. The various types of white blood cells, red blood cells, and platelets can be differentiated according to (1) the color they stain, (2) their size and configuration, (3) the structure of the nuclear chromatin, and (4) the presence or absence of nucleoli within the nucleus. An experienced hematologist, hematopathologist, or laboratory technologist can identify the various cells, their maturities, and other characteristics.

The red blood cells visible on smears may be characterized according to variations in size and shape. The term *anisocytosis* refers to an abnormal variation in the size of the cells. Abnormal variation in shape is *poikilocytosis* and may denote cells that are shaped like teardrops, pears, helmets, and ovals. Poikilocytosis may reflect defective *erythropoiesis* (formation and development of red blood cells).

Spherocytes are cells in which the diameter/thickness ratio is decreased. These cells appear spherical in shape instead of having the normal biconcave disk of the red blood cell. They have increased osmotic fragility and are seen in a congenital hemolytic anemia called congenital spherocytosis. Sickle cells are characteristic of hemoglobin S and other sickling forms of hemoglobin. The cells assume a sickle shape on deoxygenation.

Polychromasia is a term used when cells vary in their color distribution. *Normochromia* reflects a normal hemoglobin concentration in cells. *Hypochromia* denotes a cell that is pale, reflecting a decreased hemoglobin concentration as seen in iron-deficiency anemia.

Other variations in RBC structure that can be identified on a stained smear are *siderocytes* (cells containing granules of inorganic iron) and *nucleated red blood cells* or *normoblasts* (normally observed in the bone marrow but present in the peripheral blood in response to high erythrocyte demand).

The major component of the red blood cell is the protein hemoglobin (Hb). Synthesis of hemoglobin in the red blood cell extends from the erythroblast to the reticulocyte stage of development. Its major function is the transport of O_2 and CO_2. The hemoglobin concentration of blood is measured by its color intensity using a photometer and is expressed as grams of hemoglobin per hundred milliliters of blood (g per 100 ml) or grams per deciliter (g per dl).

The type of hemoglobin can also be identified. Approximately 300 genetically controlled types can be identified, mainly through variations in the structural arrangement of the amino acid groups. While most types are without clinical significance and are functionally normal, some produce marked morbidity and mortality. *Hemoglobin electrophoresis* identifies the abnormal hemoglobin. The various types move at different characteristic velocities across paper or starch gel, based on their electrical charge. Hemoglobins are identified by letters or by their place of occurrence and discovery:

Hb A: Normal adult hemoglobin

Hb F: Fetal hemoglobin

Hb S: Hemoglobin found in sickle cell disease

Hb Memphis

Another measure, the *hematocrit* (Hct) or packed cell volume, indicates the volume of the whole blood which is composed of red blood cells. This measurement is the percentage of red blood cells in the whole blood after centrifugation of the specimen and is expressed as cubic millimeters of packed cells per 100 ml of blood or in volumes per 100 ml.

Utilizing the results of the red blood cell count, the hemoglobin concentration, and the hematocrit, *red cell indices* are calculated to reflect the size of the red blood cell, its hemoglobin content, and its concentration. The simple division of the hematocrit by the red cell count gives the *mean corpuscular volume* (MCV). This is a size measurement, expressed as cubic micrometers, with the normal range being 81 to 96 μm^3. Red blood cells in that range are termed *normocytic*, being of normal cell size. An MCV less than 81 μm^3 indicates cells that are termed *microcytic* because they appear smaller than 7 μm on smears, whereas an MCV greater than 96 μm^3 indicates *macrocytic* cells that are larger than 8 μm on smears.

The *mean corpuscular hemoglobin concentration* (MCHC) measures the amount of hemoglobin in 100 ml of packed red blood cells. Determined by dividing the hemoglobin measurement by the hematocrit, it is expressed in grams per 100 ml. The normal range is 30 to 36 g per 100 ml of blood and such blood is termed *normochromic*; a finding of less than 30 per 100 ml is *hypochromic* because these cells appear pale on the smear. The *mean corpuscular hemoglobin* (MCH) measures the amount of hemoglobin present in a single red blood cell. It is determined by dividing the amount of hemoglobin in 1000 ml of blood by the number of red cells per cubic millimeter of blood. The MCH is expressed in picograms of hemoglobin per red blood cell. The normal value is about 27 to 31 pg per red blood cell.

The *reticulocyte count*, another important determination, reflects bone marrow activity. A reticulocyte is an immature nonnucleated red blood cell which contains residual RNA in its cytoplasm. Normally only 1 to 2 percent are seen in the peripheral blood. A peripheral blood smear, taken as described above, is treated with a supravital stain, which imparts a blue color to any RNA within immature red blood cells; such cells appear to have a net or "reticulum" inside, hence the name reticulocyte (see Table 15-1). The residual RNA disappears within the first day or two that the cell is outside the

TABLE 15·1

METHODS FOR EXAMINING BLOOD

Measurement	Description
Red cell count	Number of RBCs in 1 mm^3 of blood (millions per cubic millimeter)
Hemoglobin concentration	Amount of hemoglobin in a given volume of blood (expressed as g per 100 ml)
Hematocrit	Percent of blood which is made up of RBCs (volume %)
Mean corpuscular volume (MCV)	Volume of each individual RBC (μm^3): $$MCV = \frac{hematocrit, vol~\% \times 10}{red~cell~count, millions/mm^3}$$
Mean corpuscular hemoglobin concentration (MCHC)	Proportion of each RBC occupied by hemoglobin (concentration measurement): $$MCHC = \frac{hemoglobin, g/100~ml \times 100}{hematocrit, vol~\%}$$
Mean corpuscular hemoglobin (MCH)	Amount of hemoglobin present in each RBC (weight measurement): $$MCH = \frac{hemoglobin, g/100~ml \times 10}{red~cell~count, millions/mm^3}$$
White cell count	Number of WBCs in 1 mm^3 of blood
Differential count	Percent of the various types of WBCs seen on examination of a peripheral film (granulocytes—PMNs,* eosinophils, and basophils—monocytes, and lymphocytes)
Platelet count	Number of platelets in 1 mm^3 of blood
Reticulocyte count	Percent of immature nonnucleated RBCs containing residual RNA

*PMN: polymorphonuclear leukocyte.

bone marrow, and the cell becomes a mature red blood cell. An increased number of circulating reticulocytes indicates increased bone marrow activity, while a decrease or absence indicates bone marrow failure.

Normal values for these measurements are given in Table 15-2.

TABLE 15·2

NORMAL BLOOD CELL VALUES

	Men	Women
Red cell count, million cells/mm^3	4.7–6.1	4.2–5.2
Hemoglobin, g per 100 ml	13.4–17.6	12.0–15.4
Hematocrit, vol %	42–53	38–46
MCV, μm^3 per RBC	81–96	
MCHC, g per 100 ml RBC	30–36	
MCH, pg per RBC	27–31	
Total white cell count, cells/mm^3	4000–10,000	
Granulocytes*		
PMNs, %	38–70	
Eosinophils, %	1–5	
Basophils, %	0–2	
Monocytes, %*	1–8	
Lymphocytes, %*	15–45	
Platelets, cells/mm^3	150,000–400,000	
Reticulocyte count, %†	1–2	

*% of total WBCs.
†% of total RBCs.

Study of bone marrow

A *bone marrow aspiration and biopsy* are performed when the preceding studies yield insufficient data, or when diseases are suspected which may affect the hematologic system. Aspiration studies are also used to guide the dosages of chemotherapy and radiation therapy in patients with hematologic malignancies.

An accurate bone marrow specimen in an adult can be obtained from the sternum, the spinous processes of the vertebrae, or the anterior or posterior iliac crest. If a biopsy is also required, the latter is the preferred site.

Bone marrow biopsy, as well as aspiration, must be considered a minor surgical procedure and carried out under aseptic conditions. The patient is placed comfortably on his or her side with the back slightly flexed and the knees drawn toward the chest. The posterior iliac crest is cleansed and covered with antiseptic solution. The skin, subcutaneous tissue, and periosteum are anesthetized using 1 to 2% lidocaine (Xylocaine). A 2- to 3-mm incision is made to facilitate penetration with a 14-gauge 2- to 4-cm bone marrow needle and to avoid introducing a skin plug into the marrow cavity. On entry, the stylet is removed from the needle, a 10-ml syringe is attached, and, with a swift, short aspiration, approximately ¼ ml of bone marrow is withdrawn. Even though the patient experiences tremendous pressure throughout the procedure, he or she must be warned that a sudden sharp but brief pain may be felt because of the negative pressure that occurs with aspiration.

Smears are quickly made with the aspirate, and grayish-white particulate matter can usually be observed along with fat vacuoles. A portion of the specimen is allowed to clot and is sectioned for further study. Cell counts and differentials are also obtained from the aspirate.

A biopsy is usually indicated in hematologic malignancies. In this procedure a special biopsy needle (a Jamshidi needle, 11 cm long with a 3-mm diameter tapering to a 2-mm cutting edge) is used to obtain a bone spicule. This bone spicule is extruded onto a glass slide using a probe inserted through the cutting edge. Several imprints are made by gently touching the slide with the spicule, which can be stained with Wright's stain, as discussed above with the peripheral smear. One or two slides may be stained, with Prussian blue reaction depicting stored iron. The biopsy spicule is placed in Bouin's or Zenker's solution, both of which are fixatives. The specimen is then placed in paraffin blocks, sectioned, stained, and studied microsopically.

The bone marrow biopsy is used to study the marrow cellularity without destroying the architecture. Bone marrow of increased activity is termed *hypercellular* or *hyperplastic*; marrow with decreased activity is *hypocellular* or *hypoplastic*. The ratio of myeloid (bone marrow leukocytes) to erythroid (red blood cell) elements (M/E ratio) is calculated, and the presence of a normal, increased, or decreased number of megakaryocytes (platelet precursors) is noted. Cell distribution, maturation abnormalities, and neoplastic cells can be observed. Status of the bone, such as fibrosis, can also be identified.

Biochemical studies

Various studies can be utilized to measure levels of the elements necessary for cell development, especially that of red blood cells. These studies include measurements of serum iron (Fe), total iron-binding capacity (TIBC), vitamin B_{12}, and folic acid levels. The iron-binding capacity measures the ability of plasma transferrin to carry iron from the gastrointestinal tract or iron stores to the bone marrow. It is elevated in iron-deficiency anemia. Other studies related to hematology include the coagulation studies (see Chap. 18).

QUESTIONS

The composition of the blood and the monocyte-macrophage system

Directions: Answer the following questions on a separate sheet of paper.

1. Define *hematology*.

2. Describe the three major types of cells found in the cellular component of whole blood.

3. Explain the theory of hematopoiesis.

4. Describe the assessment process applied when one is diagnosing blood dyscrasias.

Directions: Circle the letter preceding each item below that correctly answers the question. More than one answer may be correct.

5. The portion of blood in which cellular elements are suspended is referred to as the:
   a. Cytoplasm of cells   *b.* Platelets   *c.* Plasma

6. The aqueous component of blood is referred to as:
   a. Globulins   *b.* Platelets   *c.* Plasma
   d. Leukocytes

7. Albumin consists of approximately what percent of the serum protein?
   a. 13   *b.* 24   *c.* 40   *d.* 53

   a. 13   *b.* 24   *c.* 40   *d.* 53

8. Fibrinogen accounts for what percent of the serum protein?
   a. 1   *b.* 4   *c.* 6   *d.* 10

9. The purpose of the red cell indices is to measure:
   a. Count of the number of normal platelets
   b. Size of the red blood cell   *c.* Hemoglobin content of the red blood cell   *d.* Morphologic content of red blood cell

10. Which of the following anatomic sites are used for a bone marrow specimen:
    a. Posterior iliac crest   *b.* Sternum   *c.* Spinous process of the sterum   *d.* Anterior iliac crest

11. Which of the following red blood cells is characteristically found in congenital hemolytic anemia:
    a. HbA   *b.* Hb Memphis   *c.* Spherocytes
    d. Hb F

Directions: Match each descriptive statement in col. A to its appropriate measurement in col. B.

Column A	Column B
12. ___ Red cell count	*a.* Percentage of packed RBCs in a sample of blood (volume percent)

13. ____ Hemato-
crit

14. ____ Mean cor-
puscular vol-
ume (MCV)

15. ____ Hemoglo-
bin concentra-
tion

16. ____ Mean cor-
puscular hemo-
globin concen-
tration
(MCHC)

17. ____ Reticulo-
cyte count

18. ____ White
cell count

19. ____ Mean cor-
puscular hemo-
globin (MCH)

20. ____ Differen-
tial count

21. ____ Platelet
count

b. Amount of hemoglobin in a
given volume of blood (g per
100 ml)

c. Number of WBCs in 1 mm³
of blood

d. Number of RBCs in 1 mm³
of blood (millions per cubic
millimeter)

e. The proportion of each RBC
occupied by hemoglobin
(concentration measurement)

f. Number of platelets in 1 mm³
of blood

g. Volume of each individual
RBC (μm³)

h. Percentage of the different
types of WBCs seen on ex-
amination of a peripheral film

i. Percentage of immature nonnucleated RBCs containing
residual RNA

j. Amount of hemoglobin present in each RBC (weight
measurement)

Directions: Circle T if the statement is true and F if it is false. Correct the false statements.

Approximate normal values:

22. T   F   Red cell count (millions per cubic
millimeter): 3.0 to 4.0 (men); 2.0 to
3.0 (women)

23. T   F   Hematocrit (volume percent): 42 to
53 (men); 38 to 46 (women)

24. T   F   Hemoglobin (g per 100 ml): 13.4 to
17.0 (men); 12.0 to 15.0 (women)

25. T   F   Total white cell count (cells per cubic
millimeter): 1000 to 3000

26. T   F   Platelets (cells per cubic millimeter):
50,000 to 100,000

27. T   F   Lymphocytes (percent of WBCs): 15
to 45

CHAPTER 6

THE RED BLOOD CELL

OBJECTIVES

At the completion of this chapter you should be able to:

1. Recognize a red blood cell (erythrocyte).
2. Describe the functions of the normal red blood cell, its major components, and their functions.
3. Explain the process of red cell production (erythropoiesis).
4. Define *anemia*.
5. List and identify the causative factors associated with classic signs and symptoms of anemia.
6. Differentiate between the morphologic and etiologic classifications of anemia.
7. Differentiate between the three morphologic classifications of anemia.
8. Describe the two major etiologic classifications of anemia.
9. Contrast an isoimmune and an autoimmune response in relation to hemolysis caused by extracorpuscular problems.
10. Identify for aplastic anemia the etiology, causative agents, signs, symptoms, treatment, and prognosis.
11. Differentiate between iron-deficiency (microcytic, hypochromic) anemia and megaloblastic (macrocytic, normochromic) anemias according to etiology, causative factors, signs and symptoms, and treatment.
12. Formulate a definition of *sickle cell disease*.
13. Identify for sickle cell disease the defect in hemoglobin structure, genetic abnormality (homozygous vs. heterozygous state), and the results of amino acid substitution.
14. Explain the cycle of a sickle cell infarctive crisis in relation to deoxygenation of red blood cells.
15. Identify for sickle cell anemia the incidence, racial group affected, criteria for diagnosis, laboratory evaluation, signs and symptoms, clinical manifestations, and treatment.
16. List the principles involved in the treatment of anemia.
17. Define polycythemia.
18. Distinguish between relative and absolute polycythemia and primary and secondary forms of polycythemia.
19. Given a case study, identify the type of anemia evident in the patient.

The red blood cell, or erythrocyte, as seen microscopically is a nonnucleated biconcave disk approximately 8 μm in diameter, 2 μm thick at its outer perimeter, and decreasing to 1 μm or less at its center (Fig. 16-1). Since the cell is soft and pliable, it changes in configuration during passage through the microcirculation. The outer protein-laden stroma comprises the blood group antigens A and B and the Rh factor identifying the individual's blood type. The red blood cell's major component is the protein hemoglobin (Hb), which transports O_2 and CO_2 and maintains normal pH through a series of intracellular buffers. The Hb molecule consists of two pairs of polypeptide chains *(globin)* and four *heme* groups, each one containing an atom of ferrous iron. This configuration allows the most expedient exchange of gases.

Red blood cells number approximately 5 million per cubic millimeter of blood in the average adult and have a life span of 120 days. A steady balance is maintained between normal daily red blood cell losses and replacement. It is postulated that red blood cell production is stimulated by a glycoprotein hormone, *erythropoietin,* believed to originate in the kidney. It is theorized that erythropoietin production is influenced by tissue hypoxia due to such factors as changes in atmospheric O_2, decreased O_2 content of arterial blood, and decreased hemoglobin concentration. The stem cells committed to erythrocyte production appear to be the targets of erythropoietin and initiate proliferation and maturation of red blood cells. Further, maturation is dependent on adequate amounts and proper utilization of nutrients (i.e., vitamin B_{12}, folic acid, proteins, enzymes, and minerals and metals, such as iron and copper).

Hemoglobin production takes place in the bone marrow through all the maturational stages. The red blood cell enters the circulation as a reticulocyte from the bone marrow. The reticulocyte is the final developmental stage of the immature red cell and contains a network of reticular strands. Small amounts of hemoglobin are still synthesized during the 24- to 48-hour maturational stage; the reticulum then dissolves and the mature red blood cell remains.

As the red cell ages, it becomes rigid and fragile and finally ruptures. The hemoglobin is phagocytosed primarily in the spleen, liver, and bone marrow and is reduced to globin and heme. Globin reenters the amino acid pool. Iron is liberated from heme, and the greater part is transported by the plasma protein transferrin to the bone marrow for red cell production. The remaining iron is stored in the form of *ferritin* and *hemosiderin* in the liver and other body tissues for future use (Guyton, 1981). The remaining heme moiety is reduced to carbon monoxide (CO) and biliverdin. The CO, carried in the form of carboxyhemoglobin, is excreted via the lungs. The biliverdin is reduced to free bilirubin; this is slowly released into plasma, where it combines with plasma albumin and is transported to the hepatic cells for excretion into the bile canaliculi (Robinson, 1983). In the presence of active red cell destruction, as in hemolysis, the rapid release of large amounts of bilirubin into the extracellular fluids causes the yellowish hue to the skin and conjunctivae called *jaundice* (Guyton, 1981).

ABNORMALITIES OF RED BLOOD CELL PRODUCTION

Alterations of the red blood cell mass produce two distinct entities. When there are insufficient numbers of red blood cells, *anemia* develops. The opposite condition, too many red blood cells, results in *polycythemia.*

Anemia

By definition, anemia is a reduction below the normal level in the number of red blood cells, the quantity of hemoglobin, and the volume of packed red blood cells (hematocrit) per 100 ml of blood. Anemia is thus not a diagnosis but a reflection of an underlying pathophysiologic alteration which is elucidated by a careful history, physical examination, and laboratory confirmation.

In anemia, since all organ systems may be involved, a wide range of clinical manifestations may result. These are dependent upon (1) the rate at which the anemia develops, (2) the age of the individual, (3) his or her compensatory mechanism, (4) his or her activity level, (5) the underlying disease state, and (6) the severity of the anemia.

As the effective number of red blood cells de-

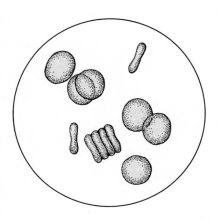

FIGURE 16-1
Erythyrocytes.

creases, less O_2 is delivered to the tissues. Sudden blood loss (30 percent or more), as in hemorrhage, results in symptomatology secondary to hypovolemia and hypoxemia. The usual signs and symptoms are restlessness, diaphoresis (cold perspiration), tachycardia, shortness of breath, and rapid progression to circulatory collapse or shock. However, a drop in red blood cell mass over a period of several months (even a 50 percent decrease) allows the body's compensatory mechanism to adapt and the patient is usually asymptomatic, except on exertion. The body's compensatory mechanism functions by (1) increasing the cardiac output and respirations, thereby increasing the delivery of O_2 to the tissues by the red blood cells, (2) increasing the release of O_2 by hemoglobin, (3) expanding plasma volume by pulling fluid from the tissue spaces, and (4) redistributing blood flow to vital organs (deGruchy, 1978).

One of the most common signs attributed to anemia is *pallor*. This generally results from decreased blood volume, decreased hemoglobin, and vasoconstriction to maximize O_2 delivery to major vital organs. As factors such as skin pigmentation, temperature, and depth and distribution of the capillary bed influence *skin color*, it is not a reliable index for pallor. The color of the nail beds, palms, and mucous membranes of the mouth and conjunctivae can be used more effectively to assess pallor.

Tachycardia and cardiac murmurs (sounds caused by increased velocity of blood flow) reflect the increased cardiac workload and output. Angina (chest pain), especially in older individuals with coronary stenosis, may result from myocardial ischemia. In severe anemia, congestive heart failure may result because the anoxic heart muscle cannot adapt to its increased workload. *Dyspnea* (difficulty in breathing), shortness of breath, and increased fatigue on exertion are manifestations of decreased O_2 delivery. Headache, dizziness, faintness, and tinnitus (ringing in the ears) may reflect the decreased oxygenation of the central nervous system. Gastrointestinal symptoms may also occur in severe anemia; they are generally associated with deficiency states. These symptoms are anorexia, nausea, constipation or diarrhea, and stomatitis (a sore tongue and mouth).

Classification of anemias

Anemias may be classified according to (1) the morphology of the red blood cell, based on its appearance on a stained smear, and the indices, or (2) the etiology.

In the classification of anemias according to morphology, *micro* or *macro* refer to size of the red blood cells and *chromic* to their color. Three major classifications are recognized. The first is the *normocytic, normochromic* anemia, wherein the red blood cells are of normal size and shape and contain the normal amount of hemoglobin (MCV and MCHC are normal or low normal) but the individual is anemic. Causes of this type of anemia are acute blood loss, hemolysis, chronic diseases including infections, endocrine disorders, renal disorders, marrow failure, and metastatic infiltrative diseases of the bone marrow.

The second major category is the *macrocytic, normochromic* anemia. Macrocytic means that the red blood cells are larger than normal but are normochromic because the hemoglobin concentration is normal (MCV increased; MCHC normal) (Fig. 16-2). This results from disordered or interrupted nucleic acid synthesis of DNA as seen in deficiency states of vitamin B_{12} and/or folic acid. This may also occur in cancer chemotherapy because the agents employed interfere with cell metabolism.

The third broad category of anemias are the *microcytic, hypochromic* anemias (Fig. 16-3). *Microcytic* means small, *hypochromic* means containing less than the normal amount of hemoglobin (MCV decreased; MCHC decreased). This generally reflects either insufficient heme (iron) synthesis, as in iron-deficiency anemia, sideroblastic states, and chronic blood loss, or impaired globin synthesis, as in thalassemia (congenital abnormal hemoglobin disease).

In classification of anemias by etiology the major causes considered are (1) increased red blood cell loss and (2) decreased or defective cell production.

Increased red blood cell loss may have two causes. (1) There may be direct loss from the circulation

FIGURE 16-2
Peripheral blood characteristic of macrocytic anemia. In the upper right, the red blood cells are not as uniformly round (poikilocytosis) as they are in Fig. 16-1 and are of different sizes (anisocytosis). Most of the cells are either of normal size or too large. The large oval red blood cells seen in the lower left are called ovalomacrocytes. These cells are characteristic of the vitamin B_{12} and folate deficiencies.

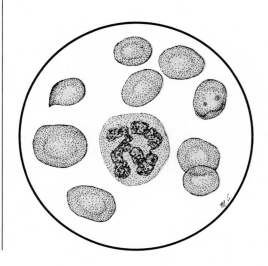

through *bleeding.* Bleeding from trauma or ulcers may remove a large volume from the circulation. Chronic bleeding from polyps in the colon, malignancy, hemorrhoids, or menstruation also causes red blood cell loss. (2) Destruction of red blood cells in circulation, known as *hemolysis,* can also occur because a defect in the red blood cell itself shortens its life or because an altered environment leads to its destruction. Conditions in which the red blood cell itself is defective include:

1. *Hemoglobinopathies,* that is, inherited abnormal hemoglobin, an example being *sickle cell disease*

2. Impaired globin synthesis, as in *thalassemia*

3. Red blood cell membrane defects, as in *hereditary spherocytosis*

4. Enzyme deficiencies, as in glucose 6-phosphate dehydrogenase (G6PD) deficiency

The foregoing are hereditary disorders. However, hemolysis can also be due to problems of the red blood cell environment, that is, extracorpuscular problems. These problems often entail an immune response. An *isoimmune* response involves different individuals within the same species and results from an incompatible blood transfusion. An *autoimmune* response consists of production of antibodies against one's own red blood cells. The condition termed *autoimmune hemolytic anemia* can occur without known cause secondary to administration of drugs (e.g., alpha-methyldopa, quinine, sulfonamides, L-dopa) or to other disease states such as lymphoma, chronic lymphocytic leukemia, lupus erythematosus, rheumatoid arthritis, and viral infections. The autoimmune hemolytic anemias are further classified according to the temperature at which the antibody reacts with the red blood cells—they may be *warm antibody type* or *cold antibody type.*

Malaria, a parasitic disease transmitted to humans by the bite of an infected female anopheline mosquito, results in severe hemolytic anemia by actual infestation of the red blood cell by a *Plasmodium* parasite. This causes an irregular surface defect in the red blood cell.

The defective red blood cells are then rapidly removed by the spleen from the circulation (Beutler, 1983).

Hypersplenism (enlarged spleen, pancytopenias, and normal or hypercellular bone marrow) can also cause hemolysis by red blood cell trapping and destruction. Severe burns, especially when the capillary bed is disrupted, can also lead to hemolysis.

The second major etiologic classification includes *decreased* or *defective red blood cell production* (dyserythropoiesis). Any condition affecting the bone marrow function would fall into this category. Included are (1) disseminated malignancies such as breast cancer, the leukemias, and multiple myeloma; toxic drugs and chemicals; and irradiation and (2) chronic diseases involving the kidneys and liver, infections, and endocrine deficiencies. Lack of essential vitamins, such as B_{12}, folic acid, and vitamin C, and lack of iron can bring about ineffective red blood cell formation leading to anemia. In order to determine the diagnosis of anemia, both the morphologic and etiologic considerations must be incorporated.

Aplastic anemia

Aplastic anemia is a condition featuring insufficient production of blood cells. This is a life-threatening disorder of the stem cell in the bone marrow. As afflicted individuals are deficient in erythrocytes, leukocytes, and thrombocytes, their condition is described as *pancytopenia.* Morphologically the red blood cells are normocytic and normochromic, the reticulocyte count is low or absent, and bone marrow biopsy indicates a "dry tap" with marked hypoplasia and replacement with fatty tissue. The major steps in treatment are identification and removal of the causative agent. However, in some instances no causative agent can be identified, and this is referred to as an idiopathic condition.

Predictable causes of aplastic anemia (temporary or permanent) can be summarized as follows:

1. Antineoplastic or cytotoxic agents

2. Radiation therapy

3. Certain antibiotics

4. Miscellaneous drugs such as anticonvulsants, thyroid medication, gold compounds, and phenylbutazone

5. Benzene

6. Viral infection (especially the hepatitis organisms)

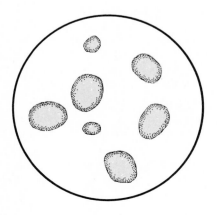

FIGURE 16-3
Erythrocytes characteristic of hypochromic anemia.

Table 16-1 identifies various drugs and their hematologic effects. In addition, the chemical benzene and viral infection have been identified as causes of aplastic anemia. Aplastic anemia following viral hepatitis is particularly severe and likely to be fatal in outcome. The symptom complex in aplastic anemia relates to the pancytopenia.

The signs and symptoms of anemia have already been discussed. Other related symptoms are attributed to deficiencies of platelets and white blood cells. The platelet deficiency may lead to (1) ecchymosis and petechiae (bleeding into the skin), (2) epistaxis (nosebleeds), (3) gastrointestinal bleeding, (4) genitourinary bleeding, and (5) central nervous system bleeding. The deficiency of white blood cells brings increased susceptibility to infection.

Severe aplasia with a decreased or absent reticulocyte count, a granulocyte count of less than 500 per cubic millimeter, and a platelet count of less than 20,000 may bring about death from infection and/or bleeding within weeks or months. However, a person less severely affected may live for years. The major focus of treatment is supportive care until bone marrow recovery occurs. Since infection and bleeding due to other cell-line deficiencies are the major causes of death, prevention of bleeding and infection becomes essential. Prevention measures may include a protected environment (laminar airflow rooms or life island) and good hygiene. In the event of bleeding and/or infection judicious use of blood component therapy (i.e., red blood cells, granulocytes, and thrombocytes) and antibiotics becomes essential. Bone marrow–stimulating agents such as androgens are thought to induce erythropoiesis, but their efficiency is uncertain. Corticosteroids are used to promote vascular integrity and as an aid against bleeding. Patients with chronic aplastic anemia adapt well and can be maintained at an Hb between 8 and 9 g with periodic blood transfusions.

Young individuals with aplastic anemia secondary to stem cell damage have responded well to bone marrow transplantation with compatible donors [siblings with matching human histocompatibility leukocyte antigens (HLA)]. This procedure involves the complete destruction of remaining bone marrow with cytotoxic agents and ionizing radiation which is followed by infusion of 700 to 800 ml of HLA-matched donor marrow.

Iron-deficiency anemia

Morphologically this condition is classified as microcytic, hypochromic anemia with a quantitative decrease in hemoglobin synthesis. Iron deficiency is the major cause of anemia in the world. It is particularly prevalent in women of childbearing age, secondary to their menstrual losses and to their increased iron demand during pregnancy. Other causes of iron deficiency include (1) inadequate iron intake, as seen in infants maintained on milk-only diets to 12 to 24 months and individuals who follow vegetarian dietary habits; (2) impaired absorption as after gastrectomy; and (3) persistent blood loss as with slow gastrointestinal bleeding from polyps, neoplasms, gastritis, esophageal varices, aspirin ingestion, and hemorrhoids.

Normally the average adult body contains 3 to 5 g of iron, depending on sex and size. Nearly two-thirds of the iron is found in hemoglobin, and it is released with cell senescence and death and transported via plasma transferrin to the bone marrow for erythropoiesis. With the exception of minute amounts in myoglobin (muscle) and in heme enzymes, the remaining one-third is stored for further needs in the liver, spleen, and bone marrow as ferritin and hemosiderin.

While the average diet contains 10 to 20 mg of iron, only about 5 to 10 percent (1 to 2 mg) is actually absorbed. As the iron stores are depleted, more is absorbed from the diet. Ingested iron is converted to ferrous iron in the stomach and duodenum and is absorbed from the duodenum and proximal jejunum. It is then transported by plasma transferrin to the bone marrow for hemoglobin synthesis or to the tissue stores.

Each milliliter of blood contains 0.5 mg of iron. Iron losses generally are minute, from 0.5 to 1 mg/day. However, menstruating females lose an additional 15 to 28 mg/month. During pregnancy, although loss to menses ceases, the daily iron requirement increases to meet the demands of the mother's increased hemoglobin mass and the formation of the placenta, umbilical cord, and fetus, as well as to compensate for blood lost during delivery.

In addition to the signs and symptoms presented for anemia, severely iron-deficient individuals (plasma iron < 40 mg per 100 ml; Hb 6 to 7 g per 100 ml) have brittle, fine hair and nails that are thin, flat, and easily broken and that may actually become spoon-shaped (koilonychia). In addition, the papillae of the tongue atrophy resulting in a pale, smooth, shiny beefy-red appearance, and they become inflamed and sore. Angular stomatitis (cracking with redness and pain at the corners of the mouth) may also occur.

Examination of the blood reveals a normal or near-normal red cell count and a reduced hemoglobin level. On peripheral smear the RBCs are microcytic and hypochromic (decreased MCV, decreased MCHC, and decreased MCH) with poikilocytosis and anisocytosis. (See Plate 27.) The reticulocyte count may be normal or decreased. The iron level is reduced while the total serum iron-binding capacity is increased.

Treatment of iron deficiency necessitates identification and resolution of the underlying cause of the ane-

TABLE 16-1

HEMATOLOGIC EFFECTS SECONDARY TO DRUGS

Generic name	Brand name*	Hemolysis	Megalo-blastosis	Aplasia	Leukopenia or agranulocy-tosis	Thrombo-cytopenia†	Thrombo-cytopathy†
Antibiotics							
Chloramphenicol	Chloromycetin	X		XX	X	X	
Erythromycin	Ilosone			X	X	X	
Penicillin	Pen-Vee K	XX		X	X	X	X
Sulfisoxazole	Gantrisin	XX		X	X	XX	
Tetracycline	Sumycin	X		X	X	X	
Anticonvulsants							
Diphenylhydantoin	Dilantin	X	X	X	X	X	
Phenobarbital	Luminal	X	X	X		X	
Mephenytoin	Mesantoin	X	X	X	X	X	
Oral hypoglycemics							
Tolbutamide	Orinase	X		XX	X	X	
Chlorpropamide	Diabinese				X	X	
Anti-inflammatory drugs							
Acetylsalicylic acid, aspirin		X		X	X	XX	XX
Colchicine				X	X	X	X
Gold compounds				X	XX	X	
Phenacetin		XX			X	XX	
Indomethacin	Indocin	X		X	X	X	XX
Phenylbutazone	Butazolidin			XX	XX	XX	XX
Antihypertensives and diuretics							
Chlorothiazide	Diuril	X		X	X	X	
Methyldopa	Aldomet	XX		X	X	X	
Antineoplastics							
Mechlorethamine hydrochloride	Mustargen			XX	XX	XX	
Cyclophosphamide	Cytoxan			XX	XX	XX	
Vincristine	Oncovin			XX	XX	XX	
Methotrexate	A-Methopterin		XX	XX	XX	XX	
Mercaptopurine	Purinethol		XX	XX	XX	XX	
Tranquilizers							
Chlordiazepoxide	Librium			X	X		X
Imipramine	Tofranil			X	XX		X
Chlorpromazine	Thorazine	X	X	X	X	X	X

Key: X = infrequently occurring: XX = frequently occurring
*This list is not all-inclusive. Other equally effective brands may exist.
†Thrombocytopenia is a decrease in platelet numbers; thrombocytopathy is an alteration in platelet function.

mia. Surgical intervention may be necessary to inhibit active bleeding that results from polyps, ulcers, malignancies, and hemorrhoids; dietary alterations may be needed for babies fed milk only or for individuals with food idiosyncracies or who are taking large doses of aspirin. While dietary modifications may increase the available iron (e.g., by adding liver), supplemental iron is needed to increase the hemoglobin and restore iron stores. Iron is available in parenteral and oral forms. The majority of patients respond well to oral compounds such as ferrous sulfate. Parenteral iron preparations are used very selectively because they are costly and have a high incidence of adverse reactions.

Megaloblastic anemias

Another major category of anemias are the *megaloblastic anemias*, which are classified morphologically as macrocytic normochromic anemias. Megaloblastic anemias are often caused by vitamin B_{12} and folic acid (folate) deficiencies, which result in disordered DNA synthesis. These deficiencies may be secondary to malnutrition, malabsorption, lack of intrinsic factor (as seen in pernicious anemia and postgastrectomy), parasitic infestations, intestinal disease, and malignancies, as well as to cancer chemotherapeutic agents. In individuals with tapeworm infections (with *Diphyllobothrium latum*) secondary to ingestion of infected fresh water fish, the tapeworm competes with its host for the vitamin B_{12} in ingested food, which leads to megaloblastic anemia (Beck, 1983).

Even though pernicious anemia is the prototype condition for the megaloblastic anemias, folate deficiency is more commonly encountered in clinical practice. Megaloblastic anemia often is seen as malnutrition in the elderly, alcoholics, or teenagers, and in pregnancy where there is an increased demand to meet the needs of the fetus and lactation. This demand is also increased in hemolytic anemias, malignancies, and hyperthyroidism. Celiac disease and tropical sprue also cause mal-

absorption, and drugs that act as folic acid antagonists interfere with utilization.

The minimum daily requirement of folate is approximately 50 mg. This must be provided by dietary sources. The most abundant sources are red meats (e.g., liver and kidney) and fresh leafy green vegetables. The average diet provides more than the needed amounts, but only with proper preparation. For example, 50 to 90 percent of the folate can be lost with cooking in large volumes of water. Folate is absorbed from the duodenum and upper jejunum, weakly bound to plasma proteins, and stored in the liver. In the absence of folate intake, folate stores are usually depleted in approximately 4 months. In addition to the symptoms described for anemias, individuals with megaloblastic anemia secondary to folate deficiency may appear malnourished and experience severe glossitis (inflamed painful tongue), diarrhea, and loss of appetite. Serum folate levels are also decreased (< 4 ng/ml). The bone marrow of a patient with megaloblastic anemia is depicted in Fig. 16-4. Plate 28 illustrates the peripheral blood findings seen in megaloblastic anemia. The reticulocyte count is usually decreased along with the hematocrit and hemoglobin.

As mentioned previously, treatment depends on identifying and removing the underlying cause. This includes correcting the dietary deficiencies and replacement therapy with folic acid or vitamin B_{12}. Alcoholic patients who are hospitalized often have a "spontaneous" response when given a nutritionally balanced diet.

Sickle cell disease

Causes

Sickle cell disease is one of the hemoglobinopathies secondary to abnormalities in hemoglobin structure. The defect in structure occurs in the globin fraction of

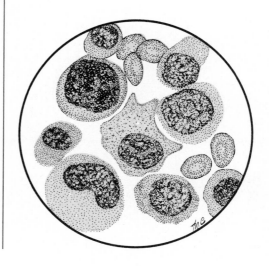

FIGURE 16-4
Bone marrow characteristic of megaloblastic anemia. In the upper right there is one red blood cell precursor which is nearly normal, with a condensed nuclear chromatin pattern. The remaining cells are very large and have an open nuclear chromatic pattern. These large cells (two to three times normal size) are also red blood cell precursors. In the lower left is a large white blood cell precursor (metamyelocyte) which is two to three times normal size. This finding indicates that all cell lines develop abnormally in this condition.

the hemoglobin molecule. Recall that globin is constructed of two pairs of polypeptide chains. For example, Hb S differs from normal Hb A in the substitution of valine for glutamic acid in one pair of chains. In Hb C, lysine is in that position. As noted previously, many abnormal hemoglobins exist with varying degrees of symptoms, ranging from none to severe.

Sickle cell disease is a recessive autosomal codominant hereditary condition whereby a homozygous state (abnormal gene inherited from both parents) is required to produce symptomatic sickle cell anemia. The heterozygous state (abnormal gene inherited from only one parent) is referred to as *sickle cell trait*. It is generally asymptomatic, and the individual has a normal life span. In patients with sickle cell trait, morbidity related to impaired oxygenation, such as that during anesthesia, at high altitudes, and with chronic obstructive pulmonary disease (COPD), has been reported but is extremely rare and not well documented (Beutler, 1983).

The amino acid substitution in sickle cell disease results in major rearrangement of the hemoglobin molecule when deoxygenation (decreased O_2 tension) occurs. The red blood cells then undergo *tactoid formation*, where they elongate and become rigid and crescent- or sickle-shaped (Fig. 16-5).

Deoxygenation can occur for many reasons. The slowed blood flow of the microcirculation serves to enhance deoxygenation. It is postulated that the Hb S erythrocytes adhere to the endothelium, further retarding blood flow. The increased deoxygenation may take the abnormal red blood cells below a critical point and bring on sickling within the microvasculature. Because

of their rigidity and irregular membrane, sickle cells clump together, leading to vascular occlusion, pain crisis, and organ infarctions (Hebbel et al., 1980). Frequent episodes of sickling and unsickling cause the cell membranes to fragment and become fragile. The cells are then hemolyzed and removed by the monocyte-macrophage system. The red cell life span is markedly reduced, and an increased demand, therefore, is put on the bone marrow for replacement. Figure 16-6 depicts the cycle of sickle cell infarctive crisis.

Sickle cell anemia is the most prevalent form of congenital hemolytic anemia. Affecting about 1 in 600 American blacks, sickle cell anemia is the most common form of sickle cell disease. Hb S accounts for 75 to 95 percent of the Hb; the remainder is Hb F, which accounts for 1 to 20 percent. The diagnosis is based on the patient's history, physical findings, and laboratory evaluation. A *sickle solubility test* is done to confirm the presence of Hb S in the red blood cell. In this test RBCs are mixed with a reducing agent and the solution becomes turbid. *Hemoglobin electrophoresis* further delineates the abnormal Hb. The anemia is generally normocytic, normochromic, with Hb ranging between 5 and 10 g per 100 ml. Peripheral smear shows anisocytosis and poikilocytosis, leukocytosis (increased WBCs), thrombocytosis, and nucleated RBCs (see Fig. 16-5). The reticulocyte count is markedly increased.

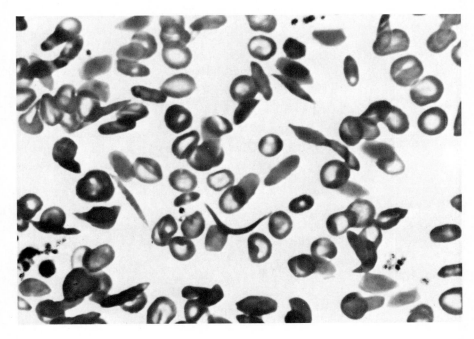

FIGURE 16-5
Sickle cells. The characteristic sickle- or crescent-shaped red blood cells are shown in a peripheral smear. (Courtesy of Dr. Koichi Maeda, Ford Hospital, Detroit, Michigan.)

Signs and Symptoms

Signs and symptoms occur as a result of the vascular occlusions that cause infarcts in various organs such as kidney, lung, and central nervous system. Infants usually are asymptomatic for 5 to 6 months because of the persistence of fetal hemoglobin (Hb F), which tends to inhibit sickling. Clinical manifestations include failure to thrive, impaired growth and development, and frequent episodes of bacterial infections, especially pneumococcal infections. Initially the spleen is enlarged, but owing to repeated infarcts it becomes atrophied and nonfunctional before the child is 8 years of age. This process is referred to as *autosplenectomy*. Susceptibility to infection persists throughout life.

Swollen, painful, inflamed hands and feet (hand-foot syndrome known as *dactylitis*) are seen in about 20 to 30 percent of children under 2 years of age. They result from ischemia and infarction of the metacarpal and metatarsal bones; the condition is accompanied by fever. Debilitating, recurrent "painful crises" are the major cause of the morbidity from sickle cell disease. The most frequent sites affected are the abdomen, back, chest, and joints. Crises are exacerbated by infection or dehydration, may mimic other acute illnesses, and last from a few hours to several days. The incidence of the crises decreases with increasing age. Aplastic crisis may also occur, especially in children, with intermittent cessation of bone marrow function and marked decrease in erythropoiesis and reticulocyte count.

Cardiac signs of anemia (i.e., tachycardia, murmurs) are usually present. Increased heart size and congestive heart failure may also occur. Renal involvement is evidenced by an impaired ability to concentrate urine, and repeated infarctions can lead to papillary necrosis and hematuria. Repeated pulmonary infections and/or infarctions impair pulmonary function. Central nervous system infarctions ("strokes"), although rare, can lead to varying degrees of hemiplegia. Chronic leg ulcers above the ankle and along the medial aspect of the tibia are encountered. Due to the increased red blood cell breakdown the patients are often *icteric (jaundiced)* and develop *cholelithiasis (gallstones)* secondary to increased bilirubin. Physical appearance ranges from the thin asthenic to that of normal development. Table 16-2 depicts the clinical manifestations of sickle cell anemia.

Treatment

Since there is no known way to prevent or reverse sickling, treatment emphasizes prevention of the disease and includes genetic counseling of individuals with known sickle cell trait. Treatment of the patient should include stressing the importance of maintenance of optimum oxygenation, good health and hygiene, and prevention of dehydration and infections. For example, pneumococcal vaccine (Pneumovax) decreases the incidence of pneumococcal infections and should be offered to sickle cell patients. Infections must be treated promptly and vigorously. Deficiencies of folic acid and iron should be remedied. However, while an anemic crisis may be managed at home, severe painful crises require hospitalization and diagnosis and treatment of the underlying cause (e.g., pneumonia, osteomyelitis). Hydration (IV or oral) is imperative, and electrolyte balance should be carefully monitored. Sedation and analgesics will provide symptomatic relief. Respiratory suppressants such as morphine should be avoided. As drug dependence and job difficulties may occur secondary to frequent crises, long-term counseling and support are indicated.

POLYCYTHEMIA

The previous discussion has focused on conditions resulting from insufficient numbers of red blood cells. In the condition called *polycythemia* there are too many red blood cells. *Polycythemia* means an excess *(poly)* of all the cell lines *(cythemia)* but is generally used for conditions in which the red cell mass exceeds normal.

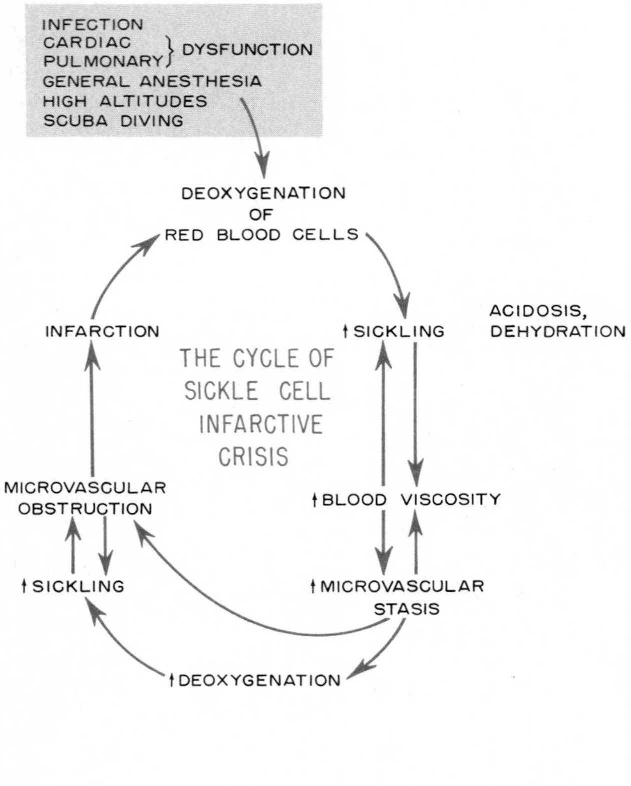

FIGURE 16-6
The cycle of a sickle cell infarctive crisis

TABLE 16-2

CLINICAL MANIFESTATIONS OF SICKLE CELL ANEMIA

System	Complications	Signs and symptoms	Related to
Cardiac system	Congestive heart failure	Cardiomegaly, systolic ejection murmur, tachycardia, shortness of breath, dyspnea on exertion, restlessness	Anemia, chronic hemolysis
Pulmonary system	Pulmonary infarction, pneumonia (especially *Haemophilus influenzae* and *Streptococcus pneumoniae*)	Chest pain, cough, shortness of breath, fever, hemoptysis, restlessness	Infarctive crisis, increased susceptibility to infection, intrapulmonary arteriovenous shunting, functional asplenia
Central nervous system	Cerebral thromboses	Hemiplegia, aphasia, drowsiness, convulsions, headache, bowel and bladder dysfunction	Infarctive crisis
Genitourinary system	Renal dysfunction	Flank pain, hematuria, isothenuria	Renal papillary necrosis secondary to microinfarcts
	Priapism	Penile engorgement and pain	Infarctive crisis and intravascular sickling
Gastrointestinal system	Cholecystitis, hepatic fibrosis, hepatic abscess	Abdominal pain, hepatomegaly, jaundice, fever	Chronic hemolysis, infarctive crisis
Ocular system	Retinal detachment, peripheral vessel disease, hemorrhage	Pain, altered vision, blindness	Microinfarcts
Skeletal system	Aseptic necrosis of femoral or humeral heads, dactylitis (usually in young children)	Pain, decreased mobility, painful and swollen hands and feet	Infarctions, infection, intramedullary infarction with or without periostitis
Skin	Chronic leg ulcers	Pain, open and draining ulcers	Infarctions, impaired circulation in capillaries and venules due to intravascular sickling

This condition results in increased whole-blood viscosity and increased blood volume.

There are both *relative* and *absolute* forms of polycythemia. *Relative* polycythemia occurs when the volume of circulating plasma is decreased (hemoconcentration) but the total volume of circulating red blood cells is normal. Therefore, the hematocrit rises in males to 53 percent and in females to 46 percent. The major cause is *dehydration*. This may be due to (1) increased fluid losses as seen with diuretic therapy, excessive vomiting, burns, and fever, (2) decreased fluid intake, or (3) redistribution of fluids from plasma to tissues due to a crush injury (deGruchy, 1978). Another form of relative polycythemia is *pseudo-* or *stress* polycythemia. While the exact cause is not known, the incidence of this condition is highest in middle-aged, obese, highly anxious males, which makes stress a highly suspected cause. Cigarette smoking seems to exacerbate this state as the chronic carbon monoxide exposure enhances erythrocytosis.

Absolute polycythemia refers to a condition where the actual circulating red cell mass is increased. This may be *primary*, as in polycythemia vera, or *secondary*, which results from underlying medical problems (e.g., cardiopulmonary diseases decrease arterial O_2 saturation which stimulates erythropoiesis; renal tumors increase erythropoietin production). This condition is also seen in individuals who live at high altitudes where atmospheric O_2 is decreased.

In *primary* or *polycythemia vera*, the pluripotential stem cell is abnormal. There is marked erythrocytosis, leukocytosis, and thrombocytosis. This is a progressive disease of middle age, equally affecting males and females. The signs and symptoms are secondary to the increased total blood volume and increased blood viscosity. The plasma volume is usually normal, and vasodilatation occurs to accommodate the increased red blood cell volume. The patient presents with a plethoric (brick-red) complexion with "bloodshot" eyes. The symptoms are nonspecific, ranging from a sensation of "fullness in the head" to headache, dizziness, difficulty in concentrating, visual blurring, and post-bathing pruritus (itching). The increased blood volume and viscosity (slow blood flow) along with the elevated platelet numbers and abnormal platelet function predispose the individual to thrombosis as well as hemorrhage. The disease progresses over a 10- to 15-year period with complications such as the bone marrow becoming increasingly fibrosed and the liver and spleen increasing in size; it terminates in a "spent," nonproductive marrow.

Laboratory studies reveal a persistently elevated hemoglobin (>18 g), hematocrit, and blood volume. The white blood cell and platelet counts are also elevated. The reticulocyte count is normal or slightly increased.

Treatment modalities for polycythemia vera include periodic phlebotomy (removal of blood by venesection), radioactive phosphorus, and chemotherapeutic agents such as busulfan. For secondary polycythemia, treatment is dependent upon the underlying cause.

QUESTIONS

The red blood cell

Directions: Answer the following questions on a separate sheet of paper.

1. What are the major components and functions of the normal red blood cell?

2. Explain the relationship of erythropoietin to red blood cell production.

3. Define *anemia.*

4. List the classic signs and symptoms of anemia.

5. State two etiologic factors related to anemia and give at least two examples of each type.

6. Describe the three morphologic classifications for anemia and give at least two examples of each type.

7. What are three major principles to consider when treating anemia?

8. What is polycythemia?

9. Describe the two classifications of absolute polycythemia. (Include an example of each type.)

10. Draw a normal red blood cell.

11. Explain the cycle of a sickle cell infarctive crisis in relation to deoxygenation of red blood cells.

Directions: Complete the following statements by filling in the blanks.

12. An anemia in which the MCV and MCHC are normal is referred to as _____.

13. An anemia referred to as a life-threatening disorder resulting from a process affecting the stem cell in the bone marrow is _____.

Directions: Circle the letter preceding each item below that correctly answers the question. More than one answer may be correct.

14. The blood cells that can be described as nonnucleated, biconcave disks are:
    a. Eosinophils   *b.* Thrombocytes   *c.* Erythrocytes   *d.* Monocytes

15. In which of the following sites does hemoglobin production occur through all the maturational stages:
    a. Bone marrow   *b.* Lymphatic tissue
    c. Spleen   *d.* Liver

16. Mr. B., a 20-year-old male, recently was diagnosed as having a fish tapeworm infection (*Diphyllobothrium latum*) after eating infected fresh-water raw fish. The type of anemia most likely to be associated with this condition is:
    a. Aplastic   *b.* Iron-deficiency   *c.* Megaloblastic
    d. Hemolytic

17. The development of autoimmune hemolytic anemia can occur secondary to:
    a. An incompatible blood transfusion
    b. Lymphoma   *c.* Administration of quinine or methotrexate   *d.* Hereditary spherocytosis

18. A microcytic, normochromic anemia usually results from:
    a. Acute blood loss   *b.* Insufficient heme (iron) synthesis   *c.* Impaired globin synthesis
    d. Disorder or interrupted nucleic acid synthesis of DNA   *e.* Sideroblastic states

19. A macrocytic normochromic anemia is usually caused by a deficiency of:
    a. Vitamin B_{12} *b.* Iron   *c.* Folic acid   *d.* Potassium

20. Mrs. B., a 36-year-old female, was diagnosed as having iron-deficiency anemia. Which one of the following red blood characteristics is most commonly found in anemia due to iron deficiency?
    a. Normocytic normochromic   *b.* Microcytic hypochromic   *c.* Macrocytic normochromic

21. Mr. M. is a 60-year-old male who has been drinking steadily since his wife died over 2 years ago. In the past year his meals consisted mainly of hamburgers. He was admitted to the hospital because of weakness and loss of appetite.

Physical assessment revealed:

> Pale, emaciated white male
>
> Pale mucous membranes and nail beds
>
> Enlarged liver
>
> Severe glossitis

Laboratory data revealed the following:

> Hemoglobin 6.2
>
> B_{12} 343 pg/ml (normal range 200–900)
>
> Folic acid 3.0 ng/ml (normal range 6–20)
>
> Hematocrit 17
>
> Many ovalomacrocytes

The most likely diagnosis is:
a. Megaloblastic anemia secondary to folate deficiency   b. Pernicious anemia
c. Polycythemia   d. Aplastic anemia

22. In sickle cell disease the most common form of hemoglobin is:
a. Hb C   b. Hb S   c. Hb A   d. Hb F

23. Which of the following describes sickle cell disease?
a. Recessive autosomal-dominant hereditary disease   b. Sex-linked recessive disorder   c. Displays increased deoxygenation within the microvasculature   d. Marked by occurrence of clumping   e. Red blood cells' life span is markedly reduced   f. Most prevalent form of congenital hemolytic anemia

24. A 6-year-old black female presents with pale mucous membranes and conjunctival icterus. Further examination revealed lymphadenopathy, cardiac enlargement, ascites, joint swelling, and splenic enlargement. Oval, cigar-shaped sickled cells were seen on a stained blood smear. Her diagnosis is sickle cell disease. The patient developed severe bone and joint pain in her extremities and an elevated temperature of 102°F (38.9°C) with leukocytosis. This syndrome is referred to as:
a. Chronic sickle cell anemia   b. Sickle cell thalassemia disease   c. Sickle cell crisis   d. Chronic normochromic anemia

25. The principles of treatment for the syndrome described in the above question include:
a. Monitoring of the blood pH   b. Administration of respiratory suppressants   c. Administration of chemotherapeutic agents to reverse the sickling process   d. Maintenance of adequate hydration and electrolyte balance

Directions: Circle T if the statement is true and F if it is false. Correct the false statements.

26. T   F   Relative polycythemia is characterized by a normal total red blood cell mass.

27. T   F   Absolute polycythemia refers to a condition in which the circulating red blood cell mass is increased.

28. T   F   Sickle cell disease affects approximately 1 in 300 American blacks.

THE WHITE BLOOD CELL

OBJECTIVES

At the completion of this chapter you should be able to:

1. Cite the five types of white blood cells normally found in peripheral blood.

2. Distinguish between the three types of granulocytes and the monocytes and lymphocytes normally found in the circulation.

3. Describe the functions of each of the cells listed in objective no. 2.

4. Explain the role of colony stimulating factor (CSF) in leukocyte cell differentiation.

5. Describe leukocytosis by identifying the type of cells and types of disease conditions related to it.

6. List the possible etiologic factors of neutropenia and agranulocytosis.

7. Explain the genetic and environmental factors associated with leukemia.

8. Describe the rationale for the FAB classification of acute leukemia.

9. Differentiate between acute and chronic myelogenous (granulocytic) leukemia, and acute lymphoblastic (lymphocytic) and chronic lymphocytic leukemia in relation to incidence, sex distribution, causal factors, survival, signs and symptoms, laboratory findings (peripheral blood, bone marrow) and complications.

10. Evaluate the signification of the characteristic Philadelphia chromosomal patterns in acute lymphoblastic (lymphocytic) and chronic myelogenous (granulocytic) leukemia.

11. Cite the significance of immunologic identification in the acute and chronic leukemias.

12. Cite the commonly used chemotherapeutic agents in the acute and chronic leukemias.

13. Differentiate between Hodgkin's and non-Hodgkin's lymphomas according to the type of cells involved, signs and symptoms, complications, age group affected, treatment, and prognosis.

14. Differentiate between multiple myeloma and Waldenström's macroglobulinemia by identifying the location of neoplasm, age group affected, presenting symptoms, diagnosis, treatment, and prognosis for each.

15. Given case studies, identify the type of plasma cell dyscrasia, leukemia, or lymphoma evident in each patient.

Defense against infection is the major role of *leukocytes* or *white blood cells*. The normal range for the white cell count is from 4000 to 10,000 per cubic millimeter. The five types identified in the peripheral blood are (1) *neutrophils* (55 percent of the total), (2) *eosinophils* (1 to 2 percent), (3) *basophils* (0.5 to 1 percent), (4) *monocytes* (6 percent), and (5) *lymphocytes* (36 percent).

Neutrophils, *eosinophils*, and *basophils* are also called granulocytes, which means cells with granules in the cytoplasm. Granulocytes range in size from 10 to 14 μm in diameter. Their identification depends on the affinity of the granules for certain dyes. Cells whose granules have an eosin affinity, staining red to red-orange, are called *eosinophils*, whereas cells with a blue or basic dye affinity are called *basophils*. The granules of the neutrophils, which are also called *segmented neutrophils* and *polymorphonuclear leukocytes* (PMN), have little affinity for either eosin or basic dyes, staining a faint pink or blue surrounded by a light pink cytoplasm. All three types of granulocytes (Fig. 17-1) seem to originate from the pluripotential stem cell in the bone marrow.

It is theorized that granulopoietin, a glycoprotein biochemically similar to erythropoietin, is the stimulating factor responsible for leukocyte cell differentiation.

This factor is referred to as *colony stimulating factor* (CSF). It is thought to be derived from monocytes and macrophages, in response to bacterial endotoxins that are released during infection, and from activated T lymphocytes and endothelial cells. It has also been detected in various body tissues and in human serum and urine (Golde, 1983; Barr and Seymore, 1982). Detectable levels of CSF have been found in the serum during periods of inflammation, viral infections, and stress. The CSF is believed to act directly upon the stem cell's colony-forming units in the bone marrow, committing them to differentiation to the neutrophil and monocyte cell lines. The cells undergo a mitotic (dividing) proliferating phase, followed by a maturation phase. The time required varies for the different leukocytes and ranges from 9 days for the eosinophil to 12 days for the neutrophil. All these phases are accelerated during periods of infection. In the bone marrow, as the cell matures it becomes smaller, and the round or oval nucleus acquires two to five lobes, surrounded by cytoplasm containing small, evenly distributed granules (Fig. 17-1). These granules contain enzymes (e.g., myeloperoxidase, muramidase, and cationic antibacterial proteins) which,

FIGURE 17-1.
Granulocytes. (A) Basophils. (B) Neutrophils. (C) Eosinophil.

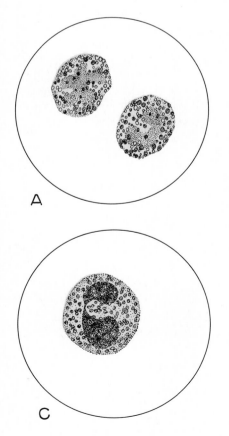

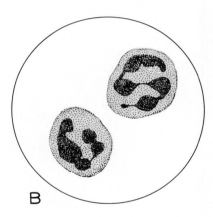

A

B

C

upon degranulation of the white cells, kill and digest bacteria.

The bone marrow contains a constant reserve pool of about 10 times the quantity of neutrophils produced daily (Schrier, 1979). In the presence of infection, the reserve pool of neutrophils is mobilized and released into the circulation, where they remain for about 6 to 8 hours. This egress from the bone marrow is believed to be regulated by a neutrophil-releasing factor (Quesenberry, 1983). Neutrophils in the circulation are divided between the circulating pool and the marginating pool (white blood cells which lie along the capillary wall). With ameboid movements, the neutrophils move by diapedesis from the marginal pool into the tissues and mucous membranes. The cells serve as the body's primary defense system against bacterial infection; their method of defense is the process of *phagocytosis*. This is discussed in detail in Chap. 4. The overall dynamic feedback mechanism controlling leukocyte production has yet to be elucidated and is not within the scope of this chapter.

Eosinophils have a weak phagocytic function which is not clearly understood. They appear to function in antigen-antibody reactions; levels are elevated during asthmatic attacks, drug reactions, and certain parasitic infestations (see Chap. 9). *Basophils* carry the histamine- and platelet-activating factors in their granules to inflamed tissues. Their actual function is poorly defined. Elevated levels of basophils (basophilia) are found in myeloproliferative disorders, that is, proliferative disorders of blood-forming cells.

The *monocyte* (Fig. 17-2) is larger than the neutrophil and has one nucleus. The nucleus is folded or in-

dented and looks lobulated with brainlike convolutions. The cytoplasm appears more abundant in relation to its nucleus and stains dull blue-gray with faint, evenly distributed granules. The differentiation, maturation, and release of the monocytes occur over 24 days, a much longer period than for granulocytes.

Monocytes leave the circulation and become tissue macrophages and are a part of the monocyte-macrophage system. The monocyte's life span is weeks to months. As monocytes, these cells also have phagocytic functions, removing injured and dead cells, cell fragments, and microorganisms (as in bacterial endocarditis).

Lymphocytes are mononuclear leukocytes in the peripheral blood. They have a round or oval nucleus surrounded by a narrow rim of blue-staining cytoplasm containing a few granules. The nuclear chromatin pattern is heavily clumped with a network of inner connections. Lymphocytes (Fig. 17-3) vary in size from small (7 to 10 μm) to large cells the size of granulocytes. They also appear to originate from a pluripotential stem cell in the bone marrow and migrate to other lymphoid tissue including the lymph nodes, spleen, thymus and the mucosal surfaces of the gastrointestinal tract and the respiratory tract. There are two types of lymphocytes, the long-lived thymus-conditioned thymus-dependent T lymphocytes and the non-thymus-dependent B lymphocytes. T lymphocytes migrate from the thymus gland to other lymphoid tissue. They are typically located in the paracortex of lymph nodes and the periarteriolar lymphoid sheets of the white pulp of the spleen. B lymphocytes are distributed in the follicles of lymph nodes, the spleen, and the medullary cords of the lymph nodes (Sweet, 1980). The T lymphocytes are responsible for cellular immune responses through the production of antigen-reactive cells while B lymphocytes, properly stimulated, differentiate into immunoglobulin-producing plasma cells, responsible for the humoral im-

FIGURE 17-2
Monocytes.

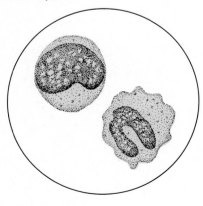

FIGURE 17-3
Mature lymphocytes.

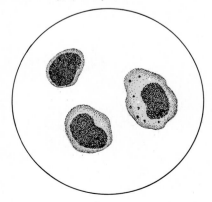

mune response. The reader is referred to Chap. 5 for a complete discussion of the functions and interrelationships of the T and B lymphocytes.

201
WHITE BLOOD CELL DISORDERS

WHITE BLOOD CELL DISORDERS

Disorders of the white blood cells can affect any or all of the cell lines and are generally related to production defects or early destruction.

Leukocytosis refers to an increase in the leukocytes generally exceeding 10,000 per cubic millimeter. *Granulocytosis* refers to an increase in granulocytes but in common usage refers only to an increase in the neutrophils; thus *neutrophilia* is the more accurate term. Leukocytes increase as a physiologic response to protect the body from invading microorganisms. In response to an acute infection or inflammation, neutrophils leave the marginating pool and enter the area of infection; the bone marrow releases its reserve pool and initiates an accelerated granulopoiesis. Because of this increased demand, an increased number of immature forms called *band* (or *stab*) *neutrophils* enter the circulation, a process referred to as a "shift to the left." As the infection subsides, the neutrophils decrease and the monocytes increase (monocytosis). With progressive resolution, the monocytes decrease and mild lymphocytosis (increased lymphocytes) and eosinophilia (increased eosinophils) occur. The term *leukemoid reaction* refers to a state of elevated leukocytes, with an increase in immature forms, reaching levels of 100,000 per cubic millimeter. This is in response to infectious, toxic, and inflammatory states and also occurs in malignancy, especially breast, kidney, lung, and metastatic carcinomas (Beck, 1977). Disorders in which there is a general increase in blood-forming cells are termed *myeloproliferative disorders*.

Neutrophilia

Neutrophilia also occurs following stress states such as severe violent exercise or injection with epinephrine. This is a "pseudoleukocytosis" as leukocytes are redistributed, released from the marginating pool to the circulating pool, and can be counted. Granulopoiesis is not initiated in the bone marrow, and so the actual numbers do not increase. Treatment with corticosteroids also results in a pseudoleukocytosis. Corticosteroids are thought to increase the release of granulocytes from the marrow reserves as well as to inhibit the margination of granulocytes. This results in a higher circulating leukocyte pool. Eosinophilia occurs with skin disorders such as mycosis fungoides and eczema, allergy states such as asthma and hay fever, drug reactions, and parasitic infestations. Eosinophilia is also seen in malignancies and myeloproliferative disorders, as is basophilia.

Monocytosis is seen during the recuperating phase of infection and in chronic granulomatous diseases such as tuberculosis and sarcoidosis. *Lymphocytosis* refers to an elevated lymphocyte count. Lymphocytes activated by viral or antigenic stimuli are transformed into larger atypical lymphocytes. These cells are present in larger numbers in infectious mononucleosis, infectious hepatitis, toxoplasmosis, measles, mumps, some allergic reactions such as serum sickness, drug sensitivities, and the malignant lymphomas (Schrier, 1979). In addition to lymphocytosis these patients may often have an enlarged liver, spleen, and lymph nodes, all areas of lymphocyte formation.

Leukopenia refers to a decreased number of leukocytes, *neutropenia* to a decrease in the absolute neutrophil count. Because of the role of neutrophils in host defense, an absolute neutrophil count of less than 1000 per cubic millimeter predisposes the individual to infection; counts under 500 per cubic millimeter, to very serious, life-threatening infections. Neutropenia may result from *ineffective* and *defective neutrophil production*. This is seen in hypoplastic or aplastic anemias secondary to cytotoxic drugs, toxic substances, and viral infection; starvation; and replacement of normal bone marrow by malignant cells (e.g., in leukemia).

Agranulocytosis is a very serious condition characterized by an extremely low leukocyte count and absence of neutrophils. The causative agent is generally a drug which interferes with cell formation or enhances cell destruction. Drugs commonly implicated are the myelosuppressive (suppress bone marrow) chemotherapeutic agents used in the treatment of hematologic and other malignancies. Increasingly, more commonly used drugs (i.e., analgesics, antibiotics, and antihistamines) have been identified as capable of causing severe neutropenia or agranulocytosis. This response to the drugs is either dose-related or an idiosyncratic reaction.

Common symptoms of agranulocytosis are infection and feelings of general malaise (discomfort, lassitude, headache, and muscle aches) followed by ulceration of the mucous membranes, fever, and tachycardia. If untreated, sepsis and death ensue. Removal of the offending agent will often inhibit and reverse the process with an increased production of the neutrophils and other normal marrow elements.

Leukemia

Classification of leukemias

Leukemia, originally described by Virchow in 1847 as "white blood," is a neoplastic disease characterized by an abnormal proliferation of the hematopoietic cells. Classification as acute or chronic is according to the cell type involved and the maturity of the cell. Accurate classification is vital as the treatment modalities and prognosis vary accordingly.

The classification of the chronic leukemias is based on the identification of the predominant mature white blood cell—a granulocyte (granulocytic/myelocytic leukemia) or a lymphocyte (lymphocytic leukemia). While various classifications of the acute leukemias exist, the French-American-British (FAB) cooperative group has proposed a morphologic classification based on the cell differentiation and maturation of predominant leukemia cells in the bone marrow, as well as cytochemical studies (Gralnick, 1977; Dabich, 1980) (Table 17-1). This classification should lead to treatment differentiation which then would maximize efforts at attaining long-term remissions and cures.

Incidence

While both sexes are affected, there is a slight male to female predominance. Acute granulocytic or myelo-

cytic leukemia is seen in adults of all ages. Acute lymphocytic leukemia is more prevalent in children under 15 years of age, with a peak between the ages of 2 and 4. Chronic granulocytic or myelocytic leukemia is most frequently seen in middle age but can occur in any age group. Chronic lymphocytic leukemia is seen in older individuals.

Etiology

While the basic cause of leukemia is unknown, both genetic predisposition and environmental factors seem to play a role. Familial leukemias are rare, but there seems to be a higher incidence of leukemia in siblings of affected children, with the incidence increasing to 20 percent in monozygote (identical) twins. Individuals with chromosomal abnormalities as in Down's syndrome seem to have a twentyfold increased incidence of acute leukemia.

Environmental factors include exposure to ionizing radiation with manifestations of leukemia occurring years later. Chemicals (e.g., benzene, arsenic, chloramphenicol, phenylbutazone, and antineoplastic agents) are being implicated with increased frequency, especially the alkylating agents. The likelihood of leukemia increases in patients treated with both radiation and chemotherapy. Any hypoplastic bone marrow state seems to predispose the individual to leukemia. Viral agents have been identified for some time as causing leukemia in animals. In early 1980, a human T-cell leukemia virus of HTLV I was isolated from the lymphocytes of a patient with cutaneous lymphoma and has since been isolated from serum samples of patients with T-cell leukemia (Jacobs and Gale, 1984).

Acute Leukemias

Acute myelogenous or granulocytic leukemia

Acute myelogenous or granulocytic leukemia (AGL) accounts for 80 percent of the acute leukemias seen in adults. The onset may be abrupt or progressive over a 1- to 6-month period. If untreated, death ensues in approximately 2 months. With treatment about 65 percent of the patients attain a complete remission (without evidence of disease) and a median survival of 1 to 1½ years. A few long-term remissions have been reported in the literature.

Clinical manifestations are related to the decrease or absence of normal hematopoietic cells. There is evidence that acute leukemia is a uniclonal neoplasm which originates in the transformation of a single or a few hematopoietic cells. The exact nature of the molecular lesion(s) responsible for the transformed cells' neoplastic properties is not clear, but the critical defect is intrinsic and inheritable by the cells' progeny (Clarkson, 1983).

TABLE 17-1

FAB* CLASSIFICATION OF ACUTE LEUKEMIA

Acute lymphoblastic leukemia	
L-1	Acute lymphocytic leukemia of childhood—homogeneous cell population
L-2	Acute lymphocytic leukemia seen in adults—heterogeneous cell population
L-3	Burkitt's lymphoma-type leukemia—large cells, homogeneous cell population

Acute myeloblastic leukemia	
M-1	Granulocytic differentiation without maturation
M-2	Granulocytic differentiation with maturation to promyelocytic stage
M-3	Granulocytic differentiation with hypergranular promyelocytes associated with disseminated intravascular coagulation
M-4	Acute myelomonocytic leukemia—both granulocytic and monocytic cell lines
M-5	Monocytes predominate and may be either well or poorly differentiated
M-6	Predominance of erythroblasts with severe dyserythropoiesis

*French-American-British Cooperative Group.
Source: Gralnick, 1977.

Signs and symptoms of the acute leukemias are related to neutropenia and thrombocytopenia. These are recurrent, severe infections with ulcerations of the mucous membranes, perirectal abscesses, pneumonias, septicemias accompanied by chills, fever, tachycardia, and tachypnea. These signs and symptoms are responsible for the high mortality associated with acute leukemia.

Thrombocytopenia results in bleeding evidenced by petechiae and ecchymosis (bleeding into the skin), epistaxis (nosebleeds), and hematomas in the mucous membranes, as well as gastrointestinal and urinary tract bleeding. Bone pain and tenderness may be present due to bone infarcts or subperiosteal (beneath the periosteum) infiltrates.

Anemia is not an early manifestation because of the long life span of the erythrocyte (120 days). When anemia is present, headaches and symptoms of fatigue and dyspnea on exertion are evident, along with marked pallor.

Diagnosis is established through peripheral blood count and bone marrow examination inclusive of chromosomal studies. Metabolic alterations are also seen with increased uric acid due to the high WBC turnover.

Therapy is directed toward elimination of the abnormal cell line; normal cell lines will regenerate themselves, with 65 percent of patients experiencing remission of the disease. Table 17-2 lists the chemotherapeutic agents commonly used in the treatment of hematologic malignancies. Most current regimens include cytosine arabinoside, doxorubicin, vincristine, and prednisone. The chemotherapeutic agents selected destroy the cells by various mechanisms such as interfering with cell metabolism and maturation. The same clinical manifestations of pancytopenia accompanying active disease are present after chemotherapy. Supportive care is the key to the increased survival of these patients. Care should include assiduous precautions against infection and bleeding, aggressive antimocrobial therapy in the case of infection, and the judicious use of blood component therapy (such as platelets, packed red blood cells, and granulocytes).

Acute lymphocytic leukemia

Acute lymphocytic leukemia (ALL) is the most common cancer affecting children. It is manifested by an abnormal proliferation of lymphoblasts in the bone marrow and extramedullary sites (those outside of the bone marrow, i.e., lymph nodes and spleen) (Fig. 17-4). Signs and symptoms, as with AGL, are related to suppression of normal bone marrow elements. Because extramedullary sites are also involved, children have enlarged lymph nodes (lymphadenopathy) and hepatosplenomegaly. Bone pain is very common. Central nervous system involvement occurs (i.e., headaches, vomiting, seizures, visual disturbance). The onset of ALL is usually abrupt with rapid progression and death if un-

treated. Improved survival with treatment has been dramatic. Not only do 90 to 95 percent achieve a full remission, but 50 percent maintain their remissions for 5 years or longer. This is achieved through combined chemotherapy, radiotherapy, and immunotherapy. Most chemotherapy programs include vincristine, prednisone, and L-asparaginase, in combination. The course of ALL for adults is similar to that for AGL.

Chronic leukemias

Chronic granulocytic leukemia

Chronic granulocytic leukemia (CGL) is seen most frequently in middle-aged adults but may occur in any age group. Unlike AGL, CGL is insidious in its onset, often discovered on routine examinations and blood screening. CGL is considered a myeloproliferative disorder because the bone marrow is hypercellular with proliferation of all the cell lines (Fig. 17-5). Granulocyte counts generally are greater than 30,000 per cubic millimeter. While maturation is disordered, most of the cells are mature and functional. In 85 percent of the cases a chromosome abnormality referred to as the Philadelphia chromosome is present. The Philadelphia chromosome is a translocation of the long arm of chromosome 22 to that of 9. It is depicted in Fig. 17-6.

Signs and symptoms are related to a hypermetabolic state—fatigue, weight loss, increased diaphoresis, and heat intolerance. The spleen is enlarged in 90 percent of the cases, which leads to a sensation of abdominal fullness and early satiety. The median survival rate, with or without treatment, is about 3 years. Treatment with intermittent chemotherapy is directed toward suppressing the excessive hematopoiesis and reducing spleen size. Invariably the patients progress to a more aggressive, resistant phase with an overwhelming production of myeloblasts ("blast transformation"). Death ensues within weeks to months after blast transformation.

Chromic lymphocytic leukemia

Chronic lymphocytic leukemia (CLL) is a lymphoproliferative disorder seen in the older age group (median age 60) with a 2:1 male predominance. It is manifested by a proliferation and accumulation of small abnormal mature lymphocytes in the bone marrow, peripheral blood, and extramedullary sites, with levels reaching 100,000 per cubic millimeter or more. The abnormal lymphocyte is generally a B lymphocyte, which leads to insufficient immunoglobulin synthesis and de-

TABLE 17-2

COMMONLY USED CHEMOTHERAPEUTIC AGENTS IN HEMATOLOGIC MALIGNANCIES

| Drug | | | | Toxicity | |
Generic name	Brand name*	Disease	Administration†	Acute	Long-term
Alkylating agents					
Mechlorethamine hydrochloride, nitrogen mustard	Mustargen	Hodgkin's	IV push	Anorexia; nausea and vomiting: nausea, 30 minutes–4 hours after injection	Myelosuppression, amenorrhea, male sterility
Cyclophosphamide	Cytoxan, Endoxan	Lymphomas Chronic lymphocytic leukemia Acute leukemia Multiple myeloma Waldenström's macroglobulinemia	PO, IV	Delayed nausea, 6–18 hours	Alopecia, hemorrhagic cystitis, myelosuppression, amenorrhea, male sterility, immunosuppression
Busulfan	Myleran	CGL Polycythemia vera Thrombocythemia	PO	Minimal nausea	Myelosuppression, skin pigmentation, pulmonary fibrosis, Addisonian syndrome
Chlorambucil	Leukeran	CLL Hodgkin's Lymphomas	PO	Mild anorexia; nausea and vomiting	Myelosuppression
Antimetabolites					
Methotrexate	A-Methopterin	ALL AGL	PO, IV, IM, IT, IP	Nausea, vomiting	Myelosuppression, stomatitis, diarrhea, alopecia, mucosal ulceration, hepatic-renal dysfunction, immunosuppression
Cytosine arabinoside (cytarabine)	Cytosar, Ara-C	AGL Acute myelomonocytic leukemia	IV, SC	Nausea, vomiting	Myelosuppression, GI mucositis, immunosuppression
6-Mercaptopurine	6MP, Purinethiol	ALL AGL	PO, IV	Nausea, vomiting	Myelosuppression, hepatocellular dysfunction, GI mucositis
6-Thioguanine, 6-TG		AGL	PO	Nausea, vomiting	Myelosuppression, photosensitivity, hepatocellular dysfuntion
Natural products, plant alkaloids					
Vincristine sulfate	Oncovin	ALL AGL Hodgkin's	IV	Nausea, local phlebitis	Peripheral neuropathy, myopathy, alopecia
Vinblastine	Velban	Hodgkin's Lymphomas	IV	Local phlebitis, mild nausea, stomatitis, glossitis	Leukopenia, rare peripheral neuropathy
Etoposide VP-16	Vepesid	AGL	IV	Orthostatic hypotension, mild nausea, vomiting, anorexia	Myelosuppression, alopecia
Antibiotics					
Doxorubicin hydrochloride	Adriamycin	Acute leukemia Lymphomas	IV	Severe vesicant with tissue necrosis, nausea	Myelosuppression, alopecia. Cardiac toxicity with cumulative doses

204

TABLE 17-2 (*continued*)

Drug		Disease	Administration†	Toxicity	
Generic name	Brand name*			Acute	Long-term
Daunorubicin hydrochloride (Daunomycin)	Cerubidine	Acute leukemia Lymphomas Hodgkin's Multiple myeloma	IV	Severe vesicant with tissue necrosis, nausea	Myelosuppression, alopecia. Cardiac toxicity with cumulative doses
Bleomycin	Blenoxane	Lymphomas	IV, IM, SC	Fever, possible anaphylaxis, acute pulmonary edema	Pulmonary fibrosis with cumulative doses. Minimal myelosuppression, skin and nail discoloration
Enzymes					
L-asparaginase	Elspar	ALL	IV, IM	Hypersensitivity with potential for anaphylaxis. Nausea, vomiting, and anorexia	Hyperglycemia, pancreatitis, hepatotoxicity, general malaise, somnolence, depression
Adrenocorticoids					
Prednisone	Orasone, Deltasone	ALL AGL Lymphomas Multiple myeloma Waldenström's macroglobulinemia	PO	GI distress, water retention	GI distress, chemical diabetes, water retention, osteoporosis, psychosis

*This list is *not* all-inclusive. Other equally effective brands may exist.
†IV: intravenous; PO: by mouth; IM: intramuscular; IT: intrathecal; IP: intraperitoneal; SC: subcutaneous.

pressed antibody response. The onset is insidious and is often discovered on routine blood work or because of painless lymphadenopathy and splenomegaly. As the disease progresses, the liver also enlarges. Patients with only lymphocytosis and lymphadenopathy may survive 10 years or longer. Early anemia and thrombocytopenia (low platelet count) reflect a poor prognosis with a median survival of 2 years.

Signs and symptoms, which are similar to those of CGL, reflect a hypermetabolic state. Massive organ en-

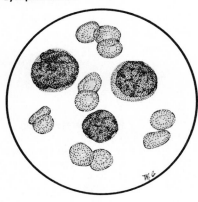

FIGURE 17-4
Lymphoblast.

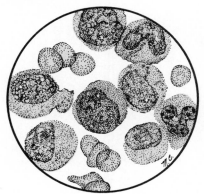

FIGURE 17-5
Bone marrow characteristic of chronic granulocytic leukemia.

205

largement causes mechanical pressure on the stomach with symptoms of early satiety, abdominal discomfort, and bowel irregularities. Infections of the skin and pneumonia may be present; these are secondary to the altered immunologic state as well as the neutropenia.

Treatment is generally indicated and directed toward reducing the lymphocytic mass, thus reversing the pancytopenia and relieving the discomfort caused by the organ enlargement. Chemotherapy with alkylating agents and corticosteroids is used.

Table 17-3 presents the differential features of the leukemias.

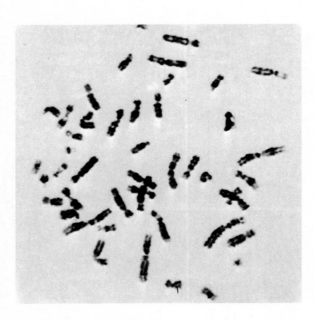

Lymphoma

General considerations

The *lymphomas* are the lymphoproliferative class of disorders. Their cause is unknown, but viruses have been implicated, especially the Epstein-Barr virus seen in Burkitt's lymphoma. The initial tumor formation in these disorders is in the secondary lymphatic tissues (i.e., lymph nodes and/or spleen), and subsequent dissemination to the bone marrow and other tissues may occur.

Two broad categories of lymphomas are identified on the basis of the microscopic histopathology of the involved lymph nodes. The categories are the lymphomas of *Hodgkin's disease* and the *non-Hodgkin's* lymphomas. While the signs and symptoms of the lymphomas overlap, the treatment and prognosis are different for each kind. Thus it is imperative to establish an accurate diagnosis. For this, one or more lymph nodes are surgically removed and studied microscopically.

The lymphomas are differentiated according to the predominant types of cells (lymphocytes vs. histiocytes) found in the lymph node, as well as their distribution. The cells may be distributed in a nodular or diffuse manner. These cells destroy the normal architecture of the lymph nodes. In general, a better prognosis is associated with the nodular distribution where there is a predominance of lymphocytes. Immunologic and cytochemical studies are done to identify the origin of the neoplastic cell as either a B or T lymphocyte.

One of the major determinants of treatment, as well as the prognosis, is the clinical stage (extent of disease) of the patient at the time of diagnosis (Table 17-4). After tissue diagnosis is established, staging procedures must be carried out. These commonly include (1) complete physical examination, (2) routine blood studies, (3) chemistries (liver and kidney function), (4) chest roentgenograms (x-ray) looking for hilar lymphadenopathy (enlarged bronchial lymph nodes), followed by full chest tomograms (laminograms) (see Chap. 38), (5) lymphangiograms to check for retroperitoneal and iliac node involvement, (6) liver-spleen scans, and (7) multiple bone marrow aspirations and biopsies. In the absence of bone marrow involvement a laparotomy (see Chap. 23) with splenectomy and liver biopsy is often done in Hodgkin's disease patients for accurate staging. This is not routinely done in non-Hodgkin's lymphoma.

FIGURE 17-6

Karyotype of a marrow cell from a female patient with chronic granulocytic leukemia. A fragment has been lost from chromosome 22 and translocated to chromosome 9. The preparation is stained with the acetic-saline-Giemsa method 1 to show banding patterns. (Reproduced with permission from Dr. Raymond Teplitz.)

TABLE 17-3

DIFFERENTIAL FEATURES OF THE LEUKEMIAS

Diagnosis	Acute myelogenous (granulocytic) leukemia	Acute lymphoblastic (lymphocytic) leukemia	Chronic myelogenous (granulocytic) leukemia	Chronic lymphocytic leukemia
Incidence (age)	Throughout adult 10% in children	Usually in children <15 years Peak 3–4 years; May occur in adults	Ages 20–60 years Peak 40 years May occur in children	Median 60 years
Sex distribution	Slight M:F predominance 3:2	M:F predominance 5:4	Slight predominance M:F	M:F predominance 2:1
Implicated causal factors	High ionizing radiation, chemical exposure, genetic aberrations (e.g., Down's)	Genetic aberrations (e.g., Down's) irradiation, virus	Ionizing radiation, chemical exposure	Unknown
Survival	3–6 months without treatment 1–3 years with treatment Some long-term survivors	3–6 months without treatment Low-risk features: >50% 5 years or more survival (null-cell; ages 2–10) High-risk High-risk features: ± 2 years survival (T & B cell; children < 2 years, teens, young adults)	1–10 years Mean 3 years	2–25 years
Signs and symptoms	Variable: ecchymosis, gum and nose bleeding, malaise, fatigue, fever, sternal tenderness, occasional hepatosplenomegaly	Variable: hepatosplenomegaly, lymphadenopathy, 10% mediastinal mass, ecchymosis, low-grade fever, weight loss, sternal tenderness, bone and joint pain, malaise, fatigue	Splenomegaly, bone tenderness, pallor, hypermetabolic symptoms, diaphoresis, weight loss, anorexia	Painless lymphadenopathy, hepatosplenomegaly, acquired hypersensitivity to insect bites
Peripheral blood	Elevated, normal, or decreased white blood with ± myeloblasts Thrombocytopenia Anemia	Markedly elevated white blood cells with lymphocytosis White count may be N or ↓ Thrombocytopenia Anemia	Markedly elevated white blood cells mainly mature granulocytes All developmental stages present including blasts Basophilia Eosinophilia Early thrombocytosis Thrombocytopenia and anemia (end stage)	Moderately elevated small mature lymphocytes; neutrophils Thrombocytopenia Anemia with progressive disease
Bone marrow	Hypercellular > 50% myeloblasts Auer rods†	Hypercellular with infiltrating lymphoblasts	Hypercellular <50% blasts megakaryocytes	>30% lymphocytes
Cytogenetics	Nonrandom chromosomal aberrations involving chromosomes 8, 7, 21	Variable chromosomal aberrations 5% Philadelphia chromosome aberrations	85% Philadelphia chromosome aberrations Other chromosomal aberrations	Random unconfirmed chromosomal aberrations

TABLE 17-3 (*continued*)

Diagnosis	Acute myelogenous (granulocytic) leukemia	Acute lymphoblastic (lymphocytic) leukemia	Chronic myelogenous (granulocytic) leukemia	Chronic lymphocytic leukemia
Immunologic identification	Not identified Lack cALLa‡ antigen (Lack T- & B-cell determinants)	85% cALLa‡ antigen (Lack B- or T-cell characteristics)	None identified	Majority have B-cell markers 1–3% have T-cell markers
Treatment (see Table 17-2)	Combination chemotherapy including: Cytosine arabinoside; Adriamycin or Daunamycin; vincristine and prednisone Blood products and antibiotic support	Combination chemotherapy including: vincristine and prednisone; methotrexate; L-asparaginase Blood products and antibiotic support	Generally single alkylating agent; Alkeran or Hydroxyurea	When symptomatic alkylating agents, corticosteroids, radiation therapy
Complications	Hemorrhage, sepsis, DIC	Hemorrhage, sepsis, CNS involvement	Myelofibrosis, pancytopenia, blast transformation, splenic infarction	Pancytopenia, hemolytic anemia, ITP viral infection

*Null cell: Lymphocytes that lack B-cell (membrane immunoglobulin) or T-cell (E-rosette formation) markers.
†Auer rods: Red-staining rods seen in cytoplasm of myeloblasts characteristic of acute myelogenous leukemia.
‡cALLa: Common ALL antigen—a distinct surface membrane glycoprotein complex carried on 70% of non-T-cell leukemia lymphoblasts.

TABLE 17-4

ANN ARBOR STAGING CLASSIFICATION (MODIFIED) OF HODGKIN'S DISEASE AND LYMPHOMAS

Stage I	Disease involves a single lymph node region located above or below the diaphragm, or one extralymphatic organ or site (I$_E$).
Stage II	Disease involves more than two adjacent or two nonadajacent regions on one side of the diaphragm, or an extralymphatic organ or site along with one or more lymph node regions on the same side of the diaphragm (II$_E$).
Stage III	Disease extends above and below the diaphragm but is limited to lymph nodes, or involves, in addition, an extralymphatic organ or site (III$_E$) or the spleen (III$_{ES}$).
Stage IV	Diffuse or disseminated involvement of one or more extralymphatic organs or tissues, such as bone marrow or liver. Further subclassification indicates absence (A) or presence (B) of systemic symptoms: weight loss exceeding 10 percent of body weight, fever, and night sweats.

Hodgkin's disease

Hodgkin's disease is seen primarily in young adults between the ages of 18 and 35 and in persons beyond 50 years of age. There is a 3:2 male-female predominance. It is classified histologically as lymphocyte predominance (LP), nodular sclerosis (NS), mixed cellularity (MC), or lymphocyte depletion (LD). The Reed-Sternberg cell, which is a malignant form of histiocyte (tissue macrophage), is a characteristic finding in Hodgkin's lymphoma (Fig. 17-7). It is a large binucleated or multinucleated cell containing large nucleoli. The

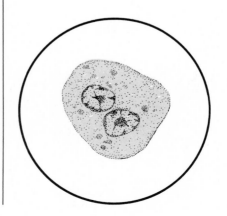

FIGURE 17-7
Reed-Sternberg cell.

younger patient generally presents with a nontender, rubbery-feeling enlarged lymph node in the low cervical or supraclavicular area, or with a dry nonproductive cough secondary to hilar lymphadenopathy. The general mode of dissemination is an orderly involvement of contiguous sites. Older patients present more often with unexplained persistent fever and/or night sweats. In certain cases the *Pel-Ebstein* fever (a cyclical pattern of elevated evening temperatures lasting a few days to weeks) is present.

Accurate clinical and pathologic staging, with appropriate treatment, has improved the prognosis of Hodgkin's disease. For example, 90 percent cures of patients with asymptomatic stages I and II disease are evident, especially of the lymphocyte predominance (LP) or nodular sclerotic (NS) types (Table 17-4). Treatments utilized include extensive radiotherapy, combination of chemotherapy and radiotherapy, or chemotherapy alone.

Non-Hodgkin's lymphomas

The median age of individuals with non-Hodgkin's lymphomas is 50 years. Classification of the non-Hodgkin's lymphomas is in a state of transition. The widely used Rappaport classification (introduced in 1956) is based on the cytology and the architectural arrangement of the malignant lymphocytes in the lymph nodes. This classification divides lymphomas according to (1) the nodular type (N), where neoplastic cells group in cohesive aggregates which stimulate lymphoid follicles, and (2) the diffuse type (D), where no aggregation occurs (Fig. 17-8).

The advancement of knowledge in the field of immunology and lymphocyte physiology, such as identifying lymphocytes as B- or T-cell type, has led to more definitive classification of the non-Hodgkin's lymphomas as reflected in the classification by Lukes and Col-

lins. Lukes and Collins demonstrated in their classification that 70 percent of the lymphomas are found to be of B-cell origin. The majority have features of cells normally found in follicular centers and thus are called *follicular-center cell lymphomas* (Ultmann, 1980). They are further classified according to their histologic features. Cells may be small or large, cleaved or noncleaved. Cleaved cells are irregular, indented, and angulated with considerable variation in nuclear configuration. Noncleaved cells have distinct nuclei, dispersed chromatin, and abundant cytoplasm (Ultmann, 1980) (see Fig. 17-8).

While constitutional symptoms (fever, weight loss, and night sweats) do occur, the incidence is lower than it is in Hodgkin's disease and does not necessarily influence prognosis. Painless lymphadenopathy is seen and may affect any or all of the peripheral lymph nodes. While hilar adenopathy is usually not seen, pleural effusions are common. Approximately 20 percent or more of the patients have symptoms related to retroperitoneal or mesenteric lymph node enlargement, presenting with abdominal pain or irregularities of bowel movements. Involvement of the stomach and small intestine is common with symptoms of pain similar to that of peptic ulcer, anorexia, weight loss, nausea, hematemesis (bloody vomiting), and melena. In diffuse histiocytic lymphoma, the tonsillar lymphatic tissue in the oro- and nasopharynx (referred to as Waldeyer's ring) is a common site of involvement.

Patients with non-Hodgkin's lymphomas of the nodular, diffuse, poorly differentiated lymphocytic type tend to present at more advanced stages initially, with about 60 to 80 percent incidence of bone marrow involvement. Staging laparotomy is generally not indicated in these individuals. Since there is usually no bone marrow involvement in the diffuse histiocytic lymphomas (10 to 15 percent), patients with presumed stages I and II should be staged surgically.

Central nervous system (CNS) diseases, while rare, do occur in the diffuse histiocytic lymphomas. The CNS is frequently the site for relapse in patients with stage IV disease along with the sites of previous involvement.

The treatment of choice for patients with localized extranodal disease is radiation, either localized or ex-

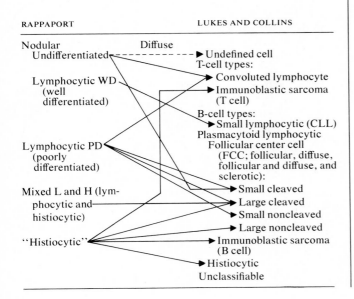

FIGURE 17-8

Comparisons of classifications. [Modified from J. Ultmann and V. DeVita, Jr., in K. Isselbacher et al. (eds.), *Harrison's Principles of Internal Medicine*, 9th ed., McGraw-Hill, New York, 1980, p. 1642.)

tended-field radiotherapy. This treatment is curative in 80 to 90 percent of the cases with diffuse histiocytic lymphoma. Patients with stage II diffuse disease require a combination of chemotherapy (utilizing three to five drugs) and radiation which is directed at the local disease. Approximately 50 percent remission or cure rates are obtained in previously untreated cases. Nodular lymphomas generally respond to nonaggressive single- or two-drug regimes. The median survival rate is 8 to 10 years for this condition (Sweet, 1980). The common chemotherapeutic agents used are listed in Table 17-2 and generally include cytoxan, prednisone, and vincristine.

PLASMA CELL DYSCRASIAS

Multiple myeloma

Multiple myeloma is a lymphoproliferative disorder associated with plasma cells. This is a malignant neoplastic disorder that arises in the bone marrow and involves primarily bone. The median age at diagnosis is 60. It is rarely seen in individuals under 40 years of age. Plasma cells are the most mature form of activated B lymphocytes and are responsible for immunoglobulin synthesis. The five main classes of immunoglobulins are IgA, IgD, IgE, IgG, and IgM (see Chap. 5).

In *multiple myeloma*, plasma cell proliferation suppresses normal marrow elements, causing the characteristic "punched out" lytic bone lesions seen on x-ray. This condition predisposes the individual to pathologic fractures. These plasma cells also produce a homogeneous immunoglobulin, as seen in electrophoresis. Most common are IgG and IgA. The excessive production of functionally abnormal immunoglobulins suppresses the normal synthesis of the other immunoglobulins. The clinical manifestations reflect the combined effects of the high tumor burden (large numbers of immature plasma cells) and abnormal globulin synthesis (Schuman and Patterson, 1975).

The symptoms generally include severe disabling bone pain, (especially in weight-bearing areas) secondary to bone destruction and pathologic fractures. Simple maneuvers such as turning in bed, coughing, or sneez-

ing can result in fractures of the arms and ribs. Compression fractures result in loss of height. Neurologic symptoms range from peripheral neuropathy to cord compression. The latter is a medical emergency, and unless treatment is promptly instituted with radiotherapy and/or chemotherapy, the patient will be paralyzed. Because of the bone destruction, calcium is mobilized, causing *hypercalcemia* (increased serum calcium levels). These patients may present with symptoms of renal failure, anorexia, confusion, and coma. If the renal failure is untreated, death ensues. In addition to hypercalcemia, renal impairment may result from the myeloma proteins (referred to as Bence Jones proteins) damaging the renal tubules. High uric acid levels secondary to the increased plasma cell turnover may also lead to renal failure. This may result from the primary disease or may be secondary to chemotherapy. Dehydration may precipitate actual renal failure.

Complications such as pneumonia, urinary tract infections, and bacteremia are common. These complications are due primarily to the decrease or lack of normal immunoglobulins as well as to the leukopenia secondary to marrow replacement or chemotherapy. Increased levels of abnormal globulins cause increased serum viscosity with visual disturbances, headache, somnolence, irritability, and confusion. Expanded plasma volume may result in congestive heart failure. The red blood cells become coated with proteins, which causes them to stick together like stacks of coins (*rouleaux*, Fig. 17-9). Bleeding manifestations occur because the protein interacts with the plasma coagulation factors as well as coating platelets, interfering with their function. One of the globulins, cryoglobulin, precipitates in cold temperatures, causing blanching, pain, and ulceration in fingertips and toes (Raynaud's phenome-

FIGURE 17-9
Peripheral blood characteristic of multiple myeloma. Peripheral blood smear depicting rouleau formation typically seen in multiple myeloma. The large cell in the center is an immature plasma cell. (Courtesy of Rita C. Pohlod, MT (ASCP) SH, Henry Ford Hospital—Special Hematology.)

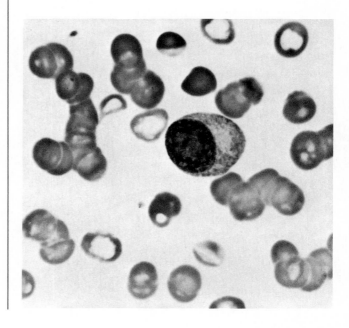

non). A normochromic, normocytic anemia is also present. Figure 17-10 depicts a peripheral blood smear in multiple myeloma, which illustrates malignant plasma cells.

Diagnosis of multiple myeloma is based on physical examination, history, and radiologic, hematologic, and chemical findings. Positive findings include an abnormal spike of protein on serum and/or urine electrophoresis and immunophoresis test and "punched out" lytic bone lesion on skeletal x-rays. Bone marrow examination usually reveals a greater than 10 percent plasmacytosis (increased number of plasmacytes in the peripheral blood) with immature plasma cells. These cells are 15 to 40 μm in diameter, basophilic, and contain an eccentrically placed nucleus with finely clumped chromatin.

Newly diagnosed patients with multiple myeloma who present with a *high tumor mass*, hemoglobin values <8.5 g, hypercalcemia, and serum IgG > 7 g or IgA >5 g carry a poor prognosis, whereas those with a *low tumor mass* have a median survival of 4 years.

Treatment is aimed at reducing the number of malignant plasma cells and preventing and controlling the complications. A solitary area of plasma cell tumor (*plasmacytoma*) is treated with local irradiation. Active disease requires combinations of radiotherapy and chemotherapy. Multiple drug combinations using three to five agents are employed; they include prednisone and an alkylating agent such as melphalan (Alkeran). These regimens are prescribed intermittently every 4 to 6 weeks for approximately 18 to 24 months. Approximately 50 percent of the patients will show a significant tumor reduction.

Impending spinal cord compression (see Chap. 52) or other tumor masses are treated with irradiation. Because immobility exacerbates bone demineralization and osteoporosis, it is imperative that the patient maintain a high level of mobility. Judicious use of analgesics, supportive garments, and walking aids will benefit. Other preventive measures such as hydration and control of infections and bleeding will limit most of the previously described complications.

Waldenström's macroglobulinemia

Waldenström's macroglobulinemia is a rare dysproteinemia which predominantly affects males over 50. Morphologically it appears as a malignant lymphoma with B lymphocytes, plasma cells, and plasmacytoid lymphocytes (resembling plasmacytes) infiltrating the bone marrow. Hepatic, splenic, and other lymphoid tissue involvements are common, resulting in enlargement of these organs. The malignant cells rarely produce bone destruction but synthesize and release large quantities of IgM into the intravascular space. This causes increased plasma volume and severe hyperviscosity. The immunoglobulin is relatively nonfunctional and may suppress production of normal immunoglobulins.

The major clinical manifestations relate to the hyperviscosity syndrome, the increased plasma immunoglobulin, and bone marrow infiltration. The symptoms of hyperviscosity are similar to those of multiple myeloma. These include marked increase in plasma volume, vision disturbances, and segmental dilatation of retinal veins with hemorrhages. Cold agglutinin disease (agglutination of RBCs at cold temperature) with hemolytic anemia has been described, as has Raynaud's phenomenon and anemia secondary to bone marrow replacement. Bleeding tendency, which is attributed to coating of the platelets and interference with the coagulation factors, is also seen and further aggravated by thrombocytopenia due to marrow replacement. Lymphadenopathy and splenomegaly may be present.

Bacterial infections are common. The bone marrow shows a plasmacytoid lymphocytosis. Blood volume and viscosity are increased. Serum protein electrophoresis depicts an IgM spike.

Treatment of Waldenström's macroglobulinemia is aimed at decreasing the IgM plasma load and bone marrow infiltration and lymphoid tissues. Since IgM is mainly a circulating intravascular protein, plasmapheresis can be used effectively to decrease the globulin and temporarily reduce the hyperviscosity symptoms. Plasmapheresis is a process whereby plasma is removed by means of a cell separator and replaced with volume expanders. In the anemic patient this procedure should be done prior to RBC infusion as the red blood cells add to the hyperviscosity syndrome. Combination chemotherapy with alkylating agents and steroids is used in-

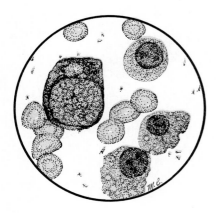

FIGURE 17-10

In the upper right field is a normal plasma cell and a plasma cell typical of multiple myeloma, while the other cells are malignant plasma cells.

termittently. Radiation is used to reduce large lymphoid aggregates. Prevention, early detection, and prompt treatment of infections are imperative because of their high incidence and increased mortality from infection. Even with appropriate treatment measures, the median survival is only 4 years.

TREATMENT OF HEMATOLOGIC MALIGNANCIES

The hallmark in the treatment of the hematologic malignancies is the use of *chemotherapeutic agents*. Current therapeutic regimes consist of multiple drugs used in combination, which result in more sustained remission rates. In select cases of Hodgkin's disease and acute lymphocytic leukemia, cures are being attained. In other diseases such as multiple myeloma, quality of life has been improved.

All cells go through a series of divisions (mitosis) and maturational stages called a cell cycle. During the mitotic phase, chromosome replication takes place, followed by the first gap or G_1 phase with RNA and protein synthesis. This is followed by the S or DNA synthesis phase and then the second gap or G_2 phase with resumed RNA synthesis. Mitosis follows, producing two daughter cells (Knopf, 1981).

In general, therapeutic regimes are developed to include drugs acting at different stages of the cell cycle. *Phase-specific* agents arrest or kill dividing cells during a specific phase of this cycle. For example, vincristine arrests cell division, cytarabine (Cytosar) interferes with DNA synthesis during the S phase. *Cycle-specific* drugs such as cyclophosphamide (Cytoxan) kill proliferating cells more effectively than resting cells and *non-cycle-*

specific agents such as nitrogen mustard and carmustine (BCNU) kill both proliferating and resting cells.

The drugs are further classified according to their mode of action. *Alkylating agents* are substances in which an alkyl radical (hydrocarbon molecule with an absent hydrogen atom) is substituted for a hydrogen atom causing cross-linking of DNA strands and abnormal base-pairing, interfering with DNA replication. This category includes nitrogen mustard, cyclophosphamide, phenylalanine mustard, and chlorambucil (Knopf, 1981; Bakemeir, 1978). The *antimetabolites*, such as methotrexate, cytosine arabinoside, and 6-mercaptopurine, interfere with the biological synthesis of DNA and RNA, and thus the cell metabolism, by either blocking the needed developmental enzymes or actually being incorporated into the DNA and/or the RNA.

The *antibiotic agents*, isolated from microorganisms, seem to inhibit DNA and RNA synthesis. Doxorubicin hydrochloride (Adriamycin) and bleomycin are only two of many antibiotic antitumor agents. *Natural products*—the vinca alkaloids, vincristine and vinblastine, derived from the periwinkle plant—interfere with the mitotic spindle formation and arrest cell division at the metaphase stage (Joss, 1980).

The *nitrosourates* are lipid-soluble alkylating agents, which inhibit nucleic acid synthesis or DNA and RNA synthesis. Drugs in this category include lomustine (CCNU) and carmustine (BCNU).

Adrenocorticosteroids are hormone preparations; while their exact action is unclear, they may influence synthetic processes related to RNA and protein synthesis (Joss, 1980). Prednisone is the one most commonly used in the hematologic malignancies and may be seen in many combinations.

The commonly used chemotherapeutic agents as presented in Table 17-2 are listed according to their classification. Their adverse reactions are divided according to acute or chronic toxicity. Acute toxicity occurs within minutes to hours after administration; chronic toxicity occurs over a longer period and is generally a cumulative, or dose-related, effect.

QUESTIONS

The white blood cell

Directions: Match the white blood cells listed in col. A with their appropriate function in col. B. More than one letter may be used in each space in col. A.

Column A
1. ____ PMNs
2. ____ Eosinophils
3. ____ Basophils
4. ____ Monocytes
5. ____ B lymphocytes
6. ____ Plasma cells
7. ____ T lymphocytes

Column B
a. Involved in phagocytosis of dead red and white corpuscles
b. Chief source of antibody production
c. Responsible for the humoral immune response
d. Present early in the acute phase of an inflammatory reaction
e. Involved in phagocytosis, killing, and/or digestion of bacteria

f. Involved in the production of antigen-reactive cells

g. Appear to function in combating acute systemic allergic reactions

h. Carry histamine and platelet-activating factors

i. Have phagocytic function, also appear to function in antigen-antibody reactions

Directions: Answer the following questions on a separate sheet of paper.

8. Explain the role of colony stimulating factor (CSF) in leukocyte cell differentiation.

9. Cite the importance of the genetic and environmental factors associated with leukemia.

10. Formulate a definition of multiple myeloma.

11. Describe the symptoms associated with Hodgkin's disease.

Directions: Circle T if the statement is true and F if it is false. Correct the false statements.

12. T F Granulopoietin is the stimulating factor responsible for leukocyte cell differentiation.

13. T F Plasma cells normally circulate in the peripheral blood.

14. T F Neutropenia is characterized by an extremely low leukocyte count and absence of neutrophils.

15. T F Granulocytes appear to originate from the pluripotential cell in the bone marrow.

16. T F The Lukes and Collins classification of non-Hodgkin's lymphomas demonstrated that 70 percent of the lymphomas are of T-cell origin.

17. T F Cells whose granules have a blue or basic dye affinity are called eosinophils.

Directions: Complete the following statements by filling in the blanks.

18. _____ refers to a neoplastic disease characterized by an abnormal proliferation and impaired functional capability of the hematopoietic cells.

19. The _____ classification of the acute leukemias is based on the predominant cell identified in the bone marrow (lymphoblast, myeloblast).

20. The cells characteristic of Hodgkin's disease are called _____.

21. _____ is a decrease below normal in the leukocyte count.

22. Certain abnormal chromosome patterns, such as the Philadelphia chromosome, are encountered in approximately 85 percent of the cases of _____.

Directions: List the type of white blood cell that is elevated in the following conditions:

23.   *Condition*   *Type of cell*

Acute bacterial   _____
infection

Allergic rhinitis   _____

Myeloproliferative   _____
disorders

Directions: Circle the letter preceding each item below that correctly answers the question. More than one answer may be correct.

24. In multiple myeloma there is an excessive production of which of the following homogeneous immunoglobulin(s):
a. IgD b. IgG c. IgE d. IgA

25. Which of the following are frequent complications encountered in patients with multiple myeloma that must be considered when planning treatment and care?
a. Pathologic fractures b. Pulmonary infections
c. Hypocalcemia d. Increased bleeding tendencies

26. Mr. B., a 60-year-old male, has been complaining of weight loss, weakness, and repeated episodes of pneumonia. Laboratory tests show very high levels of an abnormal globulin and nasal bleeding. The most likely diagnosis of Mr. B.'s condition is:
a. Chronic lymphocytic leukemia b. Lymphoma
c. Multiple myeloma d. Waldenström's macroglobulinemia

27. Mr. A., a 62-year-old male, presents with a painless lymphadenopathy, splenomegaly, and slightly enlarged liver. Diagnostic studies revealed small, abnormal, mature B lymphocytes in the bone marrow (>30 percent) with levels at 90,000 cells per cubic millimeter. The most likely condition is:
a. Acute myelogenous (granulocytic) leukemia
b. Agranulocytosis c. Chronic lymphocyte leukemia d. Chronic granulocytic leukemia

28. Which of the following reactions are seen in patients with leukemia?
    a. Growth of leukemic cells in abnormal areas
    b. Destruction of normal bone marrow   c. Increased metabolic rate   d. Production of abnormal protein

29. Your patient is an adult who complains of increasing weakness and fatigue. He has recently noticed abnormal bruising and epistaxis (nosebleeds). On admission he developed fever and pneumonia. The spleen is not palpable. Laboratory studies reveal immature-appearing cells of the neutrophilic series. The most likely diagnosis is:
    a. Acute lymphocytic leukemia   b. Acute myelogenous granulocytic leukemia   c. Chronic granulocytic leukemia   d. Chronic lymphocytic leukemia

30. Complications which are associated with chronic lymphocytic leukemia include:
    a. Pancytopenia   b. Blast transformation
    c. Hemolytic anemia   d. Splenic infarction

31. Hodgkin's disease, a lymphoproliferative disease, will usually be diagnosed by:
    a. A blood test   b. A tissue biopsy   c. Both a and b   d Neither a nor b

32. Sites of spread of Hodgkin's disease may include:
    a. Lymph nodes   b. Liver   c. Spleen   d. Bone marrow

33. Stage III Hodgkin's disease is defined as:

a. Lymphatic involvement on both sides of the diaphragm   b. Localized involvement of more than two adjacent or nonadjacent regions on one side of the diaphragm   c. Diffuse involvement of one or more extralymphatic organs or tissues such as bone marrow or liver

Directions: Match the drug in col. A with the associated toxic reaction(s) in col. B. More than one letter may be used in each space in col. A. Items may be used more than once.

Column A	Column B
34. ____ Bleomycin	a. Alopecia, hemorrhagic cystitis
35. ____ Doxorubicin	b. Severe vesicant with tissue necrosis, nausea
36. ____ Cyclophosphamide	c. Mild anorexia, nausea and vomiting
37. ____ Methotrexate	d. Delayed nausea, 6 to 18 hours
38. ____ Vincristine	e. Hypercalcemia, pancreatitis, hepatotoxicity
39. ____ Chlorambucil	f. Alopecia, peripheral neuropathy, myopathy
40. ____ L-Asparaginase	g. Myelosuppression
	h. Stomatitis, ulceration, diarrhea
	i. Pulmonary fibrosis with cumulative doses, minimal myelosuppression
	j. Immunosuppression

COAGULATION

OBJECTIVES

At the completion of this chapter you should be able to:

1. Explain the formation of platelets (thrombocytes).
2. Review the two major functions of platelets.
3. Describe the role of the liver as the major site of synthesis of plasma factors.
4. List and describe the 13 plasma clotting factors.
5. Describe the sequence of events that occurs when a blood vessel is injured by (a) identifying what enzyme is released, (b) identifying the plasma factors shared by both the extrinsic and intrinsic systems, (c) listing the plasma factors in each system, (d) explaining what causes a platelet plug, (e) identifying which factors platelets release, and (f) explaining the purpose of clot resolution.
6. Explain the difference between prothrombin time and partial thromboplastin time.
7. Cite the normal values for the following: bleeding time, platelet count, prothrombin time (PT), activated partial thromboplastin time (APTT), thrombin time (TT), and thromboplastin generation test (TGT).
8. Differentiate between the broad groups of coagulation abnormalities—primary vascular, primary platelet, and plasma factor deficiencies.
9. Differentiate between thrombocytosis and thrombocytopenia with regard to etiology, diagnosis, and treatment.
10. Describe hemophilia with regard to types, etiology, diagnosis, and treatment.
11. Formulate a definition for disseminated intravascular coagulation (DIC).
12. Explain the rationale for treatment of disseminated intravascular coagulation.

THE NORMAL COAGULATION PROCESS AND PLASMA CLOTTING FACTORS

Hemostasis and coagulation refer to a complex series of reactions which lead to the control of bleeding through the formation of a platelet and fibrin clot at the injury site. Clotting is followed by resolution or lysis of the clot and regeneration of the endothelium. In homeostatic states, hemostasis and coagulation protect the individual from massive bleeding secondary to trauma. In abnormal states, life-threatening hemorrhage or thrombosis occluding the vascular tree can occur.

At the time of injury, three major processes are responsible for hemostasis and coagulation: (1) transient vasoconstriction; (2) platelet reaction consisting of adhesion, release reaction, and aggregation of platelets; and (3) activation of the clotting factors (see Table 18-1). The initial steps occur at the exposed surfaces of the injured tissue, the subsequent reactions on surface phospholipids of the aggregated platelets.

Platelets

Platelets, or thrombocytes, are not cells but are granular, disk-shaped nonnucleated cell fragments. They are the smallest of the bone marrow cellular elements and are vital to hemostasis and coagulation. Platelets are derived from a noncommitted pluripotential stem cell, which on demand and in the presence of a platelet-stimulating factor (thrombopoietin) differentiates into the committed stem cell pool to form the megakaryoblast. This cell, through a maturation sequence, becomes a giant megakaryocyte (see Fig. 15-1). Unlike the other cellular elements, megakaryocytes undergo *endomitosis*, whereby nuclear division occurs within the cell but the cell itself does not duplicate. The cell expands as increased DNA is synthesized. The cell cytoplasm eventually breaks up into individual platelets.

Platelets measure 1 to 4 μm in diameter and have a life span of approximately 10 days. Approximately one-third are in the spleen as a reserve pool, and the remainder are in the circulation, numbering between 150,000 and 400,000 per cubic millimeter. When Wright's stain is used on a peripheral smear, these cells appear light blue with red-purple granules. Adsorbed on the platelet membrane factors V, VIII, and IX, the contractile protein actomyosin, or thrombosthenin, and various other proteins and enzymes. The granules contain the potent vasoconstrictor serotonin, the aggregating factor adenosine diphosphate (ADP), fibrinogen, platelet factors 3 and 4 (heparin-neutralizing factor), and calcium as well as enzymes. All these factors are released and activated in response to injury.

Clotting factors

The clotting factors, with the exception of factors III (tissue thromboplastin) and IV (calcium ion), are plasma proteins. They circulate in the blood as inactive molecules. Table 18-1 identifies the coagulation factors, using the internationally accepted and standardized Roman numerals, gives their synonyms, and summarizes their functions. Prekallikrein and high-molecular-weight kininogen (HMWK), along with factors XII and XI, are called *contact factors*. They are activated at the time of injury by contact with tissue surfaces. They also play a role in the dissolution of clots once they are formed.

Activation of the coagulation factors is believed to occur as an enzyme splits off a fragment of an inactive predecessor form, for this reason called a *procoagulant*. Each activated factor, except for V, VIII, XIII, and I (fibrinogen), is a protein-cleaving enzyme (serine protease), which thus activates the succeeding procoagulant.

TABLE 18-1

PLASMA CLOTTING FACTORS

I	Fibrinogen: Precursor of fibrin (polymerized protein)
II	Prothrombin: Precursor of the proteolytic enzyme thrombin and perhaps other accelerators of prothrombin conversion
III	Thromboplastin: A tissue lipoprotein activator of prothrombin
IV	Calcium: Necessary for prothrombin activation and fibrin formation
V	Plasma accelerator globulin: A plasma factor which accelerates the conversion of prothrombin to thrombin
VII	Serum prothrombin conversion accelerator: A serum factor that accelerates prothrombin conversion
VIII	Antihemophilic globulin (AHG): A plasma factor associated with platelet factor III and Christmas factor (IX); activates prothrombin
IX	Christmas factor: Serum factor associated with platelet factor III and VIII$_{AHG}$; activates prothrombin
X	Stuart-Prower factor: A plasma and serum factor; accelerator of prothrombin conversion
XI	Plasma thromboplastin antecedent (PTA): A plasma factor that is activated by Hageman factor (XII); accelerator of thrombin formation
XII	Hageman factor: A plasma factor; activates PTA (XI)
XIII	Fibrin stabilizing factor: Plasma factor; produces stronger fibrin clot that is insoluble in urea
—	Fletcher factor (prekallikrein): Contact-activating factor
—	Fitzgerald factor (high-molecular-weight kininogen): Contact-activating factor

The liver is the site of synthesis of all the coagulation factors except factor VIII and possibly XI and XIII. Vitamin K is essential for the maintenance of normal blood levels or synthesis of the prothrombin factors (II, VII, IX, and X). The available evidence suggests that factor VIII is really a complex molecule of three distinct subunits: (1) the procoagulant part, which contains the antihemophilic factor, VIII_{AHG}, absent in patients with classic hemophilia; (2) another subunit containing an antigenic site; and (3) the von Willebrand factor, VIII_{VWF}, necessary for platelet adhesion to vascular walls (Erslev and Gabuzda, 1979).

Phases of coagulation

Coagulation is initiated in homeostatic states by vascular injury. Vasoconstriction is an immediate response to the injury, followed by adhesion of platelets to collagen in the vessel wall exposed by the injury. Adenosine diphospate (ADP) is released by the platelets, causing them to aggregate. Minute amounts of thrombin (created as described below) also stimulate platelet aggregation, serving to amplify the reaction. Platelet factor III, from platelet membranes, also accelerates plasma clotting. In this way, a platelet plug forms, soon to be strengthened by the filamentous protein known as *fibrin.*

Fibrin production begins with conversion of factor X to Xa, as the activated form of a factor is designated. Factor X can be activated by means of two reaction sequences (Fig. 18-1). One requires tissue factor, or tissue thromboplastin, which is released by the vascular en-

dothelium at the time of injury. As tissue factor is not in the blood, it is an extrinsic element in coagulation, hence the name *extrinsic pathway* for this sequence.

The other sequence leading to activated factor X is the *intrinsic pathway*, given that name because it employs factors found within the vascular system of plasma. In this sequence, there is a "cascade" of reactions, one procoagulant's activation leading to activation of a successor form. The intrinsic pathway is initiated by plasma exposed to skin or collagen within a damaged vessel. Tissue factor is not required, but platelets adhering to the collagen again play a part. As Fig. 18-1 shows, factors XII, XI, and IX must be activated in succession, and factor VIII must be involved before factor X can be activated. The substances prekallikrein and high-molecular-weight kininogen are participants as well, and calcium ion is needed.

From this point coagulation proceeds along what has been called the *common pathway*. As the illustration shows, activation of factor X takes place as a result of either extrinsic or intrinsic pathway reactions. Clini-

FIGURE 18-1

Activation of factor X by the steps in the extrinsic and intrinsic coagulation pathway [Modified from H. L. Nossel, "Bleeding," in K. Isselbacher et al. (eds.), *Harrison's Principles of Internal Medicine*, 9th ed., McGraw-Hill, New York, 1980, p. 276.)

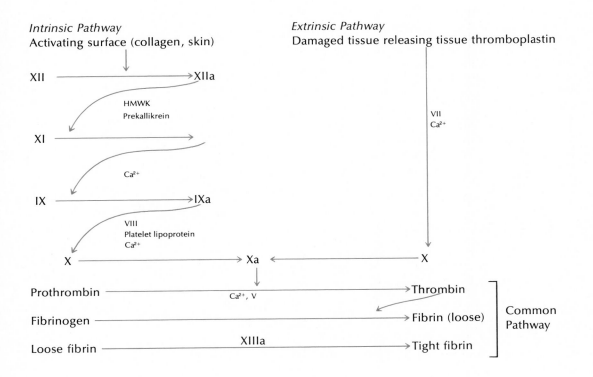

Intrinsic Pathway
Activating surface (collagen, skin)

Extrinsic Pathway
Damaged tissue releasing tissue thromboplastin

XII ⟶ XIIa

HMWK
Prekallikrein

XI ⟶

Ca²⁺

IX ⟶ IXa

VIII
Platelet lipoprotein
Ca²⁺

VII
Ca²⁺

X ⟶ Xa ⟵ X

Ca²⁺, V

Prothrombin ⟶ Thrombin

Fibrinogen ⟶ Fibrin (loose)

Loose fibrin ⟶ XIIIa ⟶ Tight fibrin

Common Pathway

cal experience suggests that both pathways participate in hemostasis (Nossel, 1980).

The next step toward fibrin production is taken when factor Xa, helped by phospholipids from activated platelets, splits prothrombin, creating thrombin. Thrombin in turn cleaves fibrinogen to form fibrin. (Small amounts of thrombin are apparently reserved to amplify platelet aggregation.) This fibrin, at first a soluble gel, is stabilized by factor XIIIa and polymerizes into a tight meshwork of fibrin, platelets, and entrapped blood cells. The fibrin strands then shorten (clot retraction), bringing together the edges of the wounded vessel wall and sealing the site.

Clot resolution

The *fibrinolytic system* refers to the sequence whereby fibrin is split by *plasmin* (also called *fibrinolysin*) into *fibrin degradation products*, leading to the dissolution of the clot. As seen diagrammatically in Fig. 18-2, several interactions are required to convert the specific inactive circulating plasma proteins into the active fibrinolytic enzyme plasmin. Circulating proteins known as *plasminogen proactivators*, in the presence of kinases (enzymes) such as streptokinase, staphylokinase and tissue kinase, as well as factor XIIa, are catalyzed to *plasminogen activators*. In the presence of additional enzymes such as urokinase, the activators convert plasminogen, a plasma protein that has been incorporated within the fibrin clot, into plasmin. Plasmin then splits fibrin and fibrinogen into fragments (fibrin-fibrin-

FIGURE 18-2
Fibrinolytic system. Antithrombin is a circulating protein that inactivates fibrin and helps to maintain blood in a fluid state.

ogen degradation products) which interfere with thrombin activity, platelet function, and fibrin polymerization, leading to the dissolution of the clot. The monocyte-macrophage and leukocyte systems also play a role in fibrinolysis through their phagocytic activities. Figure 18-3 is a graphic presentation of the sequence of events of the clotting process, as previously discussed.

Diagnostic approach

It is evident from the preceding discussion that abnormalities can occur at any stage of the hemostatic process. Evaluation then includes an in-depth history and physical and laboratory assessments. A carefully elicited history will often direct one toward the accurate diagnosis and required laboratory studies. This includes family history, coexisting medical problems, medication, exposure, prior bleeding episodes (e.g., "spontaneous" or related to surgery or tooth extractions), and the need for blood component therapy.

Careful scrutinizing of the skin and mucous membranes with attention to the type of lesions may suggest the abnormality present.

Telangiectasias are dilated capillaries and venules. They are 2- to 3-mm purple to red-purple macular spots which blanch with pressure and bleed with the slightest trauma. They are seen most commonly on the face, lips, mucous membranes, fingertips, and toes. Telangiectasias are seen as birthmarks or in a hereditary hemorrhagic disorder—Osler-Weber-Rendu disease. *Arterial spiders* are bright-red lesions with a pulsatile center and threadlike extensions radiating 5 to 10 mm in length. They are commonly seen in the face and trunk, above the waistline. These likewise blanch if pressed at their center and represent vascular anomalies, often seen in liver disease.

Petechiae are 1- to 4-mm flat, round, nonblanching, purplish hemorrhagic lesions, which may coalesce to form larger lesions called *purpura*. These are found in the mucous membranes and skin, especially in the de-

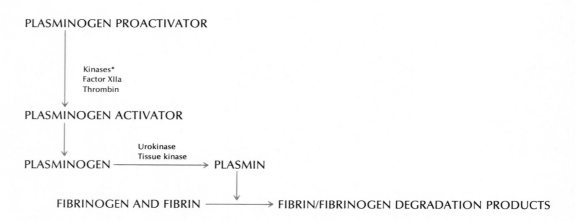

PLASMINOGEN PROACTIVATOR

Kinases*
Factor XIIa
Thrombin

PLASMINOGEN ACTIVATOR

Urokinase
Tissue kinase

PLASMINOGEN ⟶ PLASMIN

FIBRINOGEN AND FIBRIN ⟶ FIBRIN/FIBRINOGEN DEGRADATION PRODUCTS

*Includes: streptokinase, staphylokinase, tissue kinase

pendent or pressure areas. These generally reflect a platelet abnormality.

Ecchymoses, bruises or black-and-blue marks, are large macular areas of extravasated blood in the subcutaneous tissues and skin. Fresh bleeding is blue-black and fades to green-brown and yellow on resolution. While ecchymoses are commonly seen with trauma, extensive ecchymoses may reflect a platelet abnormality but are also seen in coagulation defects.

Laboratory evaluation

Laboratory evaluation will further differentiate and confirm the hemostatic defect. This should always include a peripheral blood smear and a platelet count as previously described. These studies provide morphologic platelet characteristics as well as numbers.

The *bleeding time* tests both vascular status and platelet number and function, but it does not differentiate between the two. A controlled puncture incision is made in the free-hanging earlobe (Duke method) or on the volar surface of the forearm (Ivy method). The length of time for bleeding to cease is recorded. Normal bleeding time is 3 to 7 minutes. Prolongation, such as 10 minutes, may be indicative of thrombocytopenia (platelet count of less than 100,000 per cubic millimeter), thrombocytopathy (abnormal platelet function), or both. Aspirin ingestion can interfere with platelet function for 7 to 10 days and thus should be withheld prior to testing the bleeding time. While a battery of tests is available to evaluate the coagulation status, screening tests should include the *prothrombin time* (PT), measuring the extrinsic and common pathway, and the partial *thromboplastin time* (PTT), measuring the intrinsic and common pathway.

In tests of the prothrombin time an aliquot of the patient's citrated plasma is mixed with phospholipid and tissue thromboplastin. Because calcium has been removed, coagulation does not occur. Next calcium is added, and the time required for clot formation is recorded. Normal plasma requires 11 to 13 seconds to clot

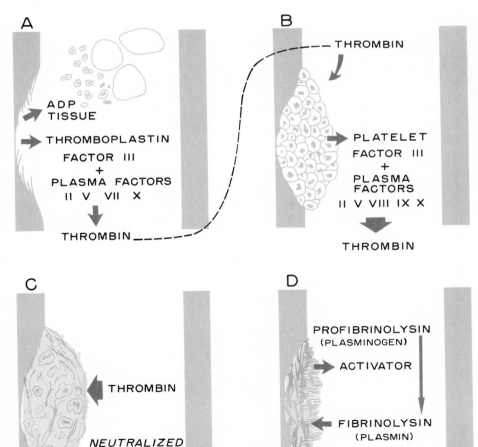

FIGURE 18-3
Sequence of events in the clotting process. [Modified from Hiss and Penner, "The Before and After of Blood Clotting," *Medical Clinics of North America*, 53 (6): Nov. 1969.]

under such conditions. Deficiencies of factors VII, X, and V, prothrombin, and fibrinogen will prolong the PT.

In tests of the PTT, phospholipid is added to the patient's citrated plasma, resulting in clot formation in 60 to 90 seconds. Adding a contact-activating agent such as kaolin reduces the variability of the study as well as the time required for clot formation. This modification gives an *activated partial thromboplastin time* (APTT). The results are compared with the APTT of normal plasma. The normal range is 26 to 42 seconds. As the PTT measures the intrinsic and common pathways, it is prolonged by deficiencies of prekallikrein, high-molecular-weight kininogen, factors XII, XI, IX, VIII, X, and V, prothrombin, and fibrinogen. If only the PT is prolonged, a deficiency or an inhibitor of factor VII can be assumed. If only the PTT is prolonged, a deficiency or an inhibitor of any intrinsic pathway factor can be assumed. With prolongation of both, a deficiency or inhibitor of the common pathway factors V and X, prothrombin, and fibrinogen can be assumed. Liver disease likewise can cause prolongation of both PT and PTT.

In tests of the *thrombin time* or thrombin clotting time (normal 10 to 13 seconds) exogenous thrombin is added to citrated plasma, and clotting time is measured. As this measures the time for transformation of fibrinogen to fibrin and detects abnormalities in fibrin polymerization or low fibrinogen level, it is used to further delineate the missing clotting factors when both PT and PTT are abnormal. Coagulation tests are depicted in Fig. 18-4 (see also Table 18-2). Heparin, a potent anticoagulant, enhances the neutralizing effects of antithrombin III on factors Xa, XIa, IXa, thrombin, and

plasmin and thus prolongs the PT, PTT, and thrombin time.

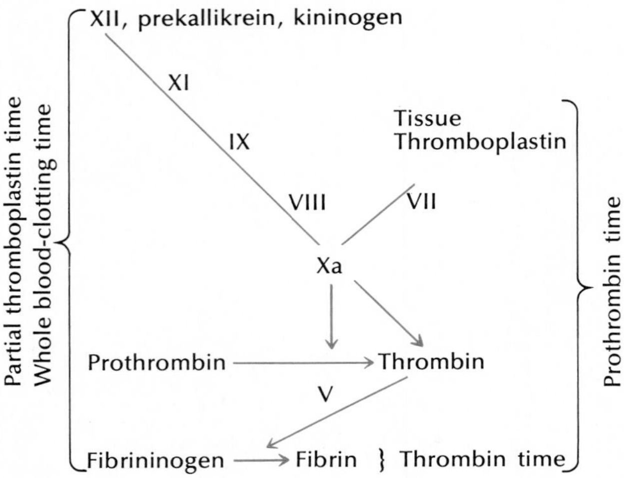

ABNORMALITIES OF HEMOSTASIS AND COAGULATION

Vascular defects

A wide variety of abnormalities can occur at any level of the hemostatic mechanism. Defects in the vascular system present with cutaneous hemorrhages, often involving the mucous membranes. They can be divided into the nonallergic and allergic purpuras. In both, platelet function and the coagulation factors are normal.

There are many forms of nonallergic purpura, that is, diseases where no true allergy is present but where various forms of vasculitis develop. The most common of these is seen in systemic lupus erythematosus. This is a collagen-vascular disease in which the patient develops autoantibodies (see Chap. 68). Vasculitis, or inflammation of vessels, occurs and destroys the integrity of the vessels, resulting in purpura.

Ineffective, deteriorating vascular supportive tissue, as seen with aging, results in *senile purpura*. Cutaneous hemorrhages are seen generally on the dorsum of the hands and forearms, aggravated by trauma. Except for the cosmetic annoyance, this is a nonthreatening condition. A similar cutaneous manifestation is seen with long-term corticosteroid therapy, believed to result from the protein catabolism in the vascular supportive tissue. Scurvy, related to malnutrition, and alcoholism likewise affect the integrity of the connective tissue of the vascular wall.

An autosomal dominant form of vascular purpura, *hereditary hemorrhagic telangiectasia* (Osler-Weber-Rendu disease), presents with profuse intermittent epistaxis and gastrointestinal bleeding. Diffuse telangiectasia is found in the buccal mucosa, tongue, nose, and lips, and probably extends throughout the gastrointestinal tract. It generally develops in adulthood. Treatment is mainly supportive.

The Ehlers-Danlos syndrome, another hereditary disease, involves decreased compliance of the perivascular tissues leading to severe hemorrhage.

The *allergic* or *anaphylactoid purpuras* are thought to result from immunologic damage to the vessels. They are characterized by petechial hemorrhages on dependent portions of the body and also involve the buttocks. Henoch-Schönlein purpura, a triad of purpura and mucosal bleeding, GI symptoms, and arthritis, is a form of allergic purpura affecting primarily children. The mech-

FIGURE 18-4
Coagulation tests. [From H. L. Nossel, "Bleeding," in I. Isselbacher et al. (eds.), *Harrison's Principles of Internal Medicine,* **9th ed., McGraw-Hill, New York, 1980, p. 277.]**

TABLE 18-2

COAGULATION STUDIES

Study	Purpose	Normal values	Clinical significance
Bleeding time	Measures platelet and vascular function	2–9½ minutes	Prolonged in thrombocytopenia, thrombocytopathy, von Willebrand's disease, aspirin ingestion, anticoagulant therapy, and uremia.
Platelet count	Assesses platelet concentration	150,000–400,000/mm³	Decreased in ITP and bone marrow malignancies; Drugs, especially chemotherapeutic agents, may cause prolonged bleeding Elevated in early myeloproliferative disorders; after splenectomy, may predispose to later thrombotic episodes
Clot reaction	Assesses platelet adequacy to form fibrin clot	Clot retracts to one-half size in 1 hour, firm clot in 24 hours if undisturbed	Poor clot retraction in thrombocytopenia and polycythemia; lysis of clot in fibrinolysis
Lee-White clotting time (coagulation)	Assesses coagulation mechanism—time required for solid clot on exposure to glass	6–12 minutes	Relatively insensitive test. Prolonged with severe deficiencies of coagulation factors, in excessive anticoagulant therapy, and with selected antibiotics. Decreased with corticosteroid therapy
Prothrombin time (PT)	Measures extrinsic and common coagulation pathway	11–16 seconds	Prolonged in deficiencies of factors VII and X and fibrinogen, excess dicumarol therapy, severe liver disease and DIC, and vitamin K deficiency
Activated partial thromboplastin time (APTT)	Measures intrinsic and common coagulation pathway	26–42 seconds	Prolonged in deficiencies of factors VIII to XII and fibrinogen, with circulating anticoagulant therapy, in liver disease and DIC, and in vitamin K deficiency. Shortened in malignancies (except liver)
Thrombin time (TT) or thrombin clotting time	Measures fibrinogen to fibrin formation	10–13 seconds	Prolonged with low fibrinogen levels, inhibitors, DIC and liver disease, anticoagulant therapy, and in dysproteinemias
Thromboplastin generation test (TGT)	Measures ability to form thromboplastin	12 seconds or less	Prolonged in thrombocytopenia, with deficiencies of factors VIII to XII, and with circulating anticoagulants
Capillary fragility test, tourniquet test, Rumpel-Leede test	Tests vascular fragility and platelet function	Occasional or no petechiae after 5 minutes of 70–90 mm pressure with blood pressure cuff	Increased petechiae with thrombocytopenia, thrombasthenia, and vasculitis
Platelet aggregation test	Tests platelet function	Platelets aggregate within a specified time when exposed to substances such as ADP, collagen, epinephrine	Decreased or absent aggregation in thrombasthenia, aspirin ingestion, myeloproliferative disorders, severe liver disease, dysproteinemias, von Willebrand's disease

anism of this disease is not well understood. Its symptoms are often preceded by an infectious state. Patients develop an inflammation of the vascular tree, at the capillary and venous levels, leading to vascular disruption, loss of red blood cells, and bleeding. Glomerulonephritis is a frequent complication. Treatment is supportive, with avoidance of aspirin and its compounds.

Thrombocytosis and thrombocytopenia

The platelets adhering to the exposed collagen of injured blood vessels, contracting and releasing ADP and platelet factor 3, are all very important in the initiation of the clotting system. Abnormalities in the numbers and/or functions of the platelets can interfere with blood coagulation. Too many or too few platelets can interfere with blood coagulation. The condition characterized by too many is known as *thrombocytosis* or *thrombocythemia*. *Thrombocytosis* is generally defined as an increase in the platelet counts above 400,000 per cubic millimeter and may be primary or secondary. Primary thrombocytosis is seen with the myeloproliferative disorders such as polycythemia vera or chronic granulocytic leukemia where there is an abnormal proliferation of the megakaryocytes, along with other cell lines, in the bone marrow. Platelet function is abnormal, which causes both bleeding and thrombosis. The bleeding time may be prolonged.

Treatment is aimed at reducing the bone marrow activity through the use of cytotoxic agents. In the presence of acute bleeding or thrombosis, plateletpheresis offers temporary relief. Antiplatelet agents such as aspirin have also been used.

Secondary thrombocytosis occurs as a consequence of other underlying causes. It may be seen temporarily after stress or exercise with storage pool release (from spleen) or may accompany increased bone marrow demand states as with hemorrhage or hemolytic anemia. An increased number of platelets is briefly seen in patients whose spleens are surgically removed. Since the spleen is the primary site of platelet storage and destruction, removal (splenectomy) without a concomitant decrease in bone marrow production will lead to thrombocytosis, often exceeding 1 million per cubic millimeter. Increased levels do not usually cause any problems until they exceed 1 million per cubic millimeter, at which point both bleeding and thrombosis can occur. The bleeding is usually mucosal, especially gastrointestinal. Thrombosis occurs mainly on the venous side but is also seen on the arterial side.

The mechanism by which the bleeding occurs is thought to be related to the increased numbers. When platelet concentration reaches this high level, sponta-

neous aggregates of platelets occur, blocking off tiny capillaries. In the process, the wall of the capillary is damaged, resulting in bleeding into the tissues. The bleeding time and other platelet function studies are generally within normal limits. Anticoagulants and antiplatelet agents have been used to avoid thrombotic episodes.

Thrombocytopenia is defined as a platelet count below 200,000 per cubic millimeter. This is due to either decreased production or increased destruction of platelets. Clinical manifestations, however, are generally absent until the count falls below 100,000 and are further influenced by other underlying or coexisting conditions such as leukemia or liver disease. Increased ecchymosis and prolonged bleeding with minor trauma are seen with levels under 50,000 per cubic millimeter. Petechiae are the major manifestation seen with platelet counts below 30,000. Mucosal, deep tissue, and intracranial bleeding are seen with counts under 20,000 and require immediate intervention to prevent exsanguination and death.

Decreased platelet production, verified by bone marrow aspiration and biopsy, is seen in any condition interfering with or inhibiting bone marrow function. This includes aplastic anemia (Chap. 16), myelofibrosis (replacement of bone marrow elements by fibrous tissue), acute leukemia (Chap. 17), and other metastatic carcinomas which replace the normal marrow elements. Deficiency states, as of vitamin B_{12} and folic acid, affect megakaryopoiesis with production of large hyperlobulated megakaryocytes. Chemotherapeutic agents (Chap. 17) are particularly toxic to the bone marrow, suppressing platelet production.

In the event of thrombocytopenia with normal platelet production, excessive destruction or sequestration is usually the cause. Any condition causing splenomegaly (markedly enlarged spleen) may be accompanied by thrombocytopenia. This includes such states as hepatic cirrhosis, lymphomas, and myeloproliferative diseases. The spleen normally holds one-third of the produced platelets, but with splenomegaly this pool may increase to 80 percent, decreasing the available circulating pool.

Platelets can also be destroyed by drug-induced antibody production as seen with quinidine and gold (Table 16-1) or by autoantibodies (antibodies acting against one's own tissues). These are seen in such disease states as lupus erythematosus, chronic lymphocytic leukemia, certain lymphomas, and idiopathic thrombocytopenic purpura (ITP). The last, seen primarily in young women, is manifested by severe life-threatening thrombocytopenia with platelet counts often below 10,000 per cubic millimeter. As described in Chap. 12, an IgG antibody is demonstrated on the platelet membrane, resulting in defective platelet aggregation and increased platelet removal and destruction by the macrophage system.

Platelet function can be altered (thrombocytopathy) in various ways, the result being prolonged bleeding. Drugs such as aspirin, indomethacin, and phenylbutazone inhibit platelet aggregation and release reaction, thus causing prolonged bleeding in spite of normal platelet numbers. The effects of a single dose of aspirin may last 7 to 10 days.

Plasma proteins as seen in macroglobulinemia and multiple myeloma coat platelets, interfering with platelet adhesion, clot retraction, and fibrin polymerization. In all these situations, correcting the underlying problem will reverse the abnormal platelet function.

INHERITED PLASMA FACTOR DISORDERS

Hemophilia

Hereditary hemorrhagic disorders can be present with a deficiency or a functional defect of any of the plasma coagulation factors except factor XII, prekallikrein, and high-molecular-weight kininogen. Absence of these three factors, while prolonging the PTT, does not cause clinical bleeding. The most common of the hereditary hemorrhagic disorders is hemophilia, an X-linked recessive disease. All the daughters of hemophiliac males become carriers. The son of a carrier female has a 50 percent chance of being a hemophiliac. Homozygous females with hemophilia (father a hemophiliac, mother a carrier) can be seen, but they are extremely rare.

Two clinically identical major types of hemophilia are (1) classic hemophilia or hemophilia A, in which antihemophilic factor VIII activity is deficient or absent, and (2) Christmas disease or hemophilia B, in which factor IX activity is deficient or absent. The degree of bleeding is related to the amount of factor activity and the severity of the injury. Spontaneous bleeding, hemarthrosis (joint bleeding), and deep tissue bleeding are seen with factor activity levels below 1 percent. However, with levels of 5 percent or more, bleeding is generally related to trauma or surgical procedures. It is usually first seen during circumcision.

Since factors VIII and IX are part of the intrinsic pathway, the PTT is prolonged while the PT, which bypasses the intrinsic pathway, is normal. Bleeding time, measuring platelet function, is normal, but delayed bleeding may occur because of inadequate fibrin stabilization. A prolonged bleeding time, in the presence of factor VIII deficiency, is indicative of von Willebrand's disease, an autosomal dominant trait occurring in males and females alike. In von Willebrand's disease, both factor VIII$_{VWF}$ and VIII$_{AHG}$ deficiency exist as well as a platelet adhesion defect.

Clinical manifestations are generally deep tissue bleeding and hemarthrosis, which are exacerbated by varying degrees of trauma. Retroperitoneal and intracranial bleeding are life-threatening.

Treatment is replacement of the deficient factor VIII or IX. In hemophilia A, cryoprecipitate containing 8 to 100 units of factor VIII per bag, or a commercially prepared concentrate, is infused. Since the half-life of factor VIII is 12 hours, the dosage must be administered at least at 12-hour intervals until bleeding ceases and the patient stabilizes. In factor IX deficiency, with a factor IX half-life of 24 hours, replacement therapy using plasma or factor IX concentrate (Konyne or Proplex) is given daily until bleeding ceases. Teaching patients and families safety measures and home infusion of concentrates at the earliest signs of bleeding has vastly improved the quality of life. Subsequently there is decreased morbidity and mortality and increased independence, as well as decreased medical costs. Hepatitis is a major risk, especially for patients with factor IX deficiency, and most adult hemophiliacs have serologic evidence of hepatitis.

Antibody inhibitors directed against the specific coagulation factor occur in 5 to 10 percent of patients with factor VIII deficiency and less often in factor IX. Subsequent infusions of the factor stimulate more antibody formation. Immunosuppressive agents, plasmapheresis to remove the inhibitor, and prothrombin complexes which bypass factors VIII and IX inhibitors are used to treat these patients. A new synthetic product, D.D.A.V.P. (1-deamino 8-D arginine vasopressin) is available for the treatment of mild to moderate hemophilia. Administered by intravenous (IV) infusion, it can induce a three- to sixfold increase in the factor VIII activity level. Since D.D.A.V.P. is a synthetic product, the risk of transmitting harmful viruses such as hepatitis or acquired immune deficiency syndrome (AIDS) is alleviated.

ACQUIRED PLASMA FACTOR DEFICIENCIES

Acquired plasma factor deficiencies may be related to decreased production of the coagulation factors, as seen in liver disease or vitamin K deficiency, or increased consumption accompanying disseminated intravascular coagulation (DIC) or fibrinolysis.

Since the liver is the major site of synthesis of factors II, V, VII, IX, and X, severe liver impairment (i.e., cirrhosis) will alter the hemostatic response. There is also a decreased hepatic clearing of the activated coagulation factors. In addition, there is an impaired vitamin K assimilation, which further impairs the synthesis of the K-dependent coagulation factors. Portal hypertension in liver disease results in congestive splenomegaly with thrombocytopenia, as well as esophageal varices. These conditions, together with coagulation defects, can lead to massive hemorrhage. The PT, PTT, and bleeding time are all prolonged.

Vitamin K, which is obtained from diet and bacterial synthesis, is required for the synthesis of factors II, VII, IX, and X. In cases of malnutrition, malabsorption, or gastrointestinal sterilization by antibiotics, vitamin K is markedly reduced with resultant decrease in the biological activity of the coagulation factors (Beck, 1977). Therapy for severe bleeding requires replacement of the coagulation factors with fresh frozen plasma (which supplies factors II, VII, IX, and X) parenteral vitamin K, and resolution of the underlying disease process.

Disseminated intravascular coagulation

Disseminated intravascular coagulation (DIC) is a multifaceted, complex syndrome in which a normally homeostatic and physiologic system of maintaining the fluidity of blood becomes a pathologic system leading to diffuse fibrin thrombi occluding the microvasculature of the body. The introduction of a procoagulant material or activity into the circulating blood initiates this syndrome. This can occur in any condition where tissue thromboplastin is liberated secondary to tissue destruction, with an initiation of the extrinsic clotting pathway. Because the placenta is a rich source of tissue thromboplastin, one of the most common causes of DIC is placental abruption (abruptio placentae, premature separation of the placenta). This condition causes retention of the conceptual products (placenta, fetus) leading to necrosis and further tissue damage. Tumor products, burns, crushing trauma, and promyelocyte leukemia all cause thromboplastin release. Initiation of the intrinsic pathway also occurs with the exposure of intrinsic procoagulants to damaged vascular endothelium as in vasculitis, sepsis, and shock. During the process of coagulation, platelets aggregate and, together with the coagulation factors, are utilized and depleted. The resultant fibrin thrombi may or may not occlude the microvasculature. Concomitantly, the fibrinolytic system is activated for the dissolution of the fibrin thrombi, which produces large numbers of fibrin and fibrinogen degradation products which interfere with fibrin polymerization and platelet function (Lewis, 1978; McKay, 1983).

The clinical manifestations depend on the extent and duration of the fibrin thrombi formation, the organs involved, and the resultant necrosis and hemorrhage. The organs most frequently involved include the kidney, brain, pituitary, lungs, and adrenals, and the mucosa of the gastrointestinal tract. Mucous membrane and deep-tissue bleeding, as well as bleeding around sites of injury, venipuncture, injection, and every orifice, are seen. Petechiae and ecchymosis are common. Other manifestations include hypotension (shock), oliguria or anuria, convulsions and coma, nausea and vomiting, diarrhea, abdominal pain, back pain, dyspnea, and cyanosis (McKay, 1983).

Diagnostic tests show an increase in the PT, PTT, TT, and level of fibrin split products. The fibrinogen level and platelet count are depressed. The peripheral blood smear may show erythrocyte fragmentation with a variety of bizarre shapes secondary to damage by fibrin strands.

Management is aimed at correcting the underlying mechanism. This may require use of antibiotics and chemotherapeutic agents, cardiovascular support, and, in the event of retained placenta, emptying the uterine contents. Replacement of plasma factors with plasma and cryoprecipitate, as well as platelet and red blood cell transfusions, may be necessary. In the presence of intense bleeding, the role of heparin, a potent antithrombin anticoagulant, is highly controversial. Heparin's role is to prevent tissue thromboplastin from activating the coagulation process and thus inhibit the consumption of the coagulation factors and fibrin deposition. The body is then able to produce enough of the various plasma factors to bring their concentration up to levels high enough to stop the hemorrhage. Low-dose heparin has been successfully used concomitantly with chemotherapeutic agents in the treatment of promyelocytic leukemia, preventing DIC secondary to thromboplastin release by the leukocytic granules.

Hypercoagulable states with an increased incidence of thrombosis also occur. These were discussed in Chap. 7 and will not be addressed here.

QUESTIONS

Coagulation

Directions: Answer the following questions on a separate sheet of paper.

1. Explain the maturation sequence of platelet cells when vascular injury occurs.

2. List in proper sequence the three ways that platelets contribute to blood coagulation.

3. What two plasma coagulation factors are shared by both the extrinsic and intrinsic systems?

4. State the mechanism that causes bleeding in primary and secondary thrombocytosis. Cite an example of each.

5. Describe the treatment goals for hemophiliacs.

6. Define disseminated intravascular coagulation (DIC).

Directions: Circle T if the statement is true and F if it is false. Correct the false statements.

7. T   F   Platelets are the primary source of immunoglobulins.

8. T   F   Treatment of hemophilia A patients is administration of immunosuppressive agents.

9. T   F   All the coagulation factors circulate in the blood as plasma proteins in a procoagulant form.

10. T   F   At the time of injury a deficiency of coagulation factor XI results in clinical bleeding.

11. T   F   Hemophilia is a sex-linked recessive genetic disorder.

12. T   F   The liver plays a vital role in the synthesis of certain plasma coagulation factors such as prothrombin and factors I, VII, X, and V.

13. T   F   The purpose of blood clotting is to stop bleeding at the site of injury.

14. T   F   Partial thromboplastin time (PTT) measures the extrinsic coagulation pathway.

Directions: Circle the letter preceding each item below that correctly answers the question. More than one answer may be correct.

15. Which of the following statements describes what occurs in blood clotting?
    a. Tissue thromboplastin is released at the site of vascular injury.   *b.* Platelets which have aggregated release factors stimulate the extrinsic system.   *c.* Fibrinolysis causes the release of factor III.   *d.* Prothrombin unites with fibrinogen to form fibrin.

16. The key initiating step in the extrinsic system is the release by tissue injury of a substance known as:
    a. Prothrombin   *b.* Thrombin   *c.* Tissue thromboplastin   *d.* Platelet factor

17. What is the normal range of bleeding time, in minutes?
    a. 2 to 4   *b.* 2 to 9½   *c.* 3 to 10   *d.* 4 to 8

18. What is the normal value for a platelet count, in platelets per cubic millimeter?
    a. 50,000 to 75,000   *b.* 100,000 to 150,000
    c. 125,000 to 300,000   *d.* 150,000 to 400,000

Directions: Match the normal range for clot formation or clotting time in column B with the appropriate screening test in column A.

Column A	Column B
19. ____ Prothrombin time (PT)	*a.* 10 to 13 seconds
20. ____ Thrombin time (TT)	*b.* 26 to 42 seconds
21. ____ Thromboplastin generation test (TGT)	*c.* 6 to 12 minutes
22. ____ Activated partial thromboplastin test (APTT)	*d.* 12 seconds or less
	e. 11 to 16 seconds

Directions: Circle the letter preceding each item below that correctly answers the question. More than one answer may be correct.

23. Thrombocytopenia may result from:
    a. Vitamin K deficiency   *b.* Disseminated intravascular coagulation (DIC)   *c.* Chronic liver disease   *d.* Antiplatelet antibodies

24. Thrombocytopenia may be considered severe and the risk of hemorrhage is great when the platelet count is below:
    a. 20,000 per cubic millimeter   *b.* 10,000 per cubic millimeter   *c.* 125,000 per cubic millimeter   *d.* 250,000 per cubic millimeter

25. A patient with classic hemophilia A has decreased activity of:
    a. Prothrombin   *b.* Factor VII   *c.* Christmas factor IX   *d.* Factor VIII

26. A hemophiliac person cannot initiate clotting at which of the following levels?
    a. Extrinsic   *b.* Intrinsic   *c.* Vascular   *d.* Platelet

27. In classic hemophilia A which laboratory findings would you expect?
    a. Normal prothrombin time (PT), abnormal partial thromboplastin time (PTT)   *b.* Abnormal PT, normal PTT   *c.* Abnormal PT, abnormal PTT

28. Mrs. A., a 23-year-old primipara, was admitted to the hospital as an obstetrical emergency with an abruptio placentae. She has been hemorrhaging profusely. Which of the following conditions would you suspect?
    a. Secondary thrombocytosis   *b.* Thrombocytopenia   *c.* Osler-Weber-Rendu disease   *d.* Disseminated intravascular coagulation (DIC)

29. An anticoagulant was ordered for Mrs. A. This treatment is expected to:

a. Release tissue thromboplastin to prevent the production of thrombin   *b.* Block tissue thromboplastin from activating the coagulation process   *c.* Inactivate the intrinsic system   *d.* Prohibit the consumption of the coagulation factors and fibrin so that the production of plasma factors is increased.

REFERENCES FOR PART III

ADAMSON, J. W.: "Polycythemia Vera," in R. J. Petersdorf et al. (eds.), *Harrison's Principles of Internal Medicine,* 10th ed., McGraw-Hill, New York, 1983, pp. 1917–1919.

BAKEMEIER, R. F., R. A. COOPER, JR., and P. RUBIN: "The Malignant Lymphomas, Multiple Myeloma, and Macroglobulinemia," in P. Rubin (ed.), *Clinical Oncology,* 5th ed., American Cancer Society, Rochester, N.Y., 1978.

BARR, R. D. and P. SEYMORE: "Hemotologic Effects of Antineoplastic Therapy," in J. F. Holland and E. Frei III (eds.), *Cancer Medicine,* 2d ed., Lea-Febiger, Philadelphia, 1982, pp. 1288–1289.

BECK, W. S.: "The Megaloblastic Anemias," in W. J. Williams et al. (eds.), *Hematology,* 3d ed., McGraw-Hill, New York, 1983, pp. 434–465.

————: (ed.): *Hematology,* 2d ed., M.I.T., Cambridge, Mass., 1977.

BERGSAGEL, D. E.: "Plasma Cell Myeloma and Macroglobulinemia," in W. J. Williams et al. (eds.), *Hematology,* 2d ed., McGraw-Hill, New York, 1977, pp. 1099–1131.

BEUTLER, E.: "Genetic Principles," in W. J. Williams et al. (eds.), *Hematology,* 3d ed., McGraw-Hill, New York, 1983, pp. 111–116.

————: "Hemolytic Anemia Due to Infections with Microorganisms," in W. J. Williams et al. (eds.), *Hematology,* 3d ed., McGraw-Hill, New York, 1983, pp. 628–629.

————: "The Sickle Cell Diseases and Related Disorders" in W. J. Williams et al. (eds.), *Hematology,* 3d ed., McGraw-Hill, New York, 1983, pp. 583–609.

BROBECK, J. R. (ed.): *Best and Taylor's Physiological Basis of Medical Practice,* 10th ed., Williams & Wilkins, Baltimore, 1979, pp. 3–115.

BUNN, H. F.: "Disorders of Hemoglobin Structure, Function and Synthesis," in R. G. Petersdorf (ed.), *Harrison's Principles of Internal Medicine,* 10th ed., McGraw-Hill, New York, 1983, pp. 1875–1885.

————: "Pallor and Anemia," in K. J. Isselbacher et al. (eds.): *Harrison's Principles of Internal Medicine,* 9th ed., McGraw-Hill, New York, 1980, pp. 262–272.

BURNS, N.: "Cancer Chemotherapy: A Systematic Approach," *Nursing, '78,* 8(2): 56–63, February 1978.

CANNELLOS, G. P. (ed.): "Lymphomas," *Clinics in Hematology,* 8(3), October 1979.

CARTER, S. K., et al.: *Chemotherapy of Cancer,* 2d ed., Wiley, New York, 1981.

CHART, I. S. and J. H. SANDERSON: "General Aspects of the Blood Coagulation System," *Pharmacology and Therapeutics,* 5(1–3): 229–233, 1979.

CLARKSON, B.: "The Acute Leukemias," in R. J. Petersdorf et al. (eds.): *Harrison's Principles of Internal Medicine,* 10th ed., McGraw-Hill, New York, 1983, pp. 798–808.

CLUFF, L. E., et al.: *Clinical Problems with Drugs,* vol. V, Saunders, Philadelphia, 1975.

CORASH, L.: "Disseminated Intravascular Coagulation," *Primary Care,* 7(3): 423–438, September 1980.

CRADDOCK, C. C., R. R. LONGMIRE, and R. MCMILLAN: "Cellular Kinetics of Lymphocytes and Plasma Cells," in W. J. Williams et al. (eds.), *Hematology,* 2d ed., McGraw-Hill, New York, 1977, pp. 902–936.

DABICH, L.: "Adult Acute Non-Lymphocytic Leukemias," *Medical Clinics of North America,* 64(4): 683–704, July 1980.

D'ERAMO, N. and M. LEVI: *Neurological Symptoms in Blood Diseases,* University Park Press, Baltimore, 1972.

DEGRUCHY, G. C.: in D. Pennington et al. (eds.), *Clinical Haematology in Medical Practice,* 4th ed., Blackwell Scientific Publications, London, 1978.

DIGGS, L. W., D. STRUM, and A. BELL: *The Morphology of Human Blood Cells,* 3d ed., Abbott Laboratories, Chicago, 1975.

ELLISON, R. R.: "Acute Myelocytic Leukemia," in J. F. Holland and E. Frei III (eds.), *Cancer Medicine,* 2d ed., Lea & Febiger, 1982, pp. 1407–1446.

ERSLEV, A., JR.: "Erythrocyte Disorders," in W. J. Williams et al. (eds.), *Hematology,* 2d ed., McGraw-Hill, New York, 1977, pp. 258–286.

———— and T. G. GABUZDA: "Pathophysiology of Hematologic Disorders," in W. Soderman, Jr., and W. Doseman, *Pathologic Physiology,* 6th ed., Saunders, Philadelphia, 1979.

FISCHBACH, F. A.: *Manual of Laboratory Diagnostic Tests,* Lippincott, Philadelphia, 1980.

FOSNOT, H. (ed.); "Sickle Cell Disease," *Patient Care,* 12(11): 164–216, June 15, 1978.

GALE, R. P.: "Advances in the Treatment of Acute Myelogenous Leukemias," *New England Journal of Medicine,* **300**(21): 1189–1197, May 24, 1979.

GOLDE, D. W.: "Neutrophil Kinetics, Production, Distribution and Fate of Neutrophils," in W. Williams et al. (eds.), *Hematology,* 3d ed., McGraw-Hill, New York, 1983, pp. 759–765.

GRALNICK, H. R., et al.: "Classification of Acute Leukemia," *Annals of Internal Medicine,* **87**(6): 740–753, December 1977.

GREEN, D.: "General Considerations of Coagulation Proteins," *Annals of Clinical and Laboratory Science,* **8**(2): 95–101, January–February 1978.

GREENSPAN, E. M. (ed.), *Clinical Interpretation and Practice of Cancer Chemotherapy,* Raven Press, New York, 1982.

GUYTON, A.: *Textbook of Medical Physiology,* 6th ed., Saunders, Philadelphia, 1981.

HARKER, L., A.: *Hemostasis Manual,* 2d ed., Davis, Philadelphia, 1979.

HART, J. D. (ed.); *French's Index of Differential Diagnosis,* 11th ed., John Wright and Sons, Chicago, 1979.

HEBBEL, R. P., et al.: "Erythrocyte Adherence to Endothelium in Sickle Cell Anemia," *New England Journal of Medicine,* **302**(18): 992–995, May 1, 1980.

HISS, R. G. and J. PENNER: "The Before and After of Blood Clotting," *Medical Clinics of North America,* **53**(6): 1309–1320, November 1969.

HOUGIE, C.: "Disorders of Hemostasis—Congenital Disorders of the Blood Coagulation Factors," in W. J. Williams et al. (eds.), *Hematology,* 3d ed., McGraw-Hill, New York, 1983, pp. 1389–1390.

JACOBS, A. and R. GALE: "Recent Advances in the Biology and Treatment of Acute Lymphoblastic Leukemia in Adults," *New England Journal of Medicine,* **311**(19): 1219–1230, November 8, 1984.

JENNINGS, B. M.: "Improving Your Management of D.I.C.," *Nursing '79,* 9(5); 60–67, May 1979.

JOSS, R. and I. H. KRAKOFF: "Cancer Chemotherapy: Park V—Natural Products—Vinca Alkaloids, Epipodophyllotoxins and Maytansine," *Hospital Formulary,* **15**(3) 194–203, March 1980.

KNOPF, M. K., et al.: *Cancer Chemotherapy, Treatment and Care,* Marion E. Morra (ed.), G. K. Hall Publishers, Boston, 1981.

KRAMER, M. S., et al.: "Pre-development in Sickle Cell Anemia," *Journal of Pediatrics,* **96**(5): 857–860, May 1980.

LAWLER, S. D.: "Significance of Chromosome Abnormalities in Leukemia," *Seminars in Hematology,* **19**(4): 257–272, October 1982.

LEWIS, J. H., et al.: *Bleeding Disorders,* Medical Examination Publishing Co., New York, 1978.

LICHTMAN, M. A. and M. R. KLEMPERER: "The Leukemias," in P. Rubin (ed.), *Clinical Oncology,* 5th ed., American Cancer Society, Rochester, New York, 1978.

LIEPMAN, M. K.: "The Chronic Leukemias," *Medical Clinics of North America,* **64**(4): 705–727, July 1980.

MARTIN, E. W.: *Hazards of Medication,* 2d ed., Lippincott, Philadelphia, 1978.

MCKAY, D. G.: "Clinical Significance of Intravascular Coagulation," *Bibliotheca Haematologica (Basel)* **49**: 63–78, 1983.

MEGLIOLA, B.: "Multiple Myeloma," *Cancer Nursing,* **3**(3): 209–218, June 1980.

MIALE, J. B.: *Laboratory Medicine—Hematology,* 6th ed., Mosby, St. Louis, 1982.

NATHWANI, B. N.: "A Critical Analysis of Classifications of Non-Hodgkin's Lymphomas," *Cancer,* **44**(2): 347–384, August 1979.

NEAME, P. B.: "Disseminated Intravascular Coagulation," in R. E. Rakel (ed.), *Conn's Current Therapy,* Saunders, Philadelphia, 1984, pp. 273–275.

NELSON, D. A. and J. B. HENRY (eds.): "Hematology and Coagulation," in Todd, Sanford, and Davidsohn, *Clinical Diagnosis by Laboratory Methods,* 16th ed., vol. 1, Saunders, Philadelphia, 1979.

NOSSEL, H. L.: "Bleeding," in K. J. Isselbacher et al. (eds.), *Harrison's Principles of Internal Medicine,* 9th ed., McGraw-Hill, New York, 1980, pp. 272–279.

PANEL OF HEMATOLOGY: *Registry on Adverse Reactions—Council on Drugs,* Charles M. Huguley, Chairman, American Medical Association, 1965–1967.

PARKS, E. D. and F. V. CHISARI, "Cellular Kinetics of Lymphocytes and Plasma Cells," in W. J. Williams (ed.), *Hematology,* 3d ed., McGraw-Hill, New York, 1983, pp. 923–933.

QUESENBERRY, P. J.: "The Concept of the Hematopoietic Stem Cell," in W. J. Williams et al. (eds.), *Hematology,* 3d ed., McGraw-Hill, New York, 1983, pp. 129–139.

RAPPAPORT, J. M. and H. F. BUNN: "Bone Marrow Failure: Aplastic Anemia and Other Disorders of the Bone Marrow," in K. J. Isselbacher et al. (eds.), *Harrison's Principles of Internal Medicine,* 9th ed., McGraw-Hill, New York, 1980, pp. 1525–1530.

ROBINSON, S. H.: "Degradation of Hemoglobin," in W. J Williams et al. (eds.), *Hematology,* 3d ed., McGraw-Hill, New York, 1983, pp. 388–395.

ROSENBERG, S. A.: "Oncology," in E. Rubenstein and D. D. Federman (eds.), *Scientific American Medicine,* Scientific American, New York, 1979–1980.

SAIDI, P.: "Diagnosis and Management of Bleeding Disorders," *American Family Physician,* **21**(1): 146–151, January 1980.

SCHRIER, S. L.: "Hematology," in E. Rubenstein and D. D. Federman (eds.), *Scientific American Medicine*, Scientific American, New York, 1979–1980.

SCHUMANN, D. and P. PATTERSON: "Multiple Myeloma," *American Journal of Nursing*, 75(1): 78–81, January 1975.

SPIVAK, J. L. (ed.), *Fundamentals of Clinical Hematology*, 2d ed., Harper & Row, Philadelphia, 1984.

SWEET, D. L. and H. M. GOLOMB: "The Non-Hodgkin's Lymphomas," *Current Problems in Cancer*, vol. IV, no. 7, Year Book, Chicago, January 1980.

ULTMANN, J. E. and V. T. DEVITA, JR.: "Hodgkin's Disease and Other Lymphomas," in K. J. Isselbacher et al. (eds.): *Harrison's Principles of Internal Medicine*, 9th ed., McGraw-Hill, New York, 1980, pp. 1633–1647.

———— and R. S. STEIN: *Non-Hodgkin's Lymphomas Monograph*, Bristol Laboratories, Chicago, 1980.

WALLACH, J.: *Interpretation of Diagnostic Test*, 3d ed., Little, Brown, Boston, 1978.

WESSLER, R.: "Care of the Hospitalized Adult Patient with Leukemia," *Nursing Clinics of North America*, 17(4): 649–663, December 1982.

WIDMANN, F. K.: *Clinical Interpretation of Laboratory Tests*, 8th ed., Davis, Philadelphia, 1979.

YATES, J. W.: "Cancer Chemotherapy Part II—Anthracycline Antibiotics—Adriamycin and Daunorubicin," *Hospital Formulary*, 14(11): 987–993, November 1979.

————: "Cancer Chemotherapy Part VII—Cytosine Arabinsoide," *Hospital Formulary*, 15(5): 398–403, May 1980.

PART IV

DANIEL J. FALL

GASTROINTESTINAL DISORDERS

Gastrointestinal disorders make up a large proportion of the illnesses which cause patients to seek medical help and are the leading cause of hospitalization in the United States. Although gastrointestinal disorders are not the direct cause of death as frequently as are cardiovascular disorders, they are among the top five causes. Cancer of the gastrointestinal tract accounts for nearly one-third of all the deaths resulting from cancer. Hepatic failure also accounts for a substantial number of deaths. Treatment for liver failure has not advanced as rapidly as treatment for renal failure; science and technology have not advanced sufficiently to allow the liver to be transplanted successfully nor to simulate its complex vital functions with an "artificial liver machine."

The gastrointestinal tract is especially vulnerable to transient disorders which produce violent symptoms but which subside within a short period of time and leave no ill effects. This feature is undoubtedly caused by the ingestion of food and drink contaminated with bacteria or various chemical substances.

This unit follows the conventional approach of gastroenterology by an anatomic classificaiton of disease. Progressing down the alimentary canal, the discussion begins with the esophagus and ends with anorectal disease. The accessory digestive organs are discussed separately.

OBJECTIVES

At the completion of this part you should be able to:

1. Describe the relationship between normal gastrointestinal anatomy and physiology and the alterations produced by disease.
2. Develop an understanding of the etiology, pathogenesis, and treatment of the various gastrointestinal diseases or disorders.

CHAPTER 9

THE ESOPHAGUS

OBJECTIVES

At the completion of this chapter you should be able to:

1. Describe the gross structure and anatomic relationships of the esophagus (including the upper and lower esophageal sphincters).

2. State the function of the esophagus.

3. Describe the structure and function of the esophageal mucosa and explain why it is vulnerable to gastric contents.

4. Describe the extrinsic and intrinsic innervation of the esophagus.

5. Explain the relationship of esophageal varices to portal hypertension.

6. Describe the transportation of a bolus of food from the mouth to the stomach (phases of swallowing, sphincter actions, primary and secondary peristaltic waves, pressure changes, and rate of transport).

7. Define dysphagia, globus hystericus, pyrosis, odynophagia, and regurgitation.

8. Describe the following diagnostic procedures and identify their value in the detection of esophageal disease: barium x-ray, endoscopy, cytology, biopsy, manometry, and acid reflux tests.

9. Contrast and compare the following esophageal motility disorders: achalasia, diffuse esophageal spasm, and scleroderma (prevalence, pathology, etiology, x-ray appearance, motility patterns, complications, common symptoms, and medical and surgical treatment).

10. Describe the effect of cholinergic drugs on the esophagus in achalasia.

11. Define tertiary peristalsis.

12. Explain why it may be difficult to differentiate between angina pectoris and diffuse esophageal spasm on the basis of symptoms.

13. Discuss the etiology, pathology, complications, and treatment of acute and chronic esophagitis.

14. Explain why chronic reflux esophagitis may be difficult to detect.

15. Illustrate the three mechanisms which operate to prevent gastric reflux.

16. Differentiate between a sliding and a rolling hiatus hernia (anatomic characteristics, complications, indications for surgery, and medical therapy).

17. Describe cancer of the esophagus (peak age, frequency, sex prevalence, symptoms, prognosis, treatment).

NORMAL ANATOMY AND PHYSIOLOGY

The esophagus is a hollow cylindrical organ about 25 cm long and 2 cm in diameter and extends from the hypopharynx to the cardiac portion of the stomach. It lies posterior to the heart and trachea, anterior to the vertebrae, and passes through a hiatus in the diaphragm just anterior to the aorta. The esophagus functions primarily to transport ingested material from the pharynx to the stomach.

Each end of the esophagus is guarded by a sphincter. The cricopharyngeus forms the upper esophageal sphincter and consists of skeletal muscle fibers. It is normally in a tonic or contracted state except during swallowing. The lower esophageal sphincter, though not anatomically distinct, behaves as a sphincter and serves as a barrier to reflux of stomach contents into the esophagus. It is normally closed except when food passes into the stomach or during belching or vomiting (see Fig. 19-1).

The wall of the esophagus consists of four layers. The inner mucosal layer is made up of stratified squamous epithelium which is continuous with the pharynx at the upper end and undergoes a sharp transition at the esophagogastric junction (z-line) to form the simple columnar epithelium of the stomach. The esophageal mucosa is normally alkaline and is not able to tolerate the highly acid contents of the stomach. The submucosal layer contains secretory cells which produce mucus. The mucus facilitates the passage of food during swallowing and protects the mucosa from chemical injury. The muscle layer is arranged in outer longitudinal and inner circular layers. The muscles of the upper one-third of the esophagus are striated, while those of the lower one-third are smooth. A transitional zone exists in the middle one-third and contains both striated and smooth muscle. The outer layer of the esophagus, unlike that of the remainder of the gastrointestinal (GI) tract, is composed not of serosa but of thickened fibrous tissue.

The major innervation of the esophagus is supplied by the sympathetic and parasympathetic fibers of the autonomic nervous system. The parasympathetic fibers are carried by the vagus nerve, which is considered to be the motor nerve of the esophagus. The function of the sympathetic fibers is poorly understood. In addition to the above extrinsic innervation, an intrinsic intra- mural meshwork of nerve fibers (Auerbach's plexus) exists between the circular and longitudinal muscle layers, and it appears to be involved in coordinating normal esophageal peristalsis.

Blood distribution to the esophagus follows a segmental plan. The upper portion is supplied by branches from the inferior thyroid and subclavian arteries. The midportion is supplied by segmental branches from the aorta and from bronchial arteries, while the subdiaphragmatic portion is supplied by the left gastric and inferior phrenic arteries.

Venous drainage also follows a segmental pattern. The cervical esophageal veins drain into the azygos and hemiazygos veins, and below the diaphragm the esophageal veins enter the left gastric vein. Communication between the portal and systemic veins allows for bypass of the liver in cases of portal hypertension. Collateral flow through the esophageal veins causes the formation of esophageal varices (varicose veins of the esophagus). These enlarged veins may rupture, causing hemorrhage which may be fatal. This complication is frequent in cir-

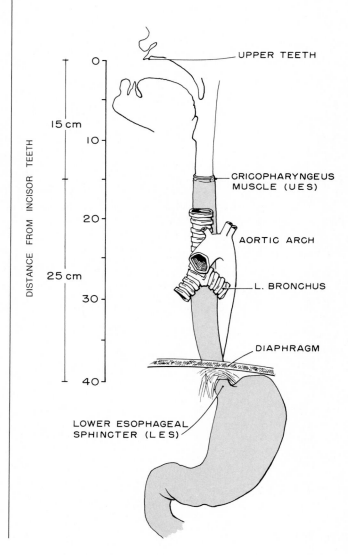

FIGURE 19-1
Gross structure and anatomic relationships of the esophagus.

rhosis of the liver and will be discussed in detail in Chap. 23.

Swallowing

Swallowing is a complex physiologic act whereby food or liquid passes from the mouth to the stomach. It is a highly coordinated muscular sequence which is initiated by a voluntary movement of the tongue and is completed by a series of reflexes in the pharynx and esophagus. The afferent side of this reflex arc involves fibers in the Vth, IXth, and Xth cranial nerves. A swallowing or deglutition center is present in the medulla. Under the coordination of this center, impulses pass outward in a flawlessly timed sequence via the Vth, Xth, and XIIth cranial nerves to the muscles of the tongue, pharynx, larynx, and esophagus.

Although swallowing is a continuous process, it occurs in three phases—oral, pharyngeal, and esophageal. In normal swallowing, a mouthful of chewed food, called a *bolus*, is thrown backward against the posterior wall of the pharynx by a voluntary movement of the tongue. The impact of the bolus against the pharynx is the stimulus that sets off the reflex movements of swallowing.

During the pharyngeal phase, the soft palate and uvula move reflexly to close off the nasal cavity; at the same time the larynx is elevated and closed off from the pharynx. Respirations are simultaneously inhibited to decrease the possibility of aspiration. In fact, it is almost impossible voluntarily to inhale and swallow at the same time.

The esophageal phase begins as the cricopharyngeus muscle relaxes briefly and allows the bolus to enter the esophagus. Following this brief relaxation, a *primary peristaltic wave*, beginning in the pharynx, is transmitted to the cricopharyngeus, causing it to contract. The peristaltic wave continues throughout the body of the esophagus, propelling the bolus to the lower esophageal sphincter, which relaxes briefly to allow entry into the stomach. The primary peristaltic wave moves at the rate of 2 to 4 cm/second, so that swallowed food reaches the stomach within 5 to 15 seconds. Beginning at the level of the aortic arch, a *secondary peristaltic wave* occurs if the primary wave fails to empty the esophagus. It is triggered by distention of the esophagus from remaining food particles. The primary peristaltic wave is essential for conveying food and liquids through the upper esophagus but is less important in the lower esophagus. The upright posture and the force of gravity are important factors in facilitating lower esophageal transport, but peristalsis makes it possible to drink water while standing on one's head.

During swallowing there are pressure changes within the esophagus which reflect the motor function of the esophagus. In the resting state pressure in the body of the esophagus is slightly below atmospheric

pressure, reflecting intrathoracic pressure. In the regions of the upper and lower esophageal sphincters, areas of high pressure exist. These high-pressure zones function to prevent aspiration and reflux of the gastric contents. The pressure decreases when each sphincter area relaxes during swallowing and then increases when the peristaltic wave passes through.

It is evident that the complex series of movements that together make up the act of swallowing may be upset by a number of pathologic processes. These processes involve interference either with transport or with the prevention of gastric reflux.

SYMPTOMS OF ESOPHAGEAL DISORDERS

Dysphagia, or the subjective awareness of an impairment in the active transport of ingested material from the pharynx, is a major symptom of disease of the pharynx or esophagus. Dysphagia should not be confused with *globus hystericus* (the feeling of a "lump in the throat"), which may be emotional in origin and present without swallowing.

Dysphagia occurs in nonesophageal disorders which result from muscular or neurologic disease. These diseases include cerebral vascular accidents, myasthenia gravis, muscular dystrophy, and bulbar polio.

Esophageal dysphagia may be of obstructive or motor origin. Obstructive causes include esophageal stricture and tumors extrinsic or intrinsic to the esophagus, resulting in narrowing of the lumen. Motor causes of dysphagia may result from diminished, absent, or disordered peristalsis or dysfunction of the upper or lower esophageal sphincters. Common motor disorders which produce dysphagia are achalasia, scleroderma, and diffuse esophageal spasm.

Pyrosis (heartburn) is another common symptom of esophageal disease. It is characterized by a hot, burning sensation usually felt high in the epigastrium or behind the xyphoid and radiates upward. Heartburn may be caused by reflux of gastric acid or bile secretions into the lower esophagus; both of these are very irritating to the mucosa. Persistent reflux is caused by incompetence of the lower esophageal sphincter and may occur with or without hiatus hernia or esophagitis. Heartburn is a common complaint during pregnancy.

Odynophagia is defined as pain induced by swallowing and may occur with dysphagia. It may be experienced as a sensation of tightness or as a burning pain, indistinguishable from heartburn, in the midchest. It may result from esophageal spasm induced by acute distention, or it may be secondary to inflammation of the esophageal mucosa.

Waterbrash refers to the regurgitation of gastric contents into the oral cavity. It differs from vomiting in that it is effortless and not accompanied by nausea. It is felt in the throat as a sour or bitter-tasting hot liquid. This effortless regurgitation is quite common in infants as a result of incomplete development of the lower esophageal sphincter. In adults, regurgitation reflects both lower esophageal sphincter incompetence and failure of the upper esophageal sphincter to serve as a regurgitation barrier.

INVESTIGATIONAL PROCEDURES

In addition to a careful history and physical examination, special diagnostic measures which are helpful in detecting esophageal disease are the barium x-ray, esophagoscopy with biopsy and possibly cytologic studies, manometric or motility studies, and acid reflux tests.

Barium x-ray

Radiologic examination of the esophagus as a routine is usually combined with that of the stomach and duodenum (upper GI tract x-ray series) using barium sulfate in a liquid or creamy suspension which is swallowed. The swallowing mechanism may be directly visualized by fluoroscopy, or the x-ray image may be recorded using motion picture techniques (cineradiography). When esophageal disease is suspected, the radiologist may place the patient in various positions to bring out in greater detail alterations in form and function. Tumors, polyps, diverticulitis, strictures, hiatus hernia, large esophageal varices, uncoordinated swallowing, and weak peristalsis may all be detected using this method.

Esophagoscopy

The direct inspection of the esophageal mucosa is an important procedure in the diagnosis of esophageal disorders. Flexible fiberoptic instruments have made this procedure much simpler and safer for the patient. Inflammation, ulcers, tumors, and esophageal varices may be visualized, photographed, and biopsied. Cell washings may be obtained for cytologic studies, which can be highly accurate in the diagnosis of eosophageal carcinoma.

Preparation for esophagoscopy includes 6 hours of fasting and various forms of premedication; among them the throat is sprayed with a local anesthetic. Endoscopic examinations of the esophagus, stomach, and duodenum are often combined in one examination.

Motility studies

Motor function of the esophagus may be studied by the use of pressure-sensitive catheters or miniature balloons placed in the stomach and then drawn back in increments. The measurement of pressure changes in the esophagus and stomach at rest and during swallowing have greatly increased understanding of esophageal activity both in health and in disease.

Figure 19-2A and B shows normal motility in a recording of the esophagus in the resting state and during swallowing. The function of the lower esophageal sphincter is of particular interest to the gastroenterologist. Normally there is a zone of high pressure (15 to 30 cm H_2O above that of the intragastric pressure) in this region; this prevents reflux of gastric contents into the esophagus. Reflux may occur if the sphincter fails to maintain a pressure above the intraabdominal pressure.

Acid reflux tests

The acid perfusion test (Bernstein test) is used to differentiate between chest pain which is cardiac in origin and pain resulting from esophageal spasm, since symptoms may be identical.

In the acid perfusion test, 0.1 N HCl is permitted to drip through a catheter at 6 to 15 ml/minute into the distal esophagus (the hydrochloric acid is of the same concentration as normal gastric acid). The patient has esophageal pain or heartburn if the test is positive. Rapid cessation of the pain after instillation of a neutral or alkaline solution confirms that the esophageal mucosa is the site of acid-induced pain. The most common finding in a positive test is reflux esophagitis, but any disease which causes a break in mucosal continuity could cause a positive test.

Other reflux tests include monitoring of the pH within the esophagus to detect reflux of acid contents from the stomach, fluoroscopic observation of the esophagus to detect reflux of barium from the stomach into the esophagus, and fluoroscopic observation of the esophagus during the ingestion of a mixture of hydrochloric acid and barium to detect momentary disorders in peristaltic activity. All the currently available tests for acid reflux have both false positives and false negatives; therefore, a combination of two or more of these studies is used for a diagnosis in difficult cases.

DISORDERS OF ESOPHAGEAL MOTILITY
Achalasia

Achalasia, formerly called cardiospasm, is an uncommon hypomotility disorder characterized by weak and uncoordinated peristalsis or aperistalsis within the body of the esophagus and by failure of the lower esophageal sphincter to completely relax during swallowing. Consequently, food and fluids accumulate in the lower esophagus and may then slowly empty as the hydrostatic pressure increases. The body of the esophagus loses its tone and may become greatly dilated (see Fig. 19-3).

The exact etiology of achalasia is unknown, but there is evidence that degeneration of Auerbach's plexus causes the loss of neurologic control. Chagas' disease of the esophagus, a disease largely confined to South America, is similar to achalasia and is caused by infection by a parasite (*Trypanosoma cruzi*) which destroys ganglion nerve cells. It is improbable, however,

FIGURE 19-2

(A) Esophageal manometric recordings. The pressure is recorded by three catheters spaced 5 cm apart. The catheters are pulled from the stomach into the esophagus. Note the zone of high resting pressure at the junction between stomach and esophagus (gastroesophageal sphincter of LES). (B) Normal swallowing. Swallowing produces a single contraction. At the same time, the sphincter zone relaxes. (C) Diffuse esophageal spasm. Repetitive nonprogressive contractions independent of water swallowing (w.s.) occur. (D) Scleroderma. The contractions produced by swallowing (s) are low in amplitude.

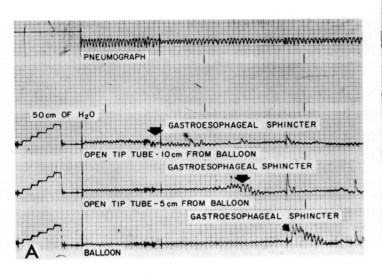

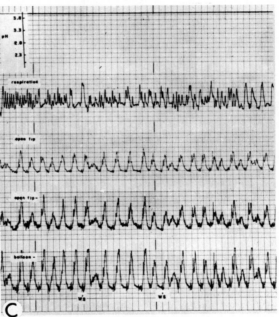

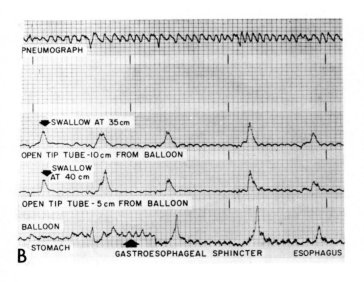

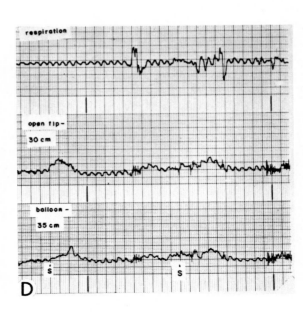

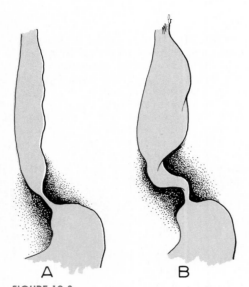

FIGURE 19-3
Esophageal achalasia. (A) Early stage, showing tapering of lower esophagus. (B) Advanced stage, showing dilatated, tortuous esophagus.

that Chagas' disease is responsible for the cases of achalasia seen in North America (Enterline and Thompson, 1984). As a result, primary peristaltic waves do not reach the lower esophageal sphincter to stimulate relaxation.

Achalasia is more common in adults than in children. The onset is usually insidious, and the most prominent symptom is dysphagia for both liquid and solid foods. Meals may be interrupted by the necessity to regurgitate. Nocturnal regurgitation may result in aspiration, resulting in chronic pulmonary infections or sudden death. The stasis of food in the esophagus may lead to inflammatory changes, erosions, and in some cases, cancer of the esophagus, although this is usually a late complication.

The diagnosis is made on the basis of the history and the characteristic appearance on x-ray. When barium is swallowed, the peristaltic wave is weak, and the collection of barium in the lower esophagus gives it a funnellike appearance. The administration of small doses of a cholinergic or parasympathomimetic drug causes marked contraction and emptying of the esophagus and confirms the diagnosis. Esophageal motility studies may be helpful in the early diagnosis of achalasia. Manometric measurements in these studies reveal that the lower esophageal sphincter fails to relax with swallowing. The resting pressure of the lower esophageal sphincter may be normal or slightly elevated.

Treatment of achalasia is palliative and consists of measures to relieve the obstruction of the lower esophagus. There is no known method of restoring normal peristalsis to the body of the esophagus. Two forms of therapy that effectively relieve symptoms are dilation of the lower esophageal sphincter and esophagomyotomy. Dilation may be achieved by passage of a mercury-filled tube called a *bougie* or, more commonly, by dilation with a pneumatic bag which is placed in the area of the lower esophageal sphincter and forcefully dilated. When dilation fails to relieve the symptoms, surgical intervention may be indicated.

The surgery most commonly performed for achalasia or esophageal stricture is the Heller myotomy, which consists of division of the muscle fibers of the gastrogesophageal junction. A pyloroplasty (enlargement of gastric outlet) frequently accompanies this procedure to allow rapid employing of stomach contents and prevent reflux into the esophagus (see Fig. 19-4).

Other helpful measures to minimize symptoms include slow eating and avoidance of alcohol and hot, cold, or spicy foods. Patients should be instructed to sleep with the head elevated to avoid aspiration.

Diffuse esophageal spasm

Diffuse esophageal spasm is a fairly common condition and is characterized by uncoordinated, nonpropulsive

FIGURE 19-4
Surgical treatment of esophageal achalasia. (A) Longitudinal incision for Heller esophagomyotomy (1) and pyloroplasty (2). (B) The esophageal incision is made through the muscle layers to allow pouching of the mucosa, thus relieving the esophageal obstruction. A gastric drainage procedure (pyloroplasty) frequently accompanies the esophagomyotomy to prevent esophageal reflux. The pyloric incision is sutered in the opposite direction to enlarge the gastric outlet.

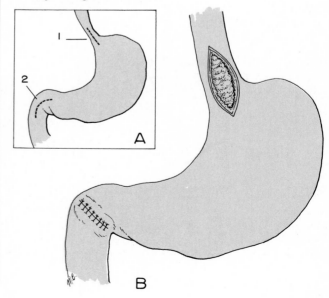

contractions (tertiary peristalsis) of the esophagus in response to swallowing. It is most prominent in the lower two-thirds of the organ but may involve the entire esophagus. The two sphincters operate normally. It is a disease of unknown cause and is seen more frequently in older patients. Similar motility disturbances may be secondary to reflux esophagitis or obstruction of the lower esophagus, as in carcinoma (usually, results of manometric studies in early carcinoma are normal).

Primary diffuse spasm of the esophagus usually occurs in patients over 50 years of age. Nonperistaltic responses to swallowing are common findings on barium x-ray and increase with aging. These x-ray findings are referred to as "corkscrew esophagus," "rosary bead esophagus," "curling," and a variety of other descriptive names which are usually of little clinical significance.

The pathogenetic basis for the diffuse spasm is poorly understood. It may represent a degeneration of local neurons, since some patients have a positive response to cholinergics as in achalasia.

Diffuse esophageal spasm is usually asymptomatic, but in a few cases the contractions may give rise to symptoms. The most common symptoms are those of intermittent dysphagia and odynophagia, which are aggravated by ingestion of cold foods and large boluses and by nervous tension. When there is intermittent chest pain, diffuse esophageal spasm may be confused with angina pectoris, especially if symptoms are not associated with eating. To add to this confusion, the pain caused by diffuse spasm is often relieved by nitroglycerin. Consequently, some patients with diffuse esophageal spasm have been misdiagnosed as having cardiac disease.

Motility studies reveal a hypermotile pattern of nonperistaltic contractions and aid in the diagnosis (see Fig. 19-2C).

Treatment consists of dietary manipulations (small meals and avoidance of cold foods), antacids, sedatives, and nitroglycerin to relieve the spasm. If symptoms are persistent and distressing, esophageal dilation may be recommended. As a last resort, a longitudinal myotomy of the distal esophagus may be performed.

Scleroderma

Esophageal motor dysfunction occurs in over two-thirds of patients with progressive systemic sclerosis (scleroderma). The basic abnormality in the GI tract is atrophy of the smooth muscle of the lower portion of the esophagus.

The diagnosis is suspected on barium swallow x-ray examination but is confirmed by manometric findings. Aperistalsis or weak peristalsis of the distal one-half to two-thirds of the esophagus and diminished pressure of the lower esophageal sphincter characterize the disease (see Fig. 19-2D).

Incompetence of the lower esophageal sphincter often leads to reflux esophagitis with subsequent stricture formation in the lower esophagus. Although gastroesophageal reflux and esophagitis are common, heartburn is not a common symptom. Dysphagia becomes a prominent symptom when esophagitis has led to stricture formation (see below).

ESOPHAGITIS

Inflammation of the esophageal mucosa may be acute or chronic and is seen in a variety of circumstances including the motility disorders just discussed. An innocuous type of esophagitis follows the ingestion of hot liquids. The substernal burning sensation is usually of short duration and may be associated with superficial edema and esophagospasm. The most common significant form of esophagitis is caused by acid reflux from the stomach, often in association with hiatus hernia. There are also infectious forms of esophagitis, including monilial esophagitis and, rarely, infections with herpes viruses.

An acute, severe form of esophagitis follows the ingestion of strong alkalis or acids. Strong alkalis are commonly found in most households in the form of drain cleaners which, if ingested, will produce a severe liquefying necrosis of the mucosa. Accidental ingestion of these substances occurs most commonly in small children, but occasionally, these substances are used in suicide attempts. Immediate symptoms include severe odynophagia, fever, toxicity, and possible esophageal perforation with consequent infection of the mediastinum and death. Long-term effects include scarring and esophageal stricture which requires periodic dilations, with bougies for the remainder of the patient's life. Treatment must be prompt and vigorous and includes the use of antibiotics, steroids, intravenous fluids, and possibly surgery.

Chronic reflux esophagitis and hiatus hernia

Chronic reflux esophagitis is the most common form of esophagitis encountered clinically. It is caused by incompetence of the lower esophageal sphincter and reflux of acid gastric or alkaline intestinal juice into the esophagus over a long period of time. The sequelae of reflux are inflammation, ulcer formation, bleeding, and scarring with stricture formation. Chronic reflux esophagitis is often associated with hiatus hernia. There is little correlation between the severity of symptoms and the degree of esophagitis. Some patients with heartburn have minimal evidence of esophagitis, while others with chronic reflux may be asymptomatic until there is stricture formation.

Mechanisms preventing reflux

Figure 19-5 illustrates the mechanisms which normally prevent reflux of gastric contents into the esophagus. The high-pressure zone at the gastroesophageal junction (or lower esophageal sphincter) is probably the most important mechanism for preventing reflux. The tone of this sphincter is affected not only by a variety of drugs but also by influences of hormones such as gastrin and secretin, which may play a very important role in maintaining the integrity of the sphincter. The acute angle between the esophagus and stomach may also be an important mechanism for preventing reflux, since this creates an arrangement like a flap valve which would prevent material from regurgitating. It has also been suggested that the short segment of the esophagus below the diaphragm is kept closed by the intraabdominal pressure. Displacement of this lower esophageal segment into the chest, as occurs in hiatus hernia, would eliminate this barrier to reflux and may well explain why there seems to be an association with reflux esophagitis.

Hiatus hernia

Hiatus hernia is defined as a herniation of a portion of the stomach into the chest through the esophageal hiatus of the diaphragm. There are two distinct types of

hiatus hernia (see Fig. 19-6). The most common form is the *direct* or *sliding hiatus hernia* in which the gastroesophageal junction slides into the thoracic cavity, especially when the patient assumes a supine position. The competency of the lower esophageal sphincter may be destroyed, resulting in reflux esophagitis. Often it is asymptomatic and is discovered only accidentally during a search for the cause of a variety of epigastric symptoms or on routine GI tract x-rays. In *paraesophageal* or *rolling hiatus hernia,* part of the gastric fundus rolls through the hiatus, and the gastroesophageal junction remains below the diaphragm. There is no insufficiency of the lower esophageal sphincter mechanism, and consequently reflux esophagitis does not occur. The major complication of paraesophageal hernia is strangulation.

Sliding and rolling hiatus hernias are diagnosed with x-ray or endoscopy. The important clinical question is whether or not there is esophageal reflux, since this has serious consequences, including esophagitis with ulceration and stricture, asthma, and aspiration penumonia. Continuous monitoring of esophageal pH with a miniaturized pH meter has been helpful in demonstrating reflux and correlating reflux with symptoms.

Treatment of sliding hiatus hernia is directed toward the prevention of reflux. The patient is instructed to eat small, frequent meals and take antacids. If overweight, the patient is instructed to reduce. Anticholinergic drugs should not be given because they cause a delay of gastric emptying and a relaxation of the lower esophageal sphincter. Metoclopramide, a derivative of procainamide, increases the tone of the lower esophageal sphincter and has usefulness in the treatment of selected cases of reflux. Nicotine, which decreases the tone, should be avoided. The patient should avoid activities which involve stooping forward, especially after meals. The head of the bed should generally be elevated

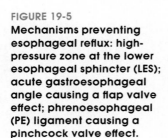

FIGURE 19-5

Mechanisms preventing esophageal reflux: high-pressure zone at the lower esophageal sphincter (LES); acute gastroesophageal angle causing a flap valve effect; phrenoesophageal (PE) ligament causing a pinchcock valve effect.

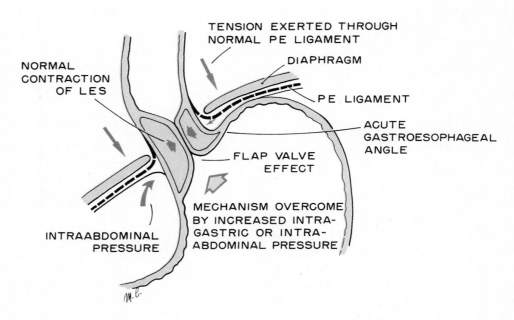

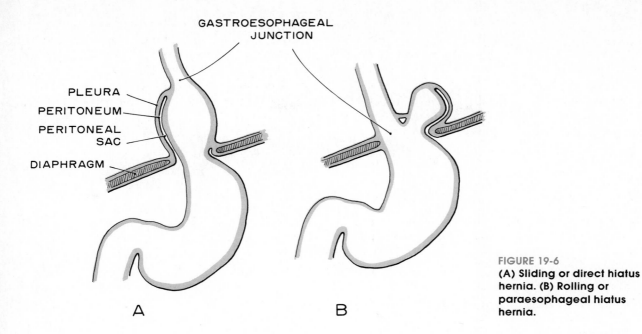

GASTROESOPHAGEAL JUNCTION

PLEURA
PERITONEUM
PERITONEAL SAC
DIAPHRAGM

A

B

FIGURE 19-6
(A) Sliding or direct hiatus hernia. (B) Rolling or paraesophageal hiatus hernia.

during sleep to prevent reflux. Surgical repair may be indicated if medical treatment fails and if there is evidence of persistent reflux esophagitis or stricture formation.

TUMORS

The most common benign tumor of the esophagus is a leiomyoma (smooth-muscle tumor), although it is rare. Leiomyomas may occasionally bleed but are usually of little clinical significance and are discovered incidentally.

Cancer of the esophagus, however, is not rare. It causes approximately 4 percent of all cancer deaths in the United States. Males between the ages of 50 and 70 years are affected most frequently. Predisposing factors include heavy smoking, alcohol abuse, and esophageal obstruction. Squamous cell carcinoma is the most common type of tumor, and it is highly malignant. Tumors can occur in any part of the esophagus, but the majority are in the lower two-thirds.

Barium x-ray, cytologic studies, and esophagoscopy with biopsy are all important in the diagnosis. The 5-year survival rate is less than 10 percent. The reason for the poor prognosis is the early lymphatic spread and the late development of symptoms. The first symptom is generally dysphagia, but this does not generally occur until the tumor involves the entire circumference of the esophagus.

Irradiation and surgical resection are the major forms of treatment. Lesions in the upper portion of the esophagus may be impossible to resect and are treated by irradiation. Bougies may be passed to dilate the lumen, or a plastic prosthesis may be inserted to enable the patient to continue eating. A newer form of palliation is the use of a laser beam to vaporize the core of the obstructing tumor to reestablish the lumen and allow passage of food.

QUESTIONS

The esophagus

Directions: Answer the following questions on a separate sheet of paper.

1. Describe the function of the esophagus.

2. Why is regurgitation more common in infants than in adults?

3. What are esophageal varices and why are they often associated with cirrhosis of the liver? Why is this condition important?

4. What is an esophagomyotomy? What is a pyloroplasty? Why are these two procedures often combined? What condition is commonly treated by esophagomyotomy and pyloroplasty?

5. What kind of instructions would you give to patients with the following conditions to minimize symptoms and prevent complications: diffuse esophageal spasm, scleroderma, sliding hiatus hernia?

6. Sketch the anatomic relations of the gastroesophageal junction and briefly describe the three mechanisms preventing reflux.

7. Describe the consequences of chronic esophageal reflux.

8. Why do patients with achalasia and sliding hiatus hernia often have chronic pulmonary infections?

9. Why is chronic reflux esophagitis sometimes difficult to identify? What test is used to assist in the diagnosis?

Directions: Circle the letter preceding each item that correctly answers the question. Only one answer is correct unless otherwise noted.

10. Which of the following statements concerning anatomy of the esophagus is false?
a. Passes through the esophageal hiatus of the diaphragm   b. Lies posterior to the heart
c. Length is about 25 cm   d. An anatomically distinct sphincter is present at the gastroesophageal junction

11. The muscle which functions as the upper esophageal sphincter is the:
a. Palatopharyngeus   b. Phrenoesophageal
c. Cricopharyngeus   d. Palatine

12. The lower esophageal sphincter is:
a. A well-differentiated zone of muscle   b. A zone of high pressure near the gastroesophageal junction   c. Normally located above the level of the diaphragm   d. A diaphragmatic muscle band externally compressing the esophagus

13. Which of the following types of epithelium is present throughout most of the length of the esophagus?
a. Simple columnar   b. Pseudostratified ciliated columnar   c. Stratified squamous

14. The extrinsic motor nerve which coordinates esophageal peristalsis is the:
a. Vagus   b. Auerbach's   c. Hypoglossal

15. The normal pH of esophageal secretions is:
a. Slight acid   b. Slight alkaline   c. Identical with the pH of gastric secretions

16. The terminal one-third of the tunica muscularis of the esophagus is composed of:
a. Smooth-muscle fibers   b. Skeletal muscle fibers   c. Both skeletal and smooth-muscle fibers

17. The second stage of swallowing is characterized by: (More than one answer is correct.)

a. Inhibition of respiration   b. Being under voluntary control   c. Closure of the vocal cords
d. Relaxation of the cricopharyngeus muscle

18. All the following cranial nerves are involved in the control of swallowing except:
a. III   b. V   c. IX   d. X   e. XII

19. Transportation of a bolus of food through the esophagus is a function of:
a. Primary peristaltic wave   b. Secondary peristaltic wave   c. Tertiary peristaltic wave
d. All the above

20. After being swallowed, food or liquids normally enter the stomach within:
a. 5 to 15 seconds   b. 30 to 40 seconds   c. 60 seconds   d. 2 minutes

21. Which of the following are required for the diagnosis of achalasia? (More than one answer is correct.)
a. Findings of weak, uncoordinated peristalsis on motility study   b. Rosary bead esophagus on barium x-ray   c. Positive response to cholinergics
d. Narrowed gastroesophageal junction

22. Achalasia is thought to be caused by:
a. Stress and nervous tension   b. Degeneration of Auerbach's plexus   c. Gastric reflux
d. Failure of the cricopharyngeus muscle to relax
e. Infection with a parasite (filaria)

23. Which of the following is the treatment of choice in achalasia?
a. Dilation with bougies (bougienage)   b. Pneumatic dilation   c. Heller esophagomyotomy
d. Anticholingeric drugs   e. Psychotherapy

24. Which of the following tests is most helpful in differentiating cardiac and esophageal pain?
a. Electrocardiogram   b. Relief of pain by nitroglycerin confirms cardiac origin of pain
c. Mecholyl test   d. 0.1 N HCl acid perfusion test

25. The portion of the esophagus primarily affected in scleroderma is the:
a. Body   b. Upper one-third   c. Lower esophageal sphincter   d. Upper esophageal sphincter

26. The most effective early treatment measures for an alkali burn of the esophagus include: (More than one answer is correct.)
a. Corticosteroid drugs   b. Immediate induction of vomiting   c. Broad-spectrum antibiotics
d. Immediate pneumatic dilation

27. Which of the following statements about hiatus hernia is true?
a. There are two distinct types   b. The paraesophageal type is the most common   c. All require surgery   d. All are associated with gastric reflux

28. Which of the following statements concerning sliding hiatus hernia is true?
a. Most frequent complication is strangulation
b. Presence of gastric reflux is principal indication for surgery   c. Should always be treated by surgery   d. Gastric fundus rolls through the hiatus, and gastroesophageal junction remains below the diaphragm

29. Which of the following statements concerning cancer of the esophagus are true? (More than one answer may be correct.)
a. Very rare form of cancer   b. More common in males   c. Associated with alcohol abuse and heavy smoking   d. More often located in the upper esophagus   e. Prognosis is generally good

Directions: Match each of the following symptoms in col. A with its proper definition or description in col. B.

Column A
30. ___ Dysphagia
31. ___ Regurgitation
32. ___ Odynophagia
33. ___ Pyrosis
34. ___ Globus hystericus

Column B
a. Hot, burning sensation usually felt high in the epigastrum
b. "Lump in the throat" present during the absence of swallowing
c. Subjective awareness of difficulty in swallowing
d. Pain in midchest induced by swallowing
e. Effortless welling-up of esophageal or gastric contents into the mouth

Directions: Match each of the following esophageal motor disorders in col. A with its common findings in motility studies in col. B.

Column A
35. ___ Diffuse esophageal spasm
36. ___ Achalasia
37. ___ Scleroderma

Column B
a. Loss of contractile power in lower distal portion of esophagus
b. Characterized by a hypermotile pattern of ineffective contractions
c. Absence of peristalsis in body of esophagus and incomplete relaxation of the lower esophageal sphincter
d. Characterized by resting pressures lower than normal at the lower esophageal sphincter
e. Characterized by resting pressure higher than normal at the lower esophageal sphincter

Directions: Circle T if the statement is true and F if it is false.

38. T F Nonperistaltic responses to swallowing increase with age.
39. T F Secondary peristalsis is important in removing food particles that remain in the esophagus after the primary peristaltic wave has passed.
40. T F The aid of gravity is essential to swallow liquids.
41. T F Cell washings for cytologic study is one of the most accurate ways to identify early cancer of the esophagus.
42. T F Endoscopic examination of the esophagus with a fiberoptic instrument requires general anesthesia.
43. T F Tertiary peristalsis consists of uncoordinated, nonpropulsive contractions of the esophagus.
44. T F Long-term effects of lye ingestion may include esophageal stricture and the necessity of periodic bougienage.

CHAPTER 20

STOMACH AND DUODENUM

OBJECTIVES

At the completion of this chapter you should be able to:

1. Identify the anatomic divisions of the stomach.
2. Identify the various types of gastric glands and their secretions.
3. Describe the layers of the stomach wall.
4. Describe the innervation of the stomach.
5. Explain the significance of the retroduodenal location of the gastroduodenal and pancreaticoduodenal arteries.
6. Describe the secretory, digestive, and motor functions of the stomach.
7. Outline and explain the three regulatory phases of gastric secretion.
8. List at least five effects of the hormone gastrin.
9. Explain the purpose of the various tests used in gastric analysis (basal analysis, stimulation analysis, and insulin hypoglycemia tests).
10. Contrast acute superficial and chronic atrophic gastritis (etiology, types of lesions, significance, symptoms, and treatment).
11. Differentiate among gastric erosions, acute ulcers, and chronic ulcers.
12. Identify the components of the gastric mucosal barrier, factors which may disturb this barrier, and the pathophysiologic consequences.
13. Explain the purpose of Brunner's glands.
14. Compare gastric and duodenal ulcers (prevalence, incidence, sex and age groups affected, pathogenesis, common sites, clinical features, and common complications).
15. Describe the complications of gastric and duodenal ulcers.
16. Describe and explain the purpose of vagotomy, antrectomy, and partial gastrectomy in the surgical treatment of peptic ulcers.
17. Differentiate between Curling's and Cushing's ulcers based on probable pathogenetic mechanisms.
18. Describe the treatment of stress ulcers complicated by hemorrhage.
19. Describe gastric carcinoma (sex and age group most commonly affected, predisposing factors, three types of lesions, symptoms, treatment, and prognosis).

The stomach lies obliquely from left to right across the upper abdomen between the liver and the diaphragm above and the transverse colon below. Its shape, size, and position vary a great deal depending on body build and posture and degree of gastric distention. When empty, the stomach resembles a J-shaped tube and when full, a giant pear. The normal capacity of the stomach is 1 to 2 liters.

The *fundus*, the *body*, and the *pylorus* or *pyloric antrum* are the three anatomic divisons of the stomach (see Fig. 20-1). The fundus is the enlarged portion to the left of and above the opening of the esophagus into the stomach. The body is the central portion, and the pyloric antrum is the lower portion. The stomach ends with the pyloric sphincter. There are two curvatures of the stomach. The upper right border presents as the concave *lesser curvature* and the lower left border as the convex *greater curvature*.

Both ends of the stomach are guarded by sphincters which regulate inflow and outflow. The *cardiac sphincter* or lower esophageal sphincter guards the opening of the esophagus into the stomach and prevents backflow of material into the esophagus, as discussed in Chap. 19. This area is known as the *cardiac region* of the stomach. The *pyloric sphincter* guards the opening between the pyloric portion of the stomach and the first portion of the small intestine (duodenum) and prevents backflow

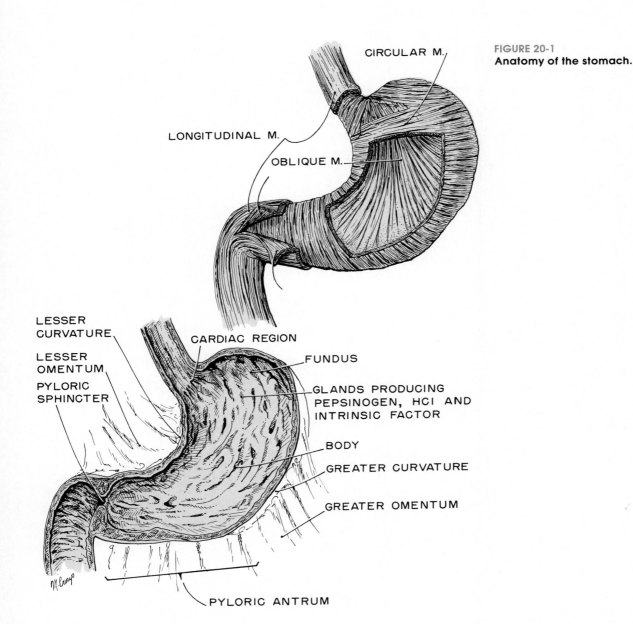

CIRCULAR M.

FIGURE 20-1
Anatomy of the stomach.

LONGITUDINAL M.

OBLIQUE M.

LESSER CURVATURE

LESSER OMENTUM

PYLORIC SPHINCTER

CARDIAC REGION

FUNDUS

GLANDS PRODUCING PEPSINOGEN, HCl AND INTRINSIC FACTOR

BODY

GREATER CURVATURE

GREATER OMENTUM

PYLORIC ANTRUM

of intestinal contents into the stomach. The pyloric sphincter is of particular clinical interest, since obstructive narrowing (stenosis) may occur as a complication of peptic ulcer disease. *Pylorospasm* is another abnormality which is very serious in infants. Spasms of these muscle fibers do not allow food to enter the duodenum properly, so that the baby vomits the food instead of digesting and absorbing it. The condition is corrected by smooth-muscle relaxants or by surgery.

The stomach is composed of four layers. The outer serous coat is formed by the peritoneum, which covers both surfaces of the stomach and is reflected off the lesser and greater curvature as the *lesser* and *greater omenta.* The lesser omentum is composed of the hepatogastric and hepatoduodenal ligaments attached to the liver, which suspend the stomach along its lesser curvature.

The three layers of muscle in the wall of the stomach are composed entirely of smooth muscle. The outermost longitudinal muscle layer extends down from the esophagus and passes mainly along the lesser and greater curvatures. The middle circular muscle layer is the most continuous and strongest of the three layers, and as it approaches the pylorus, it becomes thicker to form the muscle of the pyloric sphincter. The innermost oblique muscle is continuous with the circular muscle layer of the esophagus, is thickest in the region of the fundus, and extends to the pylorus.

The submucosa is composed mainly of loose areolar tissue and connects the muscle and mucosal layers of the stomach. It permits the mucosa to move with peristaltic motion. This layer also contains the nerve plexuses, blood, and lymph channels.

The inner mucosal layer of the stomach is arranged in temporary longitudinal folds called *rugae,* which allow for distention. Several types of glands are located in this layer and are categorized according to the anatomic portion of the stomach in which they lie. *Cardiac glands* lie near the cardiac orifice and secrete mucus. The *fundic* or *gastric glands* are located in the fundus and over the greater part of the body of the stomach. Fundic glands have three main types of cells. *Zymogenic* or *chief cells* secrete *pepsinogen,* which is converted into *pepsin* in an acid environment. *Parietal cells* secrete hydrochloric acid and water. The *neck cells* are found in the neck of the fundic gland and secrete mucus. The *pyloric glands* are located in the pyloric region of the stomach and produce *gastrin.* Other substances secreted in the stomach include enzymes and various electrolytes, especially sodium, potassium, and chloride ions. *Intrinsic factor* is secreted by the parietal cells. Intrinsic factor combines with vitamin B_{12}, enabling it to be absorbed in the small intestine. A lack of intrinsic factor results in pernicious anemia.

The stomach receives its nerve supply entirely from the autonomic nervous system. The parasympathetic nerve supply for the stomach and duodenum is conveyed to and from the abdomen through the vagus nerves (see Fig. 20-2). The vagal trunks give off gastric, pyloric, hepatic, and celiac branches. It is especially important to understand this anatomy, since selective vagotomy is of primary importance in the surgical treatment of duodenal ulcers. It will be discussed in greater detail later in this chapter.

Sympathetic innervation is supplied via the greater

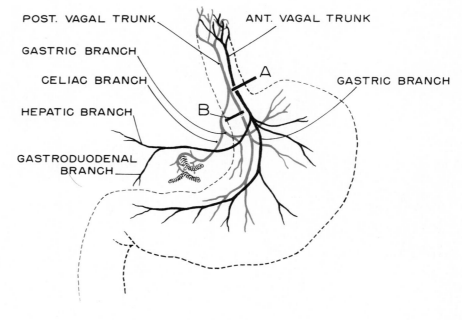

FIGURE 20-2

Parasympathetic (vagal) innervation of the stomach. It is possible to sever the vagal nerve branches supplying the stomach at points A and B, leaving intact those branches supplying other abdominal structures (selective vagotomy). Selective vagotomy is an important aspect of the surgical treatment of duodenal ulcers.

POST. VAGAL TRUNK

GASTRIC BRANCH

CELIAC BRANCH

HEPATIC BRANCH

GASTRODUODENAL BRANCH

ANT. VAGAL TRUNK

A

B

GASTRIC BRANCH

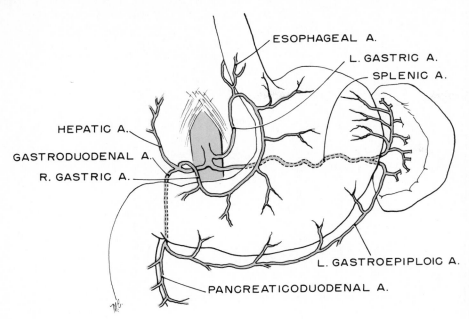

ESOPHAGEAL A.

L. GASTRIC A.

SPLENIC A.

HEPATIC A.

GASTRODUODENAL A.

R. GASTRIC A.

L. GASTROEPIPLOIC A.

PANCREATICODUODENAL A.

FIGURE 20-3
**Blood supply of the stomach
and duodenum.**

splanchnic nerves and the celiac ganglia. The afferent fibers conduct pain impulses which are stimulated by distention, muscle contraction, and inflammation and are felt in the epigastric region of the abdomen. Efferent sympathetic fibers inhibit gastric motility and secretion. *Auerbach's* and *Meissner's nerve plexuses* form the intrinsic innervation within the wall of the stomach and function to coordinate the motor and secretory activity of the gastric mucosa.

The entire blood supply of the stomach and pancreas (as well as the liver, gallbladder, and spleen) is derived mainly from the celiac artery or trunk, which gives off branches supplying the lesser and greater curvatures. Two arterial branches of particular clinical significance are the *gastroduodenal* and the *pancreaticoduodenal* (retroduodenal) arteries, which course along the posterior duodenal bulb (see Fig. 20-3). Ulcers of the posterior duodenal wall may erode into these arteries and cause hemorrhaging. The venous blood from the stomach and duodenum, as well as that from the pancreas, spleen, and the remainder of the intestinal tract, is conveyed to the liver by the portal vein.

PHYSIOLOGIC CONSIDERATIONS

The digestive and motor functions of the stomach are summarized in Table 20-1. The types of secretions have already been discussed. Motor functions include storage, mixing, and emptying *chyme* (food mixed with gastric secretions) into the duodenum. Understanding the regulation and control of gastric secretions is essential for a rational understanding of the pathogenesis and treatment of peptic ulcer disease.

TABLE 20-1

FUNCTIONS OF THE STOMACH

Motor functions	*Reservoir* function. Stores food until it can be partially digested and moved on in GI tract. Adapts to increased volume without an increase in pressure by receptive relaxation of the smooth muscle. This is mediated by the vagus nerve and induced by gastrin.
	Mixing function. Breaks food into small particles and mixes it with gastric juice through contractions of muscular coat. Peristaltic contractions controlled by a basic intrinsic electrical rhythm.
	Gastric emptying function. Controlled by opening of pyloric sphincter, which is influenced by viscosity, volume, acidity, osmotic activity, and physical state, as well as by emotions, drugs, and exercise. Gastric emptying is controlled by nervous and hormonal factors.
Digestive, secretory functions	*Digestion of protein* by pepsin and HCl is begun. Digestion of starches and fats by gastric amylase and lipase is of little importance in the stomach.
	Gastrin synthesis and release are affected by ingestion of protein, distention of the antrum, alkalinization of the antrum, and vagal stimuli.
	Intrinsic factor secretion enables the absorption of vitamin B_{12} from the distal small bowel to take place.
	Mucus secretion forms a protective shell for the stomach as well as contributing to lubrication of food for easier transport.

The control of gastric secretion

The regulation of gastric secretion may be subdivided into the cephalic, gastric or hormonal, and intestinal phases. The *cephalic phase* of gastric secretion occurs even before food enters the stomach. It results from the sight, smell, thought, or taste of food. It is mediated entirely by the vagus nerve and is eliminated by vagotomy. Neurogenic signals causing the cephalic phase may originate in the cerebral cortex or in the appetite center. Efferent impulses are then transmitted via the vagus nerve to the stomach. As a result, the gastric glands are stimulated to secrete acid, pepsinogen, and increased mucus. This phase of secretion accounts for about 10 percent of the gastric secretions normally associated with a meal.

The *gastric* or *hormonal phase* begins when food reaches the pyloric antrum. The hormone gastrin is released from the antrum and then carried by the bloodstream to the gastric glands, causing secretions. Gastrin release occurs when the vagus nerve is stimulated mechanically by distention of the antrum. This causes local and vasovagal reflexes (impulses travel to the medulla over vagal afferents and then back again to the stomach over vagal efferents; the impulses stimulate gastrin release and directly stimulate the gastric glands). Gastrin release is the primary stimulus of acid secretion. Its release is also stimulated by an alkaline pH, by bile salts in the antrum, and especially by protein foods and alcohol. Table 20-2 lists the effects of gastrin.

The gastric phase of secretion accounts for more than two-thirds of the total gastric secretion after a meal is eaten and thus accounts for most of the total daily gastric secretion of about 2000 ml. The gastric phase can be affected by surgical resection of the pyloric antrum, since this is the site of gastrin production.

The *intestinal phase* occurs when food enters the duodenum and causes the stomach to secrete small amounts of gastric juice. This phase is probably almost exclusively hormonal. Gastric secretion is probably mediated by the release of intestinal gastrin, which is probably neurally mediated. However, the role of the small intestine as an inhibitor of gastric secretion is of much greater importance.

Distention of the small intestine initiates the *enterogastric reflex*, mediated through the mysenteric plexus, sympathetic nerves, and vagus, which inhibits gastric secretion and emptying. The presence of acid (pH less than 2.5), fat, and protein breakdown products causes the release of several intestinal hormones. Secretin and cholecystokinin-pancreozymin both have a moderate inhibitory effect on gastric secretion.

TABLE 20-2

ACTIONS OF GASTRIN

Actions	Physiologic significance
Stimulates acid and pepsin secretion	Promotes digestion
Stimulates secretion of intrinsic factor	Promotes vitamin B_{12} absorption in small intestine
Stimulates pancreatic enzyme secretion	Promotes digestion
Stimulates increase in the flow of hepatic bile	Promotes digestion
Stimulates the release of insulin	Promotes glucose metabolism
Stimulates gastric and intestinal motility	Promotes mixing and propulsion of ingested food
Promotes receptive relaxation of stomach	Stomach can greatly increase volume without increasing pressure
Increases resting tone of the lower esophageal sphincter	Prevents gastric reflux during active mixing and churning
Inhibits gastric emptying	Allows time for thorough mixing of gastric contents before delivery to intestine

During the *interdigestive period* when digestion is not occurring in the gut, hydrochloric acid secretion continues at the low rate of 1 to 5 meq/hour. This is called the basal acid output (BAO) and may be measured by a 12-hour fasting gastric analysis of the secretions. The normal gastric secretions during the interdigestive period are mainly composed of mucus and contain very little pepsin and acid. Strong emotional stimuli, however, can increase the BAO via the parasympathetic (vagus) nerves and are believed to be one of the factors in the development of peptic ulcers.

DIAGNOSTIC MEASURES

Diagnostic procedures that are helpful in identifying the presence of gastric and duodenal disease include the barium x-ray, gastric analysis, and endoscopy using a flexible fiberoptic gastroscope. Photographs, biopsies, and exfoliative cytology may all be performed through the gastroscope. Exfoliative cytology, or collection of cells by lavage with normal saline solution, is a valuable technique for the identification of malignancies which may not be directly visible through the gastroscope. Malignant cells exfoliate (slough off) more readily than do normal cells. The collected solution should be placed on ice and taken to the lab immediately for analysis. Delay will result in destruction of the exfoliated cells by the digestive enzymes. Cytologic washings have about 90 percent accuracy rates in the diagnosis of cancer of the stomach.

Gastric analysis of acid secretion is another important technique in the diagnosis of gastric disease. A nasogastric tube is inserted into the stomach and the fasting contents are aspirated for analysis. The *basal analysis* measures BAO in the absence of stimulation. This test is valuable in the diagnosis of Zollinger-Ellison syndrome (a tumor of the pancreas that secretes large amounts of gastrin which, in turn, causes marked hyperacidity and multiple recurrent peptic ulcers). Duodenal ulcers are usually associated with a high BAO, while the BAO is normal to low in gastric ulcer and carcinoma.

Stimulation analysis may be performed by measurement of maximum acid output (MAO) after the administration of a drug, such as histamine, betazole hydrochloride (Histalog), or pentagastrin (synthetic gastrin), which stimulates acid secretion. *Achlorhydria* is defined as a lack of acid secretions after a maximum dose of one of the stimulating drugs (providing the analysis is accurate and there has been no reflux of duodenal contents into the stomach, which would neutralize the acid). If a patient is achlorhydric and has a gastric ulcer, the ulcer probably represents cancer and is not related to acid secretions. Patients with pernicious anemia are also achlorhydric as a result of atrophy of the secretory cells in the stomach and loss of intrinsic factor. Without intrinsic factor, vitamin B_{12} absorption is impaired, and the serum levels of vitamin B_{12} will be low.

Hypoglycemic analysis (Hollander test) is performed by inducing hypoglycemia through the injection of insulin. The gastric secretory response to insulin hypoglycemia may be used to determine the completeness of vagotomy and the likelihood of recurrent ulcers after surgery for duodenal ulcer. A drop in blood glucose to less than 50 mg per 100 ml without an increase in free hydrochloric acid indicates that the vagotomy was complete and fibers were not missed. The results are difficult to interpret and do not always correlate with ulcer recurrence. Consequently, this test is not used frequently. The significance of the surgical treatment will be discussed later in this chapter.

GASTRITIS

Gastritis is an inflammation of the gastric mucosa which may be acute, chronic, diffuse, or localized. The two most common types of gastritis—acute superficial and chronic atrophic gastritis—will be discussed.

Acute superficial gastritis

Acute gastritis is a very common, usually benign, and self-limiting disease which represents the response of the gastric mucosa to a variety of local irritants. The most common cause of acute superficial gastritis is al-

cohol. When alcohol is ingested in combination with aspirin, the effect is more deleterious than the effect of either taken alone. Diffuse hemorrhagic erosive gastritis is known to occur with heavy alcohol and aspirin abuse and may lead to the necessity of gastric resection. This serious condition will be considered with stress ulcers, since there are many similarities between the two. Destruction of the gastric mucosal barrier is believed to be the pathogenetic mechanism responsible for the injury and will be considered later.

Other causes of acute superficial gastritis include drugs such as caffeine, digitalis, iodine, aureomycin, ferrous sulfate, cinchophen, and cortisone. some spicy foods, such as those that include pepper, vinegar, or mustard, may cause symptoms suggestive of gastritis.

In superficial gastritis, the mucosa is reddened, edematous, and covered with adherent mucus; small erosions and hemorrhages are common. The degree of inflammation is highly variable.

In most cases, the diagnosis is based on the patient's history of a self-limited disorder accompanied by epigastric pain, nausea, vomiting, anorexia, and belching. In some cases, when symptoms are prolonged and resistant to treatment, additional diagnostic measures, such as endoscopy, mucosal biopsy, and gastric analysis, may be needed to clarify the diagnosis.

Acute superficial gastritis usually disappears when the offending agent is removed. Food and fluids should be withheld until the inflammation and vomiting subside. If vomiting is persistent, it may be necessary to correct fluid and electrolyte imbalance with intravenous infusions. Antiemetic drugs may help relieve the nausea and vomiting. Antispasmodics may be given to relieve smooth-muscle spasm. A bland diet and antacids may also be helpful.

Chronic atrophic gastritis

Chronic atrophic gastritis is characterized by progressive atrophy of the glandular epithelium with loss of parietal and chief cells. Consequently, there is decreased production of hydrochloric acid, pepsin, and intrinsic factor. The gastric wall becomes thin, and the mucosa presents an unusually smooth surface. This form of gastritis is frequently seen in association with pernicious anemia, gastric ulcer, and cancer.

The etiology and pathogenesis of chronic atrophic gastritis is unknown. It is more common in the elderly. Heavy alcohol intake, hot tea, and smoking may predispose to the development of atrophic gastritis.

In the case of pernicious anemia the pathogenesis

may be related to a disturbance of immunologic mechanisms. Many of these patients have circulating antibodies against parietal cells. It is not known whether the antibodies are the cause or the effect of the gastritis.

It is believed that chronic atrophic gastritis predisposes to the development of gastric ulcers and carcinoma. The incidence of gastric cancer is particularly high in patients with pernicious anemia (10 to 15 percent).

Symptoms of chronic gastritis are generally varied and vague; they include a feeling of fullness, anorexia, and vague epigastric distress. The diagnosis is suspected when there is achlorhydria or a low BAO or MAO and is confirmed by the typical histologic changes on biopsy.

The treatment of chronic atrophic gastritis varies, depending on the suspected cause of the disorder. Alcohol and drugs known to irritate the gastric mucosa are avoided. Iron-deficiency anemia (due to chronic bleeding), if present, is corrected. Vitamin B_{12} and other appropriate therapy is given in the case of pernicious anemia.

PEPTIC ULCER DISEASE

Peptic ulcers are circumscribed breaks in the continuity of mucosa, extending below the epithelium. Strictly speaking, breaks in the mucosa not extending below it are called erosions, although they are often referred to as ulcers (e.g., stress ulcers). Chronic ulcers, as opposed to acute ulcers, have scar tissue at the base (see Fig. 20-4).

By definition, peptic ulcers can be located in any part of the gastrointestinal tract exposed to the acid-pepsin gastric juice, including the esophagus, stomach, duodenum, and after gastroenterostomy, the jejunum.

Although the peptic digestive activity of gastric juice is an important etiologic factor, there is evidence that this is only one of many factors in the pathogenesis of peptic ulcer disease. Because there are many similarities and differences between gastric and duodenal ulcers, some aspects of these two entities will be considered together for convenience, while special problems relating to each will be considered separately. Gastric erosions or stress ulcers will be considered last. Table 20-3 lists some of the differences between the various types of peptic ulcers.

Pathogenesis of peptic ulcer disease

Since pure acid gastric juice is capable of digesting all living tissues, one of the major questions is, Why doesn't the stomach digest itself? Two factors seem to protect the stomach from autodigestion: the gastric mucus and the epithelial barrier.

The gastric mucosal barrier

According to Hollander's *two-component mucus barrier theory*, the thick, tenacious layer of gastric mucus constitutes the first line of defense against autodigestion. It provides protection against mechanical trauma and chemical agents. Both cortisone and aspirin produce qualitative changes in the gastric mucus which may facilitate its degradation by pepsin. However, no deficiency or abnormality of mucus has been demonstrated in patients with chronic peptic ulcer.

Davenport has emphasized the importance of a gastric mucosal barrier (see Fig. 20-5). Although the exact nature of this barrier is not understood, it probably involves the mucus lining, the lumen of the columnar epithelial cells, and the tight junctions at the apices of these cells. Normally this mucosal barrier allows very little back diffusion of H^+ from the lumen to the blood, even though there is a large concentration gradient (gastric acid with a pH of 1 versus blood with a pH of 7.4).

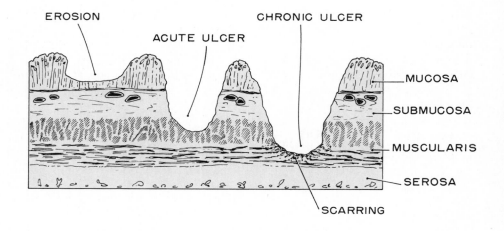

FIGURE 20-4

Peptic ulcers, illustrating an erosion, acute ulcer, and chronic ulcer. Both the acute and chronic ulcer may penetrate the entire wall of the stomach.

EROSION

ACUTE ULCER

CHRONIC ULCER

MUCOSA

SUBMUCOSA

MUSCULARIS

SEROSA

SCARRING

TABLE 20-3

DIFFERENTIATING FEATURES OF DUODENAL, GASTRIC, AND STRESS ULCERS

	Duodenal ulcer	Gastric ulcer	Stress ulcer

Incidence	Duodenal/gastric ulcer—4:1
	  Prevalence 10–12%
	  population
	Age 25–50 years
	Men/women—4:1
		Age: Usually over 50 years
		Men/women—3.5:1
			Related to severe stress, trauma,
			  sepsis, burns, head injuries
			No sex difference

Pathogenesis	Hyperacidity important factor
	Associated diseases:
	  hyperparathyroidism,
	  chronic pulmonary disease,
	  chronic pancreatitis,
	  alcoholic cirrhosis
	Ulcerogenic drugs, alcohol,
	  tobacco
	Blood group O—higher
	  frequency
	Higher frequency in those
	  subject to stress,
	  responsibility: e.g.,
	  executives, leaders
		Disruption of mucosal barrier
		  seems important factor
		Normal to low HCl production
		Presence of gastritis
		Ulcerogenic drugs, alcohol, tobacco
		Chronic bile reflux
		Not related to blood group
		More common in laboring groups
			Head injuries: hypersecretion of
			  HCl
			All others: ischemia of the
			  gastric mucosa, disruption of
			  the mucosal barrier, back
			  diffusion of HCl, acute
			  gastritis
			Hemorrhagic gastric erosions
			  may be drug-induced; alcohol
			  and aspirin most common
			  offenders

Pathology	90% in duodenal bulb	90% in antrum and lesser curvature	Usually multiple, diffuse
			  erosions; more commonly
			  located in stomach

Complications:
  Intractability
	About 10%; most respond to
	  medical therapy
		More common	

Hemorrhage	Common in posterior wall of
	  duodenal bulb
		Less common	Most frequent complication;
			  high mortality

Perforation	More common when located in
	  anterior wall of duodenum
		More common in anterior wall of
		  stomach
			Common

Obstruction	Common	Rare	
Malignancy	Almost never	Incidence about 7%	

Clinical features	Pain-food-relief pattern of pain
	  Usually well-nourished
	Seasonal exacerbations (more
	  common in spring and fall)
	Night pain common
		Pain-food-relief pattern or food-
		  pain pattern
		Anorexia, weight loss common
		Night pain uncommon
			May be asymptomatic until
			  serious complication such as
			  hemorrhage or perforation

Destruction of the gastric mucosal barrier

Aspirin, alcohol, bile salts, and other substances injurious to the gastric mucosa alter the permeability of the epithelial barrier, which allows back diffusion of hydrochloric acid with resultant injury to underlying tissues, especially blood vessels (see Fig. 20-5). Histamine is liberated, which stimulates further acid and pepsin secretion and increased capillary permeability to proteins. The mucosa becomes edematous, and large amounts of plasma proteins may be lost. The mucosal capillaries may be damaged, resulting in interstitial hemorrhage and bleeding. The mucosal barrier is unaffected by vagal inhibition or atropine, but back diffusion is inhibited by gastrin.

Destruction of the gastric mucosal barrier is believed to be an important factor in the pathogenesis of gastric ulcers. It is known that the antral mucosa is more susceptible to back diffusion than is that of the fundus, which explains why gastric ulcers are often located in the antrum. It has also been suggested that the reason for the low level of acid recovered in gastric analysis of patients with gastric ulcer is increased back diffusion, not lower production. This pathogenetic mechanism may also be important in patients with acute hemorrhagic gastritis caused by alcohol, aspirin, and severe stress.

The resistance of the duodenum to peptic ulceration is believed to be a function of *Brunner's glands* (located in the intestinal wall), which produce a highly alkaline (pH of 8), viscid, mucoid secretion which neutralizes the acid chyme. Patients with duodenal ulcer often have excessive acid secretion, which seems to be the most important pathogenetic factor. It is possible that the normal mucosal defense mechanisms are overwhelmed. The factor of decreased tissue resistance is implicated in both gastric and duodenal ulcers, although it seems to be more important in gastric ulcer.

In addition to the mucosal and epithelial barriers,

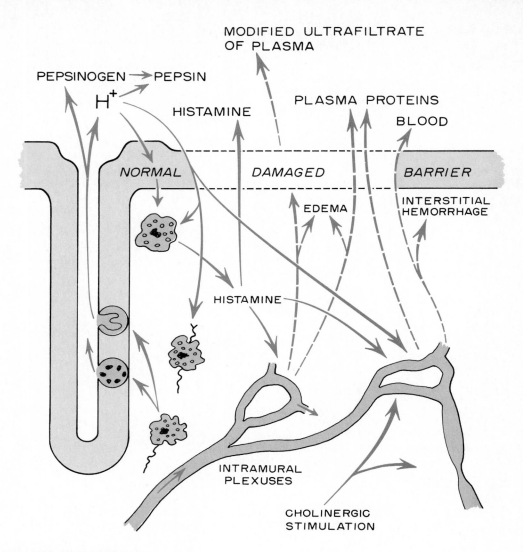

MODIFIED ULTRAFILTRATE
OF PLASMA

PEPSINOGEN → PEPSIN
H^+

HISTAMINE

PLASMA PROTEINS

BLOOD

NORMAL   *DAMAGED*   *BARRIER*

INTERSTITIAL
HEMORRHAGE

EDEMA

HISTAMINE

INTRAMURAL
PLEXUSES

CHOLINERGIC
STIMULATION

FIGURE 20-5
**Pathophysiologic consequences of back diffusion of
acid through the damaged mucosal barrier. (Redrawn
from Davenport, 1978, p. 59. Copyright 1978 by Year Book
Medical Publishers, Inc., Chicago. Used by permission.)**

tissue resistance also depends on an abundant vascular
supply and continued, rapid regeneration of epithelial
cells (normally replaced every 3 days). Failure of this
mechanism may also play a role in the pathogenesis of
peptic ulcer.

Other factors

Duodenal ulcers make up about 80 percent of all
peptic ulcers, and about 10 to 12 percent of the population is affected. Duodenal ulcers generally occur in a
much younger age group than do gastric ulcers. The
much lower incidence of peptic ulcers in women seems
to indicate a sex-linked influence.

It has been suggested that certain drugs such as aspirin, alcohol, indomethacin, phenylbutazone, and corticosteroids may have a direct irritating effect on the
gastric mucosa and produce ulceration. If they do have
an effect, it is probably caused by a disruption of one of
the protective barriers in the stomach. Other drugs,
such as caffeine, will increase acid production. Emotional stress presumably also plays a role in the pathogenesis of peptic ulcers, probably by increasing acid
production as a result of vagal stimulation.

Most peptic ulcers occur "downstream" from the
source of acid secretion. More than 90 percent of duodenal ulcers are located on the anterior or posterior wall
of the first part of the duodenum, within 2 cm of the
pyloric ring. Although gastric ulcers may occur anywhere in the stomach, 90 percent are situated along the
lesser curvature and in the pyloric gland region.

Individuals with blood group O are 35 percent
more susceptible to duodenal ulcer, which indicates that
genetic factors are involved. The incidence of gastric
ulcers does not seem to be related to blood group.

A number of diseases seem to be associated with
peptic ulcer formation; these include alcoholic liver cirrhosis, chronic pancreatitis, chronic lung disease, hyperparathyroidism, and the Zollinger-Ellison syndrome.

Finally, abnormal pyloric sphincter function resulting in bile reflux has been proposed as a pathogenetic mechanism in the development of gastric ulcer. The bile disrupts the gastric mucosal barrier, causing gastritis and increased suceptibility to ulcer formation. The damaged mucosa is ultimately eroded and digested by the action of acid and pepsin.

Clinical features

Although duodenal and gastric ulcers possibly arise from different pathologic processes, the signs and symptoms with which they commonly present are sometimes indistinguishable. The principal symptom is upper abdominal pain. This is usually located in the epigastrum and is described as a gnawing, boring, or nagging sensation. The pain usually begins about 2 hours after meals and is relieved by food or antacids. The symptoms may last for a few days, weeks, or months and then disappear for varying periods of time. The periodic nature of the symptoms is so characteristic that constant upper abdominal pain is frequently not caused by peptic ulcer. Although the food-pain-relief pattern also occurs with gastric ulcers, the symptoms seem to be more variable. In fact, with gastric ulcer, food sometimes aggravates the pain. Patients with duodenal ulcer frequently have pain in the middle of the night, but this is not as common in patients with gastric ulcer. Weight loss is frequent in patients with gastric ulcer, but persons with duodenal ulcer usually maintain normal weight.

Diagnosis

The most important criterion in the diagnosis of duodenal ulcer is a history of the typical pain-food-relief pattern. The history is not as informative in patients with gastric ulcer, since vague symptoms of epigastric distress are more common. It is not usually possible to distinguish between gastric and duodenal ulcer on the basis of history alone.

The diagnosis of peptic ulcer is usually confirmed by barium meal x-ray (see Fig. 20-6). When barium x-ray fails to reveal an ulcer in the stomach or duodenum but characteristic symptoms persist, endoscopic examination is indicated.

Benign versus malignant ulcers

Although duodenal ulcers are almost never malignant, about 7 percent of gastric ulcers turn out to be carcinoma of the stomach. It is therefore important for the gastroenterologist to differentiate between a benign and malignant gastric ulcer. In general, malignant ulcers have a shaggy, necrotic base, while benign ulcers have a smooth, clean base with a distinct margin (see Fig. 20-7). Biopsy and cytologic studies are also helpful in distinguishing a benign from a malignant ulcer.

Medical treatment

The primary objective in the medical treatment of peptic ulcer is to inhibit or buffer acid secretions in order to relieve symptoms and promote healing. Measures that achieve these ends are antacids, dietary management, anticholinergics, histamine-2 receptor antagonists

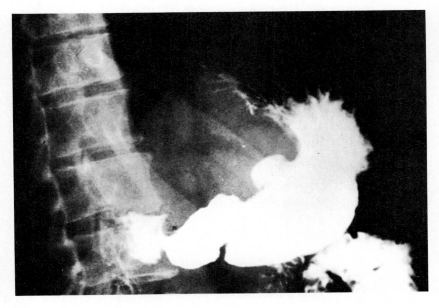

FIGURE 20-6
Barium x-ray appearance of gastric ulcer. Note the large nodular-shaped protrusion on the lesser curvature of the stomach.

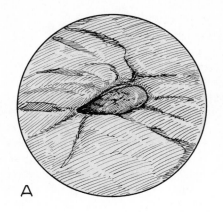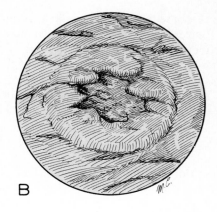

FIGURE 20-7
Gastroscopic appearance of (A) a benign gastric ulcer and (B) a malignant gastric ulcer (carcinoma). The benign ulcer has a sharp, well-defined margin. The malignant ulcer has an irregular margin which fades into the surrounding tumor mass.

(cimetidine and ranitedine), and physical and emotional rest.

Antacids are given to neutralize the acid gastric contents by keeping the pH high enough so that pepsin is not activated, thus protecting the mucosa and relieving the pain. Small, frequent meals are also important in neutralizing the gastric contents. Stimulants of acid secretion, such as alcohol and caffeine, are avoided. Anticholinergic drugs, such as propantheline bromide (Pro-Banthine) and atropine (from *Atropa belladonna*), inhibit the direct effect of the vagus nerve on the acid-secreting parietal cells. Anticholinergics also inhibit gastric motility and emptying time, and for this reason many physicians do not prescribe this kind of drug for patients with gastric ulcer. Histamine-2 receptor antagonists (cimetidine and ranitedine) have rapidly become the most common drugs used for the treatment of duodenal ulcers owing to their ability to reduce acid secretion by 70 percent. Another drug, sucralfate, not only forms an acid-impermeable membrane which adheres to injured mucosa but also accelerates mucosal cell production (a cytoprotective effect).

Physical and emotional rest are promoted by providing a quiet environment, listening to the patient's problems, and offering emotional support. Small doses of sedatives are frequently prescribed.

About 80 to 90 percent of patients with duodenal ulcer have a benign course interrupted by the necessity for medical therapy. An unknown number of patients undoubtedly treat themselves successfully with diet and antacids which are available without a prescription. The response of gastric ulcers to traditional medical therapy (diet and antacids) is not quite as successful; but using the newer histamine receptor antagonists for 12 weeks results in healing of 80 to 90 percent of gastric ulcers. Close monitoring of progress is required because drugs may relieve the symptoms of malignant gastric ulcers. These remaining patients may develop complications.

Complications

Complications of peptic ulcer disease include intractability, hemorrhage, perforation, and pyloric obstruction.

Any of these complications are indications for surgical treatment, which will be discussed subsequently.

Intractability

The most common complication of peptic ulcer disease is intractability, which simply means that the medical therapy has failed to control the symptoms adequately. Patients may have their sleep interrupted by pain, lose time from work, require frequent hospitalization, or just be unable to follow the medical regimen. Intractability is the most common reason for recommending surgery. Malignant transformation is not an important consideration in either gastric or duodenal ulcer. Those ulcers which are malignant started out as malignant, and at least by current knowledge, those that started out as benign remain benign without undergoing malignant degeneration.

Hemorrhage

Bleeding is a very common complication of peptic ulcer and occurs in at least 25 percent of the cases at some time during the course of the disease. Although ulcers in any site may bleed, the most common site of hemorrhage is in the posterior wall of the duodenal bulb, since in that location erosion into the pancreaticoduodenal or gastroduodenal arteries may occur.

The symptoms associated with bleeding ulcer depend on the rapidity of blood loss. Mild, chronic blood loss may lead to iron-deficiency anemia. The stools may be positive for occult blood (positive guaiac test) or may be black and tarry (melena). Massive bleeding may lead to hematemesis (vomiting blood) and the development of shock and may require blood transfusions and emergency surgery. Relief of pain often follows bleeding as a result of the buffering effect of blood. The mortality in these patients is from 3 to 10 percent, which represents about 25 percent of the total deaths attributable to peptic ulcer disease.

Perforation

Approximately 5 percent of all ulcers perforate, and this complication accounts for about 65 percent of deaths from peptic ulcer disease (see Fig. 4-11). The ulcers are usually on the anterior wall of the duodenum or stomach, since this area is covered only by peritoneum.

The majority of patients present in a characteristically dramatic fashion. There is a sudden onset of excruciating pain in the upper abdomen. Within minutes a chemical peritonitis develops because of the escaping gastric acid, pepsin, and food and causes intense pain. The patient fears to move or breathe. The abdomen becomes silent to auscultation and assumes a boardlike rigidity to palpation. Acute perforation can usually be diagnosed on the basis of the symptoms alone. The diagnosis is confirmed by the presence of free gas within the peritoneal cavity, presenting as a translucent crescent between the liver and diaphragm shadows. The air, of course, entered the peritoneal cavity through the perforated ulcer. The treatment is immediate surgery with gastric resection or simple suture of the perforation, depending on the patient's condition.

Occasionally a gastric or duodenal ulcer breaks through the wall but remains sealed off by a contiguous structure and is called a *penetrating ulcer*. A classic example of a penetrating ulcer is a duodenal ulcer of the posterior wall which penetrates into the pancreas and is walled off (see Fig. 20-8). Clinically, the pain becomes intractable and may radiate to the back. The patient may present with the finding of pancreatitis.

Obstruction

Obstruction of the gastric outlet as a result of inflammation and edema, pylorospasm, or scarring occurs in about 5 percent of patients with peptic ulcer. It is more common in patients with duodenal ulcer but occaisonally occurs when a gastric ulcer is located close to the pyloric sphincter.

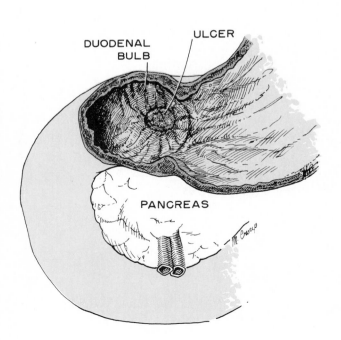

Anorexia, nausea, and bloating after eating are common symptoms. Weight loss is common. When the obstruction becomes severe, pain and vomiting may occur.

Treatment is directed toward restoring fluids and electrolytes, decompressing the stomach by insertion of a nasogastric tube, and surgical correction of the obstruction (pyloroplasty).

Surgical treatment

Patients who do not respond to medical therapy or who develop other complications such as perforation, hemorrhage, or obstruction are treated surgically. In general, surgical treatment is effected by one of two procedures, vagotomy or gastrectomy, or sometimes by both. There are many variations of these two procedures, and the type of surgery elected depends on many factors, including the nature of the pathology and the patient's age and general condition.

The common aim in the surgical treatment of duodenal ulcers is to permanently reduce the capacity of the stomach to secrete acid and pepsin. This can be achieved in at least four ways:

1. *Vagotomy* is the division of the vagus nerve branches to the stomach, thus eliminating the cephalic phase of gastric secretion. Vagotomy not only diminishes gastric secretions but also decreases gastric motility and emptying. Consequently a "drainage" procedure is required to prevent gastric retention—either a gastrojejunostomy or pyloroplasty.

2. *Antrectomy* is the removal of the entire antrum of the stomach, thus eliminating the hormonal or gastric phase of gastric secretion.

3. *Vagotomy plus antrectomy* eliminates both the cephalic and gastric phases of gastric secretion. Thus, neural stimulation is interrupted, drainage is enhanced, and the major site of gastrin production is removed. It is thought to be superior to some of the more extensive surgical procedures.

4. *Partial gastrectomy* is the removal of the distal 50 to 75 percent of the stomach, thus removing a substantial portion of the acid- and pepsin-secreting mucosa. Following gastric resection, gastrointes-

FIGURE 20-8
Duodenal ulcer of the posterior wall penetrating into the head of the pancreas, resulting in a walled-off perforation.

tinal continuity may be restored by anastomosing the gastric remnant to the duodenum (gastroduodenostomy or Billroth I procedure) or to the jejunum (gastrojejunostomy or Billroth II procedure).

Figure 20-9 illustrates some of the common surgical procedures for treating peptic ulcers.

Most surgeons treat gastric ulcer by partial gastrectomy and a gastroduodenal anastomosis. The line of resection is usually proximal to the gastric ulcer. A vagotomy is usually not performed, since these patients have normal to low gastric acid production.

Acute stress- and drug-induced ulcers

The term "stress ulcer" has been used to describe gastric or duodenal erosions which occur as a sequel to pro-

longed psychological or physiologic stress. The stress may take many forms, such as hypotensive shock following traumatic injury and major surgery, sepsis, hypoxia, severe burns (Curling's ulcers), or cerebral trauma (Cushing's ulcers). Any seriously ill patient in an intensive care setting is susceptible to the development of a stress ulcer. Acute erosive and hemorrhagic gastritis induced by an alcoholic bout, aspirin or other ulcerogenic drugs, and bile reflux are often grouped with stress ulcers, since the lesions are similar.

Acute stress ulcers are usually shallow, irregular, punched-out lesions which may be large in size, multiple, and often located in the stomach. The lesions may bleed slowly, causing melena, and are often asymptomatic or are overshadowed by the serious illness in the patient. Because these lesions are superficial, they are not usually evident on x-ray examination.

Stress ulcers are clinically apparent when there is massive gastric hemorrhage or perforation. In fact, stress ulcers account for 5 percent of all cases of peptic ulcer bleeding. Massive bleeding resulting from alcohol-induced acute erosive gastritis is also a common problem.

FIGURE 20-9

Common surgical procedures for treating peptic ulcers. (A) Vagotomy plus antrectomy (removal of the pyloric antrum). (B) Billroth I procedure (gastroduodenostomy anastomosis after resection. (C) Billroth II procedure (gastrojejunostomy anastomosis after resection).

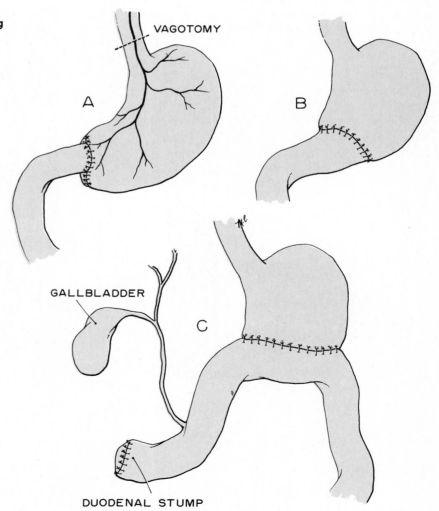

Pathogenesis

Stress ulcers are generally divided into two different groups based on probable pathogenetic mechanisms. Cushing's ulcers associated with serious brain injury are characterized by marked hyperacidity, which is possibly mediated by vagal stimulation (cerebral injury → vagal stimulation → hyperacidity → acute peptic ulcer).

On the other hand, stress ulcers associated with shock, sepsis, burns, and drugs are not characterized by gastric acid hypersecretion. The studies of Silen and Skillman (1974) suggest that disruption of the mucosal barrier function of the stomach, especially in the presence of ischemia resulting from poor vascular perfusion, may be important in the pathogenesis (see Fig. 20-10).

Treatment

Recent studies reveal that the presence of erosive gastritis (stress ulcers) is a common finding in critically ill patients. About 80 percent of the severely burned patients have evidence of occult blood in their stools. Other studies have revealed an even higher incidence of stress ulcers identified by gastroscopy in critically ill patients. Most of these patients do not have symptoms until there is massive bleeding, which occurs in about 5 percent. This has led to the prophylactic treatment of high-risk patients with cimetidine and/or antacids. The other 95 percent heal with little or no residual effects.

When bleeding occurs, attempts are made to treat the condition conservatively by blood transfusions and by ice-water lavage. When bleeding is serious, some patients have been treated successfully by continuous intraarterial perfusion with vasopressin, a powerful vasoconstrictor.

Vasopressin infusion is accomplished by inserting a catheter via the femoral artery, through the aorta and celiac trunk, and out the right or left gastric artery. The bleeding site is identified by arteriography, after which a vasopressin infusion is started. Newer and as yet experimental methods include electrocoagulation, photocoagulation (laser coagulation), and application of polymers.

When these conservative methods of treatment fail, surgery may be the only method of treatment, even though these patients are critically ill and poor surgical risks. The most effective surgical procedure is total gastrectomy, since these erosions are multiple or diffuse and tend to rebleed.

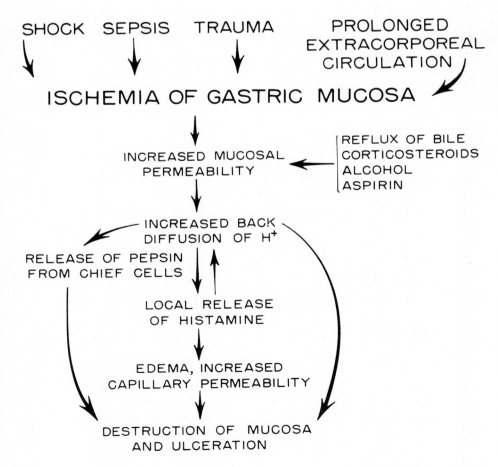

FIGURE 20-10
Pathogenesis of "stress" ulcers. (Adapted from Silen and Skillman, 1974. Copyright 1974 by Year Book Medical Publishers, Inc., Chicago. Used by permission.)

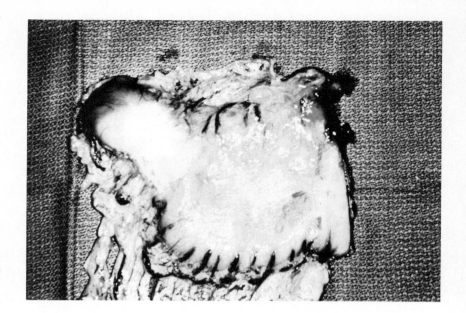

CANCER OF THE STOMACH

Carcinoma of the stomach is the most common form of gastric neoplasm and accounts for about 5 percent of all cancer deaths. Males are more frequently affected and most cases occur after the age of 40.

The cause of stomach cancer is unknown, but certain predisposing factors are recognized. Genetic factors seem to be important, since gastric cancer is more common in persons with blood group A. Geographic or environmental factors appear to be important, since gastric cancer is very common in Japan, Chile, and Iceland. For unknown reasons gastric cancer has been declining in the United States during the past 30 years. It is more common in lower socioeconimic groups. One of the most important predisposing factors is the presence of atrophic gastritis or pernicious anemia as previously discussed.

About 50 percent of gastric cancers are located in the pyloric antrum. The remainder of the lesions are distributed throughout the body of the stomach.

There are three general forms of gastric carcinoma.

Ulcerating carcinoma is the most common type and must be differentiated from a benign gastric ulcer. *Polypoid carcinoma* appears as a cauliflowerlike mass protruding into the lumen and may arise from an adenomatous polyp. *Infiltrating carcinoma* may penetrate the entire thickness of the stomach wall and is responsible for the inflexible "leather bottle stomach" (linitis plastica) (see Fig. 20-11).

Carcinoma of the stomach is seldom diagnosed in an early stage because symptoms develop late or are vague and indefinite. Early symptoms may include a mild feeling of discomfort in the upper abdomen or a feeling of fullness after eating. Eventually there is anorexia and weight loss. When the tumor is located near the cardia, dysphagia may be the first major symptom. Vomiting from pyloric obstruction may occur when the tumor is near the gastric outlet.

Radiologic studies, exfoliative cytology, and endoscopy with biopsy are all important methods in the diagnosis of gastric cancer. Surgical excision is the only effective therapy. Because of the usual late diagnosis, the prognosis is poor, with a 10 percent 5-year survival rate.

QUESTIONS

Stomach and duodenum

Directions: Answer the following questions on a separate sheet of paper.

1. Sketch the stomach and indicate the location of the following: fundus, body, pyloric antrum, pyloric sphincter, cardiac region, lesser curvature, greater curvature and glands secreting HCl and pepsin, intrinsic factor, and gastrin.

2. What are the lesser and greater omenta? Where are they located?

3. What are rugae and what is their purpose in the stomach?

4. How is pepsinogen activated in the stomach? What is the action of pepsin?

5. Describe the extrinsic and intrinsic innervation of the stomach and the function of each.

6. Name the truncal artery and its major branches supplying the stomach.

7. Why is hemorrhage a more frequent complication in duodenal ulcers of the posterior wall?

8. List three motor functions of the stomach.

9. What is the normal capacity of the adult stomach? What prevents an increase in intragastric pressure during a moderate-sized meal?

10. Why do patients become anemic when there is a deficiency or absence of intrinsic factor?

11. What controls the mixing and emptying activities of the stomach?

12. What prevents the stomach from digesting itself? Explain your answer using the theories of gastric mucosal defense formulated by Hollander and Davenport. What drugs or chemicals may alter mucosal defense? What protects the duodenum from the actions of acid and pepsin?

13. List five effects of gastrin and the physiologic significance of each.

14. What is acute superficial gastritis? Do you think you have ever had this condition? What are the symptoms?

15. Explain how gastric secretions are controlled during the three phases of gastric secretion.

Directions: *Circle the letter preceding each item below that correctly answers the question. Only one answer is correct unless otherwise noted.*

16. Gastrin is a hormone produced by:
    a. Pancreas   b. Brunner's glands   c. Duodenum
    d. Gastric antrum   e. Gastric fundus

17. Which of the following agents have been associated with an increased incidence of ulcer disease? (More than one answer may be correct.)
    a. Aspirin   b. Ethyl alcohol   c. High doses of corticosteroids   d. Phenylbutazone

18. Achlorhydria or hypochlorhydria is commonly seen in: (More than one answer may be correct.)
    a. Pernicious anemia   b. Zollinger-Ellison syndrome   c. Atrophic gastritis   d. Carcinoma of the stomach

19. Which of the following is known to cause an elaboration of gastrin from the gastric antrum? (More than one answer may be correct.)
    a. Distention of the antrum   b. Alkalinization of the antrum   c. Acidification of the antrum
    d. Distention of the fundus   e. Stimulation of the vagus

20. Which of the following phases accounts for the largest volume of gastric acid secretion?

    a. Cephalic   b. Hormonal   c. Intestinal
    d. Interdigestive

21. The enterogastric reflex: (More than one answer may be correct.)
    a. Is mediated via the mysenteric nerve plexus
    b. Stimulates gastric emptying   c. Inhibits gastric emptying   d. Inhibits gastric secretion

22. The gastric secretory pattern in duodenal ulcer is commonly in which range?
    a. Achlorhydria   b. Normal to low   c. Normal to high   d. Marked hyperacidity

23. Which of the following foods has the greatest acid secretory effect?
    a. Proteins   b. Fats   c. Carbohydrates

24. Theories regarding the pathogenesis of gastric ulcers include: (More than one answer may be correct.)
    a. Overactivity of the vagus   b. Hypersecretion of acid   c. Impaired mucosal resistance
    d. Reflux of bile into the stomach

25. Duodenal ulcer disease is:
    a. More common in women than in men
    b. Always responsive to medical treatment
    c. Very common, affecting more than 10 percent of the population   d. Associated with blood group A

26. When bleeding complicates peptic ulcer disease, pain:
    a. No longer responds to antacids   b. Radiates to the back   c. Becomes more severe   d. Usually disappears

27. Signs, symptoms, and findings indicating acute perforation of a peptic ulcer include: (More than one answer may be correct.)
    a. Boardlike rigidity of abdomen to palpation
    b. Relief from pain   c. Severe pain in upper abdomen   d. Subphrenic air bubble evident on x-ray

28. Which of the following contiguous structures would most likely be involved in a confined perforation of a peptic ulcer?
    a. Liver   b. Gallbladder   c. Pancreas   d. Lesser omentum

29. Recurrent ulcer following peptic ulcer surgery: (More than one answer may be correct.)
    a. Is related to the preoperative level of gastric acid secretion   b. Occurs most commonly after gastric ulcer   c. Is less common if vagotomy is performed

30. Which of the following statements applies to the surgical treatment of duodenal ulcer?
    a. Billroth I procedure is the surgery of choice.
    b. Billroth II procedure is the surgery of choice.
    c. A vagotomy and 75 percent gastric resection should be performed.   d. Some form of vagotomy should be performed.

31. Which of the following mechanisms would be the the most probable to explain the development of stress ulcers in a patient who developed hypotensive shock following cardiac surgery?
    a. Excess vagal stimulation → hyperacidity
    b. Gastric ischemia → disruption on the gastric mucosal barrier → increased back diffusion of H^+

32. Carcinoma of the stomach: (More than one answer may be correct.)
    a. Is most frequent after the age of 40   b. Is more common in persons with pernicious anemia
    c. Generally has a good prognosis   d. Most commonly presents as an ulcerative lesion
    e. Commonly infiltrates the stomach wall, causing it to become inflexible

33. Methods of treating acute hemorrhagic gastritis include:
    a. Electrocoagulation   b. Intraarterial vasopressin infusion   c. Ice-water lavage
    d. Total gastrectomy   e. All of the above

Directions: Match the following gastric acid analysis tests in col. A with their diagnostic value in col. B.

Column A

Column B

34. ___ Basal acid output (BAO)

a. Especially useful in the diagnosis of the Zollinger-Ellison syndrome

35. ___ Maximum acid output (MAO)

b. May be used to assess completeness of vagotomy

36. ___ Insulin hypoglycemia test

c. May be used to determine if true achlorhydria is present

Directions: Match the following differentiating features of gastric and duodenal ulcers in col. B to the type of peptic ulcer in col. A.

Column A

Column B

37. ___ Gastric ulcer

a. Symptomatically improves on antacids

38. ___ Duodenal ulcer

b. Pain in the middle of the night more common

c. Always should be treated surgically

d. Obstruction an infrequent problem

e. More common in persons with blood group O

f. Higher frequency in persons subjected to stress

Directions: Circle T if the statement is true and F if it is false.

39. T   F   The chief cells of the stomach secrete HCl.

40. T   F   The neck cells of the gastric glands secrete mucus.

41. T   F   Chronic ulcers, as opposed to acute ulcers, have scar tissue at their base.

42. T   F   A break in the gastric mucosa which does not extend beyond the mucosal layer is called an erosion.

SMALL INTESTINE

OBJECTIVES

At the completion of this chapter you should be able to:

1. Describe the following gross and microscopic anatomic features of the small intestine:
    a. Length, major divisions, inlet and outlet, position in abdomen, and anatomic relation to the ligament of Treitz
    b. Major folds of the peritoneum: mesentery and greater and lesser omenta (describe position and function)
    c. The three structural features which greatly increase the absorptive surface
    d. Major blood supply and innervation
    e. Structure and function of a villus: types of cells and their life cycle, microvilli, crypts of Lieberkühn, blood and lymphatic supply
    f. Location of appendix in relation to small and large bowel
2. List the five principal organs which produce digestive secretions and the approximate volume of their secretions.
3. List the principal digestive enzymes including source, action, and approximate optimal pH for activity.
4. Describe the function of bile in the digestion and absorption of fats and fat-soluble vitamins.
5. Identify and describe the actions of two hormones important in the regulation of intestinal digestion.
6. List the principal sites of absorption of the following nutrients: fats, sugars, amino acids, folic acid, vitamin B_{12}, and bile salts.
7. Describe and state the significance of the enterohepatic recirculation of bile salts.
8. Differentiate between maldigestion and malabsorption.
9. List at least four basic causes of the malabsorption syndrome.
10. Explain the pathophysiologic basis of the following signs and symptoms of malabsorption:
    a. Weight loss
    b. Diarrhea
    c. Steatorrhea
    d. Flatulence, abdominal distention
    e. Nocturia

    f. Weakness and easy fatigability

    g. Edema

    h. Amenorrhea

    i. Anemia

    j. Glossitis, cheilosis, peripheral neuropathy

    k. Bruising, bleeding tendency

    l. Bone pain, tetany, paresthesias

11. Describe each of the following diagnostic tests of malabsorption and indicate what each one can detect:

    a. Quantitative stool fat determination

    b. D-xylose test

    c. Schilling test

    d. Culture of small bowel contents

    e. Barium x-ray of small bowel

    f. Biopsy of small bowel

12. Describe the gross appearance and characteristics of stool in severe steatorrhea.

13. Identify the substance which causes the toxic reaction in nontropical sprue.

14. Contrast tropical and nontropical sprue with respect to proposed etiology, intestinal biopsy changes, population affected, clinical features, and treatment.

15. Identify a genetic enzyme deficiency disease common in American blacks and explain the pathophysiologic basis of the diarrhea in this condition.

16. Give four reasons why malabsorption may be a problem following extensive gastric resection.

17. Explain why postgastrectomy patients may develop vitamin B_{12} deficiency and ineffective action of bile salts.

18. Explain the basis of the theory that regional enteritis may represent a hypersensitivity reaction similar to the mechanism producing tissue damage in tuberculosis.

19. Describe regional enteritis (lesions and their distribution, clinical features, complications, treatment, and prognosis).

20. Locate the normal position of the appendix at McBurney's point.

21. Describe the anatomic features of the appendix which make it especially vulnerable to obstruction, necrosis, and perforation.

22. Describe the signs and symptoms of a classic case of acute appendicitis and explain why difficulties may be encountered in establishing the diagnosis.

23. Explain why early surgery for acute appendicitis is important.

24. Describe the reaction of the peritoneum to invasion by bacteria.

25. Differentiate between adynamic ileus and mechanical obstruction of the bowel and list the general causes of each.

26. Define the following conditions related to bowel obstruction and indicate the most common site of occurrence, relative frequency, and age groups commonly affected:

    a. Adhesions

    b. Volvulus

    c. Intussusception

    d. Malignant tumor

    e. Incarcerated hernia

    f. Strangulated bowel

27. Describe the pathophysiologic events leading to death from complete obstruction of the small bowel.
28. Describe the signs and symptoms of bowel obstruction.
29. Explain why early diagnosis and surgical intervention are important in mechanical obstruction of the small bowel.

ANATOMIC CONSIDERATIONS

The small intestine is a complex, folded tube extending from the pylorus to the ileocecal valve. It is about 12 ft long in life (22 ft in the cadaver as a result of relaxation) and is contained in the central and lower part of the abdominal cavity. The proximal end is about 3.8 cm in diameter, but the diameter gradually diminishes to about 2.5 cm at the lower end.

The small intestine is divided into the *duodenum, jejunum,* and *ileum.* This division is rather imprecise and is based on slight modifications in structure and relatively more important differences in function. The duodenum is about 25 cm long and extends from the pylorus to the jejunum. The division between the duodenum and jejunum is marked by the *ligament of Treitz,* a musculofibrous band which originates from the right crus of the diaphragm near the esophageal hiatus and attaches to the junction of the duodenum and jejunum, acting as a suspensory ligament. Approximately two-fifths of the remaining intestine is the jejunum, and the terminal three-fifths is the ileum. The jejunum lies in the left midabdominal region, while the ileum tends to lie in the right lower abdominal region. Entry of chyme into the small intestine is controlled by the pyloric sphincter, and exit of digested materials into the large intestine is controlled by the ileocecal valve. The ileocecal valve also prevents reflux of contents of the large intestine into the small intestine.

The *vermiform appendix* is a blind tube about the size of the little finger located in the ileocecal region at the apex of the cecum. Inflammation or rupture of this structure is an important cause of morbidity in young persons, although it is a less frequent cause of death now than in the preantibiotic era.

The wall of the small intestine is composed of four basic layers. The outer, or serous, coat is formed by the peritoneum. The peritoneum has a visceral and a parietal layer, and the potential space between these layers is called the peritoneal cavity. The peritoneum is reflected over and almost completely envelops the abdominal viscera.

Special names have been given to the folds of the peritoneum. The *mesentery* is a broad, fanlike fold of peritoneum which suspends the jejunum and ileum from the posterior abdominal wall and allows considerable motion of the bowel. The mesentery supports the blood and lymph vessels supplying the intestine. The *greater omentum* is a double layer of peritoneum which hangs from the greater curvature of the stomach and descends in front of the abdominal viscera like an apron. The omentum usually contains fat in considerable amounts and lymph nodes, which aid in protecting the peritoneal cavity against infection. The *lesser omentum* is the fold of peritoneum which extends from the lesser curvature of the stomach and upper duodenum to the liver, forming the hepatogastric and hepatoduodenal suspensory ligaments. One of the important functions of the peritoneum is to prevent friction between contiguous organs by secreting a serous fluid which acts as a lubricant. Inflammation of the peritoneum is called *peritonitis* and may be a serious sequel to inflammation or perforation of the bowel. Adhesions (fibrous bands) may develop following peritonitis or abdominal surgery, sometimes causing obstruction of the bowel.

The muscular coat of the small intestine has two layers: an outer, thinner layer of longitudinal fibers and an inner one of circular fibers. This arrangement aids the peristaltic action of the small intestine. The submucosal layer is composed of connective tissue, and the inner mucosal layer is thick, vascular, and glandular.

The small intestine is characterized by three structural features which greatly increase its surface area and aid in its primary function of absorption. The mucosal and submucosal layers are arranged in circular folds called *valvulae conniventes* (Kerckring's folds) which project into the lumen of the tube about 3 to 10 mm. These folds are prominent in the duodenum and jejunum and disappear near the mid-ileum. They are responsible for the feathery appearance of the small intestine on barium x-ray. The *villi* are fingerlike projections of mucosa numbering about 4 or 5 million and are present in the entire length of the small intestine (see Fig. 6-2). The villi are 0.5 to 1.5 mm long (just visible to the naked eye) and account for the velvetlike appearance of the mucosa. The *microvilli* are fingerlike projections about 1.0 μm in length along the outer surface of each individual villus. They are visible by electron microscopy and appear as a *brush border* on light microscopy. If the lining of the small intestine were smooth, the surface area would be about 2000 cm^2. The valvulae conniventes, villi, and microvilli together increase the total absorbing surface to 2 million cm^2, which is a 1000-fold increase. Diseases of the small intestine, such as sprue, which cause atrophy and flattening of the villi greatly reduce the surface area for absorption, resulting in malabsorption.

Structure of the villus

Figure 21-1 illustrates the structure of a villus, which is the functional unit of the small intestine. Each villus consists of a central lymph channel called a *lacteal* surrounded by a network of blood capillaries held together by lymphoid tissue. This, in turn, is surrounded by columnar epithelial cells. After the food has been digested, it passes into the lacteals and capillaries of the villi. The villous epithelium consists of two cell types: *goblet cells,* which produce mucus, and *absorptive cells* (with microvilli projecting from the surface), which are re-

sponsible for absorption of digested foodstuffs. Enzymes are located on the brush border and complete the process of digestion as absorption is taking place.

Surrounding each villus are several small pits called the *crypts of Lieberkühn.* These crypts are intestinal glands which produce secretions containing digestive enzymes. Undifferentiated cells in the crypts of Lieberkühn proliferate rapidly and migrate upward toward the tip of the villus, where they become absorptive cells. At the tip of the villus, they are shed into the intestinal lumen. Maturation and migration from the crypts to the tip of the villus requires only 5 to 7 days. It is estimated that 20 to 50 million epithelial cells are extruded into the intestinal lumen each minute. Because of this very high cell turnover rate (fastest in the body), the intestinal epithelium is especially vulnerable to alterations in cell proliferation. Cytotoxic drugs given for cancer or leukemia inhibit cell division, resulting in mucosal atrophy and shortening of both crypts and villi. Patients receiving these drugs often develop ulcerations of the gastrointestinal mucosa. Villi may be flattened or absent in sprue.

Blood supply and innervation

The *superior mesenteric* artery, arising from the aorta just below the celiac artery, supplies all of the small in-

FIGURE 21-1
Structure of a villus of the small intestine.

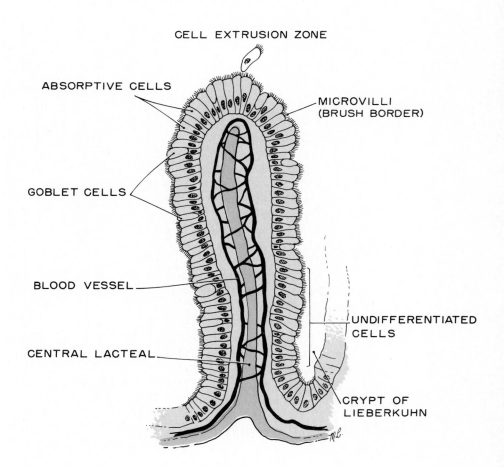

CELL EXTRUSION ZONE

ABSORPTIVE CELLS

MICROVILLI (BRUSH BORDER)

GOBLET CELLS

BLOOD VESSEL

CENTRAL LACTEAL

UNDIFFERENTIATED CELLS

CRYPT OF LIEBERKUHN

testine except the duodenum, which is supplied by the gastroduodenal artery and its branch, the superior pancreaticoduodenal artery. Blood is returned by the superior mesenteric vein, which unites with the splenic vein to form the portal vein.

The small intestine is innervated by both branches of the autonomic nervous system. Parasympathetic stimulation stimulates secretory activity and motility and sympathetic stimulation inhibits motility. Sensory fibers of the sympathetic system relay pain, while those of the parasympathetic regulate intestinal reflexes. The intrinsic nerve supply, which initiates motor function, passes through Auerbach's plexus located in the muscular layer and Meissner's plexus in the submucosal layer.

PHYSIOLOGIC CONSIDERATIONS

The small intestine has two primary functions: digestion and absorption of ingested nutrients and water. All other activities either regulate or facilitate this process. The digestive process is initiated in the mouth and stomach by the actions of ptyalin, hydrochloric acid, and pepsin on the ingested food. The process is continued in the duodenum primarily by the action of pancreatic enzymes, which hydrolyze carbohydrates, fats, and proteins into simpler substances. The presence of bicarbonate in the pancreatic secretion helps to neutralize the acid and provide an optimum pH for the action of the enzymes. The secretion of bile from the liver aids the digestive process by emulsifying fats so that a greater surface area is presented for the action of pancreatic lipase.

The action of bile results from the detergent properties of conjugated bile acids which solubilize lipid material by the formulation of micelles. *Micelles* are aggregates of bile acids and fat molecules. Fats form the hydrophobic core, and the bile acids, being polar molecules, form the surface of the micelles, with the hydrophobic end pointing inward and the hydrophilic end pointing outward toward the aqueous medium. The center of the micelle also dissolves fat-soluble vitamins and cholesterol. Thus, free fatty acids, glycerides, and fat-soluble vitamins are kept in solution until they can be absorbed by the epithelial cell surface.

The process of digestion is completed by a number of enzymes present in the intestinal juice (succus entericus). Many of these enzymes are located on the brush border of the villi and digest food substances as they are being absorbed. Table 21-1 lists the principal digestive enzymes.

Two hormones are important in the regulation of intestinal digestion. Fat, in contact with the duodenal mucosa, causes the gallbladder to contract; this is mediated by the action of *cholecystokinin*. Products of partially digested proteins in contact with the duodenal mucosa stimulate the secretion of pancreatic juice rich in enzymes; this is mediated by the action of *pancreozymin*. Pancreozymin and cholecystokinin are now believed to be the same hormone having two different effects; it is called *CCK* (some textbooks still refer to this hormone as CCK-PZ). This hormone is produced by the duodenal mucosa.

Acid in contact with the intestinal mucosa causes the release of another hormone, *secretin*, and the amount released is proportional to the amount of acid flowing through the duodenum. Secretin stimulates the secretion of the bicarbonate-containing juice from the pancreas and bile from the liver. Secretin potentiates the action of CCK.

Segmental movements of the small intestine mix ingested materials with pancreatic, hepatobiliary, and intestinal secretions, and peristaltic movements propel the contents from one end to the other at a rate suitable for optimal absorption and continuing entry of gastric contents.

Absorption

Absorption is the transfer of the end products of carbohydrate, fat, and protein digestion (simple sugars, fatty acids, and amino acids) across the intestinal wall to the vascular and lymphatic circulation for use by the body cells. In addition, water, electrolytes, and vitamins are absorbed. Absorption of the various substances takes place by both active and passive transport mechanisms which are for the most part poorly understood.

Although many substances are absorbed throughout the entire length of the small bowel, there are principal sites of absorption for specific nutrients. Knowledge of these absorption sites is necessary in order to understand how disease of the intestine may cause specific nutritional deficiencies (see Fig. 21-2).

Iron and calcium are largely absorbed in the duodenum, and calcium requires vitamin D. The fat-soluble vitamins (A, D, E, and K) are absorbed in the duodenum and require bile salts. Folic acid and the other water-soluble vitamins are absorbed in the duodenum. The absorption of sugars, amino acids, and fats is largely completed by the time the chyme reaches the jejunum. The absorption of vitamin B_{12} takes place in the terminal ileum by a special transport mechanism requiring gastric intrinsic factor. Most of the bile acids released by the gallbladder into the duodenum to aid in the digestion of fats are reabsorbed in the terminal ileum and recirculated to the liver. This circuit is termed the *enterohepatic circulation of bile salts* and is very important in maintaining the bile pool. The bile acids or salts

TABLE 21-1

THE PRINCIPAL DIGESTIVE ENZYMES

Enzyme	Source	Substrate	Products	Optimal pH	Volume of secretion*
Salivary amylase (ptyalin)	Salivary glands	Starch	Maltose (a disaccharide and smaller carbohydrate polymer); minor physiologic role	6–7	1–1½ liters daily
Pepsin	Chief cells of stomach	Protein	Proteoses, peptones	1.5–2.5	2–4 liters daily
Gastric lipase	Stomach	Fat	Fatty acids, glycerides (minor physiologic role)	—	
Enterokinase	Duodenal mucosa	Trypsinogen	Trypsin		
Trypsin	Exocrine pancreas	Denatured proteins and polypeptides	Small polypeptides (also activates chymotrypsinogen to chymotrypsin)	8.0	0.6–0.8 liter daily
Chymotrypsin		Proteins and polypeptides	Small polypeptides	8.0	
Carboxypeptidases		Polypeptides	Smaller polypeptides (removes C-terminal amino acid)	—	
Nucleases		Nucleic acids	Nucleotides	—	
Pancreatic lipase		Fat	Glycerides, fatty acids, glycerol	8.0	
Pancreatic amylase		Starch	Disaccharides	6.7–7	
Bile acids (not an enzyme)	Liver	Unemulsified fats	Emulsified fats (formation of micelles; action is physical)	7.5	0.8–1.0 liter daily
Aminopeptidases	Intestinal glands	Polypeptides	Smaller polypeptides (removes N-terminal amino acid)	8.0	2–3 liters daily
Dipeptidase		Dipeptides	Amino acids	—	
Maltase		Maltose	Glucose	5.0-7	
Lactase		Lactose	Glucose + galactose ⎱ All mono-saccharides		
Sucrase		Sucrose	Glucose + fructose ⎰		
Intestinal lipase		Fat	Glycerides, fatty acids, glycerol	8.0	
Nucleotidase		Nucleotides	Nucleosides, phosphoric acid	8.0	

*All secretions are reabsorbed except about 100 ml water normally excreted in stool per day.

thus perform their action in relation to fat digestion many times before being excreted in the feces. Disease or resection of the terminal ileum may thus cause deficiency of bile salts and interference with fat digestion. The entry of large amounts of bile salts into the colon causes colonic irritation and diarrhea.

MALABSORPTION

Diseases of the small intestine are often accompanied by alterations in function manifested by the malabsorption syndrome. Malabsorption is the condition in which there is impaired intestinal mucosal absorption of single or multiple nutrients, resulting in their excretion in the stool.

It is important to distinguish between malabsorption and maldigestion since increased loss of nutrients in the stool may be a reflection of either process. Maldigestion is failure to absorb one or more nutrients due to inadequate digestion.

Causes of malabsorption syndrome

Table 21-2 lists some of the more common causes of the malabsorption syndrome. The basic causes of maldigestion are included in the first three categories. Gastrectomy, especially the Billroth II procedure, causes poor

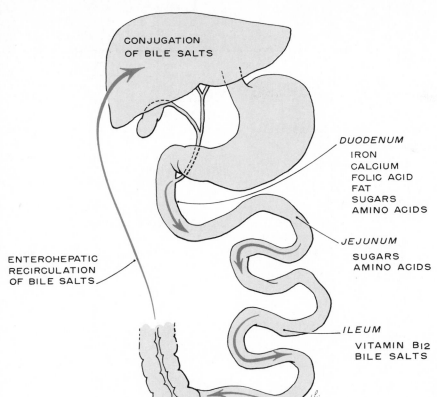

CONJUGATION
OF BILE SALTS

DUODENUM
IRON
CALCIUM
FOLIC ACID
FAT
SUGARS
AMINO ACIDS

JEJUNUM
SUGARS
AMINO ACIDS

ENTEROHEPATIC
RECIRCULATION
OF BILE SALTS

ILEUM
VITAMIN B₁₂
BILE SALTS

FIGURE 21-2
Absorption sites of the major nutrients and the enterohepatic recirculation of bile salts for reconjugation by the liver.

TABLE 21-2

SOME CAUSES OF THE MALABSORPTION SYNDROME

Prior gastric surgery
  Total gastrectomy
  Billroth II gastrectomy
  Pylorplasty
  Vagotomy

Pancreatic disorders
  Chronic pancreatitis
  Pancreatic cancer
  Cystic fibrosis
  Pancreatic resection
  Zollinger-Ellison
   syndrome

Hepatobiliary disease
  Biliary tract obstruction
  Cirrhosis and hepatitis
  Biliary fistula

Disease of the small intestine
  Primary disease of small
   bowel
    Nontropical sprue
    Tropical sprue
    Regional enteritis
    Massive bowel resection
    Bacterial overgrowth
     from stasis in afferent
     loop following Billroth
     II gastrectomy
  Ischemic disease of small
   bowel

Mesenteric
  atherosclerosis
  Chronic congestive
  heart failure

Disease of the small intestine
(continued)
  Infections and infestations of
  small bowel
   Acute enteritis
   Giardiasis
  Systemic disease involving
  small bowel
   Whipple's disease
   Amyloidosis
   Sarcoidosis
   Scleroderma

Hereditary disorders
  Primary lactase deficiency
Drug-induced malabsorption
  Neomycin
  Dilantin

mixing of chyme with gastric secretions. Hepatobiliary disease may result in insufficiency of intraluminal bile acids. Failure of the pancreas to produce or release sufficient enzymes may result from a number of pancreatic disorders. Failure of release of CCK, which stimulates pancreatic secretion, may occur in the Zollinger-Ellison syndrome as a result of excessive acidification of the duodenum or may result from disease of the intestinal mucosa itself, as in sprue. Disease of the terminal ileum or ileal resection for treatment of regional enteritis may cause insufficient bile salts by interfering with ileal resorption. Bacterial overgrowth in the duodenal stump (blind or afferent loop) causes vitamin B₁₂ malabsorption by utilizing this vitamin and causes fat maldigestion by deconjugating bile salts. Unconjugated bile salts are less effective in forming micelles and are absorbed less in the ileum. Pernicious anemia (a gastric disease) causes malabsorption of vitamin B₁₂ in the terminal ileum because of the lack of the intrinsic factor for transport. A hereditary lack of lactase causes selective malabsorption of lactose (a milk disaccharide) and is very common in American blacks. Mesenteric atherosclerosis (abdominal angina) may cause malabsorption and is a source of discomfort in elderly persons, but it is infrequently diagnosed. Chapter 23 will deal with pancreatic and hepatobiliary disorders, and this chapter will discuss a few of the more common intestinal disorders associated with malabsorption.

Signs and symptoms of the malabsorption syndrome

The signs and symptoms of malabsorption may be divided into two groups: those resulting from abnormal content in the intestinal lumen and those resulting from deficiency of dietary nutrients. Weight loss, diarrhea, steatorrhea, flatulence, and nocturia are the most common signs and symptoms and are all caused by abnormal intestinal luminal content. The signs and symptoms of malabsorption and their pathophysiologic basis are listed in Table 21-3.

Detection of malabsorption

Most of the tests useful in the diagnosis of malabsorption indicate the presence of malabsorption or maldigestion. Only a few of the tests suggest a specific diagnosis.

Stool fat

The oldest and most reliable test for documenting the presence of steatorrhea and thus malabsorption is the quantitative determination of stool fat. Normal persons excrete less than 6 g of fat in the stool per day. Fat excretion in excess of 6 g is considered excessive and is termed *steatorrhea*. In severe cases the stools are abnormal to the naked eye and appear pale, greasy, and frothy and may float. They may stick to the side of the toilet and not flush away easily.

A 72-hour stool collection for quantitative fat determination is routinely used to eliminate errors resulting from daily variations. Testing stools for fat is essential in the diagnosis of nontropical sprue, after extensive gastrectomy, and in other malabsorptive disorders. This test does not differentiate between maldigestion as in pancreatic disorders and malabsorption due to an intestinal disease such as nontropical sprue. However, there is a marked increase in undigested meat fibers in the stool in pancreatic insufficiency that is not usually present in nontropical sprue.

D-Xylose absorption test

D-Xylose is a relatively inert pentose which is absorbed in the proximal bowel without digestion, passes through the liver, and is then totally excreted by the kidneys. Measurement of the amount of D-xylose ex-

TABLE 21-3

SIGNS AND SYMPTOMS OF THE MALABSORPTION SYNDROME

Sign or symptom	Pathophysiology
Weight loss and generalized malnutrition	Impaired absorption of carbohydrate, fat, and protein → loss of calories
Diarrhea	Excess load of fluids and electrolytes introduced into colon which may exceed its absorptive capacity; bile acids and fatty acids in colon cause decreased colonic absorption of sodium and water and laxative effect from colonic irritation
Steatorrhea (bulky, frothy voluminous stools)	Excess fat content of feces
Flatulence, abdominal distention	Undigested lactose → fermentation → gas formation
	Undigested lactose → osmotic effect → shift of extracellular fluid into gut → diarrhea (may be due to primary lactase deficiency or secondary damage to brush border from intestinal lesions)
Nocturia	Delayed absorption and excretion of water (may be pooled in gut during day)
Weakness and easy fatigability	Anemia; electrolyte depletion due to diarrhea (hypokalemia, hypomagnesemia)
Edema	Impaired absorption of amino acids → protein depletion → hypoproteinemia
Amenorrhea	Protein depletion → secondary hypopituitarism
Anemia	Impaired absorption of iron, folic acid, and vitamin B_{12}
Glossitis, cheilosis	Deficiency of iron, folic acid, vitamin B_{12}, and other vitamins
Peripheral neuropathy	Deficiency of vitamin B_{12}
Bruising, bleeding tendency	Vitamin K malabsorption, hypoprothrombinemia
Bone pain	Calcium malabsorption → hypocalcemia; protein depletion → osteoporosis; vitamin D malabsorption → impaired calcium absorption
Tetany, paresthesias	Calcium malabsorption → hypocalcemia; magnesium malabsorption → hypomagnesemia
Eczema	Cause uncertain

creted in the urine therefore gives an indication of the absorptive capacity of the proximal bowel.

The test is carried out after the patient has fasted for 12 hours. At least 20 percent of D-xylose given orally should be excreted in the urine in 5 hours, provided renal function is normal. Excretion of less than this amount or blood levels of D-xylose lower than 30 mg per 100 ml indicates malabsorption. An abnormal D-xylose test is found most frequently in disorders affecting the proximal bowel, such as sprue. This test is normal in maldigestive disorders such as chronic pancreatitis.

Schilling test for vitamin B₁₂ absorption

The Schilling test is a valuable measure of vitamin B_{12} absorption and is frequently carried out in stages to determine the specific cause of the malabsorption. If urine collection is adequate, low excretion of ^{60}Co-tagged vitamin B_{12} indicates failure of absorption as a result of a lack of intrinsic factor (pernicious anemia), bacterial overgrowth in the proximal small bowel following Billroth II gastrectomy, diseased ileal mucosa as in regional enteritis, or pancreatic insufficiency. Correction of the malabsorption with intrinsic factor confirms intrinsic factor deficiency (often due to pernicious anemia). If the Schilling test returns to normal after antibiotic therapy, this helps to confirm the diagnosis of malabsorption as a result of bacterial overgrowth in the proximal bowel following Billroth II gastrectomy (the bacteria can actually take up vitamin B_{12}, thus preventing its absorption). Malabsorption of vitamin B_{12} as a result of pancreatic insufficiency may be corrected by the administration of pancreatic enzymes. Vitamin B_{12} malabsorption resulting from regional enteritis involving the terminal ileum is not corrected by any of the above measures.

Culture of duodenal and jejunal contents

The most reliable test for confirming the presence of bacterial overgrowth in the proximal bowel is aspiration and culture of the contents, but this is technically difficult and seldom used. The proximal small bowel normally contains less than 10^5 organisms per milliliter, and these are generally of the oropharyngeal variety. The most important mechanisms keeping the proximal bowel bacteriologically sterile is the normal peristalsis which sweeps bacteria distally, the gastric acid, and the secretion of immunoglobulin A (IgA) into the gut. Consequently, any condition which causes stasis of proximal intestinal contents, such as the blind loop following Billroth II surgery, may result in macrocytic anemia (because of utilization of vitamin B_{12} by organisms), diarrhea, and steatorrhea (because of deconjugation of bile salts by bacteria). Gastric achlorhydria and hypogammaglobulinemia are other conditions which may cause bacterial overgrowth.

Gastrointestinal barium x-ray studies

The x-ray appearance of the small bowel may be nonspecific or diagnostic. Characteristic features in the

malabsorption syndrome are the loss of the feathery pattern of the barium and increased flocculation of the barium with segmentation and clumping. This finding is common in sprue but is also found in other malabsorptive disorders. In regional enteritis, the ileal lumen may be narrowed (i.e., the "string sign").

Biopsy of the small intestine

The most useful test specific for the diagnosis of sprue is a biopsy of the intestinal mucosa, which reveals atrophy of villi. The biopsy may be performed through a capsule which is swallowed and located by x-ray; then the spring-activated knife is triggered.

PRIMARY SMALL INTESTINAL DISORDERS ASSOCIATED WITH MALABSORPTION

Nontropical sprue (celiac disease)

Idiopathic steatorrhea in adults and celiac disease in children are the most important causes of severe malabsorption in nontropical areas. Both these conditons are considered phases of the same disease. The disease is characterized by marked atrophy of the villi in the proximal small intestine induced by ingestion of gluten-containing foods.

Pathophysiology

Gluten is a high-molecular-weight protein found in rye, oats, barley, and especially wheat. It is, of course, found in bread, bread products, beer, and many other processed foods. Gluten and/or gluten breakdown products (especially gliadin) are toxic to patients with this disease. Symptoms disappear when gluten is withdrawn from the diet and reappear when it is reintroduced. The characteristic lesion of the bowel mucosa induced by gluten is blunting or loss of the villi and elongation of the crypts, which cause the mucosa to appear flat. The loss of villi causes a marked reduction of absorptive surface.

Although the mechanism of gluten toxicity is not understood, it has been suggested that these patients lack a specific peptidase which would normally detoxify a noxious peptide of gluten. This hypothesis is supported by the fact that there is a strong family tendency in occurrence. It has also been proposed that gluten or its metabolites cause a hypersensitivity reaction in the intestinal mucosa. This theory is supported by the fact that circulating antibodies to gliadin have been found in patients with this disease and that partial improvement of symptoms is provided by corticosteroid therapy.

Clinical features

Patients with nontropical sprue are presumably born with the disease tendency but may not develop symptoms for many years even though they include gluten in diet. Factors which precipitate the clinical onset are unknown. The onset generally occurs in infants between the ages of 6 months and 2 years and in adults between the ages of 20 and 50 years. The symptoms seldom begin during childhood or adolescence.

In infants, anorexia, irritability, and diarrhea with pale, bulky stools are soon followed by weight loss. If the infant is not treated, failure to grow is soon obvious. Lassitude, weakness, and diarrhea are the most common symptoms in adults, but patients may present with any of the signs and symptoms of malabsorption syndrome listed in Table 21-3. Adults frequently give a history suggesting sprue during childhood.

The diagnosis is established by evidence of malabsorption, typical small-bowel biopsy changes, and clinical improvement on a gluten-free diet.

Treatment

The treatment of nontropical sprue by a gluten-free diet is generally very successful, provided the patient adheres to the diet.

Tropical sprue

Tropical sprue occurs in such tropical regions as Puerto Rico, India, and the far east. The signs and symptoms are similar to those of nontropical sprue, and the biopsy changes are similar but less severe. The cause is not known. It is believed to be caused by an infectious agent, although one has not yet been identified. Most patients improve after treatment with broad-spectrum antibiotics (e.g., tetracycline).

Lactase deficiency

As indicated in the previous discussion, hydrolysis of disaccharides to monosaccharides occurs within the brush border of the intestinal mucosa. Deficiency of specific enzymes which hydrolyze disaccharides may be present as a result of a genetic defect or may be secondary to disease of the mucosa such as sprue.

Bayless and Christopher estimate that 70 percent of American blacks have a significant decrease in the activity of the enzyme lactase. Since lactose is the principal carbohydrate of milk, many persons showing milk intolerance will prove to be lactase-deficient. Orientals and African Bantus are also significantly affected, while only 5 percent of the white population is lactase-deficient.

Typical symptoms of lactase deficiency are abdominal cramps, bloating, and diarrhea following milk ingestion. The pathogenetic mechanism explaining the diarrhea is as follows. When unhydrolyzed lactose enters the large intestine, it produces an osmotic effect causing the insorption of water into the colonic lumen. Colonic bacteria also ferment the lactose, producing lactic and fatty acids which are irritating to the colon. The result is increased motility due to colonic irritation and an explosive diarrhea.

The condition is diagnosed by the history of milk intolerance and a positive lactose tolerance test. The fecal pH is also very acid (<6.0). Stool normally has a pH of 7.0 to 7.5.

Treatment consists of elimination of milk and milk products from the diet.

Postgastrectomy malabsorption

Malabsorption and weight loss are well-recognized features after a gastrectomy. They are the rule following total gastrectomy, common after the Billroth II procedure, and rare after the Billroth I procedure. Increased fat loss in the stools occurs in many patients after the Billroth II procedure, especially if the duodenal stump (afferent or blind loop) is long. The principal causes of the steatorrhea are the following: (1) poor mixing of food and enzymes due to rapid emptying of the gastric remnant (food particles too large for enzymes); (2) reduced pancreatic output because the duodenum is bypassed and has less stimulation by the acid chyme to release secretin and CCK; (3) stasis of intestinal contents in the afferent loop resulting in abnormal bacterial proliferation, which uses up vitamin B_{12} and deconjugates bile salts; (4) the loss of stomach reservoir function, which may result in a more rapid intestinal transit time with resultant diarrhea.

If the malabsorption is severe, the patient may develop anemia and symptoms as a result of any of the nutrient deficiencies listed in Table 21-3. The proper treatment of postgastrectomy malabsorption depends on identification of the mechanism responsible for the malabsorption. Broad-spectrum antibiotics (tetracycline) are given when the cause is bacterial overgrowth. Pancreatic enzyme therapy may be helpful with functional pancreatic deficiency. Smaller meals, low in carbohydrates and taken without fluids, may help delay rapid gastric emptying (dumping syndrome).

Regional enteritis (Crohn's disease)

Regional enteritis or Crohn's disease is a chronic, relapsing granulomatous inflammatory disease of the intestinal tract. Classically the terminal ileum is affected, although any portion of the gastrointestinal tract may be involved. It usually develops in young adults and affects men and women about equally.

The etiology of regional enteritis is unknown. Although no autoantibodies have been demonstrated, it has been speculated that regional enteritis may represent a hypersensitivity reaction or may be caused by an infectious agent which has not yet been identified. These theories are suggested by the granulomatous lesions, which are similar to those found in fungal and tubercular lesions of the lung.

There are some interesting similarities between regional enteritis and ulcerative colitis. Both are inflammatory diseases, although the lesions of each are distinct. Both diseases have extragastrointestinal manifestations, including uveitis, arthritis, and skin lesions which are identical. Some of these similarities and differences will be discussed under "Ulcerative Colitis" in Chap. 22.

Pathology

The terminal ileum is involved in regional enteritis in about 80 percent of the cases. In about 35 percent of the cases, lesions occur in the colon. The esophagus and stomach are less frequently affected. In some instances, "skip" lesions occur; that is, portions of diseased bowel are separated by areas of normal bowel a few inches or several feet long.

Lesions are believed to begin in lymph nodes next to the small bowel, with eventual obstruction of the lymphatic channels of drainage. The submucous coat of the intestine becomes markedly thickened as a result of the hyperplasia of the lymphoid tissue and lymphedema. With progress of the pathologic process the affected segment of the bowel becomes thickened to such a degree that it is as stiff as a garden hose (see Fig. 21-3). The lumen of the bowel may become markedly narrowed, so that it admits only a thin stream of barium, giving rise to the "string sign" on x-ray. The *entire* wall of the bowel is involved. The mucosa is commonly inflamed and ulcerated with grayish-white exudate.

FIGURE 21-3
Regional enteritis (Crohn's disease). The gut wall has been thickened by inflammation and scarring, causing marked narrowing of the lumen. At the top is more-normal mucosa. Extending downward are longitudinal ulcers which cross the transverse folds, giving the mucosa a cobblestone appearance. (Courtesy of Dr. Henry D. Appleman, Associate Professor of Pathology, University of Michigan.)

Clinical features

The signs and symptoms of regional enteritis vary a great deal according to whether the disease is early or late and according to what parts of the gastrointestinal tract are involved. Mild intermittent diarrhea (two to five stools per day), colicky pain in the lower abdomen, and malaise increasing over a period of years are usual. Sometimes there is blood in the stool. Some patients develop steatorrhea, weight loss, anemia, and other manifestations of malabsorption. Low-grade fever is common.

Certain complications are typical of regional enteritis. The development of stenosis may cause symptoms of vomiting and other signs of intestinal obstruction. An ulcerous lesion may perforate through the intestinal wall, causing peritonitis. More commonly the perforation is closed and fistulae are formed between loops of bowel, or less commonly involve the bladder or vagina. Ulcers, abscesses, and fistulae often occur in the perianal and perirectal regions. External fistulae to the anterior abdominal wall may also occur. High fever is usually as-

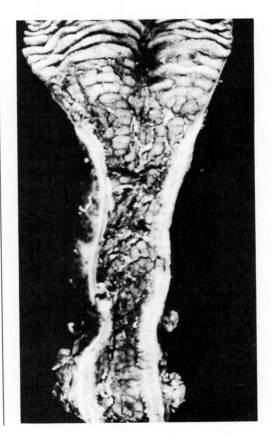

sociated with extensive inflammation or complications such as fistulae and abscesses.

Extragastrointestinal manifestations of the disease, such as arthritis, uveitis, and skin lesions, occur but are less frequent than they are in ulcerative colitis.

The diagnosis is established on the basis of the clinical presentation, the characteristic x-ray changes, and (in the case of colonic or rectal involvement) biopsy changes showing granulomatous lesions.

Treatment and prognosis

There is no specific or curative treatment for regional enteritis. The initial management of most patients is medical, supportive, and palliative, aimed at attaining remission of the disease. Corticosteroids, azathioprine, and sulfasalazine (Azulfidine) are used to promote remission and control suppurative complications. Anticholingeric drugs, such as propantheline bromide (Pro-Banthine), and antidiarrheal drugs, such as Metamucil and Lomotil, may help reduce cramping, abdominal pain, and diarrhea. Nutrient deficiencies and steatorrhea are treated by the appropriate replacements and a low-fat, low-residue diet.

Surgical treatment is generally avoided because recurrence and spread of the lesion is usual following surgical resection. Nevertheless, surgical intervention is usually necessary sometime during the course of the disease to treat complications.

When regional enteritis is characterized by an acute onset, about half the patients achieve a permanent spontaneous remission. However, regional enteritis has an insidious onset in 90 percent of patients, and the likelihood of permanent remission is only about 10 percent. Although the mortality as a direct result of the disease is low, most patients live out a miserable life with a remitting-relapsing course with intermittent hospitalization for complications.

APPENDICITIS

Appendicitis is the most common major surgical disease. Although it may occur at any age, it is most frequent in young adults. Prior to the era of antibiotics the mortality from this disease was high.

Pathogenesis

The vermiform appendix is the remnant of the apex of the cecum and has no known function in humans. It is a long, narrow tube (about 6 to 9 cm). It contains the appendicular artery which is an end artery.

In the usual position, it is located on the abdominal wall under McBurney's point. *McBurney's point* is located by drawing a line from the right anterior superior iliac spine to the umbilicus. The midpoint of this line locates the root of the appendix (see Fig. 21-4).

Appendicitis is an inflammation of the appendix involving all layers of the wall of the organ. The usual inciting event is obstruction of the lumen, usually by a *fecalith* (hardened stool). Obstruction of the outflow of mucous secretions results in swelling, infection, and ul-

FIGURE 21-4
McBurney's point, and several common positions of the appendix.

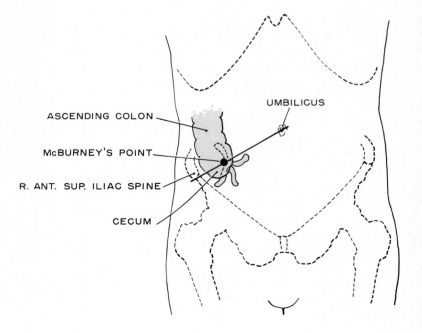

ASCENDING COLON

UMBILICUS

McBURNEY'S POINT

R. ANT. SUP. ILIAC SPINE

CECUM

ceration. The increased intraluminal pressure may cause occlusion of the appendicular end artery. If the condition is allowed to progress, necrosis, gangrene, and perforation are the usual results.

Clinical features

In the classic case of acute appendicitis, the initial symptoms are mild periumbilical pain or discomfort followed by anorexia, nausea, and vomiting. These symptoms generally develop over a period of 1 or 2 days. Within hours the pain shifts to the lower right quadrant, and there may be tenderness to palpation over McBurney's point. Later, muscle spasm and rebound tenderness may be present. A low-grade fever and moderate leukocytosis are usual findings. When rupture of the appendix occurs, there is commonly a temporary dramatic relief from pain.

Diagnostic problems

The diagnosis of even the classic case of appendicitis is complicated by the fact that many disorders present a similar clinical picture of an acute abdomen which must be differentiated from acute appendicitis. Some of these conditions are (1) acute gastroenteritis (probably the most common); (2) mesenteric lymphadenitis in children; (3) ruptured ectopic pregnancy; (4) mittelschmerz (pain due to rupture of ovarian follicle during ovulation); (5) inflammation of Meckel's diverticulum (persistence of a duct which, in the fetus, extends from the ileum to the umbilicus; present in about 2 percent of the population); and (6) regional enteritis.

Further diagnostic difficulties result from the fact that some individuals, particularly infants and the very elderly, deviate from the classic presentation. When there is doubt, it is usually safer to perform surgery, since the penalty of delay may be a ruptured appendix and peritonitis. Hospitalization is then prolonged, and some patients may die from the peritonitis.

Treatment

Once the diagnosis of appendicitis is made, the patient is prepared for surgery, and the appendix is promptly removed at any time of the day or night. If surgical removal is carried out before rupture and before the signs of peritonitis occur, the postsurgical course is generally uncomplicated and the patient is discharged from the hospital within a few days.

PERITONITIS

Inflammation of the peritoneum is a serious complication which commonly results from spread of infection from abdominal organs (e.g., appendicitis, salpingitis),

from rupture of the alimentary tract, or from penetrating abdominal wounds. The most frequent infecting organisms are the colon group in the case of a ruptured appendix, whereas staphylococci or streptococci are commonly introduced from without.

The initial reaction of the peritoneum to invasion by bacteria is the outpouring of a fibrinous exudate. Pockets of pus (abscesses) form between the fibrinous adhesions, which glue together the surrounding surfaces and thus localize the infection. The adhesions usually disappear when the infection disappears but may persist as fibrous bands which may later lead to intestinal obstruction.

If the infecting material is distributed widely over the surface of the peritoneum or if the infection spreads, generalized peritonitis may result. As generalized peritonitis develops, peristaltic activity diminishes until a state of paralytic ileus results; the intestine then becomes atonic and distended. Fluids and electrolytes are lost into the lumen of the bowel, leading to dehydration, shock, circulatory embarrassment, and oliguria. Adhesions may form between the distended loops of intestine and may impede the return of intestinal motility and result in intestinal obstruction.

Symptoms vary with the extent of the peritonitis, its severity, and the type of organisms responsible. The principal symptoms are abdominal pain (usually continuous); vomiting; and a tense, rigid, tender, and silent abdomen. Fever and leukocytosis are usual.

The prognosis is good in localized and mild forms of peritonitis and grave in generalized peritonitis due to virulent organisms.

The general principles of treatment include administration of a suitable antibiotic, decompression of the gastrointestinal tract by nasogastric or intestinal suction, intravenous repletion of fluid and electrolyte losses, removal of the septic focus (appendix, etc.) or other cause of inflammation, if possible, with drainage of pus to the outside, and measures to relieve pain.

INTESTINAL OBSTRUCTION

Intestinal obstruction may be defined as an interference (from whatever cause) with the normal flow of intestinal contents through the intestinal tract. Intestinal obstruction may be acute or chronic, partial or complete. Chronic bowel obstruction usually involves the colon as a result of a carcinoma and is slow in development. Most obstructions involve the small bowel. Complete obstruction of the small bowel is a very grave condition

and infarction (strangulation). Figure 21-5 illustrates some of the mechanical causes of bowel obstruction.

which requries early diagnosis and emergency surgical intervention if the patient is to survive.

There are two types of intestinal obstruction: (1) paralytic ileus (adynamic ileus) in which intestinal peristalsis is inhibited as a result of toxic or traumatic affectation of autonomic control of motility; and (2) mechanical obstruction, in which there is intraluminal obstruction or mural obstruction due to extrinsic pressure.

Mechanical obstruction is further classified as *simple mechanical obstruction*, in which there is only one point of obstruction, and *closed loop obstruction*, in which there are at least two points of obstruction. Because a closed loop obstruction cannot be decompressed, there is a rapid increase in intraluminal pressure leading to compression of blood vessels, ischemia,

Etiology

Nonmechanical obstruction or adynamic ileus commonly follows abdominal surgery in which there is reflex inhibition of peristalsis due to handling of the abdominal viscera. This reflex inhibition of peristalsis is often called paralytic ileus, although there is not complete paralysis of peristalsis. Another condition which is a common cause of adynamic ileus is peritonitis. Intestinal atony and gaseous distention accompany a wide variety of traumatic conditions; they especially may follow rib fracture and fracture of the spine.

The causes of mechanical obstruction are related to the age group affected and the site of the obstruction. About 50 percent of all obstructions occur in middle-aged and older people and result from adhesions from previous surgery. Malignant tumors and volvulus are the most common causes of obstruction of the large in-

FIGURE 21-5

Mechanical causes of bowel obstruction. (A) Strangulated inguinal hernia. (B) Volvulus of the sigmoid colon. (C) Ileocecal intussuception. (D) Enteroenteric intussusception due to pedunculated polyp.

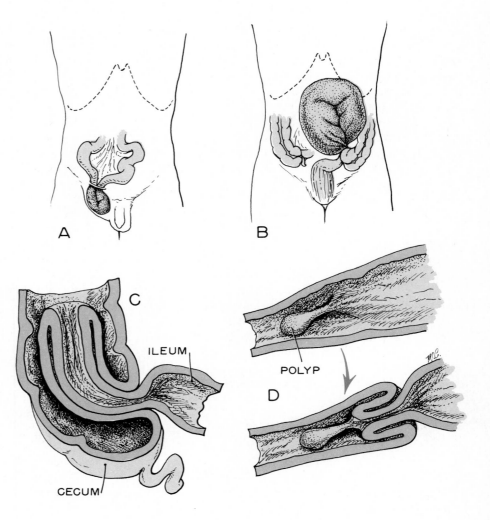

testine in middle-aged and older people. Cancer of the colon accounts for 80 percent of the obstructions. *Volvulus* is twisting of the intestine on itself. It occurs most frequently in elderly men and usually involves the sigmoid colon. Incarceration of a loop of bowel in an inguinal or femoral hernia is a very common cause of small bowel obstruction. *Intussusception* is invagination of one section of the intestine into the next section and is a cause of obstruction encountered almost exclusively in infants and young children. A common site for intussusception is invagination of the terminal ileum into the cecum. Foreign bodies and congenital anomalies are the other common causes of obstruction in infants and children.

Pathophysiology

The pathophysiologic events which occur following intestinal obstruction are similar, whether they result from mechanical or functional causes. The main difference is that in paralytic obstruction, peristalsis is inhibited from the start, while in mechanical obstruction, peristalsis is accentuated at first, is then intermittent, and is finally absent.

The obstructed bowel lumen becomes progressively distended with fluid and gas (70 percent from swallowed air) as a result of the effects of rising intraluminal pressure, which leads to a decreased flux of water and sodium ion from intestinal lumen to blood. Since about 8 liters of fluid are secreted into the gastrointestinal tract each day, nonabsorption can lead to rapid intraluminal accumulation. Vomiting and intestinal suction after treatment has begun are major sources of fluid and electrolyte loss. The net effect of these losses is contraction of the extracellular fluid compartment leading to shock—that is, hypotension, reduced cardiac output, decreased tissue perfusion, and metabolic acidosis. Continuing bowel distention results in a vicious cycle of decreased fluid absorption and increased fluid secretion into the bowel. The local effects of bowel distention are ischemia from distention and increased permeability due to necrosis, with absorption of bacterial toxins into the circulation.

Signs and symptoms

The cardinal symptoms of small bowel obstruction are pain, vomiting, absolute constipation, and abdominal distention. Pain is usually not as prominent as in adynamic ileus, although the abdomen may be tender. The pain is usually cramplike, coming in waves, and is usually located at the umbilicus. The frequency of vomiting varies with the site of obstruction. If the obstruction is high in the small bowel, vomiting is more prevalent than if the obstruction is in the ileum or large intestine. Absolute constipation is likely to occur early in large bowel obstruction, but flatus and feces may be passed early during the course of small bowel obstruction.

The abdominal x-ray is extremely important in the diagnosis of intestinal obstruction. Mechanical obstruction of the small bowel is characterized by air in the small intestine but not in the colon, while colonic obstruction is characterized by gas throughout the colon but with little or no gas in the small intestine. When the plain films are inconclusive, a barium x-ray may be performed to locate the site of obstruction.

Treatment

Treatment principles for bowel obstruction include correction of fluid and electrolyte imbalances, relief of distention and vomiting by intubation and decompression, control of peritonitis and shock if present, and removal of the obstruction to restore normal bowel continuity and function.

Many cases of adynamic ileus are cured by tubal decompression alone. A small bowel obstruction is much more serious and rapid in development than colonic obstruction. Mortality for simple obstruction is 1 to 2 percent, provided surgical intervention occurs soon enough. Delay in surgical intervention or the development of strangulation or other complications raises the mortality to about 35 or 40 percent.

QUESTIONS

Small intestine

Directions: Answer the following questions on a separate sheet of paper.

1. Why is the gastrointestinal mucosa especially vulnerable to side effects such as ulceration and bleeding from the administration of such cytotoxic drugs as cyclophosphamide (Cytoxan) and mercaptopurine?

2. Describe the function of bile in the digestion and absorption of fats and fat-soluble vitamins.

3. Differentiate between maldigestion and malabsorption.

4. Describe the appearance and characteristics of stool from a patient which would cause you to suspect steatorrhea.

5. What are the characteristics of regional enteritis which have led theorists to suspect that hypersensitivity might be responsible in its pathogenesis?

6. Name the three structures which greatly increase the absorptive surface area of the small bowel.

7. List four causes of steatorrhea in a patient following total gastrectomy or gastrojejunostomy.

8. Describe the pathophysiologic events leading to death from small bowel obstruction. Explain why early diagnosis and surgical intervention are important in mechanical obstruction of the small bowel.

Directions: Fill in the blanks with the correct word(s) in the following questions.

9. The major artery supplying the small bowel (except the duodenum) is the _____ artery.

10. The _____ sphincter controls the entry of chyme into the small bowel, and the _____ valve controls the exit of digested material into the large intestine.

11. The fanlike fold of peritoneum which suspends the jejunum and ileum from the posterior abdominal wall is called the _____.

12. The fold of peritoneum which drapes over the small bowel like an apron is called the _____. This structure has sometimes been called the policeman of the abdomen, because one of its important functions is to localize _____.

13. The musculofibrous band extending from the diaphragm to the duodenojejunal juncture which acts as a support for this portion of the small bowel is called the _____ of _____.

14. The structures which are responsible for giving the barium x-ray of the small bowel a feathery appearance are the _____.

15. The structures which account for the velvetlike appearance of the small bowel are the _____.

16. The source of the succus entericus is the _____ of _____.

17. The lymphatic vessel of the villus where fat absorption takes place is called the central _____.

18. McBurney's point is located at the midpoint on a line between the _____ and the anterior superior _____ spine. It is the point where the _____ is normally located.

Directions: Match each of the following enzymes in col. A with its secretory source in col. B and with its substrate in col. C.

Column A	Column B	Column C
19. ___ Lactase	a. Duodenal mucosa	e. Denatured proteins and polypeptides
20. ___ Ptyalin	b. Exocrine pancreas	
21. ___ Enterokinase	c. Salivary glands	f. Lactose
22. ___ Trypsin	d. Intestinal glands	g. Starch
		h. Trypsinogen

Match each of the following nutrients in col. A with its major site of absorption in col. B. (Items may be used more than once.)

Column A	Column B
23. ___ Iron	a. Stomach
24. ___ Vitamin B_{12}	b. Duodenum
	c. Duodenum and jejunum
25. ___ Sugars	d. Terminal ileum
26. ___ Fats	e. Large intestine
27. ___ Amino acids	
28. ___ Bile salts	

Match each of the following symptoms of malabsorption in col. A to its pathophysiologic basis in col. B.

Column A	Column B
29. ___ Edema	a. Impaired absorption of amino acids
30. ___ Peripheral neuropathy	b. Vitamin K malabsorption
31. ___ Bleeding tendency	c. Deficiency of vitamin B_{12}
32. ___ Diarrhea	d. Bile salts in colon
33. ___ Tetany, paresthesias	e. Lactase deficiency
34. ___ Nocturia	f. Calcium malabsorption
	g. Delayed absorption of fluid in gut

Match each of the following terms related to bowel obstruction in col. A with the proper descriptive statements from col. B.

Column A

35. _____ Adhesions
36. _____ Volvulus
37. _____ Simple bowel obstruction
38. _____ Strangulated hernia
39. _____ Intussusception

Column B

a. Twisting of a loop of bowel on itself
b. Only one point of obstruction
c. Fibrous bands which form as a result of a fibrinous exudate from peritoneum
d. Obstruction of the blood supply to a loop of bowel protruding through muscle wall
e. Almost exclusively a condition of infants and young children
f. Commonly occurs in the sigmoid colon in elderly men
g. Telescoping of the bowel
h. Most common cause of bowel obstruction in adults

Match each of the following descriptions in col. A with the correct entity from col. B.

Column A

40. _____ Usually responds to broad spectrum antibiotics
41. _____ During exacerbation is associated with very low D-xylose excretion
42. _____ Usually responds to gluten withdrawal
43. _____ Characterized by atrophy and flattening of villi

Column B

a. Nontropical sprue (celiac disease)
b. Tropical sprue
c. Both
d. Neither

Directions: Circle the letter preceding each item below that correctly answers the question. Only one answer is correct, unless otherwise noted.

44. Which of the following hormones has the primary effect of stimulating the bicarbonate component of the pancreatic juice?

a. Gastrin   b. Cholecystokinin   c. Pancreozymin   d. Secretin

45. Hydrolysis of lactose into glucose and galactose takes place:
a. In the stomach   b. Along the brush border
c. Within the lumen of the duodenum
d. Within the lumen of the jejunum

46. Mechanisms which normally keep the proximal bowel relatively sterile include which of the following? (More than one answer may be correct.)
a. Peristalsis   b. Acid chyme entering duodenum
c. Alkalinity of the pancreatic bicarbonate secretion   d. Secretion of IgA into the gut

47. The length of the small bowel in the living person is about:
a. 22 ft   b. 12 ft   c. 10 ft   d. 6 ft

48. The greatest portion of gastrointestinal gas (air) is derived from:
a. Food breakdown   b. Bacterial fermentation
c. Swallowed air

49. The diagnosis of gluten-induced enteropathy must include:
a. History of weight loss   b. Steatorrhea   c. Abnormal small bowel biopsy   d. Abnormal D-xylose excretion

50. Administration of intrinsic factor caused the Schilling test to return to normal after an initial low value in a 56-year-old woman. The probable cause of this patient's problem is:
a. Bacterial overgrowth in the proximal small bowel   b. Regional enteritis   c. Chronic pancreatitis   d. Atrophic gastritis

51. The afferent loop syndrome is characterized by: (More than one answer may be correct.)
a. Malabsorption of vitamin B_{12} b. Megaloblastic anemia   c. Heavy growth of colonic bacteria
d. Amelioration with administration of broad-spectrum antibiotics

52. The earliest sign on examination in acute appendicitis is:
a. Periumbilical hyperesthesia   b. Abdominal distention   c. Localized tenderness in the lower right quadrant   d. Rebound tenderness

53. Which of the following conditions may present difficulties in differentiation from acute appendicitis? (More than one answer may be correct.)
a. Acute gastroenteritis   b. Ruptured ectopic pregnancy   c. Regional enteritis   d. Inflammation of Meckel's diverticulum   e. Mittelschmerz

54. Bile salts are conjugated in the liver and deconjugated by bacteria in conditions of duodenal stasis.
    a. First statement is true but second is false
    b. First statement is false but second is true
    c. Both statements are true   d. Both statements are false

55. Lactase deficiency is: (More than one answer may be correct.)
    a. Always congenital   b. Only found in the western hemisphere   c. Common in the American blacks   d. A brush border disease   e. Relatively uncommon in Caucasians

56. The secretion of CCK is stimulated by: (More than one answer may be correct.)
    a. Contact of the acid chyme with the duodenal mucosa   b. Fat in contact with the duodenal mucosa   c. Alkaline chyme in contact with duodenal mucosa   d. Denatured proteins in contact with the duodenal mucosa

57. Which of the following may be a cause of intestinal malabsorption? (More than one answer may be correct.)
    a. Acute enteritis   b. Chronic hepatitis
    c. Whipple's disease   d. Mesenteric atherosclerosis

Directions: Circle T if the statement is true and F if it is false.

58. T   F   The lumen of the bowel is open and the obstruction is functional in paralytic ileus.

59. T   F   Parasympathetic fibers supplying the small bowel relay pain.

60. T   F   The daily total volume of the digestive secretions is about 8 liters.

61. T   F   Most of the enzymes of the succus entericus would be inactivated by a pH of 5.0.

62. T   F   Two factors which account for frequent obstruction and ischemic necrosis of the appendix are its narrow lumen ending in a blind pouch and its blood supply from an end artery.

CHAPTER 22

LARGE INTESTINE

OBJECTIVES

At the completion of this chapter you should be able to:

1. Identify the gross anatomic features and subdivisions of the large bowel.
2. Compare the small and large intestine with respect to size, length, sphincter control, morphologic layers, motility, and digestive and absorptive functions.
3. Describe the blood supply and innervation of the large bowel.
4. Identify the most important function of the large bowel.
5. Describe the actions of colonic bacteria.
6. Identify the source and components of flatus.
7. Explain the function of haustral churning and mass peristalsis.
8. Describe the act of defecation, including reflex and voluntary control mechanisms and factors which might interfere with control.
9. List five common anorectal disorders.
10. Explain why repeated suppression of the defecation reflex often results in chronic constipation.
11. List the important diagnostic procedures for detection of large bowel disease.
12. Define diverticulosis and diverticulitis.
13. Describe the probable pathogenetic mechanism involved in diverticulosis, including the influence of dietary factors.
14. Explain why a barium enema x-ray is generally contraindicated during an attack of acute diverticulitis.
15. Discuss the signs, symptoms, comparisons, and treatment of diverticulosis and diverticulitis.
16. Compare Crohn's disease and ulcerative colitis with respect to their pathologic and clinical characteristic features.
17. Describe the pathologic and clinical features of acute fulminating, chronic intermittent, and chronic continuous ulcerative colitis.
18. Describe the most common complications of ulcerative colitis (including three serious ones) and their treatment.
19. Describe the following types of colonic polyps: pedunculated, juvenile,

familial, and villous adenoma in terms of gross and microscopic characteristics, common sites, relative frequency, malignant potential, and treatment.

20. Rank cancer of the colon and rectum as a cause of gastrointestinal cancer and as a cause of all cancer deaths in men and women.

21. Explain why digital or proctosigmoidoscopic rectal examination is important in middle-aged and older individuals.

22. List three routes of metastasis for cancer of the large bowel.

23. Identify three predisposing factors in the pathogenesis of cancer of the large bowel.

24. Relate Burkitt's hypothesis concerning the relationship of diet to the development of cancer of the large bowel.

25. Contrast the clinical features of right- and left-sided cancer of the bowel.

26. Describe the pathologic and clinical features of internal and external hemorrhoids, including site, frequency in population, predisposing factors, symptoms, complications, and treatment.

27. Differentiate between first-, second-, and third-degree internal hemorrhoids.

28. Explain the relationship of anal fissures to the skin tags of chronic external hemorrhoids.

29. Identify four common sites of anorectal abscess formation, common causes, infecting organisms, and treatment.

30. Explain the relationship of anal cryptitis and Crohn's disease to anorectal fistulae.

31. Describe the treatment of anorectal abscesses and fistulae.

ANATOMIC AND PHYSIOLOGIC CONSIDERATIONS

The large intestine is a hollow muscular tube about 5 ft in length extending from the cecum to the anal canal. The diameter of the large intestine is noticeably larger than that of the small intestine. Its average diameter is about 2.5 in, but its diameter decreases toward the lower end of the tube.

The large intestine is divided into the cecum, colon, and rectum as illustrated in Fig. 22-1. The *cecum*, containing the ileocecal valve and with the appendix attached to its apex, comprises the first 2 or 3 in of the large intestine. The colon is subdivided into the *ascending, transverse, descending,* and *sigmoid* colon. The points at which the colon makes a sharp turn at the right and left upper abdomen are called the *hepatic* and *splenic flexures,* respectively. The sigmoid colon begins at the level of the iliac crest and describes an S-shaped curve. The lower part of the curve bends toward the left

as it joins the rectum and is the anatomic reason for placing a patient on the left side when giving an enema. In this position, gravity aids the flow of water from the rectum into the sigmoid flexure. The last major portion of the large intestine is called the *rectum* and extends from the sigmoid colon to the *anus* (opening to the outside of the body). The terminal inch of the rectum is called the *anal canal* and is guarded by internal and external sphincter muscles. The length of the rectum and anal canal is approximately 5.9 in (15 cm).

The large intestine exhibits throughout most of its length the four morphologic layers seen in the remainder of the gut. Several features, however, are peculiar to the large intestine. The longitudinal muscle coat is incomplete, being collected into three bands called the *taenia coli.* The taenia coalesce in the distal sigmoid, so that the rectum has a complete longitudinal muscle coat. The taenia are shorter than the intestine, causing it to pucker and form small sacs called *haustra.* The *epiploic appendages* are small fat-filled sacs of peritoneum

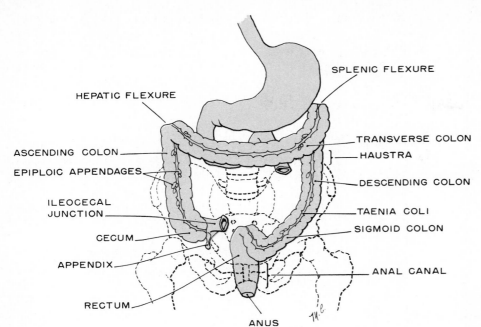

HEPATIC FLEXURE

SPLENIC FLEXURE

ASCENDING COLON

EPIPLOIC APPENDAGES

ILEOCECAL JUNCTION

CECUM

APPENDIX

RECTUM

ANUS

TRANSVERSE COLON

HAUSTRA

DESCENDING COLON

TAENIA COLI

SIGMOID COLON

ANAL CANAL

FIGURE 22-1
Anatomic relationships of the large intestine.

attached along the taenia. The mucosal layer of the large intestine is much thicker than that of the small intestine and contains no villi or rugae. The crypts of Lieberkühn (intestinal glands) are deeper and have more goblet cells than those of the small intestine.

The large intestine is clinically divided into right and left halves based on the blood supply. The superior mesenteric artery supplies the right half (cecum, ascending colon, and proximal two-thirds of the transverse colon), and the inferior mesenteric supplies the left half (distal one-third of the transverse colon, descending and sigmoid colon, and proximal part of the rectum). Additional blood supply to the rectum is provided by the middle sacral and middle and inferior hemorrhoidal arteries, which arise from the abdominal aorta and internal iliac arteries.

Venous return from the colon and superior rectum is via the superior and inferior mesenteric veins and superior hemorrhoidal veins, which become a part of the portal system delivering blood to the liver. The middle and inferior hemorrhoidal veins drain into the iliac veins and consequently are part of the systemic circulation. There are anastomoses between the superior and the middle and inferior hemorrhoidal veins, so that increased portal pressure may cause backflow into these veins, resulting in hemorrhoids.

The nerve supply to the large intestine is provided by the autonomic nervous system, with the exception that the external sphincter is under voluntary control. Parasympathetic fibers travel via the vagus to the mid-transverse colon, and pelvic nerves of sacral origin supply the distal part. Sympathetic fibers leave the spinal cord via the splanchnic nerve to reach the colon. Sympathetic stimulation causes inhibition of secretion and

contraction and stimulates the rectal sphincter, while parasympathetic stimulation has the opposite effects.

The large intestine has a variety of functions all related to the final processing of intestinal contents. The most important function is the absorption of water and electrolytes, which is largely completed in the right side of the colon. The sigmoid colon functions as a reservoir for the dehydrated fecal mass until defecation takes place.

The colon absorbs about 600 ml of water per day compared to about 8000 ml absorbed by the small intestine. The absorption capacity of the large intestine, however, is about 2000 ml/day. When this amount is exceeded by excessive delivery of fluid from the ileum, diarrhea results. The final daily excreted feces weighs about 200 g, of which about 75 percent is water. The remainder is made up of nonabsorbed food residue, bacteria, desquamated epithelial cells, and unabsorbed minerals.

Very little digestion, if any, takes place in the large intestine. The secretion of the large intestine contains much mucus, shows an alkaline reaction, and contains no enzymes. The mucus acts as a lubricant and protects the mucosa (see Fig. 6-3). In inflammatory conditions of the bowel, greatly increased mucus secretion of the bowel may be responsible for protein loss in the stool.

The bacteria of the large intestine perform many functions, including the synthesis of vitamin K and of several vitamins of the B group. There is constant putrefaction of whatever proteins are left as a result of not having been digested in the small intestine. The list of simple substances resulting from putrefaction is long and includes various peptides, amino acids, indole, skatole, phenol, and fatty acids. NH_3, CO_2, H_2, H_2S, and

CH_4 are the most important gases produced. Some of these substances are given off in the feces, while others are absorbed and carried to the liver, where they are changed to less toxic compounds and excreted in the urine.

About 1000 ml of "gas" or flatus is normally expelled from the anus each day. An excess of gas occurs with aerophagia (excessive swallowing of air, common in neurotic persons as well as in a variety of upper GI tract diseases) and when there is an increase in intraluminal gas production, which is commonly related to the diet. "Gassy foods" are those with a high content of indigestible carbohydrates. The colon bacteria attack the carbohydrates and release H_2, CO_2, and in some persons, CH_4. Presumably the gas production as a result of eating beans is due to the presence of a carbohydrate component.

In general, the movements of the large intestine are slow. A movement characteristic of the large intestine is *haustral churning*. The pouches or haustra become distended, and from time to time the circular muscles contract and cause them to empty. The movements are not progressive but cause the contents to move back and forth in a kneading action, thus allowing time for absorption. There are two types of propulsive peristalsis: (1) slow, irregular contractions which arise in a proximal segment and move forward, obliterating a few haustra; and (2) *mass peristalsis*, which is a contraction involving a large segment of the colon. Mass peristalsis moves the fecal mass from the right or transverse colon to the sigmoid colon. It occurs two or three times a day and is stimulated by the gastrocolic reflex after eating, particularly following the first meal of the day.

The act of defecation is a reflex involving the voluntary and involuntary muscles of the anal canal and terminal bowel. Figure 22-2 illustrates the basic anatomy of the rectum and anus. The entry of feces into the rectum distends its walls and stimulates mass peristaltic movements of the bowel. The principal reflex center is in the parasympathetic nerve center in the second to fourth sacral segments of the spinal cord. As the balloon-shaped rectum contracts, the levator ani muscle relaxes, causing the anorectal ring and angle to disappear. The internal and external spincter muscles relax as the anus is pulled up over the fecal mass. The act of defecation is facilitated by an increase in intraabdominal pressure brought about by voluntary contraction of the chest muscles on a closed glottis and simultaneous con-

traction of the abdominal muscles (Valsalva's maneuver or straining). Parasympathetic fibers reach the rectum via the pelvic splanchnic nerves and are responsible for contraction of the rectum and relaxation of the internal sphincter. Voluntary inhibition of defecation can be effected by contraction of the levator ani and external sphincter muscles.

The rectum and anus are the site of the most common diseases known to humans. A common cause of simple constipation is failure to empty the rectum when mass peristalsis occurs. When defecation is not completed the rectum relaxes and the desire to defecate disappears. Water continues to be absorbed from the fecal mass, causing it to become hard, so that subsequent defecation is more difficult. Excessive straining at the stool causes congestion of the internal and external hemorrhoidal veins and is one of the important causes of hemorrhoids (varicose veins of the rectum). Incontinence of stool may result from damage to sphincter muscles or from damage to the spinal cord. The anorectal area is a frequent site of abscesses and fistulae. The colon and rectum are the most frequent sites of cancer of the gastrointestinal tract.

DIAGNOSTIC PROCEDURES

Diagnosis of pathology associated with the large intestine relates mainly to symptoms associated with elimination. Constipation, diarrhea, alteration in size or color of stool, or the presence of blood in the stools are all important symptoms which focus attention on the colon and rectum. Pain of colonic origin is lateralized to the left or right sides of the abdomen, as opposed to pain of small intestinal origin, which is usually periumbilical.

History and physical exam are important diagnostic

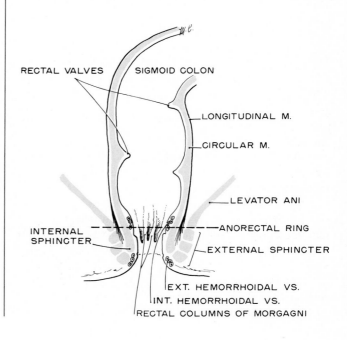

FIGURE 22-2
Anatomy of the rectum and anus.

procedures. Abdominal masses may be palpated, and digital examination is very important, since about half of all rectal carcinomas are within reach of the examining finger. Examination of the stools, sigmoidoscopy, and radiologic exam are required for a complete assessment in cases of suspected colonic disease.

The barium enema x-ray is the most common test carried out on patients with disorders of the colon. Preparation or prior cleansing of the intestine is important for a proper examination, but in the presence of an obstructing lesion or active ulcerative colitis, the use of strong cathartics may be hazardous or life-threatening to the patient. Neoplasms, strictures, diverticulosis, and polyps may all be visualized. The cecum and ascending colon may be visualized 3 to 5 hours after a barium swallow. The barium enema x-ray should always precede the barium swallow.

Direct visualization of the terminal 25 cm of the large intestine is possible through the rigid proctosigmoidoscope. Sixty percent of all the tumors of the large intestine can be visualized directly with this instrument. In addition to visual inspection of the area, bacteriologic, parasitologic, and cytologic studies can be made on washings through the instrument, and biopsy of suspicious lesions is easy to perform. The flexible fiberoptic colonoscope allows visualization and biopsy of lesions of the entire colon. Experienced examiners may be able to insert the instrument as far as the terminal ileum.

DIVERTICULAR DISEASE OF THE COLON

Diverticulosis is a condition of the colon characterized by herniation of the mucosa through the muscularis to form flask-shaped saccules. If one or more of the saccules become inflamed, the condition is called diverticulitis.

Pathophysiology

The overall incidence of diverticulosis is high; it affects about 10 percent of the population, according to most necropsy studies. It is rare below the age of 35 years but increases with age, so that at age 85 two-thirds of the population are afflicted.

The most common site for diverticula to occur is in the sigmoid colon, which is involved in about 90 percent of the cases.

Although the etiology of diverticulosis is unknown, recent motility and pressure studies have done much to support the possibility that diverticular disease may result from a disordered motility pattern of the colon. Figure 22-3 illustrates the normal motility pattern in the colon and the proposed pathogenetic mechanism of diverticulosis. Diverticula-bearing zones of the colon are prone to strong contractions of the circular muscles, which build up very high intraluminal pressures. It seems likely that these high pressures are responsible for herniations of the mucosa through the muscle coat, which become diverticula. The usual position for the diverticula is at the mesenteric attachment of the colon, where the entry of blood vessels weakens the wall. The pressure changes in diverticular disease are similar to those found in spastic or irritable colon syndrome, which is believed by many to have a basis in anxiety and emotional tension.

A factor of even greater importance in the etiology of diverticular disease relates to the amount of roughage in the diet. Diverticulosis is rare in those who eat a diet high in roughage but is very common in Europeans and North Americans (of all races) who eat a low-roughage diet. The tension or strain on the wall of a hollow organ is related to the pressure within and to the diameter of the organ. If a tube such as the colon is habitually of narrow bore (as the result of a low-fiber diet), then the strain on the wall from a buildup of pressure will be greater than would be the case if it were filled with feces.

Clinical features and complications

The majority of patients with diverticulosis suffer no symptoms, and the problem will remain unidentified unless a barium enema x-ray is performed in the investigation of some unrelated condition. When diverticula are discovered, it is important for the physician to rule out carcinoma. This differentiation is made by the x-ray appearance, colonoscopic exam, and biopsy. A barium enema x-ray is dangerous during an attack of acute diverticulitis because of the danger of perforation.

In many patients, symptoms are mild and consist of flatulence, intermittent diarrhea or constipation, and discomfort in the lower left quadrant of the abdomen. These symptoms can usually be attributed to the irritable colon syndrome which may precede the development of diverticulosis in some patients.

The complications of diverticular disease are the result of acute or chronic diverticulitis, which may result in bleeding, perforation and peritonitis, abscess and fistula formation, or intestinal obstruction from stricture (see Fig. 22-4).

In the case of acute diverticulitis, there are fever, leukocytosis, and pain and tenderness in the lower left quadrant of the abdomen. During a bout of acute inflammation, bleeding may occur from vascular granulation tissue and is usually minor. In rare instances, bleeding may be massive as a result of erosion of the large penetrating blood vessel next to the diverticula. Bleed-

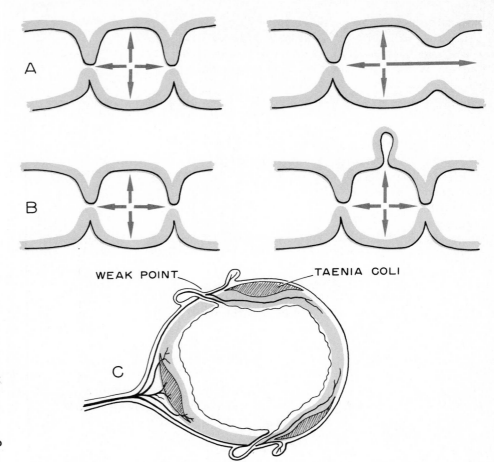

FIGURE 22-3
Pathogenesis of diverticular disease. (A) Normal motility pattern. (B Abnormal motility pattern in which there is failure of relaxation and buildup of high intraluminal pressure resulting in the formation of a diverticulum. (C) Cross section of colon showing that the weak point in the circular muscle is where a blood vessel pierces the muscle. Herniation of the lining mucosa and the formation of diverticuli develop at these points.

WEAK POINT   TAENIA COLI

C

ing is usually treated conservatively, but on rare occasions a bowel resection has been necessary.

Sometimes, acutely inflamed diverticula rupture. If the perforation is small, the result may be abscess formation next to the perforated diverticulum. If the perforation is large, fecal material may enter the peritoneum and cause a most severe form of peritonitis with a high mortality. Symptoms of perforation are similar to those of perforated ulcer except that pain, rigidity, and tenderness are most marked in the lower left quadrant.

Chronic diverticulitis applies to a bowel which is subjected to repeated attacks of inflammation. The result may be fibrosis and adhesions of the surrounding structures. When chronic inflammation has caused sig-

FIGURE 22-4
Complications of diverticulitis.

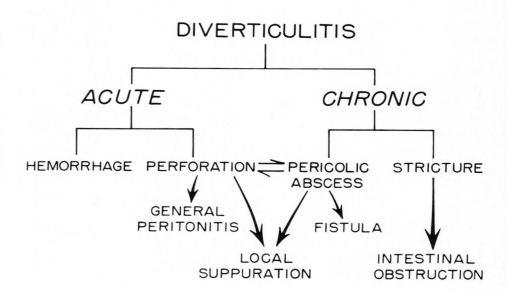

TABLE 22-1

DIFFERENTIATING FEATURES OF ULCERATIVE COLITIS AND CROHN'S DISEASE

Characteristic feature	Ulcerative colitis	Crohn's disease
Depth of involvement	Mucosa and submucosa	Transmural
Granulomatous inflammatory response	Rare	Common
Rectal involvement	95%	50%
Small bowel involvement	Usually normal	80%
Right colon involvement	Occasional	Frequent
Distribution of lesion	Continuous with rectum	Discontinuous "skip" lesions
Inflammatory mass	Rare	Commonly palpable
Diarrhea	Common	Common
Rectal bleeding	Common, continuous	Rare
Internal fistulae	Rare	Common
Anal abscess	Occasional	Common
Anorectal fissures and fistulae	Rare	Common
Cobblestone appearance of mucosa	Unusual (pseudopolyps, granular, shaggy)	Common
Toxic megacolon	Occasional	Rare
Malignant potential	High after 10 years	Very low
Extragastrointestinal manifestation (arthritis, eye and skin involvement, etc.)	Occasional	Less frequent than in ulcerative colitis
Strictures	Occasional, mild	Common
Finger clubbing	Rare	Common
Relative frequency	Five times more common than Crohn's disease	
Familial and Jewish association	Yes	Yes
Autoantibodies	Frequent	Not found

nificant narrowing of the lumen, chronic incomplete bowel obstruction may result, giving rise to symptoms of constipation, ribbonlike stools, intermittent diarrhea, and abdominal distention. The final obstructive picture may be precipitated by a superimposed acute attack, leading to a pericolic abscess which narrows the already occluded lumen. A fistula may also form as a complication of a pericolic abscess. The most common type is the vesicocolic fistula. The flow is always from the colon to the bladder, and the complaint is *pneumaturia*, or the passage of air bubbles in the urine.

Treatment

If diverticula are discovered incidentally and the patient is asymptomatic, they are not generally treated. However, 90 percent of the cases of diverticulitis are treated medically. Mild cases without signs of perforation are treated by a liquid diet, stool softeners, bed rest, and a broad-spectrum antibiotic. Antibiotics effective against gram-negative anaerobic bacteria may be given to patients with suspected perforation or abscess. Incision and drainage of abscesses may be necessary.

Surgical intervention is only needed for severe and extensive disease or in the event of complications. The essential surgical treatment is resection of the diseased colon with anastomosis to restore continuity. In the absence of complications the surgery may be carried out in one stage. In other cases the surgeon may perform a temporary colostomy (diversion of feces to the abdominal surface). Anastomosis and closure is then carried out at a later date.

INFLAMMATORY DISEASE OF THE LARGE INTESTINE

Chronic inflammatory disease of the large bowel is divided into two major entities—nonspecific ulcerative colitis and Crohn's disease of the large bowel (granulomatous colitis). Although these two conditions have many features in common, there are enough differences to separate them into two distinct clinical entities. Table 22-1 lists the differentiating features of these two diseases. There are enough overlapping features to lead some investigators to believe that both these diseases may represent variations in response to the same etiologic agent.

Ulcerative colitis

Ulcerative colitis is a nonspecific inflammatory disease of the colon generally following a prolonged course with alternating periods of remissions and exacerbations. Abdominal pain, diarrhea, and rectal bleeding are the cardinal signs and symptoms. The essential lesion is an inflammatory reaction of the subepithelial zone developing at the base of the crypts of Lieberkühn, which may eventually produce ulceration of the mucosa. The peak onset of the disease is between the ages of 20 and 40 years, and it is equally distributed between the sexes. The incidence of ulcerative colitis is about 1 per 10,000 white adults per year. Crohn's disease is about one-fifth as common. Both diseases are less common in nonwhites.

Etiology and pathogenesis

The etiology of ulcerative colitis, like that of Crohn's disease, is unknown. Genetic factors seem to be involved in the etiology, since there is a definite familial relationship between ulcerative colitis, Crohn's disease, and ankylosing spondylitis.

There is also evidence to suggest that autoimmunity is involved in the pathogenesis of ulcerative colitis. Anticolon antibodies have been found in the serum of patients with this disease. Lymphocytes from patients with ulcerative colitis damage normal colon epithelial cells in tissue culture.

The psychological aspects of ulcerative colitis have been the subject of much controversy. It now seems that psychological stress only plays a secondary role in provoking overt disease.

The initial pathologic lesion is confined to the mucosal layer and consists of abscess formation in the crypts, as opposed to Crohn's disease, which involves the entire thickness of the bowel wall. Early in the disease, edema and congestion of the mucosa occur. The edema may lead to extreme friability, so that bleeding occurs from any minor trauma, such as the surface being lightly rubbed.

In more advanced stages of the disease, the crypt abscess breaks through the wall of the crypt and spreads in the submucosa, undermining the mucosa. The mucosa is then shed into the bowel lumen, leaving areas of denuded mucosa (ulcers). Ulceration is at first scattered and shallow, but at a later stage the mucosal surface is lost over wide areas, leading to considerable loss of tissue, protein, and blood.

Clinical features

There are three common clinical types of ulcerative colitis related to frequency of symptoms. The *acute fulminating* ulcerative colitis is characterized by an abrupt onset, with severe, bloody diarrhea, nausea, vomiting, and fever, which causes a rapid depletion of fluids and electrolytes. The entire colon may be involved, with undermining and stripping of the mucosa, causing loss of considerable blood and mucus. This type of colitis occurs in about 10 percent of the patients. The prognosis is poor, and toxic megacolon is a frequent complication.

The majority of patients with ulcerative colitis have the *chronic intermittent (recurrent)* type of colitis. The onset tends to be insidious, occurring over a period of months to years. The mild form of the disease is characterized by short attacks occurring at intervals of months to years and lasting 1 to 3 months. There may be little or no fever or constitutional symptoms, and usually only the distal colon is affected. Fever and systemic symptoms may accompany the more severe form, and the attack may last 3 or 4 months, sometimes passing into the *chronic continuous* type of disease. In the chronic continuous disease, the patient continues to have diarrhea after the initial attack. As compared to the intermittent type, more of the colon tends to be involved and complications are more frequent.

In mild forms of ulcerative colitis, diarrhea may be mild and bleeding is intermittent and slight. In severe disease there are more than six stools per day with considerable blood and mucus. The chronic loss of blood and mucus may lead to anemia and hypoproteinemia. Severe colicky pain may be present in the lower abdomen and is relieved somewhat by defecation. Very few deaths occur directly from this disease, but it may be mildly or severely disabling.

The diagnosis of ulcerative colitis is usually straightforward. There is diarrhea with passage of blood, and sigmoidoscopy reveals a friable and intensely inflamed mucosa with exudate. In 95 percent of the cases the rectosigmoid area of the colon is involved. The disease may extend from this area but always in a continuous fashion, in contrast to Crohn's disease, which tends to skip. Barium x-ray studies of the colon aid in determining the extent of more proximal changes but should not be done during an acute attack, since they may precipitate toxic megacolon and perforation. Colonoscopy and biopsy can often differentiate ulcerative colitis from granulomatous colitis.

Complications

Complications of ulcerative colitis may be local or systemic. Rectal fistulae, fissures, and abscesses are not as common as they are in granulomatous colitis. Occasionally a rectovaginal fistula forms. A few patients may have narrowing of the bowel lumen as a result of fibrosis, which is generally mild compared to Crohn's disease.

One of the more serious complications is *toxic dilatation,* or *megacolon,* in which there is paralysis of the motor function of the transverse colon, with rapid dilatation of that segment of the bowel. Toxic megacolon is most frequently associated with pancolitis. The mortality is about 30 percent, and perforation of the bowel frequently results. The treatment for this complication is emergency colectomy. Massive hemorrhage is another complication sometimes requiring emergency colectomy.

Carcinoma of the colon is another significant complication which occurs with increasing frequency after the patient has had the disease for more than 10 years. After patients have had total colon involvement with ulcerative colitis for 25 years, the probability of cancer is increased to 40 percent.

The systemic complications are diverse, and it is difficult to relate some of them causally to the colonic disease. These include pyoderma gangrenosum, episcleritis, uveitis, arthritis, and ankylosing spondylitis. Disordered hepatic function is common in ulcerative colitis, and established hepatic cirrhosis is an accepted complication. The presence of severe systemic complications may be an indication for surgical treatment of the colitis, even when the colonic symptoms are mild (see Fig. 22-5).

Treatment

There is no cure or specific medical treatment for ulcerative colitis. The aims of therapy are to control the inflammation, maintain the patient's nutritional status, give symptomatic relief, and prevent infection and other complications.

Corticosteroid drugs are given to reduce inflammation and induce clinical remission. Sulfonamide drugs are given, but their mechanism of action is poorly understood. A low-residue diet causes diminution in the number of stools and thereby makes the patient more comfortable. The diet must also be high in protein to compensate for that lost in the exudative lesions, and high in vitamins as well. During exacerbations, tincture of opium and paregoric are sometimes given to control diarrhea. Anticholingeric drugs also help relieve the abdominal cramps and diarrhea. Emotional support and reassurance are important aspects of treatment.

When medical management fails and when the condition becomes intractable, surgical intervention is indicated. The most common procedure performed is total colectomy and the creation of a permanent ileostomy. Some physicians also recommend a colectomy for all patients who have had total colon involvement for more than 10 years, since the incidence of carcinoma of the colon is so high. Cancer of the colon is difficult to diagnose in these patients, since such symptoms as weight loss or bloody stools may be regarded as another exacerbation of the ulcerative colitis rather than as signs of cancer.

NEOPLASMS OF THE LARGE INTESTINE

Neoplasms of the colon and rectum may be benign or malignant. True benign neoplasms (lipomas, carcinoid tumors, and leiomyomas) are rare in the colon. Colonic polyps, however, are very common and occupy an intermediate position between benign and malignant neoplasms.

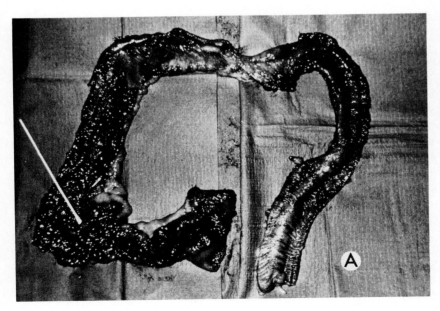

FIGURE 22-5
Some complications of ulcerative colitis (A) Hemorrhage—surgical specimen of large intestine removed from a patient with ulcerative colitis to control bleeding. The probe is at the site of a small perforation. (B) Toxic megacolon—the large dilatated colon is protruding through a surgical incision. (C) Pyoderma gangrenosum—a necrotic skin ulcer found in association with inflammatory bowel disease.

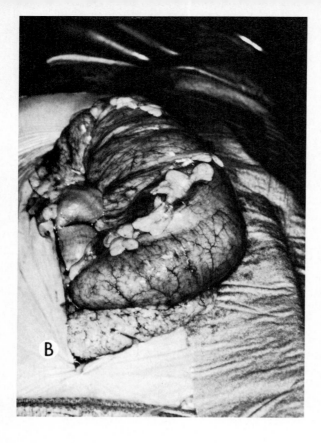

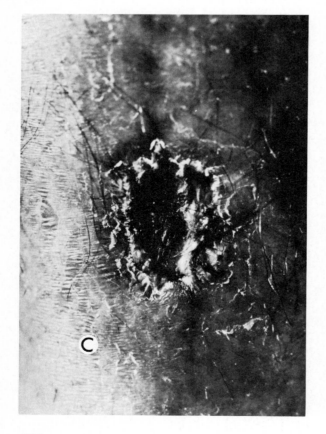

Colonic polyps

A polyp is a growth which arises from a mucosal surface and extends outward. There are three recognized patterns of colonic polyps: pedunculated adenomas, villous adenomas, and familial polyposis.

Pedunculated adenomas (also called adenomatous polyps or polypoid adenomas) are globelike structures attached to the mucous membrane by a thin stalk. This type of polyp occurs in both sexes and in all age groups, 1.89 although they become increasingly common with advancing age. Autopsy and sigmoidoscopy studies show that 7 to 10 percent of the population over the age of 45 years is afflicted. Although pedunculated polyps may occur in any part of the colon, they are more frequently located in the distal 25 to 30 cm. Pedunculated polyps may be singular or multiple; they are usually 0.5 to 1.0 cm in diameter but may be as large as 4 or 5 cm. Histologically, these polyps consist of proliferating glands. The relationship of adenomatous polyps to cancer of the colon is a subject of great controversy, since they have much the same distribution in the colon as cancer and are often associated with cancer. The prevailing opinion is that they are harmless. However, if the polyps are multiple or if the head is greater than 1.0 cm in diameter, the chances of malignancy are higher.

Another form of pedunculated polyp occurring most frequently in children under the age of 10 years is the *juvenile polyp.* Juvenile polyps are often large, vascular, and have long pedicles. They are believed to be inflammatory in origin and may present by bleeding or prolapse through the anus. Juvenile polyps occasionally occur in adults.

The *villous adenoma* (villous papilloma, sessile adenoma), in contrast to the pedunculated adenoma, is a sessile (broad-based) tumor. The surface is distinctly papillary to the naked eye and appears as a nodular mass. Histologically, the lesion is composed of fingerlike (villous) projections. It is usually solitary and located in the sigmoid colon or rectum. Villous adenomas are generally large (greater than 5 cm) and are about one-eighth as frequent as pedunculated adenomas. Malignancy is much more likely to occur in these tumors (with a 25 percent chance) than in the pedunculated adenomas.

Familial polyposis is a rare disorder transmitted genetically as a dominant trait and characterized by the presence of hundreds of adenomatous polyps, both pedunculated and sessile, throughout the entire large intestine. Both sexes are affected equally. The polyps are not present at birth but usually make their appearance about the time of puberty. The probability of the development of cancer increases with age and is almost 100 percent by the age of 40.

FIGURE 22-5
(Continued)

Clinical features

Most adenomatous polyps are asymptomatic and are found incidentally on examination by sigmoidoscopy, barium enema, or on autopsy. When polyps do give rise to symptoms, these generally consist of overt or occult bleeding. Occasionally a large polyp may initiate an intussusception and cause bowel obstruction (see Fig. 21-5D). Diarrhea and mucus discharge may be associated with large villous adenomas and familial polyposis.

Treatment

The treatment of colonic polyps is influenced by the debate concerning their malignant potential. Since there is no question about the malignant potential in familial polyposis, this condition is treated by total proctocolectomy and permanent ileostomy or subtotal resection with ileorectal anastomosis. When the rectum is preserved, it is examined periodically for cancer.

The guidelines for the treatment of pedunculated or villous adenomas are not as clear. In general, polyps which are greater than 2 cm in diameter, multiple, or villous are regarded with a high degree of suspicion and should be removed. Polyps which are pedunculated, singular, and less than 1.0 cm in diameter are rarely malignant and can be observed periodically.

Polyps may be excised from below through the sigmoidoscope or colonoscope. Larger lesions and villous adenomas are treated by laporotomy and segmental resection.

Carcinoma of the colon and rectum

The colon (including the rectum) is the most common site for malignancy of the gastrointestinal tract. Cancer of the colon is the second most frequent cause of all cancer deaths in both men and women in the United States and is led only by cancer of the lung and breast. Cancer of the large intestine is usually a disease of older people, and the peak incidence is in the sixth and seventh decades. It is rare below the age of 40, except in persons with a history of ulcerative colitis or familial polyposis. The sexes are affected about equally, although cancer of the colon is more common in women while the lesion is more common in the rectum in males. Nearly three-fourths of all the cancers of the bowel occur in the rectosigmoid portion, so that they may either be palpated during a rectal exam or viewed with a sigmoidoscope. The cecum and ascending colon are the next most common sites. The transverse colon and flexures are least likely to be affected.

The tumor may present as a *polypoid*, bulky, fungating mass projecting into the lumen and becoming ulcerated very quickly. It may extend around the bowel as an *annular*, ringlike stricture. Annular lesions are more common in the rectosigmoid portion of the bowel, while the polypoid or flat lesion is more common in the cecum and ascending colon. Histologically, almost all of the large bowel cancers are adenocarcinomas (composed of glandular epithelium) and may secrete mucus to a varying degree. The tumor may spread (1) by direct infiltration of adjacent structures, as into the bladder; (2) by lymphatics to the pericolic and mesocolic lymph nodes; and (3) by the bloodstream, usually to the liver, since the colon is drained by the portal system. The prognosis is relatively favorable when the lesion is confined to the mucosa and submucosa at the time of surgical resection and much less favorable when lymph node metastasis has occurred.

Etiology

Although the causes of cancer of the large bowel, as with other cancers, have not been established, certain predisposing factors have been identified. The relationship between ulcerative colitis, certain types of colonic polyps, and cancer of the bowel has already been discussed.

Another important predisposing factor may relate to dietary habits, since cancer of the bowel (like diverticulosis) is about 10 times more common in western populations, who eat foods high in refined carbohydrates and low in roughage, than in primitive populations (Africa), who eat foods high in roughage. Burkitt has proposed that a low-fiber, highly refined carbohydrate diet leads to alterations in fecal flora and changes in the degradation of bile salts or of the breakdown products of protein and fat, some of which may be carcinogenic. A low-fiber diet allows concentration of these potential carcinogens into a smaller volume of stool. In addition, the transit time is increased. The net result is prolonged contact time of potential carcinogens with the bowel mucosa.

Clinical features

The most common symptoms of cancer of the bowel are changes in bowel habits, bleeding, pain, anemia, anorexia, and weight loss. The signs and symptoms vary according to the location and are commonly divided into those affecting the right and left halves of the large bowel.

Carcinoma of the left colon and rectum tends to cause a change in bowel habits as a result of irritation and reflex responses. Diarrhea, crampy pain, and distention are common. Since lesions of the left colon tend to encircle, obstruction is a common problem. Stool may be narrow and ribbonlike in shape. Both mucus and gross blood are often visible on the feces. Anemia may result from chronic blood loss. A sigmoid or rectal growth may involve nerve roots, lymphatics, or veins, producing symptoms in the legs or perineum. Hemorrhoids, low back pain, rectal urgency, or urinary frequency may develop as a result of pressure on these structures.

Carcinoma of the right colon, where the bowel contents are liquid, tends to remain occult until far advanced. There is a little tendency to obstruct, since the bowel lumen is larger and the feces are liquid. Anemia due to bleeding is common, but the blood is occult and can only be detected by a guaiac test (a simple test which may be performed on the clinical unit). Mucus is likewise not visible, as it is well mixed in the stool. In the thin person a tumor of the right colon may sometimes be palpated, but this is not usual at an early stage. The patient may suffer from vague abdominal discomfort which is sometimes epigastric.

Treatment

The treatment of carcinoma of the colon and rectum is surgical removal of the tumor and its lymphatic drainage. The most common procedures performed are the right hemicolectomy, transverse colectomy, left hemicolectomy or anterior resection, and abdominoperineal resection. The results of surgical excision are fairly good compared to results with cancer in other areas of the body. The overall 5-year survival rate is approximately 50 percent.

ANORECTAL DISORDERS

Hemorrhoids

Hemorrhoids, or "piles," are varicose veins of the anal canal. They are usually arbitrarily divided into two classes, internal and external. Internal hemorrhoids are varices of the superior and middle hemorrhoidal veins, and external hemorrhoids are varices of the inferior hemorrhoidal veins. As the terms imply, the external hemorrhoids appear external to the sphincter ani muscles, and the internal hemorrhoids appear behind the sphincters.

Both types of hemorrhoids are very common and are present in about 35 percent of the population over

the age of 25 years. Although the condition is not life-threatening, it may cause considerable discomfort.

Hemorrhoids result from venous congestion caused by interference with venous return from the hemorrhoidal veins. Several etiologic factors have been implicated, including constipation or diarrhea, straining, pelvic congestion associated with pregnancy, enlargement of the prostate, uterine fibroids, and tumors of the rectum. Chronic liver disease associated with portal hypertension frequently results in hemorrhoids, since the superior hemorrhoidal veins drain into the portal system (see Fig. 23-2). In addition, the portal system is valveless, so that backflow readily occurs.

External hemorrhoids are classified as acute or chronic. The acute form presents as a bluish, rounded swelling at the anal verge and is actually a hematoma, although it is referred to as an acute external thrombosed hemorrhoid. They are often quite painful and pruritic because the nerve endings in the skin are pain receptors. Sometimes it is necessary to evacuate the clot under local anesthesia, or it may be treated by hot sitz baths and analgesics. A chronic external hemorrhoid or skin tag is usually the sequel to an acute hematoma. Anal skin tags consist of one or more folds of anal skin composed of connective tissue and a few blood vessels.

Internal hemorrhoids are classified as first, second, and third degree. First-degree (early) internal hemorrhoids do not protrude through the anal canal and can only be detected by proctoscopy. They are usually located in the right and left posterior and right anterior positions, following the distribution of the tributaries of the superior hemorrhoidal vein, and appear as globular reddish swellings. Second-degree hemorrhoids may prolapse through the anal canal after defecation; they may recede spontaneously or can be reduced manually. Third-degree hemorrhoids are permanently prolapsed. The most common symptom of internal hemorrhoids is painless bleeding, since there are no pain fibers in this area. Most cases of hemorrhoids are of the mixed variety rather than being strictly internal or external.

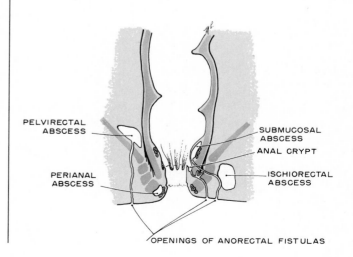

PELVIRECTAL ABSCESS

SUBMUCOSAL ABSCESS

ANAL CRYPT

PERIANAL ABSCESS

ISCHIORECTAL ABSCESS

OPENINGS OF ANORECTAL FISTULAS

FIGURE 22-6
Common sites of anorectal abscesses and fistulas. Inflammation often begins in the anal crypts.

The most common complications of hemorrhoids are bleeding, thrombosis, and strangulation. A strangulated hemorrhoid is a prolapsed one in which the blood supply is cut off by the anal sphincter.

Diagnosis of hemorrhoids is made by inspection and proctoscopy. When hemorrhoids and rectal bleeding occur in a middle-aged or older patient, it is important for the physician to rule out cancer.

The majority of patients with hemorrhoids need not undergo surgery. Medical treatment includes sitz baths, or other forms of moist heat, bed rest, stool softeners to prevent constipation, and the use of suppositories. Surgical excision may be indicated when there is persistent bleeding, prolapse, or intractable pruritis and anal pain.

Anal fissure (fissure in ano)

An anal fissure (fissure in ano) is a crack in the lining of the anus caused by stretching from the passage of hard fecal matter; therefore, constipation is a common cause. The most prominent symptom is severe burning pain following defecation, and the bowel movement is usually accompanied by a small amount of bright red blood. These patients are nearly always constipated; since the bowel movement is so very painful, the constipation becomes progressively worse because they fear to have a bowel movement. Anal fissures are often seen in association with the skin tags of external hemorrhoids. Treatment is surgical excision of the tract if local dilatations, ointments, and cleansing do not help.

Anorectal abscess and fistula in ano

An anorectal abscess is a localized infection, with the collection of pus in the anorectal area. The infecting organisms are usually *Escherichia coli*, staphylococci, or streptococci. A fistula in ano is a chronic granulomatous tract that goes from the anal canal to the skin outside the anus or from an abscess to the anal canal or the perirectal area. An anorectal fistula is often preceded by abscess formation. The sites of abscess and fistula formation are illustrated in Fig. 22-6. The perianal abscess is the most common type of anorectal abscess, followed by the ischiorectal, submucous, and pelvirectal locations. The perianal abscess is usually obvious as a red, painful swelling close to the anal verge. The pain is aggravated by sitting or coughing. A submucous or ischiorectal abscess may be palpated as a swelling on rectal examination. A pelvirectal abscess may be more difficult to identify. Discharge of pus from an anorectal fistula may be the first sign. Sometimes a fistula may be palpated or its course determined by the gentle passage of a probe from the external opening, with a finger of the other hand in the anal canal.

Anorectal abscesses commonly begin as an inflammation of the anal crypts, which are located at the lower end of the columns of Morgagni. The anal glands open into these crypts. Obstruction or trauma to their ducts gives rise to stasis and predisposes to infection. Mucosal tears from hard, constipated stools may be a predisposing factor. In a few cases a predisposing local lesion such as ulcerated hemorrhoids or anal fissure may be present.

When symptoms of diarrhea are associated with recurrent anorectal fistulae, it is important that presence of Crohn's disease be suspected, since 75 percent of patients with Crohn's disease confined to the large bowel develop a fistula in ano. Twenty-five percent of patients develop a fistula in ano when Crohn's disease is confined to the small intestine.

The treatment of anorectal abscesses and fistulae is incision and drainage of the abscess and excision of any associated fistulae.

QUESTIONS

Large intestine

Directions: Answer the following questions on a separate sheet of paper.

1. Draw a picture of the large intestine in the abdominal and pelvic cavities and label the parts with the following terms: appendix; cecum; ascending, transverse, descending, and sigmoid colon; rectum; anal canal; anus; hepatic and splenic flectures; haustra; and taenia coli.

2. What are the most important functions of the large bowel?

3. Discuss the differences in structure between the small and large bowel. How do these lead to differences in function?

4. Briefly summarize the mechanical operation of the large bowel (haustral churning, mass peristalsis).

5. List five common anorectal disorders.

6. List the most common diagnostic procedures used for the detection of disease of the large bowel. What can be detected with each?

7. Do all cases of acute diverticulitis require surgical intervention? If not, what is the medical treatment for acute diverticulitis?

8. Identify three predisposing factors in the pathogenesis of cancer of the colon or rectum.

9. What is Burkitt's hypothesis concerning the relationship of diet to the development of cancer of the bowel?

10. Why are hemorrhoids a frequent manifestation of hepatic cirrhosis and portal hypertension?

11. Define fissure in ano and fistula in ano. Is there any relationship between these two disorders and hemorrhoids? What disease of the gastrointestinal tract is often associated with anorectal fistulae?

Directions: Circle the letter preceding each item that correctly answers the question. Only one answer is correct, unless otherwise noted.

12. The right half of the colon receives its blood supply from the:
    a. Superior mesenteric artery   *b.* Splenic artery
    c. Inferior mesenteric artery   *d.* Left colic artery

13. The superior hemorrhoidal veins are part of the:
    a. Portal circulation   *b.* Systemic circulation

14. The major reservoir for feces is in which segment of the large bowel?
    a. Cecum   *b.* Transverse colon   *c.* Ascending colon   *d.* Descending colon   *e.* Sigmoid colon

15. In which segment of the colon is the greatest amount of water absorbed?
    a. Cecum and ascending colon   *b.* Descending and sigmoid colon   *c.* Rectum

16. Which of the following statements are true about colonic mucus? (More than one answer may be correct.)
    a. It is under autonomic control.   *b.* Parasympathetic stimulation causes an increase in mucus production.   *c.* The colonic mucosa maintains a layer of mucus on its surface.   *d.* The presence of visible mucus in the stools indicates overproduction.

17. Variations in intestinal gas normally depend on: (More than one answer may be correct.)
    a. How much air is swallowed   *b.* Variations in diet   *c.* Type of intestinal bacteria   *d.* Weight of the individual

18. The desire to defecate is initiated by:
    a. Contraction of the external anal sphincter
    b. Contraction of the internal anal sphincter
    c. Contraction of the rectum   *d.* Distention of the sigmoid colon   *e.* Distention of the rectum

19. Substances produced by bacterial putrefaction in the large intestine:

a. Indole   *b.* Skatole   *c.* Phenol   *d.* Amino acids and fatty acids   *e.* All of these

20. The cecum and ascending colon may be visualized on x-ray within how many hours after a barium meal?
    a. One-half   *b.* 1 to 2   *c.* 3 to 5   *d.* 10 to 12

21. Approximately what percentage of rectal and large bowel tumors may be visualized or palpated on rectal digital or proctosigmoidoscopic examination?
    a. 100 percent   *b.* 60 to 70 percent   *c.* 25 to 35 percent   *d.* 10 to 20 percent

22. Which of the following statements concerning diverticulosis is true? (More than one answer may be correct.)
    a. It is a common condition in persons over the age of 50 years in the United States.   *b.* It occurs more frequently in Africans who eat a high-fiber diet.   *c.* It is frequently associated with or preceded by the irritable colon syndrome.   *d.* Disordered colonic motility with generation of high intraluminal pressures in the colon is important in the pathogenesis.   *e.* Diverticula of the colon form most frequently at the point where arterioles penetrate the muscularis.

23. Diverticula are most common in which segment of the colon?
    a. Cecum   *b.* Ascending colon   *c.* Transverse colon   *d.* Descending colon   *e.* Sigmoid colon

24. The most common symptom of an attack of acute diverticulitis is:
    a. Pain in the lower left quadrant of the abdomen
    b. Pain in the lower right quadrant of the abdomen   *c.* Vomiting   *d.* Massive bleeding from the rectum

25. The most common complications of acute or chronic diverticulitis are: (More than one answer may be correct.)
    a. Massive bleeding requiring emergency colectomy   *b.* Perforation   *c.* Stricture causing partial bowel obstruction   *d.* Vesicocolic fistula

26. The most common site of fistula formation as a result of a perforated diverticulum is the:
    a. Peritoneum   *b.* Small intestine   *c.* Urinary bladder   *d.* Vagina

27. Which of the following is the most common clinical course of ulcerative colitis?
    a. Acute fulminating   *b.* Acute onset with full recovery   *c.* Chronic continuous   *d.* Chronic continuous with full recovery after 5 to 10 years   *e.* Chronic intermittent (relapsing-remitting course)

28. Patients with ulcerative colitis may reveal abnormalities in which of the following organ systems? (More than one answer may be correct.)
    a. Joints   *b.* Heart   *c.* Eyes   *d.* Lungs   *e.* Skin

29. The rectosigmoid segment of the large bowel is involved in what percentage of cases of ulcerative colitis?
a. 15 percent   b. 45 percent   c. 75 percent
d. 95 percent

30. Which of the following statements are true concerning toxic megacolon? (More than one answer may be correct.)
a. It is often associated with pancolitis.   b. The motor function of a bowel segment is paralyzed.
c. The transverse colon is frequently affected.
d. It is usually treated medically.   e. It is associated with a high mortality.

31. A cardinal symptom or sign of ulcerative colitis is:
a. Constipation   b. Diarrhea with blood and mucus in the stool   c. Ribbon-shaped stools
d. Periumbilical pain

32. Some of the known extracolonic manifestations of ulcerative colitis are: (More than one answer may be correct.)
a. Uveitis   b. Pyoderma gangrenosum
c. Episcleritis   d. Arthritis   e. Ankylosing spondylitis

33. Skin manifestations are associated with which of the following disorders? (More than one answer may be correct.)
a. Diverticulosis   b. Ulcerative colitis   c. Cancer of the colon   d. Granulomatous colitis
e. Regional enteritis

34. The role of adrenal steroid drugs in the treatment of ulcerative colitis is to:
a. Cure the active disease   b. Induce clinical remission   c. Prevent recurrence completely

35. The most common surgical treatment for intractable ulcerative colitis is:
a. Right hemicolectomy   b. Left hemicolectomy
c. Total colectomy with permanent ileostomy
d. Cecostomy

36. Cancer of the bowel involving which of the following sites is frequently diagnosed late in its course?
a. Cecum   b. Descending colon   c. Sigmoid colon   d. Rectum

37. The most common cause of death secondary to gastrointestinal cancer in the United States is from cancer of the:
a. Esophagus   b. Stomach   c. Small intestine
d. Colon and rectum

38. The most common symptom of cancer of the right colon is:
a. Change in bowel habits   b. Pain
c. Constipation   d. Gross blood in the stools
e. Diarrhea

39. Symptoms which commonly accompany cancer of the left colon include: (More than one answer may be correct.)

a. Change in bowel habits   b. Melena   c. Back pain   d. Abdominal cramps

40. Which statements are true with respect to adenomatous polyps? (More than one answer may be correct.)
a. It is the most common type of benign tumor in the colon.   b. They are most frequently located in the distal 25 to 30 cm of the bowel.   c. They are familial.   d. They occur more frequently in patients with cancer of the large bowel.   e. They are generally benign when singular or less than 1 cm in diameter.

41. Familial polyposis of the colon is characterized by: (More than one answer may be correct.)
a. Densely packed polyps throughout the colon
b. An inheritable recessive trait   c. Marked predisposition to cancer of the large bowel   e. Alopecia

42. The most common site of malignant lesions of the large bowel is:
a. Rectosigmoid area   b. Descending colon
c. Cecum   d. Transverse colon

Directions: Fill in the blanks with the correct word(s) or circle the correct option.

43. _____ is a condition in which there is herniation of the mucosa through the muscularis of the large bowel to form flask-shaped saccules. The condition is called _____ when the saccules become inflamed.

44. _____ adenoma or adenomatous polyp is a globelike structure on a pedicle arising from a mucosal surface. _____ polyps have very long pedicles and often occur in children.
A _____ adenoma is a broad-based tumor composed of villous projections. _____ _____ is a hereditary disease characterized by the presence of hundreds of polyps throughout the colon.

45. An encircling of _____ form of cancer growth is more common in the left colon, while the shape is more likely to be _____ in the cecum.

46. Three routes of spread of cancer of the bowel are _____, _____, and _____.

47. Internal hemorrhoids are varicosities of the _____ and _____

hemorrhoidal veins and are located (inside or outside) the anal sphincters. The _____ hemorrhoidal veins are involved in external hemorrhoids.

48. Three common complications of hemorrhoids are _____, _____, and _____.

Directions: Match each of the following characteristic features of inflammatory bowel disease in col. A with the correct disorder in col. B.

Column A

49. ____ Caused by a specific infectious agent

50. ____ Granulomatous inflammation

51. ____ Familial and Jewish association

52. ____ Transmural lesion common

53. ____ Internal fistulae common

54. ____ Lesions continuous with rectum

55. ____ High malignant potential after 10 years

56. ____ Most commonly associated with toxic megacolon

57. ____ Most common disease of the two

58. ____ "Skip" lesions common

59. ____ May represent an immunologic disorder

Column B

a. Crohn's disease

b. Ulcerative colitis

c. Both

d. Neither

60. ____ Anorectal abscesses, fissures, and fistulae common complications

61. Rank the following types of colonic polyps according to malignant potential, with 1 being the highest: a. Villous adenomal b. Familial polyposis c. Pedunculated polyp less than 1.0 cm in diameter

Directions: Circle T if the statement is true and F if it is false. Correct the false statements.

62. T F Fecal incontinence results from destruction of the second to fourth sacral segments of the spinal cord.

63. T F The external anal sphincter is under autonomic nervous control.

64. T F Diverticulitis almost always requires surgical resection.

65. T F Vitamin D is synthesized in the large bowel by the action of colonic bacteria.

66. T F Normally, about 1000 ml of flatus is expelled from the anus daily.

67. T F Barium enema x-ray is generally contraindicated during acute diverticulitis because of the danger of perforation.

68. T F First-degree internal hemorrhoids are permanently prolapsed.

69. T F Second-degree hemorrhoids prolapse following straining at the stool but recede spontaneously or can be reduced manually.

70. T F Approximately 5 percent of the population over the age of 25 years suffer from hemorrhoids.

71. T F The perianal and ischiorectal areas are the most common sites of anorectal abscess formation.

72. T F The formation of an anorectal abscess or fistula is often preceded by anal cryptitis initiated by a mucosal tear from hard feces.

73. T F Successful treatment of anorectal abscess or fistula usually requires surgery.

74. T F Medical treatment of hemorrhoids includes stool softeners, moist heat, and the use of suppositories.

CHAPTER 23

LIVER, BILIARY TRACT, AND PANCREAS

OBJECTIVES

At the completion of this chapter you should be able to:

1. Describe the anatomic relation of the liver to the biliary tract, stomach, duodenum, and pancreas.
2. Describe the gross structure, size, and shape of the liver.
3. Describe the structure and function of the liver lobule.
4. Explain why blood circulation through the liver is unusual.
5. Identify the capillary beds which drain into the portal circulation and clinically significant points of anastomosis between the portal and systemic circulations.
6. List and describe the eight major functions of the liver.
7. Identify the major components of bile.
8. Identify the major plasma proteins and coagulation factors synthesized by the liver.
9. Describe the circulatory, defense, and detoxification functions of the liver.
10. Describe the gross structure and function of the gallbladder.
11. Identify the following structures of the biliary tract: right hepatic duct, common hepatic duct, cystic duct, common bile duct, ampulla of Vater, and sphincter of Oddi.
12. Describe the gross structure of the pancreas in terms of size, shape, divisions, and ducts.
13. Describe the histology of the pancreas in relation to its functions.
14. Identify the three types of pathologic changes in diseases of the liver, gallbladder, and pancreas.
15. Explain the clinical significance of the following tests in the evaluation of liver, biliary, and pancreatic function: serum and urine bilirubin, urobilinogen, Bromsulphalein (BSP) test, serum proteins, prothrombin time, blood ammonia, serum and urine amylase, serum lipase, cholesterol, enzymes, and hepatitis B antigen.
16. Identify the radiographic techniques used in the diagnosis of liver, biliary, and pancreatic disorders and describe what each may reveal.

17. Describe a liver biopsy (preparation, contraindications, procedure, aftercare, and possible complications).

18. Describe the methods of portal pressure measurement and the significance of an elevation.

19. Define jaundice and indicate the sites of earliest detection.

20. Outline the steps of normal bilirubin metabolism.

21. Differentiate between unconjugated and conjugated bilirubin.

22. Identify the four general pathogenetic mechanisms of hyperbilirubinemia and jaundice; describe disorders associated with each.

23. Define kernicterus.

24. Explain the pathogenesis of transient jaundice common in the newborn.

25. Differentiate between intrahepatic and extrahepatic cholestasis and list the common causes of each.

26. Compare the following features of hemolytic, hepatocellular, and obstructive jaundice: skin, urine and stool color, pruritis, serum and urine bilirubin, and urine urobilinogen.

27. Contrast hepatitis A and hepatitis B with respect to the following features: common names, transmission, incubation, presence of hepatitis antigens in serum, population affected, seasonal incidence, clinical features and general prognosis, and complications.

28. Describe the morphologic changes in the liver in a mild case of hepatitis.

29. Describe the clinical features of hepatitis during the prodromal, icteric, and recovery phases.

30. Differentiate between chronic persistent and chronic active hepatitis.

31. Describe the treatment of hepatitis.

32. Describe the value of gamma globulin in the prevention and treatment of hepatitis A and B.

33. List public health and clinical measures to reduce the incidence of hepatitis.

34. Define cirrhosis of the liver and describe its consequences.

35. Identify the single most important cause of cirrhosis.

36. Distinguish among Laennec's, postnecrotic, and biliary patterns of cirrhosis on the basis of prevalence, gross and microscopic pathology, pathogenesis, and prognosis.

37. Describe the relationship between malnutrition, alcoholism, and fatty infiltration of the liver.

38. Describe alcoholic hepatitis and its possible relationship to cirrhosis.

39. Explain the relationship of primary cancer of the liver to cirrhosis.

40. Distinguish between primary and secondary biliary cirrhosis.

41. Explain the pathophysiologic basis of the following clinical manifestations of cirrhosis: jaundice, peripheral edema, hepatic coma, gynecomastia, spider angiomas, testicular atrophy, altered hair distribution, hypoalbuminemia, increased bleeding tendency, anemia, leukopenia, thrombocytopenia, and splenomegaly.

42. Define portal hypertension and identify the basic mechanism responsible for its development in cirrhosis of the liver.

43. Define ascites and identify key factors responsible for its development.

44. Explain the development of esophageal varices, prominent superficial abdominal veins, and internal hemorrhoids in cirrhotics.

45. Discuss possible complications from esophageal varices, including the treatment and prognosis.

46. Describe possible complications in the treatment of ascites with diuretics or a large paracentesis.

47. Identify the basic characteristics of hepatic encephalopathy.

48. Identify the primary source of ammonia in the body, its normal metabolism, and its excretion.

49. Describe the relationship of liver cell failure and /or portal-systemic shunting to the development of hepatic encephalopathy.

50. Identify several endogenous or exogenous factors which may precipitate hepatic encephalopathy.

51. Describe the major signs, symptoms, and electroencephalogram findings of the four stages in the progression of hepatic encephalopathy to coma.

52. Describe asterixis, how it is tested, and its significance.

53. Describe constructional apraxia and its significance in monitoring the progression of hepatic encephalopathy.

54. Explain why it is important to detect hepatic encephalopathy in its early stages.

55. Describe the treatment of hepatic encephalopathy, including measures to prevent its recurrence.

56. Explain why dietary protein restriction, removal of blood from the intestinal tract, and intestinal sterilization are important measures in the treatment of hepatic encephalopathy.

57. Compare the characteristics of bilirubin, cholesterol, and mixed cholesterol gallstones.

58. Describe cholelithiasis and cholecystitis in terms of incidence, population affected, etiology, pathogenesis, clinical features, diagnosis, complications, and treatment.

59. Define the identifying characteristics of acute and chronic pancreatitis.

60. Describe the mechanisms which protect the normal pancreas from autodigestion.

61. List the two primary etiologic factors in acute and chronic pancreatitis.

62. Describe the range of injury in acute pancreatitis and possible mechanisms causing the injury.

63. Describe the signs, symptoms, diagnosis, and treatment objectives for acute pancreatitis.

64. Differentiate between a pancreatic abscess and a pseudocyst.

65. Describe the primary features of chronic pancreatitis (pathology, etiology, clinical course, diagnosis, and treatment).

66. Discuss the prevalence, types, and general prognosis of primary cancer of the liver, gallbladder, and pancreas.

67. Explain the relationship of gallstones and cirrhosis of the liver to cancer of the gallbladder and liver.

68. Identify possible reasons why the liver is such a common site of malignant tumor metastasis.

69. Explain why cancer of the gallbladder or pancreas is usually diagnosed in an advanced stage.

ANATOMIC AND PHYSIOLOGIC CONSIDERATIONS

The liver, biliary tract, and pancreas all develop as offshoots of the fetal foregut in a region which later becomes the duodenum; all are intimately associated with the physiology of digestion. It is reasonable to consider these structures together because of their anatomic proximity, their closely related functions, and the similarity of the symptom complexes induced by many of their disorders.

Liver

The liver is the largest gland in the body, averaging about 1500 g, or 2.5 percent of the body weight in a normal human adult (see Fig. 23-1). It is a soft, plastic

FIGURE 23-1

(A) Liver, gallbladder, and pancreas. (B) Microscopic structure of hepatic functional unit (liver lobule). (C) Pancreatic acinar units.

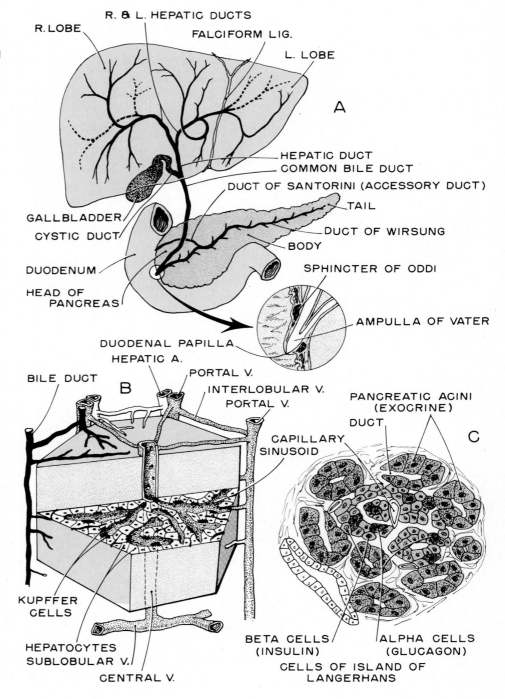

organ, which is molded by the surrounding structures. The superior surface is convex and lies beneath the right dome and part of the left dome of the diaphragm. The lower portion of the liver is concave and provides a roof over the right kidney, stomach, pancreas, and intestines. There are two principal lobes, the right and the left. The right lobe is divided into anterior and posterior segments by the right segmental fissure, not seen from the exterior. The left lobe is divided into medial and lateral segments by the externally visible *falciform ligament*. The falciform ligament passes from the liver to the diaphragm and the anterior abdominal wall. The surface of the liver is covered by visceral peritoneum, except for a small area on the posterior surface which is attached directly to the diaphragm. Several ligaments which are reflections of the peritoneum help to support the liver. Beneath the peritoneum is a dense connective tissue layer called the *capsule of Glisson*, which covers the surface of the entire organ; at the hilum or *porta hepatis* on the inferior surface, it is continued into the liver substance, forming a framework for the branches of the portal vein, hepatic artery, and bile ducts.

Microscopic structure

Each lobe of the liver is divded into structures called *lobules*, which are the microscopic and functional units of the organ (see inset of Fig. 23-1). Each lobule is a hexagonal body composed of plates of cuboidal hepatic cells arranged radially around a central vein that drains the lobule. Between the plates of hepatic cells are capillaries called *sinusoids*, which are branches of the portal vein and hepatic artery. The sinusoids, unlike other capillaries, are lined with phagocytic or *Kupffer cells*. Kupffer cells belong to the monocyte-macrophage system, and their main function is to engulf bacteria and other foreign particles in the blood. Only the bone marrow exceeds the liver in the mass of monocyte-macrophage cells; thus it is one of the principal organs of defense against bacterial invasions and toxic agents. In addition to branches of the portal vein and hepatic artery encircling the periphery of the liver lobule, bile ducts are also present. The interlobular bile ducts form very small bile capillaries called *canaliculi* (not shown), which course within the center of the liver cell plates. Bile formed in the hepatocytes is excreted into the canaliculi, which join to form larger and larger bile ducts until the common bile duct is reached.

Circulation

The liver has a dual blood supply—from the digestive tract and the spleen via the *portal vein* and from the aorta via the *hepatic artery*. About one-third of the incoming blood is arterial and about two-thirds is venous from the portal vein. A total volume of 1500 ml passes through the liver each minute and is drained via

the right and left *hepatic veins*, which empty into the inferior vena cava (see Fig. 23-2).

The portal vein is unique in that it is interposed between two capillary beds, one in the liver and the other in the digestive area which it drains. Upon entering the liver, the portal vein divides into branches which come into contact with the circumference of the liver lobules. These branches then give off interlobular veins, which run between the lobules. These give rise to the sinusoids, which run between the plates of hepatocytes to enter the central veins. Central veins from several lobules join to form the sublobular veins, which in turn join to form the hepatic veins (refer to inset of Fig. 23-1). The finest branches of the hepatic artery also empty into the sinusoids, making the blood composition unique in that it is a mixture of arteral blood from the hepatic artery and venous blood from the portal vein. Figure 23-2 illustrates the origin of blood flowing into the portal system; increased pressure in this system is a common manifestation in liver disorders, with serious consequences involving the vessels in which the portal blood originates. Several points of portacaval anastomosis are of clinical significance. In cases of obstruction to flow in the liver, portal blood may be shunted around the liver to the systemic venous system. The consequences of portal hypertension and shunting are discussed in greater detail later in this chapter.

Liver function

In addition to ranking first in size as a parenchymal organ, the liver also ranks first in the number, complexity, and variety of its functions. The liver is essential for the maintenance of life, is involved in almost every metabolic function of the body, and is specifically responsible for more than 500 separate activities. Fortunately, it has a large reserve capacity and needs only 10 to 20 percent functioning tissue to sustain life. Complete destruction or removal of the liver results in death within 10 hours. The liver has an impressive regenerative ability. Partial surgical removal will, in most cases, initiate a rapid replacement of dead or diseased cells with new liver tissue.

Table 23-1 lists the major functions of the liver. Understanding these functions is a prerequisite to understanding its pathophysiology.

The formation and excretion of bile is a major function of the liver; the bile ducts transport and the gallbladder stores and releases bile into the small intestine as needed. The liver secretes about 1 liter of yellow bile each day. the basic components of bile are water (97 percent), electrolytes, bile salts, phospholipids (mainly

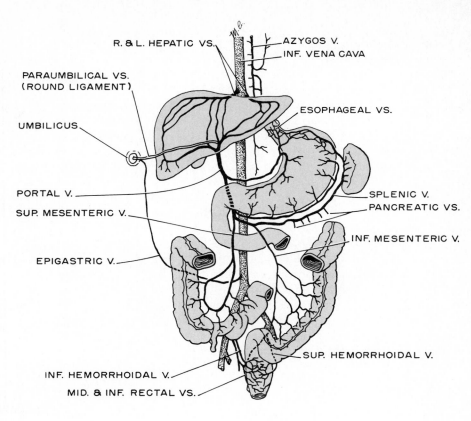

FIGURE 23-2

Hepatic-portal system. Blood is carried from the stomach, intestines, spleen, and pancreas into the liver sinusoids. Hepatic veins convey it to the inferior vena cava. Clinically significant sites of anastomosis between the hepatic and systemic circulations are (1) the esophageal veins (portal tributary) which anastomose with the azygos veins (systemic tributary); (2) the paraumbilical veins in the round ligament originate in the left branch of the portal vein which connect with the superficial veins of the anterior abdominal wall (systemic tributaries) in the area of the umbilicus; (3) the superior rectal or hemorrhoidal veins (portal tributary) which anastomose with the middle and inferior rectal veins (systemic tributaries); (4) the portal tributaries to the intestines, pancreas, and liver which anastomose with the phrenic, renal, and lumbar veins (systemic tributaries, not shown). In portal hypertension and chronic liver disease, blood may back up in these veins and be shunted around the liver through the points of anastomosis.

R. & L. HEPATIC VS.
AZYGOS V.
INF. VENA CAVA
PARAUMBILICAL VS. (ROUND LIGAMENT)
ESOPHAGEAL VS.
UMBILICUS
PORTAL V.
SUP. MESENTERIC V.
SPLENIC V.
PANCREATIC VS.
INF. MESENTERIC V.
EPIGASTRIC V.
SUP. HEMORRHOIDAL V.
INF. HEMORRHOIDAL V.
MID. & INF. RECTAL VS.

lecithin), cholesterol, and bile pigments (mainly conjugated bilirubin). Bile salts are essential for fat digestion and absorption in the small intestine. After being acted upon by bacteria in the small intestine, most of the bile salts are reabsorbed in the ileum, recirculated to the liver, and reconjugated and resecreted (see Chap. 21). Although bilirubin (bile pigment) is a metabolic end product and has no physiologically active role, it is nonetheless important as an indicator of liver and biliary tract disease, since it tends to color tissues and fluid with which it comes in contact. Normal bilirubin metabolism and jaundice as a sign of disease are discussed later in this chapter.

The liver plays an essential role in the metabolism of three types of foodstuffs delivered by the portal vein after absorption from the intestines. These are carbohydrates, proteins, and fats. Monosaccharides from the small intestine are converted into glycogen and stored as such in the liver (glycogenesis). From this storage depot of glycogen, a constant supply of glucose is released into the blood (glycogenolysis) to meet the changing body requirements. Some of the glucose is metabolized in the tissues to produce heat and energy, and the remainder is converted either into glycogen and stored in the muscles or into fat and stored in the subcutaneous tissues. The liver is also capable of synthesiz-

ing glucose from proteins and fat (gluconeogenesis). The role of the liver in protein metabolism is essential to survival. The plasma proteins, except gamma globulin, are synthesized by the liver. These include albumin, which is necessary for the maintenance of the colloid osmotic pressure, and prothrombin, fibrinogen, and other clotting factors. In addition, most degradation of amino acids begins in the liver with deamination, or the removal of an amino group (NH_2). The ammonia released is then synthesized into urea and excreted by the kidneys and intestines. Ammonia formed in the gut by the action of bacteria on protein is also converted to urea in the liver.

Other metabolic functions of the liver include fat metabolism, vitamin, iron, and copper storage; the conjugation and excretion of adrenal and gonadal steroids; and the detoxification of numerous endogenous and exogenous substances. The detoxification function is very important and is accomplished by liver enzymes which oxidize, reduce, hydrolyze, or conjugate the potentially harmful substance, rendering it physiologically inactive. Endogenous substances, such as indol, skatol, and phenol, which are produced by the action of bacteria on amino acids in the large intestine, and exogenous substances, such as morphine, phenobarbital, and other drugs, are detoxified in this manner.

TABLE 23-1

Major functions of the liver

Function	Comments
Formation and excretion of bile	
Bile salts metabolism	Bile salts are essential for the digestion and absorption of fats and fat-soluble vitamins in the intestine.
Bile pigment metabolism	Bilirubin, the main bile pigment, is a metabolic end product from the processing of old red blood cells. It is conjugated in the liver and excreted in bile.
Carbohydrate metabolism	Liver plays an important part in maintaining the normal blood glucose level and providing energy for the body. Carbohydrate is stored in the liver as glycogen.
Glycogenesis	
Glycogenolysis	
Gluconeogenesis	
Protein metabolism	
Protein synthesis	Serum proteins synthesized by the liver include albumin, and the alpha and beta globulins (not gamma globulin).
	Blood-clotting factors synthesized by liver include fibrinogen (I), prothrombin (II), and factors V, VII, VIII, IX, and X. Vitamin K is a necessary cofactor in the synthesis of II, V, IX, and X.
Urea formation	Urea is formed exclusively in the liver from NH_3, which is then excreted in the urine and feces. NH_3 is formed from deamination of amino acids and action of intestinal bacteria on amino acids.
Protein (amino acid) storage	
Fat metabolism	Triglycerides, cholesterol, phospholipids, and lipoproteins (absorbed from intestine) are hydrolyzed to fatty acids and glycerol.
Ketogenesis	
Cholesterol synthesis	Liver plays major role in cholesterol synthesis, most of which is excreted in the bile as cholesterol or cholic acid.
Fat storage	
Vitamin and mineral storage	Fat-soluble vitamins (A, D, E, K) stored in liver, also vitamin B_{12}, copper, and iron.
Steroid metabolism	Liver inactivates and excretes aldosterone, glucocorticoids, estrogen, progesterone, and testosterone.
Detoxification	Liver is responsible for biotransformation of substances that are potentially harmful (e.g., drugs) into harmless substances which are then excreted by kidneys.
Flood chamber and filter action	Liver sinusoids provide depot for blood backed up from venae cavae (right-sided heart failure); phagocytic action of Kupffer cells removes bacteria and debris from blood.

Finally, the liver functions as a "flood chamber" and "filter" because of its strategic position between the intestinal and general circulation. In cases of right-sided heart failure, the liver may become passively congested with a large amount of blood. The Kupffer cells in the sinusoids filter bacteria and other injurious materials from the portal blood by phagocytosis.

Gallbladder

The gallbladder is a pear-shaped hollow sac resting directly beneath the right lobe of the liver (see Fig. 23-1). Bile, which is secreted continuously by the liver, enters the small bile ducts within the liver. The small bile ducts join to form two larger ducts which emerge from the undersurface of the liver as the *right* and *left hepatic ducts* but which immediately join to form the *common hepatic duct*. The hepatic duct merges with the *cystic duct* from the gallbladder, forming the *common bile duct*. In many persons, the common bile duct merges with the pancreatic duct to form the *ampulla of Vater* (dilatated portion in common channel) before opening into the small intestine. The terminal parts of both ducts and the ampulla are surrounded by circular muscle fibers known as the *sphincter of Oddi.*

The principal function of the gallbladder is the storage and concentration of bile. It is capable of holding about 45 ml of bile. Hepatic bile may not immediately enter the duodenum; instead, after passing down the hepatic duct, it may be diverted into the cystic duct and gallbladder. In the gallbladder, the lymphatics and blood vessels absorb water and inorganic salts, so that gallbladder bile is about 10 times as concentrated as hepatic bile. At intervals the gallbladder contents are emptied into the duodenum by simultaneous contraction of the muscular coat and relaxation of the sphincter of Oddi. The normal stimulus of gallbladder contraction and emptying is the entry of acid chyme into the duodenum. The presence of fatty foods is the strongest stimulus to contraction. The hormone CCK mediates the contraction.

Pancreas

The pancreas is a long slender organ about 6 in in length and 1.5 in in width. It lies retroperitoneal and is divided into three major segments—the head, body, and tail (see Fig. 23-1). The head lies in the concavity formed by the duodenum, and the tail touches the spleen.

The pancreas is made up of two basic types of cells having entirely different functions (see inset of Fig. 23-1). The exocrine cells, clustered into groups called *acini*, produce the components of the pancreatic juice (see Table 21-1). The endocrine cells, or islets of Langerhans, produce the endocrine secretions insulin and glucagon, which are important for carbohydrate metabolism.

The pancreas is a compound tubuloalveolar gland. As a whole, it resembles, a bunch of grapes, the branches of which are the ducts terminating in the main pancreatic duct (duct of Wirsung). Small ducts from each acinus empty into the main ducts. The main duct, extending throughout the length of the gland, often joins the common bile duct at the ampulla of Vater before entering the duodenum. An accessory duct, the *duct of Santorini*, is frequently found extending from the head of the pancreas into the duodenum, about 1 in above the duodenal papilla.

OVERVIEW

Pathologic changes in diseases of the liver, gallbladder, and pancreas may be broadly categorized into three types: inflammatory, fibrotic, and neoplastic changes. Hepatitis, cholecystitis, and pancreatitis show evidence of acute or chronic inflammation of the involved tissues. Gallstones and biliary tract obstruction are frequently associated with cholecystitis and pancreatitis. Fibrotic changes occur with cirrhosis of the liver and in chronic inflammatory conditions. Primary tumors of the liver, pancreas, or gallbladder, whether benign or malignant, are rare. Widespread destruction of parenchymal cells resulting from inflammation, fibrosis, neoplasms, or obstruction interferes with secretory and excretory functions. Jaundice (yellow coloration of the body tissues) is a common symptom and results from interference with the excretion of bilirubin. Portal hypertension, ascites, esophageal varices, and hepatic encephalopathy are common complications in advanced cirrhosis and hepatic failure.

DIAGNOSTIC TESTS

Table 23-2 lists some of the most common diagnostic tests used to detect disordered function of the liver, gallbladder, and pancreas. It should be emphasized that no single test or procedure is capable of measuring the total function of the liver, since it is involved in nearly every metabolic process in the body and has a large functional reserve. Usually a battery of diagnostic tests is utilized.

Radiologic methods useful in the diagnosis of disorders of the liver, biliary system, and pancreas are summarized in Table 23-3. Other diagnostic methods include esophagoscopy, which allows direct visualization of esophageal varices; duodenoscopy, which allows visualization of the papilla of Vater and insertion of a catheter in order to inject contrast medium directly into the biliary or pancreatic system; peritoneoscopy (insertion of peritoneoscope through an abdominal stab wound), which allows direct visualization of the anterior surface of the liver and gallbladder; and an electroencephalogram, which may be abnormal in hepatic encephalopathy. Finally, percutaneous liver biopsy is a common procedure performed at the bedside and is described in greater detail below.

Percutaneous liver biopsy is a valuable method of diagnosing diffuse parenchymal disease such as cirrhosis, hepatitis, and drug reactions. Prior to performing the procedure, the patient's capacity to clot bood is evaluated, and cross-matched blood is provided in case of need. The procedure itself is brief. The skin is cleansed and anesthetized. As a patient holds his or her breath in expiration to bring the liver and diaphragm to the highest position, the needle is inserted into the liver in the eighth or ninth intercostal space or subcostally and withdrawn (see Fig. 23-3F). The specimen is then expelled into formalin for later histologic examination. It is vitally important that patients understand that they are to hold their breath and not move during the procedure, to prevent laceration of the liver. The procedure is contraindicated in patients who cannot meet this requirement.

After the procedure the patient lies on the right side for about 2 hours to splint the chest and remains in bed for 24 hours. Although rare, complications of liver biopsy may be dangerous. The chief danger is intraperitoneal hemorrhage (0.2 percent), which results from penetration of a large blood vessel. Bile peritonitis is a rare but serious complication requiring immediate surgical intervention. Vital signs are checked every 15 minutes until stable and then every 1 or 2 hours for the first 24 hours after the procedure. The dressing is

TABLE 23-2

Tests of liver, biliary, and pancreatic function

Test	Normal	Clinical Significance
Biliary excretion		Measures ability of liver to conjugate and excrete bile pigment
Direct serum bilirubin (conjugated)	0.1–0.4 mg per 100 ml	Elevated when excretion of conjugated bilirubin is impaired
Indirect serum bilirubin (unconjugated)	0.1–0.5 mg per 100 ml	Elevated in hemolytic conditions and Gilbert's syndrome.
Total serum bilirubin	0.2–0.9 mg per 100 ml	Both direct and total serum bilirubin elevated in hepatocellular disease.
Urine bilirubin	0	Conjugated bilirubin excreted in urine when elevated in serum, suggesting liver cell or biliary tract obstruction. Urine appears brown; foam appears yellow when shaken—simple bedside test.
Urine urobilinogen	0–4 mg/24 h	Decreased when bile excretion impaired; increased when amount produced exceeds ability of liver to reexcrete it as in hemolytic jaundice.
Dye excretion		
Bromsulphalein test (BSP)	<5% retention in 1 h	Removed from blood, stored, conjugated, and then excreted in the bile. Excretion dependent on functional liver cells, patent biliary ducts, and hepatic blood flow. BSP test is a very sensitive index of liver function, useful in detecting early liver cell damage and recovery from infectious hepatitis, but owing to occasional toxic reactions, it is not widely used.
Protein metabolism		
Total serum protein	6–8 g per 100 ml	Most of the serum proteins and coagulation proteins are synthesized by the liver and are therefore decreased in a variety of liver impairments.
Serum albumin	3.5–5.5 g per 100 ml	
Serum globulin	1.5–3 g per 100 ml	
Prothrombin time	11–16 sec	Increased with decreased prothrombin synthesis due to liver cell damage or decreased vitamin K absorption in biliary obstruction. Vitamin K essential for prothrombin synthesis.
Blood ammonia	30–70 μg per 100 ml	Liver converts NH_3 to urea. Rises in hepatic failure or in large portal-systemic shunts.
Carbohydrate metabolism	60–180 units per 100 ml	Obstruction and inflammatory disease of pancreas interfere with normal flow of amylase into intestinal tract and result in increased serum levels. Marked increase in acute pancreatitis (also increased in parotid gland disease and other conditions).
Urine amylase	<260 units/h	Urinary amylase remains high for longer than serum amylase (1 wk); >300 units/h indicates pancreatitis.
Fat metabolism		
Serum lipase	<1.5 units	Pancreatic digestive enzyme released into blood with breakdown of acinar cells in obstructive or inflammatory conditions of pancreas.
Serum cholesterol	150–280 mg per 100 ml	Increased in bile duct obstruction, decreased in liver cell damage.
Serum enzymes		
SGOT	5–40 units/ml	Enzymes serum glutamic oxaloacetic transaminase (SGOT), serum glutamic pyruvic transaminase (SGPT), and lactic dehydrogenase (LDH) are concentrated especially in heart, liver, and skeletal muscle. Released from damaged tissue (necrosis or altered cell permeability). Increased in liver cell damage and in other conditions, especially myocardial infarction.
SGPT	5–35 units/ml	
LDH	90–200 milliunits/ml (varies with units used)	
Alkaline phosphatase	2–5 Bodansky units	Manufactured in bone, liver, kidneys, intestine, and excreted in bile. Increased in biliary obstruction. Also increased in bone disease, liver metastasis.
Immunologic tests		Key diagnostic test in detecting hepatitis B antigen (HBAg or Australia antigen) in long-incubation or serum hepatitis.

TABLE 23-3

Radiologic methods in the diagnosis of liver, biliary, and pancreatic disorders

Test	Comments
Plain film of abdomen	May reveal calcific densities in the gallbladder, biliary tree (gallstones), pancreas, and liver. May also reveal splenomegaly.
Barium meal (see Fig. 23-3A)	Reveals esophageal varices in 70–90% of the cases. Tumors of the head of the pancreas often produce a displacement or irregularity of the second portion of the duodenum (reverse 3 sign common).
Oral cholecystogram	Conjugation and excretion of the dye by the liver allows visualization of the gallbladder and bile ducts, thus revealing gallstones. Poor or no visualization of the contrast medium may be caused by liver cell disease or biliary obstruction.
Intravenous cholecystogram	Visualizes the bile ducts and localizes obstructive lesions of the major ducts.
Transhepatic cholangiogram (see Fig. 23-3B)	Dye given by percutaneous puncture and blind probing for a bile duct into which dye is injected. May help to distinguish hepatic from posthepatic jaundice. Hazards involve bile leakage and hemorrhage.
Endoscopic retrograde cholangiopancreatography (ERCP) (see Fig. 23-3B)	Endoscopic insertion of a catheter into the duodenal papilla with injection of contrast medium through catheter into pancreatic or biliary ductules. Allows visualization of these structures.
Radioisotope liver scan with radio-tagged iodinated rose bengal, gold, or technetium (see Fig. 23-3C)	Reveals anatomic changes in liver tissue; lesions appear as filling defects (tumors, cysts, abscesses).
Selective celiac axis angiography (see Fig. 23-3D)	Visualization of pancreatic, hepatic, and portal circulation possible. Reveals tumor masses, disruption as in cirrhosis, and portal collateral circulation.
Portal pressure measurement (see Fig. 23-3E)	Principal procedures are percutaneous splenic pulp manometry, transhepatic puncture, and catheterization of the hepatic vein or the umbilical-portal vein. Portal pressure elevated in cirrhosis. Procedures often combined with injection of contrast medium.
Splenoportogram (see Fig. 23-3E)	Demonstrates size and patency of portal and splenic collaterals.

checked frequently for local bleeding, and a pressure dressing is applied if necessary. Severe abdominal pain may indicate bile peritonitis and should be carefully evaluated. Figure 23-3 illustrates some of the diagnostic procedures useful in liver, biliary, and pancreatic disorders.

BILIRUBIN METABOLISM AND JAUNDICE

The accumulation of bile pigments in the body causes yellow discoloration of the tissues called *jaundice*. Jaundice can usually be detected in the sclerae (whites of eyes), skin, or by a darkening of the urine when the serum bilirubin reaches 2 to 3 mg per 100 ml. The normal serum bilirubin is 0.2 to 0.9 mg per 100 ml. Surface tissues richest in elastin, such as the sclerae and the undersurface of the tongue, usually become stained first.

A consideration of the mechanisms of jaundice involves an understanding of the formation, transportation, metabolism, and excretion of bilirubin.

Normal bilirubin metabolism

In the normal individual, bilirubin formation and excretion proceeds smoothly through the steps outlined in Fig. 23-4. About 85 percent of the bilirubin is produced by the breakdown of senescent red blood cells in the monocyte-macrophage system. The average life span of a red blood cell is 120 days. Each day about 50 ml of blood is destroyed, and 200 to 250 mg of bilirubin is produced. It is now known that about 15 percent of total bile pigment does not depend on this mechanism but is derived from destruction of maturing erythroid cells in the bone marrow (ineffective hematopoiesis) and from other hemoproteins, notably those in the liver.

In the catabolism of hemoglobin (largely occurring in the spleen), globin is first dissociated from heme, after which the heme is converted to biliverdin. Unconjugated bilirubin is then formed from biliverdin. Unconjugated bilirubin, loosely bound to albumin, is transported in the blood to the liver cells. Bilirubin metabolism by the liver cell involves three steps—uptake, conjugation, and excretion. Uptake by the liver cell involves two cytoplasmic or acceptor proteins, which have been designated as Y and Z proteins. Conjugation of bilirubin with glucuronic acid takes place in the endoplasmic reticulum of the liver cell. This step is dependent on the presence of glucuronyl transferase, an enzyme which catalyzes the reaction. Conjugation of the bilirubin molecule greatly changes its characteristics. Conjugated bilirubin is lipid-insoluble, water-soluble, and incapable of being excreted in the urine. In contrast, unconjugated bilirubin is lipid-soluble, water-insoluble, and incapable of being excreted in the urine. Transport of conjugated bilirubin across the cell membrane and secretion into the bile canaliculi by an active process is the final step of bilirubin metabolism in the liver. In order to be excreted in the bile, bilirubin must be conjugated. Conjugated bilirubin is then excreted via the biliary tree into the small intestine.

Intestinal bacteria reduce conjugated bilirubin to a series of compounds called stercobilin or urobilinogen. These substances account for the brown color of stool. About 10 to 20 percent of the urobilinogen undergoes enterohepatic circulation, while a small fraction is excreted in the urine.

Pathophysiologic mechanisms in jaundice states

There are four general mechanisms by which hyperbilirubinemia and jaundice can occur: (1) excess production of bilirubin; (2) impaired hepatic uptake of unconjugated bilirubin; (3) impaired conjugation of bilirubin, and (4) decreased excretion of conjugated bilirubin into bile because of either intrahepatic or extrahepatic factors which may be functional or caused by mechanical

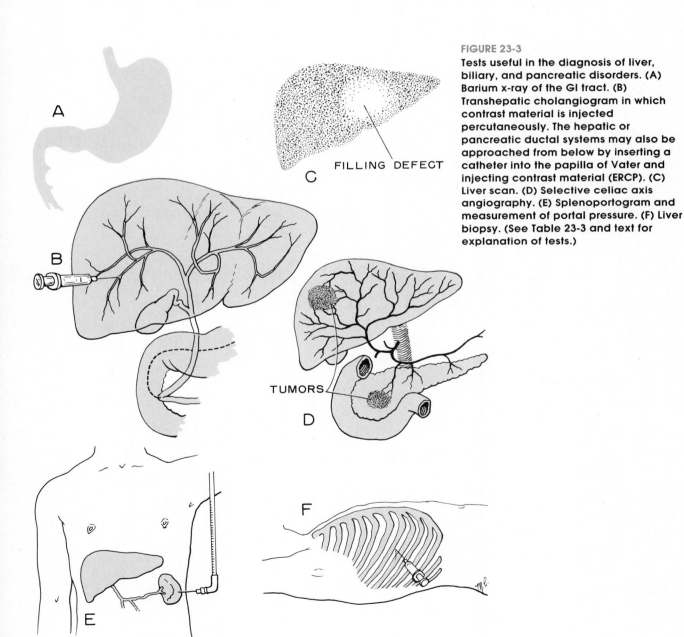

FILLING DEFECT

TUMORS

FIGURE 23-3
Tests useful in the diagnosis of liver, biliary, and pancreatic disorders. (A) Barium x-ray of the GI tract. (B) Transhepatic cholangiogram in which contrast material is injected percutaneously. The hepatic or pancreatic ductal systems may also be approached from below by inserting a catheter into the papilla of Vater and injecting contrast material (ERCP). (C) Liver scan. (D) Selective celiac axis angiography. (E) Splenoportogram and measurement of portal pressure. (F) Liver biopsy. (See Table 23-3 and text for explanation of tests.)

obstruction. The first three mechanisms result in predominantly unconjugated hyperbilirubinemia, while the fourth results in predominantly conjugated hyperbilirubinemia.

Excess bilirubin production

Hemolytic disease, or an increased rate of red blood cell destruction, is the most common cause of excess bilirubin production. The resultant jaundice is customarily called *hemolytic jaundice*. Conjugation and transfer of bile pigment proceeds normally, but the supply of unconjugated bilirubin is greater than the liver can handle.

Consequently, the level of unconjugated bilirubin in the blood rises. The serum bilirubin level, however, rarely exceeds 5 mg per 100 ml in patients with severe hemolysis, and the jaundice is a mild pale yellow. Since unconjugated bilirubin is water-insoluble, it cannot be excreted in the urine, and bilirubinuria does not occur. There is, however, increased production of urobilinogen (due to the increased bilirubin load presented to the liver and increased conjugation and excretion), which in turn results in increased fecal and urinary excretion. The urine and stool may thus be darker.

Some common causes of hemolytic jaundice are abnormal hemoglobins (hemoglobin S in sickle cell anemia), abnormal red blood cells (hereditary spherocytosis), antibodies in the serum (Rh or transfusion incompatibility or as a result of autoimmune hemolytic disease), administration of some drugs, and some lymphomas (enlarged spleen and increased hemolysis). In

FIGURE 23-4
Normal bilirubin metabolism.

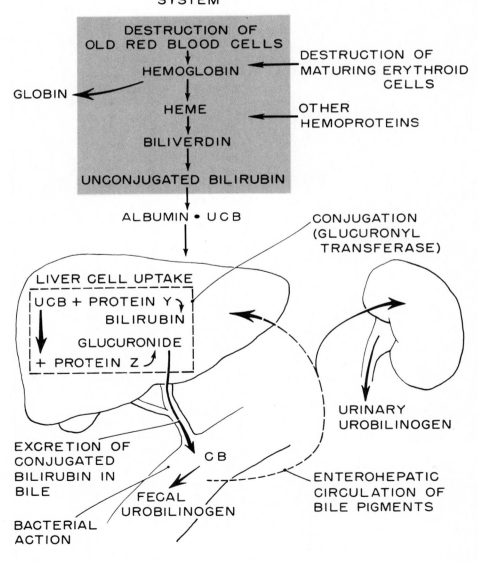

some cases hemolytic jaundice may result from increased destruction of red blood cells or their precursors in the bone marrow (thalassemia, pernicious anemia, porphyria). This process is referred to as ineffective erythropoiesis.

In the adult, chronic overproduction of bilirubin may lead to the formation of gallstones predominantly composed of bilirubin; otherwise the mild hyperbilirubinemia is not generally harmful. Treatment is directed toward correction of the hemolytic disease. However, in infancy unconjugated bilirubin levels higher than 20 mg per 100 ml may lead to *kernicterus*, a condition in which bilirubin is deposited in the lipid-rich basal ganglia of the brain, causing damage.

Impaired uptake of bilirubin

Gilbert's syndrome is a benign familial condition characterized by mild unconjugated hyperbilirubinemia (<5 mg per 100 ml) and jaundice. The degree of jaundice fluctuates, and is often aggravated by prolonged fasting, infection, stress, or trauma. The onset is most common during adolescence, and the condition is reported to affect about 5 percent of the male population. Liver function tests and fecal and urinary urobilinogen levels are normal. Bilirubinuria is absent. The underlying defect is considered to be a deficiency of the hepatic uptake of bilirubin, although impaired conjugation may also play a role. One of the most important aspects of Gilbert's syndrome is its recognition so that the affected individual can be reassured that the condition is benign.

Impaired uptake of bilirubin resulting from immaturity of the Y and Z acceptor proteins may play a role in neonatal jaundice. In other conditions, damage to these proteins by certain drugs such as novobiocin or by infection or malnutrition may also account for elevation of unconjugated serum bilirubin.

Impaired conjugation of bilirubin

The Crigler-Najjar syndrome is a rare hereditary disease in humans in which there is a complete deficiency of glucuronyl transferase from birth. Since conjugation of bilirubin cannot take place, the bile is colorless, unconjugated serum bilirubin generally exceeds 20 mg per 100 ml, and kernicterus is common. The prognosis is poor, and death usually occurs during infancy or early childhood. In a milder form of the disease in which there is only a partial deficiency of glucuronyl transferase, jaundice may not be manifested until adolescence and the prognosis is good. Phenobarbital, which is able to induce increased glucuronyl transferase activity, often causes jaundice to disappear in these patients.

The transient unconjugated hyperbilirubinemia which develops during the second and fifth days of life in the newborn is believed to result from immaturity of the hepatic enzyme system.

Decreased excretion of conjugated bilirubin

Impaired excretion of bilirubin, whether due to functional or obstructive factors, results in predominantly conjugated hyperbilirubinemia. Because conjugated bilirubin is water-soluble, it is excreted in the urine and gives rise to bilirubinuria and dark urine. Fecal and urinary urobilinogen are commonly decreased, so that the stools are pale. Elevated conjugated bilirubin levels may be accompanied by other evidence of hepatic excretory failure, such as elevated serum levels of alkaline phosphatase, SGOT, cholesterol, and bile salts. The presence of elevated bile salts in the blood adds the new dimension of itching to the jaundice. Jaundice resulting from conjugated hyperbilirubinemia is usually deeper than that resulting from unconjugated hyperbilirubinemia. The color change ranges from a mild or deep orange-yellow to a yellow-green in cases of complete obstruction of biliary outflow. These changes are evidence of *cholestatic jaundice*, which is another name for *obstructive jaundice*. Cholestasis may be either *intrahepatic* (involving the liver cell, canaliculi, or cholangioles) or *extrahepatic* (involving bile ducts outside the liver). Similar biochemical disturbances are present in both.

The most common causes of intrahepatic cholestasis are *hepatocellular diseases* in which the hepatic parenchymal cells are damaged by viral hepatitis or the various types of cirrhosis. In these diseases, swelling and disorganization of the liver cells can compress and block the canaliculi or cholangioles. Hepatocellular disease usually interferes with all phases of bilirubin metabolism—uptake, conjugation, and excretion—but since excretion is usually impaired to the greatest extent, conjugated hyperbilirubinemia predominates. Other less common causes of intrahepatic cholestasis include certain drugs and the rare hereditary disorders of the Dubin-Johnson and Rotor syndromes. In these conditions, there appears to be interference with transfer of bilirubin across the hepatocyte membrane. Common offending drugs include halothane (anesthetic), oral contraceptives, estrogens, anabolic steroids, isoniazid, and chlorpromazine.

The most common causes of extrahepatic cholestasis are impaction of a gallstone, usually at the lower end of the common bile duct; carcinoma of the head of the pancreas, producing extrinsic pressure on the bile duct; and carcinoma of the ampulla of Vater. Less common causes are strictures from previous inflammation or surgery and enlarged lymph nodes in the porta hepatis. Intrahepatic lesions such as a hepatoma may sometimes obstruct the right or left hepatic ducts.

Intrahepatic versus extrahepatic cholestasis

The most important diagnostic decision for the physician and surgeon in conjugated hyperbilirubinemia is to determine whether the obstruction to bile flow is intrahepatic or extrahepatic. Extrahepatic cholestasis may benefit from surgery, while surgery on a patient with hepatocellular disease (intrahepatic cholestasis) may exacerbate the illness and even lead to death. The differentiation is not easy, since all forms of cholestasis produce the same clinical syndrome of jaundice, itching, increased transaminases, increased alkaline phosphatase, defective excretion of cholecystographic dyes, and nonvisualization of the gallbladder. Although the ultimate judgment is a clinical one, help in making the differentiation comes from evaluating the degree of obstruction. Intrahepatic obstruction is seldom as complete as extrahepatic obstruction. Consequently, intrahepatic cholestasis generally results in only moderate elevations of alkaline phosphatase, and small amounts of pigment appear in the stools or urobilinogen in the urine as compared to these values in extrahepatic cholestasis. Liver biopsy or duodenal or transhepatic cholangiography may be utilized to clarify difficult cases.

Table 23-4 lists some of the differentiating features of the common types of jaundice.

VIRAL HEPATITIS

Acute viral hepatitis is an infectious disease which is generalized in its distribution within the body, although the predominant effect is on the liver. The best known forms of hepatitis are hepatitis A and hepatitis B. These terms are preferred to the former terminology of "infectious" and "serum" hepatitis, since both diseases may be transmitted through parenteral and nonparenteral routes. Other synonyms and the differential features of hepatitis A and B are listed in Table 23-5 and are discussed in the following pages. Newer immunologic techniques are being developed to identify other forms of viral hepatitis (non-A, non-B hepatitis). Some of the features of non-A, non-B hepatitis are also listed in Table 23-5.

Hepatitis has become an important public health problem not only in the United States but also throughout the world. More than 60,000 cases are reported to the Center for Disease Control each year in the United States, and each year the number steadily increases. Although mortality from viral hepatitis is relatively low, extensive morbidity and economic loss are associated with the disease.

TABLE 23-4

Differentiating features of hemolytic, hepatocellular, and obstructive jaundice

Feature	Hemolytic	Hepatocellular	Obstructive
Skin color	Pale yellow	Mild or deep orange-yellow	Mild to deep yellow-green
Urine color	Normal (may darken with urobilin)	Dark (conjugated bilirubin)	Dark (conjugated bilirubin)
Stool color	Normal or dark (↑ stercobilin)	Pale (less stercobilin)	Clay-colored
Pruritus	None	Not persistent	Usually persistent
Serum bilirubin, indirect or unconjugated	Increased	Increased	Increased
Serum bilirubin, direct or conjugated	Normal	Increased	Increased
Urine bilirubin	Absent	Increased	Increased
Urine urobilinogen	Increased	Slight increase	Decreased

TABLE 23-5

Differential features of viral hepatitis

	Hepatitis A	Hepatitis B	Non-A, non-B hepatitis
Synonyms	Infectious hepatitis Short-incubation hepatitis	Serum hepatitis Long-incubation hepatitis	
Tests for hepatitis antigens and antibodies (i.e., HBsAg, HBcAg, anti-HBs, anti-HBc)	Negative	Positive	Negative
Incubation period	28 to 94 days	17 to 98 days	
Age groups	More common in young children and institutional settings	All age groups affected. Drug addicts, patients on chronic hemodialysis, and medical personnel are at high risk	All ages. Occurs following blood transfusions
Season	Fall and early winter	All year	All year
Transmission	Usually fecal and oral route among persons living in close contact, contaminated water supply; shellfish; also by parenteral route	Usually by transfusion of blood and blood products or some other form of inoculation, especially parenteral drug abuse; also by fecal-oral route and sexual contact	Blood and body fluids
Clinical features	Majority of type A infections mild and anicteric; patient simply thinks it is the "flu"	Tends to be more severe and sometimes requires hospitalization for extended periods	
	Fatigue, anorexia, low-grade fever, abdominal discomfort, arthralgias, skin rashes, enlarged tender liver, light stools, dark urine, jaundice	Changes similar to hepatitis A	Changes similar to hepatitis A
	Elevated SGOT, SGPT (early), heperbilirubinemia, abnormal liver function tests		
Mortality	Less frequent	More frequent	
Incidence of chronic aggressive hepatitis as a complication	Very low	Somewhat higher	

Etiology and epidemiology

Numerous studies in human volunteers have clearly shown that hepatitis can be transmitted between persons by a bacteria-free filtrate. Recent significant discoveries have provided new insights which may eventually lead to better control of the disease. The immunologic separation of viral hepatitis into three types, A, B, and non-A, non-B, has made it possible to define and investigate the features of each. This has also led to the expectation that vaccines will become available for use in high-risk populations. Two types of circulating antigen are present in the majority of patients with type B hepatitis. Hepatitis B surface antigen (HBsAg), previously called the Australia antigen or hepatitis-associated antigen, is believed to be the outer coat of the hepatitis B virus. Hepatitis B core antigen (HBcAg) is believed to be the core of the virus that is produced and replicates in the hepatocyte nucleus, causing tissue damage. In addition, antibodies to both the surface and core antigens exist (anti-HBs, and anti-HBc). Neither the antigens nor the antibodies exist in the serum of patients with documented infections with hepatitis A. HBAg appears in the serum of patients during the incubation period, before the signs and symptoms of hepatitis appear, and usually disappears within 3 to 12 weeks. Studies of HBAg-positive blood donors have clearly shown a high frequency of hepatitis in recipients of HBAg-positive transfusions. In addition, HBAg has been found in urine, feces, saliva, nasopharyngeal washings, and semen, indicating that infection may be transmitted by nonparenteral routes. Since the presence of HBAg is the mark of infectivity, an HBAg-positive patient should be regarded as potentially infectious. HBAg occurs in about 0.1 percent of the normal population and in 5 to 10 percent of patients following recovery from hepatitis B infection. It is not clear whether these persons are carriers or have chronic anicteric hepatitis.

Classically, the incubation period for hepatitis A was believed to range from 30 to 60 days (short incubation) and that of hepatitis B from 50 to 180 days (long incubation). Recent data, however, show that the incubation period for hepatitis A ranges from 28 to 94 days and that patients with hepatitis B become HBAg-positive 17 to 98 days after exposure to the infecting agent. Viremia occurs during the incubation period and during the early phase of the illness in both hepatitis A and B. Recent studies reveal that fecal excretion of the virus occurs in hepatitis B as well as in A.

Hepatitis A occurs mainly in the fall and early winter, affecting children more often than adults. Fecal-oral transmission, primarily by person-to-person contact, is the most common mode of transmission. It is transmitted by human carriers and persons who are incubating the disease. Sporadic cases occur, and epidemics may arise from spread by contaminated water or food, especially in institutional settings. Other modes of transmission include the ingestion of uncooked clams, oysters, and other shellfish which may harbor the virus. Hepatitis A may also be transmitted parenterally.

Hepatitis B occurs all year round and affects all age groups. Parenteral transmission seems to be the major mode of spread, although recent evidence implicates fecal-oral transmission as well. Contamination of needles, syringes, lancets, and tattooing instruments has been associated with outbreaks. Drug addicts who share common needles and syringes are at high risk. Patients on chronic hemodialysis, as well as the staff who care for them, are also at high risk. The virus has been transmitted in as little as 0.00004 ml of blood. It was hoped that the elimination of HBAg-positive blood donors would eliminate the problem of posttransfusion hepatitis, but it now appears that other forms of hepatitis (non-A, non-B) are responsible. A test for the detection of hepatitis A virus is badly needed. Whole blood and blood products, with the exception of immunoglobulins, treated albumin, and the plasma protein fraction, may be contaminated with the hepatitis virus.

Pathology

The morphologic changes in the liver are identical in hepatitis A, B, and non-A, non-B. In the classic case, the liver appears normal in size and color but is sometimes slightly edematous, enlarged, and bile-stained. Histologically, there is hepatocellular disarray, varying degrees of liver cell injury and necrosis, and periportal inflammation. These changes are completely reversible when the acute phase of the disease subsides. In a few cases, submassive or massive necrosis may lead to fulminant hepatic failure and death.

Clinical features

Infection with a hepatitis virus can result in a range of effects from fulminant hepatic failure to anicteric subclinical hepatitis. The latter is more common in type A infections, and the patient often mistakes it for the "flu." Type B infections tend to be more severe than type A infections, and the incidence of massive necrosis and fulminant hepatic failure is more common.

The vast majority of both hepatitis A and B infections are mild with complete recovery, and the clinical features are similar. Prodromal symptoms occur in all patients and may be present for a week or so before the onset of jaundice (although not all patients develop jaundice). The main features at this time are malaise, lassitude, anorexia, headache, low-grade fever, and the loss of desire to smoke. Many patients experience arthralgias, arthritis, urticaria, and transient skin rashes. Rarely, glomerulonephritis occurs. These extrahepatic manifestations of viral hepatitis may represent a syndrome similar to serum sickness and may be caused by circulating immune complexes. In addition, there may be discomfort in the right upper quadrant, usually attributed to stretching of the liver capsule.

The prodromal phase is followed by the icteric phase and the onset of jaundice. This phase usually lasts 4 to 6 weeks. During this phase, there is generally an improved feeling of well-being. Appetite returns and the fever subsides as the urine becomes darker and the stool somewhat paler. The liver is moderately enlarged and tender, and the spleen is palpably enlarged in about one-fourth of the patients. A tender lymphadenopathy is often present.

The earliest biochemical abnormality is an elevation of SGOT and SGPT levels, which precedes the onset of jaundice by 1 or 2 weeks. Urine examination at the onset will reveal the presence of bilirubin and an excess of urobilinogen. The bilirubinuria persists throughout the illness, but the urine urobilinogen may disappear temporarily if there is an obstructive phase due to cholestasis; later in the course of the illness there may be a secondary rise in urine urobilinogen.

The icteric phase is associated with hyperbilirubinemia (both conjugated and unconjugated fractions), which is usually less than 10 mg per 100 ml. The serum alkaline phosphatase level is usually normal or only moderately elevated. A mild leukocytosis is usually found in viral hepatitis, and the prothrombin time may be prolonged. HBAg is found in the serum during the prodromal phase and definitely establishes type B hepatitis.

In the uncomplicated case, recovery begins 1 or 2 weeks from the onset of jaundice and lasts from 2 to 6 weeks. Easy fatigability is a common complaint. The stools rapidly regain their normal color, the jaundice lessens, and urine color lightens. Splenomegaly, if present, rapidly subsides, but hepatomegaly may return to normal only some weeks later. Abnormal laboratory findings and liver function tests may persist for 3 to 6 months.

Complications

Not every patient with viral hepatitis pursues an uneventful course. A few patients (less than 1 percent) show rapid clinical deterioration following the onset of jaundice due to fulminant hepatitis and massive liver necrosis. Death may occur within days in some patients, while others may survive for weeks if the damage is less extensive. Many of these patients are obese, middle-aged females, and there is frequently an associated acute renal failure. Fulminant viral hepatitis is more common in type B infections contracted through the parenteral route than in type A infections contracted through the fecal-oral route.

The most common complication of viral hepatitis is a more prolonged course lasting 4 to 8 months. This is called *chronic persistent hepatitis*, and it occurs in 5 to 10 percent of patients. Despite the delayed convalescence in chronic persistent hepatitis, patients almost always recover.

Approximately 5 percent of patients with viral hepatitis have a relapse following recovery from the initial episode. This is usually associated with the ingestion of alcohol or undue physical exertion. Commonly, the jaundice is not as marked, and the liver function tests do not show the same degree of abnormality. Further bed rest is usually followed by an uneventful recovery.

After acute viral hepatitis, a few patients may develop *chronic active* or *aggressive hepatitis* in which there is piecemeal destruction of the liver and the development of cirrhosis. The condition is distinguished from chronic persistent hepatitis by liver biopsy. Corticosteriod therapy may retard the progression of hepatic injury, but the prognosis is poor. Death usually occurs within 5 years as a result of hepatic failure or the complications of cirrhosis. Chronic active hepatitis is more common following type B infections than type A. There is persistence of HBAg in the serum in about one-third of the patients, which may be related to the development of chronic active hepatitis. It is possible that the chronicity or activity of the hepatitis may be related to immunologic mechanisms initiated by the acute hepatitis. Not all cases of chronic active hepatitis follow acute viral hepatitis. Drugs may be involved in the pathogenesis of this disorder. Specific drugs implicated include alphamethyldopa (Aldomet), isoniazid, sulfonamides, and aspirin.

Treatment

There is no specific treatment for viral hepatitis. Bed rest during the acute phase and a diet that is both ac-

ceptable and nutritious are the usual general measures. Intravenous feeding may be necessary during the acute phase if the patient has persistent vomiting. Some limitation of physical activity is usually necessary until symptoms have subsided and the liver function tests return to normal.

Prevention

If individuals have been in contact with or are liable to be exposed to cases of viral hepatitis, the use of human gamma globulin is recommended. The recommended dose is 0.01 ml/lb of body weight by intramuscular injection. If given early enough, gamma globulin is highly effective in reducing the incidence of hepatitis A. In cases of exposure to type B virus, there is at least some possibility that the globulin may contain sufficient quantities of hepatitis B antibody to be helpful. Gamma globulin is of no value in the treatment of overt hepatitis.

The same high-risk individuals can be protected from the disease with the use of hepatitis B vaccine which is highly effective in producing immunity. The immunity is apparently long-lasting. At this point, we do not have an effective immunization program against non-A, non-B hepatitis.

Personnel engaged in high-risk contact, as in hemodialysis, exchange transfusions, and parenteral therapy, need to exercise great care in the handling of equipment and the avoidance of needle puncture.

Community measures important in the prevention of hepatitis include the provision of a safe food and water supply as well as effective sewage disposal. Careful attention to general hygiene, handwashing, and safe disposal of the urine and feces of infected patients are important. The use of disposable catheters, needles, and syringes eliminates an important source of infection. All blood donors should be screened for the presence of HBAg before being accepted on the donor panel.

CIRRHOSIS OF THE LIVER

Cirrhosis is a chronic disease of the liver characterized by distortion of the normal hepatic architecture by bands of connective tissue and by nodules of regenerating liver cells unrelated to the normal vasculature. The regenerating nodules may be small (micronodular) or large (macronodular). Cirrhosis may interfere with intrahepatic blood circulation, and in far-advanced cases it causes gradual failure of liver function.

The incidence of this disease has increased significantly since World War II, establishing cirrhosis as one of the most prominent causes of death in the adult male. This increase is due in part to a corresponding increase in the incidence of viral hepatitis but more significantly to an enormous increase in the intake of alcohol. Alcoholism is the single most important cause of cirrhosis.

Etiology, pathology, and pathogenesis

Although the etiology of many forms of cirrhosis is poorly understood, three characteristic patterns account for the majority of cases—Laennec's, postnecrotic, and biliary cirrhosis.

Laennec's cirrhosis

Laennec's cirrhosis (also called alcoholic, portal, and nutritional cirrhosis) is a peculiar pattern of cirrhosis associated with chronic abuse of alcoholic beverages. It accounts for 50 percent or more of the cases of cirrhosis.

The exact relationship between alcohol abuse and Laennec's cirrhosis is not known, although there is a clear and unmistakable association. The first change in the liver caused by alcohol is the gradual accumulation of fat within the liver cells (fatty infiltration) see Fig. 3-3. A similar pattern of fatty infiltration is also seen in kwashiorkor (a disorder common in backward nations as a result of severe protein deficiency), hyperthyroidism, and diabetes. Most authorities agree that alcoholic beverages exert a direct toxic effect on the liver. The accumulation of fat reflects a number of metabolic disturbances, including excess formation of triglycerides, their decreased utilization in the formation of lipoproteins, and decreased oxidation of fatty acids. It is also possible that the person ingesting excess alcohol does not eat properly and fails to consume enough protein to provide a sufficient quantity of lipoprotein agents (choline and methionine) needed for the transport of fat. It is known that low-protein diets depress the activity of alcohol dehydrogenase, the principal enzyme which metabolizes alcohol. However, the primary cause of liver damage is believed to be the direct effect of alcohol on the liver cell, which is increased by malnutrition.

Uncomplicated fatty degeneration of the liver, as might be seen in early alcoholism, is reversible provided the person ceases ingestion of alcohol; very few cases of this relatively benign condition progress to cirrhosis. Grossly the liver is enlarged, fragile, and greasy in appearance and may be functionally deficient because of the large accumulation of fat.

If the habit of alcohol abuse persists, particularly when it becomes more severe, something may occur (it is not known what does it) to tip the whole process in favor of widespread scar formation. Some authorities (Helman et al., 1971) believe that the critical lesion in the development of cirrhosis of the liver may be alcoholic hepatitis. Alcoholic hepatitis is characterized histologically by hepatocellular necrosis and polymorphonuclear neutrophil leukocyte (PMN) infiltration of the liver. However, not all patients who develop the lesion of alcoholic hepatitis progress to full-blown cirrhosis of the liver.

In far-advanced cases of Laennec's cirrhosis, thick fibrous bands form at the periphery of many lobules, partitioning the parenchyma into fine nodules. These nodules may enlarge somewhat as a result of regenerative activity as the liver attempts to replace damaged cells. The liver appears to consist of tightly packed nests of degenerating and regenerating liver cells encased in thick fibrous capsules. On this basis the condition is often referred to as *fine nodular cirrhosis*. In the final stages the liver is shrunken, hard, and almost devoid of normal parenchyma, which results in portal hypertension and hepatic failure.

Postnecrotic cirrhosis

Postnecrotic cirrhosis presumably follows patchy necrosis of liver tissue, resulting in large and small degenerative nodules surrounded and partitioned by scar and interspersed with normal liver parenchyma. About 75 percent of the cases tend to progress and result in death within 1 to 5 years. Postnecrotic necrosis accounts for about 20 percent of the cases of cirrhosis. About 25 percent of the cases have a prior history of viral hepatitis. Many patients have positive test results for HBAg, indicating that chronic active hepatitis may be an essential event. A small percentage of cases stem from documented intoxication with industrial chemicals, poisons, or drugs, such as phosphorus, chloroform, and carbon tetrachloride, or poisonous mushrooms.

A peculiar feature of postnecrotic cirrhosis is that it appears to predispose the patient to the occurrence of a primary hepatic neoplasm of the liver (hepatoma). This is seen to a somewhat lower degree in Laennec's cirrhosis also.

Biliary cirrhosis

Liver cell destruction that begins around the bile ducts gives rise to a pattern of cirrhosis known as biliary cirrhosis. It accounts for about 15 percent of the cases of cirrhosis.

The most common cause of biliary cirrhosis is posthepatic biliary obstruction. Stasis of bile causes its accumulation within the liver substance with destruction of liver cells. Fibrous bands begin forming around the periphery of the lobule, but rarely do they transect a lobule as in the pattern of Laennec's cirrhosis. The liver is enlarged, firm, finely granular, and has a green hue. Jaundice is always an early and primary part of the syndrome, as are pruritis, malabsorption, and steatorrhea.

Primary biliary cirrhosis presents a pattern somewhat similar to the secondary biliary cirrhosis just described, but it is much more rare. The cause of this condition, which is associated with lesions of the intrahepatic bile ductules, is unknown. The bile capillaries and ductules contain bile plugs, and the liver cells frequently contain a green pigment. The extrahepatic biliary tract is not involved. Portal hypertension as a complication is rare.

Clinical manifestations

The clinical features and complications of cirrhosis are common to all forms of the disease regardless of the cause, although individual types of cirrhosis may have additional distinctive clinical and biochemical features. The period during which cirrhosis presents as a clinical problem is generally only a small fraction of the total life history of the disease. For many years cirrhosis is latent, the pathologic changes progressing slowly until major symptoms induce awareness of the disease. During the long latent period, there is a gradual deterioration of liver function.

Early symptons are vague and nonspecific and include lassitude, anorexia, dyspepsia, flatulence, a change in bowel habits (either constipation or diarrhea), and slight weight loss. Nausea and vomiting, especially in the morning, are common. A dull ache or heavy feeling in the epigastrum or right upper quadrant is present in about half of the patients. In most cases the liver is hard and palpable regardless of whether it is enlarged or atrophied.

The major and late manifestations of cirrhosis develop as a result of two types of disordered physiology—liver cell failure and portal hypertension. Manifestations of hepatocellular failure include jaundice, peripheral edema, bleeding tendencies, palmar erythema (red palms), spider angiomas, fetor hepaticus, and hepatic encephalopathy. Clinical features that depend primarily on portal hypertension are splenomegaly, esophageal and gastric varices, and other evidence of abnormal collateral circulation. Ascites (fluid in the peritoneal cavity) can be considered as a manifestation of both hepatocellular failure and portal hypertension. Figure 23-5 illustrates the primary clinical manifestations of cirrhosis discussed in the following pages.

Manifestations of hepatocellular failure

Jaundice occurs in at least 60 percent of patients at some time during the course of the disease and is usually minimal. Hyperbilirubinemia without jaundice is more common. The patient may become jaundiced during a phase of decompensation with reversible deterioration of liver function. For example, the patient with cirrhosis may become jaundiced after a heavy drinking bout. Intermittent jaundice is a characteristic feature of biliary cirrhosis and occurs when there is active inflammation of the liver bile ductules (cholangitis). Patients dying from hepatic failure are usually jaundiced.

Endocrine disturbances are common in cirrhosis. Hormones of the adrenal cortex, testes, and ovaries are metabolized and inactivated by the normal liver. Spider angiomas are seen on the skin, particularly around the neck, shoulders, and chest. They consist of a central arteriole from which many small vessels radiate. Spider angiomas, testicular atrophy, gynecomastia, pectoral and axillary alopecia, and palmar erythema are all considered to be caused by an excess of circulating estrogen. Increased pigmentation of the skin is believed to result from excessive activity of melanin-stimulating hormone (MSH).

Hematologic disorders common in cirrhosis include bleeding tendencies, anemia, leukopenia, and thrombocytopenia. Nosebleeds, gingival bleeding, menstrual bleeding, and easy bruising are not uncommon, and the prothrombin time may be prolonged. These manifestations are the result of decreased hepatic production of the clotting factors. The anemia, leukopenia, and thrombocytopenia are believed to be the resultants of hypersplenism. Not only is the spleen enlarged (splenomegaly) but it is also more active in the removal of blood cells from the circulation. Other mechanisms contributing to the anemia include folate deficiency, vitamin B_{12} deficiency, iron deficiency secondary to blood loss, and increased hemolysis of red blood cells. The patient is also more susceptible to infection.

The peripheral edema which generally occurs after the development of ascites may be explained by the hypoalbuminemia and abnormal salt and water retention. The failure of the liver cells to inactivate aldosterone and antidiuretic hormone contributes to sodium and water retention.

Hepatic fetor is a musty, sweetish odor which may be detected on the patient's breath, especially in hepatic coma, and is believed to result form the liver's inability to metabolize methionine.

The most serious neurologic disorder in advanced cirrhosis is hepatic encephalopathy (hepatic coma). It is believed to result from abnormalities in the metabolism of ammonia and increased cerebral sensitivity to toxins. The development of hepatic encephalopathy is often a terminal event in cirrhosis and will be discussed in greater detail later.

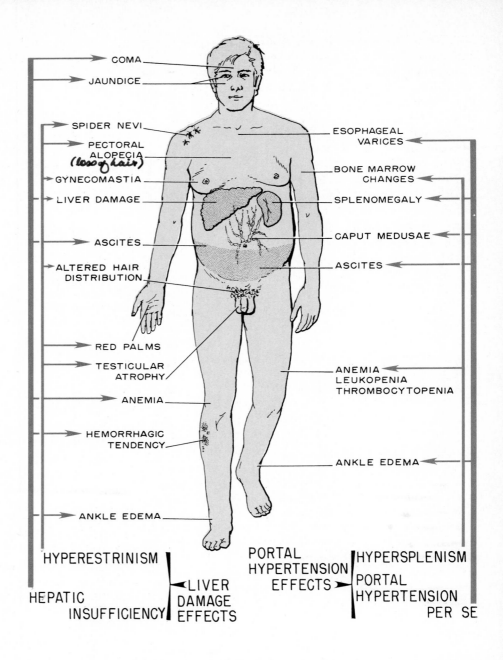

Figure labels:

COMA

JAUNDICE

SPIDER NEVI

PECTORAL ALOPECIA (loss of hair)

GYNECOMASTIA

LIVER DAMAGE

ASCITES

ALTERED HAIR DISTRIBUTION

RED PALMS

TESTICULAR ATROPHY

ANEMIA

HEMORRHAGIC TENDENCY

ANKLE EDEMA

ESOPHAGEAL VARICES

BONE MARROW CHANGES

SPLENOMEGALY

CAPUT MEDUSAE

ASCITES

ANEMIA LEUKOPENIA THROMBOCYTOPENIA

ANKLE EDEMA

HYPERESTRINISM

HEPATIC INSUFFICIENCY

LIVER DAMAGE EFFECTS

PORTAL HYPERTENSION EFFECTS

HYPERSPLENISM

PORTAL HYPERTENSION PER SE

Manifestations of portal hypertension

Portal hypertension is defined as a sustained elevation of pressure in the portal vein above the normal level of 6 to 12 cm of water. The primary mechanism for inducing portal hypertension, regardless of the disease, is increased resistance to blood flow through the liver. In addition, there is usually an increase in splanchnic arterial flow. The two factors of decreased outflow through the hepatic vein and increased inflow combine to overload the portal circuit. This overload of the portal circuit stimulates the development of collateral channels (varices) which circumvent the hepatic obstruction. The back pressure in the portal system causes splenomegaly and is partly responsible for the accumulation of ascites.

Ascites is an intraperitoneal accumulation of watery fluid containing small amounts of protein. Key factors in the pathogenesis of ascites are the increased hydrostatic pressure in the intestinal capillary bed (portal hypertension) and the decreased colloid osmotic pressure from hypoalbuminemia. Other contributing factors include the abnormal sodium and water retention and the increased synthesis and flow of hepatic lymph.

The important collateral channels which develop as a result of cirrhosis and portal hypertension are found in the lower esophagus. The shunting of blood through this circuit to the venae cavae causes dilatation of these veins (esophageal varices). These varices occur in about 70 percent of patients with advanced cirrhosis. Bleeding from these varices is a common cause of death (see Fig. 23-6).

The collateral circulation also involves the superficial veins of the abdominal wall, and its development leads to dilatated veins around the umbilicus (caput medusae). Dilatation of anastomoses between the branches of the inferior mesenteric vein and the rectal veins often leads to the development of internal hemorrhoids (see Fig. 23-2 to review points of anastomoses). Serious hemorrhage from the rupture of hemorrhoids does not usually occur, since the pressure is not as high here as in the esophagus because of the greater distance from the portal vein.

Splenomegaly in cirrhosis can be explained on the basis of chronic passive congestion due to backup and higher pressure of blood in the splenic vein.

Complications and treatment

The treatment of cirrhosis is unsatisfactory. There are no pharmacologic agents which either arrest or reverse the fibrotic process. Therapy is aimed first at dealing with any underlying cause, such as alcohol abuse or bile duct obstruction, and then at treating the various complications, including gastrointestinal hemorrhage, ascites, and hepatic encephalopathy.

Gastrointestinal bleeding

The most common and the most serious cause of gastrointestinal bleeding in cirrhosis is bleeding from esophageal varices and accounts for about one-third of all deaths. Other causes of bleeding include gastric and duodenal ulcers (there is an increased incidence in cirrhotic patients), acute gastric erosions, and a generalized bleeding tendency (as a result of prolonged prothrombin time and thrombocytopenia).

The patient presents with either melena or hematemesis. Occasionally the first sign of bleeding is hepatic encephalopathy. Depending on the amount and speed of the blood loss, there may be hypovolemia and hypotension.

A variety of measures have been used for the immediate control of bleeding. Tamponade with an apparatus such as the Sengstaken-Blakemore tube, when properly used, will stop the hemorrhage, at least temporarily (see Fig. 23-7). The veins can be visualized with fiberoptic instruments and injected with a solution that will cause a clot to form in the vein and stop the hemorrhage. Most clinicians feel that this has a temporary effect and is not effective for long-term management.

Vasopressin (Pitressin) has been used to control bleeding. The drug decreases portal pressure by decreasing splanchnic blood flow, although the effect is only temporary. In spite of these emergency measures, about 70 percent of patients die durung the first episode of bleeding.

If the patient recovers from the bleeding, either spontaneously or after emergency treatment, a portacaval shunt operation may be considered. This surgery reduces the portal pressure by anastomosing the portal vein (high pressure) to the inferior vena cava (low pressure). The shunt procedure represents drastic therapy of a major complication of cirrhosis. It lessens the chance of further esophageal bleeding but at the price of an increased risk of hepatic encephalopathy. The pa-

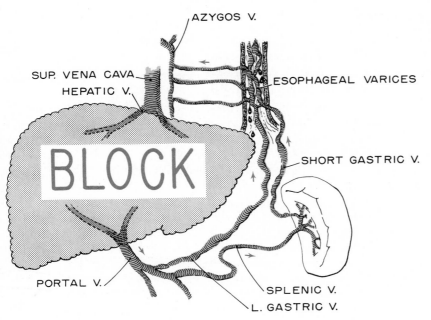

FIGURE 23-6
Hemodynamic changes in liver cirrhosis leading to the development of esophageal varices.

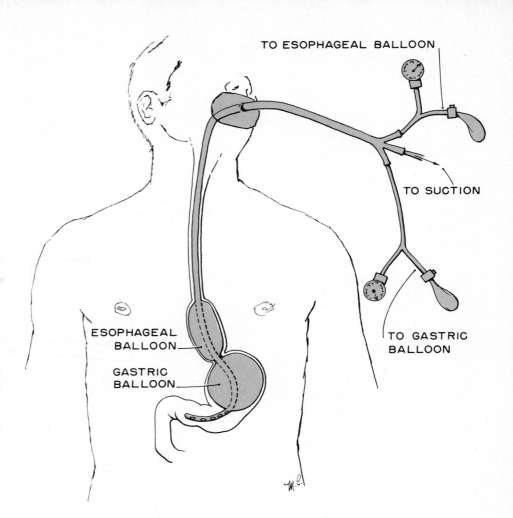

FIGURE 23-7

Sengstaken-Blakemore tube in place for the emergency treatment of hemorrhage from esophageal varices. The tube has three openings—one for gastric aspiration, one for inflating the esophageal balloon, and one for inflating the gastric balloon. The esophageal balloon is inflated to a pressure of 20 to 40 mmHg (the pressure is monitored by attachment to a gauge or a sphygmomanometer) which compresses the esophageal veins. The gastric balloon, inflated with 250 ml of air, applies pressure to the fundal veins when slight traction is applied.

TO ESOPHAGEAL BALLOON

TO SUCTION

TO GASTRIC BALLOON

ESOPHAGEAL BALLOON

GASTRIC BALLOON

tient's life expectancy is not increased but depends on the progress of the liver disease.

Gastrointestinal bleeding is one of the important precipitating causes of hepatic encephalopathy. The encephalopathy results when ammonia and other toxins enter the systemic circulation. The source of the ammonia is the bacterial breakdown of protein in the gastrointestinal tract. Hepatic encephalopathy will follow if the blood is not removed by gastric aspiration, saline cathartics, and cleansing enemas and if the bacterial breakdown of the blood protein is not prevented by the administration of neomycin or a similar antibiotic. These measures are discussed further in a later section.

Ascites

A large abdominal paracentesis is no longer considered desirable treatment for ascites because of its deleterious effects. There is danger of inducing hypovolemia, hypokalemia, hyponatremia, hepatic encephalopathy, and renal failure. Since the ascites fluid also contains 10 to 30 g of protein in each liter of fluid, there is further depletion of serum albumin, promoting the

reaccumulation of the fluid. Paracentesis is only performed when ascites causes prominent respiratory difficulty or for diagnostic purposes. Some patients with ascites also develop pleural effusions, especially in the right hemithorax. The fluid is thought to enter the chest through tears which develop in the tendinous portion of the diaphragm because of the increased abdominal pressure.

Salt restriction is a major method of treating ascites. Diuretics may also be used in conjunction with a low-sodium diet. There are a variety of diuretics and diuretic programs, but the essential feature is to introduce the diuretics gradually to avoid too brisk a diuresis. Electrolyte imbalance must be avoided, and even then diuretics may precipitate hepatic encephalopathy.

Hepatic encephalopathy

Hepatic encephalopathy (hepatic coma) is a neuropsychiatric syndrome in a patient with severe liver disease. It is characterized by mental confusion, muscle tremors, and a peculiar flapping tremor called asterixis. The mental changes may begin with mild mental clouding and may progress to death in a deep coma. Hepatic encephalopathy ending in coma is the mechanism of death in about one-third of the fatal cases of cirrhosis.

Pathogenesis

In simplest terms, hepatic encephalopathy can be described as a form of cerebral intoxication caused by intestinal contents that have not been metabolized by the liver. This condition may occur when there is liver cell damage due to necrosis or shunting (pathologic or surgically created) which permits large amounts of portal blood to reach the systemic circulation without traversing the liver.

The metabolites responsible for the encephalopathy have not been identified with certainty. The basic mechanism appears to be intoxication of the brain by breakdown products of protein metabolism produced by bacterial action in the gut. These products are able to bypass the liver because of liver cell disease or shunting. Ammonia, normally converted into urea by the liver, is one of the known toxic substances and is believed to interfere with brain metabolism (see Fig. 23-8).

Hepatic encephalopathy in chronic liver disease is usually precipitated by such events as GI bleeding, excessive protein intake, diuretics, paracentesis, hypokalemia, acute infections, surgery, azotemia, and the administration of morphine, sedatives, or ammonia-containing drugs. The harmful effects of many of these can be traced to mechanisms that result in the formation of large amounts of ammonia in the bowel. Encepahlopathy that follows potassium depletion or paracentesis is probably related to the formation of excessive ammonia by the kidneys and alterations of acid-base balance.

Clinical features

Clinical signs and symptoms of hepatic encephalopathy may arise very quickly and progress to coma when hepatic failure occurs in a fulminating hepatitis. In cirrhotic patients the progress usually is much slower and is reversible in the early stages if detected in time. Progression of hepatic encephalopathy to coma is commonly divided into four stages.

The signs in stage I are very subtle and may be easily missed. Danger signals include slight personality and behavioral changes. These may include an unkempt appearance, vacant stare, slurred speech, inappropriate laughter, forgetfulness, and inability to concentrate. However, patients may appear to be perfectly rational but uncooperative or disrespectful at times. Careful observation may reveal that they are more lethargic or sleep more than usual or that their sleep rhythms are reversed. Because of close association with such a patient, the nurse is in a strategic position to notice these

changes and should enlist the help of the family to detect subtle personality changes.

The signs in stage II are more prominent and are easily detected. Generalized muscle twitching and asterixis are characteristic findings. Asterixis, or flapping tremor, is elicited by having the patient raise both arms with forearms fixed and fingers extended. This maneuver causes involuntary rapid flexion and extension movements of the wrists (flapping) and metacarpophalangeal joints. Asterixis is a peripheral manifestation of impaired cerebral metabolism. It may also occur in the uremic syndrome. During this stage the lethargy and personality and behavioral changes become more marked.

Constructional apraxia is another prominent feature of hepatic encephalopathy. The patient cannot write clearly or draw figures such as stars or houses. A serial record of handwriting or figure construction is a useful method of determining the progress of the encephalopathy.

In state III the patient may become noisy, abusive, and violent, so that restraints may become necessary. If the patient is given a sedative at this time rather than treatment to reverse the toxic process, coma will probably ensue, and the outcome may be fatal. During this stage the patient may sleep much of the time. The electroencephalogram begins to change in stage II and is definitely abnormal in stages III and IV.

In stage IV the patient fades into a coma from which he or she cannot be aroused. Hyperactive reflexes and a positive Babinski's sign appear. At times a musty sweetish order (hepatic fetor) may be detected on the patient's breath or by just entering the room. Hepatic fetor is a grave prognostic sign, and the intensity of the odor correlates very well with the degree of somnolence and confusion. Elevation of the blood ammonia level is an additional laboratory finding which may be helpful in the detection of encephalopathy.

Treatment

The steps in treatment of hepatic encephalopathy have been suggested in discussing the mechanisms that cause it. It is most important to look for any precipitating factors, such as GI bleeding or overenthusiastic diuretic therapy, and give corrective treatment.

The initial treatment is to exclude all protein from the diet and inhibit the action of bacteria on protein substances in the bowel, since the breakdown of protein in the bowel is the source of ammonia and other nitrogenous substances. Neomycin, a nonabsorbable anti-

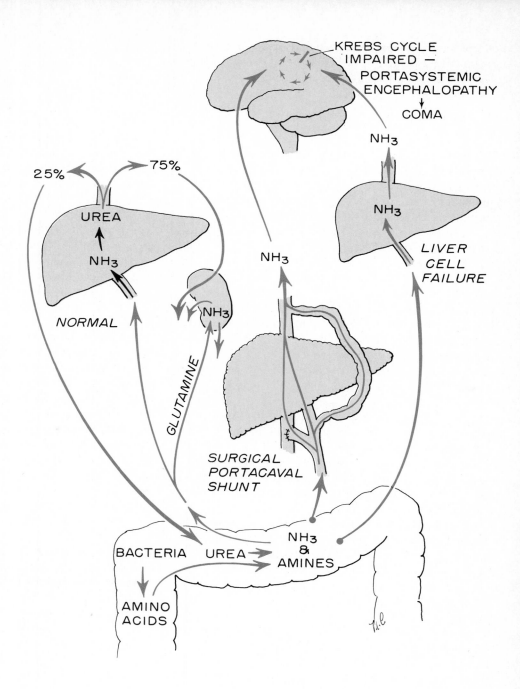

FIGURE 23-8
Normal and abnormal circulation of ammonia.

biotic, is usually the drug of choice for the inhibition of gut bacteria. The usual dose is about 4 g/day. If the patient has had recent GI bleeding (source of protein), magnesium sulfate or enemas may be given to purge the bowel. It is important to correct fluid and electrolyte imbalance, especially hypokalemia, which exacerbates encephalopathy. Barbiturates and narcotics are avoided. Nourishment is given in the form of sweetened fruit juices or intravenous glucose. These measures are usually successful if instituted early in the course of precoma and if the liver damage is not too far advanced.

A number of measures are used to prevent encephalopathy in the patient with a portacaval shunt or in one who has recovered from encephalopathy. These measures include a diet with modest amounts of protein, maintenance doses of neomycin, avoidance of potassium-depleting diuretics and ammonia-containing medication, avoidance of sedatives and narcotics, avoidance of constipation, and prohibition of all dietary protein if the symptoms should recur.

CHOLELITHIASIS AND CHOLECYSTITIS

The two most prominent diseases of the biliary tree, from the standpoint of frequency, are stone formation (cholelithiasis) and an associated chronic inflammation (cholecystitis). Although either of these conditions may occur alone, they are commonly associated and will be discussed together.

Pathology

Gallstones are essentially precipitates of one or more components of bile: cholesterol, bilirubin, bile salts, calcium, and protein (see Fig. 3-10). Of these substances, cholesterol is nearly insoluble in water and bilirubin is poorly soluble. Gallstones may be composed of pure bilirubin or pure cholesterol, or they may be mixed cholesterol stones. The latter may also contain calcium. Pure bilirubin stones are usually small, multiple, black, and associated with hemolytic disorders. These gallstones are uncommon. Pure cholesterol stones usually present as a large, solitary, round or oval structure which is pale yellow in color. Mixed cholesterol stones are the most common and are multiple and dark brown in color. Gallstones of mixed composition are frequently visible on x-ray, while those of pure composition may not be.

Etiology and pathogenesis

Gallstones are unusually common in the United States, with 10 to 20 percent of the adult population affected. Each year, several hundred thousand of these patients undergo biliary tract surgery. Gallstones are uncommon during the first two decades of life. Racial and familial factors seem to be associated with a higher incidence of gallstones. American Indians have an unusually high incidence, followed next by whites and finally blacks. Clinical conditions associated with a higher incidence of gallstones include diabetes, cirrhosis of the liver, pancreatitis, cancer of the gallbladder, and ileal disease or resection.

Gallstones are almost invariably formed in the gallbladder and rarely in other parts of the biliary tree. The etiology of gallstones is still incompletely understood; however, the most important predisposing factors appear to be metabolic disturbances causing changes in the composition of bile, bile stasis, and gallbladder infection.

Changes in the composition of bile are probably the most important factor in gallstone formation. A number of studies have indicated that the livers of patients with cholesterol gallstone disease secrete a bile that is supersaturated with cholesterol. This excess cholesterol is precipitated in the gallbladder in a manner that is not yet fully understood.

Stasis of bile in the gallbladder can lead to progressive supersaturation, changes in the chemical composition, and precipitation of the constituents. Disordered contractility of the gallbladder or spasm of the sphincter

of Oddi, or both, could cause stasis. Hormonal factors, especially during pregnancy, may be related to delayed gallbladder emptying and may account for the higher incidence in this group.

Bacterial infection within the biliary tract can play a part in stone formation by increasing cellular desquamation and mucus production. Mucus increases the viscosity of bile, and the cellular elements or bacteria may serve as a nidus for precipitation. It is probable, however, that infection is more commonly a result of the formation of gallstones than a cause of them.

Clinical features

Patients with gallstones often present with symptoms of acute or chronic cholecystitis. The acute form is characterized by the sudden onset of agonizing pain in the upper abdomen, mostly in the midepigastrium; it may radiate to the back and right shoulder. The patient may break out in a profuse sweat or walk the floor or roll from side to side in the bed. Nausea and vomiting are common. The pain may last for several hours or may recur after a partial remission. As the pain subsides, tenderness may be noted over the gallbladder. Acute cholecystitis is often associated with impaction of a stone in the cystic duct and is frequently referred to as biliary colic.

The symptoms of chronic cholecystitis are similar to those of acute cholecystitis, but the severity of the pain and the presence of physical signs are less marked. Often there is a history of vague dyspepsia, fat intolerance, heartburn, or flatulence over a prolonged period of time.

Once formed, gallstones may lie quietly in the gallbladder and cause no trouble, or they may cause complications. The most common complications are infection of the gallbladder (cholecystitis) and obstruction of the cystic or common bile ducts by a stone. Such obstruction may be temporary, intermittent, or permanent. Rarely, stones may slough through the wall of the gallbladder and cause severe inflammation, often leading to peritonitis, or may cause the walls to become thin and rupture.

Diagnosis and treatment

The diagnosis of both the acute and chronic forms of cholecystitis and cholelithiasis often rests on cholecystography or ultrasound to reveal the presence of stones or malfunctioning of the gallbladder (see Fig. 23-9).

The common treatment of these two conditions is

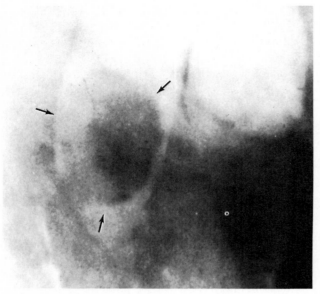

FIGURE 23-9
Gallstone.

surgical removal of the gallbladder (cholecystectomy) and/or removal of stones from the common bile duct (choledocholithotomy), which can be expected to effect a cure in about 95 percent of the cases. In cases of acute cholecystitis with severe symptoms and suspicion of pus formation, some surgeons operate at once, while others operate only if improvement does not occur within a few days. In cases of empyema or if the patient is in poor condition, the gallbladder may not be removed but merely drained (cholecystotomy).

PANCREATITIS

The pancreas is unusual in that this organ functions both as an endocrine and an exocrine gland. The chief endocrine disorder of the pancreas is diabetes; it will be discussed in the endocrinology section of this book. The exocrine products of the pancreas contain powerful enzymes which normally digest proteins, fats, and carbohydrates in ingested food. However, these potent enzymes which are so effective in digestion in the lumen of the small intestine also serve as a source of great danger to the organism if they are activated within the substance of the pancreas itself. This is essentially what happens in pancreatitis. Pancreatitis is commonly divided into acute and chronic forms.

Acute pancreatitis

Acute pancreatitis is an acute inflammatory process involving the pancreas and characterized by varying degrees of edema, hemorrhage, and necrosis of the acinar cells and blood vessels. The mortality and clinical symptoms vary with the degree of the pathologic process. When there is only pancreatic edema, mortality may be from 5 to 10 percent, while massive hemorrhagic necrosis has a mortality of 50 to 80 percent.

Etiology and pathogenesis

The main etiologic factors in acute pancreatitis are biliary tract disease and alcoholism. Less common causes include trauma, especially bullet or knife wounds, penetrating duodenal ulcer, hyperparathyroidism, hyperlipidemia, viral infection, and certain drugs such as corticosteriods and thiazide diuretics. Many times a precipitating cause cannot be found.

Pancreatitis is fairly common in adults but is rare in children. In men it is more frequently associated with alcoholism, while in women it is associated more often with gallstones.

There is virtually universal agreement that the common pathogenetic mechanism in pancreatitis is autodigestion, but the process by which the pancreatic enzymes become activated is not clear. In the normal pancreas, there are a number of protective mechanisms which act as safeguards against inadvertent activation of enzymes and autodigestion. First, the enzymes which digest protein are secreted as inactive precursors (zymogens) which must be activated by trypsin. Trypsinogen, the inactive form of trypsin, is normally converted into trypsin by the action of enterokinase in the small intestine. Once trypsin is formed, it is the key that activates all the other proteolytic enzymes. Trypsin inhibitors are present in the plasma and in the pancreas; they can bind and inactivate any trypsin inadvertently produced, so that proteolytic digestion is unlikely to occur in the normal pancreas.

Reflux of bile and duodenal contents into the pancreatic ducts has been proposed as a possible mechanism for the activation of pancreatic enzymes. This could occur when there is a common channel present and a gallstone becomes impacted at the ampulla of Vater. Atony and edema of the sphincter of Oddi might permit duodenal reflux. Obstruction of the pancreatic ducts and pancreatic ischemia may also play a role.

The two activated enzymes which are believed to play a critical role in pancreatic autodigestion are elastase and phospholipase A. Phospholipase A may be activated by trypsin or bile acids. It digests the phospholipids of cell membranes. Elastase is activated by trypsin and digests the elastic tissue of blood vessel walls, causing hemorrhage. The activation of kallikrein by trypsin is believed to play a role in the development of local damage and systemic hypotension. Kallikrein causes vasodilatation, increased vascular permeability, invasion of white blood cells, and pain.

Clinical features

The most prominent sympton of acute pancreatitis is severe abdominal pain which is sudden in onset and continuous. It is usually felt in the epigastrium but may be accentuated to the right or left of the midline. Radiation of the pain to the back is common, and the patient may obtain some relief by sitting forward. Nausea and vomiting often accompany the pain. The pain is usually severe for about 24 hours and then passes off over a period of days.

Physical examination may reveal varying degrees of shock, tachycardia, leukocytosis, and fever. There is tenderness and guarding of the abdominal muscles, but rigidity and other evidence of peritonitis occur only when the inflammation involves the peritoneum. Bowel sounds may be reduced or absent. Severe retroperitoneal bleeding may manifest as bruising in the flanks or around the umbilicus.

The diagnosis of acute pancreatitis is usually established by the finding of an increased serum amylase level. The serum amylase level is elevated during the first 24 to 72 hours, and values may be five times greater than normal. Urinary amylase levels are elevated as much as 2 weeks after an episode of acute pancreatitis. Other biochemical changes include elevation of the serum lipase level, hyperglycemia, hypocalcemia, and hypokalemia. Hypocalcemia is a common finding caused by marked fat necrosis with the formation of calcium soaps. It may be severe enough to cause tetany.

Complications of acute pancreatitis include the development of diabetes mellitus, severe tetany, pleural effusion (especially in the left hemithorax), and a pancreatic abscess or pseudocyst.

Abscesses are defined as collections of liquid secretory and necrotic products within the pancreas, while collections which occur outside the gland are called pseudocysts. Pancreatic abscesses and pseudocysts commonly occur during the second or third week after the onset of pancreatitis. A common site of a pancreatic pseudocyst is within the lesser omental sac. Secondary infection of these collections of fluid are common.

The most common sequelae of acute pancreatitis are recurrent acute attacks and the development of chronic pancreatitis.

Treatment

The primary early treatment of acute pancreatitis is medical, with surgery limited to treatment of biliary obstruction or of specific complications such as a pan-

creatic pseudocyst. Treatment objectives include relief of pain, reduction of pancreatic secretions, prevention or treatment of shock, restoration of fluid and electrolyte balance, and treatment of secondary infection. Shock and hypovolemia are treated with plasma and electrolyte infusions using the hematocrit, central venous pressure, and urine output as indices of adequate volume replacement. Meperidine (Demerol), rather than opiates, is used to relieve the pain, since it causes less spasm of the sphincter of Oddi. Elimination of all oral intake and constant gastric suction reduce intestinal distention and prevent acid contents from entering the duodenum and stimulating pancreatic secretion. Antibiotic treatment of established infection is essential, and it may be given during the first 2 weeks in the hope of preventing pancreatic abscess.

Pancreatic abscesses are treated by surgical drainage through the anterior abdominal wall or flank. Pseudocysts are managed by internal drainage between the anterior wall of the cyst and the posterior wall of the gastric antrum.

Once the acute phase of the illness subsides, oral feedings may be given beginning with carbohydrates, which stimulate pancreatic secretions least. Attempts are made to determine the cause of the inflammation. The patient is advised against alcohol for at least 3 months, and if the pancreatitis is believed to be alcohol-induced, there should be permanent and total abstinence.

Chronic pancreatitis

Chronic pancreatitis is characterized by progressive destruction of the gland, with fibrotic replacement that may result in stricture and eventual calcification. The etiologic factors are the same as those in acute pancreatitis—about one-third to one-half of patients are alcoholics. The clinical course may be one of recurrent episodes of acute pain, each leaving the patient with less functioning pancreatic mass, or a slow advance. Steatorrhea, malabsorption, weight loss, and diabetes are manifestations of advanced destruction. Chronic pancreatitis may follow acute pancreatitis, but in many patients it begins insidiously.

The most sensitive test for detecting chronic pancreatitis is the determination of bicarbonate concentration and output in the duodenum after stimulation with secretin. Other useful diagnostic measures include fecal fat determination, fasting blood glucose levels to determine islet cell damage, and arteriography and x-ray examination to detect fibrosis and calcification. Unfortunately, invasive pancreatic carcinoma can produce the same pathophysiologic findings as produced by chronic pancreatitis and consequently presents a major problem for the physician in the differential diagnosis.

The treatment of chronic pancreatitis is taxing and unsatisfacotry. Relief of pain is difficult and may require large and frequent doses of analgesics. Narcotic addiction becomes a serious problem. Steatorrhea is managed with a low-fat diet and oral administration of pancreatic enzymes. Diabetes requires control either with oral hypoglycemic agents or with insulin. Alcohol ingestion is contraindicated.

CANCER OF THE LIVER, GALLBLADDER, AND PANCREAS

Primary cancer of the liver and gallbladder are relatively uncommon tumors in the United States. However, primary cancer of the liver is quite common in Africa and Japan. Both of these malignancies have a very poor prognosis.

Malignant tumors primary to the liver arise from either parenchymal cells or bile duct epithelium. The former is known as *hepatoma* and makes up 90 percent of primary liver malignancies; the latter is called *cholangiocarcinoma*. About 75 percent of patients who develop hepatoma have underlying cirrhosis of the liver, especially the alcoholic and postnecrotic types. The most important diagnostic cues are unexplained deterioration in a cirrhotic patient and rapid enlargement of the liver.

The most common tumor of the liver is a malignant tumor which has metastasized from some other site. Metastasis to the liver can be detected in more than 50 percent of all cancer deaths. This is particularly true of gastrointestinal malignancies, but many others also show this tendency (e.g., cancers of the breast, lung, uterus, and pancreas) (see Fig. 8-8).

Most cancers of the gallbladder are adenocarcinomas, and 80 percent of these patients have gallstones. Diagnosis is generally late, since the early symptoms are insidious and resemble those of chronic cholecystitis and cholelithiasis.

Cancer of the pancreas is a relatively common tumor, with incidence now approaching that of cancer of the stomach: This tumor is more common in males than in females by a ratio of 2:1 or 3:1. The peak incidence is in the advanced years. About 60 percent arise in the head of the pancreas, usually obstructing the biliary tract and causing jaundice and a palpably enlarged gallbladder. Those arising in the body and tail often remain silent until far advanced. Other signs and symptoms include abdominal pain, weight loss, anorexia, and nausea. Differential diagnosis from chronic pancreatitis may be difficult. Because of the difficulties in diagnosis, the tumor is usually not discovered until it has already spread beyond hope of local resection.

The average life expectancy is less than 1 year after the diagnosis of cancer of the liver, gallbladder, or pancreas is established.

QUESTIONS

Liver, biliary tract, and pancreas

Directions: Answer the following questions on a separate sheet of paper.

1. Explain why blood circulation through the liver is unusual.

2. Briefly describe the structure and function of the gallbladder and pancreas. What hormones control the release of bile and the exocrine pancreatic secretions?

3. List the eight major functions of the liver. Why is the liver a major organ of defense? Why is the liver called a flood chamber? How does the liver perform its detoxification functions (mechanisms involved)? What is the role of the liver in carbohydrate, fat, and protein metabolism?

4. List the four general pathogenetic mechanisms of jaundice.

5. What is kernicterus? What is its significance?

6. Why do newborn babies often have a slight transient jaundice during the first few days after birth?

7. Does gamma globulin have any value in the treatment of existing hepatitis?

8. Enumerate measures which might help prevent the spread of viral hepatitis in the community, in the home, and in the clinical unit.

9. What percentage of liver destruction is still compatible with life? How long could you live after a total hepatectomy?

Directions: Fill in the blanks with the correct words or circle the correct word option when indicated.

10. The liver is roughly _____ in shape, weighs about (150) or (1500) g, and is located in the _____ quadrant of the abdomen. The right lobe forms a roof over the right _____; the left lobe forms a roof over two important digestive organs, the _____ and the _____. The _____ ligament divides the medial and lateral segments of the left lobe and is attached to the anterior abdominal wall. The liver is enveloped by dense connective tissue called the capsule of _____, and the stretching of this capsule in cases of hepatic enlargement is believed to cause tenderness or dull pain.

11. The chief secretory product of the liver is _____, which exits from the liver through the right and left _____ ducts, which immediately merge to form the common _____ duct; this secretory product enters the gallbladder through the _____ _____ duct and enters the duodenum through the common _____ duct. This terminal bile duct joins with the main _____ duct before entering the duodenum. The sphincter of _____ encircles the common channel and controls the entry of secretions into the duodenum.

12. Blood is supplied to the liver by the _____ artery and the _____ vein and is drained by the right and left _____ veins, which enter the inferior _____ _____. The paraumbilical veins form a potential pathway from the umbilicus to the _____ vein, allowing passage of a catheter and direct measurement of pressure in this vein. In cases of right-sided heart failure, blood may back up through the _____ veins, causing passive congestion of the liver but rarely cirrhosis. When blood flow through the liver is blocked in cirrhosis, blood may back up in the splenic vein, causing enlargement of the _____, or may be shunted around the liver through the _____veins, causing internal hemorrhoids.

13. The structural and functional unit of the liver is called the _____; it is hexagonal in shape and composed of plates of liver cells. Mixed arterial and portal venous blood flows through liver capillaries called _____, which are lined with phagocytic cells called _____ cells, and drains into a central vein at the center of the structural unit. Bile capillaries course between the hepatocytes and are called _____.

Directions: Circle the letter preceding each item below which correctly answers the question. Only one answer is correct, unless otherwise noted.

14. Which of the following clotting factors is not synthesized by the liver?
a. Prothrombin   b. Factor IV   c. Factor V   d. Factor VII   e. Factor X

15. All of the following serum proteins are synthesized by the liver except:
a. Albumin   b. Alpha globulins   c. Beta globulins   d. Gamma globulins   e. Fibrinogen

16. Which of the following hormones are catabolized by the liver? (More than one answer may be correct.)
a. Estrogen   b. Testosterone   c. Cortisone   d. Aldosterone

17. Which of the following is *not* a basic liver function?
a. Synthesis of albumin   b. Detoxification of chemicals by oxidation, reduction, and conjugation   c. Synthesis of urea from ammonia   d. Catabolism of bile   e. Phagocytosis of bacteria in portal blood

18. Which of the following functions is evidence that the liver plays a central role in lipid metabolism? (More than one answer may be correct.)
a. Chief site of bile formation   b. Synthesis of fatty acids from carbohydrate   c. Cholesterol synthesis   d. Phospholipid formation   e. Lipoprotein formation

19. The greatest value of liver scanning is in the detection of:
a. Hepatitis   b. Cirrhosis   c. Circumscribed hepatic lesions   d. Portal hypertension

20. Which of the following statements is *not* true concerning percutaneous liver biopsy?
a. The procedure is contraindicated in persons with a prolonged prothrombin time.   b. The patient must hold his or her breath and not move during needle insertion.   c. The patient must lie of the left side for 2 hours following the procedure.   d. Postbiopsy care includes frequently monitoring vital signs.   e. Significant hemorrhage is a rare complication.

21. *Direct* measurement of portal view pressure may be achieved by:
a. Percutaneous measurement of intrasplenic pressure   b. Catheterizing the hepatic vein and measuring wedged pressure   c. Passing a catheter

through the umbilical vein to the left branch of the portal vein   *d.* Percutaneous measurement of pressure in the liver ductules

22. The *chief* source of bilirubin is:
a. Senescent red blood cells   *b.* Red blood cell precursors in the bone marrow   *c.* Hemoproteins from the liver   *d.* Spleen

23. Bilirubin is formed in the monocyte-macrophage system by the reduction of:
a. Hemoglobin   *b.* Globin   *c.* Biliverdin *d.* Urobilinogen

24. The primary site of free (unconjugated) bilirubin formation is:
a. Liver   *b.* Kidneys   *c.* Spleen   *d.* Gastrointestinal tract

25. Unconjugated bilirubin is transported in the blood to the liver bound to:
a. Globulins   *b.* Red blood cell membranes *c.* Fibrinogen   *d.* Albumin

26. The enzyme responsible for the final step in bilirubin conjugation is:
a. Glucuronyl transferase   *b.* SGOT   *c.* Alkaline phosphatase   *d.* Lactate dehydrogenase

27. Conjugated bilirubin is: (More than one answer may be correct.)
a. Excreted in the bile   *b.* Water-soluble *c.* Characterized by its great affinity for lipids *d.* Capable of being excreted in the urine

28. A 21-year-old male college student is seen with the chief complaint of jaundice. His friend, a nursing student noticed that his eyes were yellow, although he had been completely asymptomatic. He also remembered that a younger brother had been icteric on several occasions. The physical exam was negative. SGOT, alkaline phosphatase, CBC, and liver scan were all normal. The test for urine bilirubin was negative. Total serum bilirubin was 4.8 mg per 100 ml (conjugated portion 0.5 mg per 100 ml). His most likely problem is:
a. Viral hepatitis   *b.* Infectious mononucleosis *c.* Hemolytic anemia   *d.* Gilbert's syndrome

29. The prognosis for the condition in question 28 is:
a. Poor   *b.* Good

30. The most likely pathogenetic mechanism causing the condition in question 28 is:
a. Transport failure of bilirubin due to defective binding to albumin   *b.* Excessive load of bilirubin presented to liver due to hemolysis   *c.* Impaired excretion of conjugated bilirubin   *d.* Impaired uptake of bilirubin by hepatocyte

31. Ms. B has been admitted to the hospital for evaluation of her jaundice. Additional findings include clay-colored stools, dark urine which forms a yellow-tinted foam when shaken, pruritus, and predominantly conjugated hyperbilirubinemia. These findings are compatible with:
a. Hemolytic jaundice   *b.* Intrahepatic cholestasis   *c.* Extrahepatic cholestasis *d.* Only *b* or *c*   *e.* All of the above

32. In hemolytic jaundice increased bilirubin will not be present *because* it is all unconjugated.
a. Both statement and reason are true.   *b.* Statement is true, reason is false.   *c.* Both statement and reason are false.   *d.* Statement is false, reason is true.

33. Pathologic changes common to diseases of the liver, gallbladder and pancreas include:
a. Fibrosis   *b.* Inflammation   *c.* Neoplasms *d.* All of the above

34. Common findings during the prodromal phase of hepatitis include: (More than one answer may be correct.)
a. Malaise   *b.* Icterus   *c.* Anorexia and loss of desire to smoke   *d.* Periportal inflammation revealed by biopsy   *e.* Low-grade fever

35. Match each of the features in col. A to the two types of hepatitis in col. B.

Column A

____ Transmitted by fecal-oral route

____ Positive test for hepatitis antigen

____ Seasonal incidence

____ Higher mortality and complications

____ Higher incidence among institutionalized

____ Especially common in drug addicts

____ Longer incubation period

____ A constant threat to patients and staff in hemodialysis units

Column B

a. Hepatitis A

b. Hepatitis B

c. Both A and B

d. Neither A nor B

_____ Epidemics common when water supply contaminated

_____ Synonym— serum hepatitis

_____ Synonym—infectious hepatitis

36. Match each of the following altered lab tests of liver, biliary, and pancreatic function in col. A to its possible clinical significance in col. B

Column A

_____ Marked increase of serum amylase

_____ Marked increase of serum alkaline phosphatase

_____ Prolonged prothrombin time

_____ Hypoalbuminemia

_____ Increased blood ammonia

_____ BSP test

_____ Urine bilirubin

_____ Hyperbilirubinemia (unconjugated)

_____ Urine urobilinogen

Column B

a. Hepatic failure or large porto-systemic shunt may be present

b. May indicate biliary obstruction; also increased in bone disease

c. Results in increased bleeding tendency; may indicate liver cell damage

d. Common in acute pancreatitis

e. Normally absent from urine; presence indicates hepatocellular disease or biliary obstruction

f. Possible hemolytic process

g. Sensitive index of liver function

h. Decreased in biliary obstruction

i. Related to edema formation in hepatic insufficiency.

Directions: Answer the following questions on a separate sheet of paper.

37. What is alcoholic hepatitis and what is its significance in relation to cirrhosis of the liver?

38. Why is cirrhosis of the liver usually not diagnosed until it is advanced?

39. What is portal hypertension? What is the basic mechanism involved in its development?

40. Describe two emergency methods of treatment for bleeding esophageal varices. Why is it so important to remove the blood from the GI tract? Describe the surgical treatment of esophageal varices to prevent recurrent bleeding. Why does the patient often develop hepatic encephalopathy after this type of surgery?

41. What is hepatic encephalopathy? How is it related to portal-systemic shunting and liver cell failure? Why is it important to detect hepatic encephalopathy in its early stages?

42. What is asterixis? How is it tested for?

43. What is constructional apraxia? Significance?

44. Make a table which outlines the four progressive stages of hepatic encephalopathy and gives the major clinical features of each stage.

45. Compare the clinical features of acute and chronic cholecystitis.

46. Why is the liver such a common site of metastasis of malignant tumors?

Directions: Circle the letter preceding each item below that correctly answers the question. More than one answer may be correct.

47. Pathologic changes present in cirrhosis of the liver include:
 a. Distortion of the liver architecture
 b. Fibrosis c. Necrosis d. Regenerative nodules e. Fatty infiltration

48. The single most important cause of cirrhosis in the United States is:
 a. Cholecystitis b. Cholestasis c. Chronic alcoholism d. Viral hepatitis

49. The major body site for the metabolism of alcohol is:
 a. Gastrointestinal tract b. Kidneys c. Brain d. Liver

50. The first morphologic change in the liver associated with alcohol abuse is:
 a. Fatty infiltration b. Cholestasis c. Necrosis d. Fibrosis

51. The hepatic lesion in severe kwashiorkor is:
 a. Cirrhosis of the postnecrotic type b. Laennec's cirrhosis c. Hepatitislike picture d. Fatty infiltration

52. Possible pathogenetic mechanisms accounting for fatty infiltration of the liver include:
 a. Excess formation of triglycerides b. Excess formation of urea by the liver cell c. Decreased oxidation of fatty acids by the liver cell d. Decreased synthesis of lipoproteins

53. The two most serious consequences of liver cirrhosis are: (Choose _two._)
 a. Hepatocellular failure b. Fatty infiltration of the liver c. Portal hypertension d. Increased production of alcohol dehydrogenase

54. The most common cause of biliary cirrhosis is:
a. Chronic active hepatitis   b. Posthepatic biliary obstruction   c. Alcoholism   d. Primary inflammatory disease of the bile ductules

55. Postnecrotic cirrhosis is characterized by:
a. Prior intoxication with chemicals in a few cases
b. A pattern of patchy necrosis   c. An enlarged firm liver with a green hue   d. An increased incidence of hepatoma

56. The incidence of esophageal varices in advanced Laennec's cirrhosis is:
a. 20 percent   b. 50 percent   c. 70 percent
d. 100 percent

57. Possible causes of anemia associated with some cases of cirrhosis include:
a. Blood loss   b. Folate and vitamin B$_{12}$ deficiency   c. Increased hemolysis in the spleen
d. All of the above

58. Common physical signs in cirrhosis include:
a. Ascites   b. Vascular spiders   c. Palmar erythema   d. Prominent superficial abdominal veins   e. All of the above

59. What percentage of cirrhotic patients die during their first episode of bleeding from esophageal varices?
a. 5 percent   b. 25 percent   c. 50 percent
d. 70 percent

60. The most important source of ammonia in the human body is the:
a. Kidney   b. Liver   c. Digestive tract
d. Central nervous system

61. In hypokalemia, there is increased production of ammonia by the:
a. Liver   b. Kidney   c. Digestive tract
d. Central nervous system

62. Asterixis may be seen in:
a. Hypoglycemic states   b. Hyperglycemic states
c. Hepatic encephalopathy   d. Uremia

63. Characteristics of hepatic encephalopathy include all of the following except:
a. Mental confusion   b. Deterioration of ability to write and construct figures   c. Abnormal EEG
d. Increased blood urea nitrogen

64. The treatment of hepatic encephalopathy usually includes:
a. High-protein diet   b. Oral neomycin
c. Intravenous penicillin   d. Corticosteroids

65. Hepatic fetor has been related to the metabolism of:
a. Bilirubin   b. Cholic acid   c. Methionine
d. Alpha-ketoglutaric acid

66. Hepatic encephalopathy may be precipitated by:
a. Vigorous diuretic therapy   b. Infection
c. Constipation   d. Paracentesis   e. Gastrointestinal bleeding

67. Prominent veins across the lateral walls of the abdomen suggest:
a. Portal hypertension   b. Inferior vena caval obstruction   c. Hepatic vein thrombosis
d. Thrombosis at the bifurcation of the iliac veins

68. Marked elevation of serum amylase (fivefold) almost invariably signifies:
a. Parotitis   b. Cancer of the pancreas   c. Intestinal obstruction   d. Pancreatitis

69. Pancreatitis may be caused by:
a. Chronic alcohol abuse   b. Common-duct gallstones   c. Excess coffee ingestion
d. Trauma to the pancreas

70. Mechanisms which protect the normal pancreas from autodigestion include:
a. Proteolytic enzymes secreted in inactive form
b. Key enzyme trypsin must be activated by enterokinase   c. Trypsin inhibitors present in plasma   d. Secretion of bicarbonate

Directions: Circle T if the statement is true and F if it is false. Correct the false statements.

71. T   F   Ascites is the accumulation of fluid within the pleural cavity.

72. T   F   Reflux of bile and/or duodenal contents into the pancreatic ducts causing activation of enzymes within the pancreas are possible mechanisms in the development of pancreatitis.

73. T   F   Hemorrhagic pancreatitis may be characterized by shock, hypovolemia, paralytic ileus, and tetany.

74. T   F   Chronic pancreatitis is most frequently associated with cholelithiasis and cholecystitis in males.

75. T   F   Abdominal pain is the most prominent symptom of pancreatitis.

76. T   F   Kallikrein, when activated within the pancreas, causes vasodilatation, increased vascular permeability, and pain.

77. T   F   Mixed cholesterol gallstones are frequently associated with hemolytic disorders.

78. T   F   A pancreatic pseudocyst is a collection of liquid secretory and necrotic products which forms within the pancreas itself during the course of acute pancreatitis.

79. T   F   Cancer of the liver and gallbladder

are common tumors in the United States, are generally detected in the early stages, and have a good prognosis.

80. T F The majority of patients with cancer of the gallbladder have gallstones.

81. T F Cancer of the head of the pancreas may be difficult to differentiate from chronic pancreatitis.

82. T F Steatorrhea, malabsorption, weight loss, and diabetes are manifestations of advanced destruction of the pancreas.

83. T F Surgical removal of the gallbladder is called choledocholithotomy.

84. Match each of the following clinical features of cirrhosis in col. A to the most likely mechanism causing them in col. B.

Column A

____ Peripheral edema

____ Jaundice

____ Spider angiomas

____ Leukopenia

____ Clotting abnormalities

____ Hemorrhoids

Column B

a. Increased circulating levels of estrogens due to failure of liver cell to inactivate them

b. Hypersplenism

c. Impaired uptake, conjugation, and excretion of bilirubin

d. Portal hypertension → increased flow and pressure through points of portal-systemic anastomoses.

e. Decreased hepatic production of fibrinogen, factor V, and other vitamin K–†ependent clotting factors

f. Liver cell failure → hypoalbuminemia → decreased colloid osmotic pressure; increased sodium and water retention

REFERENCES FOR PART IV

BAYLESS, T. M. and N. L. CHRISTOPHER: "Disaccharide Deficiency," *American Journal of Clinical Nutrition,* **22:** 181–190, 1969.

BOCKUS, H. L.: Gastroenterology, 3d ed., Saunders, Philadelphia, 1984.

BOGOCH, ABRAHAM (ed.): *Gastroenterology,* McGraw-Hill, New York, 1973.

BROOKS, F. P. (ed.): *Gastrointestinal Pathophysiology,* 2d ed., Oxford University Press, New York, 1978.

BURKITT, D. P.: "Epidemiology of Cancer of the Colon and Rectum," Cancer, **28:** 3–13, 1971.

BYNUM, T. E.: "Hepatic Mechanisms," in E. D. FROHLICH (ed.), *Pathophysiology,* 3d ed., Lippincott, Philadelphia, 1984, pp. 561–580.

DAVENPORT, H. W.: *A Digest on Digestion,* 2d ed., Year Book, Chicago, 1978.

———: "Mechanisms of Gastric and Pancreatic Secretion," in E. D. Frohlich (ed.), *Pathophysiology,* 2d ed., Lippincott, Philadelphia, 1976, pp. 481–497.

———: *Physiology of the Digestive Tract,* 3d ed., Year Book, Chicago, 1971.

———: "Salicylate Damage to the Gastric Mucosal Barrier," *New England Journal of Medicine,* **276:** 1307, 1967.

DAVIDSON, C.S.: *Liver Pathophysiology,* Little, Brown, Boston, 1970.

DIENSTAG, J. L., J. R. WANDS, and R. S. KOFF: "Acute Hepatitis," in *Harrison's Principles of Internal Medicine,* 9th ed., McGraw-Hill, New York, 1980, pp. 1459–1470.

ENTERLINE, H. and J. THOMPSON: *Pathology of the Esophagus,* Springer, New York, 1984.

GILLESPIE, I. E. and T. J. THOMPSON (eds.): *Gastroenterology,* 2d ed., Churchill Livingstone, London, 1977.

GIVEN, B. A. and S. J. SIMMONS: *Gastroenterology in Clinical Nursing,* 4th ed., Mosby, St. Louis, 1984.

GLICKMAN, R. M. and K. J. ISSELBACHER: "Diseases of the Small Intestine," in *Harrison's Principles of Internal Medicine,* 9th ed., McGraw-Hill, New York, 1980, pp. 1410–1418.

GOCKE, D. J.: "Current Status of Viral Hepatitis," *Hospital Medicine,* March 1975, pp. 8–17.

GREENBERGER, M. J. and K. J. ISSELBACHER: "Disorders of Absorption," in *Harrison's Principles of Internal Medicine,* 9th ed., McGraw-Hill, New York, 1980, pp. 1392–1409.

———: *Gastrointestinal Disorders: A Pathophysiologic Approach,* 2d ed., Year Book, Chicago, 1981.

HELMAN, R. A., et al.: "Alcoholic Hepatitis," *Annals of Internal Medicine,* **74:** 311–321, 1971.

HOLLANDER, F.: "The Two-Component Mucus Barrier, Its Activity in Protecting the Mucosa Against Ulceration," *Archives of Internal Medicine,* **93:** 107, January 1954.

HURWITZ, A. L., A. DURANCEAU, and J. K. HADDAD:

Disorders of Esophageal Motility, Saunders, Philadelphia, 1979.

IBER, F. L.: "Normal and Pathologic Physiology of the Liver," in W. A. SODEMAN, JR., and T. M. SODEMAN (eds.), *Pathologic Physiology*, 6th ed., Saunders, Philadelphia, 1979, pp. 885–927.

ISSELBACHER, K. J.: "Disturbances of Bilirubin Metabolism," in *Harrison's Principles of Internal Medicine*, 9th ed., McGraw-Hill, New York, 1980, pp. 1454–1470.

——— and J. T. LaMONT: "Diagnostic Procedures in Liver Disease," in Harrison's *Principles of Internal Medicine*, 9th ed., McGraw-Hill, New York, 1980, pp. 1450–1454.

KIRSNER, J. B. and C. S. WINANS: "The Stomach," in W. A. SODEMAN, JR., and T. M. SODEMAN (eds.), *Pathologic Physiology*, 6th ed., Saunders, Philadelphia, 1979, pp. 798–823.

LAMONT, J. T. and K. L. ISSELBACHER: "Diseases of the Colon and Rectum," in *Harrison's Principles of Internal Medicine*, 9th ed., McGraw-Hill, New York, 1980, pp. 1419–1436.

MIKKELSON. W. P.: "Portal Hypertension," *Hospital Medicine*, November 1973, pp. 56–70.

MONROE, L. S.: "Cholangitis," *Hospital Medicine*, October 1969, pp. 111–121.

NAISH, J. M. and A. E. A. Read: *Basic Gastroenterology*, Year Book, Chicago, 1974.

NETTER, F. H.: *Ciba Collection of Medical Illustrations: Vol. 3, Digestive System, Part I, Upper Digestive Tract*, Ciba Pharmaceutical Co., Summit, N.J., 1959, pp. 35–45, 49–65, 145–156, 164–187.

———: *Ciba Collection of Medical Illustrations: Vol. 3, Digestive System, Part II, Lower Digestive Tract*, Ciba Pharmaceutical Co., Summit, N.J., 1962, pp. 47–60, 77, 86–87, 170, 173.

———: *Ciba Collection of Medical Illustrations: Vol. 3, Digestive System, Part III, Liver, Biliary Tract and Pancreas*, Ciba Pharmaceutical Co., Summit, N.J., 1964.

ROBBINS, S. L. and M. ANGELL: *Basic Pathology*, 3d ed., Saunders, Philadelphia, 1981, pp. 457–546.

SCHULZE-DELRIEU, K.: "Metoclopramide," *Gastroenterology*, 77: 768–779, 1979.

SCHWARTZ, S. I.: "Liver," in S. I. Schwartz (ed.), *Principles of Surgery*, 4th ed., McGraw-Hill, New York, 1984, pp. 1257–1258.

SILEN, W.: "Acute Intestinal Obstruction," in *Harrison's Principles of Internal Medicine*, 9th ed., McGraw-Hill, New York, 1980, pp. 1437–1441.

———: "Peptic Ulcer," in *Harrison's Principles of Internal Medicine*, 7th ed., McGraw-Hill, New York, 1974, pp. 1431–1447.

——— and J. J. SKILLMAN: "Stress Ulcer, Active Erosive Gastritis, and the Gastric Mucosal Barrier," in G. H. STOLLERMAN (ed.), *Advances in Internal Medicine*, Year Book, Chicago, 1974, vol. 19.

SKINNER, D. B.: "The Esophagus," in W. A. SODEMAN, JR., and T. M. SODEMAN (eds.), *Pathologic Physiology*, 6th ed., Saunders, Philadelphia, 1979, pp. 785–797.

SLEISENGER, M. and G. FORDTRAN: *Gastrointestinal Disease*, 3d ed., Saunders, Philadelphia, 1983.

SNODGRASS., P. J.: "Pathophysiology of the Pancreas," in W. A. SODEMAN , JR., and T. M. SODEMAN (eds.), *Pathologic Physiology*, 6th ed., Saunders, Philadelphia, 1979, pp. 928–970.

TUMEN, H. J.: "Alcoholic Liver Disease," *Hospital Medicine*, September, 1974.

———: "Pitfalls in the Management of Advanced Cirrhosis," *Hospital Medicine*, April 1971.

VANTRAPPEN, G. and J. Hellemans: "Treatment of Achalasia and Related Motor Disorders," *Gastroenterology*, 79: 144–154, 1980.

WATSON, D. W. AND W. A. SODEMAN, JR.: "The Small Intestine," in W. A. SODEMAN, JR., and T. M. SODEMAN (eds.), *Pathologic Physiology*, 6th ed., Saunders, Philadelphia, 1979, pp. 824–859.

PART V

PENNY J. FORD ET AL.

CARDIOVASCULAR PATHOPHYSIOLOGY

Cardiovascular disease in the United States is epidemic in scale. Over 40 million Americans are afflicted with some disease of the heart or blood vessels; approximately 1 million deaths per year are attributable to a cardiovascular disorder. Disease of the heart and blood vessels is the leading cause of death in the country, claiming nearly as many lives as all other causes combined.

Heart attack is the major cause of cardiovascular mortality and morbidity. Approximately 550,000 deaths per year are attributable to heart attacks; many of these deaths are of middle-aged males. Of great concern is the fact that heart attack often occurs with little or no warning; the incidence of sudden death is high. Over half of the deaths from myocardial infarction occur during the first few hours after the onset of symptoms and prior to reaching the hospital. With the advent of coronary care units in the early 1960s, the hospital mortality from lethal disturbances of the cardiac rhythm has decreased significantly. However, the mortality from mechanical pump failure and shock is relatively unchanged. Efforts to mechanically assist the ventricle and reduce the size of the infarct are currently utilized in an attempt to decrease shock mortality.

Additional cardiovascular diseases with significant morbidity and mortality include rheumatic heart disease, stroke, hypertension, and congenital heart disease. The major therapeutic thrust for the control of cardiovascular disease must be primary prevention. Despite the fact that the precise pathogenesis of many cardiovascular diseases remains unknown, control of risk factors by effective screening and public education can effect a substantial reduction in cardiac morbidity and mortality. The emphasis must be upon prophylaxis rather than upon treatment of established disease; the lethal and disabling sequelae of cardiovascular disease are too pronounced to await evidence of disease.

The subsequent chapters present a detailed discussion of coronary atherosclerotic disease, valvular heart disease, heart failure, and peripheral vascular disease. Hypertension, hyperlipidemia, and rheumatic fever as they relate to the aforementioned disease entities are also considered. Techniques of circulatory assistance and cardiac transplantation will also be introduced.

OBJECTIVES

At the completion of this part you should be able to:

1. Correlate the pathophysiology of cardiovascular disease entities with the signs and symptoms of disease and the rationale for therapy.
2. Describe the influences predisposing cardiovascular structures to the development of specific disorders.

CHAPTER 24

PENNY J. FORD

ANATOMY OF THE CARDIOVASCULAR SYSTEM

OBJECTIVES

At the completion of this chapter you should be able to:

1. Describe the anatomic orientation of the heart in the thoracic cavity.
2. Locate and state the function of the following cardiac structures: atria, ventricles, semilunar valves, atrioventricular valves, and pericardium.
3. Trace the anatomic sequence of blood flow through the cardiovascular system.
4. Explain why abnormal elevations of right atrial pressure or left atrial pressure readily cause systemic venous congestion or pulmonary venous congestion, respectively.
5. Explain the relationship between the thicknesses of the right and left ventricular myocardium and the respective functions of these ventricles.
6. Identify and state the function of the sinuses of Valsalva.
7. Define automaticity, rhythmicity, conductivity, excitability.
8. Trace the normal sequence of excitation through the conduction system of the heart.
9. Describe two critical functions of the AV node.
10. State the normal intrinsic rate of impulse generation for the SA node, AV node, and ventricles.
11. Identify the layers of a blood vessel.
12. Compare the five vascular subdivisions of the systemic circulation as to structure, volume, pressure, and flow characteristics.
13. Describe the heart's blood supply, identifying the portions of the heart muscle and the conduction system supplied by each blood vessel.
14. Explain the significance of collateral circulation in the heart when occlusion of a coronary arterial branch occurs.
15. Describe the circulation of lymph and its function.
16. Contrast the systemic and pulmonic circulations.
17. Explain the influence of the autonomic nervous system upon cardiac function, including the control of heart rate, AV conduction, force of contraction, and vascular tone.

The apparent simplicity in the design of the cardiovascular system belies the intricate, yet logical, interdependence of circulatory structure and function in health and disease. Each portion of the cardiovascular system is uniquely adapted to contribute to highly integrated cardiovascular responses to disease processes. Hence, an understanding of cardiovascular anatomy is prerequisite to the examination of cardiovascular disease mechanisms and the capabilities and limitations of circulatory compensatory responses.

ANATOMIC RELATIONSHIPS

The heart lies within the mediastinal space of the thoracic cavity between the lungs. The pericardium en-

closes the heart and is composed of two layers: the inner layer, or *visceral pericardium,* and the outer layer, or *parietal pericardium.* The two pericardial layers are separated by a small amount of lubricating fluid, which reduces the friction created by the pumping action of the heart. The parietal pericardium is attached anteriorly to the sternum, posteriorly to the vertebral column, and inferiorly to the diaphragm; the visceral pericardium is in direct contact with the surface of the heart. The heart itself is composed of three layers: the outer layer or *epicardium;* the middle, muscular layer, or *myocardium;* and the inner, endothelial layer, or *endocardium* (See Fig. 24-1).

The upper chambers of the heart, the *atria,* are anatomically separated from the lower chambers, or *ventricles,* by a fibrous ring. The four cardiac valves are situated within this ring. Functionally, the heart is divided into right- and left-sided pumps, which propel venous blood into the pulmonic circulation and oxygenated blood into the systemic circulation, respectively. This functional division facilitates conceptualization of the

FIGURE 24-1

Anatomic relation of the heart to the surrounding structures. Inset shows the layers of the heart and pericardium. (Modified from G. H. Whipple et al., *Acute Coronary Care,* Little, Brown, Boston, 1972, p. 22.)

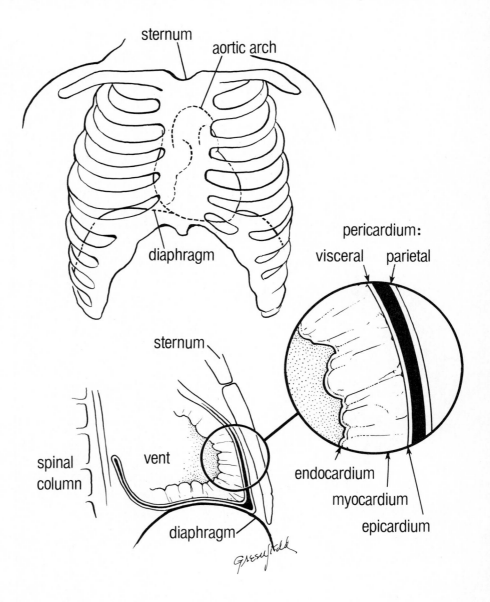

anatomic sequence of blood flow: venae cavae, right atrium, right ventricle, pulmonary artery, lungs, pulmonary veins, left atrium, left ventricle, aorta, arteries, arterioles, capillaries, venules, veins, and back to the venae cavae (see Fig. 24-2).

The schematic conception of the right and left sides of the heart shown in Fig. 24-2 is anatomically misleading however. In actuality, the heart is rotated to the left with its apex tilted anteriorly. This rotation places the right side of the heart anteriorly beneath the sternum, with the left side of the heart relatively posterior. The apex of the heart can be palpated at the midclavicular line at the fourth or fifth intercostal space (see Fig. 24-3).

Right atrium

The thin-walled right atrium functions as a reservoir and a conduit for systemic venous blood flowing to the right ventricle and lungs. Venous blood enters the right atrium via the superior vena cava, the inferior vena cava, and the coronary sinus. There are no true valves within the orifices of the venae cavae; only rudimentary valvular folds or muscular bands separate the venae cavae from the atrial chamber. Therefore, elevation in right atrial pressure as a result of right-sided congestion will be reflected backward into the systemic venous circulation.

Approximately 80 percent of the venous return to the right atrium flows passively into the right ventricle through the tricuspid valve. An additional 20 percent of ventricular filling occurs during atrial contraction; this active contribution to ventricular filling is called the

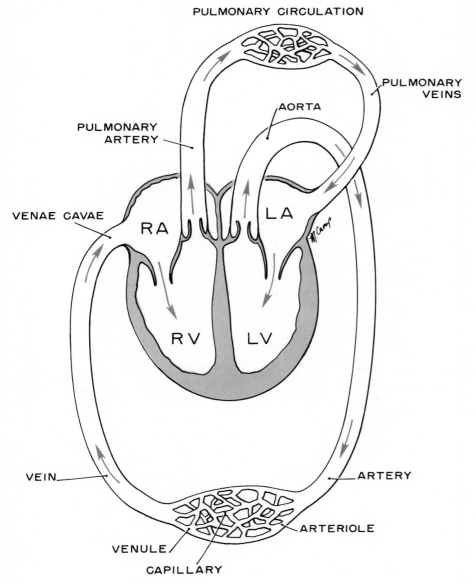

PULMONARY CIRCULATION

FIGURE 24-2
Schematic representation of blood flow through the cardiovascular system.

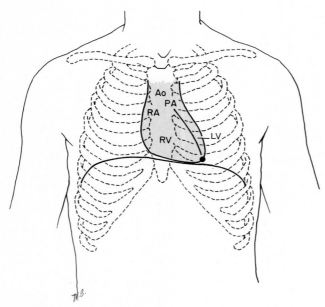

FIGURE 24-3
Orientation of the heart within the thorax. Ao, aorta; RA, right atrium; PA, pulmonary artery; RV, right ventricle; LV, left ventricle. The black dot marks the normal location of the apical impulse in the fifth left intercostal space near the midclavicular line.

"atrial kick." Loss of the atrial kick in certain cardiac arrhythmias can reduce ventricular filling and consequently decrease ventricular output.

Right ventricle

During ventricular contraction, each ventricle must generate adequate force to propel the blood received from the atrium into either the pulmonic or the systemic circulation. The right ventricle is designed in a unique crescent shape to generate a low-pressure, bellowslike contraction sufficient to propel blood into the pulmonary artery. The pulmonic circulation is a low-pressure system, offering considerably less resistance to blood flow from the right ventricle than the high-pressure systemic circuit offers to blood flow from the left ventricle. Therefore, the workload of the right ventricle is much less than that of the left ventricle. Consequently, the wall thickness of the right ventricle is only one-third that of the left ventricle (see Fig. 24-4).

In the face of gradually increasing pulmonary pressures, as with progressive pulmonary hypertension, the right ventricle undergoes muscular hypertrophy to increase its pumping force to overcome the elevated pulmonary resistance to ventricular emptying. However, in the event of an acute elevation in pulmonary resistance (such as in massive pulmonary embolization), the pumping capability of the right ventricle can be overwhelmed and death may result.

Left atrium

The left atrium receives oxygenated blood from the lungs via the four pulmonary veins. No true valves separate the pulmonary veins from the left atrium. Therefore, alterations in left atrial pressure are readily reflected retrograde into the pulmonary vasculature, and acute elevations in left atrial pressure will cause pulmonary congestion. The left atrium is a thin-walled, low-pressure chamber. Blood flows from the left atrium into the left ventricle through the mitral valve.

Left ventricle

The left ventricle must generate high pressures to overcome the resistance of the systemic circulation and sustain blood flow to peripheral tissues. The thick musculature and circular configuration of the left ventricle facilitate the development of high pressure during ventricular contraction. Even the interventricular septum separating the ventricles contributes to the powerful compression exerted by the entire ventricular chamber during contraction.

FIGURE 24-4
Schematic drawings of the heart to illustrate the differences in shape of the right and left ventricles. Top, ventricles in approximate anatomic position. Bottom, cross section illustrating the greater wall thickness and nearly circular shape of the left ventricle. (From J. W. Hurst, *The Heart,* 3d ed., McGraw-Hill, New York, 1974, p. 25.)

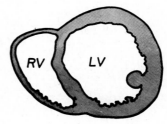
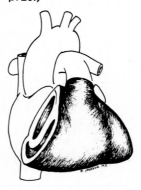

Left ventricular pressure exceeds right ventricular pressure approximately fivefold during contraction; if an abnormal communication exists between the ventricles (as with rupture of the interventricular septum after myocardial infarction), blood will be shunted from left to right through the defect. As a result, normal forward blood flow from the left ventricle through the aortic valve to the aorta will be decreased.

CARDIAC VALVES

The four cardiac valves function to maintain unidirectional blood flow through the chambers of the heart. These valves are of two types: the *atrioventricular valves* (or AV valves), which separate the atria from the ventricles, and the *semilunar valves*, which separate the pulmonary artery and the aorta from the corresponding ventricles. The valves open and close passively in response to pressure and volume changes within the cardiac chambers and vessels.

Atrioventricular valves

The leaflets of the atrioventricular valves are delicate, yet durable. The *tricuspid valve*, located between the right atrium and right ventricle, contains three leaflets. The *mitral valve*, separating the left atrium and left ventricle, is a bicuspid valve with two valve cusps or leaflets.

The cusps of both valves are attached to thin strands of fibrous tissue called *chordae tendineae*. The chordae tendineae extend to *papillary muscles*, which are muscular projections arising from the ventricular wall (see Fig. 24-5). The chordae tendineae support the valves during ventricular contraction to prevent eversion of the valve cusps into the atria. Rupture or malfunction of the chordae tendineae or papillary muscles supporting a valve would permit backflow or regurgitation of blood into the atrium during ventricular contraction.

Semilunar valves

Both semilunar valves are of similar configuration; they consist of three symmetrical cuplike cusps secured to a fibrous ring. The *aortic valve* is situated between the left ventricle and the aorta, whereas the *pulmonic valve* is positioned between the right ventricle and the pulmonary artery. The semilunar valves prevent backflow from the aorta or pulmonary artery into the ventricles during ventricular relaxation.

Immediately above the cusps of the aortic valve there are three outpouchings of the aortic wall called the *sinuses of Valsalva* (see Fig. 24-6). The orifices to

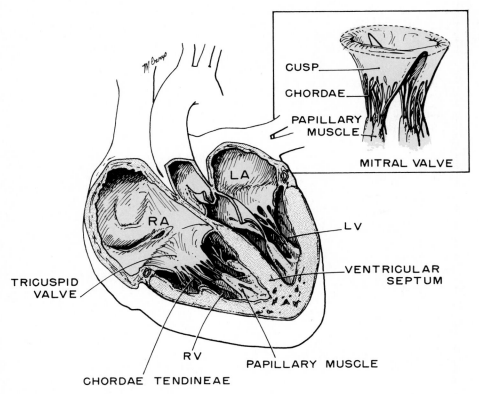

FIGURE 24-5
Anatomy of the atrioventricular valves.

CUSP

CHORDAE

PAPILLARY MUSCLE

MITRAL VALVE

LA

RA

LV

VENTRICULAR SEPTUM

TRICUSPID VALVE

RV

PAPILLARY MUSCLE

CHORDAE TENDINEAE

the coronary arteries are located within these outpouchings. These sinuses protect the coronary orifices from occlusion by the valve leaflets when the aortic valve opens.

CONDUCTION SYSTEM

The fibrous ring between the atria and ventricles isolates these chambers electrically as well as anatomically. To ensure rhythmic and synchronized excitation and contraction of the heart muscle, specialized conduction pathways exist within the myocardium. This conduction tissue exhibits the following properties:

1. Automaticity—the ability to spontaneously generate impulses.
2. Rhythmicity—the regularity of impulse generation.
3. Conductivity—the ability to transmit impulses.
4. Excitability—the ability to respond to stimulation.

As a consequence of these properties, the heart spontaneously and rhythmically initiates impulses that are transmitted throughout the conduction system to excite the myocardium and stimulate muscular contraction.

The cardiac impulse normally originates in the *sinoatrial (SA) node.* The SA node is therefore referred to as the natural pacemaker of the heart. The SA node is located in the posterior wall of the right atrium near the entrance of the superior vena cava.

The cardiac impulse then spreads from the SA node to specialized atrial conduction pathways and to the atrial muscle. An interatrial pathway, Bachmann's bundle, facilitates impulse spread from the right to the left atrium. Internodal pathways—the anterior, middle, and posterior pathways—connect the SA node with the atrioventricular node.

The electrical impulse then reaches the *atrioventricular (AV) node,* which is positioned at the top of the interventricular septum in the right atrium near the opening of the coronary sinus. The AV node is the normal route for impulse transmission between the atria and ventricles and performs two critical functions. First, the cardiac impulse is delayed here for 0.08 to 0.12 second to allow for ventricular filling during atrial contraction. Second, the AV node controls the number of atrial impulses reaching the ventricles; normally, no more than 180 impulses per minute are permitted to reach the ventricles. This protective effect is critical during certain abnormal cardiac rhythms in which atrial rates can exceed 400 beats per minute (bpm). If the ventricles were not protected from this excessive impulse bombardment, the ventricles would have inadequate time to fill and cardiac output would fall dramatically. Excessive delay or failure of impulse transmission at the AV node is known as heart block.

The wave of electrical excitation spreads from the AV node to the *bundle of His,* a thick bundle of fibers extending down the right side of the interventricular septum. The bundle divides into the *right bundle branch* and the *left bundle branch,* which descend on opposite sides of the interventricular septum. The left bundle branch bifurcates into a thin anterior and a thick posterior division. The bundle branches terminate in a complex branching network of fibers, the *Purkinje system,* which spreads throughout the inner surface of both ventricles. Spread of the wave of excitation through the Purkinje fibers is extremely rapid.

While these specialized conduction pathways speed the transmission of the cardiac impulse throughout the heart, the arrangement of myocardial cells outside the conduction system further ensures rapid impulse spread. Adjacent cells are separated by structures called intercalated disks. Within these disks are points of close intercellular membrane approximation referred to as nexuses. These nexuses facilitate rapid cell-to-cell

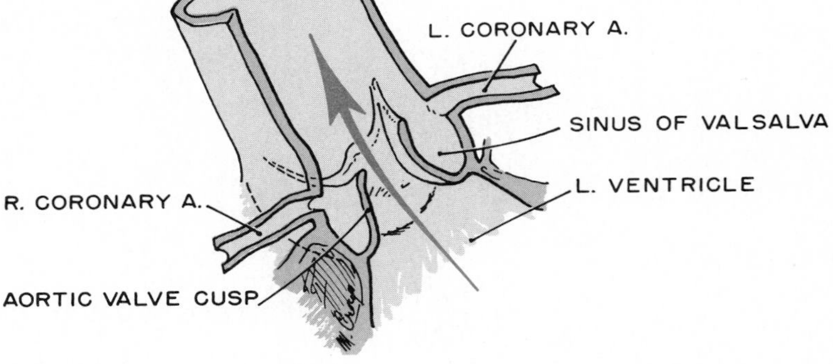

FIGURE 24-6
Sinuses of Valsalva.

AORTA

L. CORONARY A.

SINUS OF VALSALVA

L. VENTRICLE

R. CORONARY A.

AORTIC VALVE CUSP

transmission of electrical excitation, resulting in virtually simultaneous activation and contraction of the myocardial cells.

Therefore, the normal sequence of excitation through the conduction system is as follows: SA node, atrial pathways, AV node, bundle of His, bundle branches, and Purkinje fibers (see Fig. 24-7).

Anomalous anatomic connections bypassing portions of the conduction system have been identified in some individuals. These "bypass tracts" or connections can produce premature excitation of the ventricles by bypassing the intrinsic delays in conduction within the normal pathways of the conduction system. The Wolff-Parkinson-White (WPW) syndrome is an example of a preexcitation syndrome produced by impulse conduction via a bypass pathway directly connecting the atria and ventricles and bypassing the AV node.

Excitation normally originates in the SA node because the SA node exhibits the fastest intrinsic rate of impulse generation, approximately 60 to 100 bpm. However, in the event of SA node failure or its inability to generate impulses at an adequate rate, other sites can assume the role of pacemaker. The AV node is capable of generating impulses at a rate of approximately 40 to 60 bpm, and ventricular sites in the Purkinje system can generate impulses at rates of approximately 20 to 40 bpm. These lower, or "escape," pacemakers serve a critical function in the prevention of cardiac standstill (asystole) if the natural pacemaker fails.

SYSTEMIC CIRCULATION

The structural characteristics of each portion of the systemic vasculature determine its physiologic role in the integration of cardiovascular function. The vessel wall

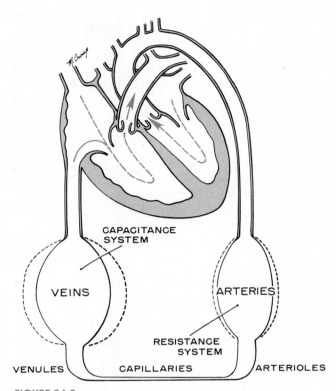

FIGURE 24-8
Schematic illustration of the systemic circulation. The arterial system may be considered as a resistance circuit (low volume, high pressure) whereas the venous system may be considered as a capacitance circuit (high volume, low pressure).

consists of three layers: the outer layer or *adventitia*; the muscular middle layer, or *medial layer*; and the inner endothelial layer, or *intima*. The systemic circulation can be subdivided into five anatomic and functional categories: (1) arteries, (2) arterioles, (3) capillaries, (4) venules, and (5) veins (see Fig. 24-8).

Arteries

The walls of the aorta and large arteries are composed of much elastic tissue and some smooth muscle. The left ventricle ejects blood into the aorta under high pressure. This sudden expulsion of blood distends the elastic arterial walls; during ventricular relaxation the elastic recoil of the walls propels blood forward throughout the circulatory system.

Peripherally, the branches of the arterial system proliferate and subdivide into smaller vessels. The relative increase in the cross-sectional area of the arterial system reduces the velocity of blood flow. This reduction in velocity of flow facilitates the eventual exchange

FIGURE 24-7
The conduction system of the heart.

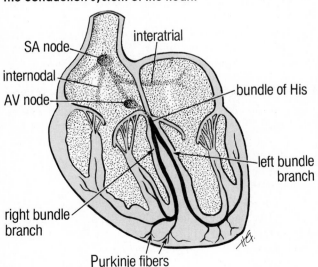

of nutrients and metabolites at the capillary level. The arterial bed contains approximately 15 percent of the total blood volume at one time. Therefore the arterial system is considered a low-volume–high-pressure circuit. Because of these volume-pressure characteristics, the arterial tree is called a *resistance circuit*.

Arterioles

At the arteriole level, the vascular wall is primarily smooth muscle with some elastic fiber. The muscular wall of the arteriole is highly responsive and can dilate or constrict to control the flow of blood to the capillary bed. As a result of this ability to significantly alter the radius of the vessel, the arterioles are the major sites of resistance to flow in the arterial tree. At the junction between the arteriole and capillary, there is a *precapillary sphincter* subject to intricate physiologic control.

Capillaries

The capillary wall is thin, consisting of a single layer of endothelial cells. Nutrients and metabolites diffuse across this thin, semipermeable membrane from areas of high concentration to areas of lower concentration. Oxygen and nutrients therefore leave the vessel to enter the interstitial space and the cell; carbon dioxide and metabolites diffuse in the opposite direction. Net fluid movement between the blood vessel and the interstitial space is dependent upon the relative balance between hydrostatic and osmotic pressures at the capillary bed.

Venules

The venules function as collecting tubules and are composed of a relatively weak, yet responsive, muscle wall. At the juncture between the capillary and venule, there is a *postcapillary sphincter*.

Veins

The veins are relatively thin-walled conduits for transport of blood from the capillary bed through the venous system to the right atrium. Venous flow to the heart is unidirectional as a result of valves strategically located within the venous channels. The veins can accommodate large volumes of blood under relatively low pressure. Because of these low-pressure–high-volume characteristics, the venous system is referred to as a *capacitance system*. Approximately 50 percent of the blood volume lies within the venous system at a given time. However, the capacity of the venous bed can be altered. Venoconstriction reduces the capacity of the venous bed, forcing blood forward to the heart and thereby increasing venous return. The movement of blood from the capillary bed toward the heart is influenced by two factors: (1) venous compression by skeletal muscles and (2) alterations in thoracic and abdominal pressures during respiration. The venous system terminates in the inferior and superior venae cavae.

CORONARY CIRCULATION

The efficiency of the heart as a pump depends on adequate oxygenation and nourishment of the heart muscle. The coronary circulation courses over the surface of the heart, carrying oxygen and nutrients to the myocardium via small intramyocardial branches. The distribution of the coronary arteries to the heart muscle and to the conduction system must be understood to recognize the consequences of coronary heart disease. The morbidity and mortality associated wth myocardial infarction depends upon the degree of both mechanical and electrical dysfunction.

Coronary arteries

The coronary arteries are the first branches of the systemic circulation. The coronary orifices are located within the sinuses of Valsalva in the aorta immediately above the aortic valve. The coronary circulation consists of the *right coronary artery* and the *left coronary artery*. The left coronary artery has two major branches: the *left anterior descending artery* and the *left circumflex artery* (see Fig. 24-9).

The arteries course around the heart in two external anatomic grooves: the *atrioventricular groove*, encircling the heart between the atria and ventricles, and the *interventricular groove*, separating the two ventricles. The juncture of these two grooves on the posterior surface of the heart is a critical anatomic landmark known as the *crux of the heart*. The AV node is located at this juncture; therefore, whichever vessel crosses the crux nourishes the AV node. The terms *right dominance* and *left dominance* simply designate whether the right or the left coronary artery crosses the crux.

The right coronary artery courses laterally around the right side of the heart in the right atrioventricular groove. In 90 percent of all hearts, upon reaching the posterior surface of the heart, the right coronary artery extends to the crux, then descends toward the apex of the heart in the posterior interventricular groove. The main left coronary artery branches shortly after its origin in the aorta. The left circumflex artery extends laterally around the left side of the heart in the left atrioventricular groove. This circumferential distribution corresponds to its designation as the "circumflex" artery. Similarly the term "left anterior descending artery" describes the anatomic pathway of this arterial branch. The left anterior descending artery (LAD) courses down the surface of the heart in the anterior interventricular groove. It crosses the apex of the heart, reversing direction and extending upward along the posterior surface of the interventricular groove to meet the distal branches of the right coronary artery.

Each major vessel gives off characteristic epicardial and intramyocardial branches. The LAD gives rise to *septal* branches supplying the anterior two-thirds of the septum and *diagonal* branches coursing over the anterolateral surface of the left ventricle. The posterolateral surface of the left ventricle is supplied by *marginal* branches of the circumflex artery.

The anatomic pathways result in the following correlations between coronary arteries and nutrient supply of cardiac muscle. Basically, the right coronary artery supplies the right atrium, right ventricle, and the inferior wall of the left ventricle. The left circumflex artery supplies the left atrium and the lateral and posterior walls of the left ventricle. The left anterior descending artery nourishes the massive anterior wall of the left ventricle.

The nutrient supply of the conduction system is another critical correlation determined by anatomic pathways. The SA node, despite its position in the right atrium, is supplied in 55 percent of individuals by the right coronary artery and in 45 percent by a branch of the left circumflex artery. The AV node, supplied by the artery crossing the crux, is nourished in 90 percent of individuals by the right coronary artery and in 10 percent by the left circumflex artery.

These correlations have significant clinical implications. For instance, a lesion of the right coronary artery would be expected to be associated with the highest incidence of AV nodal conduction disturbances, whereas a lesion of the left anterior descending artery would be more likely to interfere with the pumping function of the left ventricle.

Anastomoses between arterial branches exist within the coronary circulation. These anastomoses are of critical import as potential routes for collateral or alternative circulation to nourish myocardial regions deprived of flow by lesions obstructing normal pathways in the coronary vasculature (see Fig. 24-10).

Cardiac veins

The distribution of the coronary veins essentially parallels that of the coronary arteries. There are three subdivisions of the venous system of the heart: (1) the *thebesian veins* make up the smallest system, draining a portion of the right atrial and right ventricular myocardium; (2) the *anterior cardiac veins* are intermediate in importance, emptying a large portion of the right ventricular venous drainage directly into the right atrium; (3) the *coronary sinus and its branches* compose the largest, most significant venous system, draining the bulk of myocardial venous return into the right atrium through the coronary sinus ostium beside the orifice of the inferior vena cava.

LYMPHATIC CIRCULATION

The lymphatic capillary network in the interstitial spaces collects excess fluid and protein filtered through the systemic capillaries. This capillary filtrate is then returned to the systemic circulation via collecting vessels located in close approximation to the veins. Lymph is propelled upward through unidirectional valves by a combination of two dynamic influences: (1) external compression by muscles and arterial pulsations and (2)

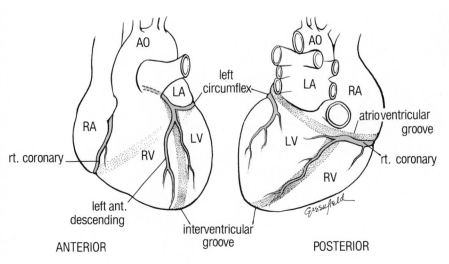

FIGURE 24-9
Coronary arteries supplying the anterior and posterior aspects of the heart.

intrinsic peristalsis. The terminal thoracic duct and right lymphatic duct empty into the subclavian veins.

PULMONIC CIRCULATION

The pulmonic circulation is described in depth in Part VI. However, significant differences between the systemic and the pulmonic circulation warrant mention. The pulmonic vasculature has thinner walls and less smooth muscle. The pulmonary circuit is therefore more distensible and offers less resistance to flow. Pressure in the pulmonic circuit is approximately one-fifth that in the systemic circuit. The walls of the pulmonary vasculature are much less reactive to autonomic and humoral influences, whereas alterations in oxygen and carbon dioxide content of the blood and alveoli profoundly

alter flow through the pulmonary vasculature. These differences make the pulmonary circuit particularly well suited to fulfill its physiologic function of oxygen uptake and carbon dioxide removal.

INNERVATION OF THE CARDIOVASCULAR SYSTEM

The cardiovascular system is richly innervated by fibers of the autonomic nervous system. The two divisions of the autonomic nervous system are the parasympathetic and sympathetic systems, which exhibit opposite effects and operate reciprocally. For instance, stimulation of the sympathetic system is usually coupled with inhibition of the parasympathetic system; conversely, parasympathetic stimulation and sympathetic inhibition are typically concurrent events. This reciprocal action increases the precision of neural regulation by the autonomic nervous system.

Autonomic nervous system regulation of the cardiovascular system requires the following components: (1) sensors, (2) afferent pathways, (3) an integration center, (4) efferent pathways, and (5) receptors.

There are two primary groups of sensors: the *baroreceptors* and the *chemoreceptors*. The baroreceptors, located in the aortic arch and carotid sinus, are sensitive to the stretch or distortion of the vessel wall caused by alterations in arterial pressure. Stimulation of these re-

FIGURE 24-10
Collateral circulation to the myocardium. (A) The bulk of blood flow to an area of myocardium is through the coronary blood vessel, with minimal flow through arterial anastomoses. (B) A lesion (e.g., an atherosclerotic plaque) in the coronary artery causes the development of increased collateral circulation, which may allow an adequate blood supply to the compromised area of myocardium.

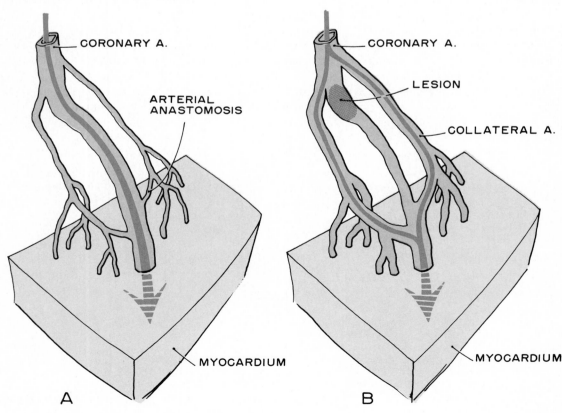

ceptors by elevation of arterial pressure signals the cardioregulatory center to inhibit cardiac activity; conversely, reduction of arterial pressure initiates reflex augmentation of cardiac activity. The chemoreceptors, located in the carotid body and aortic arch, are stimulated by reduction in arterial oxygen concentration, elevation of carbon dioxide tension, and elevation in hydrogen ion concentration (reduced blood pH). Activation of the chemoreceptors stimulates the cardioregulatory center to augment cardiac activity. Other receptors, which are sensitive to stretch resulting from alterations in blood volume, are located at the juncture between the great veins and atria. Two reflex responses occur upon stimulation of these receptors: an increase in heart rate (Bainbridge reflex) and diuresis.

Afferent pathways in the vagus and glossopharyngeal nerves carry the neural impulses from the receptors to the brain. The integration center or cardioregulatory center is located in the upper medulla and lower pons. The cardioregulatory center receives impulses from the baroreceptors and chemoreceptors and transmits impulses to the heart and vessels via the parasympathetic and sympathetic nerve fibers. Higher centers of the brain, such as the cerebral cortex and hypothalamus, can also influence autonomic nervous activity via the medulla. The efferent pathway from the cardioregulatory center to the heart is chiefly via the vagus nerves for the parasympathetic fibers, whereas the sympathetic fibers travel via the cardiac nerves. Receptors are located in the conduction system of the heart, the myocardium, and the smooth muscle of the blood vessels. Stimulation of the receptors alters the heart rate, the strength of myocardial contraction, and the diameter of blood vessels.

The parasympathetic fibers innervate the SA node, the atrial musculature, and the AV node via the vagus nerves. Parasympathetic fibers also extend to the ventricular muscle, but the functional significance of these pathways seems limited. Stimulation of parasympathetic fibers causes the release of acetylcholine. Acetylcholine mediates the transmission of the neural impulse to the cardiac receptors. Parasympathetic stimulation restrains cardiac action by reducing the heart rate, the speed of impulse conduction through the AV node, and the force of atrial and perhaps ventricular contraction. This response to parasympathetic stimulation is also referred to as a *cholinergic response* or a *vagal response*.

The sympathetic fibers extend to the entire conduction system and myocardium, as well as to the smooth muscle of the vasculature. Norepinephrine is the sympathetic neurotransmitter. Sympathetic stimulation causes the release of epinephrine and norepinephrine from the adrenal medulla. Sympathetic stimulation accelerates the heart by increasing heart rate, speed of impulse conduction through the AV node, and the force of myocardial contraction. This sympathetic response is also called the *adrenergic response*. The response of the heart to sympathetic stimulation is mediated by cardiac receptors called beta receptors. The vasculature contains two types of receptors, alpha and beta receptors. Sympathetic stimulation of vascular alpha receptors results in vasoconstriction; vascular beta receptor stimulation results in vasodilation. The cardiac and vascular beta receptors are distinguished as $beta_1$ and $beta_2$, respectively. Selective stimulation of these receptors, combined with variations in the intensity of sympathetic activity, regulates the degree of vasoconstriction, thereby controlling the capacity of the vascular bed and influencing the vascular resistance to blood flow and consequently arterial pressure. For example, arterial constriction would increase arterial pressure and the peripheral resistance to blood flow. Venoconstriction would reduce the capacity of the venous bed and increase venous return to the heart.

This cardiovascular reflex arc operates to stabilize arterial pressure and cardiac output and to mediate alterations relative to body needs. Cardiac output and arterial pressure can be increased by sympathetic stimulation and parasympathetic inhibition, resulting in an elevation of heart rate, increased force of contraction, and vasoconstriction. Conversely, abnormal elevations in blood pressure will result in reflex slowing of heart rate, reduced contractility, and vasodilation.

QUESTIONS

Anatomy of the cardiovascular system

Directions: Answer the following questions on a separate sheet of paper

1. Trace the anatomic sequence of blood flow through the cardiovascular system, naming the structures traversed.

2. Describe the two critical functions of the AV node.

3. Discuss the differences in the wall thickness of the right and left ventricles in terms of function. Relate the relative wall thicknesses to differences in the systemic and pulmonary circulations.

4. What is the function of the chordae tendineae and papillary muscles?

5. How many valve cusps are there on the valve between the left ventricle and aorta? Name this valve. Name the outpouchings above the valve cusps. What is the function of these outpouchings?

6. Identify the layers of the pericardium. What does the space between the layers contain and what is its function?

7. How is lymph propelled in lymphatic vessels?

8. Contrast the vascular effects of sympathetic stimulation of the alpha and beta receptors. Differentiate between beta$_1$ and beta$_2$ receptors.

Directions: Circle the letter preceding each item below that correctly answers the question. Only one answer is correct unless otherwise noted

9. The portion of the heart lying directly beneath the sternum is the:
a. Cardiac apex b. Left atrium c. Crux of the heart d. Right ventricle

10. The apex of the heart is normally palpated in the:
a. Fifth intercostal space to the right of the sternum at the midclavicular line b. Fifth intercostal space to the right of the sternum at the anterior axillary line c. Fifth intercostal space to the left of the sternum at the midclavicular line d. Fifth intercostal space to the left of the sternum at the anterior axillary line

11. All the valves of the heart have three cusps except:
a. Pulmonic b. Aortic c. Mitral d. Tricuspid

12. Oxygenated blood is contained within the
a. Pulmonary artery b. Pulmonary veins c. Superior vena cava d. Inferior vena cava

13. In order to generate high pressure to propel blood through the systemic circulation, the configuration of the left ventricle is:
a. Cresent-shaped b. Circular c. Elliptical

14. The outermost layer of the wall of a blood vessel is called the:
a. Intima b. Media c. Adventitia d. Serosa

15. The primary reason that blood flow through the capillaries is slow is because:
a. Capillaries are very small b. Capillary pressure is low c. Precapillary resistance is high d. Total capillary cross-sectional area is great

16. The SA node is the pacemaker of the heart because:

a. It is the only structure capable of spontaneously generating impulses. b. It is richly innervated by sympathetic nerves. c. It has the fastest intrinsic rate of impulse generation. d. It is anatomically the point of impulse origin.

17. Cardiac impulse conduction is slowest through the:
a. Purkinje fibers b. Interatrial pathways c. Bundle branches d. AV node

18. At any given time, most of the blood in the circulatory system is in the:
a. Arteries b. Veins c. Capillaries d. Heart

19. An increase in the mean arterial pressure causes: (More than one answer may be correct.)
a. Activation of baroreceptors b. Decreased sympathetic outflow to the heart c. Increased parasympathetic outflow to the heart d. Increased sympathetic outflow to vascular receptors

20. The response resulting from the above would be: (More than one answer may be correct.)
a. A decrease in the blood pressure b. An increase in the total peripheral resistance c. A decrease in the heart rate d. Reduced contractility of the heart

21. Which of the following statements concerning the cardiovascular chemoreceptors is *not* true?
a. They are located in the carotid sinus and aortic arch. b. Afferent impulses from the chemoreceptors are carried to the cardioregulatory center via the glossopharyngeal and vagus nerves. c. Chemoreceptors are stimulated by a reduction in the arterial oxygen concentration. d. Chemoreceptors are stimulated by an elevation of CO_2 tension. e. Activation of the chemoreceptors stimulates the cardioregulatory center to increase parasympathetic outflow to the heart.

Directions: Match each of the coronary arteries in col. A with appropriate items in col. B.

Column A	Column B
22. ____ Right coronary artery	a. Divides into two main branches
23. ____ Left coronary artery	b. One of its branches supplies the anterior wall of the left ventricle
	c. Supplies the AV node in 90 percent of individuals
	d. Supplies the SA node in more than 50 percent of individuals

24. Arrange the following structures to represent the normal sequence of cardiac conduction:
a. Bundle of His b. Purkinje fibers c. SA node d. Bundle branches e. Interatrial pathways f. AV node

Directions: Match each of the cardiovascular structures in col. A with its location in col. B.

Column A

25. ____ Chordae tendineae

26. ____ Interventricular septum

27. ____ Endocardium

28. ____ Epicardium

29. ____ Myocardium

30. ____ Sinuses of Valsalva

Column B

a. Separates right and left ventricles into two chambers

b. Is the muscular layer of heart

c. Attaches to AV valve leaflets on one end and to papillary muscles at the other end

d. Is the outer layer of the heart

e. Is the inner layer of the myocardial wall

f. Contains orifices of coronary arteries

Directions: Fill in the blanks with the correct word or phrase.

31. The conduction tissue of the heart exhibits the following properties: _____, the ability to spontaneously generate impulses; _____, the ability to respond to stimulation; _____, the ability to transmit impulses; _____, the regularity of impulse generation.

32. Elevations of right atrial pressure or left atrial pressure readily result in neck vein distention and pulmonary congestion, respectively, because the venae cavae and pulmonary veins, unlike most systemic veins, have no true _____.

33. In cases of coronary artery occlusion, _____ circulation may protect the involved muscle tissue from ischemia or necrosis.

34. Lesions of the _____ artery are associated with the highest incidence of AV nodal conduction disturbances. Lesions of the _____ artery are more apt to interfere with the pumping function of the left ventricle.

35. The intrinsic rate of the SA node is _____; the rate of the AV node is _____; and the ventricular rate is _____.

PHYSIOLOGY OF THE CARDIOVASCULAR SYSTEM

OBJECTIVES

At the completion of this chapter you should be able to:

1. State the relationship between the electrical and mechanical events of the cardiac cycle.
2. Define depolarization, repolarization, systole, diastole, action potential, electrocardiogram, and effective and relative refractory periods.
3. Differentiate between the slow response and fast response action potentials in terms of location, configuration, and significance.
4. Describe cardiac muscle ultrastructure and function.
5. Describe the electrical and mechanical events of the five phases of the cardiac cycle, including pressure and volume changes, valve opening and closure, and heart sounds.
6. Define cardiac output, cardiac index, stroke volume, ejection fraction, end-diastolic volume, and end-systolic volume.
7. Indicate the normal values for cardiac output and cardiac index.
8. Explain how depressed myocardial function affects stroke volume and end-diastolic volume.
9. Explain how cardiac output is related to stroke volume and heart rate.
10. Define and explain the relationship of preload, contractility, and afterload to stroke volume.
11. Explain and illustrate Starling's law of the heart and relate this to sarcomere length.
12. Describe the relationship between ventricular wall tension, intraventricular pressure, interventricular radius, and wall thickness.
13. Identify and discuss the determinants of blood flow and its distribution in the body.
14. State Poiseuille's law.
15. Define cardiac reserve in terms of compensatory mechanisms and explain the limitations of compensation.

Each cardiac cycle consists of a sequence of interdependent electrical and mechanical events. The wave of electrical excitation spreading from the SA node through the conduction system and to the myocardium stimulates muscular contraction. This electrical excitation is referred to as *depolarization*; it is followed by electrical recovery or *repolarization*. The mechanical responses are *systole*, or muscular contraction, and *diastole*, or muscular relaxation. The correlation between ventricular depolarization and ventricular contraction is illustrated in Fig. 25-1.

The electrical activity of the cell, recorded graphically via intracellular electrodes, exhibits a characteristic configuration, the *action potential* (see Fig. 25-2A). The summated electrical activity of all myocardial cells can be visualized in an *electrocardiogram* (see Fig. 25-2B). The waves on the electrocardiogram correlate with the spread of electrical excitation through the conduction system and myocardium. The significance of the waveforms is discussed in subsequent sections.

Immediately following myocardial depolarization, there is a brief interval, known as the *absolute* or *effective refractory period*, during which the myocardium is incapable of responding to any stimulus. A *relative refractory period* follows, during which the myocardium will respond only to a stimulus of greater than normal intensity. Tetanic contracture of the myocardium as a result of repetitive stimulation is therefore impossible.

Electrophysiology

The electrical activity of the heart is the result of alterations in cell membrane permeability which permit ionic movement across the cell membrane and change

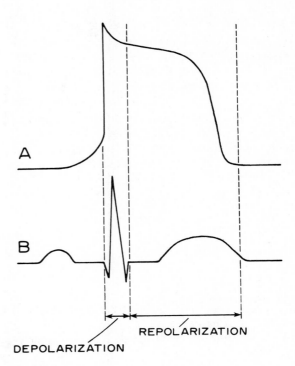

FIGURE 25-2
Electrical activity of the heart. (A) Recording of the intracellular potential of a single cardiac cell during a complete cardiac cycle. (B) A standard electrocardiographic recording from the body surface, representing the summated electrical activity of all the myocardial cells. The time periods within the dashed lines represent depolarization and repolarization of the ventricles.

FIGURE 25-1
Correlation between ventricular depolarization and ventricular contraction. (Modified from A. J. Vander, J. H. Sherman, and D. S. Luciano, *Human Physiology*, 2d ed., McGraw-Hill, New York, 1975, p. 238.)

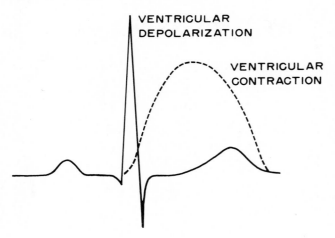

the relative electrical charge along the membrane. Ions are believed to flow through ion-specific channels situated along the membrane. These channels are described as "slow" channels or "fast" channels, distinguished by the rate of ionic flow and the mechanism activating the different channels. Three ions are of particular importance in cellular electrophysiology: potassium, sodium, and calcium ions. Potassium is the dominant intracellular cation, whereas sodium and calcium ion concentrations are highest extracellularly. Chloride ion shifts are also significant in some cardiac cells.

Recording an intracellular action potential from a typical myocardial cell produces the distinctive configuration illustrated in Fig. 25-2A. This action potential consists of five discrete phases corresponding to distinct electrophysiologic events (see Fig. 25-3):

1. *Resting phase—phase 4:* In the resting state, the cardiac cell exhibits a difference in electrical potential or voltage across the cell membrane. The inside

of the cell is relatively negative and the outside of the cell is relatively positive; thus the cell is polarized. This difference results from the relative permeability of the cell membrane to surrounding ions, particularly the positively charged sodium and potassium ions. In the resting state the cell membrane is more permeable to potassium than to sodium. Therefore, small amounts of potassium ions seep out of the cell from areas of high potassium concentration into the extracellular fluid where the potassium concentration is lower. This intracellular loss of positive potassium ions leaves the inside of the cell relatively negative in electrical charge (Fig. 25-3A).

2. *Rapid depolarization—phase 0:* Depolarization of the cell is the result of greatly increased membrane permeability to sodium. Extracellular sodium ions rush into the cell through fast channels, propelled by the sodium concentration gradient. This influx of positive sodium ions reverses the relative charge across the cell membrane; the outside of the cell becomes negative, and the inside becomes positive (see Fig. 25-3B).

3. *Partial repolarization—phase 1:* Immediately after depolarization, a small, abrupt change in ionic concentration and relative electrical charge occurs. This phase is believed to result from a transient influx of negatively charged chloride ions into the cell. The intracellular increase of negative charge leaves the inside of the cell slightly less positive (see Fig. 25-3C). In effect, the cell is partially repolarized.

FIGURE 25-3
Cellular electrophysiology. (A) Resting phase. (B) Rapid depolarization. (C) Partial repolarization. (D) Plateau. (E) Rapid repolarization.

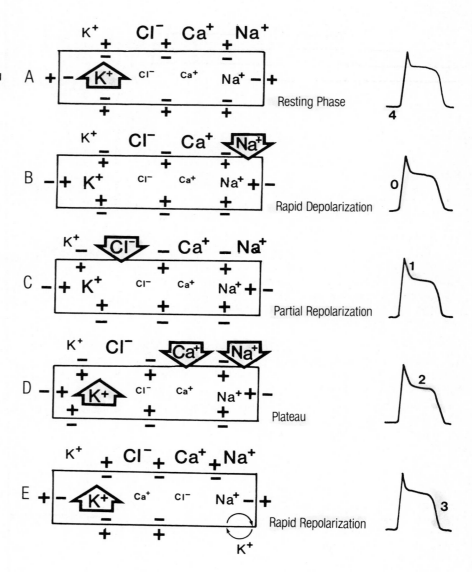

4. *Plateau—phase 2:* A sustained plateau, corresponding to the absolute refractory period of the myocardium, follows. During this period, no net change in electrical charge across the membrane occurs. A balance is maintained between the influx and efflux of positively charged ions. A slow inward flow of calcium ions is primarily responsible for this plateau; some inward movement of sodium through slow channels also contributes. This inward movement of positive charge is countered by an outward movement of potassium ions (see Fig. 25-3D).

5. *Rapid repolarization—phase 3:* During rapid repolarization, the slow inward currents of calcium and sodium are inactivated and the membrane permeability to potassium increases greatly. Potassium moves out of the cell, reducing the positive charge within the cell; eventually the inside of the cell regains its relative negativity and the outside of the cell its relative positivity (see Fig. 25-3E). The resting ionic distribution is restored by the continuous action of the sodium-potassium pump actively transporting potassium intracellularly and sodium extracellularly.

The action potential configuration just described is characteristic of that found in nonspecialized myocardial fibers located in the atria and ventricles and in specialized conducting fibers of the atrial tracts and His-Purkinje system. This type of action potential is referred to as the *fast response*. A second type of action potential, known as the *slow response*, is observed during intracellular recordings from the specialized fibers of the sinoatrial (SA) node and the atrioventricular (AV) node. The configurations of both action potentials are illustrated in Fig. 25-4. The slow response configuration is more gradual than that of the fast response; depolarization of these cells is attributed to slow inward currents of calcium and sodium ions, rather than to rapid sodium influx through the fast channels. Given the fact that the physiologic properties of these specialized cells differ distinctly from those of the conducting pathways and myocardium, electrophysiologic distinctions should not be surprising. For example, the property of automaticity, the ability to spontaneously generate impulses, results from automatic changes occurring during the resting phase of the slow response action potential. Note in Fig. 25-4B that as soon as repolarization is complete, the cell slowly and spontaneously begins to depolarize toward threshold. As soon as threshold level is reached, the cell will automatically fire. Conduction velocity is also directly attributable to the type of action potential. Slower conduction through the AV node in contrast to rapid conduction through the Purkinje fibers is due to differences in the configuration of the slow response and fast response action potentials.

Muscle ultrastructure

The *sarcomere* is the basic contractile unit of the myocardium (see Fig. 25-5). It is composed of two overlapping myofilaments, the thick *myosin* filament and the thin *actin* filament. Cross-bridges or linkages form between these myofilaments at regular intervals. In addition to the actin and myosin proteins, the sarcomere

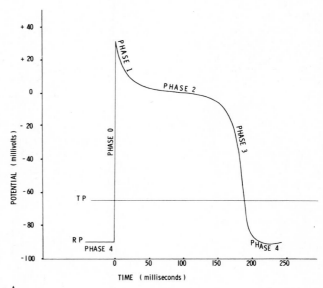

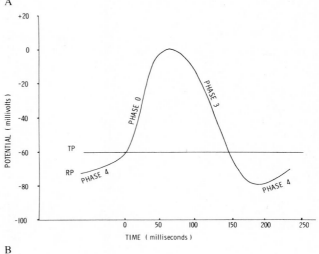

FIGURE 25-4
Configuration of action potential. (A) Fast response. (B) Slow response. (From J. Willis Hurst, R. Bruce Logue, Robert C. Schlant, and Nanette Kass Wenger, *The Heart*, 4th ed., McGraw-Hill, New York, 1978, p. 639.)

contains troponin and tropomyosin proteins. In the resting state, the troponin-tropomyosin complex inhibits cross-bridge formation.

The electrical excitation of the myocardial cell initiates muscular contraction by stimulating the release of calcium from the sarcoplasmic reticulum and other cellular sources. The calcium currents produced during the plateau phase of the action potential contribute to this release. The released calcium diffuses through the sarcoplasm to the myofilaments. Calcium then binds to the troponin protein, inactivating the inhibitory effect of the troponin-tropomyosin system upon the contractile proteins, actin and myosin. The actin and myosin myofilaments then interact to form linkages or cross-bridges that generate force to slide these overlapping myofilaments past each other, thereby shortening the sarcomere (see Fig. 25-5). The shortening of multiple sarcomere units produces muscular contraction. Relaxation of the muscle is the result of calcium uptake by the sarcoplasmic reticulum which dissociates the actin-myosin cross-bridges.

The force of myocardial contraction is dependent upon the interaction between sarcomere myofilaments. For example, administration of calcium can increase contractile force by increasing calcium availability to the sarcomere. Conversely, overstretching the sarcomere would reduce contractile force by reducing the amount of overlap and subsequent linkage formation between the actin and myosin filaments.

Phases of the cardiac cycle

The phases of the cardiac cycle can most easily be conceptualized in the following sequence: (1) middiastole, (2) late diastole (3) early systole, (4) late systole, (5) early diastole (see Fig. 25-6).

1. *Middiastole:* This is the phase of slow ventricular filling, or *diastasis*. The atrial and ventricular chambers are relaxed. Blood entering the atria through venous channels flows passively into the ventricles through the open AV valves. The semilunar valves are closed.

2. *Late diastole:* The wave of depolarization spreads through the atria and pauses at the AV node. The atrial muscle contracts, contributing an additional 20 percent to the ventricular volume.

3. *Early systole:* Depolarization spreads from the AV node through the bundle branches to the ventricular myocardium. As ventricular contraction begins, the pressure within the ventricles rises above that of the atria, causing the AV valves to close, which generates the first heart sound. The ventricular chambers continue to develop higher pressures; however, during this phase the pressures within the aorta and pulmonary artery exceed the ventricular pressures keeping the semilunar valves closed. This is termed *isovolumetric contraction*, since the ventricular volumes remain constant.

4. *Late systole:* As soon as the ventricular pressures exceed the pressures within the blood vessels, the semilunar valves open and ventricular ejection into the pulmonic and systemic circulation occurs. This ejection phase can be divided into a brief, initial phase of "rapid ejection" and a subsequent, more sustained phase of "reduced ejection."

5. *Early diastole:* The wave of repolarization then spreads through the ventricular myocardium, and the ventricular chambers relax. As the muscle relaxes, the ventricular pressures drop below the arterial pressures, causing the semilunar valves to close, which produces the second heart sound. Relaxation continues until the ventricular pressures drop below that of the atrial pressures, causing the AV valves to open. The period between semilunar valve closure and opening of the AV valves is referred to as *isovolumetric relaxation*, since ventricular volumes remain constant despite continued reduction in ventricular pressure. As the AV valves open, the ventricles fill rapidly with the venous blood that has accumulated in the atria. Almost 80

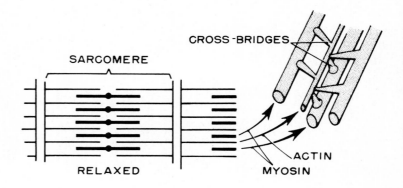

FIGURE 25-5

Muscle ultrastructure. The myofibrils are composed of thick myosin filaments and thin actin filaments. Cross-bridges are observed at regular intervals between the actin and myosin filaments, forming linkages during muscle contraction. The amount of overlap between the actin and myosin filaments is decreased during muscle relaxation and increased during contraction. This causes a corresponding increase or decrease in the sarcomere length.

percent of ventricular filling occurs during this phase.

CARDIAC OUTPUT

Definitions

The result of the synchronized, rhythmic myocardial contraction is the ejection of blood into the pulmonic and systemic circulations. The volume of blood ejected by each ventricle per minute is the *cardiac output*. An average cardiac output is 5 liters/minute. However, cardiac output varies to meet the needs of the peripheral tissues for oxygen and nutrients. Since cardiac output requirements also vary according to body size, a more accurate indicator of cardiac function is the *cardiac index*. The cardiac index is the cardiac output divided by body surface area; it ranges from 2.8 to 3.6 liters/minute/square meter of body surface.

Stroke volume is the volume of blood ejected by each ventricle per beat. Approximately two-thirds of the volume of blood in the ventricle at the end of diastole (end-diastolic volume) is ejected during systole. This portion of blood ejected is known as the *ejection fraction*; the residual ventricular volume at the end of systole is referred to as the *end-systolic volume*. Depression of ventricular function impairs the ability of the ventricle to empty, thereby reducing stroke volume and the ejection fraction with a consequent elevation of residual ventricular volumes.

Determinants of cardiac output

Cardiac output is dependent upon the relationship between two variables, heart rate and stroke volume:

Cardiac output = heart rate × stroke volume

Cardiac output can be held remarkably constant despite alterations in one variable by compensatory adjustments in the other variable. For instance, if the heart rate slows, the period of ventricular relaxation between heartbeats is longer, and ventricular filling time is thereby increased. Consequently, ventricular volumes are greater and more blood can be ejected per beat. Conversely, if stroke volume drops, cardiac output can be stabilized by increasing the heart rate. Obviously, these compensatory adjustments can only maintain cardiac output within limits. The alteration and stabilization of cardiac output depends upon control mechanisms regulating heart rate and stroke volume.

Control of heart rate

Heart rate is largely under the extrinsic control of the autonomic nervous system; parasympathetic and sympathetic fibers innervate the SA node and the AV node, influencing the rate and speed of impulse conduction. Stimulation of the parasympathetic fibers decreases the heart rate, whereas sympathetic stimulation increases it. In the normal resting heart, the influence of the parasympathetic system seems to dominate in maintaining the heart rate at approximately 80 bpm. If all neural and hormonal influences upon the heart were blocked, the intrinsic rate would be about 100 bpm. However, in the presence of heart disease, the sympathetic system predominates in the control of heart rate

FIGURE 25-6

Phases of the cardiac cycle. (Modified from M. O. Vinsant, M. I. Spense, and M. E. Chapell, *A Commonsense Approach to Coronary Care: A Program,* **Mosby, St. Louis, 1975, p. 6.)**

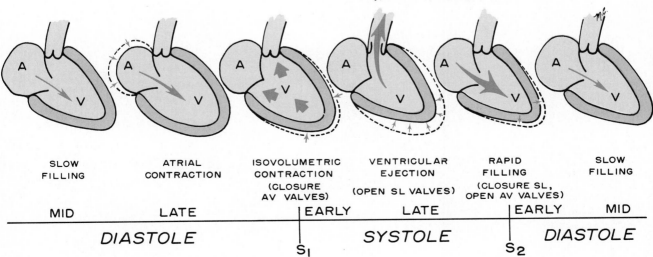

SLOW FILLING	ATRIAL CONTRACTION	ISOVOLUMETRIC CONTRACTION (CLOSURE AV VALVES)	VENTRICULAR EJECTION (OPEN SL VALVES)	RAPID FILLING (CLOSURE SL, OPEN AV VALVES)	SLOW FILLING
MID	LATE	EARLY	LATE	EARLY	MID

DIASTOLE — S₁ — *SYSTOLE* — S₂ — *DIASTOLE*

and the maintenance of cardiac compensation. Endogenous myocardial stores of norepinephrine augment the catecholamine supply available from neural sympathetic fibers and the adrenal medulla. These endogenous stores eventually become depleted in chronic heart failure.

Control of stroke volume

Stroke volume is dependent upon three variables: (1) preload, as explained by Starling's law of the heart, (2) contractility, and (3) afterload.

Starling's law of the heart states that stretching the myocardial fibers during diastole will increase the force of contraction during systole (see Fig. 25-7). An analogous example is that of increasing the stretch on a rubber band to increase the force of elastic recoil upon release. Myocardial fibers can be stretched by increasing ventricular diastolic volumes. The degree of stretch is expressed in terms of preload (i.e., diastolic fiber length prior to contraction).

The degree of fiber stretch or preload is determined by the ventricular volume. The volume of blood contained within the ventricles during diastole depends upon the amount of venous return. Venous return is influenced primarily by circulating blood volume and the venous tone. Increasing venous return, and consequently ventricular volumes, stretches the myocardial fibers. Stretching the sarcomere maximizes the number of interaction sites available for actin-myosin linkage by increasing the overlap between the myofilaments. Consequently, the force of contraction rises.

Typically, the sarcomere is stretched to 2.0 μm during diastole (see Fig. 25-8A). The optimal sarcomere length is 2.2 μm (see Fig. 25-8B). Therefore a reserve in sarcomere length and resultant force of contraction exists. Starling's law is functional within limits determined by the myocardial ultrastructure described earlier. Stretching the sarcomere to more than 2.2 μm would

FIGURE 25-7
Starling's law of the heart. (A) Normal filling during diastole causes normal fiber stretch and normal contractile force and stroke volume. (B) Increased filling during diastole causes increased fiber stretch, increased force of contraction, and increased stroke volume.

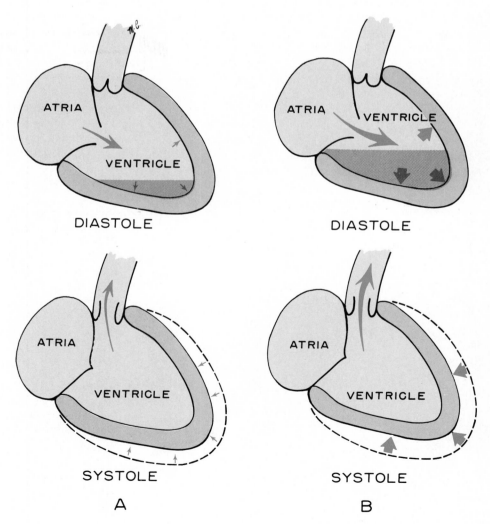

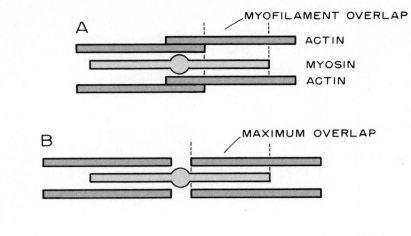

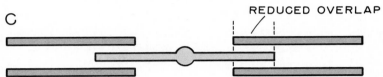

FIGURE 25-8
Effect of sarcomere length upon myofilament overlap. (A) Usual sarcomere length of 2.0 μm. (B) Optimal sarcomere length of 2.2 μm. (C) Excessive sarcomere length of 2.5 μm.

reduce the strength of contraction by reducing the number of available interaction sites (see Fig. 25-8C). Fortunately, the myocardial sarcomeres are extremely resistant to overstretching.

The relationship between myocardial fiber length and force of contraction is referred to as the *ventricular function curve* (see Fig. 25-9). Increasing ventricular end-diastolic volumes will initially increase force of contraction and stroke volume. Thus the curve demonstrates an initial ascending limb of improved function. Eventually the curve flattens or plateaus, indicating that additional increments in ventricular volume will not im-

prove function further; optimal fiber stretch has been achieved. In summary, increased preload will, up to a point, increase the force of contraction and, consequently, the volume of blood ejected from the ventricle.

Previously, it was thought that a descending limb of the ventricular function curve existed. The failing heart was believed to operate on the descending limb of this curve. The descent would correspond to ventricular volume overload, which would produce excessive myocardial dilatation by stretching the sarcomere beyond 2.2 μm, thereby depressing the force of contraction. It is now believed that only an ischemic heart seems to exhibit a true descending limb of the ventricular function curve. Heart failure is now conceptualized in terms of depression of the entire ventricular function curve.

Alterations in the position of the ventricular function curve reflect changes in *contractility or inotropic state*, the second determinant of stroke volume. Contractility by definition refers to changes in the force of contraction occurring independent of changes in myocardial fiber length. Increased contractility is the result of intensification of the interactions at the actin-myosin cross-bridges in the sarcomere. The administration of calcium or catecholamines would enhance contractility

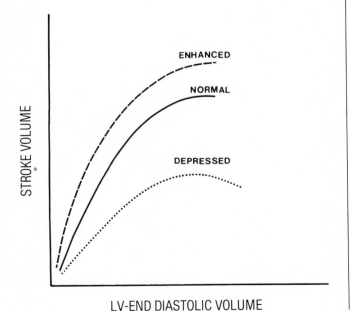

FIGURE 25-9
Ventricular function curve. The solid black line represents the normal ventricular function curve. Note that increasing end-diastolic volume increases stroke volume up to a point. Displacement of the curve upward and to the left represents improved ventricular function, as would be seen with sympathetic nervous system stimulation. Displacement of the curve downward and to the right represents myocardial depression as would be seen with acidosis, hypoxia, or cardiac failure.

by shifting the entire ventricular function curve upward and to the left. Increased contractility elevates stroke volume by increasing ventricular emptying during systole. Factors depressing myocardial function, such as acidosis or hypoxia, shift the curve downward and to the right.

new   <u>Afterload</u> is the third determinant of stroke volume. Afterload is the amount of tension the ventricle must develop during systole to open the semilunar valve and eject blood. It is primarily a function of intraventricular pressure, intraventricular size or radius, and ventricular wall thickness. The relationship between wall tension, pressure, radius, and wall thickness is expressed in this simplified version of the Laplace relationship:

$$\text{Wall tension} = \frac{\text{intraventricular pressure} \times \text{radius}}{\text{ventricular wall thickness}}$$

The Laplace equation indicates that there is a direct relationship between intraventricular pressure and chamber size and the amount of tension the ventricle must generate to eject blood during systole. An increment of either intraventricular pressure or intraventricular size elevates the amount of tension the ventricle must develop to eject blood. For example, elevation of arterial pressure will increase the resistance to ventricular ejection, thereby necessitating the development of increased intraventricular pressure and wall tension to overcome the resistance. Similarly, as the ventricular radius or chamber size increases, the ventricle must develop more tension during systole to generate a given pressure and eject blood. In other words, a dilated ventricle must develop more tension than does a normal

ventricle to generate the same systolic pressure (see Fig. 25-10). Thus, an increase in afterload can be produced by either increased arterial pressure or ventricular dilation. Excessive increases in afterload may adversely affect ventricular emptying, reducing stroke volume and consequently cardiac output.

Increases in wall thickness or myocardial hypertrophy decrease wall tension or afterload according to the Laplace relationship. In other words, as the ventricle hypertrophies, proportionally less wall tension must be developed by the ventricle to generate pressure and eject blood, because of the increase in muscle mass.

In summary, the integration of the mechanisms controlling heart rate and stroke volume determine ventricular function and cardiac output. Heart rate is primarily under extrinsic neural control. Control of stroke volume is a function of the interaction of three variables: preload, contractility, and afterload (see Fig. 25-11).

BLOOD FLOW TO THE PERIPHERY

The dynamics of peripheral blood flow is perhaps the most critical element of circulatory physiology for two reasons. First, the distribution of the cardiac output within the periphery depends upon properties of the vascular bed. Second, the volume of cardiac output depends upon the amount of blood returning to the heart. Essentially, the heart will eject a volume of blood equivalent to its venous return.

Principles of blood flow

Blood flow is dependent upon two opposing variables: (1) the pressure propelling blood and (2) the resistance to flow. Blood flow increases as the pressure propelling

FIGURE 25-10

Effect of ventricular size on afterload. The dilated ventricle on the right must generate more tension than the normal ventricle on the left to generate the same systolic pressure of 120 mmHg.

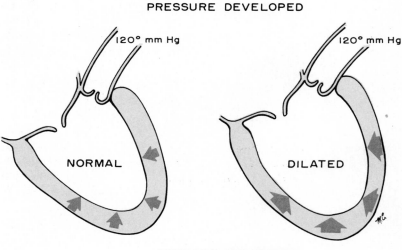

PRESSURE DEVELOPED

120° mm Hg   120° mm Hg

NORMAL   DILATED

TENSION GENERATED

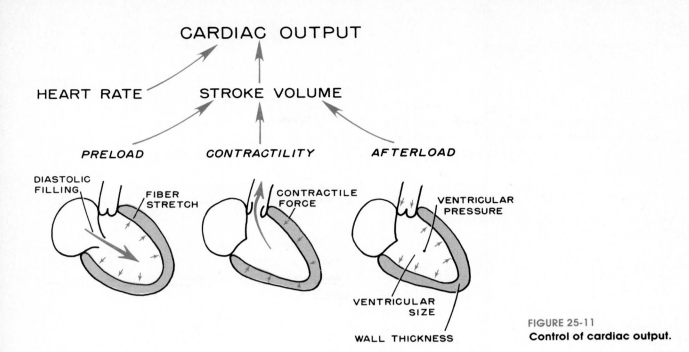

FIGURE 25-11
Control of cardiac output.

blood increases; inversely, flow decreases as resistance increases.

A pressure difference or pressure gradient must exist between two points for blood to flow between the points. The greater the pressure gradient, the greater the flow. Blood flows throughout the systemic circulation from the arterial to the venous end in response to pressure gradients. The mean arterial pressure, or average driving pressure at the arterial end of the circulation, is approximately 100 mmHg. Capillary pressure averages 25 mmHg. Pressure at the venous end of the circulation or right atrium is close to 0 mmHg. Thus pressure progressively declines throughout the systemic circulation. The pressure gradient between the arterial and venous ends of the systemic circulation is approximately 100 mmHg (mean arterial pressure − right atrial pressure or central venous pressure).

Alterations in either the *mean arterial pressure* or the *right atrial pressure* will influence blood flow by changing the pressure gradient between the two points. Mean arterial pressure will change if either the vascular contents (cardiac output) or the vascular capacity (total peripheral resistance) is altered:

Mean arterial pressure
= cardiac output
× total peripheral resistance

For example, either massive hemorrhage or extensive vasodilation (as in gram-negative sepsis) can profoundly reduce arterial pressure. However, the pressure alteration is sensed by the baroreceptors, and reflex compen-satory responses mediated by the autonomic nervous system ensue to stabilize arterial pressure. Right atrial pressure depends upon the balance between venous return to the atrium and the ability of the right atrium to empty. Disease of the tricuspid valve and impaired right ventricular function can both reduce right atrial output and abnormally elevate right atrial pressure.

Resistance, the second determinant of blood flow, is primarily determined by the radius of the blood vessel. Other factors, such as blood viscosity and vascular length, also alter resistance to flow. However, since these properties are relatively constant, their influence is normally insignificant. Resistance is extremely sensitive to alterations in the lumen of the blood vessel. Poiseuille's law demonstrates that resistance (R) is inversely proportional to the fourth power of the radius (r) of the blood vessel:

$$R \propto \frac{1}{r^4}$$

Hence, reduction of the radius by one-half will increase the resistance to flow 16-fold. The arteriole is the major site of vascular resistance. Alterations in the smooth muscle tone of the arteriolar wall regulate resistance to flow and, consequently, the amount of flow to the capillary bed.

In summary, flow (F) is directly proportional to the pressure gradient (ΔP) and inversely proportional to the vascular resistance:

$$F = \frac{\Delta P}{R}$$

The pressure gradient is determined by pressures at the arterial and venous ends of the circulation. Resistance is primarily a function of the radius of the blood vessels, altered most significantly at the arteriolar level.

Distribution of blood flow

Blood flow is distributed among the multiple organ systems according to the metabolic needs and functional demands of the tissues. Since tissue needs are continually changing, blood flow must continually be readjusted. As tissue metabolism increases, blood flow must increase to supply oxygen and nutrients and to remove the end products of metabolism. For instance, during strenuous exercise, flow to the exercising skeletal muscle must increase. Dual control of the distribution of cardiac output is possible through extrinsic and intrinsic regulatory mechanisms.

Extrinsic control

Blood flow to a given organ system can be increased either by increasing cardiac output or by shunting blood from a relatively inactive organ system to the more active organ. The activity of the sympathetic nervous system can produce both responses. First, sympathetic stimulation augments cardiac output by increasing heart rate and force of contractility. Second, sympathetic adrenergic fibers also extend to the peripheral vasculature, particularly the arteriole. Selective alterations in sympathetic discharge will stimulate alpha and beta receptors, preferentially constricting some arterioles and dilating others to redistribute blood to capillary beds according to need. Within any capillary bed there is considerable reserve for increased flow, since only a portion of the capillaries are perfused at a given time. Therefore, flow can be increased by opening nonperfused capillaries as well as by further arteriolar dilation of perfused capillaries.

Skeletal muscle vasculature is uniquely capable of vasodilation because sympathetic cholinergic fibers originating in the cerbral cortex innervate these vessels. These fibers release acetylcholine, resulting in relaxation of vascular smooth muscle. Parasympathetic cholinergic fibers innervate only selected, small portions of the peripheral vasculature; therefore, parasympathetic activity does not significantly influence the distribution of cardiac output or total peripheral resistance.

In addition to neural control, an extrinsic influence upon peripheral resistance and flow is exerted by humoral agents. The adrenal medulla secretes catecholamines, epinephrine and norepinephrine, in response to sympathetic activity. These hormones elicit sympathetic responses in the peripheral vasculature. Other bloodborne agents—vasopressin, angiotensin, serotonin, bradykinin, and histamine—are currently under investigation to establish their role in peripheral vascular control.

Intrinsic control

Local control of blood flow at the tissue level occurs through autoregulation. Autoregulation permits readjustment of blood flow relative to tissue metabolic activity. The precise mechanism for local changes in vascular resistance and blood flow is unclear. It has been suggested that tissue metabolites released when oxygen demand exceeds oxygen supply mediate this response. Tissue ischemia is an extremely potent stimulus for vasodilation. The logic of this compensatory response is obvious although the exact mechanism is unclear. The vasodilation may be a direct response to the oxygen lack, or the lack may trigger the release of chemical vasodilators, such as adenosine or prostaglandins. The direct vasodilatory effect of metabolites such as carbon dioxide and lactic acid is another possibility.

The relative strength of extrinsic and intrinsic control mechanisms varies among organ systems. In vital, flow-dependent organs, such as the heart and brain, the intrinsic mechanisms predominate, whereas in other areas, such as the skin, autonomic control predominates.

In addition to these control mechanisms designed to increase oxygen delivery to the tissues, the tissues can increase oxygen supply by extracting more oxygen from the arterial blood. In most organs, with the notable exception of the heart, only a small proportion of the oxygen available in the arterial blood is extracted by the tissue. When an oxygen deficit develops in the tissues, the concentration gradient of oxygen between the arterial blood and the tissue increases. This causes more oxygen to diffuse from the intravascular to the extravascular space, thereby increasing oxygen delivery to the cells.

When compensatory mechanisms are unable to sustain adequate peripheral perfusion, as in shock, flow must be distributed according to priority. Blood will be shunted away from "nonvital" areas, such as the skin and kidney, to maintain perfusion of the brain and heart. Consequently, early signs of shock or inadequate tissue perfusion are decreased urine output and cold, pale skin. Significant alterations in mentation and cardiac function occur much later in the shock state, when flow is compromised even to the vital organs.

CARDIAC RESERVE

Normally, the heart possesses the ability to increase its pumping capacity significantly above resting levels. This cardiac reserve enables the normal heart to increase output approximately fivefold. The increase in cardiac output can occur through increments in heart rate or stroke volume (cardiac output = heart rate × stroke volume).

Heart rate can normally increase from resting levels of between 60 to 100 bpm to approximately 180 bpm, primarily through sympathetic stimulation. Rates above this can be deleterious for two reasons. First, as heart rate increases, the duration of diastole shortens and ventricular filling time is reduced; eventually stroke volume will fall, negating the advantage of further rate increments. Second, rapid heart rates can adversely affect myocardial oxygenation because cardiac work is increased while the diastolic period, during which most coronary flow occurs, is reduced.

Stroke volume can increase either by increased ventricular emptying due to increased contractility or by increased diastolic filling and a subsequent rise in ejection volume. However, both increased force of contraction and increased ventricular volumes will elevate cardiac work and oxygen demand. In addition, the effect of increased diastolic filling upon contractility and stroke volume is limited by the degree of myocardial fiber stretch.

If the heart is subjected to chronic volume or pressure overload, the ventricular muscle may *dilate* to increase contractile force, according to Starling's law, or *hypertrophy* to increase muscle mass and pumping force. Both responses, although compensatory in nature, eventually contribute to further cardiac decompensation. Dilation increases cardiac work by increasing the amount of tension the ventricle must develop to generate a given pressure according to the law of Laplace. Furthermore, excessive dilation will eventually reduce contractile force. Hypertrophy increases the muscle mass requiring nutrient supply, thereby increasing oxygen demand.

QUESTIONS *Answers start pg 1084*

Physiology of the cardiovascular system

Directions: Answer the following questions on a separate sheet of paper.

1. What are the two major mechanical phases of the cardiac cycle and what does each represent? What does an electrocardiogram represent and how is it different from an action potential? What is the relationship between the electrical and mechanical events of the cardiac cycle?

2. State Starling's law of the heart. What is the relationship of Starling's law to the ventricular function curve?

3. State Poiseuille's law as it applies to blood circulation. How would you calculate the systemic blood pressure gradient?

4. Hemodynamic measurements on a 46-year-old woman with a body surface area of 1.5 m^2 reveal the following data: cardiac output (CO) 4.5 liters/minute; left ventricular end-diastolic volume (EDV) 100 ml; left ventricular end-systolic volume (ESV), 30 ml. What is her left ventricular stroke volume (SV)? What is her cardiac index (CI) and left ventricular ejection fraction (EF)? Are these values normal?

Directions: Circle the letter preceding each item that correctly answers the question. Only one answer is correct, unless otherwise noted.

5. The rapid depolarizing phase of an action potential in heart muscle is caused by a:
   a. Sudden increase in the permeability of the membrane to sodium   b. Decrease in the permeability of the membrane to potassium   c. Decrease in the sodium pumping rate   d. Sudden increase in the permeability of the membrane to potassium

6. Which of the following substances is released from the sarcoplasmic reticulum and diffuses to the sarcomere to produce myocardial contraction?
   a. Na$^+$ b. K$^+$ c. Ca^{2+} d. ATPase

7. Expected changes resulting from severing both vagi include: (More than one answer may be correct.)
   a. Interruption of the afferent pathways from the aortic arch baroreceptors   b. Increase in the heart rate to approximately 100 bpm   c. Increase in the cardiac output   d. Increase in the mean arterial pressure

8. When a patient was given a certain drug, the mean arterial pressure increased and the total peripheral resistance decreased. This drug probably caused:
   a. Vasoconstriction and an increase in cardiac output   b. Vasoconstriction and a decrease in the cardiac output   c. Vasodilation and an increase in the cardiac output   d. Vasodilation and a decrease in the cardiac output

9. Within limits, an increase in the end-diastolic vol-

ume of the ventricle will: (More than one answer may be correct.)
a. Increase the stroke volume of the ventricle
b. Decrease the stroke volume of the ventricle
c. Increase the force of contraction   d. Decrease the cardiac work

10. An increase in cardiac contractility results in an increased stroke volume or stroke work for a given left ventricular end-diastolic volume and is reflected by a shift of the ventricular function curve to the:
a. left   b. right

11. Cardiac muscle cannot be tetanized because:
a. The refractory period lasts throughout the period of contractions   b. The impulse spread through the conduction system is too rapid
c. The muscle fibers are relatively ischemic after each contraction   d. Intracardiac calcium levels are too low

12. The volume of blood ejected by the ventricle depends on: (More than one answer may be correct.)
a. Preload   b. Afterload   c. Contractile state

13. Which of the following statements concerning the Laplace relationship between wall tension, intraventricular pressure, and ventricular radius is *not* true? (More than one answer may be correct.)
a. The ventricle must generate increased tension to eject if ventricular size increases.   b. The ventricle must generate increased tension if the ventricular size decreases.   c. The ventricle must generate increased tension if arterial pressure increases.   d. The ventricle must generate increased tension if arterial pressure decreases.

14. The most important extrinsic control mechanism affecting the distribution of cardiac output is:
a. The parasympathetic system   b. The sympathetic system   c. Circulating neurohormones
d. Tissue ischemia

15. Distribution of blood flow to vital organs such as the heart and brain is predominantly controlled by:
a. Extrinsic mechanisms such as neural control and humoral agents   b. Intrinsic mechanisms or autoregulation

16. Coronary perfusion takes place:
a. Primarily during systole
b. Primarily during diastole
c. Equally during systole and diastole

17. Stretching myocardial fibers to the optimum sarcomere length increases the force of contraction by:
a. Increasing the overlap of the myofilaments
b. Intensifying the cross-bridge interactions
c. Increasing the volume of blood to be ejected

18. Factors that affect cardiac output include: (More than one answer may be correct.)
a. Circulating levels of hormones   b. Stimulation of the cardiac sympathetic nervous system
c. Exercise   d. Stroke volume

Directions: Match each of the hemodynamic parameters in col. A with its equivalent in col. B.

Column A	Column B
19. _d_ Cardiac output	a. End-diastolic volume — end-systolic volume
20. _C_ Mean arterial pressure	b. $\dfrac{\text{Cardiac output}}{\text{Body surface area}}$
21. _a_ Stroke volume	c. Cardiac output × total peripheral resistance
22. _e_ Ejection fraction	d. Heart rate × stroke volume
23. _b_ Cardiac index	e. $\dfrac{\text{Stroke volume}}{\text{End-diastolic volume}}$
24. _f_ Blood flow	f. $\dfrac{\text{Mean arterial pressure} - \text{central venous pressure}}{\text{Resistance}}$

25. Arrange the mechanical events of the cardiac cycle in the proper time sequence beginning with (a), the closure of the AV valves.
a. AV valves close   b. AV valves open
c. Semilunar valves close   d. Semilunar valves open   e. Ventricular filling occurs   f. Ventricular ejection occurs   g. Ventricular relaxation occurs   h. First heart sound   i. Second heart sound   a, h, d, f, g, c, i, b, e

Directions: Fill in the blanks with the correct words or circle the correct option.

26. The _absolute refractory period_ period is that time during the cardiac cycle when the myocardium will not respond to any stimulus. The myocardium is capable of responding to a strong stimulus during the _____ _relative_ refractory period.

27. In the resting state the inside of the cell is _neg._ charged with respect to the outside. During the repolarization of a cell the sodium-potassium pump moves _potassium_ into the cell and _sodium_ out of the cell.

28. During the ventricular filling phase of the cardiac cycle the AV valves are (open) (closed) and the semilunar valves are (open) (closed).

29. During the ventricular ejection phase of the cardiac cycle the AV valves are (open) (closed) and the semilunar valves are (open) (closed).

30. During the phase of ventricular filling the cardiac impulse is delayed at the _AV node_.

Directions: Circle the letter preceding each item below that correctly answers the question.

31. Choose the *false* statement concerning the slow response action potential in cardiac tissue:
a. It is the characteristic intracellular recording from the SA node.   b. Inward currents of Ca^{2+} and Na^+ are responsible for the unstable resting phase.   c. The stable resting phase results from an influx of Cl^- ions via slow channels.   d. Characteristics of this type of action potential account for the relatively slower conduction time through the AV node.

32. Automaticity of cardiac tissue may be defined as:
a. Ability to transmit impulses   b. Ability to spontaneously generate impulses   c. Ability to respond to stimulation   d. Regularity of impulse generation

33. A pacemaker cell in the SA node:
a. Has a stable phase 4 potential   b. Has a phase 0 potential primarily caused by a "fast current"   c. Has a distinct and prolonged phase 1 and 2 potential   d. Has a phase 0 depolarization which is much slower than that in nonpacemaker cardiac cells

Directions: Match each of the phases of the fast response action potential in col. A with the appropriate descriptive phrase(s) in col. B.

Column A

Column B

34. _B_ Phase 0
35. _C_ Phase 1
36. _A, D_ Phase 2
37. _F_ Phase 3
38. _E_ Phase 4

a. Slow influx of Ca^{2+} is primarily responsible for the plateau during this phase

b. Rapid decrease in electronegativity of the cell membrane due to change of permeability to Na^+ and its rapid influx into cell

c. Partial repolarization due to influx of negatively charged ions into the cell

d. This phase corresponds to the absolute refractory period

e. The inside of the cell is negative with respect to the outside, and the ionic concentrations of Na^+ and K^+ on either side of the cell membrane are maintained at a steady state by the Na/K pump

f. Rapid repolarization caused by cessation of inward currents of Ca^{2+} and Na^+ and rapid efflux of K^+ from the cell

CHAPTER
26

PENNY J. FORD
F. MICHAEL. VISLOSKY

DIAGNOSTIC PROCEDURES IN CARDIOVASCULAR DISEASE

OBJECTIVES

At the completion of this chapter you should be able to:

1. Define each of the following signs and symptoms of heart disease and state its physiologic basis: angina, dyspnea, orthopnea, paroxysmal nocturnal dyspnea, palpitations, peripheral edema, syncope, and weakness and fatigue.

2. Define the four functional categories of the New York Heart Association classification of heart disease.

3. Describe and explain the possible significance of the following findings during examination of the arterial system: pulse deficit, bounding pulse, thready pulse, irregular pulse, slow upstroke, waterhammer pulse, and alterations in pulse pressure.

4. Name and locate the peripheral pulses commonly palpated in the physical examination; explain the significance of absent, diminished, or unequal peripheral pulses.

5. Correlate the auscultated sounds of Korotkoff with arterial systolic and diastolic blood pressures.

6. State the formula for estimation of the mean arterial pressure.

7. Describe the procedure for estimation of central venous pressure by examination of the jugular veins; explain the significance of deviations from normal.

8. Explain the significance of Kussmaul's sign and a positive hepatojugular reflux test.

9. Explain the significance of the jugular venous a, c, and v waveforms and the possible significance of deviations from normal.

10. Outline the types of information that may be obtained in examination of the precordium.

11. Explain the possible significance of lateral displacement of the point of maximum impulse, a substernal heave, and precordial thrills.

12. Define and explain the possible significance of the following observations related to precordial auscultation: physiologic and paradoxical splitting of the second heart sound, ventricular and atrial gallops, opening snap, and systolic and diastolic murmurs.

13. State the standard method of grading murmur loudness.

14. Name and locate on the chest the five standard areas for heart sound auscultation.

15. Identify the waveforms of a normal electrocardiogram and give examples of abnormalities which may be detected using this diagnostic technique.

16. State the recording sites utilized for each lead of the 12-lead electrocardiogram, including the polarity of each.

17. Define electrical axis.

18. Explain how the hexaxial reference system is derived.

19. Describe the following diagnostic procedures and give examples of cardiovascular abnormalities which may be detected using each technique:
    a. Echocardiogram
    b. Phonocardiogram
    c. Chest x-ray
    d. Nuclear imaging
    e. Digital subtraction angiography
    f. Cardiac catheterization
    g. Coronary arteriography

20. Identify five categories of data obtainable during cardiac catheterization.

21. Describe the anatomic approach for catheterization of the right and left sides of the heart.

22. Contrast the diagnostic approaches for obtaining evidence of valvular stenosis and of valvular regurgitation.

23. State the indications for performing coronary angiography and the characteristics of a bypassable lesion.

24. List four hemodynamic parameters measured at the bedside with intravenous catheters.

Increasingly sophisticated diagnostic techniques are available to detect heart disease and its clinical sequelae. However, the utilization of these techniques and the interpretation of test results are adjuncts to the systematic clinical assessment of the patient, not substitutes for a thorough history and physical examination. Thus a brief overview of the systematic bedside assessment of the patient with heart disease must precede a description of common diagnostic procedures.

CLINICAL ASSESSMENT

A systematic clinical assessment includes a complete history and physical examination utilizing the techniques of inspection, palpation, percussion, and auscultation. Examination of the cardiovascular system must include the heart and the peripheral vascular system. A detailed discussion of the peripheral vascular examination and related diagnostic tests is presented in Chap. 30.

History

The history must include an assessment of the individual's life-style and the impact of heart disease upon the activities of daily living if the patient rather than the disease is to be treated. The following signs and symptoms of heart disease are commonly elicited during the history of the patient with heart disease: (1) *angina*, or chest pain, a consequence of myocardial oxygen lack or ischemia; (2) *dyspnea*, or difficulty in breathing, due to increased respiratory effort associated with pulmonary vascular congestion and alterations in lung distensibility; *orthopnea*, or difficulty in breathing in the recumbent position; *paroxysmal nocturnal dyspnea*, or an attack occurring at rest during the night, as a result of left ventricular failure; (3) *palpitations*, or an awareness of the heartbeat, due to changes in the rate, regularity, or force of cardiac contraction; (4) *peripheral edema*, or swelling caused by fluid accumulation in the interstitial spaces, usually noted in dependent areas as a result of the effect of gravity, and preceded by weight gain; (5) *syncope*, or transient loss of consciousness, a result of inadequate cerebral blood flow; and (6) *fatigue and weakness*, commonly a consequence of low cardiac output and reduced peripheral perfusion.

It must be determined what factors precipitate symptoms and what relieves the symptoms. Angina is commonly precipitated by exertion and relieved by rest. Dyspnea is commonly associated with exertion; however, changes in body position and the consequent redistribution of body fluid by gravity may precipitate dyspnea. Orthopnea, or dyspnea in the recumbent position, can be relieved by elevation of the trunk with pillows. In addition, the degree of disability associated with the elicited symptoms must be determined. The New York Heart Association has developed guidelines for the classification of patients according to the level of physical activity required to produce symptoms (see Table 26-1). The categories range from Class I patients, asymptomatic with ordinary physical exertion, to Class IV patients, symptomatic at rest.

Physical examination

Simple inspection yields a wealth of information regarding the patient's physical and psychological status. Such observations as color, body build, respiratory pattern, work of breathing, and general appearance must all be incorporated into the clinical picture. Palpation, coupled with inspection, furthers and substantiates the cumulative data base. Skin temperature, turgor, and

TABLE 26-1

NEW YORK HEART ASSOCIATION PATIENT CLASSIFICATION GUIDELINES

Class I	Asymptomatic with ordinary physical exertion
Class II	Symptomatic with ordinary physical exertion
Class III	Symptomatic with less than ordinary physical exertion
Class IV	Symptomatic at rest

moistness can be evaluated. Severity of edema can be quantified on a scale of 1+ to 4+ according to persistence of the indentation left by the palpating finger in the edematous area (1+ indicates a slight depression that disappears rapidly; 4+ indicates a deep depression that disappears slowly). Capillary refill can be evaluated by depressing the tip of the nailbed until blanching is observed, then releasing the pressure and noting the length of time required for color to return. Normally, immediate refill is observed. The following structures are systematically examined: arteries, veins, and anterior chest wall.

Arterial pulse and pressure

The arterial pulse is palpated to elicit the following information: (1) rate, (2) regularity, (3) amplitude, and (4) quality. Certain cardiac arrhythmias can be detected by alterations in the rate or regularity of the arterial pulse. Irregularities of cardiac rhythm are associated with variability in pulse amplitude. If the interval between cardiac impulses is irregular, the ventricular filling time and, consequently, the stroke volume vary with each beat. For instance, shortening the interval between beats reduces filling time and stroke volume; consequently, the amplitude of the peripheral arterial pulsation is reduced for that beat. For this reason, irregular rhythms are occasionally associated with a "radial pulse deficit," or a palpated radial rate slower than the auscultated apical rate. This simply indicates that the ventricular filling time was so short that the volume of blood ejected into the periphery for some beats was too small to be palpated in the peripheral bed.

The quality of the arterial pulses is an important index of peripheral perfusion. A consistently weak, thready pulse may indicate a low stroke volume or increased peripheral vascular resistance. Conversely, a forceful, bounding pulse correlates with high stroke volumes and reduced peripheral resistance. The contour of the arterial pulse can best be appreciated by light palpation of the carotid artery. Palpation of a small pulse with a slow upstroke would characterize aortic stenosis—a lesion which impedes blood flow through the aortic valve. This pulse is described as an *anacrotic pulse* (see Fig. 26-1); the slow upstroke is also referred to as *pulsus tardus*. The valvular lesion of aortic regurgitation produces a bounding, rapidly rising and collapsing pulse referred to as a *waterhammer pulse*.

Pulsus alternans and *pulsus bigeminus* are both characterized by alternating strong and weak pulsations. However, pulsus alternans occurs at regular intervals and reflects left ventricular failure, whereas pulsus bigeminus is produced by alteration in pulse volume due to a bigeminal (every second beat) pattern of premature beats in the cardiac rhythm (see Fig. 26-1). *Pulsus paradoxus* is an exaggerated fall in systolic pressure of greater than 10 mmHg during inspiration. Normally,

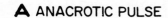

A ANACROTIC PULSE   **B** WATERHAMMER PULSE

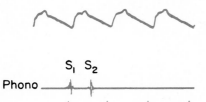
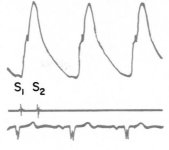

S₁ S₂   S₁ S₂

Phono

ECG

C PULSUS ALTERNANS   **D** PULSUS BIGEMINUS

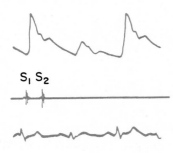
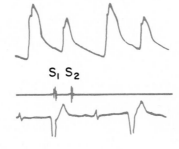

S₁ S₂   S₁ S₂

FIGURE 26-1
Characteristic arterial pulse wave sphygmograms with simultaneously recorded phonogram. (A) Anacrotic pulse. (B) Waterhammer pulse. (C) Pulsus alternans. (D) Pulsus bigeminus. (From J. M. Sana and R.D. Judge, 1975, p. 194)

systolic pressure falls slightly on inspiration because the reduction in intrathoracic pressure is transmitted to the pulmonic vasculature and produces a slight increase in pulmonary blood volume and a corresponding decrease in venous return to the left side of the heart. Cardiac tamponade, or constrictive pericarditis, can compromise cardiac filling further and exaggerate this inspiratory fall producing the paradoxical pulse.

An impression of the consistency of the arterial wall can best be obtained by rolling a peripheral artery under the examining fingers; hardening or thickening of the walls can be detected. A full cardiovascular examination includes palpation of arterial pulsations for quality and equality at multiple sites: (1) dorsalis pedis, (2) posterior tibialis, (3) popliteal, (4) femoral, (5) radial, (6) brachial, and (7) carotid.

The quality of peripheral pulses is graded on a 4-point scale (0 = absent; 1 = markedly reduced; 2 = moderately reduced; 3 = slightly reduced; and 4 = normal). Auscultation over arterial sites for bruits may be indicated if localized narrowing is suspected.

Auscultation of blood pressure concludes the arterial examination. Arterial blood pressure is measured by listening for the onset and disappearance of sounds referred to as Korotkoff sounds (sometimes spelled Korotkov) in an artery occluded by a blood pressure cuff (see Fig. 26-2). The timing of these sounds is correlated with pressure readings on a mercury manometer. Initially, the pressure in the cuff is increased to exceed systolic

pressure in the artery so that no flow through the artery occurs and no sound is heard. As pressure in the cuff is gradually reduced below systolic pressure, flow begins. However, the flow is turbulent because it occurs through a constricted lumen; turbulent flow produces sound. The onset of turbulent flow is heard as the first Korotkoff sound and correlates with systolic pressure. Further reductions in cuff pressure produce characteristic alterations in the sound as flow increases through the arterial lumen, until the sound disappears. Either abrupt muffling or disappearance of sound correlates with diastolic pressure.

The normal arterial blood pressure is approximately 120/80. In general, hypertension is designated as a diastolic pressure over 95 mmHg or a systolic pressure over 160 mmHg (see Chap. 27 for further discussion). Hypotension, for a given individual, is best evaluated in terms of adequacy of peripheral perfusion. Early signs of inadequate peripheral perfusion would be a decreased urine output and cold, pale skin with reduced peripheral pulses. The kidneys and skin are relatively nonvital organs; therefore, as arterial pressure falls, blood is shunted from these organs to the more vital organs, the heart and brain.

The *pulse pressure* is the difference between the systolic and diastolic blood pressure. For example, a blood pressure of 120/80 corresponds to a pulse pressure of 40 mmHg. If arterial pressure falls and sympathetic compensatory vasoconstriction occurs, the pulse pres-

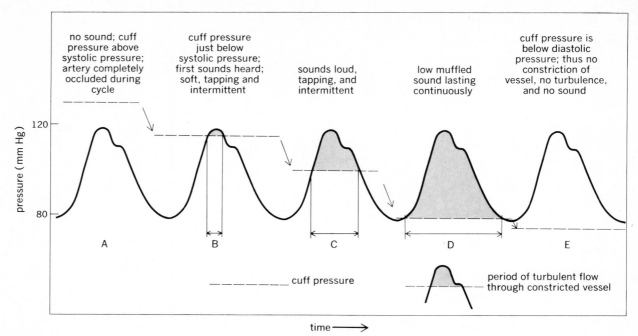

no sound; cuff pressure above systolic pressure; artery completely occluded during cycle

cuff pressure just below systolic pressure; first sounds heard; soft, tapping and intermittent

sounds loud, tapping, and intermittent

low muffled sound lasting continuously

cuff pressure is below diastolic pressure; thus no constriction of vessel, no turbulence, and no sound

pressure (mm Hg)

120

80

A   B   C   D   E

cuff pressure

period of turbulent flow through constricted vessel

time ⟶

FIGURE 26-2

Korotkoff sounds. Systolic blood pressure is recorded at B when the first sounds are heard during a blood pressure measurement. Diastolic pressure is recorded at the point of sound muffling or disappearance, D or E. (From A. J. Vander, J. H. Sherman, and D. S. Luciano, *Human Physiology,* **2d ed., McGraw-Hill, New York, 1975, p. 250.)**

sure is reduced or narrowed. A fall in pressure to 105/90 would narrow the pulse pressure to 15 mmHg. The pulse pressure is influenced most significantly by stroke volume and peripheral resistance. A narrow pulse pressure indicates a low stroke volume or a high peripheral resistance or both. A falling blood pressure and narrowing pulse pressure is an ominous sign of left ventricular dysfunction. The *mean arterial pressure* is the average peripheral perfusion pressure. This value is not simply the average of the diastolic and systolic pressures, because the duration of diastole exceeds the duration of systole at normal heart rates. Consequently, mean arterial pressure is estimated by adding the diastolic pressure to one-third of the pulse pressure.

Venous pressure and pulsations

Jugular venous pressure and pulsations reflect the function of the right side of the heart. The jugular veins are examined to estimate central venous pressure and to analyze pulsations. To estimate central venous pressure, the internal jugular veins are examined with the trunk elevated approximately 15 to 30°. Normally, the highest point of venous pulsation ascends no more than 3 cm above the sternal angle or angle of Louis (i.e., the juncture between the manubrium and body of the sternum). Abnormal elevation of the venous pressure, as in failure of the right side of the heart, can be estimated

by measuring the vertical distance between the level of jugular venous pulsation and the sternal angle. With extreme elevations of pressure, usually over 25 cm of water, the jugular veins remain distended to the angle of the jaw with trunk elevations of 90°.

Venous pressure normally fluctuates with respiration; inspiration produces a fall in venous pressure because intrathoracic pressure decreases, favoring venous return to the heart. A paradoxical increase in venous pressure with inspiration, known as *Kussmaul's sign,* indicates an impediment to venous return to the right side of the heart, as in severe right heart failure.

The *hepatojugular reflux test* is an important diagnostic clue to the presence of right heart failure. Manually sustained pressure is applied for approximately 30 to 60 seconds over the right upper quadrant of the abdomen: the neck veins are observed simultaneously. The abdominal pressure increases venous return to the heart. The normal heart is able to adapt and immediately accept the increased venous return. However, the failing right side of the heart is unable to readily accept this increased load; therefore the distention of the jugular veins will increase and the level of venous pulsations will rise in the neck. This response of the jugular veins is referred to as a positive hepatojugular reflux test.

The anatomic basis for the hepatojugular reflux test may be understood by recalling that the liver functions as a "flood chamber" in its strategic location between the intestinal and general circulation. The liver sinusoids hold a large amount of blood, which is forced into the inferior vena cava through the hepatic veins when pressure is applied over the liver during the reflux test (see Fig. 23-2 and Table 23-1).

The pulsations of the jugular veins are also analyzed to evaluate function of the right side of the heart. At normal venous pressures, maximal venous pulsation can best be observed with trunk elevation of approximately 15 to 30°. The venous waves are gentle and undulating, with three positive components: the *a*, *c*, and *v* waves (see Fig. 26-3A). The *a* wave is produced by atrial contraction; the *c* wave correlates with the onset of ventricular contraction and seems to result from the bulging of the tricuspid valve into the right atrium; the *v* wave corresponds to the period of atrial filling during ventricular ejection prior to opening of the tricuspid valve. The *c* wave is difficult to distinguish in the jugular veins because of its low amplitude.

Predictable alterations in waveform configuration result from tricuspid valve disease. Tricuspid stenosis impedes the blood flow from the right atrium into the right ventricle, forcing the right atrium to generate more pressure during contraction and creating "giant *a* waves" (see Fig. 26-3B). Tricuspid valvular regurgitation during ventricular systole produces a retrograde flow wave distorting the *c* and *v* waves, referred to as a "significant *v* wave" (see Fig. 26-3C). Certain cardiac arrhythmias also alter the configuration of the venous waves by disrupting the sequential, synchronized contraction of the atria and the ventricles.

Precordial movements

Physical examination of the anterior chest involves inspection and palpation of the precordium. The thoracic movements are inspected for symmetry and visible pulsations. The chest is then palpated for normal and abnormal pulsations. The apical impulse, produced by the thrust of the heart against the chest wall during systole, is located. Normally, the point of maximal impulse (PMI) can be palpated as a rhythmic, brief tap approximately 1 to 2 cm in diameter, located in the fifth intercostal space just medial to the midclavicular line.

With left ventricular hypertrophy, the apical impulse becomes more sustained, more forceful, and larger. The PMI is displaced laterally to the left and downward. Right ventricular hypertrophy characteristically produces a *substernal heave*, or a systolic lift of the sternum, as the contractile force of the anterior right ventricle increases. Abnormal pulsations are also noted with coronary atherosclerotic disease; damaged myocardial fibers with limited or absent contractile force bulge passively outward during systole, creating paradoxical precordial movements. In addition, the turbulent flow associated with heart murmurs can create palpable precordial vibrations known as "thrills."

Heart sounds

Auscultation of the chest permits identification of normal heart sounds, abnormal heart sounds, murmurs, and extracardiac sounds. The first and second heart sounds correlate with closure of the AV valves and the semilunar valves, respectively. Thus the first heart sound is heard at the onset of ventricular systole, as ventricular pressures rise above atrial pressures and close the mitral and tricuspid valves. An abnormal accentuation of the first heart sound is noted in mitral stenosis as a result of the stiffening of the valve leaflets.

The second heart sound is audible at the beginning of ventricular relaxation as ventricular pressure falls below the pressure within the pulmonary artery and aorta, closing the pulmonic and aortic valves. Typically, right ventricular ejection lasts slightly longer than does left ventricular ejection, resulting in asynchronous valve closure. Therefore the aortic valve closes before the

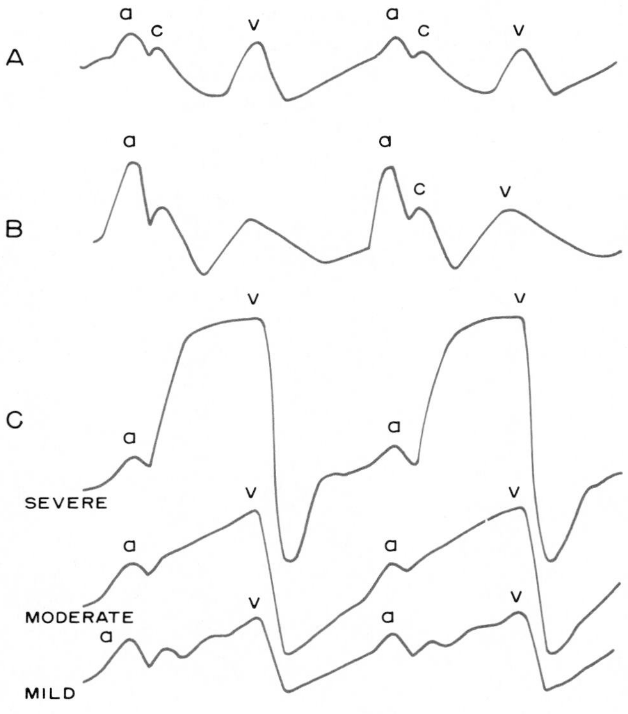

FIGURE 26-3
Jugular venous waveforms. (A) Normal waves, of low amplitude and undulating. The *a* wave is produced by atrial contraction; the *c* wave is produced by ventricular contraction and the consequent bulging of the tricuspid valve into the right atrium; the *v* wave is produced during atrial filling prior to the opening of the tricuspid valve. (B) Giant *a* waves seen in tricuspid stenosis. (C) Mild, moderate, and severe tricuspid regurgitation. In severe tricuspid regurgitation, the *c* and *v* waves summate into huge *v* waves. (Modified from J. W. Hurst, *The Heart*, 3d ed., McGraw-Hill, New York, 1974, pp. 184, 187.)

pulmonic valve, producing a normal physiologic splitting or separation of the valve closure sounds. Inspiration accentuates physiologic splitting because venous return to the right side of the heart increases, thus producing an increment in the volume of right ventricular ejection. During expiration, splitting becomes less pronounced or disappears.

Abnormal paradoxical splitting signifies closure of the pulmonic valve prior to closure of the aortic valve. A paradoxical response to respiration is noted; that is, splitting is most pronounced with expiration and subsides with inspiration. Paradoxical splitting is observed during delayed activation of the left ventricle, as in left bundle branch block, or with prolonged left ventricular ejection, as in aortic stenosis.

Two additional heart sounds can occasionally be heard during ventricular diastole. The third and fourth heart sounds can be physiologic manifestations but are usually heard in conjunction with heart disease; the pathologic appearance of the third or fourth heart sound is referred to as a *gallop rhythm*. This term is applicable because the addition of another heart sound simulates the rhythm of a horse's gallop. The third heart sound occurs during the period of rapid ventricular filling and is consequently referred to as a *ventricular gallop* when it is abnormal. This sound can occur normally in children and young adults. However, it is usually a pathologic finding produced by cardiac dysfunction, particularly ventricular failure.

The fourth heart sound occurs during atrial systole and is referred to as an *atrial gallop*. Normally it is faint or inaudible, occurring immediately prior to the first heart sound. The atrial gallop is audible when ventricular resistance to atrial filling increases, as a result of either reduced ventricular wall distensibility or increased ventricular volumes.

Heart murmurs are the result of turbulent flow within the cardiac chambers and vessels. Turbulent flow is produced either by flow through structural abnormalities (narrowed valvular orifices, incompetent valves, or dilated arterial segments) or by high velocity flow through normal structures. Murmurs are described

according to (1) timing relative to cardiac cycle, (2) intensity, (3) location or region of maximum audibility, and (4) characteristics.

Diastolic murmurs occur after the second heart sound during ventricular relaxation. The murmurs of mitral stenosis and aortic regurgitation occur during diastole. Systolic murmurs are designated as either ejection murmurs, occurring during midsystole after the early phase of isovolumetric contraction, or regurgitant murmurs, occurring throughout systole. Murmurs occurring throughout systole are referred to as pansystolic or holosystolic. The murmur of aortic stenosis would typify an ejection murmur, whereas mitral regurgitation produces a pansystolic murmur.

The loudness of a murmur is graded on a scale of I to VI, with grade I representing a faint murmur and grade VI representing a murmur audible with the stethoscope off the chest wall. Five standard areas of the chest wall, illustrated in Fig. 26-4 as aortic, tricuspid, pulmonic, mitral (or apical) regions and Erb's point, are commonly utilized to localize the region of maximum murmur audibility. Specification of unique sound characteristics such as pitch, quality, duration, or radiation is also included in the description of a heart murmur.

Finally, identification and description of extracardiac sounds are essential. For instance, the stiff, thickened valve cusps in mitral stenosis produce an audible "opening snap" in early diastole. A pericardial "friction rub," caused by pericardial inflammation, is audible as a rough sandpaper sound.

NONINVASIVE DIAGNOSTIC PROCEDURES

Surface electrocardiogram

The electrocardiogram (ECG) is the graphic recording of the heart's electrical activity. Characteristic waveforms on the ECG, arbitrarily designated as P, QRS,

FIGURE 26-4

Position for auscultation of heart sounds. Aortic area (second right interspace close to sternum). Pulmonic area (second left interspace close to sternum). Third left interspace close to sternum (sometimes called Erb's point) where murmurs of both aortic and pulmonic origin may be heard. Tricuspid area (fifth left intercostal space close to sternum). Mitral (apical) area (fifth left intercostal space just medial to the midclavicular line).

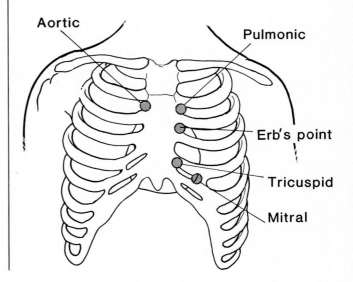

and T waves, correlate with the spread of electrical excitation and recovery through the conduction system and myocardium (see Fig. 26-5A). These waves are recorded on graph paper with a horizontal time scale and a vertical voltage scale (see Fig. 26-5B). The significance of the waveforms and intervals on the ECG is as follows:

1. *P wave:* The P wave corresponds to atrial depolarization. The normal stimulus for atrial depolarization originates in the sinus node; however, the magnitude of electrical current associated with excitation of the sinus node is too small to be visualized on the ECG. The P wave is normally gently rounded and upright in most leads. Atrial enlargement may increase the amplitude or width of the P wave and alter its configuration. Cardiac arrhythmias can also change the P wave configuration. For instance, rhythms originating near the AV junction may cause inversion of the P wave because the direction of atrial depolarization is reversed.

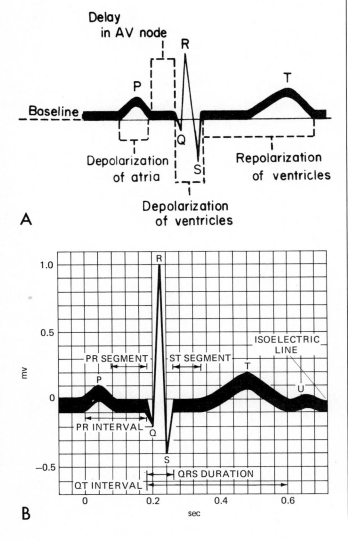

A

B

2. *PR interval:* The PR interval is measured from the beginning of the P wave to the onset of the QRS complex. This interval includes impulse transmission time through the atria and the delay of the impulse at the AV node. The normal interval is 0.12 to 0.20 second. Abnormal prolongation of the PR interval is indicative of an impulse conduction disturbance, referred to as *first-degree heart block.*

3. *QRS complex:* The QRS complex represents ventricular depolarization. The amplitude of this wave is great as a result of the large muscle mass traversed by the electrical impulse. However, impulse spread is rapid; normally, the duration of the QRS complex is between 0.06 and 0.10 second. Prolongation of impulse spread through the bundle branches, known as *bundle branch block,* widens the ventricular complex. Abnormal cardiac rhythms originating in the ventricles, such as ventricular tachycardia, also widen and distort the QRS complex because the specialized pathways that speed impulse spread through the ventricles are bypassed. Ventricular hypertrophy would increase the amplitude of the QRS complex as the muscle mass enlarges.

Atrial repolarization occurs during the period of ventricular depolarization. However, the magnitude of the QRS complex obscures any electrocardiographic evidence of atrial recovery.

4. *ST segment:* This interval is interposed between the wave of ventricular depolarization and repolarization. The initial phases of ventricular repolarization occur during this period; however, the changes are too subtle to be apparent on the ECG. Abnormal depression or elevation of the ST seg-

FIGURE 26-5
(A) Correlation between the waves of the electrocardiogram and impulses that spread through the heart. (B) The normal recording of the electrocardiogram on graph paper. Amplitude (in millivolts) is represented on the vertical axis while the horizontal axis represents time (in seconds). Each small square represents 0.04 second with 5 small squares equaling 0.2 second. Normal intervals are: PR, 0.12 to 0.20 second; QRS, 0.06 to 0.10 second; QT, 0.36 to 0.44 second. The ventricular rate may be calculated by counting the number of R waves in 6 seconds and multiplying by 10 or counting the number of small squares between two complexes (R to R) and dividing this number into 1500. (A, from J. Constant, *Learning Electrocardiography,* Little, Brown, Boston, 1973, p. 3. B, reproduced with permission, from W. F. Ganong, *Review of Medical Physiology,* 8th ed., Lange Medical Publications, Los Altos, Calif., 1977, p. 405.)

ment are associated with myocardial ischemia and infarction, respectively. Digitalis administration characteristically produces sagging of the segment.

5. *T wave:* Ventricular repolarization generates the T wave. Normally, the T wave is slightly asymmetrical, rounded, and upright in most leads. Inversion of the T wave is associated with myocardial ischemia. Hyperkalemia, or serum potassium elevation, will cause peaking and elevation of the T wave.

6. *QT interval:* This interval is measured from the beginning of the QRS complex to the end of the T wave, encompassing ventricular depolarization and repolarization. The average QT interval is 0.36 to 0.44 second for normal heart rates. The QT interval is prolonged with the administration of certain antiarrhythmic drugs, such as quinidine.

The electrical currents generated within the heart during depolarization and repolarization are conducted to the body surface where they can be recorded by electrodes in contact with the skin. By convention, nine recording electrodes are placed on the extremities and chest wall with a ground electrode, utilized to reduce

electrical interference, attached to the right leg. Varying combinations of these electrodes produce 12 standard leads. Each of the 12 leads records the electrical events of the entire cardiac cycle. However, each lead views the heart from a slightly different perspective; therefore, waveforms will look slightly different in each lead. Three categories of leads are commonly designated (see Fig. 26-6):

1. *Standard limb leads (leads I, II, III):* These leads measure the difference in electrical potential between two points; thus the leads are bipolar, with one negative and one positive pole. Electrodes are placed on the right arm, left arm, and left leg. Lead I views the heart from the axis connecting the right arm and left arm, with the left arm as the positive pole; lead II, from the right arm and left leg, with the left leg positive; and lead III, from the left arm and left leg, with the left leg positive (Fig. 26-6A).

2. *Augmented limb leads (leads aVR, aVL, aVF:* These leads are electrically adjusted to measure the absolute electrical potential at one recording site, that of a positive electrode placed on the extremities, creating, in essence, a unipolar lead. This is accomplished by electrically canceling out the effect of the negative pole and establishing an "indifferent" electrode at zero potential. Adjustments are made automatically within the ECG machine to

FIGURE 26-6

Electrode positions for the standard 12-lead electrocardiogram. (A) Standard limb leads (I, II, III). (B) Augmented limb leads (aVR, aVL, aVF). (C) Precordial leads (V₁ to V₆).

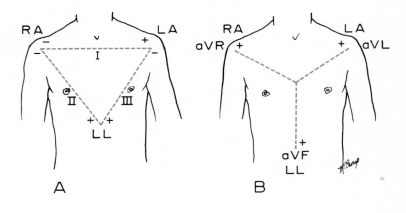

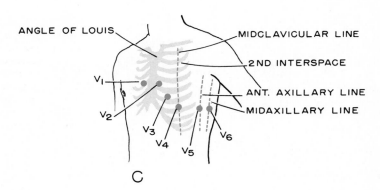

join the other limb electrodes creating a common indifferent electrode with essentially no effect on the positive recording electrode. The voltage recorded from the positive electrode is then amplified or "augmented" to produce a selected, unipolar limb lead tracing. There are three augmented limb leads: aVR, recording from the right arm; aVL, from the left arm; and aVF, from the left leg. (The aVF location can be easily remembered by associating the "F" with "foot") (Fig. 26-6B).

3. *Precordial or chest leads* (V_1 to V_6): These leads are unipolar leads recording the absolute electrical potential of sites on the anterior chest wall, or precordium. Identification of the following landmarks facilitates accurate placement of the precordial electrodes: (1) angle of Louis, the sternal protuberance at the juncture between the manubrium and body of the sternum; (2) the second intercostal space, adjacent to the angle of Louis; (3) the left midclavicular line; and (4) the anterior and midaxillary lines (Fig. 26-6C). Electrodes are placed sequentially on the chest wall at six different sites:

V_1—located in the fourth intercostal space to the right of the sternum

V_2—located in the fourth intercostal space to the left of the sternum

V_3—located midway between V_2 and V_4

V_4—located in the fifth intercostal space in the midclavicular line

V_5—horizontal to V_4 in the anterior axillary line

V_6—horizontal to V_5 in the midaxillary line

The standard limb leads and augmented limb leads view the heart in the frontal plane. The relative perspective of each lead is conceptualized most easily utilizing a schematic diagram, known as the *hexaxial reference system*. This reference system is derived in the following manner (see Fig. 26-7): (1) Connecting the lead axes of leads I, II, and III forms an equilateral triangle, referred to as *Einthoven's triangle*. The heart is considered the electrical center of the triangle. (2) Positioning the lead axes so that each radiates from the

center of the triangle creates a second diagram, known as the *triaxial reference system*. (3) Combining the triaxial reference system diagram with the schematic representation of the augmented limb leads radiating from the electrical center of the thorax produces the *hexaxial reference system*. The hexaxial reference system is an invaluable aid to electrocardiographic interpretation, permitting calculation of the average direction of electrical activity within the heart. The average direction of electrical activation, calculated from the ECG is referred to as the *electrical axis* of the heart.

Other modified leads are often used in special situations. A modified lead V_1 (MCL$_1$) is frequently used for bedside monitoring to facilitate arrhythmia detection and analysis. This lead is a bipolar lead, with the positive electrode positioned in the standard V_1 position (fourth intercostal space to the right of the sternum) and the negative electrode positioned near the left shoulder beneath the clavicle.

The waveform configurations apparent in each lead will depend upon the orientation of the particular lead relative to the path of cardiac electrical activity. The leads of the hexaxial reference system view the heart in the frontal plane; the six precordial leads offer another perspective from the horizontal plane. Waves will be positive (i.e., deflected upward) if the electrical activity of the heart approaches the positive electrode of a given lead. For example, in Fig. 26-8 the P wave and QRS complex of lead II are positive because the wave of depolarization approaches the positive left leg electrode of

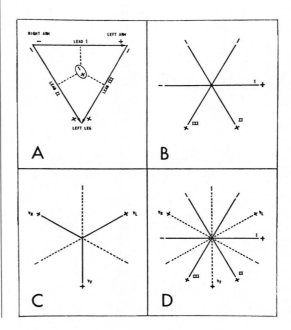

FIGURE 26-7
Derivation of the hexaxial reference system. (A) The Einthoven triangle, showing the axes of the standard limb leads with the heart at the center of the triangle. (B) The axes of the limb leads are moved to the center of the triangle forming a triaxial reference system. (C) The axes of the augmented (unipolar) limb leads. (D) The axes of the standard and unipolar limb leads are superimposed, forming a hexaxial reference system. (From H. H. Friedman, *Outline of Electrocardiography*, McGraw-Hill, New York, 1963, p. 28.)

lead II. Conversely, the same waves in lead aVR are negative because the path of electrical activity is moving away from the positive right arm electrode. In addition, the amplitude of waves varies among leads. As a rule, wave amplitude will be greatest in a lead lying parallel to the path of depolarization. Notice that lead II in Fig. 26-8 demonstrates the greatest wave amplitude, indicating that lead II most closely parallels the path of depolarization in this ECG.

The ECG permits detection of abnormalities in cardiac rate and rhythm, chamber enlargement, myocardial ischemia or infarction, drug and electrolyte effects, and shifts in the direction of electrical activation.

Conventional bedside monitoring techniques have been extended to ambulatory monitoring (telemetry) and continuous 24-hour electrocardiographic recording (Holter monitoring).

Echocardiogram

Echocardiography is a cardiac diagnostic technique utilizing ultrasound as the examination medium. A transducer transmitting ultrasonic waves (high-frequency sound waves beyond the limit of human hearing) is applied to the patient's chest wall and directed at the heart (see Fig. 26-9). As the ultrasonic beam traverses the heart, ultrasonic waves are reflected back to the transducer whenever the beam crosses a boundary between cardiac structures or substances (e.g., blood) with different acoustic impedance. These reflected ultrasonic waves, or "cardiac echoes," are then converted to electrical impulses, amplified, and recorded, documenting the dimensions and motion of cardiac structures. The precordium can be scanned by moving the transducer in several directions.

Conventional echocardiography records a one-dimensional sequential display of tissues traversed by the ultrasonic beam (see Fig. 26-9). Since this display is recorded for a period of time, characteristic patterns of tissue movement are inscribed permitting identification of structures and analysis of function. This technique is referred to as M-mode (or motion mode) echocardiography. Echocardiography is useful in the diagnosis of valvular and congenital heart disease. M-mode echos are of particular value in clinical situations with characteristic alterations in tissue movement or boundaries, such as in mitral stenosis or pericardial effusion. Figure 26-10 illustrates the normal motion of the anterior and posterior mitral valve leaflets relative to the restricted motion of stenotic, immobile mitral leaflets.

The recent advent of two-dimensional (2D) echocardiography has expanded the applications of echocardiography. Two-dimensional echos (see Fig. 26-11) detect structures along the entire plane of the ultrasonic beam so that a full transverse section can be displayed. Doppler techniques have also been applied to echocardiography. By directing an ultrasonic beam onto the moving cardiac structures and determining the difference between the frequency of the emitted beam and that subsequently received, the velocity of flow or movement of the structures can be determined (using

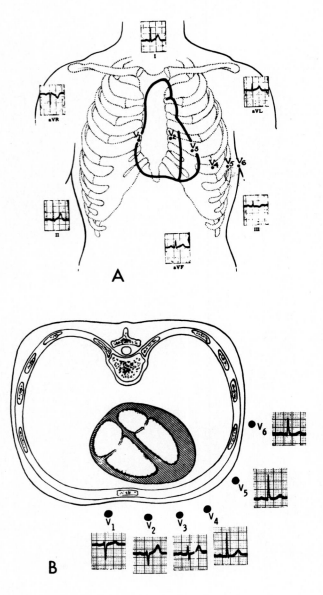

FIGURE 26-8

A, normal ECG patterns in the frontal plane (standard leads I, II, and III and augmented unipolar leads aVR, aVL, and aVF). B, normal ECG patterns in the horizontal plane (precordial leads V_1 to V_6). (Reproduced with permission, from M. J. Goldman, *Principles of Clinical Electrocardiography*, 9th ed., Lange Medical Publications, Los Altos, Calif., 1976.)

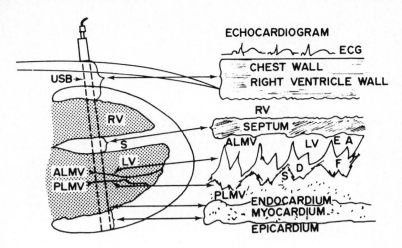

FIGURE 26-9

Normal echocardiogram. Path of ultrasound beam (USB) is shown schematically on the left. On the right is a diagram of the corresponding echocardiogram for this direction of the transducer. Abbreviations: RV, right ventricle; S, septum; LV, left ventricle; ALMV, anterior leaflet of the mitral valve; PLMV, posterior leaflet of the mitral valve; S, systole; D, diastole, E, peak of rapid anterior opening of mitral valve during beginning of diastole; A, peak of anterior movement of leaflet into the ventricle produced by atrial systole: F, position of leaflet during rapid ventricular filling. (From Peter C. Gazes, *Clinical Cardiology,* copyright © 1975 by Year Book Medical Publishers, Inc., Chicago, used by permission. (Modified from R. L. Popp, et al., *American Journal of Cardiology,* 24:528, 1969.))

the Doppler principle). By combining various Doppler methods with echocardiography, two-dimensional views of cardiac structures as well as their velocity of movement can be evaluated.

Phonocardiogram

A phonocardiogram is the graphic recording of the sounds, both normal and abnormal, generated during the cardiac cycle. It is usually recorded in conjunction with the ECG and an external pulse tracing, such as the carotid or apical pulsation (see Fig. 26-12). A microphone positioned on the chest wall receives the sound waves, which are then amplified and recorded. Simultaneously, a pressure transducer senses the external pulsations of the carotid artery or cardiac apex. The ECG is obtained from body surface electrodes.

The phonocardiogram provides documentation and confirmation of auscultated heart sounds and murmurs. Simultaneous recording of the phonocardiogram, ECG, and pulse tracing permits correlation of the timing of recorded sounds with the mechanical and electrical events of the cardiac cycle. This facilitates accurate interpretation of abnormal cardiac sounds.

Systolic time intervals (STI), useful in the evaluation of ventricular performance, can also be determined at this time. For example, left ventricular ejection time (LVET) can be calculated by measuring the distance from the upstroke of the carotid pulse to the dicrotic

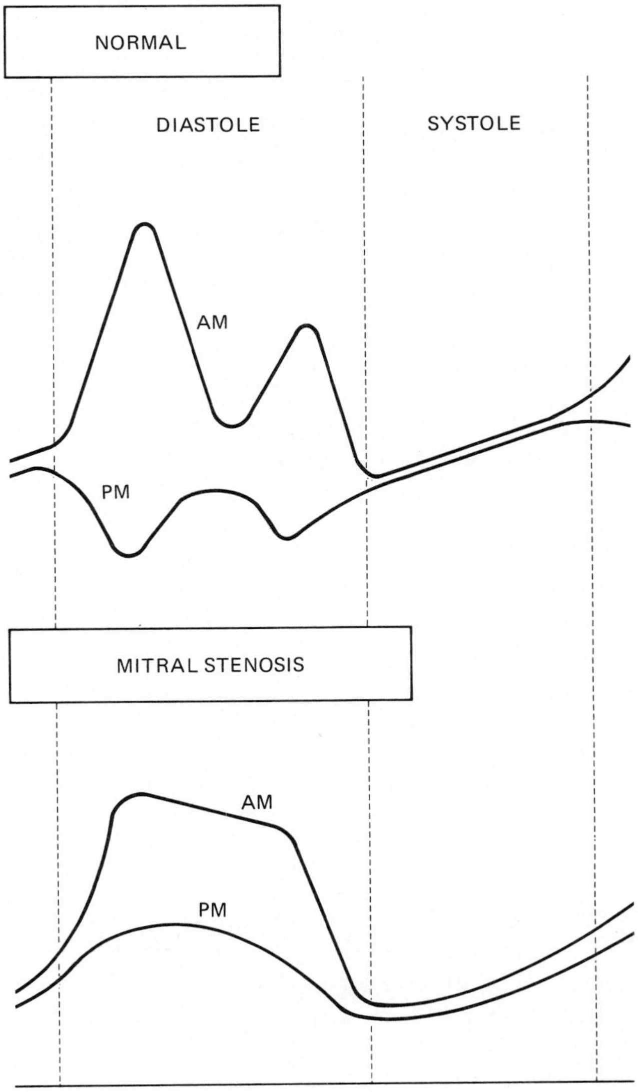

FIGURE 26-10

Mitral valve echocardiogram. Above, normal leaflet motion (AM, anterior mitral valve leaflet; PM, posterior mitral valve leaflet). Below, abnormal leaflet motion with mitral stenosis. (Adapted from J. M. Duchak, S. Chang, and H. Feigenbaum, "The Posterior Mitral Valve ECHO and the Electrocardiographic Diagnosis of Mitral Stenosis," *American Journal of Cardiology,* 29: 631, 1972.)

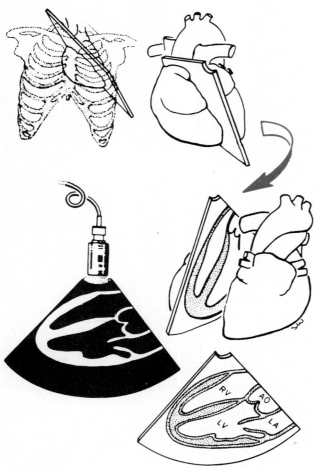

FIGURE 26-11

Two-dimensional (2D) echocardiogram. In contrast to the M-mode one-dimensional "ice-pick" view, two-dimensional echocardiography simultaneously detects all cardiac structures lying within the plane of examination, displaying the image on a video screen. (From Ream and Fogdall, 1982, p. 109.)

notch, which corresponds to aortic valve closure and the onset of diastole. LVET would be prolonged by conditions interfering with the ejection of blood from the ventricle, such as aortic stenosis. The total duration of electromechanical systole, measured from the onset of the QRS to the recording of the second heart sound or aortic valve closure (i.e., the QS_2 interval), can be deter-

FIGURE 26-12

Characteristic normal arterial pulse wave with simultaneous recording of a phonocardiogram and electrocardiogram. (Adapted from Sana and Judge, 1975, p. 192.)

mined. This interval includes all the electrical and mechanical events of ventricular systole.

Radionuclide imaging

Radionuclide imaging involves the intravenous injection of small quantities of radioactive isotopes, referred to as tracers, into a peripheral vein. The tracer either binds to the blood or is selectively taken up by normal or infarcted myocardium. The tracer's affinity for blood or myocardium depends on the properties of the radioactive substance selected. The distribution of the tracer can be detected by sensitive nuclear cameras which record a *nuclear image* of the heart in various positions.

Three radionuclide techniques are currently utilized: (1) *myocardial imaging* with thallium 201 to evaluate regional myocardial perfusion; (2) *acute myocardial infarction imaging* with technetium 99m pyrophosphate to detect acute myocardial necrosis or injury, and (3) *multiple gated blood pool scanning* with technetium-labeled red blood cells to evaluate ventricular function.

Myocardial imaging with thallium is useful in the evaluation of ischemia and coronary artery disease since thallium distribution within the myocardium depends primarily on blood flow. Thallium, a potassium analogue, concentrates in normally perfused myocardial cells; consequently thallium uptake will be diminished or absent in regions of ischemia or infarction. These regions of poor tracer uptake will appear as defects or "cold spots" on the recorded image. Ischemia can be distinguished from infarction if the defect disappears on serial scans as thallium is redistributed into ischemic zones. A persistent defect suggests infarction.

Thallium imaging is usually performed in combination with exercise electrocardiography. Serial images are recorded in multiple projections during exercise and at rest, since perfusion abnormalities may not be apparent at rest.

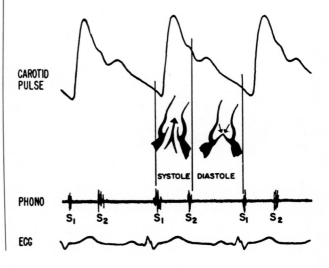

Imaging with technetium pyrophosphate differs from that with thallium in that this radioisotope accumulates selectively in acutely damaged myocardium permitting identification of the site and evaluation of the extent of necrosis. Areas of concentrated uptake appear as "hot spots" on the scan. This pattern of tracer uptake can be observed within 12 to 72 hours after infarction and persists for 10 to 14 days.

Radiolabeled antibody fragments against cardiac myosin are currently being studied as infarct-specific radionuclide imaging agents. These antibodies attach themselves to cardiac myosin, which becomes exposed as myocardial cellular membrane integrity is destroyed during progressive myocardial ischemia. This methodology offers advantages over other infarct-imaging agents in that these antibodies are thought to be necrosis-specific and therefore allow more accurate quantification of infarct size.

The combination of infarct-imaging with cardiac computed tomography also expands the usefulness of these diagnostic procedures. By obtaining multiple images in projections of 360°, computer reconstruction then allows a three-dimensional view of infarct size and may also help to delineate zones of myocardial ischemia and infarction.

Blood pool scanning is invaluable in the evaluation of ventricular function. This technique involves labeling red blood cells or albumin with technetium so that the blood volume or blood pool can be visualized as outlined by the cardiac chambers and vessels. "First pass" blood pool scanning is used to record the initial passage of the radioactive tracer through the heart. This technique is useful to detect and quantify degrees of valvular regurgitation and intracardiac shunting.

A more sophisticated and widespread application of the blood pool scan is the *multiple gated blood pool scan* (GBPS or MUGA). With this method of scanning, images are recorded over multiple cardiac cycles and then summated or superimposed to improve the resolution of the nuclear image (see Fig. 26-13). To accurately synchronize the camera with the cardiac cycle, the camera is "gated" or "triggered" by the ECG. The gated blood pool scan permits noninvasive determination of ejection fraction, ventricular volumes, and regional patterns of wall motion.

Nuclear magnetic resonance (NMR) is a new imaging technique which does not require the administration of radioisotopes. Tomographic or three-dimensional images (i.e., multiple images obtained in projections of 360° with subsequent computer reconstruction) as well as metabolic information may be obtained.

FIGURE 26-13

Multigated blood pool imaging uses a computer in association with the scintillation camera to sort the scintillation information arising from the patient into multiple time segments. Although any number of time segments (n) can be recorded, the cycle is usually divided into less than 30. In any one cycle the amount of scintillation information is too little to permit an adequate view of the heart to the recorded. However, by recording data for n cycles, the quality of the image may build up to a point where sufficient detail can be seen to observe small wall motion abnormalities. (From Johnson, Haber, and Austen, 1980, p. 1058.)

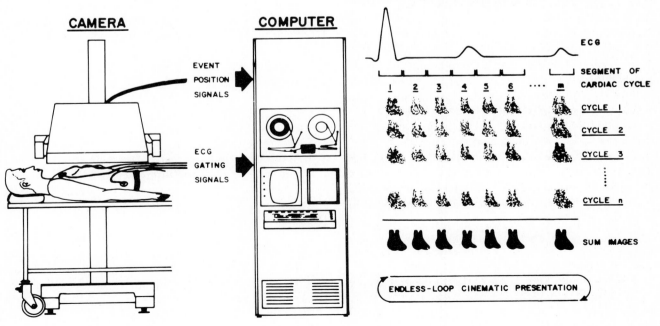

This technique involves the emission of radiofrequency pulses which disturb the total magnetization of the organs or tissues under investigation. Total magnetization of the organs or tissues occurs because cell nuclei are charged and possess an intrinsic spin. This moving spin generates a magnetic field, and the response of the charged cell nuclei to radiofrequency pulses allows assessment of the metabolic activity of living cells. It may be possible to distinguish ischemic versus infarcted myocardium based on the different patterns of metabolic activity of these tissue states.

Exercise testing

Exercise testing with a treadmill or bicycle ergometer permits evaluation of exercise-induced symptoms and/or electrocardiographic changes. Multiple ECG leads are monitored continuously and blood pressure is measured frequently during the test. Patients are requested to report any symptoms immediately. Exercise testing can also be used in conjunction with radionuclide imaging to detect change in myocardial perfusion during exercise. This combination is referred to as *stress imaging*. Comparisons are made between the nuclear image obtained at rest and during exercise.

Digital subtraction angiography

Digital image-processing computers have now assumed cardiovascular applications. The computers enhance radiographic images, yet require a smaller amount of contrast material than do standard angiography techniques, which will be discussed in the section on cardiac catheterization. Left ventricular volumes and ejection fraction can be accurately assessed using this method. This is accomplished by converting radiographic images into a digital format by image subdivision. A matrix of small picture elements (pixels) is created. Signals are assigned a pixel number corresponding to their intensity. This method helps eliminate soft tissue and bone densities in the image, enhancing visualization.

This procedure is much safer than cardiac catheterization, requiring only venous injection of small amounts of contrast material, and may be performed at the bedside. This technique may also be employed for peripheral angiography.

Chest x-ray

A series of chest x-rays in four standard positions is useful in the cardiac diagnostic workup (see Fig. 26-14): (1) posteroanterior or frontal position; (2) left lateral posi-

tion with left side forward; (3) right anterior oblique position with the body rotated approximately 60° to the left, which places the right shoulder anterior; and (4) left anterior oblique position with the left shoulder anterior. In each position, a different anatomic perspective of the heart is visible. The contour of the heart contrasts with the radiolucent air-filled lungs.

The following findings can be detected on the chest x-ray: (1) generalized cardiac enlargement, or cardiomegaly; (2) localized chamber enlargement; (3) calcification in valves or coronary arteries; (4) pulmonary venous congestion; (5) interstitial or alveolar edema; and (6) enlargement of the pulmonary artery or dilation of the ascending aorta.

An impression of generalized cardiac enlargement can be noted in chest x-rays; however, precise estimation of the degree of enlargement is of questionable accuracy. In contrast, chamber enlargement distinctly alters the contour of the heart, permitting specification of the involved chamber. In the posteroanterior position, the right border of the heart consists of the superior vena cava with the right atrium below. An angle appears at the juncture between the two. The structures comprising the left border, from top to bottom, are the aorta, pulmonary artery, and left ventricle. This projection permits identification of right atrial, left ventricular, and pulmonary arterial enlargement. Right atrial enlargement, for example, displaces the right boundary outward to the right, rounding the curvature of the cardiac contour.

In the left lateral position, the anterior border is primarily the right ventricle, with the posterior border consisting of the left atrium superiorly and the posterior wall of the left ventricle inferiorly. The esophagus lies behind the posterior boundary. Right ventricular and left atrial enlargement are best appreciated in this view. Outlining the esophagus with swallowed barium facilitates the diagnosis of left atrial enlargement, which produces an esophageal indentation with posterior displacement.

Radiologic examination of the lungs demonstrates the effects of cardiac dysfunction upon the pulmonary vasculature. Left heart failure or mitral valve disease increases pulmonary venous congestion, dilating the pulmonary veins in characteristic patterns. Excessive elevation of venous pressure results in transudation of fluid into the interstitial space and eventually into the alveoli. Fluid seepage from the intravascular space, or pulmonary edema, produces a clouding, or haziness, of the vascular shadows, progressively whitening the normally dark shadows of the radiolucent lungs.

Characteristic findings typify particular cardiac lesions. For example, in mitral stenosis (a lesion impeding blood flow from the left atrium to the left ventricle) left atrial enlargement and pulmonary venous congestion would be noted. Valvular calcification might also be observed.

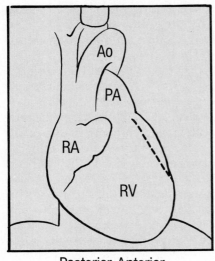

Posterior-Anterior

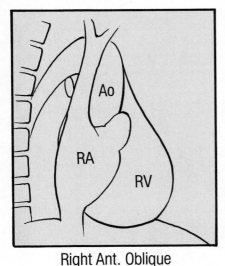

Right Ant. Oblique

Left Lateral

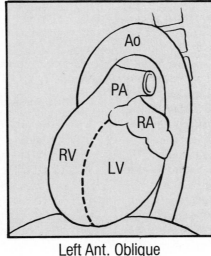

Left Ant. Oblique

FIGURE 26-14
Orientation of the heart in four standard positions for cardiac roentgenography. In the posteroanterior position, the borders of the right atrium and left ventricle are displayed. The right ventricle and the left atrium are not visible on the borders of the silhouette. In the left lateral position, the silhouette of the right ventricle is seen anteriorly and the left atrium posteriorly. In the right anterior oblique position the right ventricle and left atrium are again seen in silhouette. In the left anterior oblique position the right and left ventricle are seen in silhouette. The left atrium can be discerned in this projection. (Modified from R.F. Rushmer, *Cardiovascular Dynamics*, 3d ed., Saunders, Philadelphia, 1970, p. 336.)

INVASIVE DIAGNOSTIC PROCEDURES

Electrophysiology studies

Intracardiac electrocardiographic techniques, or electrophysiology (EP) studies, permit a more detailed analysis of the mechanisms of cardiac impulse formation and conduction than do standard electrocardiographic recordings. The body surface electrocardiogram (ECG) records the summated signals of atrial and ventricular activation, represented by the P wave and QRS complex, respectively. The amplitude of the signals generated by the formation of the impulse within the sinus node and its conduction through specialized conduction pathways are too small to be detected. Positioning intracardiac recording electrodes in close proximity to the conduction system and myocardium amplifies these signals.

Detailed information regarding the genesis and conduction of impulses is required for many reasons, including the following: (1) to evaluate sinus node dysfunction and/or AV conduction delays, (2) to identify the site of and/or mechanism for complex arrhythmias, such as reentrant supraventricular tachycardias or refractory ventricular tachycardias, and (3) to assess the efficacy of pharmacologic or pacemaker therapy for refractory arrhythmias.

The testing protocol utilized and the sites selected for recording depend upon the indication for study. However, the following general principles apply to the majority of studies. One or more catheters with multiple electrodes are advanced through the peripheral veins under fluoroscopic guidance to the desired intracardiac site or sites. Figure 26-15 illustrates catheter placement for EP testing for refractory ventricular tachycardia. These electrodes can be used for intracardiac recording and/or pacing. Electrical stimulation of the atria or ventricles with an external programmable pulse generator may be indicated to induce and/or terminate tachyarrhythmias or to evaluate sinus node response or conduction delays. The intracardiac recordings obtained during spontaneous and/or paced rhythms are then analyzed. For example, His bundle recordings are used to localize the site of AV block. For this study, the recording catheter is positioned across the tricuspid valve beside the membranous interventricular septum. Three electrodes on this catheter record deflections from the low right atrium, His bundle, and right ventricle. These intracardiac deflections are illustrated in Fig. 26-16 in comparison with the body surface ECG. Delays in conduction in the AV node can be readily distinguished from delays in the His-Purkinje system. The utilization of EP testing for refractory ventricular arrhythmias will be discussed in depth in Chap. 27.

Cardiac catheterization

Cardiac catheterization is the insertion of catheters into the cardiovascular system to study the anatomy and function of the heart in the presence of suspected or documented heart disease. Depending on the location of a suspected lesion and the degree of myocardial dysfunction, selected studies are performed, including (1) measurement of pressures in the cardiac chambers and vessels, (2) analysis of the waveform configuration of recorded pressures, (3) sampling of the oxygen content in selected regions, (4) opacification of the cardiac cham-

bers and/or coronary arteries with contrast material, and (5) determination of cardiac output. Normal pressures, waveform configurations, and oxygen contents are illustrated in Fig. 26-17.

Two general approaches to the heart are currently utilized; right-sided heart catheterization and left-sided heart catheterization. Right-sided heart catheterization requires insertion of a catheter into the venous system, usually via an antecubital vein in the right arm or the femoral vein. The catheter is progressively advanced through the peripheral venous system to the vena cava and into the right atrium, right ventricle, and pulmonary artery. Advancing the catheter further into a distal segment of the pulmonary arterial bed eventually produces a "wedging," or lodging, of the catheter tip in the vessel lumen. This wedge position is referred to as the pulmonary capillary position. Left-sided heart catheterization involves the retrograde passage of the catheter through the arterial system to the aorta, across the aortic valve, and into the left ventricle. The catheter is commonly inserted in either the brachial or femoral artery. Passage of the catheter into the aorta also permits selective cannulation and study of the coronary arteries.

Catheterization in coronary atherosclerotic disease

Coronary angiography, or injection of contrast material into the coronary arteries, is most commonly utilized to determine the feasibility and timing of coronary artery bypass grafting for a given patient. Additional indications for coronary angiography include evaluation of atypical angina and coronary revascularization results. The catheterization procedure involves the opacification of both coronary arteries, followed by a left ventriculogram, or injection of the contrast medium into the left ventricle, to evaluate left ventricular function.

Coronary angiography provides the following information: (1) the location of the lesion or lesions, (2) the degree of obstruction, (3) the presence of collateral circulation, and (4) the extent of disease in the distal arterial bed. Certain lesions identified at the time of catheterization are considered high-risk lesions. One example of a high-risk lesion is significant stenosis of the main left coronary artery; relatively urgent surgery may be advised when this is found.

The evaluation of left ventricular function is an important adjunct to coronary angiography. Injection of contrast material into the left ventricle permits visualization of ventricular wall movement and chamber size; areas of absent motion (akinesis), reduced motion (hypokinesis), or asynchronous contraction (dyskinesis) or

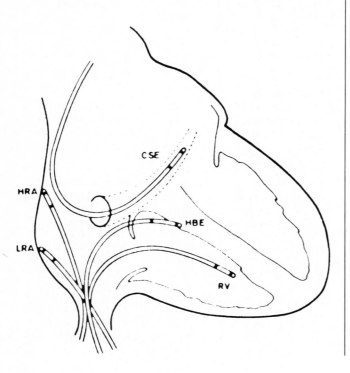

FIGURE 26-15
Catheter placement for electrophysiologic (EP) testing.

bulging are noted. Rupture of a necrotic interventricular septum after myocardial infarction would also be detected during left ventriculography. Since the pressures are higher on the left side of the heart than on the right, blood would be shunted through the interventricular defect, opacifying the right ventricle. In addition, oxygen sampling would demonstrate abnormal elevation of oxygen content in the right ventricle as a result of the recirculation of oxygenated blood through the defect. Measurement of left ventricular pressure, arterial pressure, cardiac output, and ejection fraction completes the overall assessment of left ventricular function.

Catheterization in valvular heart disease

Catheterization is useful to confirm the presence of valvular stenosis or regurgitation, to estimate the severity of the lesion, and to establish or exclude the presence of associated lesions. The approach to the two lesions—stenosis, or valvular obstruction to blood flow, and regurgitation, or backward flow through the valve—differs.

Valvular regurgitation is documented by injection of contrast material into the chamber beyond the diseased valve; if regurgitation is present, opacification of the chamber proximal to the valve will occur when the valve fails to close securely. For example, with mitral regurgitation, the contrast medium injected into the left ventricle would appear in the left atrium during the next ventricular contraction as blood and contrast material flow backward through the diseased valve. The severity of the regurgitation is estimated according to the degree of left atrial opacification and the time required for the contrast material to disappear from the left atrium. Aortic regurgitation is detected by injection of contrast material into the ascending aorta, with subsequent opacification of the left ventricle during ventricular relaxation.

Regurgitation is also associated with abnormalities in the pressures within the cardiac chambers and alterations in waveform configuration. Mitral regurgitation creates a volume overload for the left atrium, elevating left atrial and pulmonary pressures. In addition, the typ-

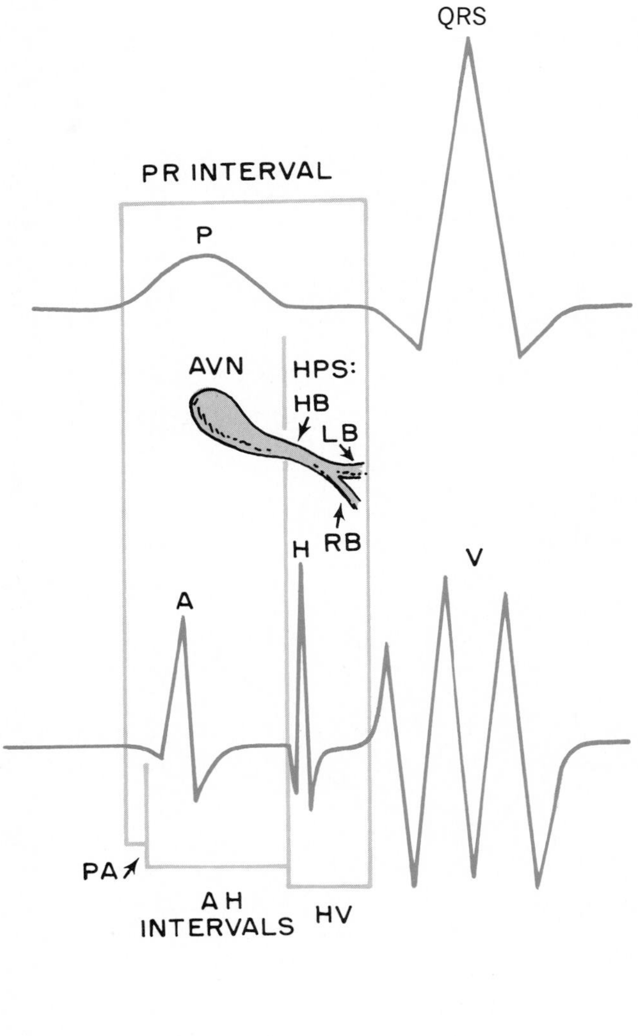

FIGURE 26-16

Surface versus intracardiac ECG: Depicted are simultaneously recorded surface (top) and intracardiac (bottom) electrocardiograms along with the anatomic structures of the atrioventricular specialized conduction system involved in normal impulse transmission. The surface electrocardiogram shows a P wave (atrial muscle depolarization) and a QRS complex (ventricular muscle depolarization). A PR interval can be measured and represents the following conduction times: intraatrial; atrioventricular nodeal (AVN), His bundle (HB), right bundle (RB), and left bundle (LB) branches; and Purkinje fiber. In contrast, the single intracardiac tracing from the atrioventricular junction shows three deflections: A (low atrial muscle depolarization), H (His bundle activation) and V (ventricular muscle depolarization). Three intervals can be measured when the surface and intracardiac electrocardiograms are compared: (1) the PA interval—measure of intraatrial conduction time, as impulse tranverses from its exit from the sinus node (near superior vena cava) to the intracardiac recording site low in the right atrium at the AV junction; (2) the AH interval—approximation of AVN conduction time (penetration of the AVN is assumed to occur simultaneously with arrival of the impulse at the low right atrium, anatomic site of the AVN), and (3) the HV interval—measure of conduction time through the His-Purkinje system (HPS = His bundle, right and left bundles, and Purkinje network) to its exit at the ventricular muscle. From the aforementioned three intervals, conduction delays which exhibit as first-degree AV block (prolonged PR interval) can be differentiated as due to delay in the atria, AVN, or HPS. Sites of higher degrees of AV block can also be determined and isolated to one of those areas (From Gilbert and Ashtar, 1980, p. 86.)

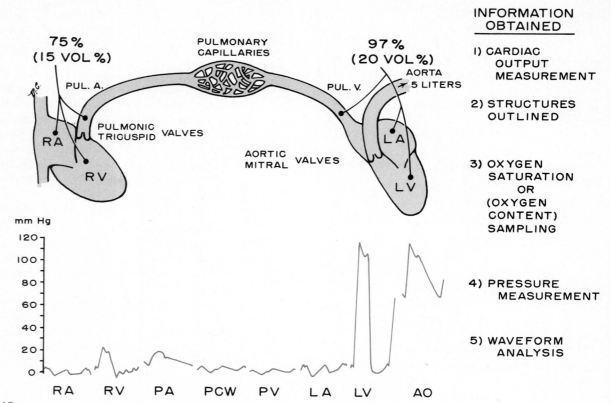

1) CARDIAC OUTPUT MEASUREMENT

2) STRUCTURES OUTLINED

3) OXYGEN SATURATION OR (OXYGEN CONTENT) SAMPLING

4) PRESSURE MEASUREMENT

5) WAVEFORM ANALYSIS

FIGURE 26-17
Data obtained during cardiac catheterization.

ical low-amplitude undulating left atrial waveform exhibits an abrupt increase in amplitude during ventricular contraction as blood flows backward through the valve.

Valvular stenosis can be visualized by injecting contrast material into the chamber proximal to the diseased valve; as the opacified blood flows through the restricted orifice, the valve boundaries are outlined. Typical alterations in pressures and waveforms are seen with valvular stenosis. For instance, the aortic pressure tracing associated with aortic stenosis demonstrates a slow upstroke and delayed peak as a result of the resistance to ventricular ejection into the aorta (see Fig. 26-18). Elevations in pressure in the chambers proximal to a stenotic lesion also occur. For example, mitral stenosis elevates left atrial and pulmonary venous pressures. These pressure elevations are reflected retrograde through the lungs and detected most easily via a catheter in the wedge position in the pulmonary artery. This pressure measurement is known as the *pulmonary capillary wedge pressure* and accurately reflects left atrial pressure.

Valvular stenosis produces a pressure gradient, or difference in pressure, between the chambers on either side of the valve. The pressure gradient results because the chamber proximal to the lesion must generate increased pressure to force blood through the obstructed

valve. An example of a pressure gradient resulting from severe aortic stenosis is illustrated in Fig. 26-19. Notice the large pressure discrepancy, with the left ventricle generating pressures up to 210 mmHg to force blood through the aortic valve to sustain an aortic systolic pressure of 130 mmHg. The pressure gradient in this example is 80 mmHg; normally the pressure gradient is less than 5 mmHg.

In addition to the measurement of the pressure gra-

FIGURE 26-18
Carotid artery pressure tracing. (A) normal; (B) aortic stenosis.

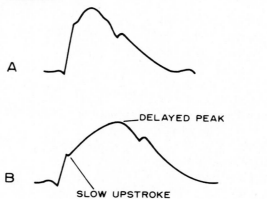

A

B

DELAYED PEAK

SLOW UPSTROKE

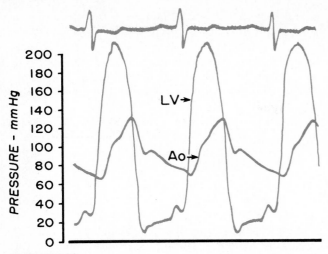

FIGURE 26-19
Left ventricular (LV) and aortic (Ao) pressure tracings in severe aortic stenosis. (Adapted from W. Grossman, *Cardiac Catheterization and Angiography,* **Lea & Febiger, Philadelphia, 1980, p. 315.)**

dient, it is necessary to utilize a formula calculating the area of the valve orifice. The determination of the pressure gradient across the valve and estimation of the valve area are the two most critical indices of the severity of stenosis.

Hemodynamic monitoring

Bedside monitoring of selected intracardiac and intravascular pressures permits ongoing evaluation of cardiovascular status. The following hemodynamic parameters can be monitored in critical care units: (1) right atrial or central venous pressure (RAP or CVP) and left atrial pressure (LAP), (2) right ventricular pressure (RVP) and (indirectly) left ventricular end-diastolic pressure (LVEDP), (3) pulmonary artery pressure (PAP) and pulmonary capillary wedge pressure (PCWP), (4) arterial pressure, and (5) cardiac output (CO).

The basic components of the pressure monitoring system (see Fig. 26-20) include (1) intravascular catheter, (2) fluid-filled extension tubing and stopcocks, (3) continuous flush device, (4) pressure transducer, and (5) pressurized flush solution. Depending on the pressure(s) to be monitored, the catheter may be either of a single-lumen design, such as a radial arterial catheter, or of a multiple-lumen design, such as the Swan-Ganz balloon-tipped pulmonary arterial catheter.

The most commonly used pulmonary arterial catheter contains four separate lumens (see Fig. 26-21). One lumen is for the inflation of the balloon at the tip of the catheter, which is used for positioning the catheter. The distal and proximal lumens are used for the monitoring of pulmonary arterial or pulmonary capillary wedge

pressures and the right atrial pressure, respectively. The final lumen is for cardiac output measurement.

The catheter is connected to the pressure transducer by stopcocks and a noncompliant pressure tubing filled with fluid. The hemodynamic pressures and pulsations are transmitted through this fluid column to the pressure transducer. The pressure transducer converts the mechanical pulsation to an electrical signal which can be displayed on the bedside monitor.

To maintain the patency of the catheter, a continuous flush device is interposed between the catheter and the transducer. The continuous flush device is designed in a Y configuration to permit simultaneous pressure recording via the transducer and continuous flush-

FIGURE 26-20
Basic components of pressure monitoring system. (Modified from M. A. Boldt, *Acute Coronary Care,* **Wiley, New York, 1983, p. 115.)**

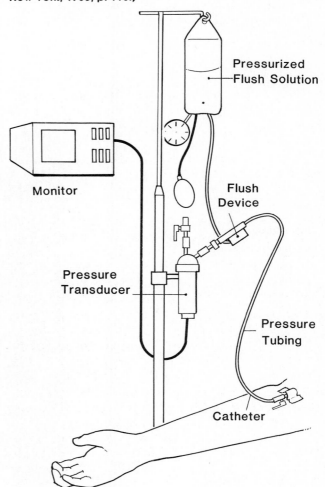

ing with solution. The device is connected to a bag of heparinized saline solution surrounded by an inflatable bag used to pressurize the solution so that it can flow against the higher intravascular or intracardiac pressures.

To interpret the significance of recorded hemodynamic pressures and waveform configurations, it is necessary to refer back to the electrical and mechanical events of the cardiac cycle discussed in depth in Chap. 25. The interdependent relationship between electrical stimulation of the myocardium and the mechanical response is illustrated in Fig. 25-1. The five mechanical phases of the cardiac cycle are reviewed there as well. Each of these mechanical phases produces characteristic alterations in the contour of the waveforms recorded within the cardiovascular system. The relationship between the phases of the cardiac cycle and the characteristic waveforms of the left side of the heart are summarized in Fig. 26-22.

Atrial waveforms are normally of low amplitude, given the low pressures generated by these chambers. Right atrial pressures average from 0 to 10 mmHg, with

left atrial pressures approximating 3 to 15 mmHg. Left heart pressures normally exceed right heart pressures owing to the higher resistance to ejection posed by the systemic circuit relative to the pulmonic circulation. Direct measurement of left atrial pressure is usually restricted to postoperative cardiac surgical intensive care units.

Atrial pressures reflect changes in the volume status of the heart as well as alterations in cardiac function and structure. A reduction in atrial pressure would be produced by hypovolemia; conversely, hypervolemia would elevate atrial pressure. Atrial pressures are also valuable in the assessment of ventricular function, in the absence of AV valve dysfunction. As the ventricles fill during diastole, the atrial and ventricular chambers are in direct communication. At the end of diastole, the pressures between these two chambers have equilibrated; therefore, atrial pressures are equal to ventricular pressures at the end of diastole. Right or left ventricular failure produces increases in right ventricular end-diastolic pressure (RVEDP) or left ventricular end-diastolic pressure (LVEDP) as residual ventricular volumes rise owing to impaired ventricular function. A change in ventricular end-diastolic pressure is immediately reflected backward to the atrium, where a corresponding rise in atrial pressure is observed.

Atrial waveforms are characterized by three positive components—the a, c, and v waves—corresponding to three events in the mechanical cycle that increase atrial pressure (see Fig. 26-3). The a wave corresponds to atrial contraction, the c wave is produced by the

FIGURE 26-21
Pulmonary artery catheter. (From S. Millar (ed.), *Methods in Critical Care*, Saunders, Philadelphia, 180, p. 58.)

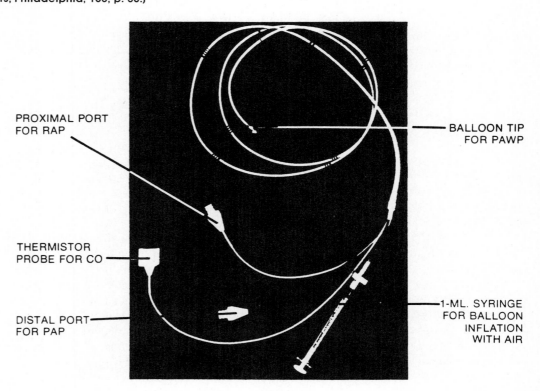

PROXIMAL PORT
FOR RAP

BALLOON TIP
FOR PAWP

THERMISTOR
PROBE FOR CO

DISTAL PORT
FOR PAP

1-ML. SYRINGE
FOR BALLOON
INFLATION
WITH AIR

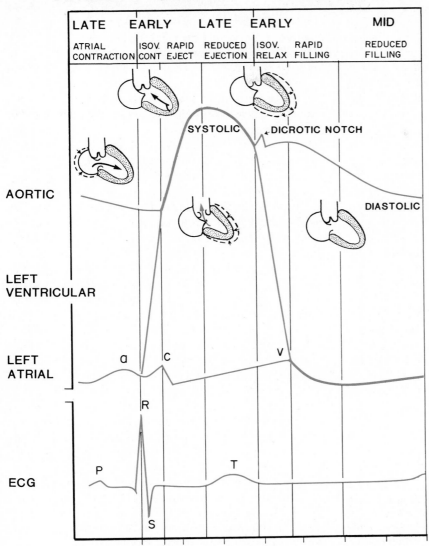

DIASTOLE		SYSTOLE				DIASTOLE	
LATE	EARLY		LATE	EARLY		MID	
ATRIAL CONTRACTION	ISOV. CONT	RAPID EJECT	REDUCED EJECTION	ISOV. RELAX	RAPID FILLING	REDUCED FILLING	

SYSTOLIC

DICROTIC NOTCH

AORTIC

DIASTOLIC

LEFT VENTRICULAR

LEFT ATRIAL

a   c   v

ECG

R

P   T

S

FIGURE 26-22
Correlation between the events of the cardia cycle and waveforms observed in hemodynamic and ECG tracing.

backward bulging of the atrioventricular valve with the onset of isovolumetric contraction, and the v wave is due to atrial filling during ventricular ejection (note that the AV valves normally remain closed at this time).

Predictable alterations in the atrial configuration are observed with changes in cardiac function and/or structure as discussed earlier in this chapter. For example, loss of atrial contraction during atrial fibrillation is manifested as loss of a waves. Asynchronous contraction of the ventricles and atria, as with complete heart block, intermittently superimposes the a wave on the c and v waves producing large "cannon" a waves (Fig. 26-23). Increased resistance to atrial contraction, as with AV valve stenosis or ventricular failure, increases the size of the a wave. Regurgitation of blood through an incompetent AV valve during ventricular systole superimposes an abnormal pulsation on the c and v waves referred to as a "significant v wave" (see Fig. 26-3). The

characteristic changes of AV valve dysfunction will be apparent in either the right atrial or left atrial trace depending on whether the tricuspid or mitral valve is affected.

Ventricular pressures and waveforms are not routinely monitored at the bedside. In certain settings, such as right ventricular failure secondary to chronic obstructive lung disease, a multilumen pulmonary artery catheter with a right ventricular (RV) lumen rather than the right atrial lumen described earlier can be inserted for direct RV pressure monitoring. However, familiarity with the RV trace is required during monitoring with the pulmonary artery catheter so that backward displacement of the catheter into the ventricle can be detected immediately (see Fig. 26-24).

Pulmonary arterial pressures and pulmonary capillary wedge pressures are measured with the balloon-tipped multiple-lumen catheter described earlier. The

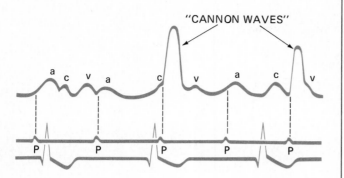

FIGURE 26-23
Cannon waves in complete heart block, schematic jugular venous and heart sound tracings, and electrocardiogram. Note the irregularly occurring cannon waves produced by atrial systole when atrial contraction occurs with the tricuspid valve closed by ventricular systole. When atrial systole occurs during the phase of rapid ventricular filling, the *a* waves are smaller than usual. (From J. W. Hurst, B. Logue, R. Sclant, and N. Wenger (eds.), *The Heart,* 4th ed., McGraw-Hill, New York, 1978, p. 197.)

FIGURE 26-24
Intracardiac pressure waveforms recorded from a fluid-filled catheter. Right side of the heart and pulmonary artery wedge pressures are on the borderline of being elevated, but the contours are normal. Sys, peak systolic pressure; ed, end-diastolic pressure; RF, rapid-filling wave; SF, slow-filling wave; I, incisura. Also shown are *a, c,* and *v* waves and the *x* and *y* descents. (From Eugene Braunwald (ed.), *Heart Disease: A Textbook in Cardiovascular Medicine,* 1st ed., Saunders, Philadelphia, 1980, p. 289.)

catheter is advanced into the pulmonary artery via a peripheral vein and the right side of the heart. With the balloon deflated, pressures in the pulmonary artery can be measured. Periodically, the balloon is inflated. With inflation of the balloon, blood flow propels the catheter distally into the pulmonary vasculature until the tip "wedges" in a small arterial branch. In this position, the pressure transmitted backward from the left side of the heart through the pulmonary vasculature is sensed by the catheter tip. Therefore the pulmonary capillary wedge pressure reflects left atrial and, consequently, left ventricular end-diastolic pressure (Fig. 26-25). This relationship is distorted by mitral valve or pulmonary vascular abnormalities.

Pulmonary artery pressures average 25/10 mmHg. Pulmonary hypertension may be observed in conditions such as chronic obstructive lung disease, chronic mitral valve disease, and pulmonary emboli. As mentioned, pulmonary capillary wedge (PCW) pressures approximate left atrial (LA) pressures. The contour of the PCW pressure trace is similar to that of the LA pressure trace, although the low-amplitude *c* wave may be more difficult to visualize.

Arterial pressures are usually monitored via the radial artery, although femoral lines are not uncommon. Brachial, axillary, pedal, or temporal sites can also be used. Constant monitoring of arterial pressure is particularly valuable during the intravenous administration of vasoactive drugs, such as sodium nitroprusside or dopamine, used to regulate blood pressure. In addition to recording systolic and diastolic blood pressures, mean arterial pressure (MAP) is measured. This pressure represents the average driving pressure perfusing the tissues. Mean arterial pressure is a function of cardiac output (CO) and total peripheral resistance (TPR).

The following alterations in the arterial pulse have been discussed earlier in this chapter: (1) pulsus tardus produced by aortic stenosis, (2) waterhammer pulse as-

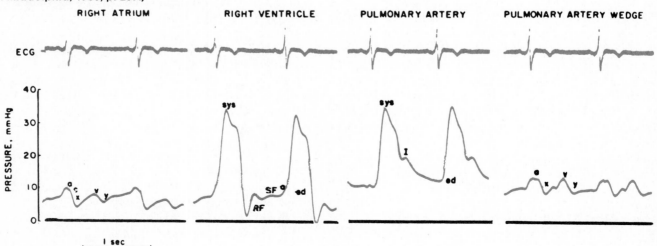

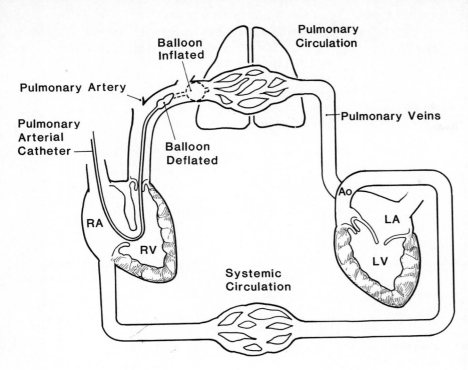

FIGURE 26-25
Pulmonary artery catheter position.

sociated with aortic regurgiation, (3) pulsus alternans due to ventricular failure, (4) pulsus bigeminus caused by premature beats in a bigeminal rhythm, and (5) pulsus paradoxus associated with caridac tamponade.

Cardiac output can be measured at the bedside by two techniques: dye dilution or thermal dilution (see Fig. 26-26). The dye dilution technique involves the injection of a known quantity and concentration of dye into the venous end of the circulation, usually via a central venous line. The dye mixes with the blood and is progressively diluted. Downstream, a sample of arterial blood is gradually withdrawn and analyzed for dye concentration. A dilution curve (i.e., dye concentration against time), is recorded permitting calculation of cardiac output.

The thermal dilution technique substitutes a known quantity of fluid at a given temperature as the injectate. This technique requires insertion of the four-lumen pulmonary artery catheter. A lumen opens into the right atrium for injection of a cold solution, and a thermistor at the catheter tip in the pulmonary artery senses temperature changes. The catheter is connected

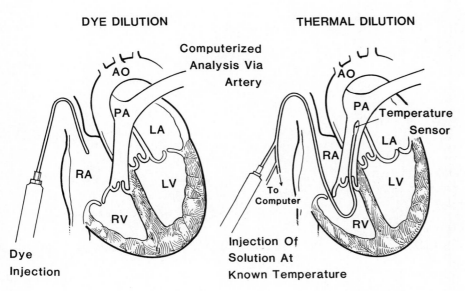

FIGURE 26-26
Cardiac output measurement techniques. (Modified from Vinsant and Spense, 1981, p. 265.)

to a bedside computer so that outputs can be calculated immediately upon injection. Calculation of cardiac out-put also permits determination of pulmonic or systemic vascular resistance (i.e., systemic vascular resistance equals the difference between mean arterial pressure and right atrial pressure divided by cardiac output, times a correction factor of 80). Calculation of systemic vascular resistance is valuable in the administration of vasodilators and vasoconstrictors.

QUESTIONS

Diagnostic procedures in cardiovascular disease

Directions: Answer the following questions on a separate sheet of paper.

1. Mr. H. is a 59-year-old accountant who has been diagnosed as having atherosclerotic heart disease. Recently he found it necessary to resign from the manufacturing firm where he worked because of weakness, fatigue, and inability to climb the stairs to his second floor office without precipitating an episode of chest pain. At home, Mr. H. is able to perform light housework but experiences shortness of breath and/or chest pain if he attempts to mow the lawn with a power mower. How would this patient's heart disease be categorized according to the New York Heart Association guidelines?

2. Palpation of the carotid arteries on a 68-year-old female with a blood pressure of 178/100 reveals that the left carotid pulse has a much lower amplitude than does the right. Explain the possible significance of this finding. What is this patient's mean arterial pressure?

3. How is the hepatojugular reflux test performed? How would you determine if the test were positive? What is the possible significance of a positive test?

4. What is a hexaxial reference system and how is it derived?

5. Discuss the type of data and evaluation of the cardiovascular status that may be obtained from cardiac catheterization.

6. List the indications for performing coronary angiography and the characteristics of a bypassable lesion.

Directions: Circle the letter preceding each item below that correctly answers the question. Only one answer is correct unless otherwise noted.

7. The symptoms of weakness and easy fatigability in patients with myocardial failure are probably a consequence of:
a. Low cardiac output   b. Increased contractility of the heart muscle   c. Decreased peripheral perfusion   d. Only a and c   e. All of the above

8. Hypertension in the adult is defined as blood pressure greater than:
a. 120/80 mmHg   b. 130/80 mmHg   c. 160/95 mmHg   d. 145/85 mmHg

9. A decreased pulse pressure may indicate: (More than one answer may be correct.)
a. Decreased stroke volume   b. Decreased peripheral resistance   c. Increased peripheral resistance   d. Decreased blood viscosity

10. A slow-rising and sustained carotid pulse is characteristic of:
a. Mitral stenosis   b. Aortic stenosis   c. Mitral regurgitation   d. Aortic regurgitation

11. A quick-rising and collapsing (waterhammer) pulse is characteristic of:
a. Mitral stenosis   b. Aortic stenosis   c. Mitral regurgitation   d. Aortic regurgitation

12. Jugular venous distention to the level of the jaw angle in a person sitting with the trunk elevated 90° correlates with a central venous pressure of at least:
a. 10 cm water   b. 15 cm water   c. 20 cm water   d. 25 cm water

13. In the normal adult lying with the trunk elevated 30°, the pulsation within the jugular vein should rise above the sternal angle no more than:
a. 1 to 2 cm   b. 2 to 3 cm   c. 5 to 6 cm   d. 7 to 8 cm

14. A large, early v wave in the jugular venous pulse is most likely to be present in:
a. Mitral regurgitation   b. Tricuspid regurgitation   c. Mitral stenosis   d. Tricuspid stenosis

15. A giant a wave in the jugular venous pulse is most likely to be present in:
a. Mitral regurgitation   b. Tricuspid regurgitation   c. Mitral stenosis   d. Tricuspid stenosis

16. In the cardiovascular examination, the chest is inspected and palpated for: (More than one answer may be correct.)
   a. Apical impulse   b. Thrills   c. Symmetry of thoracic movements   d. Lifts or heaves

17. A thrill is a palpable:
   a. Pericardial friction rub   b. Heart sound
   c. Apical impulse   d. Murmur

18. The apical impulse is normally located:
   a. At the fifth intercostal space near the left midclavicular line   b. Adjacent to the angle of Louis
   c. At the lower left sternal border in the fourth intercostal space   d. At the fourth intercostal space at the anterior axillary line

19. In cases of left ventricular hypertrophy, the PMI will: (More than one answer may be correct.)
   a. Comprise an area less than 2 to 3 cm in diameter   b. Comprise an area greater than 2 to 3 cm in diameter   c. Shift laterally to the left and downward   d. Shift to the mediastinal area producing a substernal heave

20. The precordium refers to the area of the chest overlying the:
   a. Lungs   b. Sternum   c. Heart   d. Mediastinum

21. A lift or heave is the rise with each heartbeat of the:
   a. Precordium   b. Cardiac apex   c. Sternum
   d. Rib cage

22. A heart sound that occurs in early diastole and is considered normal in children and young adults but pathologic in older adults is the:
   a. First heart sound   b. Second heart sound
   c. Third heart sound   d. Fourth heart sound

23. Sounds occurring early in systole are most likely:
   a. Atrial gallops   b. Ventricular gallops   c. Systolic ejection murmurs   d. Opening snaps of the mitral valve

24. The heart sound normally heard best over the aortic area is the:
   a. First heart sound   b. Second heart sound
   c. Third heart sound   d. Fourth heart sound

25. Murmurs occurring in diastole follow the:
   a. First heart sound   b. Second heart sound

26. During auscultation of the blood pressure, systolic pressure correlates with the:
   a. Onset of sound in the occluded artery
   b. Abrupt muffling of sound   c. Disappearance of sound   d. Persistent tapping

27. The ECG monitor strip represents:
   a. Mechanical activity of the heart   b. Electrical activity of the heart   c. Both a and b   d. Neither a nor b

28. Normally, ventricular depolarization:
   a. Occurs at the T wave   b. Occurs after ventricular contraction   c. Indicates ventricular diastole   d. Stimulates ventricular contraction

29. By convention, a positive wave on the ECG indicates:
   a. The path of electrical activity is approaching a negative electrode   b. The path of electrical activity is approaching a positive electrode   c. The path of electrical activity is moving away from a negative electrode   d. The path of electrical activity is moving away from a positive electrode

30. The ECG leads measuring the horizontal plane of the heart are the:
   a. Standard limb leads   b. Augmented limb leads
   c. Precordial leads   d. Bipolar leads

31. In standard lead II of the ECG, the electrical potential difference is recorded between the:
   a. Right arm and left leg   b. Right arm and left arm   c. Right arm and right leg   d. Left arm and right leg

32. Which of the following leads is *not* unipolar?
   a. aVR   b. aVF   c. V_6 d. II

33. A normal QRS electrical axis is characterized by:
   a. Large positive QRS deflections in leads II, III, and aVF   b. Large positive QRS deflections in lead aVR   c. Large negative QRS deflections in leads II, III, and aVF   d. Large positive QRS deflections in leads I and aVL

34. A catheter wedged in a branch of the pulmonary artery measures a pressure correlating most directly with:
   a. Right atrial pressure   b. Right ventricular pressure   c. Left atrial pressure   d. Pulmonary arterial pressure

35. Which of the following vessels is commonly used for right heart catheterization?
   a. Femoral artery   b. Brachial artery   c. Jugular vein   d. Antecubital vein

36. The correct identification of the aortic and pulmonic components of the second heart sound on the phonocardiogram is aided by the simultaneous recording of the:
   a. Electrocardiogram   b. Jugular venous pulse
   c. Carotid arterial pulse   d. Radial pulse

37. Echocardiography utilizes the principle of:
   a. Hydrodynamics   b. Ultrasound   c. Radioemission   d. Electromagnetic force

38. A noninvasive procedure for analyzing cardiac structures and wall motion is:
   a. Phonocardiography   b. Electrocardiography
   c. Echocardiography   d. Vectorcardiography

Directions: Match each of the terms in col. A with its definition in col. B.

Column A

39. ____ Angina
40. ____ Palpita-
    tions
41. ____ Orthop-
    nea
42. ____ Syncope
43. ____ Dyspnea
44. ____ Edema

Column B

a. Awareness of increased breathing effort
b. Difficulty in breathing in the recumbent position
c. Chest pain due to myocardial ischemia
d. Heartbeats sensed by the patient
e. Accumulation of fluid in the interstitial spaces
f. Transient loss of consciousness
g. Abnormal chest pulsations noticed by the patient

Directions: Match each of the jugular venous waveforms in col. A with its cause in col. B.

Column A

45. ____ a wave
46. ____ v wave
47. ____ c wave

Column B

a. Produced by bulging of the tricuspid valve into the right atrium during ventricular contraction
b. Produced by increased right atrial pressure during atrial filling prior to the opening of the tricuspid valve
c. Produced by atrial contraction

Directions: Match each of the abnormal heart sounds in col. A with its probable cause in col. B.

Column A

48. ____ Midsys-
    tolic murmur
49. ____ Pansys-
    tolic murmur
50. ____ Middias-
    tolic murmur
51. ____ Opening
    snap in early
    diastole

Column B

a. May be produced by aortic stenosis
b. May be produced by pulmonic regurgitation
c. May be produced by mitral stenosis
d. May be produced by mitral regurgitation

Directions: Match each area of transmission of the cardiac valvular sounds in col. A with its anatomic location on the chest in col. B.

Column A

52. ____ Mitral
53. ____ Tricuspid
54. ____ Aortic
55. ____ Pulmonic

Column B

a. Second intercostal space, left sternal border
b. Second intercostal space, right sternal border
c. Fifth intercostal space, mid-clavicular line
d. Lower left sternal border

Directions: Match the ECG waveform in col. A to the electrical events in col. B.

Column A

56. ____ P wave
57. ____ QRS com-
    plex
58. ____ T wave

Column B

a. Ventricular repolarization
b. Atrial depolarization
c. Ventricular depolarization
d. Atrial repolarization

Directions: Match each of the ECG intervals in col. A with its normal duration in col. B.

Column A

59. ____ PR inter-
    val
60. ____ QRS com-
    plex
61. ____ QT inter-
    val

Column B

a. 0.36 to 0.44 second
b. 0.12 to 0.20 second
c. 0.06 to 0.10 second

Directions: Match each ECG abnormality in col. A with its possible cause in col. B.

Column A

62. ____ Depres-
    sion of the ST
    segment
63. ____ Elevation
    of the ST seg-
    ment
64. ____ Inversion
    of the P wave
65. ____ Inversion
    of the T wave
66. ____ Peaking of
    the T wave
67. ____ Prolonged
    PR interval
68. ____ Prolonged
    QT interval

Column B

a. Slow conduction time through the AV node
b. Myocardial ischemia
c. Hyperkalemia
d. Myocardial necrosis
e. AV nodal arrhythmia
f. Quinidine effect

Directions: Match each of the cardiac diagnostic techniques in col. A with its purpose in col. B.

Column A

69. _____ Flow-directed balloon-tipped catheter

70. _____ Electrophysiology study

71. _____ Phonocardiography

72. _____ Echocardiography

73. _____ Thermodilution pulmonary artery catheter

74. _____ Catheter tip lies in the right atrium or superior vena cava inserted via an antecubital vein

75. _____ Chest roentgenogram

76. _____ Nuclear imaging

Column B

a. Records intracardiac electrical impulses to evaluate mechanisms of impulse generation and conduction

b. Murmurs heard during heart auscultation may be documented

c. Cardiac output may be calculated at the bedside with data obtained

d. Size and location of an area of necrosis may be estimated

e. Abnormal valve motion may be detected

f. Pulmonary wedge pressure may be measured

g. Central venous pressure may be measured

h. Enlargement of the heart and great vessels may be detected

Directions: Circle T if the statement is true and F if it is false.

77. T F The dorsalis pedis pulse may be palpated at the back of the knee.

78. T F Left atrial enlargement is detected best in the lateral view of the chest x-ray.

79. T F Kussmaul's sign is a decrease in the central venous pressure during inspiration.

80. T F A patient with an apical heart rate of 78 and a radial rate of 70 has a pulse deficit.

81. T F Physiologic splitting of the second heart sound is caused by asynchronous closure of the aortic and pulmonic valves and is always considered pathologic.

82. T F Paradoxical splitting of the second heart sound is heard on expiration and disappears on inspiration and may be caused by left bundle branch block.

83. T F The sounds of Korotkoff are produced by turbulent blood flow through the aortic valve during blood pressure measurement.

84. T F Paroxysmal nocturnal dyspnea is a symptom of left ventricular failure.

Directions: Fill in the blanks with the correct words.

85. During cardiac catheterization, contrast material is injected into the heart chamber distal to the diseased valve to confirm the diagnosis of valvular _____.

86. The pressure gradient between the left ventricle and the aorta is normally less than _____. A large pressure gradient indicates _____.

87. Heart murmurs are the result of _____ blood flow within the cardiac structures.

PENNY J. FORD
F. MICHAEL VISLOSKY
MADELINE M. O'DONNELL

CORONARY ATHEROSCLEROTIC DISEASE

OBJECTIVES

At the completion of this chapter you should be able to:

1. Describe the interaction between myocardial oxygen supply and demand and identify the determinants of each.
2. Differentiate between myocardial infarction and ischemia and describe the relationship between them; explain why the left ventricle is most vulnerable to ischemia and infarction.
3. Describe the progressive pathologic changes in a coronary blood vessel in the development of clinically significant atherosclerotic lesions.
4. Identify the most common sites of coronary atherosclerotic lesions.
5. Identify and describe the modifiable and nonmodifiable factors that increase the likelihood of an individual developing coronary atherosclerotic disease.
6. List the metabolic, physiologic, hemodynamic, electrocardiographic, and clinical changes associated with myocardial ischemia.
7. Define and explain the common terms used to describe myocardial infarction: subendocardial, transmural, anterior, and inferior.
8. Describe the sequential changes associated with myocardial healing after myocardial infarction.
9. Describe the functional changes resulting from myocardial infarction and the factors affecting the degree of functional impairment.
10. Define vasovagal response.
11. Identify the characteristic diagnostic triad associated with myocardial infarction.
12. Define and describe the physiologic consequences of the following complications of myocardial infarction:
    a. Congestive heart failure
    b. Cardiogenic shock
    c. Papillary muscle dysfunction
    d. Rupture of the ventricular septum
    e. Rupture of the ventricular free wall
    f. Ventricular aneurysm
    g. Thromboembolism

> *h.* Pericarditis
> *i.* Dressler's syndrome
> *j.* Arrhythmias

13. Identify eight factors which predispose to arrhythmias in coronary atherosclerotic disease.

14. Explain how abnormal rates of impulse generation resulting in tachycardia or bradycardia compromise cardiac function.

15. Differentiate between premature and escape beats.

16. Identify the most common arrhythmia.

17. Identify and place on a rate continuum atrial and ventricular arrhythmias.

18. Differentiate between first-, second-, and third-degree heart block; describe bundle branch block.

19. List eight risk factors which may increase the incidence of atherosclerotic heart disease.

20. Identify three hemodynamic factors which may be modified to reduce oxygen demand in the treatment of myocardial ischemia.

21. Describe the mechanisms of action of the following drugs in the treatment of ischemic heart disease: propanolol (Inderal), digitalis, antihypertensive agents, vasodilators, and sedatives.

22. Explain why the benefit of treating myocardial ischemia by increasing the coronary blood flow and oxygen supply is limited.

23. Describe the effects of hypoxemia, hypotension, and arrhythmias on coronary oxygen supply and how these problems are treated.

24. State the rationale for rest in the treatment of acute myocardial infarction.

25. Describe the general principles of treatment for the following arrhythmias: tachycardia, bradycardia, escape rhythms, ventricular irritability, atrial irritability, atrial tachycardia, ventricular fibrillation, and heart block.

26. Describe the treatment for congestive heart failure, acute pulmonary edema, and cardiogenic shock.

27. Compare saphenous vein bypass graft as a method of coronary revascularization with an internal mammary artery bypass graft.

28. List the indications for coronary revascularization, the cardiac catheterization findings indicating operable disease, and the two most important factors affecting the success of surgery.

29. Describe the following cardiac surgical procedures: aneurysmectomy, septal defect repair, infarctectomy, mitral valve replacement, and heart transplantation.

30. Explain the importance of rehabilitation in the treatment of patients with atherosclerotic heart disease.

A critical balance exists between myocardial oxygen supply and demand; oxygen supply must equal demand (see Fig. 27-1). A reduction in oxygen supply or an increase in oxygen demand can disturb this balance and threaten myocardial function.

There are four major determinants of myocardial

oxygen demand: heart rate, contractile force, muscle mass, and ventricular wall tension (see Table 27-1). Wall tension or afterload is a function of variables identified in the Laplace equation: intraventricular pressure, ventricular radius, and ventricular wall thickness. Therefore, cardiac work and oxygen demand are elevated by tachycardia (rapid heart rates), increased force of contraction, hypertension, ventricular dilation and hypertrophy.

If myocardial oxygen demand increases, oxygen supply must increase concurrently. To significantly increase oxygen supply, coronary flow must increase, since myocardial oxygen extraction from the arterial blood is almost maximal under resting conditions. The most potent stimulus to dilating the coronary arteries and increasing coronary flow is local tissue hypoxia. The normal coronary vasculature can dilate and increase flow approximately five to six times above resting levels. However, stenotic, diseased vessels are unable to dilate, and therefore a state of oxygen deficit can result when oxygen demand exceeds the capacity of the vasculature to increase flow. *Ischemia* is a transient, reversible state of oxygen lack. Prolonged ischemia will lead to muscle death, or *necrosis*. Clinically, necrosis of the myocardium is referred to as *myocardial infarction*.

The left ventricle is the chamber most susceptible to myocardial ischemia and infarction by virtue of

TABLE 27-1	
DETERMINANTS OF MYOCARDIAL OXYGEN DEMAND	
Heart rate	Wall tension
	Intraventricular pressure
Contractile force	
Muscle mass	Ventricular radius

unique myocardial oxygenation characteristics. First, left ventricular oxygen demand is great as a result of the high systemic resistance to ejection and the large muscle mass. In addition, coronary flow is phasic in nature. The branches of the coronary arteries are deeply embedded in the myocardium. During systole, these intramyocardial branches are compressed, which increases the resistance to flow. Coronary flow therefore occurs primarily during diastole. Contraction of the thick left ventricular wall essentially terminates systolic flow through its intramyocardial branches, especially in the innermost or subendocardial region; some systolic flow continues in the vessels of the thinner-walled right ventricle.

PATHOGENESIS

Pathology

Coronary atherosclerosis is the most common cause of coronary artery disease. Atherosclerosis causes a localized accumulation of lipid and fibrous tissue within the coronary artery, progressively narrowing the lumen of the vessel. As the lumen narrows, resistance to flow increases and myocardial blood flow is compromised. As the disease progresses, the luminal narrowing is accompanied by vascular changes that impair the ability of the diseased vessel to dilate. Thus the balance between myocardial oxygen supply and demand becomes precarious, threatening the myocardium beyond the lesion.

Considerable controversy has arisen regarding the pathogenesis of coronary atherosclerosis. However, the pathologic changes within the affected vessel can be summarized as follows (Fig. 27-2):

1. Deposition of small amounts of lipid material, apparent as "fatty streaks," in the intima

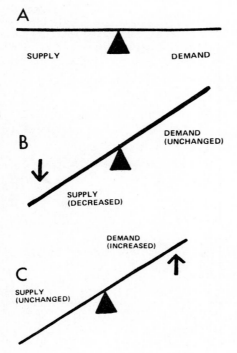

FIGURE 27-1
Balance between myocardial oxygen supply and demand. (A) Normally, myocardial oxygen supply and demand are in balance. (B) Imbalance due to decreased coronary blood supply (e.g., low blood pressure) while the demand for oxygen remains unchanged. (C) Imbalance due to increased demand (e.g., exercise) while the blood supply to the myocardium remains unchanged (e.g., coronary atherosclerosis limits ability of blood vessels to increase supply). (Adapted from M. C. Clark, "Chest Pain," *Heart & Lung*, 4: 956, 1975.)

2. Accumulation of lipid, especially cholesterol-rich β-lipoprotein, in the intima and inner media

3. Fibrous encapsulation of the lesion, creating *fibrous plaques*

4. Development of *atheromas*, or complex atherosclerotic plaques consisting of lipid, fibrous tissue, collagen, calcium, cellular debris, and capillaries

5. Degenerative changes in the arterial wall

Despite this progressive luminal narrowing and the concurrent loss of vascular responsiveness, clinical manifestations of disease do not appear until the atherogenic process is well advanced. This preclinical phase can last 20 to 40 years. Clinically significant lesions, producing myocardial ischemia and dysfunction, usually obstruct over 75 percent of the vessel lumen. The final step in the pathologic process producing the clinical insult can occur in the following ways: (1) progressive luminal narrowing by plaque enlargement, (2) hemorrhage into the atheromatous plaque, (3) thrombus formation initiated by platelet aggregation, (4) embolization of a thrombus or plaque fragment, or (5) coronary arterial spasm. Despite the variety of causes leading to acute coronary occlusion, autopsy studies suggest intraluminal thrombosis as the major causative event, superimposed on preexisting atherosclerotic lesions. Whether thrombotic occlusion is a primary or a secondary event has yet to be determined. Some investigators feel that coronary arterial spasm superimposed on an atherosclerotic plaque increases intraplaque pressure with subsequent rupture of capillaries within the plaque, leading to plaque rupture and thrombosis. Still others feel that a combination of mechanisms mentioned previously results in the final occlusive process.

Notably, atherosclerotic lesions usually develop in the proximal, epicardial segments of the coronary artery at sites of abrupt curvature, branching, or attachment. The lesions tend to be localized and focal in distribu-

TABLE 27-2

RISK FACTORS

Nonmodifiable	Modifiable
Age	Major
Sex	Elevated serum lipids
Family history	Hypertension
Race	Cigarette smoking
	Impaired glucose tolerance
	Diet high in saturated fat, cholesterol, and calories
	Minor
	Sedentary life-style
	Psychological stress
	Personality type

tion; however, in advanced disease, areas of diffuse involvement become pronounced.

RISK FACTORS

It is no longer contended that atherosclerosis is simply a result of the aging process. The appearance of "fatty streaks" in the coronary arterial wall as early as childhood is a natural phenomenon and does not necessarily progress to atherosclerotic lesions. It is now believed that many factors interact to accelerate the atherogenic process. A number of so-called risk factors have been identified that increase susceptibility to the development of coronary atherosclerosis in a given individual (Table 27-2).

There are four nonmodifiable biological risk factors: age, sex, race, and family history. Susceptibility to coronary atherosclerosis increases with age; the development of significant disease before age 40 is unusual. However, the correlation between age and disease onset may simply reflect the longer duration of exposure to other atherogenic factors. Females seem relatively immune until after menopause and then become as susceptible as males. The protective effect of estrogen has

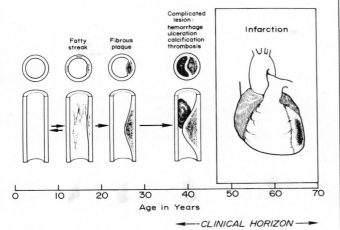

FIGURE 27-2
Progressive pathologic changes in coronary atherosclerotic disease. Fatty streaks are found as one of the earliest lesions of atherosclerosis. Many fatty streaks regress, whereas others progress to fibrous plaques and eventually to atheromas. These may then become complicated by hemorrhage, ulceration, calcification, or thrombosis and may produce myocardial infarction. (From J. W. Hurst, *The Heart,* 3d ed., McGraw-Hill, New York, 1974, p. 989.)

been postulated as an explanation for early female immunity. Blacks are more vulnerable to atherosclerosis than are whites. Finally, a positive family history for coronary heart disease (i.e., siblings or parents developing disease before age 50) increases the likelihood of the premature development of atherosclerosis. The relative contribution of genetic and environmental influences is unknown. A genetic component can be linked with some pronounced, accelerated forms of atherosclerosis, as in familial lipid disorders. However, family history may also reflect a strong environmental component, perhaps a life-style that produces tension or obesity.

Additional risk factors are amenable to modification, potentially retarding the atherogenic process. Major risk factors are elevated serum lipid levels, hypertension, cigarette smoking, impaired glucose tolerance, and diets high in saturated fats, cholesterol, and calories.

Hyperlipidemia

The plasma lipids—cholesterols, triglycerides, phospholipids, and free fatty acids—are derived from exogenous dietary sources and endogenous lipid synthesis. Cholesterol and triglyceride are the two lipids of major clinical significance relative to atherogenesis. The association between serum cholesterol elevation and increased prematurity and severity of atherosclerosis is well established. The relationship between triglycerides and coronary disease is suggestive, yet inconclusive. The higher the serum cholesterol level, the greater the coronary risk. According to the American Heart Association, levels over 250 mg per 100 ml increase coronary risk threefold in contrast to levels under 194 mg per 100 ml. The relationship between serum cholesterol elevation and coronary risk is particularly strong in younger patients.

The term *hyperlipidemia* denotes an elevation of serum cholesterol and/or triglycerides above normal limits. Designation of "normal" lipid values is complicated by the fact that no absolute serum level can be cited as the critical threshold for abnormality in a given individual. Normal limits are defined relative to plasma lipid values representative of the general population. The upper limit of normal is considered to be the 90th to 95th percentile; these values are age- and sex-dependent. Clinical application of these limits must be done cautiously, in that "normal" values may not be "ideal" relative to coronary risk.

Hyperlipidemia can be primary or secondary to another underlying condition, such as hypothyroidism or poorly controlled diabetes mellitus. The differential diagnosis and treatment of lipid disorders are facilitated by considering lipid elevations in terms of lipoproteins. Since lipids are insoluble in plasma, lipids are bound to proteins as a mechanism for serum transport. This bonding produces four major classes of lipoproteins: (1) chylomicrons, (2) very low-density lipoproteins (VLDL), (3) low-density lipoproteins (LDL), and (4) high-density lipoproteins (HDL). The relative concentrations of lipid and protein vary among classes. Of the four lipoprotein classes, the chylomicrons and VLDL are richest in triglyceride, whereas LDL and HDL contain the largest proportion of cholesterol.

Distinguishing the pattern of lipoprotein elevation can be extremely significant not only to medical management but also to coronary risk predictions. For example, serum cholesterol elevation would reflect elevation of either LDL or HDL. However, only LDL elevation is associated with increased coronary risk; HDL elevation correlates with decreased risk. For this reason, HDL cholesterol has been referred to as "benevolent" cholesterol. This observation has stimulated interest in the potential "protective" effect of HDL elevation.

Lipoprotein elevations, or *hyperlipoproteinemias*, are described according to specific patterns of elevation. Five patterns or types have been identified—I, II (A and B), III, IV, and V; each corresponds to a characteristic elevation of one or more lipoproteins. These patterns are not specific indicators of particular lipid disorders; however, the type of elevation is useful as a therapeutic guide. Only three types of hyperlipoproteinemia are associated with premature atherosclerosis—I, III, and IV.

The term *familial hyperlipoproteinemia* is used to describe a group of primary lipid disorders resulting from inborn abnormalities in lipid metabolism. Four disorders known to be associated with coronary atherosclerosis are listed in Table 27-3. Untreated familial hypercholesterolemia carries a particularly ominous prognosis—a 50 percent probability of developing premature atherosclerosis before 50 years of age.

The therapy of acquired or secondary hyperlipidemia is directed at correcting the underlying cause. However, the therapy of primary hyperlipidemia is controversial in that there is no conclusive evidence that

TABLE 27-3

PRIMARY HYPERLIPOPROTEINEMIAS ASSOCIATED WITH CORONARY ATHEROSCLEROSIS

Familial hypercholesterolemia

Familial hypertriglyceridemia

Familial combined hyperlipidemia (multiple lipoprotein-type hyperlipidemia)

Familial dysbetalipoproteinemia

the reduction of blood lipid levels decreases coronary risk. Therapeutic guidelines have been established based upon presumptive evidence. Initial therapy consists of dietary management. A reduction of serum cholesterol can usually be accomplished with restriction of cholesterol and saturated fat intake. Consumption of cholesterol-rich foods, such as organ meats, shrimp, scallops, egg yolk, and saturated animal fats, should be reduced; substitution of lean meats, fish, and polyunsaturated vegetable fats should be encouraged. The value of dietary cholesterol restriction in the reduction of serum cholesterol levels is currently controversial yet widely accepted. If triglycerides are elevated, restriction of alcohol consumption and weight normalization are essential.

If dietary therapy is unsuccessful or lipid elevations are severe, hypolipemic drugs are recommended, although the long-term benefits of such therapy are not conclusive. For hypercholesterolemia, cholestyramine or colestipol is indicated with the addition of nicotinic acid or clofibrate if necessary. Hypertriglyceridemia is usually most sensitive to clofibrate or nicotinic acid. For highly selected patients, partial ileal bypass surgery has been recommended to reduce serum cholesterol levels secondary to bile acid depletion.

Routine lipid screening tests must be recommended for relatives of individuals with familial hyperlipidemia or premature atherosclerotic heart disease so that appropriate therapy can be instituted, in the hope of retarding atherogenesis and its consequences.

Hypertension

Hypertension is recognized as the leading cause of death in the United States. Approximately one-quarter of the adult population is hypertensive, and the incidence is even greater among blacks. The risk of developing not only cardiac disease but also neurologic, renal, and vascular disease is significantly increased among hypertensive individuals. The higher the blood pressure, the greater the risk.

Hypertension is defined as an abnormal elevation of systolic and/or diastolic blood pressure. The precise delineation of abnormality is somewhat arbitrary; acceptable values vary with age and sex. In general, systolic values ranging from 140 to 160 mmHg and diastolic values from 90 to 95 mmHg are considered indicative of borderline hypertension. The diagnosis of hypertension is unequivocal with values in excess of 160 mmHg systolic and 95 mmHg diastolic pressure. These values are consistent with a conceptual definition of hypertension as a pressure elevation associated with an increase in cardiovascular mortality of over 50 percent.

The course of hypertensive disease is particularly insidious; hypertensive individuals can remain asymptomatic for many years. This latent period masks disease progression until significant organ damage occurs.

Symptoms, if present, are typically nonspecific, such as headache or dizziness. If hypertension remains undetected and untreated, death results from heart failure, myocardial infarction, stroke, or renal failure. However, early detection and effective treatment of hypertension can significantly decrease associated morbidity and mortality. Consequently, routine blood pressure screening is of paramount importance in hypertension control.

The cause of hypertension is unknown in approximately 90 percent of the cases. This idiopathic form of hypertension is referred to as *primary* or *essential* hypertension. The precise pathogenesis appears to be extremely complex with interaction of multiple variables. Proposed mechanisms include alterations in the following: (1) renal excretion of sodium and water, (2) baroreceptor sensitivity, (3) vascular responsiveness, and (4) renin secretion. The remaining 10 percent of hypertensive disease is secondary to some other underlying disease process, such as renal parenchymal disease or primary aldosteronism.

The mechanism by which hypertension produces disability and death relates directly to its effect upon the heart and blood vessels. The elevation in systemic blood pressure increases the resistance to left ventricular ejection; consequently, cardiac workload is increased. In response, the ventricle hypertrophies to increase the force of contraction. However, the ability of the ventricle to sustain cardiac output via compensatory hypertrophy is eventually exceeded, and cardiac dilation and failure result. The heart is further compromised by an associated acceleration of coronary atherosclerosis. As coronary atherosclerosis progresses, myocardial oxygen supply is reduced. Angina or myocardial infarction can result since a concurrent rise in myocardial oxygen demand occurs secondary to the ventricular hypertrophy and increased cardiac work. Approximately one-half of hypertensive deaths are due to myocardial infarction or failure.

Hypertensive vascular damage is apparent thoughout the periphery. Retinal vascular changes, easily observed and quantified during ophthalmoscopic examination, are useful in both the evaluation of disease progression and response to therapy. Accelerated atherosclerosis and medial necrosis of the aorta predispose to the formation of aneurysms and dissections. Structural changes in the small arteries and arterioles cause progressive occlusive vascular disease. As the vascular lumen narrows, arterial flow is compromised and tissue microinfarction can result. The consequences of these vascular changes are most striking in the brain and kidneys. Cerebral vascular occlusion or rupture accounts for approximately one-third of hypertensive deaths.

Progressive sclerosis of the renal vasculature with resultant organ dysfunction and renal failure can also be fatal. (See also Parts VII and VIII.)

The therapy of mild to moderate essential hypertension remains controversial in that, despite the obvious benefits of hypertension control, antihypertensive therapy may involve some disagreeable side effects and long-term patient compliance is difficult to achieve. Therapy initially consists of restriction of dietary sodium intake and weight reduction to ideal body weight. If this approach is unsuccessful, pharmacologic therapy with diuretics, sympatholytic agents, vasodilators, or a combination of these may be indicated. Hypertension secondary to another cause is treated by reversing the underlying process.

Other modifiable factors

The risk of cigarette smoking is related to the number of cigarettes smoked per day, not to the length of time that the patient has smoked. An individual smoking more than a pack a day is twice as susceptible to coronary atherosclerotic disease as a nonsmoker. The effect of nicotine on catecholamine release by the autonomic nervous system seems to be the mechanism responsible. The effect, however, is noncumulative; ex-smokers seem to revert to the low risk of nonsmokers.

Diabetics evidence a greater prevalence, prematurity, and severity of coronary atherosclerosis. The mechanism is as yet unresolved, but perhaps an abnormality in lipid metabolism or a predisposition to vascular degeneration associated with the impaired glucose tolerance is responsible. The American diet—high in calories, total fat, saturated fat, sugar, and salt—contributes to the development of hyperlipoproteinemia and obesity. Obesity increases cardiac work and oxygen demand.

The list of minor risk factors expands as additional biological-environmental correlates with coronary heart disease are identified. At present, a sedentary life-style and psychosocial stress seem contributory. An interesting relationship between the so-called type A behavior pattern and accelerated atherogenesis has been popularized by Rosenman and Friedman. The type A personality manifests intense competitiveness, ambition, aggressiveness, and a sense of time urgency. It is commonly acknowledged that catecholamine release accompanies stress; however, the question arises as to whether stress is atherogenic or simply precipitates the attack. A theory of stress-induced atherogenesis might postulate neuroendocrine influences upon circulatory dynamics, serum lipids, or blood clotting.

Hence, the speculation continues. However, the fact remains that coronary atherosclerosis is a multifactorial disease and there is substantiated evidence that certain risk factors accelerate atherogenesis. The complexity of the process is highlighted by the fact that in the presence of more than one risk factor, the susceptibility to atherogenesis is not simply additive; the factors are synergistic. The interaction of multiple factors significantly accelerates the disease process.

PATHOPHYSIOLOGY

Ischemia

Oxygen demand in excess of the capacity of the diseased vessels to supply oxygen results in localized myocardial ischemia. Transient ischemia causes reversible changes at the cellular and tissue levels, depressing myocardial function.

The oxygen lack forces the myocardium to shift from aerobic metabolism to anaerobic metabolism. Anaerobic metabolism via glycolytic pathways is a much less efficient means of energy production than is aerobic metabolism via oxidative phosphorylation and the Krebs cycle; the production of high-energy phosphate is reduced considerably. The end product of anaerobic metabolism, lactic acid, accumulates, reducing cellular pH.

The combination of hypoxia, reduced energy availability, and acidosis rapidly impairs left ventricular function. The strength of contraction in the affected myocardial region is reduced; the fibers shorten inadequately with less force and velocity. In addition, the wall motion of the ischemic segment is abnormal; the segment passively bulges outward with each ventricular contraction (see Fig. 27-3).

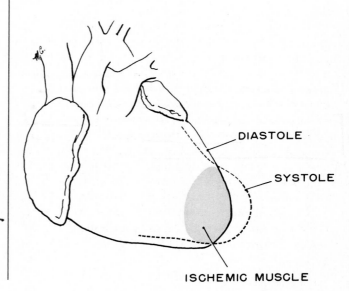

FIGURE 27-3
Ischemic wall bulging during systole.

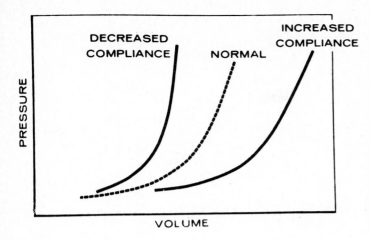

FIGURE 27-4

Ventricular compliance, or the pressure-volume relationship of the ventricles. The dotted line in the center indicates the typical relationship between pressure and volume. As volume is increased initially, there is only a small rise in pressure. As volume increase continues, the rise in pressure is greater. Each solid line indicates an alteration in pressure-volume relationships—decreased compliance on the left and increased compliance on the right. This represents a greater or lesser degree of stiffness of the ventricle in relation to the filling volume. Ventricular compliance is a dynamic phenomenon, and this property can change rapidly. (From W. A. Sodeman, Jr. and W. A. Sodeman (eds.), *Pathologic Physiology*, 5th ed., Saunders, Philadelphia, 1974, p. 276.)

The reduced contractility and impaired wall motion alter hemodynamics. The hemodynamic response is variable, depending upon the size of the ischemic segment and the degree of reflex compensatory response by the autonomic nervous system. Depression of left ventricular function may lower cardiac output by reducing stroke volume (the amount of blood ejected per beat). Reduction in systolic emptying increases ventricular volumes. As a result, left-sided pressures will rise; the left ventricular end-diastolic pressure and pulmonary capillary wedge pressure will be elevated. This pressure elevation is magnified by changes in wall compliance or distensibility induced by ischemia. A reduction in compliance occurs, accentuating the elevation in pressure for a given ventricular volume (see Fig. 27-4).

During ischemia, the manifest hemodynamic pattern is commonly that of mild increments in blood pressure and heart rate prior to the onset of pain. Apparently, this represents a sympathetic compensatory response to the depression of myocardial function. With the onset of pain a further catecholamine stimulation frequently occurs. A depression of blood pressure would suggest ischemic involvement of a large area of myocardium or a vagal response.

Myocardial ischemia is typically associated with two characteristic electrocardiographic changes resulting from alterations in cellular electrophysiology: T wave inversion and ST segment depression (see Fig. 27-5). A variant form of angina, Prinzmetal's angina, is associated with ST segment elevation.

Ischemic attacks usually subside within minutes if the imbalance between oxygen supply and demand is corrected. The metabolic, functional, hemodynamic, and electrocardiographic changes are reversible.

Angina pectoris is the chest pain associated with myocardial ischemia. The exact mechanism by which ischemia produces pain is unclear. It seems that neural pain receptors are stimulated by the accumulated metabolites, by an unidentified chemical intermediary, or by local mechanical stress resulting from abnormal myocardial contraction. Typically, the pain is described as a substernal pressure, occasionally radiating down the medial aspect of the left arm. A clenched fist placed upon the sternum graphically illustrates the classic pattern (Fig. 27-6). However, many patients never experience typical angina; anginal pain may mimic indigestion or a toothache. Classically, angina is precipitated by activities increasing myocardial oxygen demand, such as exercise, and is relieved within minutes by rest or nitroglycerin. The less common Prinzmetal's angina typically occurs at rest rather than during exertion. The role of coronary spasm in precipitating such pain is under investigation.

Infarction

Prolonged ischemia of over 30 to 45 minutes causes irreversible cellular damage and muscle death, or necrosis. Permanent cessation of contractile function occurs in the necrotic or infarcted area of the myocardium. The infarct is surrounded by a zone of ischemic, potentially viable tissue (see Fig. 27-7). The ultimate size of the infarct depends upon the fate of this ischemic zone; necrosis of this marginal area will extend the infarct size, whereas reversal of the ischemia minimizes the residual necrosis.

Myocardial infarction usually affects the left ventri-

FIGURE 27-5

Classic ECG changes with ischemia. (A) T-wave inversion. (B) T-segment depression.

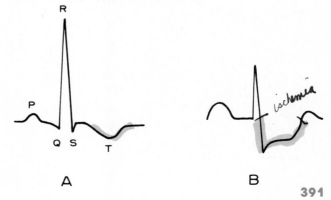

391

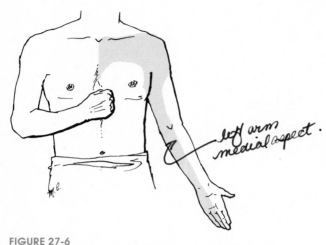

FIGURE 27-6
Typical pattern of referred pain in angina pectoris.

left arm medial aspect.

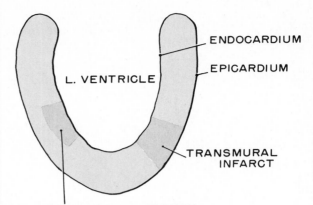

FIGURE 27-8
Transmural and subendocardial infarction.

cle. A *transmural infarction* involves the full thickness of the wall; a *subendocardial* infarction is limited to the inner half of the myocardium (see Fig. 27-8). Infarctions are described further according to location on the ventricular wall (see Fig. 27-9). For instance, an anterior myocardial infarction involves the anterior wall of the left ventricle. Other common infarct sites are designated as inferior, lateral, posterior, and septal. Extensive infarctions involving large portions of the ventricle would be described accordingly, that is, as anteroseptal, anterolateral, or inferolateral. Infarction of the posterior wall of the right ventricle is also observed in approximately one-quarter of left ventricular inferior wall in-

FIGURE 27-7
Zones of necrosis and ischemia.

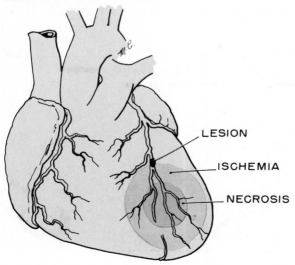

farctions. Biventricular compromise should be anticipated in this situation.

Obviously, the infarct location correlates with disease in a particular region of the coronary circulation (see Table 27-4). For example, anterior wall infarctions result from lesions in the left anterior descending artery. Knowledge of the infarct location and the coronary anatomy is of critical importance in the anticipation of complications associated with myocardial infarction. For example, inferior wall infarction, usually the result of right coronary artery lesions, can be associated with variable degrees of heart block. This is to be expected, because the AV node receives its nutrient supply from the same vessel that nourishes the inferior wall of the left ventricle.

The infarcted muscle undergoes a sequence of changes during the healing process. Initially, the infarcted muscle appears bruised and cyanotic as a result of regional stagnation of blood. Cellular edema and an inflammatory response with leukocytic infiltration ensue within 24 hours. Cardiac enzymes are released from the cells. Tissue degradation and removal of all necrotic fibers begins by the second or third day. During this phase, the necrotic wall is relatively thin. By about the third week, scar formation begins. Gradually, fibrous connective tissue replaces the necrotic muscle and undergoes progressive thickening. By the sixth week, the scar is well established.

Myocardial infarction significantly depresses ventricular function as a result of the loss of contracility in the necrotic muscle and the impaired contractility in the surrounding ischemic muscle. Functionally, myocardial infarction results in changes similar to those noted with ischemia: (1) reduced contractility, (2) abnormal wall motion, (3) altered ventricular wall compliance, (4) reduced stroke volume, (5) diminished ejection fraction, (6) elevated ventricular end-systolic and end-diastolic volumes, and (7) increased left ventricular end-diastolic pressure.

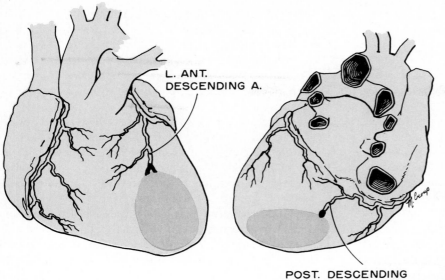

L. ANT.
DESCENDING A.

POST. DESCENDING
BRANCH R. CORONARY A.

FIGURE 27-9
Localization of infarcts on the ventricular wall. Left, infarct of the anterior wall due to occlusion of the left anterior descending artery. Right, inferior wall infarction due to occlusion of the posterior descending branch of the right coronary artery.

A wide spectrum of left ventricular dysfunction is apparent after myocardial infarction. The degree of functional impairment depends upon a number of factors:

1. *Infarct size*—infarcts of over 40 percent of the myocardium are associated with a high incidence of cardiogenic shock.

2. *Infarct location*—anterior wall infarction is more likely to significantly depress mechanical function than is inferior wall damage.

3. *Function of uninvolved myocardium*—old infarcts would compromise residual myocardial function.

4. *Collateral circulation*—collateral circulation, via either preexisting arterial anastomoses or new channels, can develop in response to chronic ischemia and regional hypoperfusion, improving blood flow to the threatened myocardium.

5. *Cardiovascular compensatory mechanisms*—reflex

TABLE 27-4

CORRELATION BETWEEN VENTRICULAR SURFACES, ECG LEADS, AND CORONARY ARTERIES

Surface of left ventricle	ECG leads	Coronary artery usually involved
Inferior	II, III, aVF	Right coronary
Lateral	I, aVL	Left circumflex
Anterior	V_2–V_4	Left anterior descending
Septal	V_1–V_2	Left anterior descending
Apical	V_5–V_6	Left anterior descending
Posterior	V_1–V_2 (reciprocal changes)	Left circumflex

compensatory mechanisms operate to maintain cardiac output and peripheral perfusion.

Reflex sympathetic augmentation of the heart rate and contractility can improve ventricular function. Generalized arteriolar constriction increases total peripheral resistance, thereby increasing mean arterial pressure. Venoconstriction reduces venous capacity, increasing venous return to the heart and ventricular filling. Increased ventricular filling elevates the force of contraction and subsequent ejection volumes. This is best illustrated by comparing the normal ventricular function curve with that of the compromised myocardium (see Fig. 27-10). With depression of ventricular function, higher diastolic filling pressures are necessary to maintain stroke volume. Elevation of diastolic filling

FIGURE 27-10

Depression of the ventricular function curve. The dotted line represents the relationship of stroke volume to left ventricular end-diastolic volume for the normal heart shown previously in Fig. 25-9. The failing heart (solid line) must increase the end-diastolic volume to maintain stroke volume. Therefore, cardiac dilatation occurs.

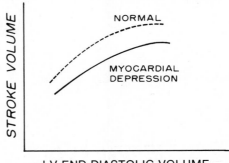

pressure and ventricular volume stretches myocardial fibers, increasing the force of contraction according to Starling's law. Circulatory filling pressures can be increased further by renal retention of sodium and water. As a result, myocardial infarction is commonly associated with transient left ventricular enlargement caused by compensatory cardiac dilation. If necessary, compensatory cardiac hypertrophy can also occur to increase the force of contraction and ventricular emptying.

In summary, a battery of reflex responses are available to forestall deterioration of cardiac output and perfusion pressure: (1) augmentation of heart rate and contractility, (2) generalized vasoconstriction, (3) sodium and water retention, (4) ventricular dilation, and (5) ventricular hypertrophy. However, all compensatory responses can eventually contribute to further myocardial deterioration by increasing myocardial oxygen demand.

The hemodynamic presentation after myocardial infarction is variable. Cardiac output may be slightly reduced or maintained at normal levels. Heart rate is usually not persistently elevated unless extensive myocardial depression occurs. Blood pressure is a function of the interaction between myocardial depression and autonomic reflexes. The autonomic response to myocardial infarction is not always the predictable sympathetic

support of the compromised circulation. Pain or stimulation of parasympathetic ganglia in the myocardium, especially in the inferior wall, complicates the hemodynamic response. Parasympathetic stimulation reduces the heart rate and blood pressure, adversely affecting cardiac output and peripheral perfusion. This type of response is known as vasovagal.

Myocardial infarction is classically associated with a characteristic diagnostic triad. First, the typical clinical picture consists of severe, prolonged chest pain frequently associated with sweating, nausea, vomiting, and a sense of impending doom. However, a small proportion of myocardial infarctions are "silent" or asymptomatic. Second, serum levels of the cardiac enzymes released by the necrotic myocardial cells are elevated. The released enzymes include creatine phosphokinase (CK or CPK), glutamic oxaloacetic transaminase (GOT or SGOT), and lactic dehydrogenase (LDH). The pattern of enzyme elevations follows a characteristic time course after myocardial infarction (Fig. 27-11). Although it is a valuable adjunct to diagnosis, enzyme interpretation is limited by the fact that the measured enzyme elevations are not specific indicators of myocardial damage—coexisting processes can produce misleading enzyme elevations. Measurement of isoenzymes, enzyme fractions specifically released by the damaged myocardium, increases diagnostic accuracy. Release of the MB-CK isoenzyme is the most specific enzymatic indication of myocardial infarction. Finally, electrocardiographic changes, consisting of pronounced Q waves, ST segment elevation, and inverted T waves, are evident during acute infarction (see Fig. 27-12). These changes are apparent in the leads overlying the area of myocardial necrosis. Over time, the ST segment and T wave changes revert to normal; only the abnormal Q waves persist as electrocardiographic evidence of an old infarction.

Complications of ischemia and infarction

Congestive heart failure

Congestive heart failure is a state of circulatory congestion produced by myocardial dysfunction. The location of the congestion depends upon the ventricle involved. Left ventricular dysfunction, or left heart failure, produces pulmonary venous congestion, whereas right ventricular dysfunction, or right heart failure, results in systemic venous congestion. Failure of both

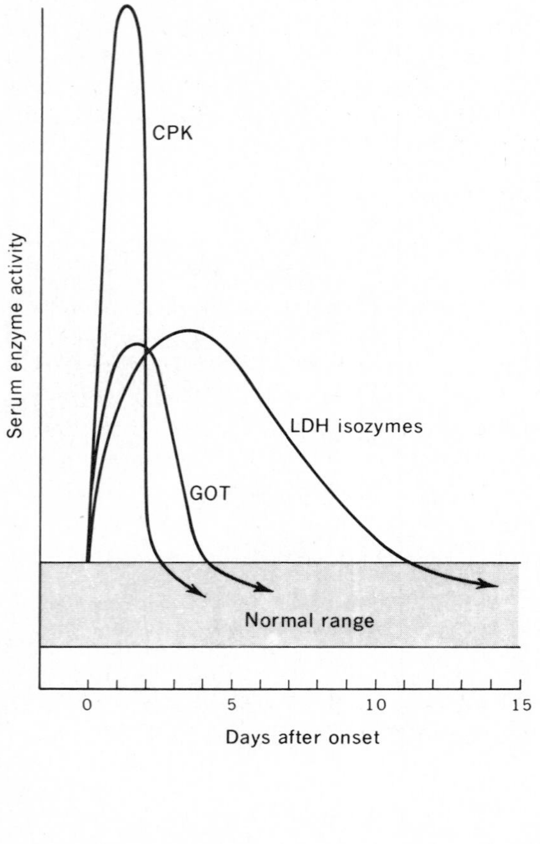

FIGURE 27-11

Characteristic pattern of serum enzyme elevations after myocardial infarction. CPK, creatinine phosphokinase; GOT, glutamic oxaloacetic transaminase; LDH, lactic dehydrogenase. (From E. Braunwald, J. S. Alpert, and R. S. Ross, *Harrison's Principles of Internal Medicine*, 9th ed., McGraw-Hill, New York, 1980, p. 1126.)

CPK

Serum enzyme activity

LDH isozymes

GOT

Normal range

0   5   10   15

Days after onset

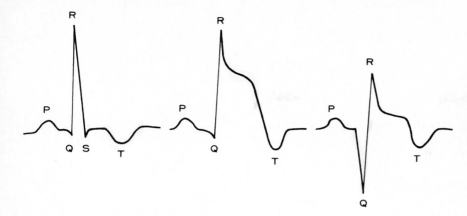

FIGURE 27-12
ECG changes overlying an area of myocardial infarction. T-wave inversion (left), ST-segment elevation (middle), pronounced Q waves (right). The Q waves indicate myocardial necrosis and are irreversible. The ST- and T-wave changes result from ischemic injury and disappear over time.

ventricles is referred to as biventricular failure. Failure of the left side of the heart is the most common mechanical complication following myocardial infarction, occurring approximately 50 percent of the time.

Myocardial infarction compromises myocardial function by reducing contractility, producing abnormal wall motion, and altering chamber compliance. As the ability of the left ventricle to empty effectively lessens, stroke volume falls and residual ventricular volumes rise. Consequently, left ventricular pressures rise. This pressure elevation is transmitted backward into the pulmonary venous circuit. If the hydrostatic pressure in the pulmonary capillary bed exceeds the vascular oncotic pressure, fluid transudation into the interstitium results. Further elevation of pressure eventually causes pulmonary edema due to fluid seepage into the alveoli.

The fall in stroke volume elicits a compensatory sympathetic response. Heart rate and contractile force increase to maintain cardiac output. Peripheral vasoconstriction occurs to stabilize arterial pressure and redistribute blood flow away from the nonvital organs, such as the kidney and skin, to maintain perfusion of the vital organs. Venoconstriction increases venous return to the right side of the heart, further augmenting contractile force according to Starling's law of the heart. Activation of the renin-angiotensin-aldosterone system in response to the fall in renal blood flow and glomerular filtration rate results in renal retention of sodium and water. This further increases venous return.

The clinical manifestations of heart failure reflect the degree of myocardial compromise and the efficacy and magnitude of compensatory responses. The following findings are commonly noted during left heart failure:

1. *Signs and symptoms:* Dyspnea, oliguria, weakness, fatigue, pallor, weight gain
2. *Auscultation:* Rales, third heart sound (due to dilation and noncompliance of the ventricle during rapid filling)
3. *Electrocardiogram:* Tachycardia

4. *Chest x-ray:* Cardiomegaly, pulmonary venous congestion, vascular redistribution to the upper lobes.

Failure of the left side of the heart can progress to failure of the right as pulmonary vascular pressures rise, stressing the right ventricle. In addition to this indirect route of compromise via the pulmonary vasculature, left ventricular dysfunction directly affects right ventricular function via shared anatomic and biochemical features. The two ventricles share a common wall, the interventricular septum, and lie within the pericardium. In addition, biochemical changes, such as depletion of myocardial stores of norepinephrine during failure, can adversely affect both ventricles. Finally, infarction of the right ventricle can occur, particularly in association with inferior wall infarction of the left ventricle. Right ventricular infarction obviously predisposes the right side of the heart to failure. The systemic venous congestion produced by right heart failure is manifested by findings such as engorged neck veins, hepatomegaly, and peripheral edema.

Cardiogenic shock

Cardiogenic shock results from profound left ventricular dysfunction following massive infarction, usually involving over 40 percent of the left ventricle. A vicious, self-perpetuating cycle of progressively irreversible hemodynamic changes ensues: (1) reduced peripheral perfusion, (2) reduced coronary perfusion, and (3) increased pulmonary congestion. Hypotension, metabolic acidosis, and hypoxemia further depress myocardial function. The incidence of cardiogenic shock is 10 to 15 percent. The associated mortality is approximately 80 to 90 percent.

Papillary muscle dysfunction

Closure of the mitral valve during ventricular systole is dependent upon the functional integrity of the left ventricular papillary muscles and chordae tendineae. Ischemic dysfunction or necrotic rupture of a papillary muscle impairs mitral valve function and permits varying degrees of leaflet eversion into the atria during systole (see Fig. 27-13). Valvular incompetence results in retrograde flow from the left ventricle into the left atrium with two consequences: a reduction in forward aortic flow and an elevation in left atrial and pulmonary venous congestion. The volume of regurgitant flow depends upon the extent of papillary muscle disease; ischemia commonly causes mild to moderate congestive heart failure. However, papillary muscle necrosis and rupture is a catastrophic event with rapid deterioration into pulmonary edema and shock.

Ventricular septal defect

Necrosis of the interventricular septum can result in rupture of the septal wall, which creates a ventricular septal defect. Since the septum receives a dual blood supply from arteries descending the anterior and posterior surfaces of the interventricular groove, septal rupture indicates extensive coronary artery disease involving more than one artery.

Essentially, the rupture establishes a second outflow tract from the left ventricle. During each ventricular contraction, there is competitive outflow through the aorta and the septal defect (see Fig. 27-14). Since pressures on the left side of the heart are far greater than pressures on the right side of the heart, blood will be shunted through the defect from left to right, from the area of greater pressure to the area of lesser pres-

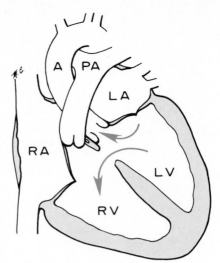

FIGURE 27-14
Ventricular septal defect.

sure. Great volumes of blood can be shunted over to the right side of the heart, reducing the amount of blood available to be ejected via the aorta. Significant reductions in cardiac output with concurrent elevations in right ventricular work and pulmonary congestion result.

Cardiac rupture

Although rare, rupture of the ventricular free wall may occur early in the course of transmural infarction during the phase of necrotic tissue removal prior to scar formation. The thin, necrotic wall ruptures, resulting in massive bleeding into the pericardial sac. The relatively inelastic pericardial sac is unable to distend. Thus the blood-filled pericardial sac compresses the heart, producing cardiac tamponade (see Fig. 27-15). Cardiac tamponade reduces venous return and cardiac output. Death usually occurs within a few minutes.

Ventricular aneurysm

Transient paradoxical myocardial bulging of the ischemic myocardium is common, and a sustained ventricular aneurysm occurs in approximately 15 percent of patients. The aneurysm is usually on the anterior or apical surface of the heart. Ventricular aneurysms balloon outward with each systole, passively distended by a portion of the stroke volume (see Fig. 27-16). Ventricular aneurysms can produce three problematic consequences: (1) chronic congestive heart failure, (2) systemic embolization of mural thrombi, and (3) refractory ventricular arrhythmias.

Thromboembolism

Necrosis of the ventricular endothelium roughens the endothelial surface, predisposing to thrombus for-

FIGURE 27-13
Papillary muscle rupture.

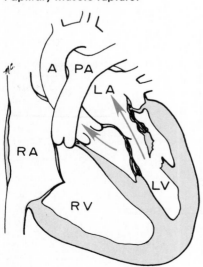

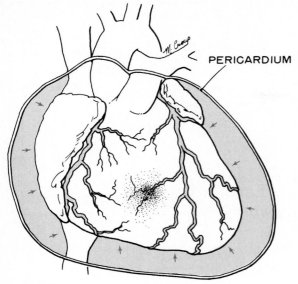

FIGURE 27-15
Cardia tamponade.

mation. A fragment of an intracardiac mural thrombus can dislodge and embolize systemically. A second potential site of thrombus formation is the systemic venous system: venous embolization would cause pulmonary embolism, a complication discussed in Part VI.

Pericarditis

Transmural infarction can roughen the epicardial layer in contact with the pericardium, irritating the pericardial surface and resulting in an inflammatory reaction; rarely, a pericardial effusion, or fluid accumula-

FIGURE 27-16
Ventricular aneurysm.

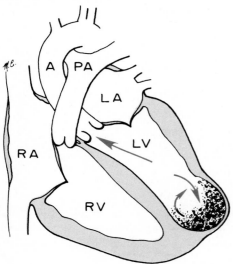

tion between the layers, occurs. Fluid accumulation is rarely significant enought to cause cardiac tamponade.

Dressler's syndrome

This post-myocardial infarction syndrome is a benign inflammatory response with pleuropericardial pain. It is postulated that the syndrome might represent a hypersensitivity reaction to the necrotic myocardium.

Arrhythmia

A disturbance of cardiac rhythm, or arrhythmia, is the most common complication during myocardial infarction, having an incidence of approximately 90 percent. Arrhythmias result from alterations in myocardial cellular electrophysiology. The electrophysiologic alteration is manifested by a change in the configuration of the action potential, which is the graphic recording of cellular electrical activity. For instance, sympathetic stimulation increases the slope of spontaneous depolarization, thereby increasing the heart rate (see Fig. 27-17). Clinically, arrhythmia diagnosis is based upon interpretation of the electrocardiogram.

Multiple predisposing factors account for the high incidence of arrhythmias in the setting of coronary atherosclerotic disease: (1) tissue ischemia, (2) hypoxemia, (3) autonomic nervous system influences (e.g., parasympathetic stimulation that decreases heart rate), (4) metabolic derangements (e.g., lactic acidosis due to compromised tissue perfusion), (5) hemodynamic abnormalities (e.g., reduction in coronary perfusion associated with hypertension), (6) drugs (e.g., digitalis toxicity), and (7) electrolyte imbalance (e.g., hypokalemia with excessive diuresis).

Cardiac rhythm abnormalities can be categorized according to the following basic mechanisms: abnormal automaticity, abnormal conduction, or a combination of the two.

The normal heart rate is between 60 and 100 bpm. A heart rate under 60 bpm is referred to as a *bradycardia*, whereas a *tachycardia* indicates a heart rate over 100 bpm (see Fig. 27-18). Both rate abnormalities can adversely affect cardiac function. Since heart rate is a primary determinant of cardiac output [cardiac output (CO) = heart rate (HR) × stroke volume (SV)], extreme increments or reductions in heart rate can lower cardiac output. Tachycardias lower it by reducing ventricular filling time and stroke volume, and bradycardias lower it by reducing the frequency of ventricular ejection. As cardiac output falls, arterial pressure and peripheral perfusion decrease. Furthermore, tachycardias

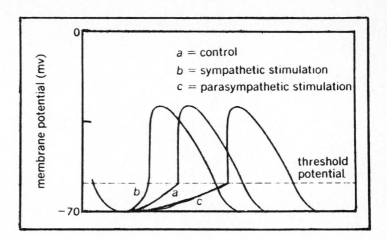

FIGURE 27-17

**Effects of sympathetic and parasympathetic
stimulation on the slope of the action potential of
an SA-node cell. (From A. J. Vander, J. H. Sherman,
and D. S. Luciano, *Human Physiology,* 1st ed.,
McGraw-Hill, New York, 1970, p. 258.)**

can aggravate myocardial ischemia by increasing myocardial oxygen demand while simultaneously reducing
the duration of diastole, the period of greatest coronary
flow, thereby compromising coronary oxygen supply.

Any cardiac impulse originating outside of the sinus
node is considered abnormal and is referred to as an *ectopic beat.* Ectopic beats can originate in the atria, the
atrioventricular junction, or the ventricles under two
conditions: (1) failure or excessive slowing of the sinus
node, or (2) premature activation of another cardiac site.
Ectopic beats resulting from sinus node failure serve a
protective function by initiating a cardiac impulse before prolonged cardiac standstill can occur (see Fig. 27-
19). These beats are called *escape beats.* If the sinus
node fails to resume normal function, the ectopic site
will assume the role of pacemaker and sustain the cardiac rhythm. This is referred to as an *escape rhythm.*

FIGURE 27-18

**Sinus rhythms. (A) Normal sinus rhythm. (B) Sinus
bradycardia. (C) Sinus tachycardia. (Reprinted with
permission of Macmillan Publishing Co., Inc., from
P-QRS-T: A Guide to Electrocardiographic Interpretation,
5th ed., copyright © by Joseph E. F. Riseman, 1968, p. 63.)**

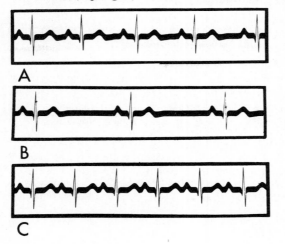

A

B

C

Once the sinus node resumes normal function, the escape focus is suppressed.

Premature activation of cardiac sites other than the
sinus node disrupts the normal cardiac cycle; impulses
occur prematurely before the sinus node recovers sufficiently from one beat to initiate another (see Fig. 27-20).
These beats are referred to as *premature beats.* Premature beats are produced by two basic mechanisms: (1)
increased automaticity or (2) reentry, a form of abnormal conduction. Reentry is by far the more common
mechanism. During reentry, illustrated in Fig. 27-21, a
single cardiac impulse reenters and excites a myocardial
region previously activated, producing a premature
beat. These sites can produce isolated premature beats
or sustained tachycardias; arrhythmias can develop in
the atria, atrioventricular junction, or ventricles and are
designated accordingly. For instance, an "atrial premature beat" originates in the atria, whereas "ventricular
tachycardia" is ventricular in origin.

Ventricular premature beats are the most common
form of arrhythmia (see Fig. 27-22A). However, ventricular irritability can degenerate into life-threatening ventricular tachycardia or ventricular fibrillation (see Figs.
27-22B and C). *Ventricular tachycardia* severely reduces cardiac output as a result of the rapid rate, usually
over 120 bpm, and the loss of mechanical synchrony between atrial and ventricular contraction. *Ventricular fibrillation* results in the abrupt cessation of effective ventricular contraction; the ventricles quiver without
coordination.

Atrial arrhythmias can be conceptualized along a
continuum of rate acceleration associated with progressive reduction in atrial function: (1) *premature atrial
beat,* (2) *atrial tachycardia*—atrial rate approximately
150, (3) *atrial flutter*—atrial rate approximately 300, and
(4) *atrial fibrillation*—quivering, uncoordinated atrial
activity (see Fig. 27-23). To protect the ventricles from
responding to extremely rapid atrial stimulation, the
AV node does not normally conduct atrial impulses at
rates greater than 180 bpm. For instance, in atrial flutter
with an atrial rate of 300, only every second or third

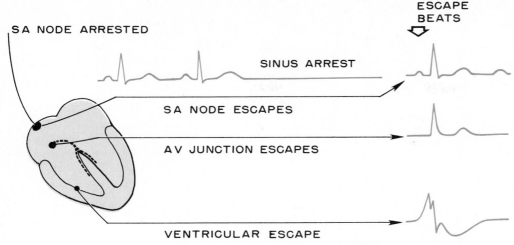

SA NODE ARRESTED

SINUS ARREST

ESCAPE BEATS

SA NODE ESCAPES

AV JUNCTION ESCAPES

VENTRICULAR ESCAPE

FIGURE 27-19

Escape beats. A period of cardiac asystole may result when the SA node fails to send impulses to the atria unless lower pacemakers, or escape pacemakers, take over to maintain the cardiac rhythm. (If the first beat after the sinus arrest originates in the AV node, it is called a functional escape beat. If the impulse after sinus arrest originates in the ventricles, it is called a ventricular escape beat. (Modified from F. H. Netter, *The Ciba Collection of Medical Illustrations, vol. 5, The Heart,* Ciba Pharmeceutical Company, Summit, N.J., 1969, p. 67.)

atrial impulse is conducted; consequently the ventricular rate is 100 to 150. The hemodynamic response to atrial arrhythmias depends upon the ventricular rate and the efficacy of atrial contraction. For instance, in atrial fibrillation, the atrial musculature is unable to contract effectively and actively contribute to ventricular filling; thus, cardiac output may fall.

Heart block is a delay or interruption in impulse conduction between the atria and the ventricles. The cardiac impulse normally spreads from the sinus node along internodal pathways to the AV node and ventricles within 0.20 second (normal PR interval); ventricular depolarization occurs within 0.10 second (normal QRS duration). Heart block occurs in three progressively more serious forms. In *first-degree heart block,* all impulses are conducted through the AV junction; however, conduction time is abnormally prolonged. In *second-degree heart block,* some impulses are conducted to the ventricles, but some impulses are blocked. There are two types of second-degree heart block. Wenckebach (Mobitz I) is characterized by repetitive cycles of progressively lengthening AV conduction time, culminating in the nonconduction of one beat. The second type, Mobitz II, involves conduction of some impulses with a constant AV conduction time and nonconduction of other impulses. In *third-degree heart block, no impulses are conducted to the ventricles.* Unless *escape pacemakers,* either junctional or ventricular in origin, to function, cardiac standstill results (see Fig. 27-24). *Bundle branch block* is an interruption of conduction in the bundle branches which prolongs ventricular depolarization time beyond 0.10 second.

THERAPEUTIC INTERVENTION

Primary prevention

The most critical therapeutic intervention in the setting of coronary atherosclerosis is the primary prevention of

the disease. Disease prevention is essential for many reasons:

1. Clinically apparent disease is preceded by a long latent period with silent progression of disease, apparently in early adulthood. Lesions considered to

FIGURE 27-20

Premature beats. (A) Atrial premature beat. (B) AV-junctional premature beat with P hidden in the QRS. (C) Ventricular premature beat. (Reprinted with permission of Macmillan Publishing Co., Inc., from *P-QRS-T: A Guide to Electrocardiographic Interpretation,* 5th ed., copyright © by Joseph E. F. Riseman, 1968, pp. 68, 83.)

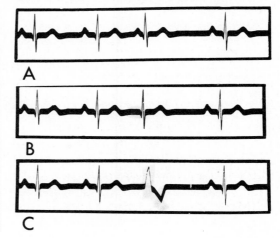

A

B

C

REENTRY

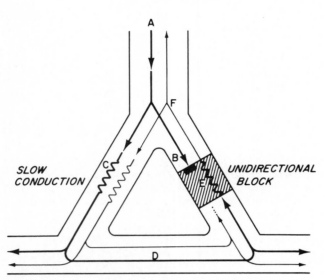

FIGURE 27-21
Features of reentry. An impulse is shown entering both limbs of an available circuit at point A. The impulse encounters antegrade (unidirectional) block in the shaded area at point B because the effective refractory period of this region exceeds that of the tissue in region C. The impulse is conducted with delay through region C, traverses region D distal to the site of unidirectional block, and retrogradely penetrates this region (E), resulting in completion and perpetuation of the reentry circuit. Slow conduction in region C or E allows sufficient time for recovery of excitability to occur in region F following its previous depolarization by the initiating (antegrade) impulse. A delicate balance of conduction delay and differential refractoriness must coexist in two limbs of the circuit in order for reentry to be initiated and sustained. Exit into and excitation of the surrounding myocardium by the reentrant impulse may occur at any point in the circuit. The rate of the resulting arrhythmia is determined both by the conduction time within the reentry circuit and by the refractory period of the surrounding myocardium. (From Johnson, Haber, and Austen, 1980, p. 154.)

be precursors of atherosclerotic disease have been identified in the coronary arterial walls of children and young adults.

2. There is no curative therapy for coronary atherosclerotic disease; once the disease is recognizable clinically, therapy is essentially palliative, undertaken to minimize the severity of clinical sequelae and to potentially slow disease progression.

3. The consequences of coronary atherosclerosis can be catastrophic. Myocardial infarction often occurs with little or no warning; the incidence of sudden

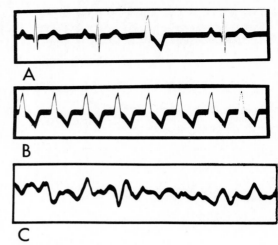

FIGURE 27-22
Ventricular arrhythmias. (A) Ventricular premature beat. (B) Ventricular tachycardia. (C) Ventricular fibrillation. (Reprinted with permission of Macmillan Publishing Co., Inc., from *P-QRS-T: A Guide to Electrocardiographic Interpretation,* 5th ed., copyright © by Joseph E. F. Riseman, 1968, pp. 69, 71, 99.)

death is high. Over half of the deaths associated with myocardial infarction occur during the first few hours of infarction, prior to hospitalization.

4. Coronary atherosclerosis is the leading cause of death in the country; approximately 550,000 deaths were attributable to myocardial infarction in 1981.

FIGURE 27-23
Atrial arrhythmias. (A) Atrial premature beats from different foci. (B) Atrial tachycardia with P superimposed in T. (C) Atrial flutter (4:1). (D) Atrial fibrillation. (Reprinted with permission of Macmillan Publishing Co., Inc., from *P-QRS-T: A Guide to Electrocardiographic Interpretation,* 5th ed., copyright © by Joseph E. F. Riseman, 1968, pp. 67, 71.)

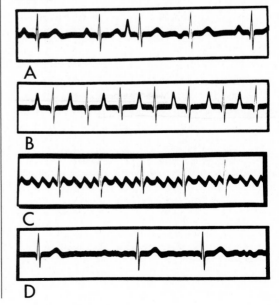

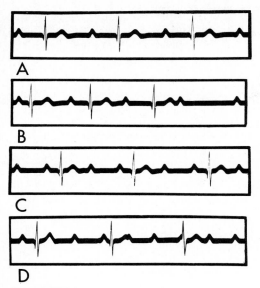

FIGURE 27-24

Heart block. (A) First-degree heart block. (B) Second-degree heart block—Wenckebach or Mobitz. I (C) Second-degree heart block—Mobitz II. (D) Third-degree heart block or complete heart block. (Reprinted with permission of Macmillan Publishing Co., Inc., from *P-QRS-T: A Guide to Electrocardiographic Interpretation,* 5th ed., copyright © by Joseph E. F. Riseman, 1968, p. 81.)

Since the precise pathogenesis of atherosclerosis is still undefined, the control of risk factors known to increase susceptibility to atherogenesis is the crux of disease prophylaxis. The risk factors amenable to modification are (1) hyperlipidemia, (2) hypertension, (3) smoking, (4) obesity, (5) dietary intake high in calories, total fat, saturated fat, cholesterol, and salt, (6) diabetes, (7) sedentary life-style, and (8) psychosocial stress. Measures should be initiated to eliminate or control these risk factors in every individual, with major emphasis upon the first three.

The question arises of when to initiate risk factor surveillance and control. Currently, the concept of disease prophylaxis has been applied primarily to "coronary-prone" adults, those with identified risk factors, and individuals with evidence of disease. However, control of risk factors earlier in life seems more likely to prevent atherogenesis or retard disease progression so that a substantive reduction in cardiac morbidity and mortality can be achieved. The emphasis must be upon health education with early detection and control of risk factors rather than upon treatment of the clinical sequelae of established disease.

Treatment

Ischemia and infarction

General principles

The therapeutic aim with myocardial ischemia is to correct the imbalance between myocardial oxygen de-

mand and oxygen supply. Restoration of oxygen balance can be accomplished by two mechanisms: reduction of oxygen demand and elevation of oxygen supply (see Table 27-5).

To reduce oxygen demand, the physiologic variables determining myocardial oxygen requirements must be controlled. Three major determinants of oxygen demand are amenable to therapy: (1) heart rate, (2) contractile force, and (3) afterload (arterial pressure and ventricular size). Reducing heart rate, force of contraction, arterial pressure, and ventricular size reduces cardiac work and oxygen demand.

Nitroglycerin, the therapeutic mainstay for reversal of ischemia, relieves angina primarily by peripheral vasodilation of the arterial and venous beds and secondarily by improving the distribution of coronary blood flow to ischemic areas. Arterial vasodilation reduces arterial pressure, thereby decreasing the systemic resistance to ventricular ejection and afterload. Dilation of the veins increases the capacity of the venous bed with pooling of blood in the periphery. As a result, venous return to the heart falls, decreasing ventricular volume and ventricular size. Thus, peripheral vasodilation reduces preload. Consequently, oxygen demand is reduced. Long-acting nitrites, still the subject of controversy, exhibit similar effects.

Propranolol (Inderal), a beta-adrenergic blocking agent, interrupts ischemia by selectively inhibiting the effects of the sympathetic nervous system upon the

TABLE 27-5

MEDICAL THERAPY OF MYOCARDIAL ISCHEMIA

1. Reduction of oxygen demand
   a. Pharmacologic reduction in cardiac work
      (1) Nitroglycerin
      (2) Nitrites
      (3) Propranolol (Inderal)
      (4) Digitalis
      (5) Diuretics
      (6) Vasodilators
      (7) Sedatives
      (8) Calcium antagonists
   b. Physical reduction in cardiac work
      (1) Bed rest
      (2) Restful environment
2. Increment in oxygen supply
   a. Nitroglycerin
   b. Oxygen administration
   c. Vasopressors
   d. Antiarrhythmics
   e. Anticoagulants and fibrinolytic agents
   f. Calcium antagonists

heart; these effects are mediated by beta receptors. Beta stimulation increases heart rate and force of contraction. Propranolol blocks these effects, reducing heart rate and force of contraction and thereby diminishing myocardial oxygen requirements. The reduced contractile force does produce a mild increment in ventricular size by lowering stroke volume. However, in the absence of heart failure, this slight increment in oxygen demand is greatly outweighed by the reduced demand prompted by blockade of the sympathetic effects upon heart rate and contractility.

Digitalis can relieve angina associated with heart failure by increasing the force of contraction and, as a result, stroke volume. As ventricular emptying increases, ventricular size is reduced. Despite the increased oxygen demand associated with increased contractile force, the net effect of digitalization in heart failure is a reduction of myocardial oxygen demand.

Other pharmacologic interventions similarly act upon the determinants of myocardial oxygen demand to correct the oxygenation imbalance. Diuretics reduce blood volume and venous return to the heart, thereby reducing ventricular volume and size. Vasodilators or antihypertensive agents decrease arterial pressure and resistance to ventricular ejection. Consequently, afterload is diminished. Sedatives and antidepressants can also reduce angina induced by stress or depression.

The impaired ability of the diseased coronary vasculature to dilate and increase blood flow limits the available therapeutic measures to increase coronary oxygen supply. Although nitroglycerin is known to dilate the major epicardial branches of the coronary circulation, total coronary blood flow does not increase. However, nitroglycerin does improve flow to the ischemic area apparently by vasodilation of collateral vessels.

Two potential consequences of myocardial dysfunction that can further the reduction in myocardial oxygen supply are hypoxemia and hypotension. In the setting of hypoxemia, oxygen administration can increase the oxygen content of arterial blood and, consequently, myocardial oxygen delivery. Hypotension reduces coronary perfusion pressure. This is particularly worrisome because diseased coronary vessels, unable to dilate to increase flow, are "pressure-dependent" to maintain flow. A reduction in coronary perfusion pressure can perpetuate the ischemic imbalance. Therefore, vasopressors to maintain arterial pressure or volume administration to maintain adequate ventricular filling pressures and stroke volume may be indicated. Arrhythmias can also adversely affect coronary perfusion by reducing cardiac output and arterial pressure; therefore, antiarrhythmics may be beneficial.

The value of anticoagulants and fibrinolytic agents, such as streptokinase, in the prevention or dissolution of coronary thrombi and protection of myocardium remains the subject of much controversy. The use of calcium antagonists to relax vascular smooth muscle and relieve angina due to coronary spasm is under investigation.

After myocardial infarction, rest is the primary therapeutic principle. The objectives are to allow for healing of the infarcted tissue, thus reducing the incidence of complications, and to salvage the ischemic zone surrounding the infarct, thereby reducing the ultimate size of the infarct.

Revascularization

The aim of revascularization is to increase the blood flow and oxygen supply to ischemic regions beyond an obstructive coronary arterial lesion. Two techniques are currently utilized: saphenous vein bypass graft and internal mammary artery bypass graft.

The technique of saphenous vein bypass grafting involves anastomosing a reversed segment of the saphenous vein to the ascending aorta and to the coronary artery beyond the area of obstruction (see Fig. 27-25). Thus, a vascular conduit is created to shunt blood around the lesion to the ischemic myocardium. Internal mammary artery grafting requires anastomosis of the distal segment of the internal mammary artery to the coronary artery.

Vein bypass grafting is the more common procedure. However, a small proportion of these grafts gradually occlude as a result of a fibrous overgrowth of the intimal wall of the vein. It is postulated that this process of fibrous intimal hyperplasia might be the result of subjecting a vein to arterial pressures. Although the internal mammary artery does not seem vulnerable to the same incidence of occlusion, certain disadvantages are associated with this procedure relative to vein bypass grafts. For example, the anterior anatomic location of the internal mammary artery limits its application to lesions of the left anterior descending artery and proximal lesions of other vessels. In addition, the diameter of the vessel is smaller, limiting blood flow.

The indications for revascularization are not standardized nor is the precise impact of surgical intervention upon the natural history of coronary artery disease known. However, the following indications seem to warrant surgical intervention: (1) disabling angina refractory to medical therapy, (2) unstable or preinfarction angina (i.e., recurrent angina at rest despite maximal medical therapy), (3) ongoing ischemia after myocardial infarction, and (4) lesions threatening major portions of the myocardial wall (i.e., main left coronary artery lesions). Early revascularization after myocardial infarction to salvage the ischemic zone surrounding the infarct is the subject of speculation, as is the value of

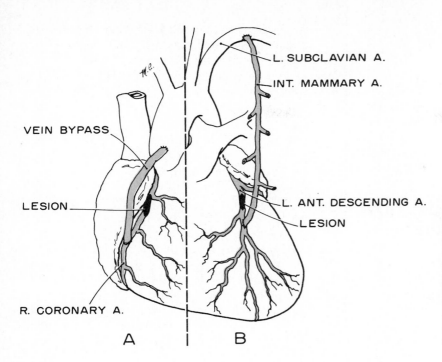

FIGURE 27-25
Coronary artery revascularization procedures. (A) Saphenous vein bypass graft. The vein is sutured to the ascending aorta and to the right coronary artery at a point distal to the blockage so that flow distal to the blockage is again established. (B) In the internal mammary artery procedure, the internal mammary artery is shown anastomosed to the anterior descending branch of the left coronary artery, bypassing the lesion.

surgery in cardiogenic shock. It must be emphasized that revascularization cannot reverse necrosis; only ischemic areas of myocardium benefit from the increased blood flow and oxygen supply.

Prior to revascularization, cardiac catheterization is necessary to determine the location and extent of disease. The following findings characterize operable disease: (1) a bypassable lesion (i.e., one located proximally in the artery), (2) a significant or "high-grade" lesion (i.e., one obstructing over 75 percent of the vessel lumen), and (3) a patent distal vessel, which ensures a site beyond the lesion to which to anastomose the graft. Revascularization is performed in some patients with endarterectomy of the distal bed if diffuse distal disease is noted. Endarterectomy is the removal of the inner atherosclerotic core of the vascular lumen.

At the time of catheterization, the function of the left ventricle is also assessed. The success of surgery seems to correlate most directly with two factors: the degree of left ventricular dysfunction and the magnitude of flow achieved through the bypass graft.

Angioplasty

Percutaneous transluminal coronary angioplasty (PTCA) is currently used for the treatment of coronary atherosclerosis. A narrow catheter with a radiopaque, inflatable balloon mounted on the tip is inserted percutaneously or through a small incision into a peripheral artery. The catheter is threaded via the aorta into the coronary artery to the atherosclerotic lesion using fluoroscopic guidance. The balloon, once in the appropriate position relative to the lesion, is inflated for a moment in an attempt to dilate the coronary lumen (see Fig. 27-26). The histologic mechanism for this dilation includes compression and splitting of the atherosclerotic plaque, as well as stretching and disruption of the arterial wall layers.

Patient selection for PTCA is usually confined to those individuals with discrete atherosclerotic lesions in proximal coronary locations which are easily accessible to the balloon-dilating catheter. This procedure is generally limited to select patients with angina refractory to maximal medical therapy. If dilation is unsuccessful or complications arise, revascularization of the coronary artery is undertaken.

Fibrinolytic therapy

Acute reperfusion of an acutely occluded coronary artery has gained widespread interest in recent years. This interest has stemmed from the realization that reducing the ultimate size of acute myocardial infarction is associated with improved prognosis.

Based on the premise that acute myocardial infarction is caused by coronary thrombosis in the majority of cases, interventions have been aimed at dissolving coronary thrombi soon after the onset of acute infarction. A time frame of 3 to 5 hours has been the limiting factor for the application of these interventions because permanent myocardial necrosis will occur if coronary reperfusion is not carried out before such permanent damage occurs.

The mainstay of acute coronary reperfusion rests with a group of agents called *fibrinolytics*. These agents activate the fibrinolytic system, thereby producing clot lysis. The agents include such drugs as streptokinase, urokinase, and tissue plasminogen activator.

The basic mechansim of action of these agents is to induce fibrinolysis. By various mechanisms, these agents promote the conversion of plasminogen to plasmin, a proteolytic enzyme capable of lysing fibrin clot. By fibrin degradation induced by plasmin, clot lysis occurs, and flow is reestablished to the acutely occluded coronary artery. Angioplasty may be performed in conjunction with fibrinolytic therapy to reduce occurrence of rethrombosis. After the conclusion of fibrinolytic therapy, anticoagulation is usually carried out to prevent rethrombosis.

Complications

General principles

Early detection and prevention of complications is of utmost importance. Two categories of complications must be anticipated: electrical instability or arrhythmias and mechanical dysfunction or pump failure. Electrocardiographic monitoring is initiated immediately. Arrhythmia management follows logical principles:

1. Tachycardias are decelerated by parasympathetic stimulation (e.g., carotid sinus massage), antiar-

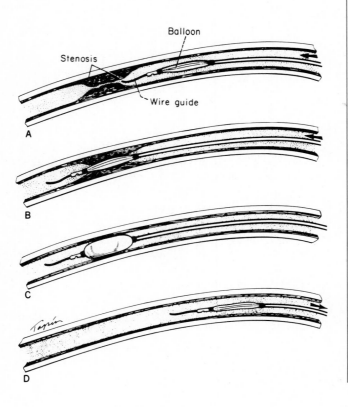

rhythmic drugs, or electrical cardioversion, if necessary. Bradycardias can be accelerated by drugs that either stimulate sympathetic beta receptors (such as propranolol) or inhibit parasympathetic effects (such as atropine). Electrical pacing may be indicated if hemodynamic deterioration is pronounced and drugs are ineffective.

2. "Escape beats," which result from sinus node failure, must be differentiated from "premature beats" to effectively treat rhythm disturbances originating in sites other than the sinus node. To treat escape rhythms, drugs are administered to speed the normal pacemaker, the sinus node; obviously, drugs must not be given to suppress the escape pacemaker, since cardiac standstill could result.

   Ventricular arrhythmias usually respond to antiarrhythmic agents such as lidocaine (Xylocaine) and procainamide. Ventricular fibrillation requires immediate defibrillation with cardiopulmonary resuscitative maneuvers. The management of refractory ventricular arrhythmias will be reviewed in the next section.

   Atrial arrhythmias are best controlled by administering an antiarrhythmic drug, such as quinidine, to suppress the irritability. Digoxin administration is required with atrial tachycardias to slow conduction through the AV node and control the ventricular rate response. This combination of drugs may convert the abnormal rhythm to a normal one. Electrical cardioversion may be indicated to restore the normal rhythm if the arrhythmia persists and is poorly tolerated.

3. Therapy of heart block is directed at restoring or simulating normal conduction, either through the administration of drugs speeding conduction and heart rate, such as atropine or isoproterenol (Isuprel), or by electrical pacing.

Mechanical dysfunction produces a clinical spectrum ranging from mild congestive heart failure to cardiogenic shock. Congestive heart failure prompts efforts to (1) reduce intravascular volume and congestion and associated fluid transudation, (2) improve myocardial function, and (3) reduce cardiac work. Mild to moderate congestive heart failure is managed with restrictions of salt intake, and with diuretics, digitalis, and rest. The

FIGURE 27-26

Schematic drawing of percutaneous transluminal angioplasty. The catheter is positioned proximal to the stenosis (A) and then passed through the stenotic segment so that the dilation balloon lies within the area of stenosis (B). The balloon is inflated (C), deflated, and (D) removed; repeat angiography is performed to evaluate the size of the improved lumen. (From Johnson, Haber, and Austen, 1980, p. 426.)

development of pulmonary edema necessitates the addition of more aggressive measures. Morphine, in addition to its sedative and respiratory depressant effects, dilates the periphery with pooling of blood in the veins and reduction in venous return. The administration of vasodilators, such as nitroglycerin or sodium nitroprusside (Nipride), to reduce the resistance to ejection may be indicated to facilitate ventricular emptying. Severe pulmonary edema may require the application of rotating tourniquets or rarely phlebotomy, the withdrawal of 100 to 500 ml of blood, to reduce the volume overload. Aminophylline can be administered to relieve associated bronchospasm and, secondarily, to increase cardiac output by increasing contractile force. Administration of oxygen and possibly mechanical ventilation are required to correct hypoxemia.

Progression of left ventricular dysfunction to cardiogenic shock, characterized by inadequate tissue perfusion, is an ominous development. This syndrome, with a mortality approaching 100 percent, remains a therapeutic dilemma. Efforts are directed at the maintenance of tissue perfusion and the simultaneous reduction of cardiac work. Vasopressors are frequently needed to maintain arterial pressure. Metabolic acidosis, caused by lactic acid accumulation, must be reversed by the administration of sodium bicarbonate. Emergency intraaortic balloon pumping may be indicated.

Pacing therapy

The utilization of pacemakers has become increasingly sophisticated. Both temporary and permanent, implantable pulse generators have been developed with a variety of pacing characteristics. Current pulse generators are capable of pacing either the atria or the ventricles, or pacing both atria and ventricles in a sequential fashion. Pacing stimuli can be delivered in demand or fixed-rate modes. Demand pacing can be further classified according to two modes of response: (1) inhibited and (2) triggered. In the inhibited mode, the pacer shuts off when an intrinsic cardiac impulse is sensed. In the triggered mode, the pacer fires during the refractory period of the sensed beat, without generating a paced beat. By contrast, fixed-rate pacing delivers a stimulus at a predetermined, fixed rate. An international classification system has been developed to standardize pacemaker coding (see Fig. 27-27).

Management of refractory ventricular arrhythmias

The presence of recurrent, malignant ventricular arrhythmias unresponsive to standard pharmacologic therapy is an indication for electrophysiologic (EP) evaluation. Such arrhythmias are usually seen in the setting of chronic ischemic heart disease. Ventricular aneu-

FIGURE 27-27
Three-letter identification code presently in international use. (From Johnson, Haber, and Austen, 1980, p. 233.)

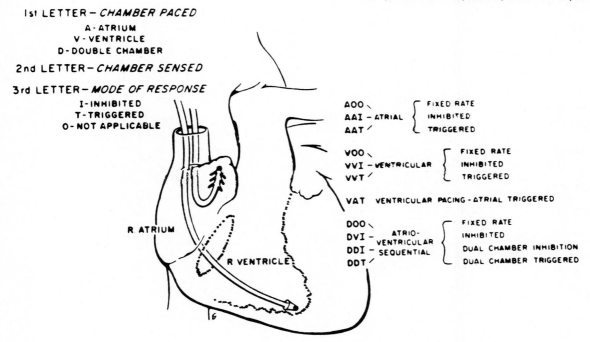

rysms or previous ventricular surgery may predispose to the development of refractory ventricular arrhythmias.

The purposes of EP testing are to identify an effective drug regimen to control the arrhythmia and/or to localize the arrhythmogenic site. Prior to the initial EP study, all antiarrhythmic drugs are discontinued if at all possible. Catheters with multiple electrodes are then positioned within the heart under fluoroscopic guidance (see Fig. 26-15 for catheter placement). A stimulation protocol is followed to induce ventricular tachycardia (VT); this programmed stimulation can consist of progressively more premature ventricular stimuli, double ventricular extra-stimuli, or bursts of rapid ventricular pacing. Intracardiac recordings of the arrhythmia are obtained. The arrhythmia is terminated with another burst of rapid ventricular pacing or countershock if required.

Upon completion of the study, a transvenous right ventricular pacing catheter is left in place for serial testing. Oral or intravenous antiarrhythmic drugs are then administered alone or in combination. After adequate blood levels of the drugs are achieved, programmed electrical stimulation is repeated to determine whether or not the arrhythmia can be induced. If conventional antiarrhythmics—quinidine, procainamide, disopyramide, phenytoin, propranolol—are not effective, then investigational drugs such as mexiletine or amiodarone may be tried until an optimal regimen is identified on which the tachycardia can no longer be induced or is slowed.

If drug trials are ineffective, alternative therapies, such as pacemaker therapy or surgery, are considered. Electrode catheter ablation or implantation of an automatic implantable defibrillator can be used in some highly selected cases.

Two basic mechanisms of pacemaker therapy have been identified. The first, "overdrive suppression," is used to prevent the occurrence of the arrhythmia. With overdrive pacing, the pacer stimulates the heart at a rate slightly faster than its intrinsic rate, thus suppressing the arrhythmogenic focus. This is most effective if the underlying heart rate is relatively slow. The second type of pacing is "interruption pacing," whereby the pacer delivers a brief burst of rapid ventricular pacing to interrupt the reentrant pathway or suppress the site of arrhythmia origin once the arrhythmia occurs.

Surgery is the third therapeutic option. The application of surgical techniques to the correction of electrical rather than mechanical abnormalities is still relatively new, yet promising. Surgery has been successfully applied to the treatment of recurrent paroxysmal supraventricular tachycardia due to reentry of the cardiac impulse via an accessory atrioventricular pathway. Figure 27-28 illustrates the surgical technique for division of this anomalous pathway, the Kent bundle, in the treatment of Wolff-Parkinson-White (WPW) syndrome.

FIGURE 27-28
Surgical procedure for treatment of WPW syndrome. The left-hand panel represents a cross section of the left side of the heart at the level of the AV groove. Possible Kent bundle locations are shown in black. Successful surgical ablation of the HIS bundle is accomplished working from inside the atrium through an incision at the annulus. Epicardial structures are pushed back, leaving a denuded left ventricular surface. (From J. D. Fisher, *Progress in Cardiovascular Disease*, 24(1): 63, 1981, p. 63. By permission.)

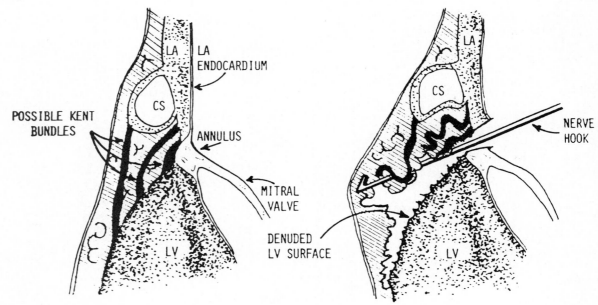

This type of surgery established a precedent for developing surgical approaches for the treatment of refractory arrhythmias.

The potential efficacy of application of recently developed surgical approaches to refractory ventricular tachycardia rests with observations that these arrhythmias seem to originate in the endocardial layer of the left ventricle and are usually due to reentry. Previously, aneurysmectomy or coronary artery bypass grafting were performed alone or in combination, with limited success in the control of refractory ventricular arrhythmias. Now these procedures are commonly performed in conjunction with newer techniques of endocardial resection or encircling endocardial ventriculotomy.

Preoperatively, EP testing is performed in an attempt to localize the origin of the ventricular tachycardia. Intracardiac recordings are obtained from multiple sites within the ventricle after the induction of ventricular tachycardia as described earlier. A "map" of electrical recordings from the surface of the heart is constructed. The recordings are analyzed, and the site evidencing the earliest activation is identified; this site is considered the point of origin of the arrhythmia. This technique is referred to as "cardiac mapping."

Intraoperatively, mapping is repeated. Epicardial mapping can be obtained via a manual probe or fingertip electrode or by using a net containing multiple electrodes for simultaneous recording. Epicardial mapping is not considered to be as accurate a method of localizing the site of origin as is endocardial mapping. Once the ventricle is opened, an endocardial map can be recorded.

Once the site has been localized, the endocardium is resected to eliminate the point of origin of the ventricular tachycardia. If endocardial resection is not possible, an encircling endocardial ventriculotomy may be employed. With this technique, an incision is made around the involved area, usually encompassing an aneurysm or region of endocardial fibrosis. The incision extends through the endocardium to the epicardium, electrically isolating the site from the normal myocardium. The incision is then enclosed with sutures.

Electrode catheter ablation consists of the fluoroscopic placement of a catheter electrode at the endocardial focus of tachycardia which has been previously mapped. A posterior defibrillator paddle is placed, and an electric countershock is delivered through the catheter electrode. This, in effect, ablates the focus of tachycardia, creating a small endocardial infarction.

Surgical repair of mechanical defects

Aneurysmectomy is the removal of the noncontractile, paradoxically bulging scar. There are three indications for aneurysm resection: (1) chronic congestive heart failure, (2) systemic embolization of mural thrombi, and (3) recurrent ventricular arrhythmias.

Aneurysms are associated with a high incidence of malignant, refractory ventricular arrhythmias, perhaps resulting from the persistent mechanical strain at the boundary between the normal myocardium and the scarred, outpouching segment. The aneurysm is excised through the left ventricular scar with removal of mural thrombi. Removal of the aneurysm and subsequent reduction of ventricular size improves the mechanical efficiency of the heart. Intraoperatively, the site causing recurrent ventricular arrhythmias can be localized and excised or sectioned.

A *ventricular septal defect* can be repaired either by simple closure of the hole in the septum or by insertion of a patch graft; access to the septum is gained via the infarct in the ventricle. Upon closure of the left ventricular incision, a portion of the noncontractile left ventricular scar is frequently excised, a procedure referred to as *infarctectomy*.

Dysfunction of the mitral valve resulting from papillary muscle rupture or malfunction necessitates *replacement of the mitral valve* with excision of the papillary muscles.

Cardiac transplantation can be lifesaving for patients considered inoperable or unsalvageable with less aggressive surgical intervention. Patients with end-stage heart disease are considered for cardiac transplantation. The operation involves removal of the diseased heart and replacement with a normal donor heart. Technically, the operation is uncomplicated, requiring reanastomoses of the separated vessels with the donor heart. Cardiac transplantation will be discussed in more detail in Chap. 28.

Rehabilitation

The ultimate goal of therapeutic intervention in coronary atherosclerotic disease is to restore the cardiac patient to a productive and satisfying existence. The long-term consequences of myocardial infarction—physical, psychological, social, and vocational invalidism—have long been ignored with devastating impact. The complications of myocardial disease are not restricted to the hospital setting, nor does the responsibility of health professionals for the ultimate well-being and coping ability of patients terminate upon their discharge from the hospital. As early as clinically feasible, patients should be enrolled in an in-patient cardiovascular rehabilitation program that will continue after hospital discharge.

Cardiac rehabilitation, as defined by the American Heart Association and the Task Force on Cardiovascular Rehabilitation of the National Heart, Lung, and

Blood Institute, is the process of restoring and maintaining the physical, psychological, social, educational, and vocational potentials of the patient.

Patients must be assisted to progressively resume a level of activity consistent with physical limitations and to be relatively unhampered by psychological stressors. Many patients can resume all normal activities. Explicit, individualized patient and family education, covering diet, medications, activity progression, and risk factor reduction/modification, is essential. Every patient and family require guidance and education during the transition from the dependence of illness to the independence of health.

QUESTIONS *Answers begin on pg 1087*

Coronary atherosclerotic disease

Directions: Answer the following questions on a separate sheet of paper.

1. Explain why the left ventricle is most vulnerable to ischemia and infarction.

2. What are the most common sites of coronary arterial occlusion?

3. Name five factors affecting the degree of functional impairment following an acute myocardial infarction.

4. What is a vasovagal response and what might cause this response following an acute myocardial infarction? How does it affect the compensatory response?

5. Name three important diagnostic findings associated with myocardial infarction.

6. Explain hemodynamically why either tachycardias or bradycardias impair cardiac function.

7. Identify three hemodynamic factors which may be modified to reduce oxygen demand in the treatment of myocardial ischemia.

8. Explain why medical efforts to treat myocardial ischemia by increasing coronary blood flow and oxygen supply are of little value.

9. State the primary objective of rest in the treatment of acute myocardial infarction.

10. Describe the treatment of congestive heart failure, pulmonary edema, and cardiogenic shock.

11. Why is rehabilitation an important aspect of the treatment of patients with atherosclerotic heart disease?

Directions: Circle the letter preceding each item below that correctly answers the question. Only one answer is correct unless otherwise noted.

12. The most potent stimulus to increasing coronary blood flow is:
    a. Systemic lactic acidosis   *b.* Local myocardial hypoxia   *c.* Sympathetic stimulation   *d.* Increased arterial pressure

13. In the normal heart, how many times can coronary blood flow increase above resting levels?
    a. 1 to 2   *b.* 5 to 6   *c.* 8 to 10   *d.* 15 to 20

14. The earliest pathologic change apparent in the coronary blood vessel in the development of coronary atherosclerosis is:
    a. Fibrous encapsulation of the lesion   *b.* Fatty streaks in the adventitia   *c.* Fatty streaks in the intima   *d.* Accumulation of β-lipoprotein in the media

15. Myocardial infarction may result from: (More than one answer may be correct.)
    a. Hemorrhage into the coronary atheromatous plaque   *b.* Platelet aggregates in the coronary blood vessel   *c.* Coronary artery spasm   *d.* Embolization of a thrombus or plaque fragment

16. Major modifiable risk factors for coronary atherosclerotic disease include all of the following except:
    a. Hyperlipidemia   *b.* Hypertension   *c.* Family history   *d.* Cigarette smoking

17. Optimal serum cholesterol levels should be no greater than what level to reduce the risk of coronary atherosclerotic disease?
    a. 150 mg per 100 ml   *b.* 200 mg per 100 ml   *c.* 250 mg per 100 ml   *d.* 300 mg per 100 ml

18. A form of angina in which there is ST segment elevation is:
    a. Preinfarction angina   *b.* Prinzmetal's angina   *c.* Dressler's angina   *d.* Unstable angina

19. Which of the following changes does not commonly occur before or during an attack of angina pectoris?
    a. An increase in blood pressure   *b.* A decrease in heart rate   *c.* An increase in myocardial oxygen demand   *d.* An increase in left ventricular end-diastolic pressure   *e.* A decrease in myocardial wall compliance

20. Depressed left ventricular function resulting from an area of ischemia or necrosis always necessitates:
    a. An increase in end-diastolic volume to maintain stroke volume   b. A decrease in end-diastolic volume to maintain stroke volume   c. An increase in heart rate to maintain cardiac output   d. An increase in blood pressure to maintain tissue perfusion

21. Complete occlusion of the left anterior descending coronary artery would result in:
    a. Anterior wall infarct   b. Inferior wall infarct   c. Complete heart block   d. Posterior wall infarct

22. Which of the following functional changes would be least expected in patients with acute myocardial infarction?
    a. A decrease in cardiac output   b. A decrease in left ventricular end-diastolic pressure   c. An increase in pulmonary wedge pressure   d. An increase in the central venous pressure

23. Impending left-sided heart failure following myocardial infarction can be detected earliest by monitoring the:
    a. Systemic blood pressure   b. Central venous pressure   c. Pulmonary wedge pressure   d. Pulse pressure

24. The earliest stage of lung involvement in left ventricular failure is:
    a. Interstitial edema   b. Alveolar edema   c. Pleural effusion   d. Pulmonary congestion

25. In patients who develop cardiogenic shock, the percentage of left ventricular mass which is infarcted is generally at least:
    a. 10 percent   b. 20 percent   c. 40 percent   d. 60 percent

26. Characteristic hemodynamic abnormalities in cardiogenic shock include: (More than one answer may be correct.)
    a. Decreased peripheral perfusion   b. Decreased coronary perfusion   c. Hypotension   d. Decreased cardiac output

27. Left ventricular papillary muscle rupture following myocardial infarction results in: (More than one answer may be correct.)
    a. Mitral regurgitation   b. A systolic murmur   c. A diastolic murmur   d. Death in a high percentage of cases   e. Pulmonary congestion

28. Which of the following statements regarding ventricular rupture is *not* correct?
    a. The peak incidence is during the healing phase of necrotic tissue removal.   b. Rupture is a complication of transmural myocardial infarction.   c. The peak incidence is about 6 weeks following infarction.   d. Rupture is associated with cardiac tamponade.

29. The major effect of cardiac tamponade is to:
    a. Produce atelectasis   b. Distend the pericardium   c. Compress the heart   d. Increase the pulse pressure

30. The myocardial scar following myocardial infarction is well established after approximately:
    a. 3 weeks   b. 6 weeks   c. 3 months   d. 6 months

31. A ventricular aneurysm may give rise to:
    a. Chronic congestive heart failure   b. Systemic emboli   c. Refractory ventricular arrhythmias   d. All of the above

32. The most frequent complication following myocardial infarction is:
    a. Congestive heart failure   b. Cardiogenic shock   c. Left ventricular papillary muscle dysfunction   d. Dressler's syndrome   e. Arrhythmias

33. Factors predisposing to the development of arrhythmias in coronary atherosclerotic disease are: (More than one answer may be correct.)
    a. Myocardial ischemia   b. Lactic acidosis   c. Hypokalemia   d. Digitalis toxicity

34. An ectopic beat may originate in all of the following sites except:
    a. Atria   b. Ventricles   c. AV junctional tissue   d. SA node

35. Which of the following is the most common arrhythmia associated with myocardial infarction?
    a. Atrial tachycardia   b. Atrial fibrillation   c. Ventricular premature beats   d. Ventricular fibrillation   e. Left bundle branch block

36. Left bundle branch block results in:
    a. Absence of all P waves   b. Absence of every other P wave   c. Prolongation of the PR interval   d. Widening of the QRS complex

37. Which of the following drugs used for the treatment of myocardial ischemia improve cardiac function by decreasing arterial resistance to ventricular ejection? (More than one answer may be correct.)
    a. Propranolol   b. Digitalis   c. Diuretics   d. Vasodilators   e. Nitroglycerin

38. Which sign or symptom would occur latest in the course of left-sided heart failure?
    a. Orthopnea   b. Lung congestion   c. Decreased urine output   d. Distended neck veins

39. Factors which result from and compound the problem of myocardial ischemia include: (More than one answer may be correct.)

a. Hypoxemia   *b.* Hypotension   *c.* Arrhythmias   *d.* Acidosis

40. Which of the following statements concerning atherosclerotic heart disease is not true?
a. Lesion precursors may be found in children and young adults.   *b.* The disease begins abruptly in susceptible middle-aged adults.   *c.* It is the leading cause of death in the United States.   *d.* Hypertension, hyperlipidemia, and smoking are major predisposing factors.

41. The arrhythmia with the least effective ventricular action is:
a. Atrial flutter   *b.* Ventricular tachycardia   *c.* Ventricular fibrillation   *d.* Complete heart block

42. Which of the following ECG monitor strip tracings is typical of second-degree heart block?
a. P waves without a QRS complex   *b.* PR interval longer than 0.2 second   *c.* Widening of the QRS complex   *d.* Inversion of the T wave

43. Pacemakers are *not* used to:
a. Suppress ventricular ectopic beats   *b.* Suppress sinus tachycardia   *c.* Treat third-degree heart block   *d.* Treat sinus bradycardia

44. Coronary bypass surgery is generally indicated for patients with:
a. Preinfarction angina   *b.* Cardiogenic shock   *c.* Stable angina pectoris   *d.* Acute myocardial infarction   *e.* Ventricular aneurysm

45. The removal of an atherosclerotic plaque in coronary atherosclerotic disease is called:
a. Infarctectomy   *b.* Endarterectomy   *c.* Septal defect repair   *d.* Aneurysmectomy

Directions: Circle T if the statement is true and F if it is false. Correct the false statements.

46. T   F   Atherosclerotic heart disease is more common in diabetics than in nondiabetics.

47. T   F   In postmyocardial infarction syndrome (Dressler's syndrome), the pain is characteristic of pericarditis rather than of infarction.

48. T   F   An internal mammary artery bypass graft is associated with a significant incidence of subintimal fibrous hyperplasia.

49. T   F   Ventricular hypertrophy decreases myocardial oxygen demand.

50. T   F   Escape beats are caused by myocardial tissue irritability.

Directions: Fill in the blanks with the correct word or circle the correct word.

51. In myocardial infarction, an area of _____ surrounds the area of infarction.

52. A reduction in ventricular wall compliance (increases) (decreases) pressure for a constant ventricular volume.

53. Arrange in correct order the following changes that occur after an acute myocardial infarction.
a. Removal of necrotic tissue   *b.* Bruised and cyanotic tissue   *c.* Scar formation   *d.* Polymorphonuclear neutrophil infiltration

Directions: Match the characteristics in col. A with the disorders in col. B.

Column A

54. ____ ST segment depression is typical

55. ____ ST segment elevation is typical

56. ____ Deep Q waves

57. ____ Pain relieved by nitroglycerin

58. ____ Muscle death

59. ____ Muscle hypoxia

60. ____ If prolonged, results in necrosis

61. ____ Reversible

62. ____ Irreversible

Column B

a. Myocardial ischemia
b. Myocardial infarction

Directions: Match the type of heart block in col. A with the ECG pattern in col. B.

Column A

63. ____ First-degree heart block

64. ____ Wenckebach or Mobitz I block

Column B

a. No impulses conducted
b. All impulses conducted with prolonged PR interval
c. Some impulses nonconducted in repetitive pattern with progressive prolongation of the PR interval

65. ____ Mobitz II block

66. ____ Complete heart block

d. Some impulses nonconducted but conducted impulses have a constant PR interval

Directions: Match each of the arrhythmias in col. A to its possible therapeutic intervention in col. B.

Column A

67. ____ Sinus bradycardia

68. ____ Atrial tachycardia

69. ____ Multiple premature ventricular beats

70. ____ Ventricular fibrillation

Column B

a. Carotid sinus massage

b. Defibrillation

c. Lidocaine

d. Atropine

Directions: Match each of the drugs used to treat coronary atherosclerotic disease in col. A with its effect in col. B.

Column A

71. ____ Propranolol

72. ____ Lidocaine

73. ____ Atropine

74. ____ Nitroglycerin

75. ____ Digitalis

Column B

a. Suppression of ventricular irritability

b. Increased heart rate

c. Decrease of heart rate and force of contraction

d. Increase of force of myocardial contraction

e. Vasodilation of coronary collaterals and peripheral vessels

Directions: Circle the letter preceding each item that correctly answers the question. Only one answer is correct unless otherwise noted.

76. A decreased risk of developing coronary heart disease is believed to be associated with an elevation of:
a. LDL   b. HDL   c. VLDL   d. Chylomicrons

77. In untreated familial hypercholesterolemia the probability of developing premature atherosclerosis before the age of 50 years is approximately:
a. 10 percent   b. 30 percent   c. 50 percent
d. 70 percent

78. Patterns or types of hyperlipoproteinemias associated with premature atherosclerosis include which of the following? (More than one answer may be correct.)
a. I   b. II   c. III   d. IV   e. V

79. Initial treatment of primary hyperlipidemia will most likely include all the following measures except:
a. Restriction of alcohol   b. Restriction of saturated fats   c. Clofibrate   d. Weight reduction

80. Which of the following statements is *not* true regarding hypertension?
a. Approximately 25 percent of the adult population is hypertensive   b. A lower prevalence of hypertension is found among blacks   c. A clearcut increase in the risk of coronary heart disease is associated with hypertension   d. The usual course of hypertensive disease involves an asymptomatic latent period of many years duration

81. All the following statements concerning the pathophysiology of essential hypertension are true *except*:
a. The primary hemodynamic alteration in essential hypertension is an increased vascular resistance.   b. Left ventricular ejection pressure is increased secondary to the increased vascular resistance.   c. Myocardial hypertrophy increases myocardial oxygen demand.   d. Excessive salt intake has been demonstrated to have no significant role in the development of essential hypertension.

82. An elevation of which of the following enzymes is the most specific indication of a myocardial infarction?
a. GOT or SGOT   b. CK   c. LDH
d. MB-CK

83. All the following functional changes would be expected following a transmural myocardial infarction of the anterior myocardial wall except:
a. Increased left ventricular end-systolic and end-diastolic volume   b. Increased left ventricular end-diastolic pressure   c. Increased ejection fraction   d. Decreased contractility

84. Which of the following statements is false concerning the reentry phenomenon?
a. Reentry is the most common mechanism producing a premature beat.   b. The reentry mechanism refers to increased automaticity.   c. One or more areas in the heart where the refractory period is longer than others may account for the reentry phenomenon.   d. The reentry mechanism explains the temporal dependence of certain ectopic beats.

VALVULAR HEART DISEASE

OBJECTIVES

At the completion of this chapter you should be able to:

1. Identify the characteristics of normal valvular function, including the mechanism of opening and closure.
2. Describe the functional effects of valvular stenosis and regurgitation.
3. Identify and briefly describe five causes of valvular heart disease.
4. Compare the frequency of lesions for the four heart valves.
5. Describe the pathogenesis of valvular damage in rheumatic fever.
6. List the major and minor manifestations of acute rheumatic fever according to the revised Jones criteria.
7. Describe the morphologic changes in valvular stenosis and regurgitation.
8. Define functional regurgitation.
9. Describe the pathophysiology of the following valvular disorders: mitral stenosis and regurgitation, aortic stenosis and regurgitation, tricuspid stenosis and regurgitation.
10. Indicate and contrast the auscultatory, electrocardiographic, roentgenographic, and hemodynamic findings for the valvular disorders listed in objective 9.
11. Describe the etiology and functional disturbances in pulmonic valvular disease.
12. Predict and give examples of functional alterations resulting from compound valvular lesions.
13. Describe the preventive therapy for rheumatic fever and bacterial endocarditis.
14. Describe the medical therapy for mitral valve disease.
15. Define mitral commissurotomy.
16. Describe the indications, contraindications, and surgical procedure for a mitral commissurotomy and a mitral valve replacement.
17. Explain how a ball and cage prosthetic heart valve operates.
18. Explain why prompt surgical intervention is important after the onset of symptoms in the treatment of aortic stenosis.
19. Indicate the surgical treatment of aortic stenosis and regurgitation.

Valvular disease causes abnormalities in blood flow across the cardiac valves. Normal valves demonstrate two critical flow characteristics: unidirectional flow and unimpeded flow. The valves open when the pressure in the chamber proximal to the valve exceeds the pressure in the chamber or vessel beyond the valve. Closure occurs when the pressure beyond the valve exceeds pressure in the proximal chamber. For instance, the atrioventricular valves open when atrial pressures exceed ventricular pressures and close when ventricular pressures exceed atrial pressures. The valve leaflets are so responsive that even a slight pressure difference (less than 1 mmHg) between chambers will open and close the leaflets.

A diseased valve can produce two types of functional derangements: (1) *valvular regurgitation*—the valve leaflets fail to close securely, permitting backward flow (*valvular insufficiency* and *valvular incompetence* are synonymous terms); and (2) *valvular stenosis*—the valve orifice becomes restricted, impeding forward flow. Regurgitation and stenosis can occur together in the same valve as a "mixed lesion," or either one can occur alone as a "pure lesion."

Valvular dysfunction increases cardiac work. Valvular regurgitation forces the heart to pump the additional regurgitant volume of blood, thus producing an increment in *volume work*. Valvular stenosis necessitates the generation of increased pressure to overcome the increased resistance to flow, thereby elevating *pressure work*. The characteristic myocardial responses to volume work and pressure work are, respectively, chamber dilation and muscular hypertrophy. Myocardial dilation and hypertrophy are compensatory mechanisms intended to increase the pumping capability of the heart.

PATHOGENESIS

Valvular heart disease was once considered to be almost entirely rheumatic in origin. Despite the declining incidence of rheumatic fever, rheumatic damage is still the most common cause of valvular deformity requiring surgical correction. Acute rheumatic fever is a sequel of a group A beta-hemolytic streptococcal pharyngitis. Rheumatic fever develops only if a significant immunologic or antibody response to the antecedent streptococcal infection occurs. Approximately 3 percent of pharyngeal streptococcal infections are followed within 2 to 4 weeks by attacks of rheumatic fever. Initial attacks of rheumatic fever are typically observed during childhood and the early teenage years. The incidence of streptococcal infection, and therefore of rheumatic fever, is directly related to factors predisposing to the development and transmission of infection; socioeconomic factors, such as living conditions and access to medical care and antibiotic therapy, are foremost in this regard.

The precise pathogenesis of rheumatic fever is unknown. Two possible mechanisms are (1) a hyperimmune response, either autoimmune or allergic in nature, and (2) a direct effect of the streptococcal organism or its toxins. An immunologic explanation is considered most plausible, although the latter mechanism cannot be entirely ruled out. An autoimmune reaction to a streptococcal infection would hypothetically produce tissue damage, or manifestations of rheumatic disease, as follows: (1) group A streptococcus would produce pharyngeal infection, (2) streptococcal antigen would result in antibody production in a hyperimmune host, (3) antibodies would react with the streptococcal antigen and with host tissues that are antigenically similar to streptococcus (i.e., antibodies are unable to distinguish streptococcal antigen from cardiac tissue antigen), and (4) autoantibodies reacting with host tissues would produce tissue damage.

Whatever the pathogenesis of this disease, the presentation of acute rheumatic fever is that of a diffuse, inflammatory process affecting the connective tissue of many organs, particularly the heart, joints, and skin. Signs and symptoms are nonspecific and include fever, migratory arthritis, arthralgia, skin rash, chorea, and tachycardia. Cardiac involvement is most significant for two reasons: (1) mortality during the acute phase, although extremely low, is attributed exclusively to cardiac failure; and (2) residual disability results primarily from valvular deformity.

Acute rheumatic fever can produce inflammation of all cardiac layers, referred to as *pancarditis*. Endocardial inflammation typically involves the valvular endothelium, causing leaflet swelling and erosion of the cusp edges. Beadlike vegetations are deposited along the leaflet borders (see Fig. 28-1). These acute changes may interfere with effective valve closure, producing valvular regurgitation; stenosis is not encountered as an acute lesion. The appearance of a murmur is the most common clinical manifestation of acute valvular involvement.

With myocardial involvement, characteristic nodular lesions, referred to as *Aschoff's bodies*, appear in the cardiac walls. Myocarditis may result in cardiac enlargement or congestive heart failure; however, clinical progression to failure is unusual during initial attacks. When present, failure is usually associated with concomitant valvular involvement. Pericarditis, usually observed with myocarditis and valvulitis, is relatively uncommon. An exudative pericarditis with thickening of the pericardial layers is characteristic of acute rheumatic fever. Pericarditis typically presents with a friction rub, although pericardial effusions may develop. Progression to cardiac tamponade is rare.

Initial attacks of rheumatic carditis usually subside

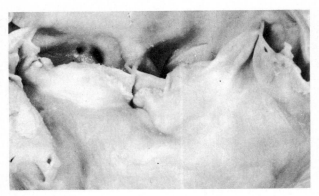

FIGURE 28-1
Acute rheumatic endocarditis of the aortic valve. The vegetations form a beadlike row of deposits which tends to conform to the line of closure. (From J. W. Hurst, *The Heart,* 3d ed., McGraw-Hill, New York, 1974, p. 795.)

with little residual damage. However, recurrent attacks produce progressive valvular deformity. The pathologic changes of chronic rheumatic valvular disease are the product of healing with scar formation, recurrent inflammatory insults, and progressive deformity with hemodynamic stress and aging.

Given the gradual progression of chronic rheumatic valvular disease, symptoms generally do not appear for years after the initial attack; this latent period can last into the third, fourth, or fifth decade. The eventual deformity producing valvular stenosis is characterized by cusp thickening and leaflet fusion along the commissures (the junction between the leaflets). These changes narrow the valvular orifice and reduce leaflet motion, thus producing an obstruction to forward blood flow. The chordae tendineae of the AV valves may also thicken and fuse (see Fig. 28-2) creating a fibrous tunnel below the cusps further impeding flow.

The lesion associated with valvular regurgitation consists of shrunken, retracted cusps that inhibit cusp contact and shortened, fused chordae tendineae that restrain the AV valve leaflets (see Fig. 28-3). These changes impair valve closure, thereby permitting backward flow through the valve.

Calcification and sclerosis of valvular tissue with aging contribute to the ultimate deformity in valves with rheumatic malformation. Chronic disease with ventricular failure and enlargement can also disrupt the function of the AV valves. As the ventricular shape alters, the ability of the papillary muscles to approximate the valvular leaflets during valve closure is reduced. In addition, the valve orifice can enlarge, further compromising valve closure. Valvular regurgitation can result.

This type of valvular regurgitation occurring secondary to chamber enlargement is known as functional regurgitation.

The incidence of valvular disease is highest in the mitral valve, followed by that in the aortic valve. The predominance of left-sided valvular disease is attributed to the relatively greater hemodynamic stress experienced by these valves. It is postulated that hemodynamic stress increases the degree of acquired valvular deformity. The incidence of tricuspid disease is relatively low. Pulmonic disease is rare. Disease of the tricuspid or pulmonic valves is usually associated with other valvular lesions, whereas aortic or mitral disease is frequently seen as an isolated lesion.

In addition to rheumatic disease, other causes of valvular deformity and malfunction are being recognized with increasing frequency. Other significant causes of valvular heart disease are (1) valve destruction by infective endocarditis, (2) inborn defects of connective tissue, (3) dysfunction or rupture of the papillary muscles as a result of coronary atherosclerosis, and (4) congenital malformations.

Infective endocarditis can be caused by many organisms, including bacteria, fungi, and yeast. Bacterial infections are the most common; consequently, the entity is frequently referred to as bacterial endocarditis. Endocarditis may present in an acute or subacute form. Acute endocarditis is due to infection with a highly virulent organism, such as staphylococcus, and typically follows a rapidly fulminating course with early valvular destruction. Normal valves may be affected. Subacute

FIGURE 28-2
Mitral valve viewed from below in a case of mitral stenosis. The valve is converted into a funnel-shaped structure, the apex of which is in the left ventricle. (From J. W. Hurst, *The Heart,* 3d ed., McGraw-Hill, New York, 1974, p. 798.)

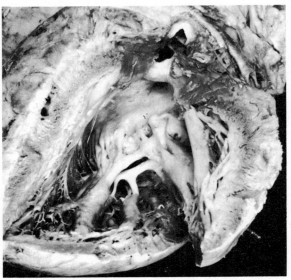

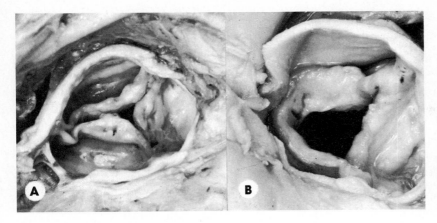

FIGURE 28-3

Two examples of rheumatic endocarditis with aortic insufficiency. (A) The valve leaflets are thickened and shortened to a relatively minor degree. The shortening creates a small triangular-shaped orifice in the center of the aortic valve, which persists during diastole. (B) The aortic valve leaflets are significantly reduced in size, producing a wide triangular-shaped orifice. (From J. W. Hurst, *The Heart,* 3d ed., McGraw-Hill, New York, 1974, p. 803.).

bacterial endocarditis (abbreviated SBE if bacterial in origin) is caused by organisms of less virulence, such as streptococci, and has a more gradual presentation and course. Nonspecific signs and symptoms, including fever, joint pain, myalgias, and skin manifestations, are commonly reported. Typically, valves with preexisting abnormalities or mechanical prosthetics are involved. Endocarditis produces vegetations along the cusp edges; vegetations may extend to involve the valve and even the myocardium. Subsequently, the cusps may fibrose, erode, or perforate, causing valvular dysfunction which is typically regurgitant in nature.

Mitral valve prolapse is a congenital syndrome characterized by redundancy of the valve leaflets and elongation of the chordae tendineae. The cusps prolapse or balloon into the atrium to varying degrees during ventricular systole; mitral regurgitation may or may not result. These functional changes are due to alterations in the collagen structure of the cusp. The exact incidence of mitral valve prolapse is not known; it has been reported to be as high as 28 percent in women. The course of this syndrome can be benign although endocarditis prophylaxis is usually indicated.

Papillary muscle dysfunction or rupture can lead to a wide spectrum of valvular dysfunction. Papillary muscle abnormalities may be intermittent, secondary to ischemia, and may produce only episodic mild regurgitation. However, if rupture of a necrotic papillary muscle occurs, acute mitral regurgitation results. Acute mitral regurgitation is poorly tolerated.

Congenital malformations can occur in any valve. For example, approximately 1 to 2 percent of aortic valves are bicuspid rather than tricuspid in structure.

Certain valvular lesions strongly suggest the underlying cause of dysfunction. For example, isolated mitral stenosis is usually rheumatic in origin, whereas isolated aortic stenosis usually results from premature calcification of a congenitally bicuspid valve. Isolated tricuspid or pulmonic disease is almost invariably a congenital defect. Combined valvular lesions suggest rheumatic causation.

PATHOPHYSIOLOGY

Mitral stenosis

Mitral stenosis impedes blood flow from the left atrium to the left ventricle during ventricular diastole (see Fig. 28-4). To adequately fill the ventricle and maintain cardiac output, the left atrium must generate more pressure to propel blood beyond the valvular obstruction. Therefore the pressure difference, or pressure gradient, between the chambers rises; normally the pressure gradient is minimal.

The left atrial musculature hypertrophies to increase its pumping force. The active contribution of atrial contraction to ventricular filling becomes increasingly important. The primary function of the left atrium ceases to be that of a passive reservoir and conduit for blood flowing to the ventricle. Atrial dilation occurs as the left atrial volume rises owing to the inability of the chamber to empty normally.

The rise in left atrial pressure and volume is reflected backward into the pulmonary vasculature—pressure in the pulmonary veins and capillaries rises. A spectrum of pulmonary congestion, ranging from mild venous congestion to interstitial edema with occasional fluid transudation into the alveoli, results.

Eventually, pulmonary arterial pressure must rise in response to the chronic elevation of pulmonary venous resistance. This response ensures an adequate pressure gradient for blood flow through the pulmonary vasculature. However, pulmonary hypertension increases the resistance to right ventricular ejection into the pulmonary artery. The right ventricle responds to this increased pressure work with muscular hypertrophy.

Gradually, the pulmonary vasculature undergoes anatomic changes apparently designed to protect the pulmonary capillaries from excessively high right ventricular pressures and pulmonary flow. The mechanism mediating this anatomic response is unclear. Structural changes—medial hypertrophy and intimal thickening—occur in the walls of the small arteries and arterioles.

415

These changes narrow the vessel lumen, elevating pulmonary vascular resistance. Pulmonary pressure can progressively climb to systemic levels.

The right ventricle is ill-suited to perform as a high-pressure pump over long periods of time. Therefore, the right ventricle eventually fails as a pump. Right ventricular failure is reflected backward into the systemic circulation, producing systemic venous congestion and peripheral edema. The right-sided failure can be compounded by functional regurgitation of the tricuspid valve as a result of right ventricular enlargement.

Over a period of years the lesion of mitral stenosis narrows the valve orifice. Symptoms characteristically do not appear until the valve orifice has been reduced by more than 50 percent, from a normal area of 4 to 6 cm^2 to less than 1.5 cm^2. With this degree of valvular restriction, left atrial pressure rises to maintain ventric-

ular filling and cardiac output; consequently, pulmonary venous pressure rises, producing dyspnea. A diastolic heart murmur, indicative of abnormal flow through the restricted orifice, is usually noted much earlier in the course of the disease. Valvular dimensions of 0.5 to 1 cm^2 reflect critical mitral stenosis.

The clinical picture can differ depending upon the underlying hemodynamics; however, the earliest symptom is usually dyspnea on exertion. Two hemodynamic changes associated with exertion are poorly tolerated in mitral stenosis: (1) tachycardia (rapid heart rate) and (2) elevated left atrial pressure. Tachycardia reduces the duration of diastole, the period of ventricular filling from the atria. The duration of diastole is critically important in mitral stenosis because the lesion itself impairs ventricular filling and, consequently, atrial emptying. Therefore, cardiac output is essentially "fixed" and cannot be increased because of the valvular obstruction to blood flow into the ventricle. As ventricular filling time falls with tachycardia, cardiac output is reduced further, and pulmonary congestion increases. The elevation of left atrial pressure with exertion due to increased venous return further compounds the pulmonary congestion. Since forward flow is restricted, the pressure elevation is transmitted backward to the lungs. Thus, dyspnea upon exertion is the result of pulmonary congestion. Weakness and fatigue are also prominent early symptoms as a result of the fixed, and eventually reduced, cardiac output.

As the disease progresses, respiratory symptoms become more pronounced. Susceptibility to pulmonary infection is high. Orthopnea and paroxysmal nocturnal dyspnea at rest may be noted. Transmission of the elevated pulmonary vascular pressures to the bronchial capillaries may result in capillary rupture and mild hemoptysis. Eventually, the lungs become fibrotic and noncompliant. The distribution of blood flow within the lungs shifts. Normally, there is relatively greater perfusion of the lower lobes than of the upper lobes because of the effect of gravity upon blood flow. In mitral stenosis, flow predominates in the upper lobes, presumably as a result of greater pulmonary vascular disease and interstitial edema in the lower lobes.

Atrial fibrillation frequently develops as a result of chronic atrial hypertrophy and dilation. With the onset of atrial fibrillation, severe exacerbation of symptoms can occur. The quivering atrial musculature is incapable of coordinated muscular contraction. This loss of the active "atrial kick" reduces ventricular filling. Ventricular filling is further reduced by the rapid ventricular

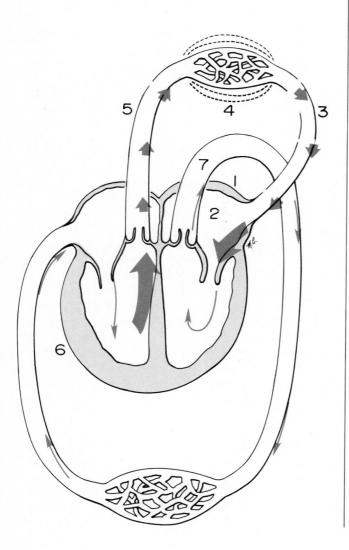

FIGURE 28-4

Pathophysiology of mitral stenosis: 1, left atrial hypertrophy; 2, left atrial dilatation; 3, pulmonary venous congestion; 4, pulmonary congestion; 5, pulmonary hypertension; 6, right ventricular hypertrophy; 7, fixed cardiac output.

response to atrial fibrillation (heart rates approximate 150 bpm unless treated). The abrupt onset of rapid atrial fibrillaiton can result in low cardiac output and pulmonary edema. Hemodynamic adaptation occurs, usually with pharmacologic assistance (i.e., with digoxin). However, the onset of atrial fibrillation exacerbates the risk of thrombus formation and systemic embolization due to stasis of blood in the left atrium proximal to the stenotic valve. Palpitations may also be noted with atrial fibrillation.

End-stage mitral stenosis is associated with right heart failure with consequent systemic venous engorgement, hepatomegaly, peripheral edema, and ascites. Right heart failure and chamber dilation can result in functional tricuspid regurgitation. However, mitral stenosis need not progress to this extreme. With the onset of symptoms, the disease can be managed medically, with eventual surgical correction.

The following findings are commonly noted in mitral stenosis:

1. *Auscultation:* diastolic murmur and accentuated first heart sound (AV valve closure) and opening snap resulting from the loss of leaflet pliability

2. *Electrocardiogram:* left atrial enlargement (widened and notched P wave, known as "P mitrale"), if rhythm is normal sinus; atrial fibrillation; right ventricular hypertrophy

3. *Chest x-ray:* left atrial and right ventricular enlargement; pulmonary venous congestion; interstitial pulmonary edema; pulmonary vascular redistribution to the upper lobes; mitral valve calcification

4. *Hemodynamic findings:* elevated pressure gradient across the mitral valve; elevated left atrial pressure and pulmonary capillary wedge pressure with prominant *a* waves; elevated pulmonary artery pressure; low cardiac output; elevated right-sided heart pressures and jugular venous pressure with significant *v* waves in right atrial trace or jugular veins if tricuspid regurgitation is present

Mitral regurgitation

Mitral regurgitation permits retrograde blood flow from the left ventricle to the left atrium as a result of incomplete valve closure (see Fig. 28-5). During systole, the ventricle simultaneously ejects blood forward into the aorta and backward into the left atrium. The work of

both the left ventricle and the left atrium must increase to preserve cardiac output.

The left ventricle must pump a sufficient volume of blood to maintain a normal forward flow into the aorta and the regurgitant flow through the mitral valve. For instance, the normal ventricular output per beat (stroke volume) is 70 ml. If the regurgitant flow is 30 ml per beat, the ventricle must pump 100 ml per beat to maintain a normal stroke volume. The additional volume load created by the regurgitant valve prompts ventricular dilation. According to Starling's law of the heart, ventricular dilation increases myocardial contractility. Eventually, the ventricular wall hypertrophies to further increase contractile force.

In the early stages of mitral regurgitation, the wall compliance or distensibility of the dilated left ventricle is increased. Increased wall compliance affects the rela-

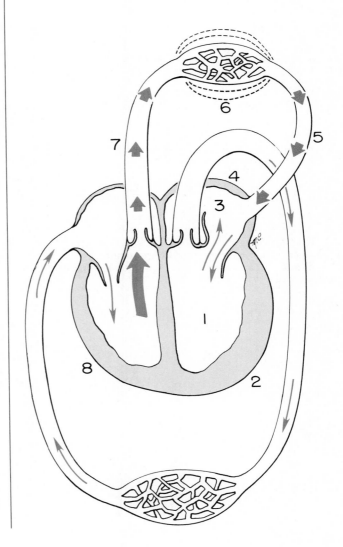

FIGURE 28-5
Pathophysiology of mitral regurgitation: 1, left ventricular dilatation; 2, left ventricular hypertrophy; 3, left atrial dilatation; 4, left atrial hypertrophy; 5, pulmonary venous congestion; 6, pulmonary congestion; 7, pulmonary artery hypertension; 8, right ventricular hypertrophy.

tionship between ventricular volume and pressure (wall compliance = volume/pressure), enabling the ventricle to accommodate increased diastolic volumes without abnormal elevations in pressure. However, when the left ventricle begins to fail, left ventricular end-diastolic pressure and consequently left atrial pressure rise, reflecting inadequate ventricular emptying.

Regurgitation creates a volume load not only for the left ventricle but also for the left atrium. The left atrium dilates to accommodate the increased volume and to increase the force of atrial contraction. Subsequently, the atrium hypertrophies to further increase atrial contractile force and output. Initially, increased left atrial compliance permits accommodation of increased volume without significant pressure elevation. Thus, for a while, the left atrium buffers the effect of the regurgitant volume, protecting the pulmonary vasculature and limiting pulmonary symptoms.

However, mitral regurgitation is a self-perpetuating lesion. As ventricular volumes and dimensions increase, valve function worsens. Chamber enlargement increases the degree of regurgitation by displacement of the papillary muscles and dilation of the mitral orifice, reducing leaflet contact during valve closure.

As the lesion worsens, the ability of the left atrium to distend and protect the lungs is exceeded. Left ventricular failure is usually the prelude to accelerated cardiac decompensation. The left ventricle becomes over-burdened, and forward flow through the aorta falls, with a simultaneous rise in backward congestion. Gradually, the predictable sequence of pulmonary and right heart involvement ensues: (1) pulmonary venous congestion, (2) interstitial edema, (3) pulmonary arterial hypertension, and (4) right ventricular hypertrophy. These changes are less pronounced than changes with mitral stenosis. Mitral regurgitation can culminate in right heart failure, although this occurs less frequently than it does in mitral stenosis.

The course of the disease is profoundly altered if the onset of mitral regurgitation is acute, as in papillary muscle rupture, rather than chronic. Acute mitral regurgitation is poorly tolerated. Normally, the left atrium is relatively noncompliant and therefore unable to abruptly distend and accommodate the regurgitant volume (see Fig. 28-6). Thus the sudden increase in volume and pressure is transmitted directly to the pulmonary vasculature. Within hours, fulminating pulmonary edema and shock can develop.

The earliest symptoms of mitral regurgitation are (1) weakness and fatigue caused by the reduction in forward flow, (2) exertional dyspnea, and (3) palpitations. Severe symptoms are precipitated by left ventricular failure with consequent low cardiac output and pulmonary congestion. The following findings are associated with mitral regurgitation:

1. *Auscultation:* murmur throughout systole (holosystolic or pansystolic murmur)

2. *Electrocardiogram:* left atrial enlargement (P mitrale), if rhythm normal sinus; atrial fibrillation; left ventricular hypertrophy

3. *Chest x-ray:* left atrial enlargement; left ventricular enlargement; variable pulmonary vascular congestion

4. *Hemodynamic findings:* increased left atrial pressure with significant v waves; elevated left ventric-

FIGURE 28-6

(A) Acute and (B) chronic mitral regurgitation. Note that in chronic mitral regurgitation there is greater dilatation and hypertrophy of the left atrium and ventricle. Acute mitral regurgitation causes greater pulmonary congestion because the left atrium is less compliant or distensible.

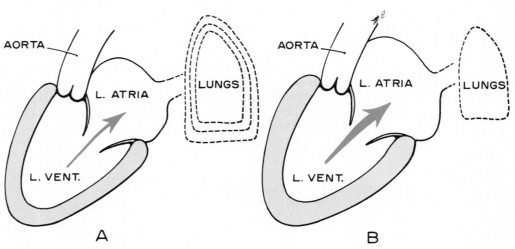

ular end-diastolic pressure; variable elevations of pulmonary pressures

Aortic stenosis

Aortic stenosis obstructs blood flow from the left ventricle into the aorta during ventricular systole. As the resistance to ventricular ejection increases, the pressure work of the left ventricle rises. In response, the left ventricle hypertrophies to generate more pressure and maintain peripheral perfusion; a marked pressure gradient develops between the left ventricle and the aorta (see Fig. 28-7). Hypertrophy reduces ventricular wall compliance and the wall becomes relatively stiff. Thus, despite the maintenance of normal cardiac output and ventricular volumes, ventricular end-diastolic pressure is slightly elevated.

The reserve pumping capability of the left ventricle is considerable. For instance, the left ventricle, which normally generates a systolic pressure of 120 mmHg, can develop pressure up to approximately 300 mmHg during ventricular contraction. To compensate

and maintain cardiac output, the left ventricle not only generates higher pressure but also prolongs the duration of ejection. Therefore, despite the progressive restriction of the aortic orifice and a consequent elevation of ventricular work, the mechanical efficiency of the heart is maintained for long periods. Eventually, however, the adaptive ability of the left ventricle is overwhelmed. The onset of progressive symptoms heralds a critical point in the course of aortic stenosis. Critical aortic stenosis corresponds to a reduction in valvular orifice from 3 to 4 cm^2 to less than 0.5 cm^2; generally a pressure gradient does not develop across the valve until this orifice is reduced approximately 50 percent.

A characteristic triad of symptoms is associated with aortic stenosis: (1) angina, (2) syncope, and (3) left ventricular failure. If unheeded, these symptoms indicate a poor prognosis, with an average survival of less than 5 years. The onset of left ventricular failure, indicating cardiac decompensation, is particularly ominous. Angina is produced by an imbalance in myocardial oxygen supply and demand; demand increases with hypertrophy and increased myocardial work, while supply is potentially reduced by the powerful systolic compression of the coronary arteries by the hypertrophied muscle. In addition, with myocardial hypertrophy, the ratio of capillaries to muscle fiber mass is reduced. The oxygen diffusion distance is therefore increased, potentially limiting myocardial oxygen supply. The subendocardial layer of the left ventricle is the most vulnerable. Syncope occurs primarily with exertion, as a result either of arrhythmias or an inability to increase cardiac output sufficiently to maintain cerebral perfusion.

Progressive ventricular failure impairs ventricular emptying. Cardiac output falls and ventricular volumes rise. Ventricular dilation, occasionally associated with functional mitral regurgitation, ensues. Advanced aortic stenosis is associated with severe pulmonary congestion. Right ventricular failure and systemic venous congestion are indicative of end-stage disease. It is uncommon for aortic stenosis to progress to this extreme. That the occurrence of right heart failure is unusual is probably caused by the high mortality associated with left heart failure earlier in the course of the disease. In addition, there is a significant incidence of sudden death in symptomatic patients with severe aortic stenosis. The pathogenesis of sudden death is controversial; however, it is usually precipitated by strenuous exertion.

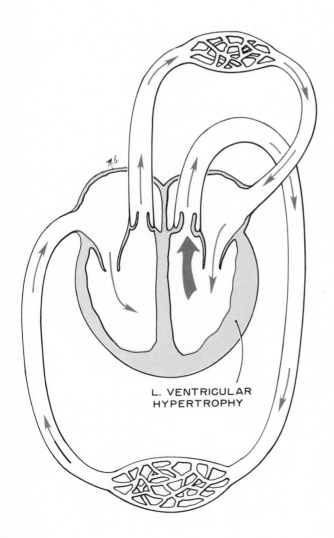

L. VENTRICULAR HYPERTROPHY

FIGURE 28-7
Pathophysiology of aortic stenosis.

The signs of aortic stenosis are as follows:

1. *Auscultation:* systolic ejection murmur; paradoxical splitting of S_2
2. *Electrocardiogram:* left ventricular hypertrophy
3. *Chest x-ray:* poststenotic proximal aortic dilatation (resulting from local trauma from blood ejected under high pressure striking the aortic wall); valvular calcification
4. *Hemodynamic findings:* significant aortic gradient (50 to 100 mmHg); elevated left ventricular end-diastolic pressure; delayed carotid upstroke

Aortic regurgitation

Aortic regurgitation produces a reflux of blood from the aorta into the left ventricle during ventricular relaxation (see Fig. 28-8). In essence, the peripheral bed competes with the left ventricle for the blood ejected by the ventricle during systole. The magnitude of forward flow, or "runoff," into the periphery relative to retrograde flow into the ventricle depends upon the degree of valve closure and the relative resistance to flow between the periphery and the ventricle. Characteristically, peripheral vascular resistance is low in aortic regurgitation, apparently as a compensatory mechanism to maximize forward flow. However, late in the course of the disease, peripheral resistance rises, increasing retrograde flow through the aortic valve and accelerating the disease progression.

The clinical course of aortic regurgitation is the least understood and the most variable of the valvular lesions. However, the disease obviously imposes a severe volume load upon the left ventricle. With each contraction, the ventricle must eject a quantity of blood equal to the normal stroke volume plus the regurgitant volume. The left ventricle dilates greatly and eventually hypertrophies, assuming a distinctive globular shape. An associated increase in wall compliance enables the ventricle to tolerate increased diastolic volumes without abnormal pressure elevations.

The marked left ventricular compensatory ability in combination with a competent mitral valve maintains ventricular function for a long time. Symptoms rarely develop until left ventricular decompensation, oc-

casionally compounded by functional mitral regurgitation, occurs. Irreversible left ventricular damage, resulting from the prolonged ejection of the volume overload against systemic resistance, can be sustained. The point of significant deterioration is ill-defined. Early symptoms are fatigue, dyspnea on exertion, and palpitations. Angina may also be noted with left ventricular hypertrophy and low arterial diastolic pressures, which increase oxygen demand and decrease oxygen supply, respectively. Heart failure precipitates a downhill course of falling cardiac output and rising ventricular volume with retrograde left atrial and pulmonary congestion.

The following signs are associated with aortic regurgitation:

1. *Auscultation:* diastolic murmur; characteristic Austin-Flint murmur or diastolic rumble; systolic murmur caused by increased ejection volume
2. *Electrocardiogram:* left ventricular hypertrophy
3. *Chest x-ray:* left ventricular enlargement; dilation of proximal aorta

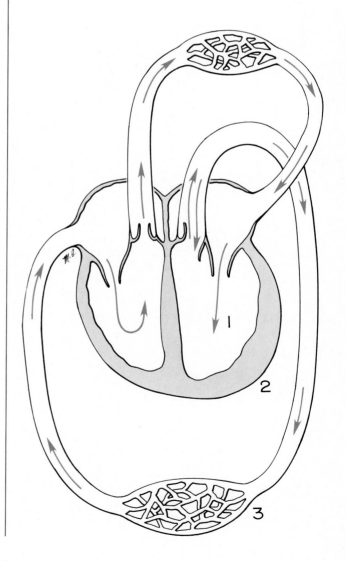

FIGURE 28-8

Pathophysiology of aortic regurgitation: 1, left ventricular dilatation; 2, left ventricular hypertrophy; 3, hyperdynamic peripheral circulation.

4. *Cardiac catheterization:* opacification of the left ventricle during injection of contrast material into the aortic root

Characteristic findings are noted in the peripheral circulation as a result of the hyperdynamic myocardial action and the low peripheral resistance. The forceful, high-volume, left ventricular ejection followed by the rapid forward runoff of blood into the periphery and backward into the left ventricle through the diseased valve creates a rapid distention of the vasculature followed by a sudden collapse. These cardiovascular dynamics can be manifested by (1) waterhammer pulses, characterized by a rapid rise and collapse of the arterial pulse; (2) pistol-shot pulses, audible upon auscultation of femoral artery; (3) Quincke's capillary pulsation, visible as alternating flushing and paling of the nail-bed capillaries: (4) systolic head bobbing as the collapsed neck vessels fill rapidly; and (5) widened pulse pressure with a low diastolic pressure.

Tricuspid valve disease

Stenosis of the tricuspid valve restricts blood flow from the right atrium into the right ventricle during diastole. This lesion is usually associated with disease of the mitral and aortic valves secondary to severe rheumatic heart disease. Tricuspid stenosis increases the work of the right atrium, forcing the chamber to generate more pressure to maintain flow across the obstructed valve. The right atrium has a limited ability to compensate and therefore dilates rapidly. As right atrial volumes and pressures rise, systemic venous engorgement and pressure elevation result (see Fig. 28-9).

The classic findings of right heart failure ensue: (1) venous distention with large *a* waves, (2) peripheral edema, (3) ascites, (4) hepatic enlargement, and (5) nausea and anorexia resulting from gastrointestinal engorgement. The following signs are associated with tricuspid stenosis:

1. *Auscultation:* diastolic murmur
2. *Electrocardiogram:* right atrial enlargement (tall, peaked P waves known as P pulmonale)
3. *Chest x-ray:* right atrial enlargement
4. *Hemodynamic findings:* pressure gradient across the tricuspid valve and elevated right atrial and central venous pressures with large *a* waves.

Pure tricuspid regurgitation is usually the consequence of advanced left heart failure or severe pulmonary hypertension resulting in right ventricular deterioration. As the right ventricle fails and enlarges, functional regurgitation of the tricuspid valve is produced. Tricuspid regurgitation is associated with right heart failure and the following findings:

1. *Auscultation:* murmur throughout systole
2. *Electrocardiogram:* right atrial enlargement (tall and narrow P wave known as P pulmonale), if rhythm is normal sinus; atrial fibrillation; right ventricular hypertrophy
3. *Chest x-ray:* right atrial and ventricular enlargement
4. *Hemodynamic findings:* elevated right atrial pressure with significant *v* waves.

Pulmonic valve disease

The incidence of pulmonic valvular lesions is extremely low. Pulmonic stenosis is usually congenital, rather than

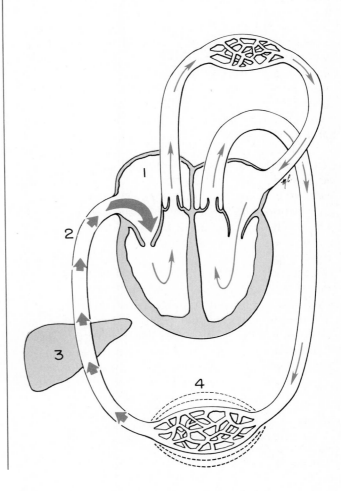

FIGURE 28-9
Pathophysiology of tricuspid stenosis. 1, right atrial dilatation; 2, venous congestion; 3, hepatomegaly; 4, systemic congestion.

rheumatic, in origin. Stenosis of the pulmonic valve increases right ventricular pressure work, producing right ventricular hypertrophy. Symptoms result when right ventricular failure occurs, producing systemic venous engorgement and its clinical sequelae.

Functional pulmonic regurgitation can occur as a sequela to left-sided valvular dysfunction with chronic pulmonary hypertension and dilation of the pulmonic valve orifice. However, this lesion is seen rarely.

Compound valvular disease

Mixed lesions, consisting of stenosis and regurgitation in the same valve, commonly occur. This is to be expected because a stenotic, immobile valve is often unable to close completely. *Combined lesions*, or multivalvular disease, are often seen because rheumatic heart disease commonly afflicts multiple valves.

Mixed lesions and combined lesions compound the valvular dysfunction described for isolated or *pure lesions*, altering to a variable degree the physiologic consequences. Compound lesions can either magnify or buffer a physiologic consequence of a pure lesion. For instance, mixed aortic regurgitation and aortic stenosis increase the volume load and pressure work of the left ventricle and greatly intensify the left ventricular strain. As a result, this combination is associated with a rapidly progressive downhill course.

However, the combination of aortic stenosis and mitral stenosis, in essence, protects the left ventricle from the magnitude of left ventricular strain associated with isolated aortic stenosis. This protective effect results from the reduction in left ventricular filling caused by the restriction to blood flow through the mitral valve. Diminished ventricular filling reduces the volume of the blood that the left ventricle must force through the restricted aortic orifice.

THERAPEUTIC INTERVENTION

Rheumatic fever and subacute bacterial endocarditis are two disease processes afflicting the heart valves that can be prevented, thus reducing the incidence or severity of acquired valvular lesions. Rheumatic fever can be prevented by early detection and treatment of group A beta-hemolytic streptococcal infections with penicillin. Early diagnosis and treatment of acute rheumatic fever are also essential. The diagnosis of acute rheumatic fever can be complicated in that no single clinical or laboratory finding is pathognomonic for this disease entity; many of the findings are nonspecific. The modified

TABLE 28-1

JONES CRITERIA (REVISED)

Major manifestations	Minor manifestations
Carditis	Fever
Polyarthritis	Arthralgia
Erythema marginatum	Previous rheumatic fever or rheumatic heart disease
Subcutaneous nodules	Elevated erythrocyte sedimentation rate (ESR) or positive C-reactive protein (CRP)

Supporting evidence of preceding streptococcal infection: history of recent scarlet fever; positive throat culture for group A streptococcus; increased ASO titer or other streptococcal antibodies.

Source: American Heart Association, 1965.

Jones criteria, illustrated in Table 28-1, are useful in the diagnosis of acute rheumatic fever. These criteria are designated as major or minor according to their relative importance as diagnostic indicators. The presence of two major criteria or one major and two minor criteria indicates a high probability of acute rheumatic fever. Evidence of an antecedent streptococcal infection is also prerequisite to the diagnosis; elevated antistreptolysin levels (ASO) are frequently used to establish the presence of streptococcal antibodies.

Treatment of acute rheumatic fever is palliative and includes (1) antibiotics, such as penicillin or erythromycin, to eliminate any residual streptococcal organisms; (2) anti-inflammatory agents, such as salicylates or corticosteroids; (3) analgesics, if indicated for arthritic pain; and (4) restriction of physical activity according to the degree of carditis. Associated cardiac failure might necessitate salt restriction, digoxin, and diuretics.

After the initial attack of rheumatic fever, susceptibility to recurrent attacks is extremely high. Consequently, antibiotic prophylaxis must begin as soon as the diagnosis is established. Single monthly injections of penicillin are effective and offer a distinct advantage over daily oral therapy in terms of patient compliance. Antibiotic prophylaxis must continue at least into adulthood to avoid potentially crippling deformity of heart valves produced by recurrent attacks of rheumatic fever. Emphasis must be upon prevention rather than treatment of streptococcal infections because recurrent rheumatic fever is frequently preceded by asymptomatic streptococcal infection. In addition, difficulty is often encountered in preventing recurrent attacks after the onset of a streptococcal infection.

Heart valves with congenital malformations or acquired deformity are particularly vulnerable to infection, or endocarditis, from systemic infections or even from the transient septicemia associated with minor surgical procedures (e.g., dental extractions). Appropriate prophylactic antibiotic coverage during substantiated or potential systemic infection is critical to prevent further valvular deterioration. Once valvular damage has been sustained, the course of the disease and medical therapy varies according to the site and severity of the lesion.

Mitral valve disease produces symptoms earlier in the course of the disease than does aortic valve disease. This earlier onset of symptoms results from the fact that the diseased mitral valve imposes a burden primarily upon the left atrium, whereas the diseased aortic valve burdens the left ventricle. The thin-walled left atrium is poorly suited to maintain its pumping capability in the face of an ever-increasing pressure or volume load. In addition, since no true valves separate the pulmonary veins from the left atrium, left atrial congestion is readily transmitted retrograde to the lungs, producing pulmonary symptoms. With aortic valve disease, the left ventricle compensates well for a long period of time, resulting in a long asymptomatic phase. The left atrium is protected from the left ventricular strain as long as the mitral valve remains competent and the left ventricular pumping capability is sustained.

Mitral valve disease

The clinical progression of mitral valve disease is gradual and prolonged. Dyspnea is usually the most prominent and disabling symptom. However, symptoms are initially responsive to medical therapy consisting of (1) diuretics to reduce congestion, (2) digoxin to increase contractile force in the presence of mitral regurgitation, which increases left ventricular work, (3) antiarrhythmics, if atrial fibrillation occurs, and (4) anticoagulants, if systemic embolization becomes a threat. Eventually, surgical intervention becomes necessary to control the progressively disabling symptoms. Occasionally, surgical intervention is precipitated by an abrupt deterioration associated with arrhythmias, embolization, or pulmonary infection.

Selected patients with pure mitral stenosis are considered for mitral commissurotomy, or surgical splitting of the valve leaflets fused along the commissures, when their symptoms have progressed to functional Class II heart disease (i.e., symptomatic with ordinary physical exertion). Mitral commissurotomy is contraindicated in patients with mitral regurgitation or with significant valvular calcification; splitting the commissures under these two conditions would either worsen the regurgitation or prompt calcific embolization.

Mitral commissurotomy (see Fig. 28-10) is performed by introducing a dilator through the apex of the left ventricle, guiding it by a finger inserted through the left atrium into the mitral orifice. The commissures are then split by blunt pressure as the dilator tip is opened. This procedure separates the fused leaflets, dilating the mitral orifice. This procedure usually results in relief or reduction of symptoms for a period of years. However, the procedure is palliative; eventually mitral valve replacement is considered as disease progression produces further disability. In carefully selected cases, mitral commissurotomy can be a valuable therapeutic adjunct, postponing the need for valve replacement.

Mitral valve replacement is considered when symptoms have progressed to functional Class III heart disease (i.e., symptoms with less than ordinary physical exertion). At this point, symptoms are less responsive to medical therapy, and the resultant disability is considered significant. Pulmonary hypertension, indicative of significant disease progression, substantiates the decision to replace the mitral valve. Further disease progression to functional Class IV is associated with a

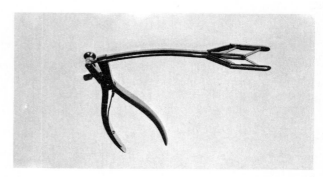

A

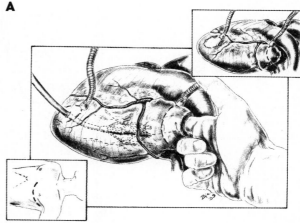

B

FIGURE 28-10
Mitral commissurotomy. (A) Tubb's mitral valve dilator, used for closed mitral commissurotomy. (B) Transventricular mitral valvulotomy. It is important to advance the dilator into the mitral valve under control by the right index finger. (From J. W. Hurst, _The Heart,_ 3d ed., McGraw-Hill, New York, 1974, p. 973.)

FIGURE 28-11
Prosthetic valves: (A) Starr-Edwards ball and cage valve.
(B) Björk-Shiley tilting disk valve. (C) Carpentier-Edwards
tissue valve. (A, courtesy of American Edwards
Laboratories, division of American Hospital Supply Corp.,
Santa Ana, Calif. B and C, from Johnson, Haber, and
Austen, 1980, pp. 533, 556.)

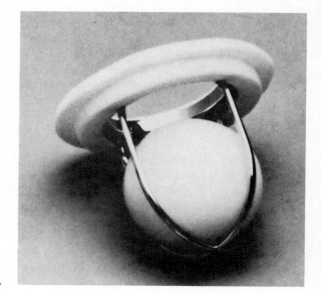

A

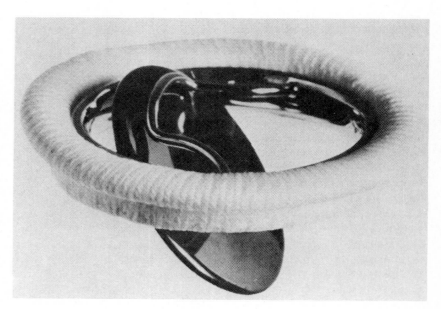

B

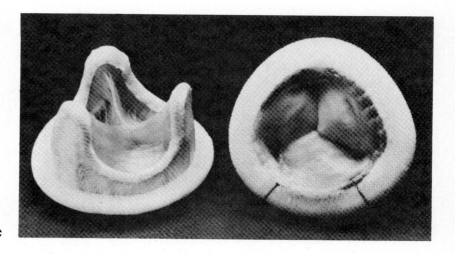

C

higher operative mortality and morbidity as a result of residual myocardial and pulmonary dysfunction.

Mitral valve replacement involves excision of the valve, chordae tendineae, and papillary muscles. A prosthetic valve, designed to simulate normal valve function, is inserted. Three types of prosthetic valves are illustrated in Fig. 28-11. All these valves open and close in response to pressure changes on either side of the valve. For example, with the ball and cage valve in the mitral position the ball rests in the bottom of the cage during ventricular relaxation permitting the blood to flow from the atrium to the ventricle. During ventricular contraction, as ventricular pressure exceeds atrial pressure, the ball is propelled upward in the cage to seal the mitral orifice, preventing backward flow.

Aortic valve disease

The management of aortic valve disease is in distinct contrast to that of mitral valve disease. The onset of significant symptoms—angina, syncope, failure—usually correlates with left ventricular decompensation, signaling a need to consider surgical intervention. The risk of operation for most symptomatic patients is less than the risk of prolonged medical therapy. Once the patient is symptomatic, the course of aortic disease is progressively downhill. Severe aortic stenosis is potentially unpredictable, lethal entity; sudden death can occur without warning. Aortic regurgitation poses somewhat of a therapeutic dilemma; the timing of surgery is less well-defined. Close surveillance of patients with aortic valve disease is essential to detect early signs of clinical deterioration. Surgical intervention in both aortic regurgitation and aortic stenosis requires replacement of the valve.

QUESTIONS

Valvular heart disease

Directions: Answer the following questions on a separate sheet of paper.

1. List and briefly describe five causes of valvular heart disease.
2. What is functional AV regurgitation?
3. Comment on the following statement: "Before rendering any treatment that may result in even the slightest release of bacteria into the bloodstream, one is obligated to make absolutely sure that the patient is not affected by any kind of heart deformity. If it is known or suspected that the patient has a deformity of the heart, it is absolutely necessary to administer prophylactic antibiotics."
4. What is the medical treatment for each of the following problems associated with mitral valve disease: pulmonary congestion, atrial fibrillation, and systemic emboli?
5. What is a mitral commissurotomy?
6. List the revised Jones criteria. What is their purpose? Illustrate.

Directions: Circle the letter preceding each item below that correctly answers the question. Only one answer is correct unless otherwise noted.

7. Mitral valve closure occurs when:
   a. Left ventricular pressure exceeds left atrial pressure   *b.* Left atrial pressure exceeds left ventricular pressure   *c.* Left ventricular pressure exceeds aortic pressure   *d.* Left atrial pressure equals left ventricular pressure

8. Arrange the heart valves in correct order according to relative frequency of involvement in valvular heart disease.
   a. Pulmonic   *b.* Aortic   *c.* Mitral   *d.* Tricuspid

9. The organism which precedes the development of rheumatic heart disease is:
   a. Group A beta-hemolytic streptococcus
   b. Streptococcus viridans   *c.* Staphylococcus aureus   *d.* Staphylococcus albus

10. Progressive valvular lesions in rheumatic fever are primarily a result of:
    a. A single episode of rheumatic carditis
    b. Chronic infective carditis   *c.* Recurrent episodes of rheumatic carditis   *d.* Subacute bacterial endocarditis

11. The primary site of vegetations in rheumatic carditis is:
    a. On the papillary muscles   *b.* Diffuse distribution over the endocardium   *c.* Along the chordae tendineae   *d.* Along the valve leaflets at their lines of contact

12. Morphologic changes which characterize pure rheumatic valvular stenosis include all of the following except:
    a. Leaflet fusion along the commissures
    b. Shrunken, retracted cusps   *c.* Thickening of

the chordae tendineae   *d.* Thickening of valvular cusps

13. Morphologic changes which characterize pure rheumatic valvular regurgitation include all of the following except:
    a. Shrunken, retracted cusps   *b.* Shortened, fused chordae tendineae   *c.* Rupture of the papillary muscles   *d.* Enlargement of the valvular orifice

14. Dilation and hypertrophy of the left atrium are the initial compensatory response in:
    a. Aortic stenosis   *b.* Tricuspid stenosis   *c.* Mitral stenosis   *d.* Acute rheumatic fever

15. Dilation and hypertrophy of the left ventricle occur in:
    a. Mitral stenosis   *b.* Mitral regurgitation   *c.* Tricuspid regurgitation   *d.* Pulmonary stenosis

16. Which of the following is the earliest symptom in patients with mitral stenosis?
    a. Palpitations   *b.* Dyspnea on exertion   *c.* Orthopnea   *d.* Angina

17. Symptoms with mild exertion appear when the orifice of the mitral valve (normally 4 to 6 cm^2) is reduced to:
    a. 3 to 4 cm^2 *b.* 2 to 3 cm^2 *c.* 1 to 2 cm^2 *d.* Less than 1 cm^2

18. Which of the following disorders is *least* likely to result in left ventricular strain?
    a. Systemic hypertension   *b.* Aortic regurgitation   *c.* Mitral stenosis   *d.* Ventricular aneurysm

19. Atrial fibrillation complicating mitral stenosis creates the following problem or problems: (More than one answer may be correct.)
    a. Loss of atrial contraction   *b.* Potential systemic embolization   *c.* Potential right ventricular failure   *d.* Decreased ventricular filling time

20. Chronic mitral stenosis may result in all of the following except:
    a. Enlargement of the left atrium   *b.* Increased pressure in the left ventricle   *c.* Redistribution of pulmonary blood flow to the upper lobes   *d.* A fixed cardiac output   *e.* Pulmonary hypertension

21. Mitral valve insufficiency will result in blood regurgitating from the:
    a. Right ventricle back to the right atrium
    b. Pulmonary artery back to the right ventricle
    c. Left ventricle back to the left atrium

d. Right atrium back to the superior and inferior venae cavae

22. The most likely cause of *acute* mitral regurgitation would be:
    a. Recurrent episodes of rheumatic endocarditis   *b.* Chest trauma   *c.* Bacterial endocarditis   *d.* Ruptured papillary muscle complicating myocardial infarction

23. In differentiating acute mitral regurgitation from chronic mitral regurgitation, all of the following statements are correct except:
    a. Fulminating pulmonary edema is more common in acute mitral regurgitation   *b.* Left ventricular hypertrophy is common in chronic mitral regurgitation   *c.* A dilated left atrium is common in acute and chronic mitral regurgitation   *d.* Atrial fibrillation is common in chronic mitral regurgitation, but normal sinus rhythm is more likely in the acute form

24. Isolated aortic stenosis usually results from:
    a. A congenital bicuspid valve   *b.* Rheumatic valvular disease   *c.* Atherosclerotic heart disease   *d.* Progressive calcification with aging

25. The primary response to aortic stenosis is:
    a. Right ventricular hypertrophy   *b.* Left ventricular hypertrophy   *c.* Pulmonary hypertension   *d.* Enlargement of the left atrium

26. Atrial fibrillation is *least* likely to be associated with:
    a. Mitral regurgitation   *b.* Mitral stenosis   *c.* Aortic stenosis   *d.* Coronary atherosclerotic disease

27. Which of the following findings would *not* be expected in a patient with severe aortic stenosis?
    a. Paradoxical splitting of the second heart sound   *b.* Poststenotic dilation of the aorta on chest x-ray   *c.* Enlarged and sustained apical impulse on palpation   *d.* A pressure gradient of 100 mmHg between the aorta and left ventricle on cardiac catheterization   *e.* A widened pulse pressure

28. Potential symptoms and signs in moderate aortic stenosis include all of the following *except*:
    a. Angina pectoris   *b.* Effort syncope   *c.* Peripheral edema   *d.* Paroxysmal nocturnal dyspnea

29. In aortic stenosis, life expectancy after the onset of significant symptoms averages:
    a. Less than 5 years   *b.* 5 to 8 years   *c.* 9 to 11 years   *d.* 12 to 15 years

30. Characteristic signs of severe aortic regurgitation include: (More than one answer may be correct.)
    a. Pistol-shot pulses heard over the femoral artery   *b.* Corrigan (waterhammer) pulses   *c.* Austin Flint murmur   *d.* Systolic head bobbing   *e.* Al-

ternating flushing and paling of nail-bed capillaries
(Quincke's capillary pulsation)

31. Which of the following statements concerning tricuspid stenosis is not true?
    a. There is an increased pressure gradient between the right ventricle and right atrium on cardiac catheterization.   b. Electrocardiographic findings include tall, peaked P waves and right atrial enlargement.   c. Central venous pressure is usually normal.   d. There is accentuation of the a wave of the jugular venous pulse.   e. Hepatomegaly and ascites are common findings on physical examination.

32. Pure tricuspid regurgitation is usually:
    a. Associated with rheumatic heart disease
    b. A functional disorder associated with right heart failure   c. Associated with acute myocardial infarction   d. A functional disorder associated with left ventricular hypertrophy

33. Which of the following findings is not associated with tricuspid regurgitation?
    a. Positive hepatojugular reflux test   b. Water-hammer pulse   c. Prominent v wave of the jugular venous pulse   d. Distended neck veins
    e. Opacification of the right atrium when the right ventricle is injected with contrast media

34. Which of the following combinations of valvular disease would probably be the most lethal?
    a. Aortic stenosis + mitral stenosis   b. Tricuspid regurgitation + mitral stenosis   c. Aortic regurgitation + mitral regurgitation   d. Aortic regurgitation + aortic stenosis

35. The x-ray findings of right ventricular hypertrophy in the absence of pulmonary arterial hypertension are suggestive of:
    a. Tricuspid stenosis   b. Mitral stenosis   c. Pulmonic stenosis   d. Aortic regurgitation

36. Pulmonic stenosis is usually the result of:
    a. Rheumatic fever   b. Coronary atherosclerotic disease   c. Congenital deformity of the valve
    d. None of the above

37. Subacute bacterial endocarditis in a susceptible host may be prevented by: (More than one answer may be correct.)
    a. Replacement of diseased valves   b. Use of antibiotics prior to and after dental surgery   c. Antibiotic prophylaxis throughout adolescence
    d. Antibiotic prophylaxis for genitourinary tract instrumentation

38. Replacement of the mitral valve is indicated when the patient's disability is classified, according to the New York Heart Association, as:
    a. Class I   b. Class II   c. Class III   d. Class IV

39. A suitable candidate for mitral commissurotomy is a patient with a mitral valve that is:
    a. Heavily calcified   b. Stenotic and regurgitant
    c. Stenotic and flexible   d. Stenotic and immobile

40. The most common complication of mitral commissurotomy in the setting of significant valvular calcification is:
    a. Mitral regurgitation   b. Calcific embolization
    c. Re-stenosis   d. Valve perforation

41. Which statements regarding the function of a prosthetic ball and cage heart valve in the mitral position are correct? (More than one answer may be correct.)
    a. During systole the ball is propelled upward to seal the orifice and prevent backflow.   b. The prosthetic valve is sutured to the papillary muscles which regulate valve opening and closure.
    c. During diastole the ball rests on the bottom of the cage.   d. The fact that atrial pressure exceeds ventricular pressure accounts for the upward propulsion of the ball.

42. Which of the following criteria is an indication for consideration of imminent aortic valve replacement in aortic stenosis?
    a. Arterial pulse pressure of 50 mmHg   b. Aortic valve calcification on chest x-ray   c. Onset of symptoms of angina pectoris, effort syncope, and left heart failure   d. An increased left ventricular end-diastolic pressure at cardiac catheterization

Directions: Match the functional valvular disorder in col. A to its effects in col. B.

Column A	Column B
43. ____ Valvular regurgitation	a. Increased cardiac volume work
44. ____ Valvular stenosis	b. Increased cardiac pressure work
	c. Backward flow
	d. Resistance to forward flow
	e. Chamber dilation
	f. Muscle hypertrophy

Directions: Circle the letter preceding each item that correctly answers each question. More than one answer may be correct.

45. An indication of active rheumatic carditis is the presence of:
a. Valvular stenosis   *b.* Aschoff bodies   *c.* Calcification of vascular tissue   *d.* Perivascular fibrosis of the myocardium

46. Possible causes of valvular heart disease include:
a. Rheumatic fever   *b.* Rupture of the papillary muscle secondary to coronary atherosclerosis
c. Congenital malformations   *d.* Bacterial endocarditis

47. Which of the following would be considered major manifestations of acute rheumatic fever according to the revised Jones criteria?
a. Polyarthritis   *b.* Fever   *c.* Erythema marginatum   *d.* Abnormal erythrocyte sedimentation rate   *e.* Carditis

CHAPTER 29

PENNY J. FORD
MADELINE A. O'DONNELL
F. MICHAEL VISLOSKY

CARDIAC MECHANICAL DYSFUNCTION AND CIRCULATORY SUPPORT

OBJECTIVES

At the completion of this chapter you should be able to:

1. List the three determinants of stroke volume and describe the significance of each determinant in the setting of congestive heart failure.

2. Describe the ventricular function curve characteristic of the failing left ventricle.

3. Contrast the following terms:
   a. heart failure
   b. myocardial failure
   c. circulatory failure
   d. congestive heart failure
   e. circulatory congestion

4. State the physiologic consequences associated with an increase in LVEDP due to left ventricular failure.

5. Name the primary compensatory mechanisms associated with a reduction in stroke volume.

6. Contrast the clinical syndromes of forward versus backward failure and failure of the right side versus the left side of the heart.

7. List the clinical symptoms of left heart failure and of right heart failure.

8. Discuss the primary etiologic factors producing heart failure and identify precipitating factors.

9. Compare the three types of cardiomyopathies relative to changes in cardiac structure and function.

10. Identify the three general principles of therapy in heart failure and give specific examples of commonly used modalities.

11. Define the term *shock state*.

12. Describe the factors perpetuating the shock cycle.

13. State the systemic effects of shock.

14. Identify the hemodynamic profile characteristic of the patient in cardiogenic shock.

15. Discuss the general therapeutic approach to the patient in cardiogenic shock.

16. State the indications, hemodynamic and physiologic effects, and possible complications of:
    a. the intraaortic balloon pump,
    b. the left atrial–arterial assist device,
    c. the left ventricular–arterial assist device

17. Describe the operation of the heart-lung machine (cardiopulmonary bypass).

18. Contrast the indications and methodology for total cardiac replacement with the total artificial heart versus cardiac transplantation.

There is a wide spectrum of cardiac mechanical dysfunction ranging from mild, compensated heart failure to cardiogenic shock. The intent of this chapter is to provide an overview of this spectrum and an introduction to the techniques of circulatory assistance and cardiac transplantation. Heart failure, as the most common complication of acquired and congenital heart disease, will be discussed at length. However, it should be noted that heart failure poses a surprising paradox in that it is simultaneously relatively straightforward as a clinical syndrome yet extremely variable and complex as a pathophysiologic state. The fact that heart failure can be caused by a wide variety of disease entities contributes to its complexity. The discussion in this chapter will focus on the common forms of heart failure occurring as a complication of ischemic heart disease, valvular heart disease, and hypertension.

The spectrum of mechanical dysfunction and the methods of circulatory assistance will be considered relative to their effects upon the three primary determinants of myocardial function: preload, contractility, and afterload. This framework will be utilized because heart failure and/or the associated compensatory responses produce abnormalities in each of the determinants. Specific therapeutic modalities are selected to improve myocardial function by selective manipulation of a given determinant or determinants.

CONGESTIVE HEART FAILURE

Fundamental concepts

The three primary determinants of mechanical performance of the heart are preload, contractility, and afterload. (Please refer to Chap. 25 for a review of the introductory concepts.) *Preload* is the degree of myocardial fiber stretch at the end of ventricular filling or diastole. Increasing preload, up to a point, optimizes the overlap between actin and myosin filaments, increasing the force of contraction and cardiac output. This relationship is expressed by Starling's law of the heart. Starling's law states that stretching the myocardial fibers during diastole will increase the force of contraction during systole (refer back to Fig. 25-7). Preload is increased by elevation of ventricular diastolic volume, as would occur with retention of fluid; a reduction in preload would result from diuresis.

The relationship between increasing ventricular end-diastolic volume (EDV) and improved ventricular performance is illustrated in Fig. 29-1 as the *ventricular function curve*. The normal curve exhibits an initially steep, ascending limb where increments in volume and fiber stretch produce a corresponding improvement in ventricular function and cardiac output. The normal ventricle operates along the steep ascending limb where there is considerable reserve for improving ventricular function before the point on the curve where no further improvement is possible is reached.

At the summit of the curve, a plateau or flattening is observed where additional increments in ventricular volume are not associated with improved performance. This physiologic limit results from the rise in ventricular end-diastolic pressure produced by the increased volume. Excessive pressure elevation produces pulmonary or systemic congestion and edema from fluid transudation, negating the value of further increments in volume and pressure.

The precise relationship between the change in volume and the resultant change in pressure depends upon the compliance or distensibility of the cardiac chambers (see Fig. 29-2). An extremely compliant or distensible chamber can accommodate relatively large changes in volume without significantly increasing pressure; conversely, significant elevations in pressure can result from small changes in volume in a noncompliant chamber. A useful analogy for understanding the effect of chamber compliance on volume and pressure relationships is that of blowing up a child's balloon. Initially, balloons are extremely noncompliant and difficult to inflate; one must generate high pressures to inflate

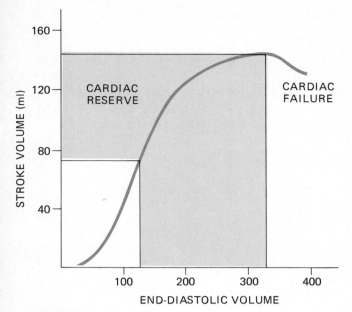

FIGURE 29-1

Starling's law of the heart. As the end-diastolic volume increases, so does the force of ventricular contraction. Thus, the stroke volume becomes greater, up to a critical point after which stroke volume decreases. (From L. F. Langley, *Review of Physiology,* **3d ed., McGraw-Hill, New York, 1971, p. 264.)**

the balloon with even small volumes of air. However, once a balloon has been repeatedly inflated and deflated, it becomes more compliant and easily distensible. One can then easily inflate the balloon with high volumes without exerting much pressure.

The ventricular function curve characteristic of the failing ventricle is depressed and flattened (see Fig. 29-3). The curve does not exhibit a descending limb caused by sarcomere overstretch, as was once believed. Depression of the curve signifies that the failing ventricle requires higher volumes to achieve the same improvement of ventricular function and cardiac output that the normal ventricle achieves with lower ventricle volumes. In other words, a given increment in ventricular volume is not associated with as great an improvement in ventricular function in the failing ventricle as would be expected in the normal ventricle.

In addition, the pronounced flattening of the curve seen with failure indicates limited cardiac reserve; once the curve flattens, no further improvement of function can be achieved with elevations of volume and pressure. It is presumed that the curve flattens suddenly because the distended, hypertrophied ventricle is relatively noncompliant; therefore small increases in volume result in significant pressure elevation and the development of congestion and edema.

Contractility, the second determinant of myocardial function, refers to changes in the force of contraction or inotropic state occurring independently of

changes in fiber length. Changes in contractile function shift the position of the ventricular function curve (see Fig. 29-3). The administration of positive inotropic drugs, such as catecholamines or digoxin, enhances contractility, shifting the curve upward and to the left. Factors depressing contractility, such as hypoxia or acidosis, shift the curve downward and to the right. As indicated, the fundamental abnormality in most forms of heart failure is depression of the ventricular function curve; this downward shift of the curve represents an intrinsic depression of myocardial contractility.

Finally, *afterload* is the amount of wall tension the ventricle must develop during systole to eject blood. According to the law of Laplace, three variables affect wall tension: intraventricular size, intraventricular pressure, and wall thickness.

$$\text{Wall tension} = \frac{\text{intraventricular pressure} \times \text{radius}}{\text{ventricular wall thickness}}$$

Factors increasing the pressure the ventricle must generate during systole (such as arterial vasoconstriction,

FIGURE 29-2

Ventricular compliance, or the pressure-volume relationship of the ventricles. The dotted line in the center indicates the typical relationship between pressure and volume. As volume is increased initially, there is only a small rise in pressure. As volume increase continues, the rise in pressure is greater. Each solid line indicates an alteration in pressure-volume relationships: decreased compliance on the left and increased compliance on the right. This represents a greater or lesser degree of stiffness of the ventricle in relation to the filling volume. Ventricular compliance is a dynamic phenomenon, and this property can change rapidly. (From W. A. Sodeman, Jr. and W. A. Sodeman (eds.), *Pathologic Physiology,* **5th ed., Saunders, Philadelphia, p. 276.)**

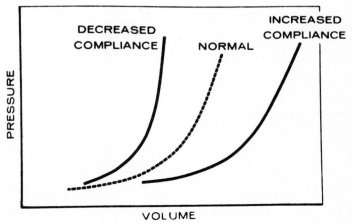

which increases the resistance to ventricular ejection) or increasing the ventricular radius (as by fluid retention) increase afterload. The failing heart is particularly sensitive to the increased workload imposed by an increase in afterload owing to its limited cardiac reserve. Reduction of afterload can be achieved with interventions such as the administration of vasodilators. Ventricular hypertrophy, another consequence of heart failure, also decreases afterload according to the law of Laplace. The increased muscle mass facilitates the work of ejection.

Definitions

Heart failure or *cardiac failure* is the pathophysiologic condition in which the heart as a pump is unable to meet the metabolic requirements of the tissues for blood. The critical features of this definition are first, that failure is defined relative to the metabolic needs of the body and second, that emphasis is placed upon the overall failure of the pumping function of the heart. *Myocardial failure* refers specifically to abnormalities in myocardial function; myocardial failure commonly leads to heart failure, but circulatory compensatory mechanisms can delay or even prevent failure of the heart as a pump. The term *circulatory failure* is even more general than the term heart failure; circulatory failure refers to the inability of the cardiovascular system to adequately perfuse the tissues. This definition encompasses any abnormality of the circulation responsible for the inadequacy in cardiac output, including alterations in blood volume, vascular tone, and the heart. *Congestive heart failure* is the state of circulatory congestion resulting from heart failure and its compensatory mechanisms. Congestive heart failure is defined in contradistinction to the more general term *circulatory congestion*, which is simply circulatory overload due to excess blood volume from cardiac failure or from noncardiac causes, such as overtransfusion or anuria.

Pathophysiology

The intrinsic defect in myocardial contractility characteristic of heart failure impairs the ability of the ventricle to empty effectively. Depressed contractility of the left ventricle reduces stroke volume and elevates residual ventricular volumes. As ventricular end-diastolic volumes rise, there is a corresponding increase in left ventricular end-diastolic pressure (LVEDP). The degree of pressure elevation depends on the compliance of the ventricle. As LVEDP rises, there is a corresponding elevation of left atrial pressure (LAP), since the atrium and ventricle communicate directly during diastole. The increase in LAP is transmitted backward into the pulmonic vasculature, elevating pulmonary venous and pulmonary capillary pressures. If hydrostatic pressure in the pulmonary capillary bed exceeds the vascular oncotic pressure, fluid transudation into the interstitium occurs. When the rate of fluid transudation exceeds the rate of lymphatic drainage, interstitial edema results. Further elevation of pressure may cause fluid seepage into the alveoli and the development of pulmonary edema (see Fig. 29-4). See also Chap. 36 for a discussion of pulmonary edema.

Pulmonary arterial pressure may rise in response to chronic elevation of pulmonary venous pressure. Pulmonary hypertension increases the resistance to right ventricular ejection. A sequence of events parallel to that affecting the left side of the heart can then result, culminating in systemic congestion and edema.

The development of systemic or pulmonic congestion and edema can be exacerbated by the development of functional regurgitation of the tricuspid or mitral valves, respectively. Functional regurgitation can result from dilation of the atrioventricular valve annulus or changes in the orientation of the papillary muscles and chordae tendineae secondary to chamber dilation.

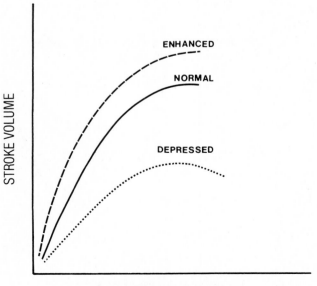

FIGURE 29-3

Ventricular function curve. The solid black line represents the normal ventricular function curve. Note that increasing end-diastolic volume increases stroke volume up to a point. Displacement of the curve upward and to the left represents improved ventricular function, as would be seen with sympathetic nervous system stimulation. Displacement of the curve downward and to the right represents myocardial depression, as would be seen with acidosis or hypoxia, or with cardiac failure.

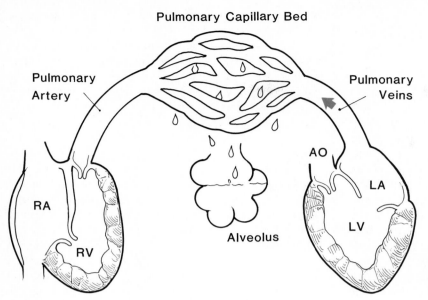

Pulmonary Capillary Bed

Pulmonary Artery

Pulmonary Veins

AO

LA

LV

RA

RV

Alveolus

FIGURE 29-4
**Pulmonary edema in left heart failure.
(Modified from Vinsant and Spense, 1981,
p. 249.)**

The fall in stroke volume with heart failure elicits a compensatory sympathetic response. Heart rate and contractile force increase to maintain cardiac output. Peripheral vasoconstriction occurs to stabilize arterial pressure and redistribute blood volume away from the relatively nonvital organs, such as the skin and kidney, to maintain perfusion to the more vital organs, such as the brain. Venoconstriction increases venous return to the right side of the heart, further augmenting contractile force according to Starling's law of the heart. Activation of the renin-angiotensin-aldosterone system in response to sympathetic stimulation and the fall in renal blood flow results in renal retention of sodium and water (see Fig. 29-5). This further increases venous return.

In response to heart failure, three primary compensatory responses are observed: (1) increased preload, (2) increased sympathetic adrenergic activity, and (3) ventricular hypertrophy. All three represent physiologic attempts to maintain cardiac output. Preload is increased immediately by the venoconstriction noted above and subsequently by renal retention of sodium and water. The exact mechanism responsible for activation of the renin-angiotensin-aldosterone system in heart failure is unknown. However, a number of factors have been implicated, including sympathetic adrenergic stimulation of the beta receptors within the juxtaglomerular apparatus, macula densa receptor response to changes in sodium delivery to the distal tubule, and baroreceptor responses to changes in circulating blood volume and pressure.

Whatever the precise mechanism, the fall in cardiac output with heart failure initiates the following events: (1) activation of the sympathetic nervous system, (2) fall in renal blood flow and eventually of glomerular filtration rate, (3) release of renin from the jux-

taglomerular apparatus, (4) renin interaction with circulating angiotensinogen to produce angiotensin I, (5) conversion of angiotensin I to angiotensin II, (6) stimulation of aldosterone secretion from the adrenal gland, and (7) retention of sodium and water in the distal tubule and collecting duct. (See Chap. 40 on renal pathophysiology for further clarification.)

This fluid retention is augmented in severe heart failure by impaired hepatic metabolism of aldosterone due to hepatic dysfunction secondary to systemic venous congestion and diminished perfusion of the liver. Antidiuretic hormone levels are also elevated in severe heart failure, which increases the absorption of water in the collecting ducts.

FIGURE 29-5
Renin-angiotensin system.

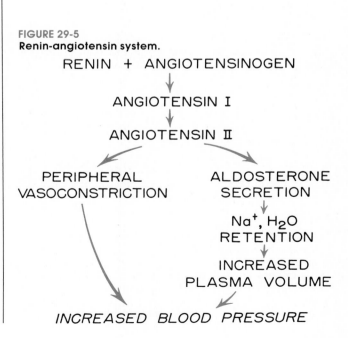

RENIN + ANGIOTENSINOGEN

↓

ANGIOTENSIN I

↓

ANGIOTENSIN II

PERIPHERAL VASOCONSTRICTION

ALDOSTERONE SECRETION

↓

Na^+, H_2O
RETENTION

↓

INCREASED PLASMA VOLUME

INCREASED BLOOD PRESSURE

The increased activity of the sympathetic adrenergic system stimulates release of catecholamines from the cardiac adrenergic nerves and adrenal medulla. As would be expected, the level of circulating catecholamines is elevated in heart failure, particularly during exercise. However, the degree of circulatory response is variable. Initially, augmentation of the heart rate and contractility is produced, as is vasoconstriction; the heart becomes increasingly dependent upon circulating catecholamines to maintain ventricular performance. Eventually, however, the myocardial response to sympathetic stimulation lessens; the catecholamines have less effect on ventricular performance. This change can best be conceptualized by referring to the ventricular function curve (Fig. 29-3). Normally, catecholamines produce a positive inotropic effect on the ventricle, shifting the curve upward and to the left; as the failing ventricle becomes less responsive to catecholamine stimulation, the degree of shift in response to stimulation lessens. This change may be related to the observation that the myocardial stores of norepinephrine become depleted with heart failure.

The vasoconstrictive effect of the adrenergic sympathetic system is augmented by activation of the renin-angiotensin-aldosterone system. Angiotensin II is a potent vasoconstrictor.

The final compensatory response to failure is myocardial hypertrophy or increased wall thickness. Hypertrophy increases the number of sarcomeres within the myocardial cell; depending upon the type of hemodynamic load producing the failure, sarcomeres develop either in parallel or in series. For example, a pressure load, as caused by aortic stenosis, is associated with increased numbers of sarcomeres arranged in parallel producing an increase in wall thickness without increasing the internal chamber size. The myocardial response to volume loads, as in aortic regurgitation, is characterized by dilation as well as increased wall thickness. This combination is believed to result from increased numbers of sarcomeres arranged in series. These two patterns of hypertrophy are referred to as concentric hypertrophy and eccentric hypertrophy (see Fig. 29-6). Whatever the precise sarcomere arrangement, myocar-

dial hypertrophy increases the force of ventricular contraction.

In addition to these three compensatory mechanisms designed to maintain cardiac output, additional mechanisms operate at the tissue level to facilitate the delivery of oxygen to the tissues. Plasma levels of 2,3-diphosphoglycerate (DPG) increase, reducing the affinity of hemoglobin for oxygen. As a result, the oxygen-hemoglobin dissociation curve shifts to the right, facilitating the release and uptake of oxygen by the tissues. (See Part VI, "Respiratory Pathophysiology," for further discussion of the oxygen-hemoglobin dissociation curve.) Oxygen extraction from the blood is increased to maintain oxygen supply to the tissues in the presence of a low cardiac output.

These mechanisms may be sufficient to maintain cardiac output at normal or near normal levels, particularly early in the course of failure and in the resting state. Typically, however, some degree of abnormality in ventricular performance and cardiac output appears in the failing heart during exercise. As the failure progresses, compensation can be expected to become less effective.

Initially, the compensatory response of the circulation is beneficial; however, eventually the compensatory mechanisms can produce symptoms, increase cardiac work, and worsen the degree of failure. The fluid retention intended to augment contractile force causes pulmonic and systemic venous congestion and edema formation. Arterial vasoconstriction and redistribution of blood flow from the nonvital organs produces signs and symptoms such as skin pallor and coolness as well as weakness and fatigue. Arterial vasoconstriction in-

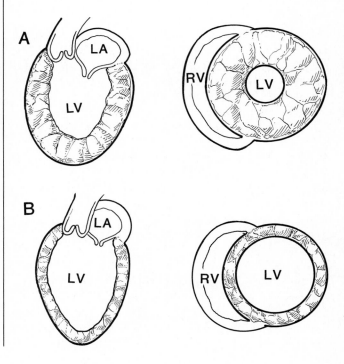

FIGURE 29-6

Patterns of ventricular hypertrophy. (A) Concentric hypertrophy secondary to a pressure load is characterized by increased wall thickness with minimal or no change in chamber size. (B) Eccentric hypertrophy secondary to a volume load is characterized by a proportional increase in wall thickness and chamber size. (Modified from Rushmer, 1976, p. 538.)

creases afterload by increasing the resistance to ventricular ejection; afterload is also increased by dilation of the cardiac chambers. Consequently, cardiac work and myocardial oxygen demand increase. Myocardial hypertrophy and sympathetic stimulation also increase myocardial oxygen demand. If the increase in myocardial oxygen demand cannot be met by a corresponding increase in myocardial oxygen supply, myocardial ischemia and further myocardial compromise can result. The end-result of these interrelated events is an increased myocardial burden and perpetuation of the underlying failure.

Clinical manifestations

Two methods of conceptualizing failure are useful in the description of clinical manifestations: (1) forward versus backward failure, and (2) right heart failure versus left heart failure. Forward versus backward failure allows distinction of symptoms resulting from inadequate cardiac output or forward blood flow from symptoms due to the backup of blood behind the failing ventricle. For example, weakness and fatigue would be produced by forward failure, whereas pulmonary congestion and edema would be due to backward failure.

The terms right heart failure versus left heart failure imply that the ventricles function as independent pumps. While this distinction can be useful as a means of categorizing symptoms, the interdependence of the ventricles must be noted. The ventricles are anatomically interdependent in that they share a common wall, the interventricular septum, and the muscle fibers composing the ventricular walls are continuous, encircling both ventricles. Not only does anatomic interdependence exist between the ventricles but so does functional interdependence, in that the ventricles are components of a continuous circuit and the volume of blood ejected from each ventricle depends on the volume received by that ventricle. It is physiologically impossible for ventricular stroke volumes to be imbalanced for a prolonged period of time. For example, the left ventricle cannot sustain an increase in cardiac output unless there is a corresponding increase in cardiac output in the right ventricle. Impaired function of one ventricle eventually interferes with function of the other ventricle. For example, a reduction in right heart output reduces filling of the left ventricle and consequently reduces cardiac output into the systemic circuit. Similarly, left heart failure is recognized as the most common cause of right heart failure, owing to the phenomenon of backward failure described above.

The fact that both ventricles are enclosed within the pericardium increases the physiologic interaction; extreme dilation of one ventricle progressively compresses the other ventricle within the pericardium. In addition, the ventricles share common biochemical changes in failure; for example, the depletion of norepinephrine stores mentioned earlier does not seem to be isolated to a single chamber. In sum, the interdependence of the ventricular pumps must be recognized. However, the terms right and left heart failure can be used to refer to a complex of symptoms corresponding to failure of a particular ventricle. For example, right heart failure produces systemic venous congestion and edema (see Fig. 29-7), whereas left heart failure produces pulmonic venous congestion and edema (see Fig. 29-4).

The clinical manifestations of heart failure should be considered relative to the degree of physical exertion associated with the appearance of symptoms. Initially, symptoms typically appear only with exertion; however, as failure progresses, exercise tolerance diminishes and symptoms are manifest earlier with lesser degrees of activity. The New York Heart Association functional classification is commonly used to express the relationship between onset of symptoms and degree of physical exertion:

Class I: Asymptomatic with ordinary physical exertion

Class II: Symptomatic with ordinary physical exertion

Class III: Symptomatic with less than ordinary physical exertion

Class IV: Symptomatic at rest

Dyspnea, or the sensation of difficulty in breathing, is the most common manifestation of heart failure. Dyspnea results from the increased work of breathing produced by pulmonary vascular congestion and alterations in lung compliance. Just as a spectrum of pulmonary congestion exists, ranging from pulmonary venous congestion to interstitial edema, and finally to alveolar edema, dyspnea presents in progressively more serious forms. *Dyspnea on exertion* (DOE) represents the earliest presentation. *Orthopnea*, or dyspnea in the recumbent position, is due primarily to the redistribution of blood volume from the dependent portions of the body to the central circulation. *Paroxysmal nocturnal dyspnea* (PND) is sudden awakening with dyspnea. It is a more specific manifestation of left ventricular failure than is either dyspnea or orthopnea. *Cardiac asthma* is PND with prominent wheezing. A nonproductive *cough* may also occur secondary to the pulmonary congestion. The development of *rales* due to pulmonic fluid transudation is characteristic of heart failure; initially rales are audible over the lung bases because of

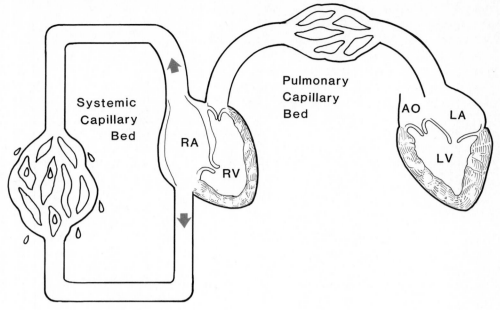

FIGURE 29-7
Systemic edema in right, heart failure. (Modified from Vinsant and Spense, 1981, p. 251.)

the effects of gravity. All of these signs and symptoms may be ascribed to backward failure of the left side of the heart.

Backward failure of the right side of the heart produces signs and symptoms of systemic venous congestion. *Elevation of jugular venous pressure* is noted; the neck veins become engorged and elevated. If tricuspid valve regurgitation develops, pulsatile *v* waves may be apparent in the jugular vein. A *positive hepatojugular reflux test* can be elicited; manual compression of the right upper quadrant of the abdomen produces jugular venous pressure elevation because the failing right side of the heart is unable to accommodate the associated increase in venous return. *Hepatomegaly*, or liver enlargement, appears; liver tenderness may be noted because of stretching of the hepatic capsule. Other *gastrointestinal symptoms*, such as anorexia, fullness, or nausea, may result from hepatic and intestinal congestion.

Peripheral edema develops secondary to fluid accumulation in the interstitial spaces. The edema is initially apparent in dependent regions of the body and is greatest at the end of the day; *nocturia*, or diuresis at night, may occur, lessening the degree of fluid retention. Nocturia results from fluid redistribution and reabsorption in the recumbent position as well as a reduction in the degree of renal vasoconstriction at rest. Advanced failure may be associated with the development of *ascites* or *anasarca*. Although the signs and symptoms of fluid accumulation in the systemic venous circuit noted above are classically considered to be secondary to right heart failure, it should be noted that the earliest manifestations of systemic congestion are usually due simply

to fluid retention rather than to overt right heart failure. All of the manifestations described above are typically preceded by *weight gain*, which simply reflects the retention of sodium and water.

Forward failure of the left ventricle produces signs of diminished organ perfusion. Since blood is shunted from nonvital organs to maintain perfusion of the heart and brain, the earliest manifestations of forward failure reflect diminished perfusion of organs such as the skin and skeletal muscles. *Skin pallor* and *coolness* result from peripheral vasoconstriction; further reductions in cardiac output associated with increased oxygen extraction and elevated levels of reduced hemoglobin produce *cyanosis*. The cutaneous vasoconstriction interferes with the body's ability to lose heat; therefore a low-grade *fever* may be noted. Underperfusion of the skeletal muscles produces *weakness* and *fatigue*. These symptoms can be exacerbated by fluid and electrolyte imbalances or anorexia. Further reduction in cardiac output can be associated with *changes in mental status*, such as the development of insomnia, restlessness, or confusion.

Examination of the arterial pulse during heart failure reveals a rapid, weak pulse. The rapid heart rate, or *tachycardia*, represents a response to sympathetic nervous stimulation. A significant fall in stroke volume and the associated peripheral vasoconstriction reduces pulse pressure (the difference between systolic and diastolic pressure), producing a weak or thready pulse. Systolic *hypotension* is noted with more severe heart failure. In addition, severe left ventricular failure may be associated with the development of *pulsus alternans*, an alternation in the strength of the arterial pulse. Pulsus alternans indicates severe mechanical dysfunction with a repetitive beat-to-beat variation in stroke volume.

Common findings upon auscultation of the chest

are *rales*, as noted earlier, and a *ventricular gallop* or S₃. The ventricular gallop occurs during the early diastolic period of rapid ventricular filling and is produced by the increased residual volumes within the ventricle and the reduction in ventricular compliance. Chest x-ray reveals the following: (1) pulmonary venous congestion, (2) vascular redistribution to the upper lobes of the lung, and (3) cardiomegaly.

Characteristic changes in blood values are also apparent. For example, alterations in fluid and electrolyte concentrations are reflected in serum levels. Typically, dilutional hyponatremia is observed; potassium levels may be normal or reduced secondary to diuretic therapy. Hyperkalemia may occur late in the course of heart failure because of renal impairment. Similarly, blood urea nitrogen (BUN) and creatinine levels may be elevated secondary to changes in glomerular filtration rate. Urine is concentrated, with a high specific gravity and reduced sodium content. Elevations of bilirubin and liver enzymes, serum glutamic oxaloacetic transaminase (SGOT) and serum alkaline phosphatase (SGPT), may result from hepatic dysfunction.

Etiology

Heart failure is the most common mechanical complication of virtually all forms of acquired and congenital heart disease. Physiologic mechanisms producing heart failure include conditions which increase preload, increase afterload, or reduce myocardial contractility. States which increase preload include aortic regurgitation and ventricular septal defect; afterload is increased by conditions such as aortic stenosis and systemic hypertension. Myocardial contractility can be depressed by myocardial infarction and cardiomyopathies. In addition to these three physiologic mechanisms causing heart failure, other physiologic factors can cause the heart to fail as a pump. Factors interfering with ventricular filling, such as atrioventricular valve stenosis, can produce failure. Conditions such as constrictive pericarditis and cardiac tamponade produce failure by a combination of physiologic effects, including impairment of ventricular filling and ventricular ejection. It should be apparent that no single physiologic mechanism or combination of mechanisms is responsible for the development of heart failure; the effectiveness of the heart as a pump can be compromised by any number of pathophysiologic states (see Table 29-1).

Similarly, no unifying biochemical explanation can be identified as the fundamental mechanism producing heart failure. The precise defect producing the impairment in myocardial contractility is unknown. It is postulated that an abnormality in the synthesis or function of the contractile proteins or in the delivery of calcium within the sarcomere may be responsible.

A number of factors can precipitate the development of heart failure by acutely stressing the circulation. These factors include (1) arrhythmias, (2) systemic

TABLE 29-1

CAUSES OF OVERALL HEART PUMP FAILURE

1. Mechanical abnormalities
   a. Increased pressure load
      (1) Central (aortic stenosis, etc.)
      (2) Peripheral (systemic hypertension, etc.)
   b. Increased volume load (valvular regurgitation, shunts, increased preload, etc.)
   c. Obstruction to ventricular filling (mitral or tricuspid stenosis)
   d. Pericardial tamponade
   e. Endocardial or myocardial restriction
   f. Ventricular aneurysm
   g. Ventricular dyssynergy
2. Myocardial (muscular) abnormalities
   a. Primary
      (1) Cardiomyopathy
      (2) Myocarditis
      (3) Metabolic abnormalities
      (4) Toxicity (alcohol, cobalt, etc.)
      (5) Presbycardia
   b. Secondary
      (1) Dysdynamic abnormalities (secondary to mechanical abnormalities)
      (2) Oxygen deprivation (coronary heart disease)
      (3) Metabolic abnormalities
      (4) Inflammation
      (5) Systemic disease
      (6) Chronic obstructive lung disease
3. Altered cardiac rhythm or conduction sequence
   a. Standstill
   b. Fibrillation
   c. Extreme tachycardia or bradycardia
   d. Electrical asynchrony, conduction disturbances

Source: Hurst, Logue, Schlant, and Wenger (eds.), 1982, p. 383.

and pulmonic infection, and (3) pulmonary embolism. Arrhythmias interfere with the mechanical function of the heart by altering the electrical stimulus initiating the mechanical response; an effective, synchronized mechanical response cannot occur without a stable cardiac rhythm. The body's response to infection stresses the myocardium by increasing metabolic demands on an already compromised circulation. Pulmonary embolism acutely increases the resistance to right ventricular ejection, precipitating right heart failure. Effective management of heart failure requires recognition and treatment of not only the underlying physiologic mechanism and disease state but also any factors precipitating heart failure.

One cause of heart failure warranting special consideration as background for the section "Cardiac Transplantation" is cardiomyopathy. *Cardiomyopathies* are diseases of the heart muscle. The key to distinguishing cardiomyopathies from other cardiac disorders is that the underlying abnormality involves the ventricular myocardium as opposed to any other myocardial structure, such as the valves or coronary arteries. Cardiomyopathies are classified as either primary or secondary; primary cardiomyopathies are idiopathic in origin, whereas secondary cardiomyopathies are associated with some other systemic disease.

Cardiomyopathies can be classified according to three types of abnormalities in structure or function: (1) hypertrophic, (2) congestive (dilated), or (3) restrictive or obliterative (see Fig. 29-8). Hypertrophic cardiomyopathy is characterized by a hypertrophied and hyperdynamic heart. The increase in muscle mass is not associated with significant myocardial dilation. Although hypertrophic cardiomyopathy can cause heart failure, congestive cardiomyopathy is the more significant entity relative to cardiac transplantation.

Congestive cardiomyopathy, in contrast to hypertrophic cardiomyopathy, is characterized by a grossly dilated and hypodynamic ventricle. There may be a lesser degree of myocardial hypertrophy. The hypodynamic ventricle contracts poorly, producing the predictable sequence of backward and forward failure described earlier. It is noteworthy that all four chambers become dilated secondary to the increased ventricular volumes and pressures. Thrombus commonly develops within these chambers owing to blood pooling and stasis; thus, embolization is a potential threat. Typically,

the onset of disease is insidious; however, progression to end-stage, refractory heart failure can result. The prognosis for refractory heart failure is extremely poor and may necessitate consideration of cardiac transplantation. The exact cause of congestive cardiomyopathy is unknown; however, autoimmune and/or viral causation has been posed. Alcoholic and peripartal cardiomyopathies have been identified. Multifactorial causation is the most plausible explanation.

Finally, restrictive cardiomyopathy represents an impairment in ventricular filling due to reduced ventricular compliance. Endocardial or myocardial fibrosis or disease can result in this restriction to filling. The restriction reduces ventricular cavity size; progression to a more severe form of cavity restriction is referred to as obliterative cardiomyopathy.

Management of heart failure

Three general principles guide the treatment of heart failure: (1) improve myocardial contractility, (2) reduce cardiac work, and (3) reduce intravascular volume and congestion and associated fluid transudation. Initial measures to achieve these objectives include the administration of digitalis to increase the force of myocardial contraction, restriction of strenuous exertion to reduce cardiac work, and restriction of dietary salt intake to reduce fluid retention. If necessary, oral diuretics are added to counter retention of sodium and water. Activity restriction and sodium restriction are intensified as the failure progresses, and more potent diuretics may be administered.

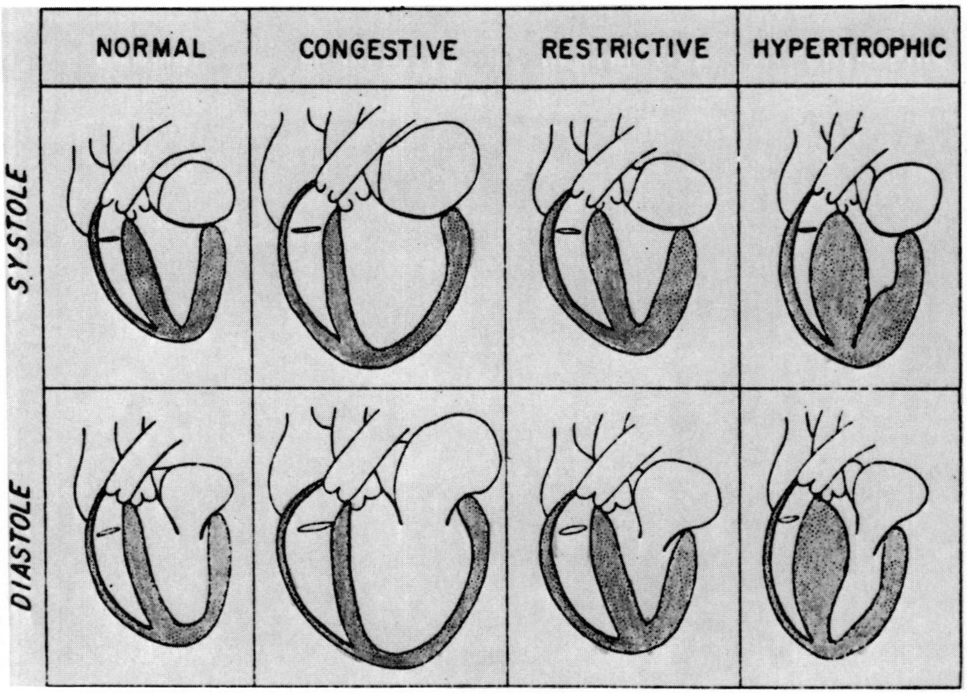

FIGURE 29-8
Types of cardiomyopathies. (From M. R. Goldman and C. A. Boucher, "Value of Radionuclide Imaging Techniques in Assessing Cardiomyopathy," *American Journal of Cardiology,* **46: 1235, 1980. Used by permission of the American Heart Association, Inc.)**

Severe heart failure, functional class III or IV, may be treated with newer modalities, such as vasodilators, nonglycoside inotropic drugs, or inhibitors of angiotensin-converting enzymes. Vasodilators reduce arterial pressure and consequently the resistance to ventricular ejection. Since the ventricle does not have to generate as high a systolic pressure to eject blood, afterload decreases. As a result, the ventricle can eject more easily and completely, as reflected by a reduction in cardiac work and a rise in cardiac output. Drugs such as hydralazine, prazosin, and nitrates are administered to dilate the vasculature and reduce afterload. Amrinone, a new nonglycoside inotropic drug, may be used to increase the force of contraction. Captopril inhibits the conversion of angiotensin I to angiotensin II, thereby reducing the circulating blood levels of angiotensin II. Since angiotensin II is a potent vasoconstrictor and increases arterial pressure, captopril reduces afterload and myocardial work by reducing arterial pressure. Captopril also inhibits aldosterone production and the associated retention of fluid.

Acute exacerbations of failure or the development of severe heart failure might necessitate hospitalization and more aggressive treatment. More aggressive measures to increase contractility include maximum digitalization and intravenous administration of inotropic drugs such as sympathetic amines. Preload is decreased by potent diuretics and, if necessary, physical removal of fluid through dialysis or other measures. Reduction of afterload may be accomplished by the administration of intravenous vasodilators or inhibitors of converting enzymes. Circulatory assistance or cardiac transplantation might be considered if warranted, given the clinical situation. These interventions will be discussed in subsequent sections.

SHOCK

Definitions

Shock does not constitute a single disease entity. It is a complex clinical syndrome encompassing a group of conditions with variable hemodynamic manifestations. Acute circulatory failure, defined earlier as the inability of the cardiovascular system to adequately perfuse the tissues, is referred to as the *shock state*. Regardless of the etiology of shock, the common denominator in all forms of shock is the reduction of blood flow to vital organs. This impairment in tissue perfusion compromises oxygen delivery to the tissues. The reduced blood flow may be due to (1) a reduction in cardiac output, (2) a maldistribution of blood flow, or (3) both of these. Most shock states are characterized by low cardiac output and increased peripheral resistance. Typically, shock is associated with profound hypotension, impaired renal and cerebral blood flow, and some degree of respiratory distress.

Etiology

A variety of conditions can culminate in shock. These conditions can be categorized according to four etiologic mechanisms (see Table 29-2). These mechanisms include cardiogenic mechanisms, obstructive mechanisms, alterations in circulatory volume, and alterations in circulatory distribution. This section will focus upon cardiogenic shock after myocardial infarction as illustrative of the shock state.

The incidence of cardiogenic shock after myocardial infarction approximates 15 percent. As a result of the infarction process, left ventricular contractility and performance may be severely impaired. The left ventricle fails as a pump and does not provide adequate cardiac output to maintain tissue perfusion. A self-perpetuating cycle then ensues (see Fig. 29-9). The cycle begins with the infarction and subsequent myocardial dysfunction. Profound myocardial dysfunction leads to reduced cardiac output and arterial hypotension. Metabolic acidosis and reduced coronary perfusion result, further impairing ventricular function and predisposing to the development of arrhythmias. As can be deduced, this cycle of cardiogenic shock must be interrupted early in the shock state to salvage left ventricular myocardium and prevent progression to an irreversible stage which is incompatible with survival. The mortality of cardiogenic shock treated with conventional interventions, such as those described for congestive heart failure, approaches 100 percent. More aggressive modalities to be discussed later in this chapter, such as intraaortic balloon pumping, have reduced this mortality.

Cardiogenic shock due to acute myocardial infarction is typically associated with a loss of approximately 40 percent of the left ventricular myocardium. In addition to such massive loss of the left ventricular musculature, focal areas of necrosis may also be found throughout the ventricle. This is thought to be due to the severe reduction in coronary blood flow and the increase in cardiac work and oxygen demand associated with compensatory responses such as sympathetic stimulation.

Mechanical defects caused by myocardial infarction can also produce significant myocardial dysfunction and shock. These defects include the following: (1) Acute mitral regurgitation due to rupture of a necrotic papillary muscle. This produces a reduction in forward blood flow or cardiac output, and large amounts of backward or regurgitant blood flow into the left atrium and pulmonary circuit. (2) Acquired ventricular septal defect due to rupture of an infarcted septum. This reduces forward blood flow into the aorta and produces shunting of

TABLE 29-2

ETIOLOGIES OF SHOCK

Cardiogenic shock

1. Secondary to arrhythmias
   a. Bradyarrhythmias
   b. Tachyarrhythmias
2. Secondary to cardiac mechanical factors
   a. Regurgitant lesions
      (1) Acute mitral or aortic regurgitation
      (2) Rupture of interventricular septum
      (3) Massive left ventricular aneurysm
   b. Obstructive lesions
      (1) Left ventricular outflow tract obstruction, e.g., congenital or acquired valvular aortic stenosis and hypertrophic obstructive cardiomyopathy
      (2) Left ventricular inflow tract obstruction, e.g., mitral stenosis, left atrial myxoma, atrial thrombus
3. Myopathic
   a. Impairment of left ventricular contractility, as in acute myocardial infarction or congestive cardiomyopathy
   b. Impairment of right ventricular contractility due to right ventricular infarction
   c. Impairment of left ventricular relaxation or compliance, as in restrictive or hypertrophic cardiomyopathy

Obstructive* shock

1. Pericardial tamponade
2. Coarctation of aorta
3. Pulmonary embolism
4. Primary pulmonary hypertension

Oligemic shock

1. Hemorrhage
2. Fluid depletion or sequestration due to vomiting, diarrhea, dehydration, diabetes mellitus, diabetes insipidus, adrenal cortical failure, peritonitis, pancreatitis, burns, ascites, villous adenoma, or pheochromocytoma

Distributive shock

1. Septicemic
   a. Endotoxic
   b. Secondary to specific infection, such as dengue fever
2. Metabolic or toxic
   a. Renal failure
   b. Hepatic failure
   c. Severe acidosis or alkalosis
   d. Drug overdose
   e. Heavy metal intoxication
   f. Toxic shock syndrome (possibly due to a staphylococcal exotoxin)
   g. Malignant hyperthermia
3. Endocrinologic
   a. Uncontrolled diabetes mellitus with ketoacidosis or hyperosmolar coma
   b. Adrenal cortical failure
   c. Hypothyroidism
   d. Hyper- or hypoparathyroidism
   e. Diabetes insipidus
   f. Hypoglycemia secondary to excess exogenous insulin or a beta-cell tumor
4. Microcirculatory, due to altered blood viscosity
   a. Polycythemia vera
   b. Hyperviscosity syndromes, including multiple myeloma, macroglobulinemia, and cryoglobulinemia
   c. Sickle cell anemia
   d. Fat emboli
5. Neurogenic
   a. Cerebral
   b. Spinal
   c. Dysautonomic
6. Anaphylactic

*Due to factors extrinsic to cardiac valves and myocardium.
Source: Braunwald (ed.), 1984, p. 579.

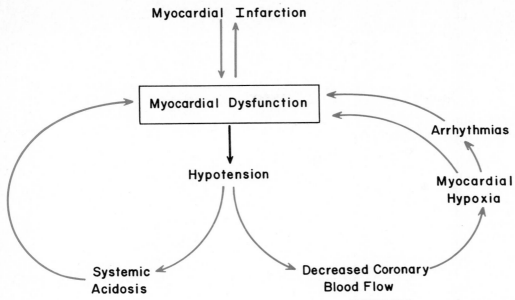

Myocardial Infarction

Myocardial Dysfunction

Hypotension

Arrhythmias

Myocardial Hypoxia

Systemic Acidosis

Decreased Coronary Blood Flow

FIGURE 29-9

Self-perpetuating cycle of cardiogenic shock. (From W. B. Dunkman et al., "Clinical and Hemodynamic Results of IABP and Surgery for Cardiogenic Shock," *Circulation*, **46**: 474, 1972. Used by permission of the American Heart Association, Inc.).

blood from the high-pressure left ventricle to the lower-pressure right ventricle. (3) Ventricular aneurysms secondary to weakening and bulging of the infarcted region. Large left ventricular aneurysms reduce left ventricular output by becoming a reservoir for blood during ventricular ejection. Also, because portions of the left ventricular musculature are rendered ineffective, the portion of ventricular volume ejected, or the ejection fraction, is reduced further, compromising cardiac output.

Pathophysiology and systemic effects

Cardiogenic shock can be viewed as a severe form of left ventricular failure. The pathophysiologic events and compensatory responses parallel that of failure, but they have progressed to a more severe form. Cardiogenic shock is characterized by left ventricular dysfunction, leading to a severe impairment of tissue perfusion and of oxygen delivery to the tissues. The depression of myocardial contractility reduces cardiac output and increases left ventricular volumes and end-diastolic pressure, leading to pulmonary congestion and edema.

As systemic arterial pressure falls, stimulation of the baroreceptors in the aorta and carotid sinus occurs. Sympathoadrenal stimulation produces reflex vasoconstriction, tachycardia, and increased contractility to augment cardiac output and stabilize blood pressure. Contractility is augmented further according to Starling's law by renal retention of sodium and water. Thus, the depressed contractility of cardiogenic shock elicits compensatory responses increasing afterload and preload. Although these protective mechanisms initially enhance arterial blood pressure and tissue perfusion, their effect on the myocardium is deleterious owing to the

increase in cardiac work and myocardial oxygen demand. Since coronary flow is inadequate, as evidenced by the infarction, the imbalance between myocardial oxygen supply and demand increases. Further myocardial dysfunction ensues secondary to ischemia and focal necrosis, perpetuating a vicious cycle of myocardial compromise. As left ventricular performance continues to deteriorate, the shock state rapidly progresses until such profound circulatory failure exists that every major organ system is affected.

The systemic affects of the shock state contribute to its eventual irreversibility. Some organs are affected more quickly and more profoundly than others. As noted, the myocardium suffers deleterious effects early in the shock state. In addition to the increases in myocardial work and oxygen demand, other significant changes occur. Because of the anaerobic metabolism induced by the shock state, the myocardium cannot maintain its normal level of high-energy phosphate stores, and ventricular contractility is further impaired. Hypoxia and acidosis inhibit energy production and contribute to further destruction of myocardial cells. These two factors also shift the ventricular function curve downward and to the right depressing contractility further.

Respiratory compromise develops secondary to the shock state. A potentially lethal complication is profound respiratory failure. Pulmonary congestion and intraalveolar edema lead to hypoxia and deterioration of arterial blood gases. Atelectasis and pulmonary infection may also occur. These factors predispose to the development of "shock lung," now frequently referred to as *adult respiratory distress syndrome* (see Chap. 37). Tachypnea, dyspnea, and moist rales are noted, as well as other symptoms described earlier as manifesting backward heart failure.

Reduced renal perfusion results in oliguria with a urine output generally less than 20 ml/hour. With further reductions in cardiac output, an associated fall in urine output will usually be observed. Because of the compensatory retention of sodium and water, urine sodium levels will be reduced. Along with the reduction in glomerular filtration rate, an increase in the blood urea nitrogen (BUN) and creatinine will be noted. With prolonged, severe hypotension, acute tubular necrosis with ensuing acute renal failure may result (see Chap. 45).

Shock of prolonged duration results in hepatic cellular dysfunction. Cellular damage may be localized to isolated zones of hepatic necrosis, or massive hepatic necrosis may occur with profound shock. Marked derangements of liver function become apparent. This is usually manifested by elevations of liver enzymes, SGOT and SGPT. Hepatic hypoxia appears to be the etiologic mechanism initiating these complications.

Prolonged ischemia of the gastrointestinal (GI) tract typically results in hemorrhagic necrosis of the bowel. Bowel injury may exacerbate the shock state by sequestering fluid in the gut and by the absorption of bacteria and endotoxins into the circulation. A decrease in GI motility is almost always noted in association with shock.

Normally, cerebral blood flow displays the property of autoregulation of flow, with dilation occurring in response to diminished flow or ischemia. Cerebral autoregulation fails to maintain adequate flow and perfusion when the mean arterial pressure falls below 60 mmHg. During prolonged periods of hypotension, symptoms of neurologic deficit may be observed. These deficits are not usually sustained if recovery from the shock state occurs, unless a cerebrovascular accident has resulted concomitantly.

During sustained shock, intravascular aggregation of cellular components of the hematologic system may occur, increasing peripheral vascular resistance further. Diffuse intravascular coagulation (DIC) may occur during the shock state, further compromising the clinical situation.

Hemodynamic profile

Criteria for the diagnosis of cardiogenic shock have been established by the Myocardial Infarction Research

Units (MIRU) of the National Heart, Lung, and Blood Institute (NHLBI). Cardiogenic shock is characterized by:

1. A systolic arterial pressure less than 90 mmHg or 30 to 60 mmHg below the previous baseline level.

2. Evidence of decreased blood flow to major organ systems:
   a. Urine output less than 20 ml/hour, usually with decreased sodium content.
   b. Peripheral vasoconstriction associated with cold, clammy skin.
   c. Impaired mental function.

3. Cardiac index* less than 2.1 liters/(minute/m²)

4. Evidence of left-sided heart failure with LVEDP/PCWP greater than 18 to 21 mmHg.

These criteria reflect severe left-sided heart failure with evidence of forward and backward failure. The systolic hypotension and evidence of impaired tissue perfusion is characteristic of the shock state. Extreme depression of the cardiac index to less than 0.9 liter/(minute/m²) may be observed with profound cardiogenic shock.

In cardiogenic shock with acute mitral regurgitation, large *v* waves are observed in the PCW trace (see Fig. 29-10). This significantly increases LA and PCW pressures and the degree of pulmonary compromise. The development of severe pulmonary edema is common in the setting of acute mitral regurgitation.

With the development of a ventricular septal defect (VSD), there is shunting and mixing of blood between the left and right ventricles. Consequently, the oxygen content of the blood in the right ventricle increases. Pressures of the right side of the heart also rise, owing to the recirculation of blood through the right side of the heart and pulmonic circuit. Insertion of a pulmonary arterial catheter is indicated to detect these alterations through blood sampling and pressure measurement in the right side of the heart. Measurement of cardiac output by dye dilution (see Chapter 26, "Diagnostic Procedures") is useful to document the presence and degree of shunting with VSD or of regurgitant flow with mitral regurgitation, as well as to measure cardiac output.

Calculated systemic vascular resistance (i.e., the difference between mean arterial pressure and central venous pressure, divided by cardiac output and multiplied

---

*Cardiac index is the cardiac output in liters per minute per square meter of body surface area (BSA). The normal resting average is 2.8 liters/(minute·m²). Average BSA for a 150-lb man is 1.75 m².

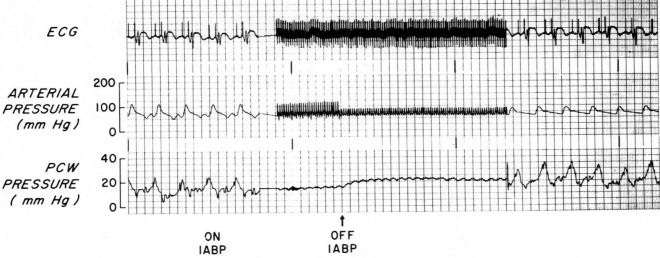

ECG

ARTERIAL
PRESSURE
(mm Hg)

200
100
0

PCW
PRESSURE
(mm Hg)

40
20
0

ON
IABP

OFF
IABP

FIGURE 29-10

The effect of intraaortic balloon pumping (IABP) on acute mitral regurgitation. At the arrow, the balloon pump is turned off. The increase in systolic arterial pressure is accompanied by a prompt rise of PCW pressure and an increase in the amplitude of systolic regurgitation *v* waves. (From H. K. Gold et al., "IABP for Ventricular Septal Defect or Mitral Regurgitation Complicating Acute Myocardial Infarction," *Circulation*, 47: 1191, 1973. Used by permission of the American Heart Association, Inc.)

by 80) will be markedly increased in cardiogenic shock owing to the intense peripheral vasoconstriction.

Management of cardiogenic shock

The support of cardiac output is essential to the management of cardiogenic shock. Ultimate survival depends upon the reduction of cardiac work and myocardial oxygen demand and the limitation of the extent of infarction and the degree of ventricular dysfunction. This is generally accomplished by administration of agents that reduce preload and afterload as well as by efforts to augment contractility.

Positive inotropic agents are administered to augment contractility. Agents commonly used are digitalis glycosides, dobutamine, and a newer inotropic agent, amrinone. Preload is decreased by reduction of intravascular volume with diuretics. Pulmonary capillary wedge pressure (PCWP), the clinical measure of LVEDP, is used to guide the administration of diuretics or volume in these acutely ill patients.

Vasodilating agents reduce both preload and afterload. Reduction of preload is accomplished with venous dilators, such as nitrates; venodilation decreases venous return to the heart. Arterial vasodilators, such as sodium nitroprusside, dilate the smooth muscle of the arterial system, reducing arterial pressure. The reduction of arterial pressure reduces the resistance to ventricular ejection and improves cardiac output. Intraaortic balloon pumping, described in the next section, also decreases afterload and may be indicated if cardiogenic shock is unresponsive to conventional measures.

Vasopressor agents which constrict the vasculature are generally avoided, since they increase afterload and myocardial oxygen demand further. The use of vasopressors is usually limited to those patients whose hy-

potension is so profound that no other means of therapy provides blood pressure support. Most vasopressor agents, for example, epinephrine or levarterenol bitartrate (Levophed), stimulate both alpha and beta receptors, although to varying degrees. Increases in afterload and cardiac work therefore cannot be avoided. Agents with beta activity also are potentially arrhythmogenic, which further hinders myocardial performance. Support of cardiac output may be indirectly improved by the administration of antiarrhythmic drugs if indicated. Restoration of sinus rhythm generally improves cardiac output and blood pressure.

Oxygenation is supported with the administration of supplemental oxygen therapy and the initiation of mechanical ventilation if indicated. Correction of metabolic acidosis is accomplished with adjustments in ventilation or the administration of sodium bicarbonate. Treatment of acute pulmonary edema involves reduction of preload with vasodilators and diuretics as described and the administration of morphine sulfate.

Invasive monitoring of the cardiovascular system is generally performed to provide continuous information relative to the patient's blood pressure and intracardiac filling pressures. Placement of an indwelling arterial catheter and a Swan-Ganz pulmonary arterial catheter is usually accomplished soon after the patient is admitted to the intensive care unit.

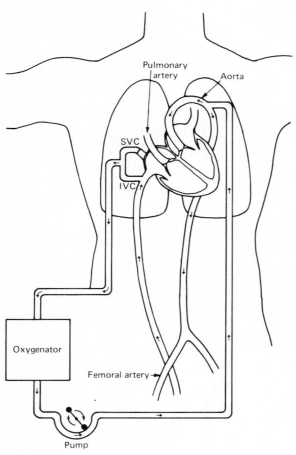

FIGURE 29-11

Total cardiopulmonary bypass. Venous blood is shunted from the right atrium to the assist device via catheters inserted into the superior vena cava (SVC) and inferior vena cava (IVC). The blood is oxygenated by the device and returned to the arterial system through a cannula in the aorta. (From M. Kinney (ed.), *AACN's Clinical Reference for Critical Care Nurses,* **McGraw-Hill, New York, 1981, p. 929.)**

CIRCULATORY ASSISTANCE

Development and evolution

Circulatory assistance was initially used for cardiopulmonary support during cardiac surgical procedures in the early 1950s. During open heart surgery, the oxygenation and systemic circulation of blood is sustained by a heart-lung machine, referred to as *cardiopulmonary bypass* (see Fig. 29-11). Catheters or cannulas are inserted into the superior vena cava and inferior vena cava to shunt venous blood away from the right side of the heart into the cardiopulmonary bypass machine. Additional blood is returned to the bypass machine by a me-

diastinal "sucker," which is placed in the operative field to collect blood lost during the surgical procedure. The bypass machine performs the following functions: (1) oxygenation of the blood, (2) cooling of blood to induce systemic hypothermia, which consequently reduces the amount of oxygen consumed by the tissues, and (3) filtration of blood to remove air and particulate matter. The blood is then pumped into the patient's arterial circulation via a cannula positioned in either the aortic arch or the femoral artery. Just prior to weaning the patient from cardiopulmonary bypass, the heat exchanger in the bypass unit rewarms the blood.

During the late 1960s, less invasive forms of circulatory assistance, such as the intraaortic balloon pump, were used to support patients in cardiogenic shock. It was hoped that circulatory assistance would interrupt the vicious cycle of cardiogenic shock by elevating arterial blood pressure, improving peripheral perfusion, and reducing cardiac work, thereby preserving ischemic, salvageable zones of the myocardium. Circulatory assistance is currently used in various forms to provide support for a variety of cardiovascular mechanical problems which will be discussed in the ensuing pages.

Intraaortic balloon counterpulsation

The intraaortic balloon is positioned in the descending thoracic aorta just distal to the left subclavian artery. It is inserted via either a percutaneous approach or a femoral arteriotomy and is threaded retrograde through the descending abdominal aorta (see Fig. 29-12). The bal-

FIGURE 29-12

Insertion and location of the aortic balloon. (From P. J. Ford and R. W. Weintraub, *Intra-Aortic Balloon Pumping,* **Aristrocrat Press, Cambridge, 1974, p. IV-2.)**

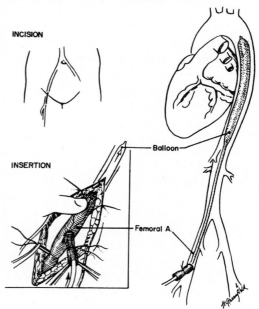

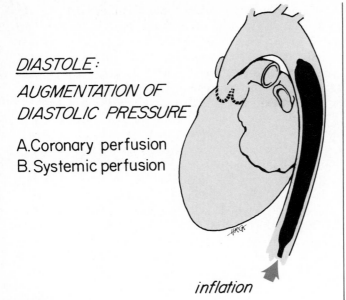

DIASTOLE:
AUGMENTATION OF
DIASTOLIC PRESSURE

A. Coronary perfusion
B. Systemic perfusion

inflation

FIGURE 29-13
Effect of intraaortic balloon inflation.

loon is inflated and deflated in synchrony with the mechanical events of the cardiac cycle. Obviously, during left ventricular ejection or systole, the balloon must be deflated. During ventricular diastole, the balloon is inflated.

Inflation of the balloon with helium occurs just as the aortic valve closes at the end of systole; balloon inflation raises aortic volume, elevating aortic pressure. This effect is referred to as *augmentation of diastolic pressure*. The physiologic effect of diastolic augmentation is twofold (see Fig. 29-13): (1) the perfusion pressure at the coronary orifices is increased during diastole, the period of greatest coronary flow, potentially increasing coronary flow; (2) systemic perfusion may also improve through elevation of mean arterial pressure.

Balloon deflation occurs rapidly, immediately prior to ventricular ejection, just before the aortic valve opens. As helium is removed from the balloon, intraaortic volume is lowered, and therefore aortic pressure is reduced. This reduction in aortic pressure lowers the resistance against which the left ventricle must eject blood; consequently, this produces reduction in wall tension during isovolumetric contraction. In other words, balloon deflation *reduces afterload*. The physiologic effects (see Fig. 29-14) are as follows: (1) reduction in cardiac work, (2) reduction in oxygen demand and myocardial oxygen consumption per unit time ($M\dot{V}O_2$), and (3) increase in cardiac output.

Balloon pumping is particularly effective in the reversal of cardiogenic shock resulting from mechanical defects, such as ventricular septal defect and mitral regurgitation. Initiation of balloon pumping in these patients reduces aortic pressure and resistance to ejection, thereby increasing forward flow through the aorta and

reducing abnormal flow through the defect. Refractory myocardial ischemia is also responsive to balloon pumping; physiologically, the intraaortic balloon pump can influence both the supply and the demand determinants of the myocardial oxygenation balance. Coronary blood flow increases with diastolic augmentation, and myocardial oxygen demand falls as a result of the reduction of afterload.

Assist devices for left side of heart

Assist devices for the left side of the heart are generating much interest as a means of temporarily supporting the failing left ventricle. Two types of such devices are currently used.

Left atrial–arterial assistance

This type of left heart assist device (LHAD) is used intraoperatively for patients who develop cardiogenic shock and cannot be weaned from cardiopulmonary bypass. It is a temporary measure aimed at supporting the circulation until the depressed myocardium is able to resume its normal function.

In this circulatory assist system, oxygenated blood is directed from the left atrium via a biosilastic cannula, through a roller pump, and back into the ascending aortic arch (Fig. 29-15). This device can provide a cardiac output of up to 5 liters/minute. After the patient has been weaned from the device, biosilastic obturators are

FIGURE 29-14
Effect of intraaortic balloon deflation.

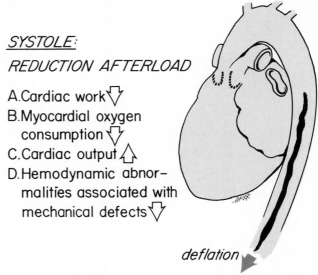

SYSTOLE:
REDUCTION AFTERLOAD

A. Cardiac work ▽
B. Myocardial oxygen
   consumption ▽
C. Cardiac output △
D. Hemodynamic abnor-
   malities associated with
   mechanical defects ▽

deflation

pumping chamber encased in a titanium housing. The device may be external to the body or implanted into the patient's abdomen. This abdomen–left ventricular assist device is abbreviated as ALVAD. Oxygenated blood is diverted from the left ventricle via a conduit attached to the ventricular apex and is led into a pumping chamber. Blood is then returned via a conduit attached to either the thoracic or the abdominal aorta (see Fig. 29-17). A pneumatic drive tube, external to the device, is connected to a drive system. This device can deliver cardiac outputs of up to 6 liters/minute and provide total circulatory assistance during periods of cardiac arrest (see Fig. 29-18). The disadvantage of this device, as compared with the left atrial-arterial assist device, is that reoperation is required for device removal. Failure of patients to be weaned from these devices may present a unique set of moral and ethical problems relating to the ultimate management of care.

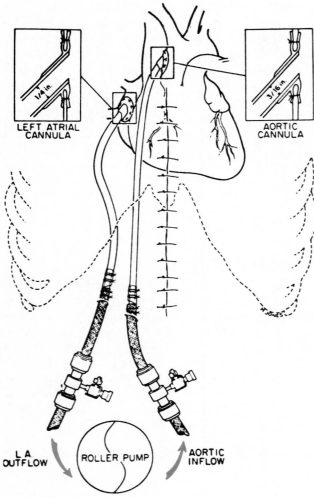

FIGURE 29-15

The cannula pump left heart assist device. (From R. S. Litwak et al., "Use of a Left Heart Assist Device after Intracardiac Surgery: Technique and Clinical Experience," *Annals of Thoracic Surgery* **21(3): 191, 1976.)**

placed through the cannulas and the circuit is sealed with silicone adhesive. This obviates the need for reoperation for device removal. The cannulas remain in situ permanently (see Fig. 29-16).

Left ventricular–arterial assistance

The application of this circulatory assist device is similar to that of the left atrial–arterial assist device, with the exception that it may be infrequently employed to support the circulation of critically ill patients awaiting cardiac transplantation.

The device is egg-shaped, with a polyurethane

FIGURE 29-16

Separation of the patient from the left heart assist device is accomplished by exposing the distal cannula tips in their subcutaneous location through a small incision (bottom inset). The pump connections are separated from the cannulas, and the obturators are slipped into place and secured with ligatures and silicone elastomer glue. They are left permanently in situ. (From R. S. Litwak et al., "Use of the Left Heart Assist Device after Intracardiac Surgery: Technique and Clinical Experience," *Annals of Thoracic Surgery,* **21(3): 191, 1976.)**

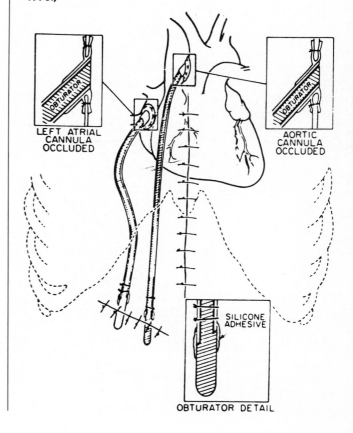

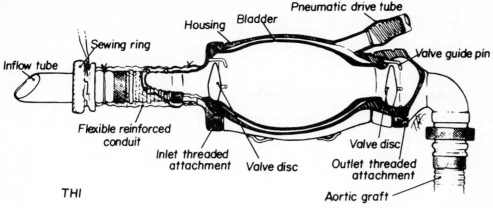

THI

FIGURE 29-17

The abdominal left ventricular assist device. (From Bregman (ed.), 1977, p. 66.)

The artificial heart

Artificial replacement of the heart has been of interest since the late 1950s. Since that time, many advances have made the artificial heart clinically applicable to human beings. The first implantation of the total artificial heart was performed in 1982 at the University of Utah.

This system employs biosynthetic pumping chambers which provide for total support of the circulation. The artificial heart contains ventricular pumping chambers, porcine valves, and conduit grafts for attachment to the great vessels (see Fig. 29-19). A pneumatic drive system operates the artificial heart, driving the internal pumping chambers. Implantation of the heart is accomplished by excising the recipient's ventricular chambers

and anastomosing the recipient's atria and great vessels to the artificial device. It is hoped that eventually the artificial heart will completely replace cardiac function on a long-term basis. This is difficult to accomplish, since the drive mechanism for the system is quite cumbersome and limits the patient's mobility. Some centers are investigating the use of nuclear-powered or electrically driven hearts to circumvent this limitation.

FIGURE 29-18

Operation of ALVAD during ventricular fibrillation and defibrillation to support aortic pressure. Note fall in aortic pressure when ALVAD is turned off for approximately two seconds. (From Bregman, 1977 (ed.), p. 108.)

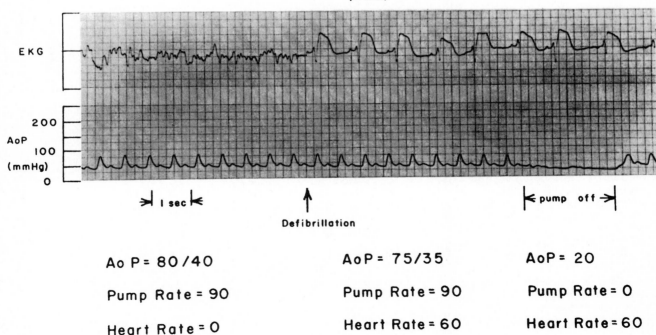

AoP = 80/40	AoP = 75/35	AoP = 20
Pump Rate = 90	Pump Rate = 90	Pump Rate = 0
Heart Rate = 0	Heart Rate = 60	Heart Rate = 60

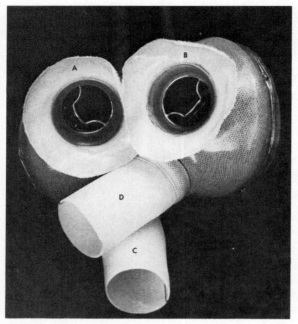

FIGURE 29-19

Artifical ventricles with quick connectors in place. A, right atrial; B, left atrial; C, pulmonary artery; D, aorta. (From Susan J. Quaal (ed.), *Comprehensive Intra-aortic Balloon Pumping,* The C.V. Mosby Co., St. Louis, 1984, p. 354; photographs by Brad Nelson, Division of Medical Illustrations, University of Utah.)

Cardiac transplantation

The first human cardiac transplant was performed in 1967 by Barnard in South Africa. After an initial period of enthusiastic response, interest waned owing to poor success. Rejection seemed an unsurmountable problem. Over the years, refinements in immunosuppressive therapy, immunological monitoring techniques and organ preservation techniques have resulted in significant improvements in patient survival. The most extensive clinical and laboratory experience with cardiac transplantation exists in the United States at Stanford University, California.

Cardiac transplantation is considered for end-stage heart disease refractory to conventional medical and surgical therapy. Class IV heart failure (i.e., the patient is symptomatic at rest) must be evident, with a life expectancy of weeks to months. The two most common conditions producing such myocardial compromise are congestive cardiomyopathy and advanced coronary artery disease. Recipients who meet these criteria for selection undergo an extensive clinical and psychosocial evaluation. Factors that would complicate the postoperative course or affect long-term survival must be ruled out. These factors include systemic infection or disease, pulmonary hypertension, peptic ulcers, insulin-dependent diabetes mellitus, irreversible liver or renal failure, pulmonary emboli or infarction, and psychosocial problems. If no contraindications are identified, a search for a potential donor is undertaken.

Potential donors are typically young trauma victims with no evidence of cardiac damage or disease and no systemic infection. Tissue matching of the donor to the recipient includes matching of the ABO system and usually human lymphocyte antigen (HLA) typing (see

FIGURE 29-20

Technique for heart transplant. The operation is performed as a conventional open-heart procedure with the usual equipment and instrumentation. It does not present any particular mechanical difficulties. The patient is prepared routinely and a median sternotomy is preformed. The patient is then connected to a cardiopulmonary bypass machine, after systemic heparization. The donor heart is excised following arrest obtained by infusion of cold cardioplegia solution. It is then placed in cold saline solution for transfer to the recipient's operating room. The heart of the recipient is excised simultaneously. (A) The aorta and pulmonary artery are divided immediately above their respective valves. Atrial walls and the interatrial septum are divided near the atrioventricular groove, leaving two

(Legend continued on next page.)

A

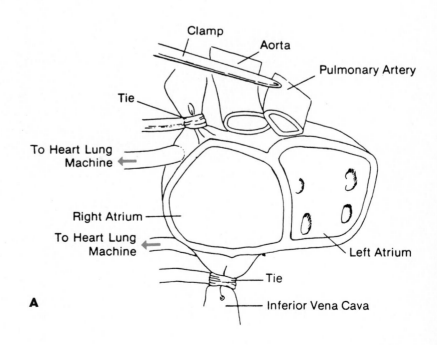

large right and left atrial cuffs. (B) Orthotopic graft is performed by anastomosing recipient and donor atrial walls and interatrial septum. (C) and (D) Major vessels of donor and recipient. The aorta and pulmonary artery are trimmed and sutured, reestablishing anatomic continuity. The cardiac transplantation procedure is terminated like any conventional open-heart procedure, with great care to prevent hemostasis and to eliminate entrapped air in the graft. The donor heart often starts beating spontaneously in sinus rhythm when perfusion is reestablished and rewarming is achieved. (From Leslie Flickinger Kern, "Surgical Treatment of Underlying Heart Disease: Coronary Artery Bypass, Heart Valve Replaement, Heart Transplant," in Cydney R. Michaelson (ed.), *Congestive Heart Failure*, The C. V. Mosby Co., St. Louis, 1983, pp. 435–436.) (*Legend continues on next page.*)

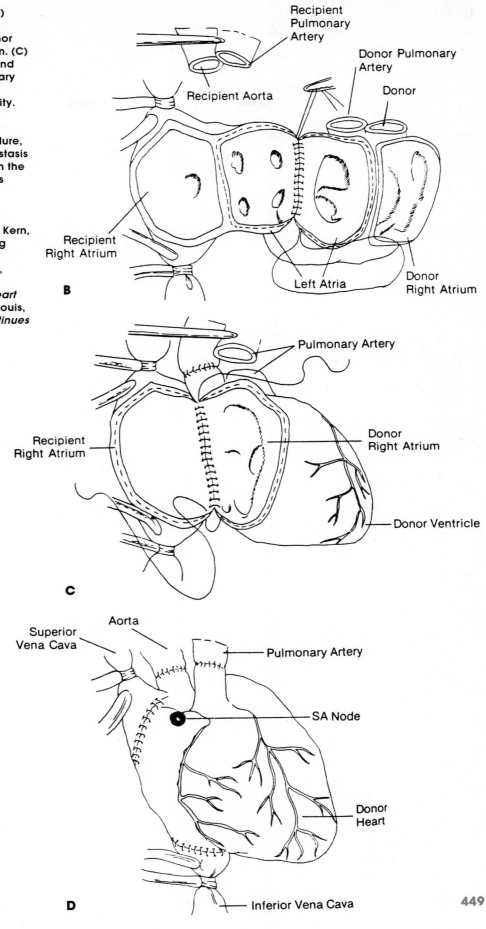

449

the discussion of renal transplantation immunology in Chap. 44). An appropriate size match is also important.

The surgical technique for cardiac transplantation is relatively straightforward, as illustrated in Fig. 29-20. A small portion of the recipient's atria remains in situ for anastomosis to the donor heart; the donor heart is then sutured to the recipient's pulmonary artery and aorta.

The greatest challenge is transplantation is the management of rejection. The body's attempt to reject foreign tissue is a fundamental biological process. Immunosuppressive therapy with cyclosporin A and ste-

roids is initiated preoperatively and continued after surgery. The advent of cyclosporin A has significantly improved survival after transplantation. Close immunologic monitoring for the signs of rejection, including decreased ECG voltage or increased levels of T lymphocytes, is instituted. Endomyocardial biopsies are performed at regular intervals and as indicated. This technique involves insertion of a biopsy catheter, or bioptome, through the right internal jugular or subclavian vein into the right ventricle to remove a portion of the endocardium for analysis. This is a very sensitive means for the detection of rejection. Immunosuppressive therapy can then be adjusted accordingly. In addition to potential rejection, infection is a significant problem, given the immunosuppressive therapy. Appropriate prophylactic and therapeutic measures are utilized.

QUESTIONS

Cardiac mechanical dysfunction and circulatory support

Directions: Circle the letter preceding each item below that correctly answers the question. Only one answer is correct unless otherwise noted.

1. The relationship between left ventricular end-diastolic volume and left ventricular performance is illustrated in the:
   a. Cardiac output curve *b.* Ratio of *dp/dt*
   c. Frank-Starling curve *d.* Arterial-alveolar gradient

2. The ventricular function curve characteristic of the failing heart is usually:
   a. Depressed and flattened *b.* Elevated and curved *c.* Gradually sloping *d.* None of the above

3. The primary compensatory responses to a reduction in stroke volume include all of the following *except:*
   a. Increased sympathetic activity *b.* Increased afterload *c.* Increased preload *d.* Ventricular hypertrophy

4. Which myocardial substance may become depleted during chronic heart failure?
   a. Epinephrine *b.* Myocardial lactate
   c. 2,3-Diphosphoglycerate *d.* Norepinephrine

5. Deleterious effects of compensatory mechanisms include: (More than one answer may be correct.)
   a. Reduced preload *b.* Increased cardiac work
   c. Improvement of heart failure *d.* Worsening of heart failure

6. A classic symptom of forward heart failure would be:

   a. Weakness and fatigue *b.* Pulmonary edema
   c. Anemia *d.* Hypovolemia

7. A classic symptom of backward heart failure would be:
   a. Weakness and fatigue *b.* Pulmonary edema
   c. Anemia *d.* Hypovolemia

8. Backward failure of the right side of the heart may produce all of the following *except:* (More than one answer may be correct.)
   a. Elevated jugular venous pressure *b.* Rales and rhonchi *c.* Peripheral edema *d.* Weight gain *e.* Hepatomegaly *f.* Ascites *g.* Orthopnea

9. The typical chest x-ray of heart failure reveals all of the following *except:*
   a. Cardiomegaly *b.* Retrocardiac densities
   c. Pulmonary venous congestion *d.* Upper lobar vascular redistribution

10 Which of the following laboratory findings may be useful in the diagnosis and management of heart failure? (More than one answer may be correct.)
   a. Serum electrolytes *b.* Platelet count
   c. BUN and creatinine *d.* Urine electrolytes
   e. Serum lipids *f.* Liver function tests

11. All of the following may precipitate heart failure *except:*
   a. Arrhythmias *b.* Infection *c.* Disseminated intravascular coagulation (DIC) *d.* Pulmonary embolism

12. The form of end-stage cardiomyopathy most frequently considered for cardiac transplantation is:

a. Hypertrophic   b. Restrictive   c. Congestive
d. All of the above

13. Measures to improve myocardial contractility may include all of the following *except:*
a. Digitalis glycosides   b. Intraaortic balloon pumping   c. Amrinone   d. Dobutamine

14. Measures to reduce cardiac work include all of the following *except:*
a. Arterial vasodilators   b. Digitalis glycosides
c. Intraaortic balloon pumping   d. Venodilators

15. The incidence of cardiogenic shock following acute myocardial infarction is approximately:
a. 10 to 15 percent   b. 30 to 35 percent   c. 80 to 90 percent   d. None of the above

16. Conventional medical management of cardiogenic shock is associated with a mortality rate approaching:
a. 25 percent   b. 50 percent   c. 75 percent
d. 100 percent

17. Cardiogenic shock may be secondary to: (More than one answer may be correct.)
a. Atrial fibrillation   b. Acute myocardial infarction   c. Acute mitral regurgitation
d. Pericarditis   e. Ventricular septal defect
f. All of the above

18. The effects of cardiogenic shock upon the myocardium include: (More than one answer may be correct.)
a. Decreased coronary blood flow
b. Arrhythmias   c. Increased afterload   d. Systemic acidosis   e. Hypoxia   f. All of the above

19. The hemodynamic profile of cardiogenic shock is characterized by all of the following *except:*
a. Cardiac index of less than 2.1 liters/(minute/m^2)
b. Evidence of organ hypoperfusion   c. LVEDP less than 18 mmHg   d. Hypotension

20. The following interventions all reduce preload *except:*
a. Vasodilators   b. Vasopressors   c. Diuretics

21. The following interventions all reduce afterload *except:*
a. Vasodilators   b. Vasopressors   c. Intraaortic balloon pumping

22. Which of the following agents does *not* increase contractility?
a. Calcium   b. Digitalis glycosides
c. Dobutamine   d. Propranolol

23. During intraaortic balloon pumping, the balloon is: (More than one answer may be correct.)
a. Deflated during ventricular systole   b. Inflated during ventricular systole   c. Inflated during ventricular diastole   d. Deflated during ventricular diastole

24. Physiologic effects of the intraaortic balloon include all of the following *except:*
a. Decreased myocardial oxygen demand   b. Increased cardiac output   c. Decreased cardiac work   d. Increased afterload

25. The artificial heart is used primarily to:
a. Offer temporary support of the circulation
b. Treat end-stage heart disease

26. The *two* most common causes of end-stage heart disease in which cardiac transplantation may be considered are:
a. Congestive cardiomyopathy   b. Papillary muscle rupture   c. Lown-Ganong-Levine syndrome
d. Advanced coronary artery disease

Directions: Circle the correct word(s) within the parentheses or fill in the blank with the correct word for each statement.

27. Congestive heart failure is the state of (pulmonary) or (circulatory) congestion resulting from failure of the heart as a (reservoir) or (pump).

28. An increase in left ventricular end-diastolic pressure, LVEDP, usually causes a concomitant increase in (RAP) or (LAP) which, in turn, increases (pulmonary venous) or (systemic venous) pressures, which leads to (pulmonary edema) or (hepatomegaly).

29. The most common mechanical complication of acquired and congenital heart disease is _____ _____.

30. Cardiogenic shock is typically associated with approximately _____ percent loss of ventricular myocardium.

31. During circulatory support with assist devices for the left side of the heart, venous blood is oxygenated by the (machine) or (patient). Oxygenated blood flows into the left side of the heart, which acts as a (pump) or (reservoir).

32. During cardiopulmonary bypass, venous blood flows through catheters placed in the _____. This venous blood is diverted to the _____ where diffusion of gases takes place. The oxygenated blood is returned to the body by a catheter placed in the _____ or _____.

33. Arrange the following events in correct chronological order:
_____ Renin release from the juxtaglomerular apparatus

_____ Conversion of angiotensin I to angiotensin II
_____ Sympathetic activation
_____ Sodium and water retention in the distal tubule and collecting duct
_____ Reduced renal blood flow and reduced GFR
_____ Interaction of renin with circulating angiotensinogen to produce angiotensin I
_____ Adrenal secretion of aldosterone

Directions: Match each clinical syndrome in col. A with its corresponding symptoms in col. B.

Column A

34. _____ Right heart failure
35. _____ Left heart failure

Column B

a. Rales
b. Dependent edema
c. Pulmonary edema
d. Third heart sound
e. Increased jugular venous pressure
f. Hepatomegaly

Directions: Match each symptom in col. A with its definition in col. B.

Column A

36. _____ Paroxysmal nocturnal dyspnea (PND)
37. _____ Cardiac asthma

Column B

a. Difficulty in breathing
b. Sudden awakening with shortness of breath
c. Shortness of breath in the recumbent position

38. _____ Dyspnea on exertion (DOE)
39. _____ Dyspnea
40. _____ Orthopnea
41. _____ Rales

d. Auscultatory findings of pulmonary congestion
e. PND with wheezing
f. Shortness of breath with physical exertion

Directions: Match the following types of cardiomyopathy in col. A with their corresponding structural abnormalities in col. B.

Column A

42. _____ Hypertrophic
43. _____ Congestive or dilated
44. _____ Restrictive or obliterative

Column B

a. Grossly enlarged, hypodynamic ventricle
b. Impeded ventricular filling
c. Increased ventricular muscle mass

Directions: Match the following interventions in col. B. with their primary physiologic effect(s) in col. A.

Column A

45. _____ Reduced preload
46. _____ Reduced afterload
47. _____ Increased contractility
48. _____ Change in vascular tone

Column B

a. Vasopressors
b. Inotropic agents
c. Intraaortic balloon pumping

CHAPTER

30

PENNY J. FORD
ELLEN KINNEALY
NANCY REIDY MACDONALD

VASCULAR DISEASE

OBJECTIVES

At the completion of this chapter you should be able to:

1. Identify the anatomic relationships between the following vessels: ascending aorta, aortic arch, descending aorta, brachiocephalic vessels, aortic bifurcation, iliac arteries, femoral arteries, popliteal arteries, and saphenous veins.

2. Define: arteriosclerosis, atherosclerosis, cystic medial necrosis, thromboangiitis obliterans, Raynaud's phenomenon, arteriosclerosis obliterans, Leriche syndrome, and saddle embolus.

3. Differentiate between thrombosis and embolization.

4. Contrast the pathophysiology of atherosclerotic occlusive and aneurysmal disease.

5. List the clinical manifestations of arterial insufficiency to the lower extremities.

6. Describe the following diagnostic procedures: Doppler ultrasonography, segmental plethysmography, segmental extremity pressure measurement, arteriography, phlebography, and iodine 125 fibrinogen testing.

7. Discuss the following surgical techniques: aortobifemoral bypass grafting, endarterectomy, saphenous vein bypass grafting, and aortic aneurysm resection with tube graft.

8. Define: true aneurysm, fusiform aneurysm, saccular aneurysm, false aneurysm, and aortic dissection.

9. Describe the clinical manifestations and complications of aortic aneurysm and aortic dissection.

10. Classify dissecting aneurysms according to the DeBakey system.

11. Distinguish the deep venous system, superficial venous system, and communicating system relative to anatomy and function.

12. Define: thrombophlebitis, phlebothrombosis, deep venous thrombosis, varicose veins, chronic venous insufficiency, and postphlebitic syndrome.

13. List three major factors predisposing to the development of venous thrombosis.

14. Identify the clinical manifestations of deep venous thrombosis.

15. Enumerate methods of vena caval interruption for prevention of pulmonary embolization.

16. Discuss the principles of medical therapy for arterial and venous disease.

INTRODUCTION

Disease processes can affect both systemic arteries and systemic veins, impairing tissue perfusion and interfering with venous return to the heart. Atherosclerosis is the most common disease affecting the arterial vasculature. Given the diffuse and progressive nature of the atherosclerotic process, multiple segments of the vasculature tend to be involved. Consequently, multisystem compromise is common; for example, peripheral vascular disease is commonly associated with cerebral and coronary disease. Treatment of the peripheral disease without regard for potential complications due to vascular compromise in the coronary or cerebral beds could be catastrophic.

This chapter will focus upon common arterial and venous diseases. The arterial section will emphasize atherosclerotic disease of the aorta and its major branches; occlusive and aneurysmal presentations will be described in detail. Disease of the coronary and cerebral circulations is included in Chapters 27 and 48. The venous disease section will include thrombophlebitis, deep venous thrombosis, varicose veins, and chronic venous insufficiency.

ARTERIAL DISEASE

Anatomy

Arterial wall

The arterial wall consists of three layers: the outer layer or *adventitia*, the middle layer or *media*, and the inner layer or *intima*. The compositions of the layers vary. The adventitia is composed primarily of connective tissue and contains nerve fibers and the blood vessels supplying the arterial wall. This vascular supply is referred to as the *vasa vasorum*, "vessel of vessels." The media contains collagen, smooth-muscle fibers, and elastin maintaining arterial strength and elasticity. The intima is a smooth, nonthrombogenic layer of endothelial cells.

Aorta and its major branches

The aorta traverses the thoracic and abdominal cavities and its segments are distinguished accordingly.

The *thoracic aorta* is divided into the following anatomic segments: (1) ascending thoracic aorta, (2) transverse aortic arch, and (3) descending thoracic aorta. The *ascending aorta* originates at the aortic valve and extends to the orifices of the vessels supplying the head, neck, and upper extremities. These vessels, collectively referred to as *brachiocephalic vessels,* arise from the *aortic arch.* As illustrated in Fig. 30-1, the brachiocephalic vessels include the innominate artery (brachiocephalic trunk), the left common carotid artery, and the left subclavian artery. The innominate artery divides into the right common carotid and the right subclavian arteries. The axillary arteries arise from the subclavians and extend to the brachial arteries, which branch into the radial and ulnar arteries.

The *descending thoracic aorta* begins distal to the left subclavian artery and extends to the diaphragm. The *abdominal aorta* begins beneath the diaphragm and branches within a few centimeters to supply the abdominal organs. The major *visceral branches* of the abdominal aorta are illustrated in Fig. 30-1 and include the celiac axis, superior mesenteric artery, and renal arteries. The inferior mesenteric artery branches off the aorta below the renal arteries. The abdominal aorta extends to the aortic bifurcation at the level of the pelvis. The *terminal aorta* is the aortic segment between the renal arteries and the bifurcation; the inferior mesenteric artery is the major branch of the terminal aorta.

The aorta bifurcates into the common iliac arteries. The common iliac arteries divide into the external iliac arteries and the hypogastric or internal iliac arteries. The external iliac arteries become the common femoral arteries. The common femoral gives off multiple branches, including the superficial femoral artery and the deep femoral artery or profunda femoris. The superficial femoral artery extends to the popliteal artery, which in turn branches into the posterior tibial artery, the peroneal artery, and the anterior tibial artery. The anterior tibial artery extends to the dorsal pedal artery.

In the event of obstruction within the arterial system, important *collateral networks* develop to bypass the involved segment and maintain blood flow. Arteries that are particularly important as potential routes for collateral flow to the lower extremeties include the inferior mesenteric artery and the profunda femoris or deep femoral artery. For example, the inferior mesen-

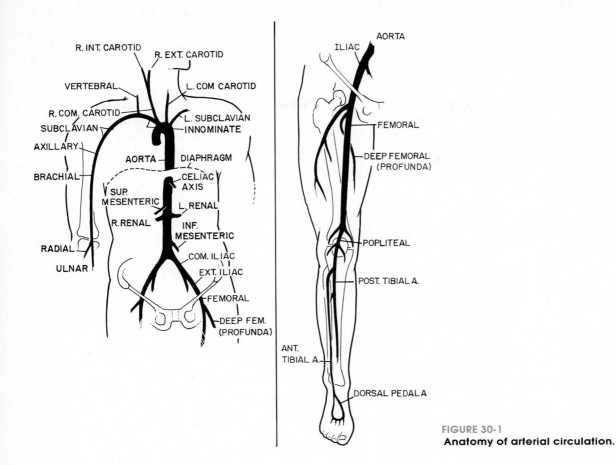

FIGURE 30-1
Anatomy of arterial circulation.

teric artery becomes enlarged to provide collateral flow in the setting of bilateral occlusion of the common iliacs (see Fig. 30-2).

Etiology and pathology of arterial disease

Arteriosclerosis includes any disease process producing degeneration, hardening, or thickening of the arterial wall. *Atherosclerosis*, the most common cause of arteriosclerosis, is characterized initially by lipid deposition on the initimal layer of the artery. Subsequently, calcification, fibrosis, thrombosis, and hemorrhage can occur, contributing to the development of a complex atherosclerotic plaque or atheroma. Eventually, the media begins to degenerate. These pathologic processes progressively occlude the vessel lumen and weaken the arterial wall. The risk factors for atherogenesis include smoking, hyperlipoproteinemia, diabetes, and hypertension. The clinical manifestations of atherosclerosis result either from vascular occlusion due to intimal deposition or from aneurysm formation due to medial degeneration. Arterial occlusive and aneurysmal disease due to atherosclerosis will be discussed in subsequent sections.

Nonatherosclerotic causes of arterial disease include (1) cystic medial necrosis, (2) arteritis or arterial inflammation, (3) arteriospastic disorders, (4) infection,

FIGURE 30-2
Collateral blood flow via inferior mesenteric artery owing to bilateral occlusion of common iliac arteries.

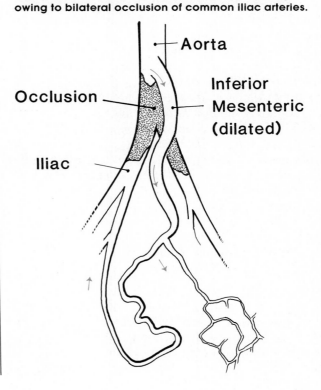

455

(5) trauma, and (6) congenital anomalies. *Cystic medial necrosis* is a pathologic process resulting in degenerative changes in the medial layer of the artery. Medial degeneration can result in aneurysm formation, aortic dissection, and spontaneous arterial rupture. A variety of conditions can produce cystic medial necrosis, including Marfan's syndrome. *Marfan's syndrome* is an inherited disorder of the connective tissue.

Inflammatory disorders of the aorta or peripheral arteries can result in arterial occlusion. *Thromboangiitis obliterans*, or Buerger's disease, is a chronic occlusive disease of the medium and small arteries and veins. The inflammation and subsequent healing and thrombosis of lesions produces vascular obstruction. Ischemic ulceration and gangrene result. Smoking appears directly related to the etiology and course of this disease.

Arteriospastic conditions can also produce transient arterial occlusion. *Raynaud's phenomenon* is produced by vasospasm of the small cutaneous and subcutaneous arteries and arterioles. It is characterized by phasic changes in skin color, usually precipitated by exposure to cold or emotional upset. An initial phase of pallor due to vasoconstriction is followed by a cyanotic phase and finally by a phase of rubor from reactive vasodilation. Raynaud's phenomenon may occur in association with other diseases; however, if no other cause can be identified and the episodes persist, the condition is referred to as *Raynaud's disease*. Given the intermittent nature of vasospasm, the course of Raynaud's phenomenon is typically benign, in contrast to that of thromboangiitis obliterans.

Arterial infection typically results from septicemia. Sources of infection include bacterial endocarditis, gastroenteritis, particularly caused by salmonella, and vascular infection from intravenous drug abuse. Syphilis is no longer a common cause of vascular damage. Arterial infection tends to localize on roughened endothelial surfaces, such as atherosclerotic plaques. Vascular trauma and congenital anomalies, such as coarctation of the aorta, are also major nonatherosclerotic causes of vascular abnormality.

Occlusive arterial disease

Definitions and pathology

The term *chronic occlusive arterial disease* encompasses disorders causing ischemia due to arterial obstruction. The most common cause of occlusive disease is atherosclerosis. Chronic occlusive disease due to atherosclerosis is referred to as *arteriosclerosis obliterans*. Atherosclerosis can occur throughout the arterial system; however, lesions tend to develop at points of branching, bifurcation, abrupt curvature, or vascular narrowing. The *Leriche syndrome* is progressive occlusion of the terminal aorta, including the bifurcation and iliacs, from atherosclerosis and thrombosis. Lesions occur more frequently in the lower extremities than in the upper extremities and tend to be localized involving segments of the artery. Common sites of involvement include (1) aortoiliac vessels, (2) femoropopliteal vessels, (3) popliteal-tibial vessels, and (4) combinations of the above.

The second most common cause of chronic occlusive disease is *thromboangiitis obliterans*; occlusion is produced by inflammation and thrombosis, as described earlier.

Acute arterial occlusion can be produced by thrombosis or embolization. *Thrombosis* is the formation of a blood clot, or *thrombus*, within the vascular system. Arterial thrombosis usually occurs at the site of an atherosclerotic plaque or within an arterial aneurysm. Detachment of a thrombus into the bloodstream is referred to as *embolization*. The *embolus* is propelled downstream to lodge in the smaller branches of the arterial system, occluding the vascular lumen. Most arterial emboli originate in the left side of the heart. Mitral stenosis and atrial fibrillation predispose to the development of atrial thrombi. Transmural myocardial infarction roughens the endothelial surface of the left ventricle, potentiating the formation of mural ventricular thrombi. Depending on the size and destination of the clot, dislodgment of thrombi from the cardiac chambers is potentially catastrophic. Emboli tend to lodge in regions of bifurcation or branching. The term *saddle embolus* refers to acute occlusion of the aortic bifurcation and iliacs.

Pathophysiology

Chronic occlusive disease progressively narrows the arterial lumen, increasing the resistance to blood flow. As the resistance to flow increases, blood flow to the tissue beyond the lesion is reduced. If the oxygen needs of the tissue exceed the ability of the vessel to supply oxygen, tissue ischemia results. A single lesion must reduce the vessel lumen by approximately 50 percent in diameter or 75 percent in cross-sectional area to produce clinically significant interference with blood flow. However, multiple stenoses occurring in sequence, as commonly seen with atherosclerosis, compound the interference with flow; in other words, less significant lesions can, in combination, seriously impair flow.

The severity of ischemia distal to an obstructive lesion depends not only upon the site and extent of occlusion but also upon the degree of collateral flow around the lesion. Fortunately, the tendency of atherosclerotic lesions to be localized and to enlarge gradually favors the development of collateral circulation. With localized lesions, the distal artery remains patent, thus alternative routes of arterial flow can bypass the lesion to perfuse the tissue beyond. As resistance to flow increases at the site of obstruction, pressure increases proximal to the lesion with a proportionate drop in pressure distal to the lesion. This pressure gradient across the obstruction promotes flow through collateral vessels. These collateral vessels gradually enlarge. Increased velocity of flow through the collateral vessels also stimulates collateral development. Severe ischemia can result from acute occlusion because collateral networks have not had time to develop. The adequacy of collateral flow is also compromised by disease in collateral vessels.

Clinical manifestations

The clinical manifestations of chronic occlusive disease progress slowly over a period of years. The signs and symptoms result from tissue underperfusion and ischemia. The primary sympton is *intermittent claudication* due to muscle ischemia. Typically, intermittent claudication occurs with exercise, when metabolic demands increase, and subsides within minutes with rest. The location of the pain correlates closely with the site of arterial disease; the arterial segment involved is always proximal to the region of ischemic muscle. For example, intermittent claudication of the hips would correlate with aortoiliac disease, whereas disease of the external iliac or common femoral vessels would be associated with thigh or calf pain. Bilateral claudication is consistent with occlusion at or above the aortic bifurcation.

Pain occurring at rest is indicative of advanced occlusive disease. Ischemic rest pain typically occurs in the foot and is severe and unremitting. Leg dependency or walking may provide some relief. Ischemic neuropathy occasionally results, particularly in diabetics, producing shocklike pain in the foot and leg.

Pulses below the occlusion are diminished or absent. The change in pulses is magnified by exercise because the vasodilation induced by exercise and ischemia increases the pressure gradient across the lesion. A bruit, indicative of turbulent flow, may be audible over the diseased arterial segment.

Significant arterial disease of the lower extremities is characterized by postural changes in skin color. Elevation of the extremity produces pallor, followed by redness or rubor with dependency. These changes occur because blood flow across the obstructive lesion is pressure-dependent and therefore extremely sensitive to the effects of gravity. The elevation pallor is the result of gravitational effects which reduce arterial pressure and consequently lower the blood volume in the capillary bed. As the extremity is lowered beneath heart level and perfusion pressure increases, color returns. The rubor results from a reactive hyperemia or maximal vascular dilation in response to tissue hypoxia. The

veins of the dependent leg also take longer to fill owing to the interference with arterial inflow.

The following tissue changes result from severe, chronic ischemia of the lower extremities: (1) trophic changes of the skin and nails with thickening of the nails and drying of the skin, (2) loss of hair, particularly on the dorsum of the feet and toes, (3) development of a temperature gradient between colder regions of poor perfusion and warmer regions of adequate perfusion, and (4) wasting of the leg muscles and soft tissues. Severe ischemia culminates in ulceration and gangrene, usually beginning on the toes or heel and progressing proximally.

Acute occlusion is characterized by sudden onset of severe ischemia. Typical manifestations are severe pain, loss of pulses, collapse of superficial veins, coldness and pallor, and impaired motor and sensory function. However, the presentation can be gradual and less dramatic.

Diagnostic findings

Physical examination yields much information relative to the degree of arterial disease. Pulses are palpated at multiple sites, compared, and graded as follows: zero, pulse absent; 1, pulse present but markedly reduced; 2, pulse present but moderately reduced; 3, pulse present but slightly reduced; 4, pulse present and normal. Leg elevation and dependency tests to elicit the characteristic postural pallor and rubor described above are utilized. The degree of occlusion is estimated according to the length of time required for elevation pallor and dependent rubor to occur; normally no pallor is observed during 60 seconds of leg elevation, and color returns within 10 seconds. Venous filling time in the dependent position is also determined; normal venous filling time is less than 15 seconds. Sensation, muscle strength, and skin temperature are also evaluated; bruits and trophic changes are noted.

Given the subjective nature of the physical examination, noninvasive testing may be indicated for further evaluation. Doppler ultrasonography and segmental plethysmography are commonly utilized. Doppler techniques utilize ultrasound to detect and quantitate the velocity of flow within a given arterial segment. A probe emitting ultrasonic waves is placed over an arterial pulse (see Fig. 30-3). The frequency of the waves reflected back to the probe from the pulsating vessel is proportionate to the flow velocity within the vessel and generates an audible signal. Since analysis of an audible signal is somewhat subjective, B-mode ultrasound can be used to simultaneously generate a visual image or tracing permitting analysis of waveforms.

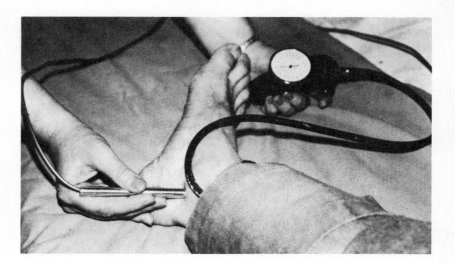

FIGURE 30-3
Method of recording ankle systolic pressure. (From James S. T. Yao, "Noninvasive Techniques of Measuring Lower Limb Arterial Pressures," in Eugene F. Bernstein (ed.) *Noninvasive Diagnostic Techniques in Vascular Disease*, 3d ed., The C. V. Mosby Co., St. Louis, 1985, in press.)

Segmental plethysmography measures pulse volume. Pneumatic cuffs are placed around the thigh and upper calf and above the ankle. The cuffs are automatically or manually inflated to approximately 65 mmHg to ensure optimal cuff contact. A transducer senses changes in cuff pressure during systole as the blood volume in the vessel increases. A pulse volume recording is generated for each site, and the cuffs are deflated. In the vascular laboratory, this technique is commonly performed simultaneously with segmental extremity pressure measurement. First the brachial blood pressure is measured to establish a baseline for comparison. Then the Doppler flow probe or a stethoscope is placed over the arterial pulse and the pneumatic cuffs on the thigh, calf, and ankle are sequentially inflated to a pressure above the brachial systolic pressure. The onset of flow during systole at each site is detected by the probe, and cuff pressure is recorded. Lower-extremity pressures are compared with brachial systolic pressure and with each other. Systolic pressures at each site should equal or exceed the brachial systolic pressure. A pressure difference or gradient of 20 to 30 mmHg between lower-extremity sites is indicative of arterial occlusion. Analysis of pulse volume recordings and obtained pressures permits estimation of disease severity. Fig. 30-4 illustrates the abnormalities in pulse volume recordings observed with moderate and severe vascular occlusion.

Segmental plethysmography and pressure measurement are commonly performed during rest and exercise. With exercise, flow abnormalities increase. Pulses distal to the occlusion are reduced or disappear, and pressure gradients increase. Exercise evaluation usually involves walking on a treadmill for 5 minutes or for as long as tolerated, with repeat measurements after exercise.

Arteriography, or opacification of the artery with contrast material, may be indicated to determine the precise location and extent of disease, particularly in the lower extremities. Collateral circulation and the condition of the proximal and distal vasculature can also be evaluated.

Management

Medical therapy

Control of risk factors is important to the treatment of arterial occlusive disease. Smoking should be stopped, given its strong association with occlusive disease, particularly with thromboangiitis obliterans. Medical therapy of associated diabetes, hyperlipoproteinemia, and hypertension is indicated, particularly dietary measures. Physical exercise seems to afford the greatest benefit in the treatment of intermittent claudication. A progressive exercise program should be developed and maintained. It is felt that the therapeutic response to physical exercise sustained over a period of time is primarily due to increased collateral development.

Foot care is crucial in the setting of lower extremity vascular disease to prevent infection and traumatic ulceration. Measures include meticulous attention to cleanliness and nail care, application of talc and lanolin to dry skin, and avoidance of trauma and temperature extremes.

The pain of intermittent claudication usually sub-

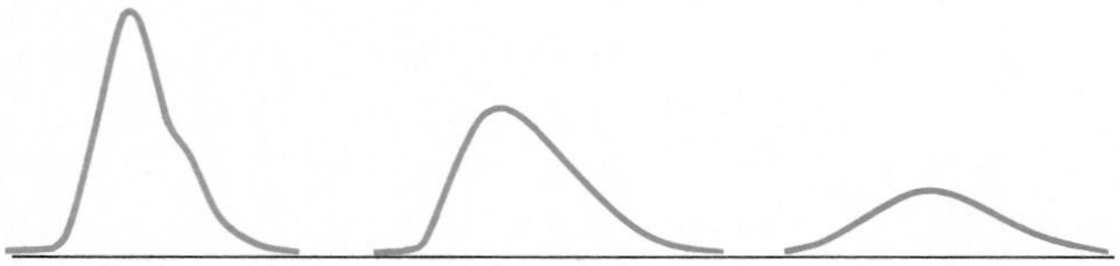

Normal   Moderate   Severe

FIGURE 30-4
Pulse volume recordings. (A) Normal. (B) Moderate stenosis. (C) Severe stenosis.

sides with rest. Ischemic rest pain can be relieved somewhat by dependency of the extremity or elevation of the head of the bed. Leg dependency increases perfusion pressure, thus relieving ischemia; elevation of the extremity is contraindicated because arterial flow would be further compromised. Analgesics may be necessary for pain control.

Management of ischemic ulcers and gangrene is problematic. In addition to instituting the measures described above, foot soaks and topical antibiotic agents may be indicated. Bed rest, with elevation of the head of the bed, reduces oxygen demand and improves flow. Pressure points should be padded to avoid further breakdown. Preventive measures to avoid injury are important, since the ability to heal is retarded by the arterial insufficiency. In addition, susceptibility to injury is increased since sensory function may be impaired. Arterial reconstruction or amputation may be necessary.

Surgical therapy

In general, surgery is considered for chronic occlusive disease if symptoms become disabling or threaten limb viability and are unresponsive to medical therapy. The precise indications for surgery and the choice of procedure vary according to the site of disease. Surgical intervention will be discussed relative to the following anatomic sites: (1) aortoiliac disease with patent femoropopliteal arteries, (2) aortoiliac with femoropopliteal disease, and (3) femoropopliteal disease.

Surgery for chronic aortoiliac disease with patent femoropopliteal vessels is usually performed for disabling intermittent claudication. Given the patency of the vessels distal to the site of disease, collateral networks develop around the aortoiliac vessels preserving limb viability. Surgical correction involves either placement of a bypass graft to shunt blood around the obstruction or endarterectomy to remove atheromatous plaque (see Figs. 30-5 and 30-6).

Bypass grafting with a knitted polyester (Dacron) bifurcation graft is the most common procedure; bifurcation grafts divide into two limbs to be sutured to both extremities. The proximal end of the graft is anastamosed to the side of the abdominal aorta beneath the renal arteries. The distal ends are anastamosed to either the external iliac or the common femoral arteries, depending on the extent of the disease. This aortobifemoral graft shunts blood around the diseased aortoiliac system to the lower extremities (see Fig. 30-5).

Endarterectomy consists of circumferential dissection and removal of the atheromatous plaque from the

arterial lumen, as illustrated in Fig. 30-6. This is performed through an arteriotomy in the vessel wall. Endarterectomy of localized disease may be performed in conjunction with aortobifemoral bypass grafting. Generally, bypass grafting is preferred to endarterectomy, since endarterectomy offers no distinct advantage and is more complicated and time-consuming.

Combined aortoiliac and femoropopliteal disease necessitates a combination of interventions. In this setting, surgery is usually indicated for limb salvage given the extent of disease and the severity of ischemia. The proximal aortoiliac lesion must be corrected first to ensure adequate arterial inflow into the femoropopliteal region. Aortobifemoral grafting is usually indicated. Subsequently, the distal femoropopliteal disease requires either endarterectomy or bypass grafting to obtain good flow to the distal vessels.

Despite controversy as to the efficacy of sympathectomy, sympathectomy may be performed simulta-

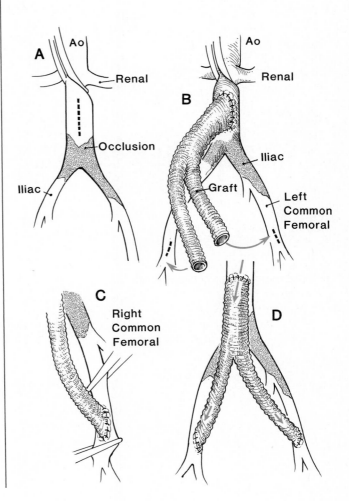

FIGURE 30-5
Aortobifemoral bypass graft. (A) Aortic incision. (B) Proximal anastomosis (C) Distal anastomosis. (D) Completed graft. (Modified from Chung, 1983, p. 336.)

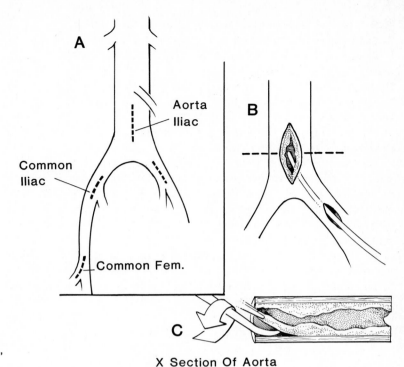

X Section Of Aorta

FIGURE 30-6
Endarterectomy. (A) Arteriotomy. (B) and (C)
Technique for circumferential dissection and
removal of plaque. (Modified from Gasper, 1981,
pp. 235, 236, 244.)

neously to reduce sympathetic tone to the lower extremities and produce peripheral vasodilation. It is hoped that blood flow through the grafts will thereby be improved. In highly selected cases, transluminal angioplasty may be attempted to dilate the iliac vessels. A balloon-tipped catheter is advanced into the iliac system via the femoral artery under fluoroscopic and pressure guidance. The balloon is inflated within the diseased segment to compress the lesion and dilate the vessel. The role of angioplasty in vascular disease is still being defined. Angioplasty can be particularly useful if sur-

gery is contraindicated or if the disease is restricted to short, isolated arterial segments.

Arterial reconstruction for femoropopliteal disease is usually performed for limb salvage. Occasionally, disabling intermittent claudication will necessitate surgery. Bypass grafting is usually preferred over endarterectomy; however, concomitant endarterectomy may be utilized for localized disease. The graft of choice is the autogenous saphenous vein, owing to high graft failure rates with prosthetic materials such as Dacron in the lower extremity. A segment of vein is removed from

FIGURE 30-7
Femoral-popliteal bypass graft. (A)
Saphenous vein graft. (B) Composite
graft. (C) Sequential femoral-
popliteal-tibial graft. (D)
Profundaplasty with patch graft.
(Modified from Gasper, 1981, pp.
274, 284, 293.)

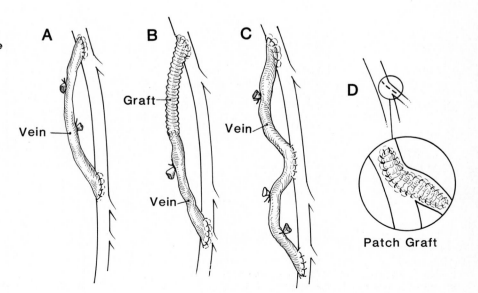

the leg and reversed before arterial anastamosis, so that the venous valves will not impede flow through the vein graft. The proximal end of the reversed graft is anastamosed to the side of the common femoral artery (see Fig. 30-7A), and the distal end to the vessel beyond the obstruction, ideally to a branch of the popliteal artery. Distal bypass grafting to regions beneath the popliteal artery is not as successful, owing to the smaller caliber of the vessel, poor flows, and the mechanical effects of knee bending and potential graft compression.

If the saphenous vein is not long enough to extend around the diseased segment, composite grafts of vein and prosthetic material can be used (see Fig. 30-7B). Sequential grafting may be utilized to provide flow at multiple points for branches of an extensively diseased segment (see Fig. 30-7C).

If femoropopliteal disease involves the profunda femoris, or deep femoral artery, profundaplasty is performed in conjunction with bypass grafting. This usually involves endarterectomy through an arteriotomy. If necessary, a patch graft may be inserted within the vessel wall to dilate the vessel (see Fig. 30-7D). Profundaplasty is important because of the profunda's importance as a collateral network for the lower extremities. In high-risk patients, profundaplasty may be performed alone under local anesthesia as a palliative procedure.

Amputation is considered in chronic occlusive disease for irreversible gangrene or uncontrolled pain. Amputation is performed as far distally as possible to minimize resultant disability.

Acute aortoiliac occlusion necessitates immediate intervention. Anticoagulation is initiated in addition to standard measures such as relief of pain and elevation of the head of the bed. Fibrinolytic therapy with agents such as streptokinase or urokinase may be considered. Embolectomy via a femoral arteriotomy may be performed for embolic disease, whereas thrombosis generally necessitates bypass grafting or thromboendartarectomy.

Aneurysmal arterial disease

Definitions and classifications

An *aneurysm* is a localized dilation of the arterial wall (see Fig. 30-8). A *true aneurysm* consists of a dilation with an intact arterial wall. Although intact, the arterial wall of a true aneurysm is distorted and composed primarily of fibrous tissue. True aneurysms can be fusiform or saccular in shape. The more common atherosclerotic *fusiform aneurysm* is a uniform, circumferential dilation, whereas the *saccular aneurysm* is a saclike

outpouching connected to the arterial wall by a narrow neck. A *false aneurysm* is an extravascular accumulation of blood with disruption of all three vascular layers; the wall of the false aneurysm is thrombus and adjacent tissue. Aneurysms can occur anywhere in the aorta or peripheral vessels. Aortic aneurysms are classified as abdominal, thoracic, or thoracoabdominal, depending on their location. Aortic dissection will be discussed in the next section.

Pathophysiology

Aneurysm formation results from degeneration and weakening of the medial layer of the artery. Medial degeneration can result from either acquired or congenital conditions, such as atherosclerosis or Marfan's syndrome. Vascular dilation can also result from the jet effect of blood streaming across an obstructive vascular plaque, creating turbulence distal to the lesion; this poststenotic dilation weakens the arterial wall.

The aneurysm becomes progressively larger according to the law of Laplace. Wall tension or stress is directly related to the radius of the vessel and the intraarterial pressure. As the vessel dilates and the radius increases, the wall tension rises, further dilating the vessel. In addition, the vast majority of individuals with aneurysms are hypertensive, further contributing to wall stress and aneurysm enlargement.

The potential contribution of arterial size to aneurysm formation is also being considered. Individuals

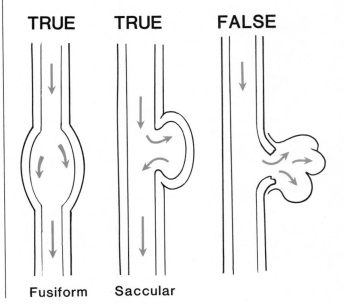

FIGURE 30-8
Aneurysm types. (A) True fusiform aneurysm. (B) True saccular aneurysm (C) False aneurysm.

with large main arteries, or *arteriomegaly*, and larger body surface areas tend to have an increased incidence of aneurysms. It has been suggested that increased aortic blood flow may affect the development of aneurysms.

Aneurysms commonly develop layers of clot along their walls owing to stagnant flow. Mural thrombi are a potential source of emboli and spontaneous aneurysm thrombosis.

Etiology and common sites

The most common site for aneurysm formation is the abdominal aorta. Abdominal aortic aneurysms (AAA) typically originate beneath the renal arteries and extend to the aortic bifurcation, occasionally involving the iliac arteries. Rarely does the aneurysm extend above the renal arteries to involve the major visceral branches of the aorta. Most abdominal aneurysms are atherosclerotic in origin.

Thoracic aneurysms can affect the descending thoracic aorta beyond the left subclavian artery, the ascending aorta above the aortic valve, and/or the aortic arch. The descending aorta is affected most frequently. Atherosclerosis and trauma are the most common causes. Deceleration trauma to the chest can rupture the intimal and medial layers of the descending aorta at the ligamentum arteriosus. The ligamentum arteriosus stabilizes the aorta at one point, while the thoracic structures move forward when the chest abruptly decelerates; this may shear the vascular layers. The adventitial layer may remain intact, although rupture or the development of false aneurysms may result. Disease of the arch is usually due to atherosclerosis. Cystic medial necrosis, as in Marfan's syndrome, is most severe in the ascending aorta and frequently results in aneurysm formation. Syphilis also damages the ascending aorta to the greatest extent.

Multiple aneurysms are frequent and may involve the peripheral and visceral arteries. The popliteal is the most commonly affected peripheral artery; visceral aneurysms are rare. Most peripheral and visceral aneurysms are atherosclerotic in origin; however, trauma and infection are also etiologic factors.

Clinical manifestations

Aneurysms are frequently asymptomatic. The first sign of disease may be a serious, potentially life-threatening complication, such as rupture, acute thrombosis, or embolization. Abdominal aneurysms may be detected during an abdominal examination as a palpable, expansile abdominal mass usually located in the umbil-

ical region to the left of midline. The appearance of symptoms is usually ominous, indicating aneurysm expansion, chronic retroperitoneal bleeding, or impending rupture. Severe abdominal or back pain may be noted. Duodenal obstruction from large aneurysms may present as epigastric discomfort or difficulties with digestion. Impotence may be reported and infrequently visceral dysfunction is noted if orifices of major visceral branches are involved. Bruits may be audible but are of little diagnostic value. Femoral pulses are diminished in some patients.

Thoracic aortic aneurysms may similarly be discovered incidentally by chest film. Aneurysms must be quite large to produce symptoms. Symptoms are usually due to expansion and compression of adjacent structures. Esophageal compression produces dysphagia; recurrent laryngeal nerve compression presents as hoarseness; neck vein distention and edema of the head and arms may indicate compression of the superior vena cava. The pain associated with thoracic aneurysms occurs in the chest.

Aneurysm rupture is catastrophic and associated with a poor prognosis. Rupture into the pericardial cavity results in exsanguination; however, rupture is usually into the retroperitoneal space where adjacent structures exert a tamponade effect. Rupture typically presents with acute abdominal or back pain occurring in association with signs of hemorrhagic shock. A pulsatile abdominal mass may be palpable, although after rupture detection may not be possible. Immediate surgical resection is necessary.

Diagnostic findings

An abdominal aneurysm can be detected by palpation. Anteroposterior and lateral abdominal x-rays are useful to confirm the clinical findings. B-mode ultrasound is indicated for noninvasive determination of aneurysm size. Newer techniques of computed tomography and radionuclide imaging are occasionally used but offer no obvious advantage over ultrasound. Arteriography is performed in selected cases, particularly if suprarenal extension or involvement of the visceral vessels is suspected. However, arteriography can underestimate aneurysm size, since the contrast material opacifies only the blood-filled portion of the aneurysm and mural thrombi can occupy a significant portion of the aneurysm.

A thoracic aneurysm may be detected as mediastinal widening on a chest x-ray. Arteriography is necessary to confirm the diagnosis and determine the degree of vascular involvement.

Management

Small, asymptomatic abdominal aneurysms may not warrant immediate surgical intervention. The size of these aneurysms is monitored carefully at regular intervals using palpation, abdominal x-rays, and ultrasound. Aneurysmal enlargement to 4 to 6 cm is considered an indication for elective aneurysm resection. If the aneurysm becomes symptomatic, surgery is considered on a more urgent basis. The technique and type of graft utilized for abdominal aneurysm repair depends upon the extent of vascular involvement. If the aneurysm is confined to the aortic region below the renal arteries and above the aortic bifurcation, a tube graft is utilized. The aneurysm is resected (see Fig. 30-9A), preserving its external layer (see Fig. 30-9B); the tube graft is then anastomosed to the aorta (see Fig. 30-9C). If collateral flow to the inferior mesenteric artery is inadequate, it is implanted into the side of the tube graft (see Fig. 30-9D). The aneurysmal shell is then wrapped around the graft to minimize blood loss. If the aneurysm extends beyond the bifurcation or if the iliac arteries are diseased, a bifurcation graft is used. The distal limbs of

the bifurcation graft can be anastomosed end-to-end or end-to-side to the distal vessels, as shown in Fig. 30-10. Endarterectomy may be necessary.

Thoracic aneurysms require surgical correction. If the aneurysm is large or compressing adjacent structures, surgery is considered on an urgent basis. The grafting technique is similar to that of abdominal aneurysm repair, and involves aneurysmal resection and replacement with a tube graft placed within the aneurysmal wall. Involvement of the arch necessitates reimplantation of the brachiocephalic vessels into the graft or utilization of aortic patch grafts. Ascending aortic aneurysms may involve the aortic valve, requiring replacement or resuspension of the aortic valve. Periph-

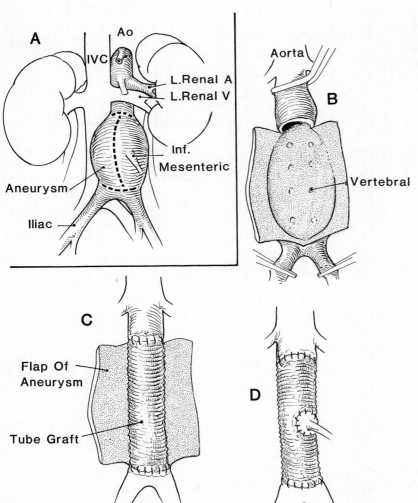

FIGURE 30-9
Repair of abdominal aneurysm. (A) Abdominal aortic aneurysm (B) Preservation of external layer (C) Insertion of tube graft. (D) Implantation of internal mesenteric artery. (Modified from Gasper, 1981, pp. 185, 189, 196.)

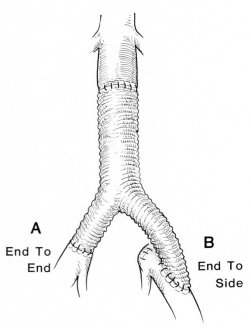

FIGURE 30-10
Aortobifemoral graft. (A) End-to-end anastomosis.(B) End-to-side anastomosis. (Modified from Gasper, 1981, p. 186.)

eral perfusion is maintained during thoracic aneurysm resections by cardiopulmonary bypass, bypass of the left side of the heart, or a vascular shunt (see Fig. 30-11).

Aortic dissection

Definitions and pathology

Aortic dissection is separation of the vascular layers by a column of blood (see Fig. 30-12A). This vascular separation creates a false arterial lumen which communicates with the true lumen via a tear in the intima. The dissection does not extend around the circumference of the vessel; rather it extends along the length of the vessel. This extension can partially or totally occlude any vessel in the path of the dissection by separating the vessel orifice from the true arterial lumen. Occasionally, the dissecting column of blood may reenter the true lumen or terminate; however, rapid progressive dissection is usually observed. Eventually the false lumen may produce aneurysmal enlargement of outer vascular layers; however, aneurysm formation does not characterize the early phase of dissection. The term *dissecting aneurysm* is therefore a misnomer, although it is used frequently as a synonym for aortic dissection.

Occasionally an intimal tear cannot be demon-

strated. In such cases, rupture of the vasa vasorum is suspected. Consequently, the relationship between the intimal tear and the development of aortic dissection is a subject of debate.

Classification and common sites

Aortic dissections are commonly described according to the DeBakey classification system. This system distinguishes three types of dissections according to site of origin and extent of dissection (see Fig. 30-12B). Type I aneurysms originate in the ascending aorta just above the aortic valve and extend distally into the abdominal aorta. Type II aneurysms are confined to the ascending aorta. Type III aneurysms begin in the descending aorta just distal to the left subclavian artery and can extend distally to the aortic bifurcation. Another common system for classifying aneurysms simply groups Type I and II aneurysms together as *proximal aneurysms* originating in the ascending aorta and distinguish Type III aneurysms as *distal aneurysms* beginning in the descending aorta.

Proximal dissections are frequently associated with cystic medial necrosis, as in Marfan's syndrome. Atherosclerosis is common with distal dissections. Deceleration trauma, as mentioned earlier with aortic aneurysms, can also cause aortic dissections by disrupting the intimal and medial layers, allowing blood to enter the vessel wall.

Clinical manifestations and diagnostic findings

The clinical manifestations vary, depending on the site and extent of dissection; however, the onset tends to be sudden and intense. Typically, severe, tearing pain is experienced. The pain can localize intially in the chest, abdomen, or back; however, as the dissection extends, the pain radiates to the back and distally toward the lower extremities. Signs of shock often develop even though arterial pressure tends to be elevated owing to underlying hypertension.

Retrograde dissection toward the aortic valve can produce aortic regurgitation manifested by a diastolic murmur and signs of congestive heart failure. As the dissection progresses, arterial branches become occluded with loss of pulses and signs of organ dysfunction; anuria may result from renal artery involvement, or lower extremity ischemia may result from iliac occlusion. Rupture is the most frequent cause of death.

Chest x-ray may evidence a widened mediastinum. Aortography is indicated to determine the location and extent of dissection.

Management

Early surgical intervention is usually indicated for proximal dissections originating in the ascending aorta

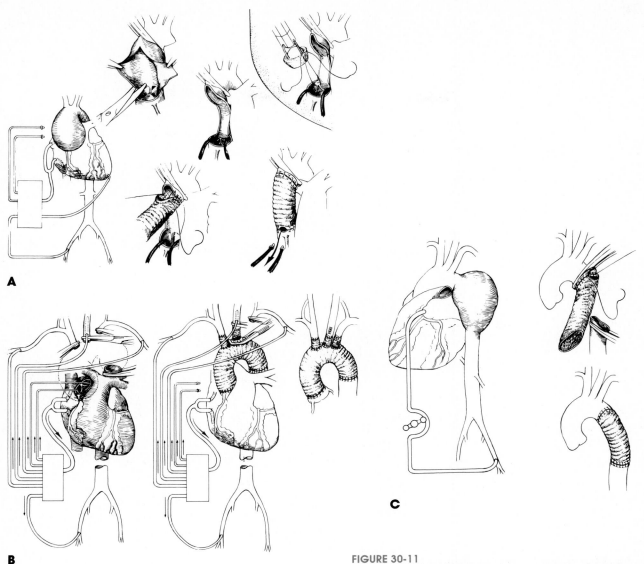

A

B

C

FIGURE 30-11

Types of surgical treatment for aneurysms of the thoracic aorta. (A) Method of resection and graft replacement of aneurysm of the ascending aorta with cardiopulmonary bypass. Insert illustrates prosthetic replacement of aortic valve, in patients with associated aortic valve insufficiency . (B) Method of resection and graft replacement of aneurysm of the arch that involves major vessels, using cardiopulmonary bypass and extracorporeal perfusion of the brain. (C) Method of resection and graft replacement of aneurysm of the descending thoracic aorta, using left-arterial—femoral-artery pump bypass. (From Hurst, Logue, Schlant, and Wenger (eds.), 1982, p. 1438.)

and arch. Distal dissections originating in and limited to the descending aorta are usually treated medically first to control the dissection and stabilize the patient. However, if the dissection progresses or if complications such as arterial occlusion or hemodynamic instability arise, surgery is indicated.

Medical therapy involves the reduction of arterial pressure with such drugs as trimethaphan camsylate (Arfonad) or sodium nitroprusside, to reduce stress on the aortic wall. The force of left ventricular contraction is reduced by administration of such drugs as propranolol, in an attempt to lower the velocity of ventricular ejection. Pain is controlled with analgesics and sedation. Hemodynamics and peripheral pulses are monitored carefully to detect complications. Serial chest x-rays are performed to monitor the size of the dissection.

Surgical repair usually involves the resection of the involved segment and replacement with a graft. Other surgical techniques include repair and reconstruction of the aorta with sutures or patch grafts. Repair of an ascending aortic dissection may involve aortic valve replacement or annuloplasty and valve resuspension. As with aneurysm repair, the peripheral circulation can be supported with total or partial cardiopulmonary bypass or vascular shunts.

465

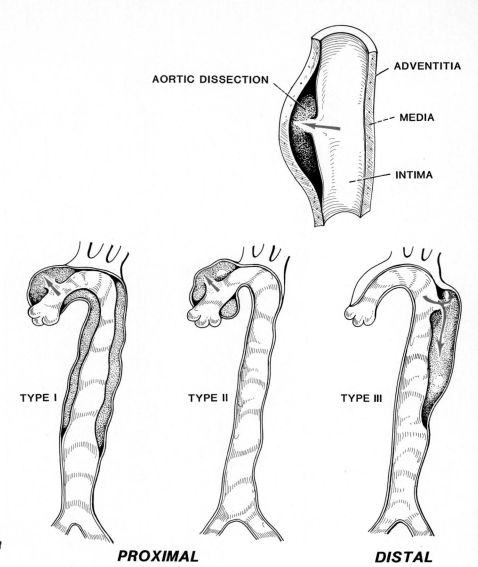

FIGURE 30-12
Aortic dissection. (A) Separation of vascular layers. (B) Classification of aortic dissection.

Labels in figure: AORTIC DISSECTION, ADVENTITIA, MEDIA, INTIMA, TYPE I, TYPE II, TYPE III, PROXIMAL, DISTAL

VENOUS DISEASE

Anatomy and physiology

In comparison to arteries, veins are thinner-walled and more distensible. Approximately 70 percent of the blood volume is contained within the venous circuit under relatively low pressure. The low-pressure–high-volume venous circuit functions as a capacitance circuit, in contrast to the high-pressure–low-volume resistance circuit of the arterial side. The capacity and volume of the venous circuit is an important determinant of cardiac output since the volume of blood ejected by the heart depends upon its venous return.

The venous system in the lower extremities (Fig. 30-13) is divided into three subsystems: (1) the superficial venous subsystem, (2) the deep venous subsystem, and (3) the communicating (perforating) subsystem. The superficial veins are situated in the subcutaneous tissues of the leg and receive venous flow from smaller vessels within the skin, subcutaneous tissue, and feet.

The superficial system consists of the greater saphenous vein and the lesser saphenous vein. The greater saphenous vein is the longest vein in the body; it extends from the malleolus of the ankle, up the inner aspect of the calf and thigh, to empty into the femoral vein just below the groin. The point of juncture between the two veins, the saphenofemoral junction, is an important anatomic landmark. The greater saphenous vein drains the anteromedial aspects of the calf and thigh. The lesser saphenous vein extends along the lateral aspect of the calf from the ankle to the knee, draining the posterolateral aspects of the calf, and empties into the popliteal vein. The junction between the saphenous and the popliteal veins is the saphenopopliteal junction. Multiple anastomoses exist between the greater and lesser saphenous veins; these anastomoses are important potential routes of collateral flow in the event of venous obstruction.

The deep venous system carries the greater part of the venous blood in the lower extremities and is situated within the muscle compartments. The *deep veins* receive flow from small venules and intramuscular vessels. The deep venous system tends to parallel the arterial vessels of the lower leg, and many vessels are named accordingly. Consequently, the system includes the anterior and posterior tibial veins, peroneal vein, popliteal vein, femoral vein, profunda femoris vein, as well as unnamed calf vessels. The iliac veins are also included in the deep venous system of the lower extremity, since venous drainage from the legs to the vena cava depends upon the patency and integrity of these vessels.

The superficial and deep venous subsystems are connected by vascular channels referred to as *perforating veins*. The perforating veins make up the communicating subsystem of the lower extremities. Flow is normally shunted from the superficial veins to the deep veins and subsequently to the inferior vena cava.

One-way semilunar valves are distributed throughout the venous system of the lower extremities. The valves are folds of the intimal layer of the vessel and consist of endothelium and collagen. These venous valves prevent retrograde flow, and they direct flow proximally from the lower extremities to the vena cava and from the superficial system to the deep system via the perforators. The competency of these valves is critical, since the flow of blood from the extremities to the heart is against gravity.

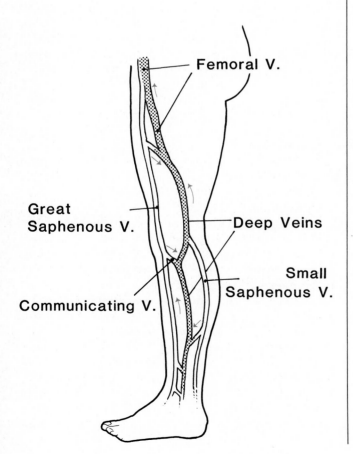

Great Saphenous V.

Femoral V.

Deep Veins

Small Saphenous V.

Communicating V.

The physiology of venous flow against gravitational forces involves the interaction of multiple factors referred to as *the venous pump*. There are peripheral and central components to the venous pump. The peripheral venous pump depends upon compression of venous channels during muscle contraction. Muscle contraction propels flow forward within the deep venous system; the venous valves prevent retrograde flow or reflux of blood during muscle relaxation. In addition, small valveless venous sinuses or venules located deep within the soleus and gastrocnemius muscles function as reservoirs of blood and empty into the deep veins during muscle contraction; the contribution of these intramuscular channels is particularly important to venous return. Central forces promoting venous return include the reduction in intrathoracic pressure with inspiration and the fall in right ventricular and right atrial pressure following ventricular ejection.

Thromboembolic venous disease

Definitions

The term *thromboembolic disease* reflects the relationship between thrombosis, the process of blood clot formation, and the ever-present risk of embolization. Frequently, the first sign of venous thrombosis is pulmonary embolism. In addition, given the morbidity and mortality associated with pulmonary embolism (see Chap. 36), the primary emphasis in the treatment of deep venous thrombosis is upon prevention of embolization.

A distinction used to be made between thrombophlebitis and phlebothrombosis based upon the degree of inflammation accompanying the thrombotic process. *Thrombophlebitis* was characterized by acute inflammatory signs, including pain, tenderness, and redness along the course of the vein. *Phlebothrombosis* was said to represent venous thrombosis without overt inflammatory signs and symptoms. The distinction was considered important in determining the risk of pulmonary embolism. Inflammation was felt to increase the adherence of the clot to the vessel wall, reducing the risk of pulmonary embolism. It is now recognized that a clear distinction between these terms cannot be made; inflammation occurs to some degree with thrombosis. Therefore, these states simply represent different degrees of an underlying process. In addition, pulmonary

FIGURE 30-13
Anatomy of the venous system.

embolism is always a risk even when the presentation of venous thrombosis is silent.

The term thrombophlebitis is best used to refer to inflamed superficial veins. The term *deep venous thrombosis* is best used to describe thromboembolic disease of the deep veins of the lower extremity. Superficial thrombophlebitis and deep venous thrombosis will be described in subsequent sections.

Pathology and pathophysiology

The precise mechanism initiating thrombosis is poorly understood. Three categories of contributing factors, referred to as the Virchow triad, are commonly recognized: (1) stasis of blood flow, (2) endothelial injury, and (3) hypercoagulability of blood. The relative contributions of each factor and the interrelationships among them are debated.

Stasis or sluggish blood flow predisposes to thrombosis and appears to be a contributing factor in the setting of immobilization or prolonged limb dependency. Immobilization, such as that occurring during the perioperative period or with paralysis, eliminates the effect of the peripheral venous pump, promoting stagnation and pooling of blood in the lower extremities.

Although endothelial injury is known to initiate thrombus formation, overt endothelial lesions cannot always be demonstrated. However, subtle endothelial changes due to chemical changes, ischemia or anoxia, or inflammation may be implicated. Overt causes of endothelial damage include direct trauma to the vessel, as with fractures and soft tissue injury, and intravenous infusion of irritating substances, such as potassium chloride, chemotherapy, or high-dose antibiotics.

Blood coagulability depends upon complex interactions between a multitude of variables including the vascular endothelium, platelets and clotting factors, and the composition and flow characteristics of blood. In addition, the intrinsic fibrinolytic system balances the coagulation system by lysis and dissolution of clot to maintain vascular patency (see Chap. 18). Hypercoagulable states result from alterations in any of these variables. Hypercoagulability has been recognized with advanced malignancy and the use of estrogen contraceptives.

A variety of risk factors have also been identified on the basis of either clinical observations or an obvious relationship to the three contributing factors identified above. Risk factors include previous history of thromboembolism, marked immobility, chronic congestive heart failure, malignancy, use of estrogen contraceptives, blood dyscrasias, advancing age, leg or pelvic trauma or surgery, and obesity. As would be expected, there is little consensus regarding the relative significance of potential risk factors.

Venous thrombosis, whatever the underlying stimulus, increases the resistance to venous outflow from the lower extremities. As resistance increases, venous emptying is impaired, with a resultant elevation of venous blood volume and venous pressure. Thrombosis can involve the valve pockets and disrupt valve function. Valve dysfunction or incompetence promotes further stasis and pooling of blood within the extremity.

The thrombus becomes more organized and adherent to the vessel wall as it matures. Consequently, the risk of embolization is greatest in the earliest phases of thrombosis; however, the tail of the clot can still become detached and embolize during the organization phase. The other potential threat of thrombosis is extension proximally or into the deep venous system depending upon the site of origin. The therapy of deep venous thrombosis is directed at avoiding embolization or further extension of clot. Ultimately, patency of the vessel lumen may be reestablished (referred to as recanalization) by clot retraction and lysis via the endogenous fibrinolytic system. Typically, some degree of residual damage persists.

Superficial thrombophlebitis

Superficial thrombophlebitis involves the subcutaneous vessels of the upper and lower extremities. The most common cause of upper-extremity thrombophlebitis is intravenous infusions, particularly of acidotic or hypertonic solutions. Superficial thrombophlebitis of the lower extremities is commonly due to varicose veins or trauma. If no obvious cause of superficial thrombophlebitis can be determined, the possibility of underlying disease processes, such as thromboangiitis obliterans or malignancy, should be considered.

The typical presentation is acute with aching or burning pain and superficial tenderness. The skin may be erythematous and warm along the length of the vein. Slight swelling may be noted. The vein may be palpable as a subcutaneous cord. System manifestations of inflammation, such as fever and malaise, may occur.

The course of superficial thrombophlebitis is usually benign and self-limiting. Embolization is unusual; however, thrombus extension into the deep venous system can occur, particularly if the thrombus is close to major communicating channels or to the junctions between the saphenous veins and the popliteal or femoral veins.

Treatment of superficial thrombophlebitis of the lower extremities includes the following interventions to reduce stasis and promote venous return: (1) external support with compression stockings or elastic bandages, (2) ambulation or lower extremity exercises, (3) periodic extremity elevation, and (4) avoidance of prolonged limb dependency with sitting or standing. Warm compresses and anti-inflammatory agents, such as aspirin, may be administered to reduce discomfort. If extension into a major vessel of the deep venous system is threatened, ligation or interruption of the involved superficial vein at the saphenofemoral junction may be indicated.

Deep venous thrombosis

Deep venous thrombosis poses significant problems relative to the risk of pulmonary embolism and long-term disability due to chronic venous insufficiency. Most thrombi originate in the calf veins; many resolve spontaneously, others propagate or embolize. The overwhelming majority of pulmonary emboli are due to deep venous thrombosis of the veins of the pelvis and lower extremity.

Clinical manifestations and diagnosis

Deep venous thrombosis is a particularly insidious problem because it is typically asymptomatic; pulmonary embolism may be the first clinical indication of thrombosis. The diagnosis is particularly troublesome in that the clinical signs and symptoms associated with deep venous thrombosis (DVT) are nonspecific and their severity does not correlate with the extent of disease.

The most reliable sign is swelling and edema of the involved extremity. Swelling results from the increased intravascular volume caused by venous pooling of blood; edema reflects fluid seepage across the capillary membrane into the interstitium because of elevated hydrostatic pressure. The superficial veins may also be dilated owing to the obstruction of flow into the deep system or shunting of blood from the deep to the superficial systems. Although unilateral swelling is typically noted, ileofemoral obstruction can produce bilateral swelling.

Pain is the most common symptom; it is typically described as aching or throbbing and may be severe. Walking may aggravate the pain. Tenderness of the involved extremity may be noted. Two techniques for eliciting limb tenderness are dorsiflexion of the foot and the inflation of an air-filled cuff over the extremity. Calf tenderness upon dorsiflexion of the foot is referred to as Homans' sign and is considered an unreliable sign of DVT; calf or thigh pain with cuff inflation is called Lowenburg's sign. Other signs include increased tissue turgor with swelling, increased skin temperature with dilation of superficial veins, mottling and cyanosis due to stagnant flow, increased oxygen extraction, and reduction of hemoglobin. Secondary arterial compromise may occur with massive venous thrombosis due to vascular compression or spasm; diminished arterial pulses and pallor may result.

Venous valve incompetence can be evaluated clinically by tests of venous filling time. The *Brodie-Tren-delenburg test* involves emptying the saphenous vein by leg elevation and reducing arterial inflow by occlusion. With valve incompetence, rapid venous filling is noted upon release of occlusion pressure and assumption of the standing position. Another technique is the manual compression test, which involves proximal compression of the vein as the vein is palpated distally to evaluate retrograde venous filling due to valve reflux.

Because of the unreliability of clinical signs, non-invasive and invasive methods of evaluation assume greater importance. The techniques of Doppler ultrasound and plethysmography described for evaluation of arterial disease are also utilized for venous disease. Doppler techniques are used to determine the velocity and direction of flow and to detect abnormal flow responses to respiration, Valsalva manuever, and venous compression. For example, venous flow in the lower extremities is typically increased during expiration. With venous obstruction, phasic respiratory variations are blunted.

Plethysmography can also be used to evaluate changes in venous volume with respiration and with segmental application of air-filled cuffs. For example, proximal application of cuff pressure above the segment under evaluation increases venous volume and pressure. Upon release of the cuff, the rate of venous emptying can be evaluated. Resistance to outflow by a venous thrombus would delay emptying.

Fibrinogen iodine 125 testing can be utilized to detect developing thrombi, particularly below the knee. Iodine 125 is a radioisotope used to tag the fibrinogen, which is then incorporated into the growing thrombus. However, this technique is not commonly used since the technique is expensive and complex and frequently detects clinically insignificant thrombi.

In the setting of venous disease, phlebography or venography is the standard to which all other techniques are compared. A bolus of contrast material is injected into the venous system to opacify the veins of the lower extremity and pelvis. It is the most reliable technique for the evaluation of the location and extent of venous disease.

Management

Given the morbidity and mortality associated with deep venous thrombosis and pulmonary embolism and the difficulties encountered in diagnosis and management, the therapeutic emphasis is upon prophylaxis rather than treatment of established thrombosis. However, controversy exists as to the appropriate form of prophylaxis and the identification of high risk patients.

Physical methods to minimize venous stasis and

pharmacologic methods of anticoagulation are commonly utilized for prophylaxis. External support with compression stockings or elastic bandages continues to be recommended to reduce venous stasis despite a lack of evidence demonstrating its effectiveness in the prevention of thrombosis and subsequent embolization. Pressure gradient stockings which promote venous return by exerting decreasing amounts of pressure from the ankle to the calf or thigh are currently being evaluated. Caution must always be exercised with all types of stockings and bandages to avoid a tourniquet effect due to poor fit or careless application.

Devices are available to simulate or stimulate the mechanical pumping action of the calf muscles. External pneumatic compression of the lower extremities is accomplished by enclosing the calves in air-filled plastic boots that are periodically inflated and deflated. Pneumatic boots have been utilized most extensively in the neurosurgical setting. Electrical stimulation of the calf muscles to initiate contraction has been utilized intraoperatively but is considered unacceptable in the majority of clinical settings owing to patient discomfort.

Venous return to the heart is improved by active and passive leg exercises and early ambulation after surgery. Elevation of the foot of the bed above heart level or periodic elevation of the lower extremities are simple manuevers to reduce venous hydrostatic pressure and facilitate venous emptying.

The administration of low-dose heparin is advocated by some to prevent thrombosis. Lower doses of heparin are felt to minimize the risk of complications while permitting adequate anticoagulation. The efficacy of this practice is again controversial.

The treatment of established deep venous thrombosis incorporates the physical principles noted above with slight modification. Bed rest is indicated initially to allow time for clot organization and adherence to the vessel wall; it is hoped that bed rest minimizes the risk of pulmonary embolization. The foot of the bed should be elevated slightly to maximize venous drainage; external compression at knee level from the bed or pillows should be avoided. Bed rest is typically continued until signs and symptoms, particularly edema, subside. Progressive ambulation with external compression stockings is then indicated.

The goal of anticoagulation therapy is to prevent thrombus propagation, extension, or embolization. The anticoagulant of choice during the acute phase of deep venous thrombosis continues to be heparin. Typically, heparin is administered by continuous infusion for approximately 7 to 10 days. This is usually followed by oral anticoagulation with warfarin (Coumadin), although the value of long-term warfarin therapy is debatable.

Since platelet adhesion and aggregation are the basis for the development of the primary hemostatic plug in the coagulation schema, antiplatelet agents, such as aspirin and low-molecular-weight dextran (Rheomacrodex), are administered by some to retard thrombosis. Similarly, fibrinolytic agents, such as streptokinase and urokinase, may be administered during the early stages of acute thrombosis to activate the endogenous fibrinolytic system. Ideally fibrinolytic therapy should be initiated within 24 to 48 hours, since mature clot is more resistant to lysis. The fibrinolytic system is responsible for clot lysis and dissolution. The role of antiplatelet and fibrinolytic drugs in the therapy of deep venous thrombosis is still being investigated.

Surgical intervention in deep venous thrombosis involves either venous thrombectomy or vena caval interruption to prevent pulmonary embolism. Thrombectomy is indicated for selected cases of massive ileofemoral thrombosis or extensive venous thrombosis threatening limb survival. Thrombectomy involves insertion of a balloon-tipped Fogarty catheter through a venotomy. The balloon is then inflated and the catheter is withdrawn, removing the clot.

A variety of techniques have been used to prevent passage of lower extremity emboli through the vena cava to the heart. Venous flow through the inferior vena cava can be either totally or partially interrupted with specially designed clips (see Fig. 30-14A) or suturing techniques (see Fig. 30-14B). With total interruption venous return is then shunted around the obstructed vena cava via smaller collateral networks; this reduction in vessel caliber limits the potential size of an embolus reaching the heart. Vena caval clips or sutures divide the vessel into smaller compartments, preventing passage of large emboli. Devices can also be inserted transvenously to interrupt flow through the inferior vena cava. The designs of the Modin-Uddin umbrella, the Greenfield filter, and the Hunter balloon are illustrated in Fig. 30-14C.

Varicose veins

The term *varicose veins* signifies venous dilation; the dilation is typically accompanied by vessel elongation and tortuosity (see Fig. 30-15). The exact cause of varicose veins is unknown. Varicosities are distinguished as primary or secondary. The cause of primary varicosities appears to be an inherent structural weakness in the vessel wall, producing dilation of the wall. Dilation can be accompanied by venous valve incompetence due to inability of the valve cusps to overlap and prevent reflux of blood. Primary varicosities tend to involve the superficial veins because of the lack of external support or resistance within the subcutaneous tissue. Secondary varicosities are due to acquired or congenital pathology of the deep venous system which produces dilation of superficial veins, perforators, or collateral channels.

A number of factors predispose to the development of varicose veins. A familial tendency has been documented; it is possible that the inherent wall weakness is inherited. In addition, factors increasing the hydrostatic pressure and blood volume within the leg, such as prolonged standing or pregnancy, contribute to venous dilation.

The primary sign of varicose veins is cosmetic disfigurement. Varicosities may be associated with dull aching of the legs, particularly pronounced at the end of the day. Discomfort is typically relieved by leg ele-

vation. The diagnosis of varicose veins is straightforward and based on observation and palpation of dilated veins.

Complications are unusual. Superficial thrombosis or hemorrhage with ecchymoses may occur. The most common complication is superficial thrombophlebitis which may necessitate surgical removal of varicosities.

Physical methods, described earlier, to reduce ve-

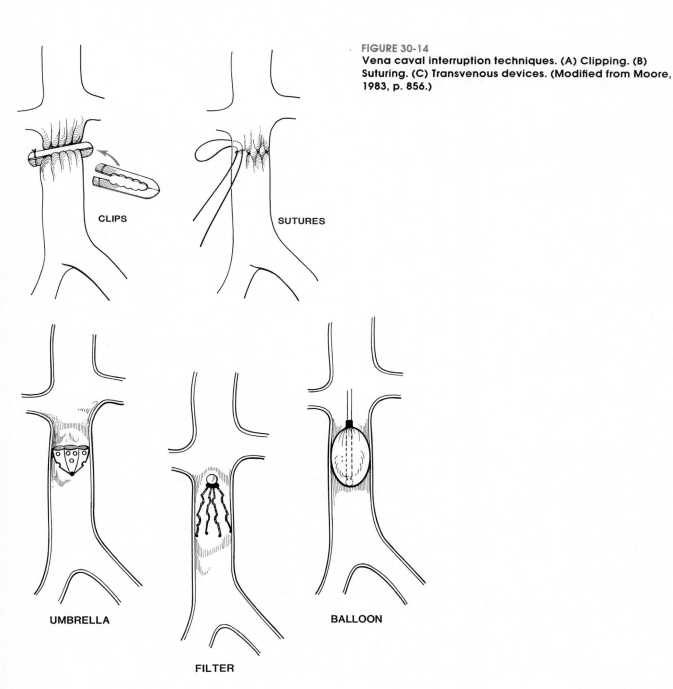

FIGURE 30-14
Vena caval interruption techniques. (A) Clipping. (B) Suturing. (C) Transvenous devices. (Modified from Moore, 1983, p. 856.)

CLIPS

SUTURES

UMBRELLA

FILTER

BALLOON

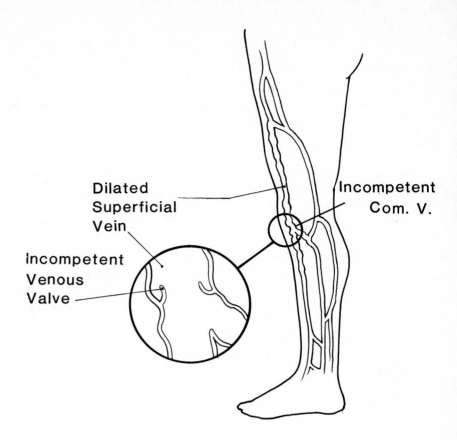

Dilated Superficial Vein

Incompetent Venous Valve

Incompetent Com. V.

FIGURE 30-15
Varicose veins.

nous stasis should be employed in the treatment of varicose veins. Injection of a sclerosing agent may be considered for small, asymptomatic varices; however, sclerotherapy presently has a limited role in the treatment of varicose veins. Surgery may be indicated to improve appearance of the lower extremity, relieve discomfort, or to avoid recurrent superficial thrombophlebitis. Surgery usually involves high ligation and stripping of the greater or lesser saphenous veins. The affected vein is ligated at either the saphenofemoral or saphenopopliteal junction and an intraluminal stripper is inserted to remove the entire vessel.

Chronic venous insufficiency

Chronic venous insufficiency is usually produced by extensive deep venous thrombosis and venous valve insufficiency; it can develop months or years after the initial episode. Milder degrees of chronic venous insufficiency can develop from longstanding varicose veins with valve insufficiency. The common denominator is chronic venous stasis and elevation of venous pressures. The term *postphlebitic syndrome* is commonly used to describe advanced chronic venous insufficiency.

The chronic elevation of venous pressure produces characteristic and progressive clinical signs of venous stasis. The increased hydrostatic pressure at the capil-

lary level results in fluid transudation into the interstitium and edema formation. Pathologic changes in the skin and subcutaneous tissue of the ankle and lower leg follow. These changes include development of a brown pigmentation due to hemosiderin deposition, induration from subcutaneous fibrosis, and dermatitis with eczematous, scaly skin. Tissue ulceration and necrosis may occur, particularly around the medial malleolus. The extremity is swollen and painful, especially after prolonged dependency.

As with thromboembolic venous disease, prevention is more readily accomplished than treatment of established chronic venous insufficiency. Prevention is directed at adequate treatment of acute thrombophlebitis, deep venous thrombosis, and varicose veins; the control of edema is particularly important since the presence of edema indicates elevated venous pressure. The medical treatment of chronic venous insufficiency includes the physical methods described earlier. In addition, it should be remembered that the tissue is extremely vulnerable to trauma; the foot should be protected whenever possible.

Lanolin or topical steroid or antibiotic ointments may be necessary to treat the dermatitis and local inflammation or infection. Stasis ulcers are particularly difficult to treat; continual compression with the premedicated Unna boot may be indicated. On occasion skin grafting is necessary in conjunction with vein ligation and stripping.

Vascular disease

1. Label the diagram below (Fig. 30-16) by matching the number of the structure on the diagram with the appropriate term from the list.

    Vessel Names

    a. _____ Ascending aorta

    b. _____ Aortic arch

    c. _____ Aortic bifurcation

    d. _____ Iliac arteries

    e. _____ Descending aorta

    f. _____ Popliteal arteries

    g. _____ Innominate artery

    h. _____ Femoral arteries

Directions: Answer the following questions on a separate piece of paper.

2. What are varicose veins and what causes them? Where are they generally located? What are some possible complications?

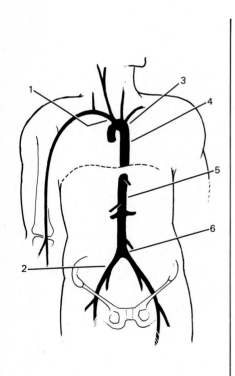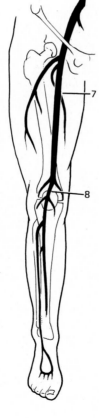

3. Is deep vein thrombosis or superficial vein thrombosis potentially the more serious? Why? Why do the superficial veins often become dilatated when there is deep vein thrombosis?

4. List several recommendations for preventing recurrent thrombophlebitis.

5. What is an aneurysm and what causes it? What are the dangers of an aneurysm?

6. What causes brownish pigmentation around the ankles and feet in patients with chronic venous insufficiency?

7. List three major conditions predisposing to venous thrombosis and embolism.

Directions: Circle the letter preceding each item below that correctly answers the question. Only one answer is correct unless otherwise noted.

8. Which of the following is usually the earliest sign or symptom of chronic occlusive arterial disease in the extremities?
   a. Intermittent claudication   b. Muscle atrophy
   c. Loss of hair over dorsum of foot   d. Digital ulceration of the involved extremity   e. Gangrene of the toes

9. Intermittent claudication resulting from chronic occlusive disease of the superficial femoral arteries commonly causes pain in the:
   a. Arch of the foot   b. Calf   c. Thigh   d. Buttocks

10. A delayed venous filling time when a leg is moved from an elevated to a dependent position occurs with which of the following conditions?
    a. Varicose veins   b. Chronic venous insufficiency   c. Peripheral arterial insufficiency
    d. Lymphedema

11. Which of the following physical findings is *not* present in patients with sudden arterial occlusion?
    a. Absence of one or more arterial pulses
    b. Loss of muscular strength   c. Decreased skin temperature in the extremity   d. Dilated superficial veins   e. Pallor and mottling of skin

12. Which of the following is the most common source of arterial emboli?
    a. Pulmonary artery   b. Aorta   c. Right atrium
    d. Left atrium   e. Peripheral artery

FIGURE 30-16
Arterial anatomy.

13. A stimulus for the development of collateral circulation is:
a. Hypertension b. Peripheral vasodilation
c. Mild chronic ischemia d. Inflammation of the arteries

14. Which of the following statements are true concerning true and false aneurysms? (More than one answer may be correct.)
a. False aneurysms are caused by entry of blood between the intima and medial layers of the blood vessel causing separation. b. A true aneurysm is a dilation enclosed by an intact arterial wall.
c. A false aneurysm consists of a localized area of clot and blood caused by a gap in the arterial wall.
d. True aneuryms only form in the aorta.

15. The formation of a blood clot within the vascular system is called:
a. Embolization b. Embolus c. Thrombus
d. Thrombosis

16. Which of the following signs and symptoms might indicate that a postoperative patient has thrombophlebitis of the leg? (More than one answer may be correct)
a. Decreased hair growth over involved area
b. Aching of extremity c. Positive Homans' sign
d. Pain and tenderness along course of superficial vein e. Oral temperature 103°F

17. The initial treatment of an acute thrombophlebitis generally consists of: (More than one answer may be correct).
a. Bed rest with the feet elevated b. Leg exercises c. Venous thrombectomy d. Warm moist compresses to the extremity e. Anticoagulant therapy

18. Which of the following statements regarding Raynaud's phenomenon is *incorrect*?
a. It results from episodic vasoconstriction of the small arteries in an extremity b. Symptoms are more frequent in a warm environment.
c. Changes in skin color caused by pallor, cyanosis, and hyperemia occur sequentially during an episode. d. Ulceration and gangrene of the digits may occur.

19. The presence of deep vein thrombosis can be detected noninvasively by:
a. Thermography b. Impedance measurements
c. Venography d. Monitoring blood pressure along the affected limb e. Monitoring skin color changes

Directions: Fill in the blank with the correct word.

20. _____ means inflammation of the vein accompanied by the formation of a clot; _____ means the formation of a clot in a vein in which there is little or no inflammation.

21. An arterial disease which starts in the smaller arteries of the hands and feet and has an intense inflammatory component is _____ _____.

Directions: Match each of the terms in col. A to its best description in col. B.

Column A

22. ____ Atherosclerosis

23. ____ Raynaud's syndrome

24. ____ Cystic medial necrosis

25. ____ Thromboangiitis obliterans

Column B

a. Episodic attacks of vasoconstriction of the arteries and arterioles in response to cold and emotional stimuli

b. Degenerative changes in the medial layer of the artery

c. Chronic occlusive disease of the medium and small arteries and veins due to inflammation and thrombosis

d. Focal intimal accumulation of lipids, carbohydrates, blood products, fibrous tissue, and calcium

Directions: Match each of the diagnostic methods in col. A to the most appropriate statement in col. B.

Column A

26. ____ Arteriography

27. ____ Doppler ultrasound detector

28. ____ Segmental plethysmography

29. ____ Radioactive fibrinogen scanning

Column B

a. Noninvasively measures the velocity of flow in a vessel

b. Visualization of arterial anatomy by injection of contrast material directly into an artery

c. Measures pulse volume

d. Injection intravenously of radioactive isotope which is detected by a counter at the site of actively forming thrombi

Directions: Match each of the blood vessel disease processes in col. A to the most appropriate surgical treatment in col. B.

Column A

30. ____ Abdominal aortic aneurysm (AAA)

Column B

a. Aortobifemoral bypass graft

b. Saphenous vein graft

31. ___ Complete aortoiliac occlusion

32. ___ Femoral-popliteal occlusion

33. ___ Deep femoral arterial occlusion

c. Aortic tube graft insertion

d. Profundaplasty

Directions: Match the type of arterial dissection in col. B with the appropriate category of the DeBakey classification in col. A.

Column A

34. ___ Type I
35. ___ Type II
36. ___ Type III

Column B

a. Aneurysms beginning beyond left subclavian and extending distally

b. Aneurysms confined to the ascending aorta

c. Aneurysms originating in the ascending aorta above aortic valve and extending distally

Directions. Circle T if the statement is true and F if it is false. Correct the false statements.

37. T F The insertion of a balloon-tipped catheter into a blood vessel in order to remove a blood clot is called an endarterectomy.

38. T F Patients with arterial occlusive disease of the lower extremities should keep the extremities slightly elevated to improve circulation.

39. T F The superficial veins are connected to the deep veins by perforating or communicating veins.

40. T F Detachment of a blood clot into the arterial circulation is called arterial thrombosis.

REFERENCES FOR PART V

AKUTSA, TETSUZO: *Artificial Heart—Total Replacement and Partial Support*, Excerpta Medica, Amsterdam, 1975.

American Heart Association: *Heart Facts: 1984*, New York, 1984.

APPLETON, D. and J. LAQUAGLIA: "Vascular Disease and Postoperative Management." *Unpublished manuscript*, 1984.

BATES, BARBARA: *A Guide to Physical Examination*, 2d ed., Lippincott, Philadelphia, 1979.

BERGAN, J., W. FLINN, and J. YAO: "Operative Therapy of Peripheral Vascular Disease," *Progress in Cardiovascular Diseases*, 26: 4, 1984.

——— and J. YAO: *Venous Problems*, Year Book, Chicago, 1978.

BERGER, EDWARD C.: *The Physiology of Adequate Perfusion*, Mosby, St. Louis, 1979.

BERNE, ROBERT and MATTHEW LEVY: *Cardiovascular Physiology*, 4th ed., Mosby, St. Louis, 1981.

BERNHARD, V., F. MADDISON, F. MOORE, et al.: *Vascular Surgery*, Saunders, Philadelphia, 1977.

BERNHARD WILLIAM F., JAMES G. CARR, and VICTOR L. POIRIER: "A Paracorporeal Left Ventricular Assist Device," *Modern Techniques in Cardiac/Thoracic Surgery*, 28, Futura Publishing Co., Mt. Kisco, New York, 1980.

BERNSTEIN, EUGENE (ed.), *Noninvasive Diagnostic Techniques in Vascular Disease*, Mosby, St. Louis, 1982.

BLANKERHORN, D., J. RODNEY, and P. CURRY: "Noninvasive Assessment of Atherosclerosis," *Progress in Cardiovascular Diseases*, 26: 4, 1983.

BRAUNWALD, EUGENE (ed.),: *Heart Disease: A Textbook in Cardiovasular Medicine*, 2d ed., Saunders, Philadelphia, 1984.

——— "Heart Failure: Pathophysiology and Treatment," *American Heart Journal*, 102(3): 486–490, 1981.

BREGMAN, DAVID (ed.): *Mechanical Support of the Failing Heart and Lungs*, Appleton-Century-Crofts, New York, 1977.

BREU, CHRISTINE S., JANE E. LINDENMUTH, and JAN H. FILLISCH: "Treatment of Patients with Congestive Cardiomyopathy during Hospitalization: A Case Study," *Heart and Lung*, 11(5): 229–235, 1982.

BULKLEY, BERNADINE H.: "The Cardiomyopathies," *Hospital Practice*, 19(6): 59–73, 1984.

CHUNG, E.: *Quick Reference to Cardiovascular Disease*, 2d ed, Lippincott, Philadelphia, 1983.

COLLINS, G.: *Medical Surgical Management*, Futura Publishing Co., Mt. Kisco, New York, 1981.

COVNER, AUDREY L. and JULIE A. SHINN: "Cardiopulmonary Transplantation: Initial Experience," *Heart and Lung*, 12(2): 131–135, 1983.

DAILEY, ELAINE K. and JOHN S. SCHROEDER: *Hemodynamic Waveforms—Exercise in Identification and Analysis*, Mosby, St. Louis, 1983.

DAVIES, M. J.: *Pathology of Cardiac Valves*, Butterworth, London and Boston, 1980.

DERIU, G., E. BALLOTTA, F. GRECO, et al.: "Abdominal

Aortic Aneurysms and Associated Peripheral Occlusive Disease," *Vascular Surgery*, May–June, 1984, pp. 146–156.

FISHER, JOHN D.: "Role of Electrophysiological Testing in Diagnosis and Treatment of Patients with Known and Suspected Bradycardias and Tachycardias," *Progress in Cardiovascular Diseases*, 24(1): 25–90, 1981.

FISHMAN, ALFRED P.: *Heart Failure*, Hemisphere Publishing Corp., Washington, 1978.

FOUAD, FETNAT M.: "Vasodilator Therapy for Congestive Heart Failure," *Cardiovascular Clinics*, 12(2): 127–135, 1981.

FOWLERS, ROBERT E. and JAY W. MASON: "Endomyocardial Biopsy," *Annals of Internal Medicine*, 97: 885–894, 1982.

GALLAGHER, JOHN J. and JAMES L. COX: "Status of Surgery for Ventricular Arrhythmias," (editorial), *Circulation* 60(7): 1440–1442, 1979.

GASPER, M. and W. BARKER: *Major Problems in Clinical Surgery*, Saunders, Philadelphia, 1981, pp. 176–227.

GERSTENBLITH, GARY: "Congestive Heart Failure," *Cardiovascular Clinics*, 12(1): 131–144, 1981.

GILBERT, CAROL J. and MASGOOD ASHTAR: "Right Heart Catheterization for Intracardiac Electrophysiologic Studies: Implications for the Primary Care Nurse," *Heart and Lung*, 9(1): 85–92, 1980.

GUYTON, ARTHUR C.: *Textbook of Medical Physiology*, 6th ed., Saunders, Philadelphia, 1981.

HACKETT, THOMAS P. and NED H. CASSES: *Massachusetts General Hospital Handbook of General Hospital Psychiatry*, Mosby, St. Louis, 1978.

HAIMOVICI, HENRY: *Vascular Surgery: Principles and Techniques*, 2d ed., Appleton-Century-Crofts, Norwich, Conn., 1984.

HARTZLER, GEOFFREY O.: "Electrode Catheter Ablation of Refractory Focal Ventricular Tachycardia," *Journal of the American College of Cardiology*, 2(6): 1107–1113, 1983.

HEIMBECKER, RAYMOND O., N. McKENZIE, C. STILLER, W. J. KOSTUK, and M. D. SILVER: "Heart and Lung Transplantation," *Heart and Lung*, 13(1): 1–4, 1984.

HURST, J. WILLIS, B. LOGUE, R. SCHLANT, and N. WENGER: *The Heart*, 5th ed., McGraw-Hill, New York, 1982.

ISERI, LLOYD T. and D. J. BENVENUTI: "Pathogenesis and Management of Congestive Heart Failure—Revisited," *American Heart Journal*, 102(2): 346–350, 1983.

JAMESON, STUART W., E. B. STINSON, P. E. OYER, J. C. BALDWIN, and N. E. SHUMWAY: "Operative Technique for Heart-Lung Transplantation," *Journal of Thoracic and Cardiovascular Surgery*, 87: 903–935, 1984.

JETT, MARY F. and LARRY E. LANCASTER: "The Inflammatory-Immune Response: the Body's Defense against Invasion," *Critical Care Nurse*, 3(6): 64–84, 1983.

JOHNSON, ROBERT A., EDGAR HABER, and W. G. AUSTEN: *The Practice of Cardiology*, Little, Brown, Boston, 1980.

JOSEPHSON, MARK E., and STUART F. SEIDES: *Clinical Cardiac Electrophysiology: Techniques and Interpretations*, Lea & Febiger, Philadelphia, 1979.

——— and LEONARD M. HOROWITZ: "Electrophysiological Approach to Therapy of Sustained Ventricular Tachycardia," *American Journal of Cardiology*, 43: 631–641, 1979.

———, ALDEN H. HARKEN, and LEONARD M. HOROWITZ: "Endocardial Excision: A New Surgical Technique for the Treatment of Recurrent Ventricular Tachycardia," *Circulation*, 60(7): 1430–1438, 1979.

JUERGENS, JOHN, JOHN SPITTEL, and JOHN FAIRBAIRN (eds.): *Peripheral Vascular Diseases*, Saunders, Philadelphia, 1980.

KARLINGER, JOEL S. and GABRIEL GREGORATOS (eds.): *Coronary Care*, Churchill Livingstone, New York, 1981.

KATZ, ARNOLD M.: "Heart Failure: New Opportunities and a New Series" (editorial), *Hospital Practice*, 18(3):13–18, 1983.

KAYE, WILLIAM: "Invasive Monitoring Techniques: Arterial Cannulation, Bedside Pulmonary Artery Catheterization, and Arterial Puncture," *Heart and Lung*, 12(3): 395–427, 1983.

LEWIS, S. M. and COLLIER, I. G.: *Medical-Surgical Nursing: Assessment and Management of Clinical Problems*, McGraw-Hill, New York, 1983.

LITWALK, ROBERT S., R. M. KOFFSKY, R. A. JURADO, et al.: "Support of Severely Impaired Cardiac Performance with Left-Heart Assist Device following Intracardiac Operation," *Heart and Lung*, 7(4): 622–626, 1978.

LOFGREN, E. and LOFGREN, K.: "The Surgical Treatment of Thrombophlebitis," *Surgery*, 90: 1, 1981.

LOWE, L.: "Venous Thrombosis and Embolism," *The Journal of Bone and Joint Surgery*, 63B: 2, 1981.

MANNICK, J.: *Surgical Clinics of North America*, 59: 4, Saunders, Philadelphia, 1979.

MARRIOTT, HENRY J. L. and MARY H. BOUDREAU CONOVER: *Advanced Concepts in Arrhythmias*, Mosby, St. Louis, 1983.

MASERI, ATTILIO, A. L'ABBATE, S. CHIERCHIA, et al.: "Significance of Spasm in the Pathogenesis of Ischemic Heart Disease," *American Journal of Cardiology*, 44: 788–792, 1979.

MASON, DEAN: *Congestive Heart Failure*, Yorke Medical Books, New York, 1976.

——— and JOHN J. COLLINS (eds.): *Myocardial Revascularization: Medical and Surgical Advances in Cor-*

onary Disease, Yorke Medical Books, New York, 1981.

MICHAELSON, CYDNEY R. (ed.): *Congestive Heart Failure*, Mosby, St. Louis, 1983.

MOORE, W.: *Vascular Surgery: A Comprehensive Review*, Grune & Stratton, Orlando, 1983.

MOSER, K. and FEDULLO, P.: "Venous Thromboembolism: Three Simple Decisions," *Chest*, **83**(1): 117–121, 1983.

NELSON, KRISTINE M.: "Cardiac Rehabilitation: An Overview," *Occupational Health Nursing*, 93–96, Feb., 1984.

NORMAN, JOHN C.: Intracorporeal Partial Artificial Hearts: Initial Clinical Trials," *Heart and Lung*, 7(5): 788–802, 1978.

———: *Coronary Artery Medicine and Surgery: Concepts and Controversies*, Appleton-Century-Crofts, New York, 1975.

OLSEN, E. G. J.: "The Pathology of Cardiomyopathies: A Critical Analysis," *American Heart Journal*, 98(3): 385–389, 1979.

QUAAL, SUSAN J. (ed.): *Comprehensive Intra-Aortic Balloon Pumping*, Mosby, St. Louis, 1984.

REAM, ALLEN K. and RICHARD P. FOGDALL (eds.): *Acute Cardiovascular Management: Anesthesia and Intensive Care*, Lippincott, Philadelphia, 1982.

RICHARDSON, DANIEL R.: *Basic Circulatory Physiology*, Little, Brown, Boston, 1976.

RUBIN, STANLEY A. and HAROLD J. C. SWAN: "Vasodilatory Therapy for Heart Failure," *Journal of the American Medical Association*, **425**(7): 761–763, February 20, 1981.

RUSHMER, ROBERT F.: *Cardiovascular Dynamics*, Saunders, Philadelphia, 1976.

RUSSELL, S.: "Prophylaxis of Postoperative Deep Vein Thrombosis and Pulmonary Embolism," *Surgery of Gynecology and Obstetrics*, **157**, July 1983.

RUTHERFORD, ROBERT, (ed.): *Vascular Surgery*, Saunders, Philadelphia, 1977.

SANA, JOSEPHINE M. and RICHARD D. JUDGE: *Physical Appraisal Methods in Nursing Practice*, Little, Brown, Boston, 1975.

SCHAFER, H. and HANDIN, R.: "The Role of Platelets in Thrombotic and Vascular Disease," *Progress in Cardiovascular Disease*, 22: 1, 1979.

SCHARITH, LEO: *The Electrocardiography of Coronary Artery Disease*, 2d ed., Blackwell Scientific Publications, London, 1975.

SCHROEDER, JOHN S. and ELAINE KIESS: *Techniques in Bedside Hemodynamic Monitoring*, 2d ed., Mosby, St. Louis, 1980.

SODEMAN, WILLIAM A. and LYNN SKELTON: "Oxygen Consumption of the Heart: Physiologic Principles and Clinical Implications," *Modern Concepts of Cardiovascular Diseases*, **XL**: 9–15, 1971.

SONNENBLICK, EDMUND H.: "Myocardial Ultrastructure in the Normal and Failing Heart," *Hospital Practice*, 5(4): 35–43, 1970.

STINSON, EDWARD B., R. B. GRIEPP, J. SCHROEDER, et al.: "Hemodynamic Observations One and Two Years After Cardiac Transplantation in Man," *Circulation* **XLV**: 1183–1194, 1972.

TOBIS, JONATHAN M., O. NALCIOGLU, and W. L. HENRY: "Cardiovascular Applications of Digital Subtraction Angiography," *Modern Concepts of Cardiovascular Disease*, **53**(4): 31–36, 1984.

UNDERHILL, SANDRA L., E. S. HALPENNY, and C, JEAN: *Cardiac Nursing*, Lippincott, Philadelphia, 1982.

URK, F., and OAKES, A.: "Assessing a Patient with Acute Aortic Dissection," *Focus on Critical Care*, 10 (2): 15–18, April 1983.

VANDER, ARTHUR, J. SHERMAN, and D. LUCIANO: *Human Physiology*, 3d ed., McGraw-Hill, New York, 1980.

VINSANT, MARIELLE O., and M. I. SPENSE: *Commonsense Approach to Coronary Care*, 3d ed., Mosby, St. Louis, 1981.

WAGNER, G. S., (ed.): *Myocardial Infarction: Measurement and Intervention*, Martinus Nijhoff Publishers, The Hague, 1982.

WEBER, KARL T., J. S. JANICKI, W. C. HUNTER, et al.: "The Contractile Behavior of the Heart and Its Functional Coupling to the Circulation," *Progress in Cardiovascular Diseases*, **XXIV**(5): 375–397, 1982.

——— and ———: "The Heart as a Muscle Pump System and the Concept of Heart Failure," *American Heart Journal*, 98(3): 371–384, 1979.

WEISS, GEORGE B., (ed.): *New Perspective on Calcium Antagonists*, American Physiological Society, Bethesda, Md., 1981.

WERNER, WENDY and ALEXANDRA CHRZANOWSKI: "Streptokinase Intracoronary Thrombolysis in Acute Myocardial Infarction," *Journal of Emergency Nursing*, 8(6): 277–284, 1982.

WINKLE, ROGER A.: "The Implantable Defibrillator in Ventricular Arrhythmias," *Hospital Practice*, 18(3): 149–165, 1983.

WOLD, BARBARA: "Dilated (Congestive) Cardiomyopathy: Considerations for the Coronary Care Nurse," *Heart and Lung*, 12(5): 544–553, 1983.

YANG, SING SAN, L. G. BENTIVOGLIO, V. MARANHAO, and H. GOLDBERG: *Cardiac Catheterization Data to Hemodynamic Parameters*, 2d ed., F. A. Davis Company, Philadelphia, 1978.

ZAK, RADOVAN: "Cardiac Hypertrophy: Biochemical and Cellular Relationships," *Hospital Practice*, 18 (3): 85–97, 1983.

ZIMMERMAN, T. and RUPLINGER, J.: "Thromboabdominal Aneurysms: Treatment and Nursing Interventions," *Critical Care Nurse*, Nov.–Dec. 1983, pp. 54–63.

PART VI

LORRAINE M. WILSON
SYLVIA A. PRICE

RESPIRATORY PATHOPHYSIOLOGY

Disorders of the respiratory system are a major cause of morbidity and mortality. Respiratory tract infections are more frequent than infections of any other organ system and range from the common cold with its relatively mild symptoms and inconvenience to a fulminant pneumonia. In 1983, approximately 135,000 persons died of lung cancer. In fact, cancer of the lung is the leading cause of male cancer deaths in the United States; it has increased at an alarming rate and is now about 25 times more prevalent than it was 45 years ago. The death rate due to lung cancer is also rising steadily for women, so that it may soon equal that of breast cancer (Koop, 1984). The incidence of chronic respiratory disease, notably chronic pulmonary emphysema and bronchitis, has also been increasing and is now a leading cause of chronic disability among the male population.

Because of the physical, social, and economic impact of respiratory diseases on the population as a whole, the prevention, diagnosis, and treatment of respiratory disorders are of paramount importance.

This section includes a brief review of respiratory tract anatomy and physiology, a discussion of the common diagnostic tests used to detect respiratory dysfunction, cardinal signs and symptoms of respiratory disease, manifestations of respiratory insufficiency and failure, and a discussion of the common respiratory diseases.

OBJECTIVES

At the completion of this part you should be able to:

1. Describe the relation between normal respiratory tract anatomy and physiology and the effects of respiratory dysfunction as a disease process.
2. Identify the etiology, pathogenesis, and treatment principles in the various respiratory diseases or disorders.

CHAPTER
31

NORMAL RESPIRATORY FUNCTION

OBJECTIVES

At the completion of this chapter you should be able to:

1. List three disorders of the respiratory system which are a major cause of morbidity and mortality.
2. Define *respiration*.
3. Name the air-conducting passages.
4. Describe the structure and identify the functions of the epithelial surfaces of the airways.
5. Describe the functions of the larynx.
6. Differentiate anatomically between the right and left mainstem bronchi.
7. Explain the clinical implications of the anatomic differences in the mainstem bronchi.
8. Identify the relation between the following anatomic structures: lobar and segmental bronchi, terminal bronchioles, acinus, respiratory bronchioles, alveolar ducts, terminal alveolar sacs, alveolar septa, and pores of Kohn.
9. Describe the microscopic structure and function of an alveolar duct and surrounding alveoli.
10. Differentiate between a respiratory bronchiole and a terminal bronchiole on the basis of structure and function.
11. Identify the function of surfactant and the conditions necessary for its production.
12. Identify the relation between the following anatomic structures of the thoracic cavity: mediastinum, hilus, lobar and segmental divisions of both lungs, apex and base of lungs, diaphragm muscle, and pleura and pleural space.
13. Differentiate between the parietal and visceral pleura.
14. Construct and label a diagram showing the relation between the heart and lungs and the circulation between them.
15. List the unique features of the lung's circulatory system and identify the significance of each feature.

16. Explain the pathogenesis of pulmonary edema.
17. Describe briefly the mechanical process of ventilation.
18. Explain the mechanism of regulation of respiration and identify the important variables.
19. List the defense mechanisms of the respiratory tract.
20. Describe the unique characteristics of the alveolar macrophage.
21. Identify the three main stages by which oxygen is transferred from the air to the tissues and carbon dioxide is excreted in the expired air.
22. Describe the mechanical process of ventilation, including thoracic pressure-volume and airflow dynamics.
23. Describe the process by which the diffusion of gases occurs across the alveolar-capillary membrane.
24. State the ventilation-perfusion requirements necessary for the transfer of gas between the alveolus and the pulmonary capillary bed.
25. Differentiate between a dead space and a shunt-producing respiratory unit.
26. Compute the volume of anatomic dead space for a given body weight.
27. Identify the two mechanisms by which oxygen is transported from the lungs to the tissues.
28. Describe oxygen transportation in relation to the oxyhemoglobin dissociation curve.
29. List the factors which may either increase or decrease the affinity of hemoglobin for oxygen.
30. Define the P_{50} and state its normal value.
31. Describe the process of carbon dioxide transport in the blood.
32. Identify the relation between ventilation, carbon dioxide homeostasis, and the acid-base balance of the body.
33. State the relation between hemoglobin concentration, hemoglobin saturation, the partial pressure of oxygen in the arterial blood, and actual oxygen delivered to the tissues.
34. Describe at least three examples of situations which may result in respiratory insufficiency and identify in each case the altered physiologic mechanism that interferes with adequate respiration.

ANATOMIC CONSIDERATIONS

Respiration may be defined as the combined activity of the various mechanisms that are involved in supplying oxygen to all the cells of the body and removing carbon dioxide (the product of cell combustion). The respiratory system accomplishes the task of respiration. Essentially, the respiratory system consists of a series of air passages which bring outside air into contact with a large expanse of specialized respiratory membrane. This membrane lies in close proximity to the capillaries, and the interface between the membrane and the cap-

illaries is the location for exchange of oxygen and carbon dioxide.

Anatomy of the respiratory tract

The air-conducting passages that bring air into the lungs are the nose, pharynx, larynx, trachea, bronchi, and bronchioles (see Fig. 31-1). The respiratory tract from the nose to the bronchioles is lined with ciliated mucous membranes. As air enters the nasal cavity, it is filtered, warmed, and humidified. These three processes are primarily functions of the respiratory mucosa, which

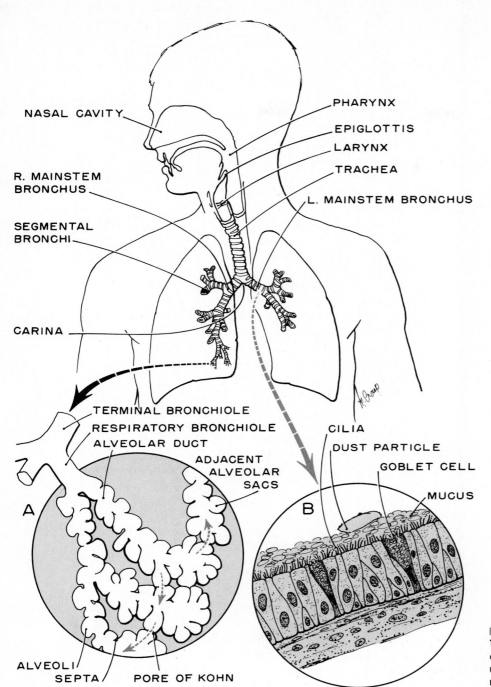

NASAL CAVITY

PHARYNX

EPIGLOTTIS

LARYNX

TRACHEA

R. MAINSTEM BRONCHUS

L. MAINSTEM BRONCHUS

SEGMENTAL BRONCHI

CARINA

TERMINAL BRONCHIOLE
RESPIRATORY BRONCHIOLE
ALVEOLAR DUCT

ADJACENT ALVEOLAR SACS

CILIA

DUST PARTICLE

GOBLET CELL

MUCUS

A

B

ALVEOLI
SEPTA
PORE OF KOHN

FIGURE 31-1
The respiratory system. Inset A, acinus or pulmonary functional unit. Inset B, ciliated mucous membrane.

consists of pseudostratified ciliated columnar epithelium and goblet cells (see inset B, Fig. 31-1). The epithelial surface is covered by a mucous blanket which is secreted by both the goblet cells and the serous glands. Coarse dust particles are filtered by hair in the nares, while fine particles are trapped in the mucous blanket. Ciliary action propels the mucous blanket posteriorly in the nasal cavity and superiorly in the lower respiratory tract toward the pharynx, from which it is swallowed or expectorated. Water for humidification is given up by the mucous blanket, and heat is supplied to the inspired air by a rich underlying vascular network. Inspired air

is thus conditioned so that it reaches the pharynx nearly dust-free, at body temperature, and 100 percent humidified.

Air passes from the pharynx into the *larynx*, or voice box. The larynx consists of a series of cartilaginous rings united by muscles and contains the vocal cords. A triangular space between the vocal cords opens into the trachea and is called the *glottis*. The glottis forms the division between the upper and lower respiratory tracts. Although the larynx has been thought of chiefly in relation to phonation, its protective functions are of much more importance. During swallowing, the rising action of the larynx, the closure of the glottis, and the doorlike action of the leaf-shaped *epiglottis*, at the entrance of the larynx all serve to guide food and fluids into the esophagus. If foreign substances do get beyond the glottis, the cough function of the larynx assists in expelling these substances as well as secretions from the lower respiratory tract.

The trachea is supported by horseshoe-shaped cartilaginous rings and is about 5 in long. The structure of the treachea and bronchi is analogous to a tree, and it is therefore called the *tracheobronchial tree*. The posterior surface of the trachea is flattened rather than round (since its cartilaginous rings are incomplete) and lies immediately in front of the esophagus. Consequently, when a round, rigid endotracheal tube with inflated cuff is inserted during mechanical ventilation, erosion may occur posteriorly through the membrane to form a tracheoesophageal fistula. Anterior erosion through the cartilaginous rings may also occur but is less common. The point where the trachea branches into the right and left mainstem bronchi is known as the *carina*. The carina is heavily innervated and can produce severe bronchospasms and coughing when stimulated.

Note in Fig. 31-1 that the right and left mainstem bronchi are not symmetric. The right bronchus is shorter and wider and continues from the trachea in a nearly vertical course. In contrast, the left bronchus is longer and narrower and continues from the trachea at a more acute angle. This anatomic peculiarity has important clinical implications. An endotracheal tube which has been placed to secure a patent airway may easily slip down into the right mainstem bronchus unless well secured at the mouth or nose. If it did slip, air would not be able to enter the left lung, which would collapse (atelectasis). However, the more vertical course of the right bronchus makes it easier to introduce a catheter for deep suctioning. Also, foreign bodies which are aspirated are more apt to lodge in the right bronchial tree because of its vertical course.

The right and left mainstem bronchi divide to become the *lobar* and then the *segmental bronchi*. This branching in ever-decreasing sizes continues down to the *terminal bronchioles*, which are the smallest airways that do not contain alveoli (air sacs). Terminal bronchioles are about 1 mm in diameter. Bronchioles are not supported by cartilaginous rings but are surrounded by smooth muscle, which allows alterations in size. All the airways down to the level of the terminal bronchioles are called *conducting airways*, since their main function is to serve as air conduits to the gas-exchanging areas of the lung.

Beyond the terminal bronchiole is the *acinus*, which is the pulmonary functional unit where gas exchange takes place (see inset A, Fig. 31-1). The acinus consists of (1) *respiratory bronchioles*, which have occasional small air sacs or alveoli arising from their walls; (2) *alveolar ducts*, completely lined with alveoli, and (3) *terminal alveolar sacs*, the final structures of the lung. The acinus, or *primary lobule* as it is sometimes called, is about 0.5 to 1.0 cm in diameter. There are about 23 generations of branching from the trachea to the terminal alveolar sac. The individual alveolus (in the grapelike cluster of alveolar sacs that make up the terminal sac) is separated from its neighbor by a thin wall, or *septum*. Small openings in the septum, called the *pores of Kohn*, allow communication between terminal alveolar sacs. The alveolus has only one layer of cells, which is less than the diameter of a red blood cell in thickness. There are about 300 million alveoli in each lung, with a surface area about the size of a tennis court.

Figure 31-2 shows the microscopic structure of an alveolar duct and the surrounding alveoli, which are polygonal in shape. Since the alveolus is essentially a gas bubble surrounded by a capillary network, the liquid-gas interface creates a surface tension which tends to resist expansion on inspiration and favors collapse on expiration. The alveoli, however, are lined with a lipoprotein substance called *surfactant* which lessens the surface tension, lowers the resistance to expansion on inspiration, and prevents collapse of the alveoli on expiration. The production of surfactant by the alveolar lining (Type II) cells depends on several factors, including maturity of the alveolar cells and their biosynthetic enzyme systems, a normal turnover rate, adequate ventilation, and blood flow to the alveolar walls. A deficiency of surfactant is believed to be an important factor in the pathogenesis of a number of lung diseases.

The thoracic cavity

The lungs are elastic, cone-shaped organs which lie within the thoracic cavity, or chest. They are separated by the central mediastinum, which contains the heart and great vessels (Fig. 31-3). Each lung has an apex (top of lung) and a base. Pulmonary and bronchial blood vessels, bronchi, nerves, and lymphatics enter each lung at the hilus to form the root of the lung. The right lung is larger than the left and is divided into three lobes by the interlobar fissures. The left lung is divided into two lobes.

Lobes are further divided into segments corresponding to the segmental bronchi. The right lung is divided into 10 segments and the left lung into 9 (see Fig. 31-3, Bronchopulmonary Segments). Pathologic processes such as atelectasis and pneumonia are often localized to individual lobes and segments. Knowledge of the segmental anatomy of the lung is important not only for the radiologist, bronchoscopist, and thoracic surgeon but also for the nurse and physical therapist,

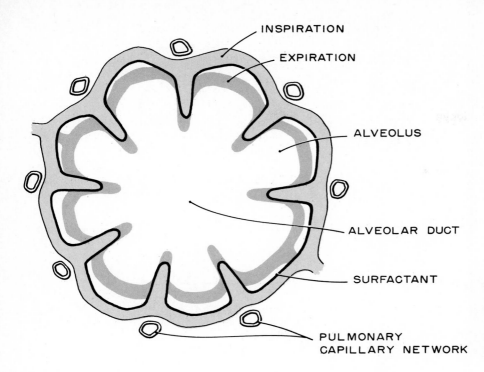

INSPIRATION

EXPIRATION

ALVEOLUS

ALVEOLAR DUCT

SURFACTANT

PULMONARY
CAPILLARY NETWORK

FIGURE 31-2
Structural changes in the terminal alveolar sac (cross section) during the respiratory cycle. (Modified from L. Gluck, "Pulmonary Surfactant and Neonatal Distress," *Hospital Practice,* **November 1972.)**

who must know with accuracy the location of the lesion in order to apply their skills.

A continuous thin sheet of collagen and elastic tissue, known as the *pleura*, lines the thoracic cavity *(parietal pleura)* and encases each lung *(visceral pleura)*. Between the parietal and visceral pleura is a thin film of pleural fluid which allows the two surfaces to glide over each other during respiration and prevents the separation of the thorax and lungs, as when two glass slides are stuck together with water: the slides can glide over each other, but they cannot easily be pulled apart. The same is true of the pleural fluid between the lungs and thorax. Since no actual space separates the parietal and visceral pleurae, the so-called pleural spaces or cavities are potential spaces only. The pressure within the pleural space is below that of the atmosphere and thus prevents the collapse of the lung. In disease, the pleura may become inflamed or air or fluid may enter the pleural space, causing compression or collapse of the lung. Three factors maintain this normal negative pressure. First, the elastic tissue of the lungs exerts a continuous force which tends to pull the lungs away from the thoracic cage; i.e., the lungs have a tendency to recoil to their smaller original size before the first expansion after birth. However, the visceral and parietal pleural surfaces in contact with each other cannot separate, so the continuous force which tends to separate them persists. This force is popularly known as the *negative pressure* of the pleural space. Intrapleural pressures vary continuously throughout the respiratory cycle (see "Ventilation," below) but are always negative. The second major factor in maintaining negative intrapleural pressure is the osmotic forces exerted across the pleural

membranes. Fluid normally moves from the capillaries in the parietal pleura into the pleural space and then is reabsorbed through the visceral pleura. The movement of the pleural fluid is believed to be governed by Starling's law of transcapillary exchange (Light, 1983); that is, fluid movement depends on a net gradient between the hydrostatic pressure of the blood tending to push fluid out and the oncotic pressure of the plasma proteins tending to hold the fluid within. Because the net gradient for pleural fluid absorption through the visceral pleura is greater than the net gradient for fluid formation by the parietal pleura, and because the surface area of the visceral pleura is greater than that of the parietal pleura, the pleural space normally contains only a few milliliters of fluid. The third factor which supports a negative intrapleural pressure is the force of the lymphatic pump. A small amount of protein normally enters the pleural space but is removed by the lymphatics in the parietal pleura; the accumulation of protein in the intrapleural space would upset the normal osmotic balance without lymphatic removal. These three factors, then, regulate and maintain the normal negative intrapleural pressure. The *diaphragm* is a dome-shaped muscle that forms the floor of the thoracic cavity and separates it from the abdominal cavity.

Pulmonary circulation

The blood supply to the lungs is unique in several respects. First, the lung has a dual blood supply from the bronchial and pulmonary arteries. The bronchial circulation provides oxygenated blood from the systemic circulation and serves to meet the metabolic needs of the

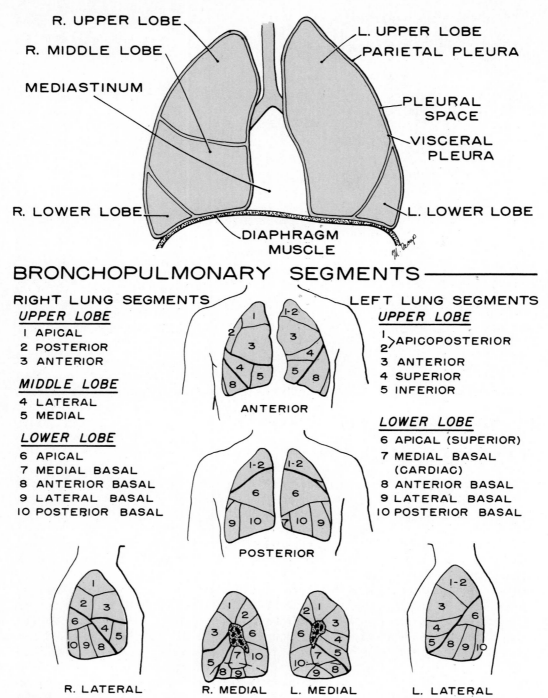

FIGURE 31-3
The thoracic cavity and the bronchopulmonary segments.

lung tissue. The bronchial arteries arise from the thoracic aorta and travel along the posterior walls of the bronchi. The larger bronchial veins empty into the azygos system, which empties into the superior vena cava and returns blood to the right atrium. The smaller bronchial veins drain into the pulmonary veins. Since the bronchial circulation does not take part in gas exchange, the unoxygenated blood accounts for a shunt which is normally about 2 to 3 percent of cardiac output.

The pulmonary artery arising from the right ventricle provides mixed venous blood to the lungs, where the blood is involved in gas exchange. A vast network of pulmonary capillaries surrounds and envelops the alveoli, providing the intimate contact necessary for the exchange of gases between the alveoli and the blood. Oxygenated blood is then returned through the pulmonary veins to the left ventricle, which distributes it

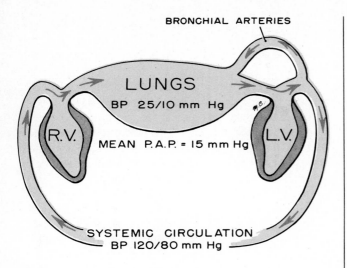

BRONCHIAL ARTERIES

FIGURE 31-4
Functional position of the lungs in the pulmonary circulation.

25 mmHg, fluid would leave the pulmonary capillaries and enter the interstitium or alveoli, causing pulmonary edema. Pulmonary edema interferes with gas exchange by interfering with the diffusion pathway between the alveolus and the capillary. Pulmonary edema is a common complication of congestive heart failure, pneumonia, and many other lung disorders.

Control of respiration

A number of mechanisms contribute to bringing air into the lungs so that exchange of gases can occur. The mechanical function of moving air in and out of the lungs is termed *ventilation* and is accomplished by a number of interacting components. Of particular importance is a reciprocating pump called the *respiratory bellows*. This bellows has two volume-elastic components: the lung itself and the chest wall surrounding the lung. The chest wall consists of the skeleton and tissues of the thoracic cage, as well as the diaphragm, abdominal contents, and abdominal wall. The respiratory muscles, which are a part of the thoracic wall, provide the driving force for the operation of the bellows. The diaphragm (assisted by those muscles that elevate the ribs and sternum) is the principal muscle involved in increasing the volume of the lung and thoracic cage dur-

to the cells via the systemic circulation. Figure 31-4 shows the functional position of the lungs in the pulmonary circulation.

Another feature of the pulmonary circulation is that it is a low-pressure, low-resistance system in comparison to the systemic circulation. Systemic blood pressure is about 120/80 mmHg, while pulmonary blood pressure is about 25/10 mmHg, with a mean pressure of about 15 mmHg. These features of the pulmonary circulation have several important consequences. The great distensibility and low resistance of the pulmonary vascular beds allows the workload of the right ventricle to be much lighter than that of the left and also allows a great increase in pulmonary blood flow during exercise without significantly increasing the pulmonary blood pressure.

As shown in Fig. 31-5 if the normal mean pulmonary hydrostatic pressure of about 15 mmHg should exceed the colloid osmotic pressure of the blood of about

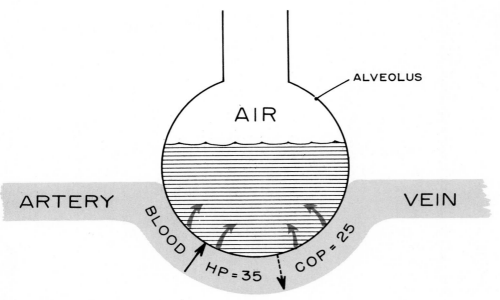

FIGURE 31-5
Pathogenesis of pulmonary edema.

ing inspiration; expiration is a passive process during quiet breathing. The mechanics of ventilation are discussed in greater detail in Chap. 32.

The respiratory muscles are controlled by the respiratory center, which is composed of neurons and receptors located in the pons and medulla (see Fig. 31-6). The respiratory center is the part of the nervous system that controls all aspects of breathing. The prime factor in the control of breathing is the response of the central chemoreceptors in the respiratory center to the partial pressure of carbon dioxide (Pa_{CO_2}) and the pH of the arterial blood. An increase in the Pa_{CO_2} or a decrease in the pH stimulates breathing.

A decrease of the partial pressure of oxygen in the arterial blood Pa_{O_2} can also stimulate ventilation. Peripheral chemoreceptors located in the carotid bodies at the bifurcation of the common carotid arteries and in the aortic bodies at the aortic arch are senstive to a de-

crease in the Pa_{O_2}. The Pa_{O_2}, however, must fall from the normal level of about 90 to 100 mmHg to a level of about 60 mmHg before ventilation is significantly stimulated.

There are also mechanisms which control the amount of air taken into the lungs. As the lung is inflated, these receptors signal the respiratory center to stop further inflation. Signals from the stretch receptors cease at the end of expiration when the lung is deflated and the respiratory center is free to initiate another inspiration. This mechanism is known as the *Hering-Breuer reflex*. Movements of joints and muscles (e.g., during exercise) also stimulate an increase in ventilation. Voluntary control input from the cerebrum can modify output from the respiratory centers, thus allowing interruption of the normal breathing cycle for laughing, crying, and speaking. The pattern and rhythmic control of breathing are exercised through the interaction of the respiratory centers located in the pons and medulla. Final motor output is transmitted via the spinal cord and phrenic nerve, which supplies the diaphragm, the principal muscle of ventilation. Other major nerves involved are the spinal accessory and tho-

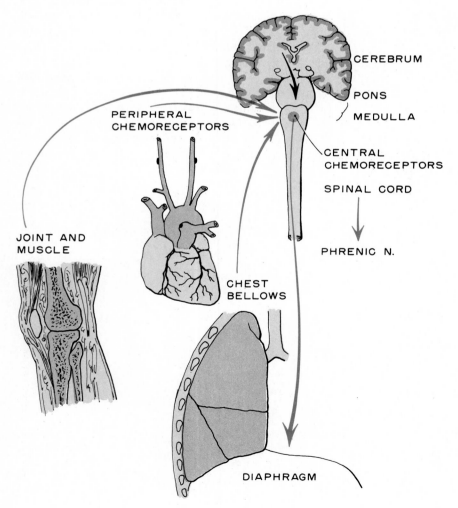

FIGURE 31-6
The control of respiration.

CEREBRUM

PONS

MEDULLA

PERIPHERAL
CHEMORECEPTORS

CENTRAL
CHEMORECEPTORS

SPINAL CORD

JOINT AND
MUSCLE

PHRENIC N.

CHEST
BELLOWS

DIAPHRAGM

racic intercostal nerves, which supply the accessory muscles of respiration and the intercostal muscles.

Defenses of the respiratory tract

The large surface area of the lung, which is separated only by a thin membrane from the circulatory system, makes a person theoretically vulnerable to invasion by foreign bodies (dust) and bacteria in the inhaled air. However, the lower respiratory tract is normally sterile. Several defense mechanisms maintain this sterility. The swallowing or gag reflex, which prevents entry of food or fluid into the trachea, and the action of the "mucociliary escalator," which traps dust and bacteria and transports them to the throat, have already been mentioned. Furthermore, the mucous blanket contains factors which may be effective in defense, including immunoglobulins (especially IgA), polymorphonuclear leukocytes, interferon, and specific antibodies. The cough reflex provides another, more forceful, mechanism to expel secretions upward so that they may be swallowed or expectorated. The *alveolar macrophage* provides the final and most important defense against bacterial invasion of the lung. The alveolar macrophage is a phagocytic cell with unique migratory and enzymatic characteristics. It moves freely over the alveolar surface and engulfs inert particulate matter and bacteria. After a microbial particle is engulfed, lytic enzymes within the macrophage kill and digest the microorganism without producing any obvious inflammatory reaction. The dust particle or microorganism is then transported by the macrophage to the lymphatics or to the bronchioles, where it is removed by the mucociliary escalator. Alveolar macrophages can clear the lung of inhaled bacteria with amazing speed. Ethyl alcohol ingestion, cigarette smoking, and corticosteroid drugs interfere with this defense mechanism.

PHYSIOLOGIC CONSIDERATIONS

The physiologic process of respiration by which oxygen is transferred from the air to the tissues and carbon dioxide is excreted in the expired air may be divided into three main stages, as illustrated in Fig. 31-7. The first stage is ventilation, which is the flow of a mixture of gases into and out of the lungs. The second stage, transportation, must be considered from several aspects: (1) the diffusion of gases between the alveolus and pulmonary capillary (external respiration) and between the systemic blood and tissue cells; (2) the distribution of blood in the pulmonary circulation and its match with the distribution of air in the alveoli; and (3) the chemical

and physical reactions of oxygen and carbon dioxide with the blood. Cell respiration, or internal respiration, is the final stage of respiration, during which metabolites are oxidized to obtain energy and carbon dioxide is produced as a waste product of cell metabolism and excreted by the lungs.

Ventilation

Air moves in and out of the lungs because pressure gradients are created between the atmosphere and the alveoli by muscular mechanical means. As mentioned previously, the thoracic cage functions as a bellows. The changes in the intrapleural and intrapulmonary (airway) pressures and lung volumes during ventilation may be followed on the graph in Fig. 31-8. During inspiration, the volume of the thorax increases because of the descent of the diaphragm and the elevation of the ribs caused by the contraction of several muscles. The sternocleidomastoids lift upward on the sternum, while the serratus, scalene, and external intercostal muscles are all involved in elevation of the ribs. The thorax enlarges in three directions: anteroposteriorly, laterally, and vertically. This increase in volume causes the intrapleural pressure to decrease from about -4 mmHg (relative to atmospheric pressure) to about -8 mmHg as the lungs are pulled to a more expanded position during

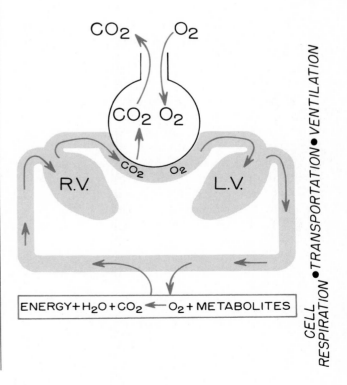

FIGURE 31-7
Principal stages of the respiratory process.

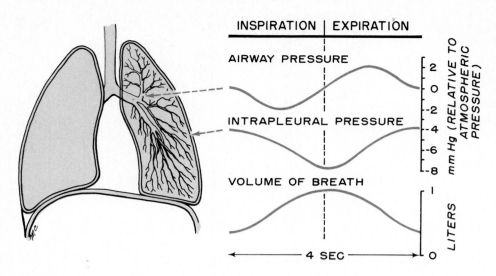

FIGURE 31-8

Changes in intrapleural and intrapulmonary (airway) pressures during inspiration and expiration. (Modified from A. J. Vander, J. H. Sherman, and D. S. Luciano, Human Physiology, 2d ed., McGraw-Hill, New York, 1975, p. 290.)

inspiration. At the same time intrapulmonary or airway pressure decreases to about -2 mmHg (relative to atmospheric pressure) from 0 mmHg at the beginning of inspiration. The pressure gradient between the airways and the atmosphere causes air to flow into the lungs until airway pressure at the end of inspiration is again equal to atmospheric pressure.

During quiet breathing, expiration is a passive movement produced by the elastic recoil of the chest wall and lungs. As the external intercostal muscles relax, the rib cage is lowered and the dome of the diaphragm ascends into the thoracic cavity, causing the volume of the thorax to decrease. The internal intercostal muscles may forcefully pull the ribs downward and inward during active, forceful expiration, coughing, defecating, or vomiting. In addition, the abdominal muscles may contract, increasing the intraabdominal pressure and pushing the diaphragm upward. This decrease in volume of the thorax causes both the intrapleural and intrapulmonary pressures to increase. The intrapulmonary pressure now rises to about 1 or 2 mmHg above that of the atmosphere. The pressure gradient between the airways and the atmosphere is now reversed, causing air to flow out of the lungs until airway and atmospheric pressure are again equal at the end of expiration. Note that intrapleural pressure is always below atmospheric pressure during the respiratory cycle. Alterations in ventilation are assessed by pulmonary function tests. The alterations, their significance, and additional complexities of mechanical ventilation are discussed in Chap. 32.

Transportation

Diffusion

The second stage in the respiratory process involves the diffusion of gases across the thin (less than 0.5 μm in thickness) alveolar-capillary membrane inter-

face. The driving force for this transfer is the partial pressure gradients between the blood and gas phases. The partial pressure of oxygen in the atmosphere at sea level is about 149 mmHg (21 percent of 760 mmHg). By the time oxygen is inspired and reaches the alveoli, its partial pressure is reduced to about 103 mmHg. This decrease in partial pressure is accounted for by the fact that inspired air is mixed with old anatomic dead-space air from the conducting airways and with water vapor. The anatomic dead space normally holds a volume of about 1 ml of air per pound of body weight (150 ml per 150-lb male). Only the fresh air which reaches the alveolus is effective ventilation. As seen in Fig. 31-9, the partial pressure of oxygen in the mixed venous blood ($P_{V_{O_2}}$) in the pulmonary capillary is about 40 mmHg. Since the partial pressure of oxygen in the capillary is less than that in the alveolus ($P_{A_{O_2}} = 103$ mmHg), oxygen diffuses readily into the bloodstream. A much smaller pressure gradient (6 mmHg) between the blood and alveolar CO_2 causes carbon dioxide to diffuse into the alveolus. The carbon dioxide is then expired into the atmosphere, where its concentration is essentially zero. The carbon dioxide gradient between blood and alveolus, even though very small, is adequate, since it diffuses about 20 times more readily than oxygen across the alveolar-capillary membrane because of its greater solubility.

Ventilation-perfusion relationships

The effective transfer of gas between the alveolus and pulmonary capillary bed requires an even distribution of air in the lungs and perfusion (blood flow) in the capillaries. In other words, the ventilation and perfusion of a pulmonary unit must be evenly matched. In the normal upright person at rest, ventilation and perfusion are nearly evenly matched except at the apex of the lung. The low-pressure, low-resistance pulmonary circulation results in a greater flow of blood at the base of

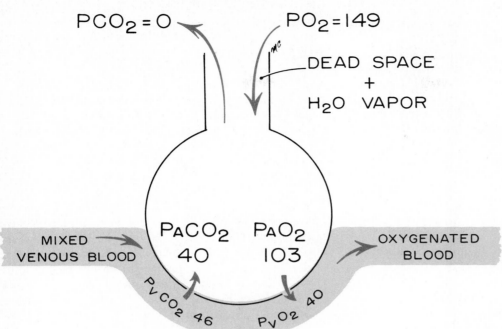

FIGURE 31-9

Diffusion of gases across the alveolarcapillary membrane.

the lung than at the apex as a result of the influence of gravity. Ventilation, however, is fairly evenly distributed. The mean value for the ratio of ventilation to perfusion ($\dot{V}/\dot{Q}$) is 0.8. This figure is obtained by taking the ratio of the normal rate of alveolar ventilation (4 liters per minute) and dividing it by the normal cardiac output (5 liters/minute). Figure 31-10 illustrates the normal state of evenly matched ventilation and perfusion in the lung, which is near unity, at 0.8.

Ventilation-perfusion inequalities occur in most respiratory diseases. Three theoretical abnormal respiratory units are illustrated in Fig. 31-11. Figure 31-11A

depicts a *dead-space unit* in which there is normal ventilation but no perfusion, causing ventilation to be wasted ($\dot{V}/\dot{Q} =$ infinity). The second abnormal respiratory unit (Fig. 31-11B) is a *shunt unit* in which there is normal perfusion but no ventilation, so that perfusion is wasted ($\dot{V}/\dot{Q} = 0$). The last unit (Fig. 31-11C) is a

FIGURE 31-11

Three theoretical respiratory units: A, dead-space unit—normal ventilation but no perfusion; B, shunt unit—normal perfusion but no ventilation: C, silent unit-no ventilation, no perfusion.

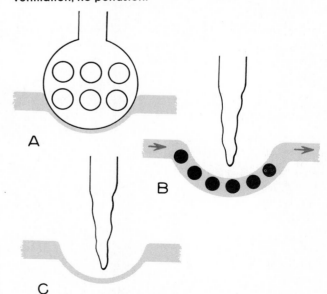

FIGURE 31-10

Even match of ventilation and perfusion in an ideal respiratory unit (normal $\dot{V}/\dot{Q} = 0.8$).

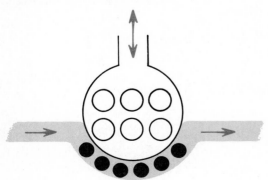

silent- unit in which there is neither ventilation nor perfusion. There are, of course, variations between the three extremes depending on the overall balance between ventilation and perfusion in the lungs. Lung diseases and functional respiratory disorders may be classified physiologically according to whether they are largely shunt-producing ($\dot{V}/\dot{Q} < 0.8$) or dead-space-producing ($\dot{V}/\dot{Q} > 0.8$) diseases.

Oxygen transport in the blood

Oxygen can be transported from the lungs to the tissues via two routes: it can be physically dissolved in the plasma or chemically combined with hemoglobin as oxyhemoglobin (HbO_2). The chemical combination of oxygen with hemoglobin is reversible, and the actual amount carried in this form is related in a nonlinear fashion to the Pa_{O_2} (partial pressure of oxygen in the arterial blood), which is determined by the amount of oxygen physically dissolved in the blood plasma. In turn, the amount of oxygen physically dissolved in the plasma is directly related to the partial pressure of oxygen in the alveolus (Pa_{O_2}). It also depends on the solubility of oxygen in plasma. The amount of physically dissolved oxygen is normally very small because of its low solubility in plasma. Only about 1 percent of the total oxygen transported to the tissues is transported in this manner. This method of transport is not sufficient to support life even at rest. The great bulk of oxygen is carried by hemoglobin, which is located inside the red blood cells. Under certain circumstances (e.g., carbon monoxide poisoning or massive hemolysis in which there is insufficient hemoglobin), sufficient oxygen to support life may be transported in physical solution by subjecting the patient to oxygen under greater than atmospheric pressure *(hyperbaric oxygen chamber)*.

The relationships involved in oxyhemoglobin transportation are illustrated in Fig. 31-12. A gram of hemoglobin can combine with 1.34 ml of oxygen. Since the average hemoglobin concentration in the blood for the adult male is about 15 g per 100 ml, 100 ml of blood can carry (15×1.34) 20.1 ml of oxygen when it is completely saturated (Sa_{O_2} = 100 percent). However, a small amount of mixed venous blood from the bronchial circulation is added to the oxygenated blood leaving the pulmonary capillaries (see Fig. 31-9). This dilution accounts for the fact that only about 97 percent of the blood leaving the lungs is saturated and (0.97×20.1) 19.5 volume percent is carried to the tissues.

At the tissue level, oxygen dissociates from hemoglobin into the plasma and diffuses from the plasma into the tissue cells in order to supply tissue needs. Although tissue needs are highly variable, normally about 75 percent of hemoglobin is still combined with oxygen when it returns to the lungs as mixed venous blood. Thus, only about 25 percent of the oxygen in the arterial blood is used to supply the tissues. Hemoglobin which has dissociated from oxygen at the tissue level is called *reduced hemoglobin* (Hb). Reduced hemoglobin is purple in color and accounts for the bluish color of venous blood which is observed in the superficial veins, as in the hands, whereas oxyhemoglobin (hemoglobin combined with oxygen) is bright red in color and accounts for the color of arterial blood.

Oxyhemoglobin dissociation curve

A clear understanding of the respiratory process requires that one understand the affinity of oxygen for hemoglobin, since tissue oxygen supply, as well as pulmonary oxygen uptake, depends critically on this relationship. This knowledge is necessary in order to interpret blood gas measurements correctly and to apply therapeutic measures for respiratory insufficiency. If whole blood is exposed to different partial pressures of oxygen and the percent saturation of hemoglobin is measured, an S-shaped curve is obtained when these

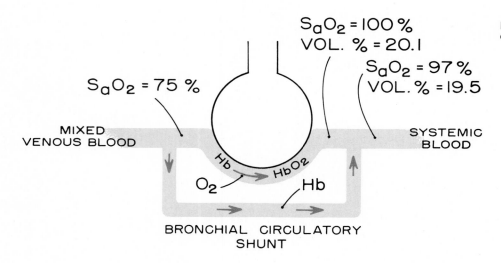

FIGURE 31-12
Oxyhemoglobin transportation.

two measurements are plotted. This curve is known as the *oxyhemoglobin dissociation curve* and demonstrates the affinity of hemoglobin for oxygen at various partial pressures. In Fig. 31-13, the middle curve represents the affinity relation between oxygen and hemoglobin under normal conditions of body temperature (98.6°F) and a blood pH of 7.4.

One fact of great physiologic importance to be noted about the curve is that there is a flat upper portion, known as the arterial portion (A), and a lower, steeper venous portion (V) which is shifted slightly to the right. At the flat upper portion of the curve, large changes in oxygen tension are associated with very small changes in oxyhemoglobin saturation. This implies that relatively constant quantities of oxygen can be supplied to the tissues even at high altitudes where the P_{O_2} may be 60 mmHg or less. It also implies that the administration of oxygen in high concentrations (normal air = 21 percent) to patients with mild hypoxemia (Pa_{O_2} 60 to 75 mmHg) is wasted, since oxyhemoglobin can be increased by only a small amount. In fact, the administration of high concentrations of oxygen may be toxic to the lung tissues and may produce other harmful effects. The release of oxygen to the tissues is augmented by the relation of the P_{O_2} to oxygen saturation on the steep venous portion of the curve, where large changes in oxyhemoglobin saturation are associated with small changes in the P_{O_2}. The normal differences in oxyhemoglobin saturation and P_{O_2} between arterial and mixed venous blood are indicated by the arrows on Fig. 31-13.

The affinity of oxygen for hemoglobin is influenced by many other factors which accompany tissue metabolism and which may be modified by disease. Some of these factors and their effect on the affinity of hemoglobin for oxygen are listed in Table 31-1.

TABLE 31-1

FACTORS AFFECTING OXYHEMOGLOBIN AFFINITY

HbO_2 dissociation curve	
Shift to left ($\downarrow P_{50}$)	*Shift to right* ($\uparrow P_{50}$)
1 $\uparrow$ pH	1 $\downarrow$ pH
2 $\downarrow$ Pco_2	2 $\uparrow$ Pco_2
3 $\downarrow$ temperature	3 $\uparrow$ temperature
4 $\downarrow$ 2,3-DPG	4 $\uparrow$ 2,3-DPG

The oxyhemoglobin curve is shifted to the right (see Fig. 31-13) in cases of a decrease in blood pH or a rise in the Pco_2. In this state, hemoglobin has less affinity for oxygen at a given P_{O_2}, so less oxygen can be transported in the blood. Pathologic conditions which cause metabolic acidosis, such as shock (production of excess lactic acid from anaerobic metabolism) or the retention of carbon dioxide (as in many pulmonary diseases), will cause a shift of the curve to the right. A slight shift of the curve to the right, represented by the venous portion of the normal curve (pH 7.38), assists the release of oxygen to the tissues. This shift is called the *Bohr effect*. The slight increase in acidity results from the effect of carbon dioxide being released from the tissues. Other factors causing a shift of the curve to the right are an increase in temperature and increased 2,3-diphosphoglycerate (2,3-DPG), which is an organic phosphate in red blood cells that binds hemoglobin and

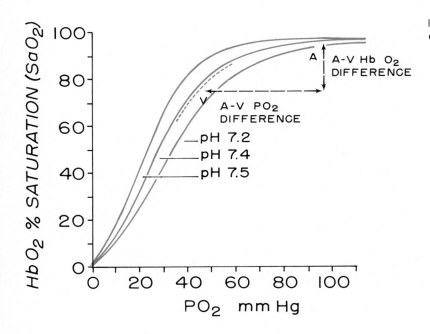

FIGURE 31-13
Oxyhemoglobin dissociation curve.

decreases its affinity for oxygen. Red blood cell 2,3-DPG is increased in conditions of anemia and chronic hypoxemia. It is important to appreciate that while the oxygen transport capability of the hemoglobin is decreased with a rightward shift of the curve, hemoglobin release of oxygen to the tissues is facilitated. Therefore, in conditions of anemia and chronic hypoxemia, the rightward shift of the curve is compensatory. A rightward shift of the curve with a rise in temperature, reflecting increased cell metabolism and a greater need for oxygen, is also adaptive and causes more oxygen to be released to the tissues for a given blood flow.

Conversely, an increase in blood pH (alkalosis) or a decrease in P_{CO_2}, temperature, and 2,3-DPG causes a leftward shift in the oxyhemoglobin dissociation curve (see Fig. 31-13). The shift to the left causes hemoglobin to have a greater affinity for oxygen. Thus there is increased oxygen uptake in the lung when there is a leftward shift, but release of oxygen to the tissues is impaired. Therefore it is theoretically possible to have hypoxia (insufficient tissue oxygen to meet metabolic needs) in severe conditions of alkalosis, especially if accompanied by hypoxemia. This condition could occur during mechanical overventilation with a respirator or at high altitudes as a result of hyperventilation. Since hyperventilation is also known to decrease cerebral blood flow as a result of the decrease in the Pa_{CO_2}, cerebral ischemia might also account for symptoms of light-headedness common under such conditions. Stored blood loses 2,3-DPG activity and causes a greater affinity of hemoglobin for oxygen. Therefore patients who receive transfusions of massive amounts of stored blood may also have impaired oxygen release to the tissues because of the leftward shift in the oxyhemoglobin dissociation curve.

The affinity of hemoglobin is popularly defined by the P_{O_2} required to produce 50 percent saturation and is readily measured in modern laboratories. Normally, P_{50} is about 27 mmHg. It is evident that with the shift of the dissociation curve to the right (decreased hemoglobin affinity for oxygen), P_{50} will be increased, whereas it is reduced with a shift of the curve to the left (increased hemoglobin affinity for oxygen).

Carbon monoxide has an affinity for hemoglobin that is about 250 times greater than that of oxygen. When this gas is inhaled, it combines with hemoglobin to form carboxyhemoglobin. When oxygen combines with carboxyhemoglobin, the reaction is not reversible, so the amount of hemoglobin available for oxygen transport is reduced. In addition, there is a leftward shift of the remaining normal hemoglobin, resulting in deficient unloading of oxygen to the tissues.

Carbon dioxide transport in the blood

Carbon dioxide homeostasis is also a necessary aspect of respiratory sufficiency. The transportation of carbon dioxide from the tissues to the lungs for elimination is accomplished in three ways. About 10 percent of the CO_2 is physically dissolved in plasma, because CO_2, unlike O_2, is highly soluble in plasma. About 20 percent of the CO_2 is combined with the amino groups on hemoglobin (carbaminohemoglobin) in the red blood cell, and about 70 percent is transported as plasma bicarbonate. Carbon dioxide combines with water as shown in the following reaction:

$$CO_2 + H_2O \rightleftharpoons H_2CO_3 \rightleftharpoons H^+ + HCO_3^-$$

This reaction is reversible and is known as the bicarbonate-carbonic acid buffer equation. The acid-base balance of the body is greatly affected by pulmonary function and carbon dioxide homeostasis. (This subject is not discussed in detail in this book. The reader is referred to the many fine books which explore fluid and electrolyte homeostasis in depth.) In general, *hyperventilation* (alveolar ventilation in excess of metabolic needs), causes alkalosis (increases in blood pH above the normal 7.4) as a result of the excess excretion of CO_2 from the lungs; *hypoventilation* (alveolar ventilation insufficient to meet metabolic needs) causes acidosis (decrease of the blood pH below the normal 7.4) as a result of the retention of carbon dioxide by the lungs. It is evident from examining the buffer equation that lowering the P_{CO_2}, as in hyperventilation, would cause the reaction to proceed to the left, with consequent lowering of the H^+ concentration (elevated pH) and that, raising the P_{CO_2} causes the reaction to proceed to the right, producing an increase in H^+ (decreased pH). Hypoventilation occurs in many conditions that affect the respiratory bellows. Carbon dioxide retention is also associated with emphysema and chronic bronchitis caused by trapped air in the lungs.

Just as the amount of O_2 transported in the blood is related to the P_{O_2} to which the blood is exposed, so the amount of CO_2 in blood is related to the P_{CO_2}. Unlike the S-shaped oxyhemoglobin dissociation curve, the carbon dioxide dissociation curve is nearly linear in the physiologic range of P_{CO_2}. This means that the carbon dioxide content of the blood is directly related to the P_{CO_2}. In addition, there is never any significant barrier to CO_2, diffusion. Therefore the Pa_{CO_2} provides a good index of the adequacy of ventilation.

Assessment of the respiratory status

It is important to point out that knowledge of the blood gases (the P_{O_2}, P_{CO_2}, and pH of the arterial blood) alone does not give enough information about the transport of O_2 and CO_2 to be sure that a patient's tissues are

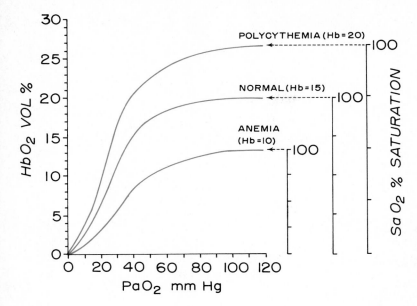

FIGURE 31-14
Relationship of hemoglobin content to oxygen content of blood at various oxygen tensions. (From N. Balfour Slonim and Lyle H. Hamilton, *Respiratory Physiology*, 3d ed., The C. V. Mosby Co., St. Louis, 1976, p. 84.)

being oxygenated properly. Many other factors are involved in the transport process, such as the adequacy of cardiac output and tissue perfusion as well as diffusion of gases at the tissue level. For example, in shock there may be inadequate tissue perfusion as a result of shunting of blood past the tissue cells, stagnation of blood caused by pooling, and inadequate cardiac output. Tissue edema may also interfere with the diffusion pathway at the tissue level. Consequently the detection of tissue hypoxia must always involve clinical observations as well as the interpretation of blood gases.

Another important piece of information that is needed for the assessment of a patient's respiratory status is the hemoglobin concentration, as well as the percent saturation of that hemoglobin. The correlation between the Pa_{O_2}, Sa_{O_2}, and oxyhemoglobin in volume percent for a patient with anemia (Hb = 10 g per 100 ml), one with a normal Hb of 15 g per 100 ml, and another with polycythemia (Hb = 20 g per 100 ml) is shown in Fig. 31-14. All the information illustrated is necessary for a proper assessment of oxygen transport. Note that the percent saturation of hemoglobin is independent of the hemoglobin concentration, while the oxygen content in volume percent is directly related to hemoglobin concentration. The volume percent reveals how much oxygen can be delivered to the tissues at a given Pa_{O_2}. For example, at a Pa_{O_2} of 100 mmHg and

100 percent saturation of hemoglobin with oxygen, the polycythemic patient can transport 26.8 ml of oxygen in every 100 ml of blood (oxygen content = 26.8 volume percent), while the anemic patient can deliver only 13.4 ml at the same oxygen tension and saturation. This is a twofold variation and illustrates the point that knowledge of the blood gases alone is insufficient information for respiratory assessment. Hemoglobin concentration, oxygen saturation, and cardiac status are also vital data.

It is obvious from the previous discussion of the structure and function of the respiratory system that adequate respiration can be inhibited on a number of levels. For example, brain injury or barbiturate overdose in an attempted suicide may interfere with control by the respiratory centers in the central nervous system. A decrease in the P_{O_2} of inspired air as a result of high altitudes or airway obstruction interferes with respiration. Neuromuscular diseases and skeletal deformities of the chest result in inadequate bellows performance. Respiratory difficulty occurs at the alveolar-capillary interface when there is thickening of the diffusion pathway, as in pulmonary fibrosis or edema. Transport of gases in the blood may be interfered with in many respects, including the limiting factor of the amount of hemoglobin. The pulmonary, cardiovascular, and hematologic systems are thus intimately associated with tissue oxygenation.

QUESTIONS

Normal respiratory function

Directions: Answer the following on a separate sheet of paper.

1. List three disorders of the respiratory system which are a major source of morbidity and mortality.

2. Define *respiration.*

3. Draw and label the epithelial surface of the airways and discuss the function of the mucosal lining in respiration. (See inset of Fig. 31-1 if you have for-

gotten the structure of the mucosal lining of the airways.)

4. Why are foreign bodies, when aspirated, usually found in the right mainstem bronchus?

5. What would happen if the pressure within the pleural space were to become equal to that of the atmosphere?

6. Sketch the position of the lungs in the circulatory system and describe some of the unique features of blood supply to the lungs. (Review Fig. 31-4 if you have forgotten the functional position of the lungs in the circulation.)

7. If the mean pulmonary artery pressure is 30 mmHg and the colloid osmotic pressure of the blood is 20 mmHg, is pulmonary edema likely to occur? Why or why not?

Directions: Complete the following statements by filling in the blanks.

8. The structure which forms the division between the upper and lower respiratory tracts is the _____.

9. The alveoli are lined by a lipoprotein substance called _____. During inspiration, expansion is facilitated, and during expiration, collapse is prevented as this substance functions to lower the _____.

10. The movement of air in and out of the lungs is called _____. To accomplish this function, the thoracic cage and lungs have been compared to a reciprocating pump or _____. The muscle which provides the main driving force during inspiration is the _____.

11. A reflex which controls the amount of air taken into the lungs is known as the _____ reflex.

12. Centers which control the pattern and rhythmicity of breathing are located in the _____ and _____ of the brain.

Directions: Circle the letter preceding each item below that correctly completes the statement. Choose the one best answer.

13. Respiration is most affected by:
    a. Body heat   b. pH   c. Pa_{CO_2} d. Pa_{O_2}
    e. Reflexes from moving limbs

14. The tracheobronchial tree divides repeatedly in a dichotomous fashion and in ever-decreasing sizes until the final pulmonary functional unit is reached. The generations of subdivisions involved number:
    a. 64   b. 32   c. 23   d. 10

15. The right lung has:
    a. 10 lobes   b. 8 lobes   c. 3 lobes   d. 2 lobes

16. Each bronchus divides into functional subunits which include:
    a. Lobar bronchi   b. Segmental bronchi
    c. Terminal bronchioles   d. Respiratory bronchioles   e. All the above

17. The functional unit of the lung (acinus) consists of all of the following except:
    a. Terminal bronchioles   b. Respiratory bronchioles   c. Alveolar duct   d. Alveolar sac
    e. Alveoli

18. The pores of Kohn:
    a. Are located between pulmonary capillaries
    b. May provide collateral ventilation   c. Are artifacts and do not really exist   d. Provide a communication between right and left lungs

19. Alveolar macrophages:
    a. Move freely over the alveolar surface   b. Are phagocytic cells   c. Contain lytic enzymes
    d. Are inhibited by cigarette smoking, alcohol ingestion, and corticosteroid drugs   e. All the above

20. The left mainstem bronchus is:
    a. Symmetric with the right   b. Shorter and broader than the right   c. Nearer to the vertical in its course than the right   d. More angulated than the right

21. All the following structures are closely associated with the larynx except the:
    a. Epiglottis   b. Glottis   c. Carina   d. Vocal cords

22. Protective functions of the larynx include all the following except:
    a. Swallowing reflex   b. Cough   c. Major role in humidification of inspired air

23. Label the diagram in Fig. 31-15 by matching the number of the structure on the diagram with the appropriate term from the following list:

    a. ___ Diaphragm   g. ___ Trachea
    b. ___ Carina   h. ___ Mainstem bronchus
    c. ___ Epiglottis   i. ___ Segmental bronchus
    d. ___ Medias-   j. ___ Apex of lung
           tinum   k. ___ Visceral pleura
    e. ___ Pharynx   l. ___ Parietal pleura
    f. ___ Larynx

24. Label the diagram in Fig. 31-16 by matching the number of the structure with the appropriate term from the following list:

a. ____ Pores of Kohn
b. ____ Alveolar duct
c. ____ Respiratory bronchiole
d. ____ Terminal bronchiole
e. ____ Acinus
f. ____ Alveolus
g. ____ Septum

Directions: Answer the following on a separate sheet of paper.

25. Why is the alveolar P_{O_2} as low as 103 mmHg when it is 149 mmHg in the inspired air?

26. What is the volume of your own anatomic dead space?

27. What is the chief mechanism of gas movement in the respiratory zone of the lung? What provides the driving force?

28. Are ventilation and perfusion perfectly matched in the healthy person at rest in the upright position? Why or why not?

29. If alveolar ventilation is 3 liters per minute and cardiac output (perfusion) is 6 liters per minute, what is the $\dot{V}/\dot{Q}$ ratio? Is this value normal, or does a person with this value have dead-space or shunt-producing disease?

FIGURE 31-15
The respiratory tract.

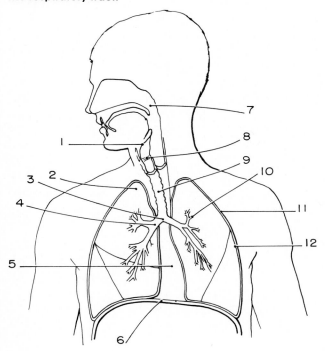

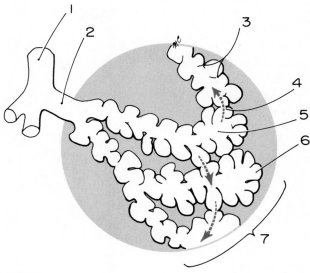

FIGURE 31-16
Pulmonary functional unit.

30. What advantage would be gained, if any, by placing a patient with severe hemolytic anemia in a hyperbaric chamber?

31. If a patient is breathing fresh air at sea level, the $P_{A_{O_2}}$ is about 103 mmHg, the arterial blood is 97 to 98 percent saturated with oxygen, and the oxygen content is 20 volume percent, will it be advantageous to increase the oxygen concentration of the inspired air? Why or why not?

32. Explain why the P_{O_2} can vary over a wide range and have little effect on the hemoglobin saturation.

33. What is the Bohr effect? What is its significance in terms of tissue oxygenation?

34. When a person hyperventilates, why is there no significant increase in the O_2 content of the arterial blood, yet there is a significant decrease in the Pa_{CO_2}? Explain this phenomenon in terms of the O_2 and CO_2 dissociation curves.

35. Why does an elevated Pa_{CO_2} never result from impaired diffusion?

36. Does knowledge of the blood gases alone provide all the information necessary to accurately assess the respiratory status? If not, what other data are necessary?

37. Beginning with inspired air, list at least three altered mechanisms or conditions which may interfere with normal respiration.

38. The respiratory process may be divided into three stages. List and describe each briefly.

39. Which muscles are used during normal quiet breathing? During breathing of maximum effort?

40. How many milliliters of oxygen are utilized by tissue cells each minute if the hemoglobin concentration is 12.0 g per 100 ml of blood, there is 100 percent saturation of the hemoglobin, cardiac output is 5000 ml per minute, and 25 percent of the oxygen delivered is utilized? (1.34 ml of oxygen combines with each gram of hemoglobin. Ignore the oxygen which is transported physically dissolved in blood plasma.)

41. Account for the fact that hemoglobin is 100 percent saturated with oxygen upon leaving the pulmonary capillary bed yet is 97 to 98 percent saturated in the systemic arteries.

42. If alveolar ventilation doubles and CO_2 production remains constant, what are the effects on arterial P_{CO_2} and the blood pH? What happens to the oxyhemoglobin dissociation curve and what are the consequences?

43. What is the partial pressure of oxygen in the inspired air of a climber on the summit of Mount Everest if the atmospheric pressure is 247 mmHg and water vapor pressure at body temperature is 47 mmHg? Do you think the mountain climber could walk very far?

Directions: Circle the letter preceding each item below that correctly answers the question. More than one answer may be correct.

44. In what form is most of the CO_2 carried in the venous blood?
a. Bicarbonate   b. Physically dissolved in the plasma   c. Carbaminohemoglobin

45. Which of the following shift the oxyhemoglobin dissociation curve to the left?
a. Decrease in temperature   b. Increase in pH
c. Decrease in 2,3-DPG   d. Increase in P_{CO2}

46. During normal quiet breathing what will the intrapleural pressure be?
a. Equal to atmospheric pressure   b. Below atmospheric pressure   c. Above atmospheric pressure

Directions: Circle the word which correctly completes each sentence.

47. During inspiration, muscular contraction causes the size of the thorax to (increase) (decrease). This size change causes a(n) (increase) (decrease) in the intrapleural pressure. Since pressure in the alveoli is (less) (more) than atmospheric pressure, air moves (into) (out of) the lungs.

48. During expiration, when the diaphragm muscle relaxes, the diaphragm (ascends) (descends), thus (increasing) (decreasing) the volume of the thoracic cavity.

49. During normal quiet expiration, the size change in the thoracic cavity causes a(n) (increase) (decrease) in the intrapleural pressure. Since pressure in the alveoli is now (more) (less) than atmospheric pressure, air moves (into) (out of) the lungs.

50. A person is accidentally exposed to carbon monoxide which combines with half the hemoglobin in the arterial blood. The Pa_{O_2} will be (normal) (high) (low). The Sa_{O_2} will be (normal) (high) (low). The arterial oxygen content will be (normal) (high) (low).

51. In general, hyperventilation causes a(n) (increase) (decrease) in the P_{CO_2} and a(n) (increase) (decrease) in the blood pH, resulting in a condition of (alkalosis) (acidosis).

52. A P_{50} of 34 mmHg means that the oxyhemoglobin curve is shifted to the (right) (left) and there is a(n) (decreased) (increased) hemoglobin affinity for oxygen.

CHAPTER

32

DIAGNOSTIC PROCEDURES IN RESPIRATORY DISEASE

OBJECTIVES

At the completion of this chapter you should be able to:

1. List the six most common methods used to detect pulmonary disease and adequacy of pulmonary function.
2. List six types of radiologic technique used to detect pulmonary disease.
3. Describe four aspects of what is depicted on a routine chest x-ray.
4. State the purpose of chest fluoroscopy and tomography.
5. Describe a bronchography, including radiopaque materials used, purpose, and potential hazards.
6. Differentiate between angiography of the pulmonary vessels and a lung scan according to material and techniques used, purpose, and major risks involved.
7. Describe bronchoscopy by identifying procedures, purposes, precautions, and potential hazards.
8. Describe the techniques used to obtain lung tissue specimens for biopsy studies.
9. State the purpose and procedure for sputum studies.
10. State the purpose and limitations of ventilatory function tests and blood gas measurements.
11. List and differentiate between the four primary static lung volumes and the four lung capacities.
12. Describe the structure and function of a spirometer.
13. Describe the following indices of ventilatory measurements in terms of the procedures used for measurement, the amount of air being measured, and the calculations required to determine the measurement:
    a. Minute volume ($\dot{V}_E$)
    b. Respiratory frequency (f)
    c. Tidal volume (V_T)
    d. Physiologic dead space (V_D)
    e. Alveolar ventilation ($\dot{V}_A$)
14. Give an example that illustrates the relation between minute ventilation, breathing pattern, and effective alveolar ventilation.

15. State the relation of the V_D/V_T ratio to effective alveolar ventilation.

16. Define *work of breathing*.

17. Differentiate between the elastic and nonelastic resistances to ventilation.

18. Define *pulmonary compliance* and list common causes of its decrease.

19. Give the compliance formula and explain each of its components.

20. Describe the direct measurement of the airway resistance of the upper airways of the lung.

21. Differentiate between the forced vital capacity and forced expiratory volume measurements.

22. Describe the significance of the forced expiratory volume/forced vital capacity (FEV_1/FVC) ratio.

23. Explain the significance of the maximum midexpiratory flow rate (MMFR).

24. Explain the significance of an increased closing volume/vital capacity (CV/VC) or closing capacity/total lung capacity (CC/TLC) ratio.

25. State the purpose of the maximum breathing capacity (MBC) or maximum voluntary ventilation (MVV) test.

26. Identify the relation between the mechanical work of breathing and the respiratory pattern in patients with restrictive or obstructive pulmonary disorders.

27. Describe the technique used for the collection of blood to measure the arterial blood gases, including the following: artery of choice, positioning of the patient's arm, procedure for puncture, syringe used, conditions under which specimen should be delivered to the laboratory.

28. List the normal values for the arterial blood gases.

29. List the causes of hypoventilation and hyperventilation and their relation to the Pa_{CO_2}

30. Summarize the acid-base changes that occur in both acidosis and alkalosis.

31. List four mechanisms in respiratory disease which may lead to hypoxemia.

32. Contrast the following in regard to changes in ventilatory function and blood gases in restrictive and obstructive patterns of pulmonary disease: vital capacity, residual volume, functional residual capacity, total lung capacity, forced expiratory volume, forced vital capacity, FEV_1/FVC, maximum breathing capacity, compliance, blood gases.

MORPHOLOGIC METHODS

Diagnostic procedures used for the detection of pulmonary disease may be classified as primarily morphologic or physiologic. Morphologic methods include radiologic techniques, endoscopy, biopsy studies, and sputum studies. Blood gas measurements and ventilatory function tests are tests which reveal physiologic function.

Radiologic techniques

The thorax is an ideal region for a radiologic examination. The aerated lung parenchyma offers little resistance to the passage of x-rays and therefore produces very radiant shadows. The soft tissues of the chest wall, the heart and great vessels, and the diaphragm do not permit the rays to pass through as readily as the lung parenchyma and therefore appear denser on the x-ray film. The bony structures of the thorax, including the ribs, sternum, and vertebrae, are even less readily penetrated, and their shadows are even denser. Radiologic methods commonly used to detect pulmonary disease include the routine chest x-ray, tomography, fluoroscopy, bronchography, angiography, and perfusion and ventilation lung scanning.

Routine chest x-ray

The routine chest x-ray is taken at a standard distance following maximum inspiration and breath holding to stabilize the diaphragm. Films are taken from the posteroanterior perspective, and sometimes lateral and oblique views are taken as well. These films provide the following information:

1. The status of the thoracic cage, including the ribs, the pleura, and the contour of the diaphragm and of the upper airway as it enters the chest
2. The size, contour, and position of the mediastinum and hilus of the lung, including the heart, aorta, lymph nodes, and root of the bronchial tree
3. The texture and degree of aeration of the lung parenchyma
4. The size, shape, number, and location of pulmonary lesions, including cavitation, fibrous markings, and zones of consolidation.

The appearance of the normal chest x-ray varies somewhat according to sex and age in different subjects and to varying conditions of respiration in the same subject. The correct interpretation of a chest film is a skill that takes considerable time to acquire. It is an invaluable aid to the physician when correlated with other observations.

Tomography

Tomography is a radiographic technique by which a series of x-rays, each representing a "slice of the lung," is taken so that a detailed picture of an area of interest can be built up. It is of particular value for identifying abnormalities in configuration of the trachea or major bronchi, defining lesions of the pleura or mediastinum (nodes, tumors, vascular structures), and in general revealing the nature and extent of abnormal shadows in the lungs and other tissues of the thorax.

Computerized tomography (CT) scanning of the thorax has resulted in a significant increase in the detection of mass lesions in the mediastinum and pleura.

Fluoroscopy

Fluoroscopy is an x-ray technique which enables the roentgenologist to view the thorax and all its contents in motion. Information can be obtained about how various zones of the lung behave during the respiratory cycle. The diaphragm can be studied particularly well using this method. In spite of its usefulness, this type of study is discouraged because of the radiation hazards to the patient and to the examiner.

Bronchography

An x-ray film of the chest taken after radiopaque material is introduced into the tracheobronchial tree is called a *bronchogram*. Substances commonly used as radiopaque material are iodized oils and, more recently, tantalum, which is inhaled as a fine powder with the help of positive pressure equipment. The bronchogram reveals in great detail the size and appearance of the tracheobronchial tree and therefore is a particularly useful technique for confirming the diagnosis of bronchiectasis and for detecting other forms of bronchial distortion. Postoperative care is the same as after bronchoscopy (discussed in the following pages). In addition, percussion and postural drainage should be used to assist in the evacuation of the contrast medium.

Angiography of the pulmonary vessels

The pulmonary arterial pattern and flow can be demonstrated by injecting radiopaque fluid through a catheter inserted via an arm vein into the right atrium and right ventricle and then into the main pulmonary artery. This technique is used to locate the site of a massive embolism or to determine the extent of a pulmonary infarction. Anomalies such as aneurysms and alterations in vascularity common in emphysema are also detectable. However, simpler diagnostic techniques are preferred for the detection of pulmonary disease whenever possible. The major risk during angiography is the development of cardiac arrhythmia as the catheter is passed through the heart chambers.

Lung scan

The isotope lung scan, though a less reliable method for the detection of pulmonary embolism, is a safer procedure. Pulmonary perfusion and sometimes ventilation scanning are carried out. A *perfusion scan* is obtained by the injection of albumen microspheres, usually labeled with technetium 99m, into a peripheral vein; these particles appear as transient emboli in the pulmonary capillaries in proportion to the active blood flow. The radioactivity distribution is counted with a scintiscanner, and the image is recorded with a camera. The pattern is almost always abnormal in embolism (area with absent radioactivity) but is not highly specific, since abnormalities are also present in other conditions, such as emphysema and pneumonia. The *ventilation scan* utilizes the inhalation of a bolus of radioactive gas, usually xenon 133. The ventilation lung scan is usually normal in embolism but abnormal in infarction, pneumonia, and emphysema.

Bronchoscopy

Bronchoscopy is a technique which allows direct visualization of the trachea and its major subdivisions. It is used most frequently to confirm the diagnosis of bronchogenic carcinoma but can be used to remove a foreign body. The conventional bronchoscope is a hollow metal tube containing a lighted mirror-lens system which is passed readily into the tracheobronchial tree after administration of local anesthesia. The newer fiberoptic bronchoscope is a flexible instrument which can transmit light and a clear image around corners. Because of its flexibility and smaller diameter, its use causes far less trauma than the conventional metal bronchoscope. The fiberoptic bronchoscope may also be passed through the nose, and inspection of the smaller bronchial subdivisions is possible. Tissue biopsy can be obtained by using a tiny forceps or flexible brush at the tip of the bronchoscope. Suction tubes may also be passed through the bronchoscope to obtain secretions for culture and cytologic studies. The fiberoptic bronchoscopy can be performed at the bedside, although the location of choice is the operating room.

Following bronchoscopy, food and fluids are withheld for at least 2 or 3 hours until the gag reflex returns; otherwise the patient may aspirate material into the tracheobronchial tree. The return of the gag reflex can be tested by touching a cotton applicator to the back of the patient's throat. When this causes the patient to gag, swallowing may be permitted. Other complications which may follow bronchoscopy are bleeding and pneumothorax caused by a ruptured bronchus. Common procedures following bronchoscopy to detect these complications are the monitoring of vital signs for a period of several hours, a chest film, and the collection of all sputum for 24 hours. The nurse should also be aware that laryngeal spasm or edema may be a delayed complication and may require endotracheal intubation and the administration of oxygen.

Biopsy studies

Tissue specimens for biopsy study may be obtained from the upper or lower airways by endoscopic techniques using either the laryngoscope or the broncho-

scope. Biopsy specimens of the pleura or lung tissue may also be obtained by either open or closed techniques. The open technique consists of a limited thoracotomy; a small intercostal incision is made after administration of anesthesia, and a tissue specimen is excised under direct visualization. A cylinder of tissue can also be obtained by the newer techniques of percutaneous needle biopsy using an air-turbine drill. The main value of lung biopsy is in diffuse lung disease not diagnosable by other means. Pneumothorax and bleeding are encountered in a substantial number of patients following this procedure.

Biopsy of the lymph nodes in the mediastinum is accomplished during *mediastinoscopy*. This involves the insertion of a lighted mirror-lens system through an incision at the base of the anterior portion of the neck. The instrument is advanced under visual control into the mediastinum, where inspection and biopsy can be accomplished. Mediastinoscopy is the major preoperative method for pathologic evaluation of regional spread to the hilar lymph nodes in lung cancer.

Sputum studies

Gross, microscopic, and bacteriologic examination of the sputum are important in the etiologic diagnosis of many respiratory diseases. The color, odor, and presence of blood provide valuable clues. Microscopic examination may reveal the causative organism in many bacterial pneumonias, in tuberculosis, and in some fungus infections. Exfoliative cell studies of the sputum may also be helpful in the diagnosis of lung carcinoma. The best time for collection of sputum is shortly after awakening, since abnormal bronchial secretions tend to accumulate during sleep. Sometimes it is necessary to induce sputum production by the use of a nebulizer. Considerable quantities of sputum are also unknowingly swallowed; the gastric contents may then be aspirated in order to obtain sputum. This procedure is carried out shortly after the patient awakens in the morning after a period of fasting.

PHYSIOLOGIC METHODS: PULMONARY FUNCTION TESTS

During the past generation, numerous tests and techniques related to the study of respiratory physiology have evolved. These pulmonary function tests fall into two broad categories: those related to ventilatory function of the lungs and chest wall and those related to gas exchange. Ventilatory function tests include measurements of lung volumes under static and dynamic conditions as well as pressure measurements. Tests related to gas exchange include analysis of gases in the expired air and in the blood. Blood gas measurements of the arterial blood commonly include the P_{O_2}, P_{CO_2}, and pH and reflect cardiopulmonary physiology.

Pulmonary function tests are becoming an increasingly important part of routine clinical evaluation and are taking their place among other diagnostic aids such as the chest x-ray and electrocardiogram. It is important to realize, however, that these tests only show the effects of disease on function and cannot be used to give a diagnosis on the basis of a pathologic change. Some diseases, however, have a characteristic pattern of disordered function, and it is possible to distinguish an obstructive pattern of ventilatory abnormality from a restrictive pattern. Obstructive ventilatory disorders affect the ability to exhale, while restrictive disorders affect the ability to inhale. Two major patterns of functional disorders which also emerge from blood measurements are disorders in which there is increased dead space or shunting.

It is essential to realize that no single test of pulmonary function can measure all possible attributes. Nevertheless, pulmonary function tests give valuable information. Ventilatory function tests give quantitative data so that the progress of a lung disease, as well as response to treatment, may be followed. In cases of pulmonary disability in which surgery is planned, such tests help to assess the patient's ability to tolerate anesthetics, narcotics, or the removal of lung tissue and help to prescribe the postoperative care needed. Since only one aspect of pulmonary function may be altered by some diseases, these studies occasionally assist in establishing the diagnosis. Blood gas measurements are an invaluable aid in assessing the severity of respiratory insufficiency and guiding the appropriate therapy. In this chapter, discussion will be confined to those tests of pulmonary function which are most widely used and most helpful in patient management.

Ventilatory function tests

Static lung volumes

Lung volumes and capacities are anatomic measurments that are affected by exercise and disease. There are four lung volumes and four lung capacities. Lung capacities always consist of two or more lung volumes. The relation between these measurements and the average values for a young, healthy, adult male are shown in Fig. 32-1. Symbols and a description of the lung capacities and volumes are listed in Table 32-1. The following five lung capacities and volumes (designated by the symbols listed in the table) can be measured directly on an instrument called the spirometer: V_T, IRV, ERV, VC, and IC. The FRC is measured by indirect means using helium or nitrogen washout methods or by using the body plethysmograph. The TLC and RV are then derived arithmetically (i.e., TLC = FRC + IC and RV = TLC − VC).

A *spirometer* is a simple instrument containing a bellows or bell which is displaced as the patient breathes into it through a valve and connecting tube, as shown in Fig. 32-2. As the spirometer is used, a graphic record of the measurment is made on a rotating drum with a recording pen.

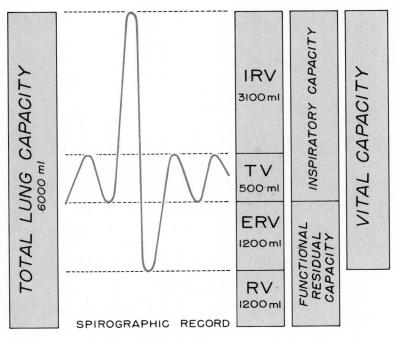

FIGURE 32-1
Relationship of the lung volumes and capacities (see Table 32-1 for explanation of symbols).

TABLE 32-1

LUNG CAPACITIES AND VOLUMES

Measurement	Symbol	Adult male average value (ml)	Definition
Tidal volume	V_T	500	Amount of air inhaled or exhaled with each breath (value listed is for resting conditions)
Inspiratory reserve volume	IRV	3100	Amount of air that can be forcefully inhaled after a normal tidal volume inhalation
Expiratory reserve volume	ERV	1200	Amount of air that can be forcefully exhaled after a normal tidal volume exhalation
Residual volume	RV	1200	Amount of air left in the lungs after a forced exhalation
Total lung capacity	TLC	6000	Maximum amount of air that can be contained in the lungs after a maximum inspiratory effort: $TLC = V_T + IRV + ERV + RV$
Vital capacity	VC	4800	Maximum amount of air that can be expired after a maximum inspiration: $VC = V_T + IRV + ERV$ (should be 80% TLC)
Inspiratory capacity	IC	3600	Maximum amount of air that can be inspired after a normal expiration: $IC = V_T + IRV$
Functional residual capacity	FRC	2400	Volume of air remaining in the lungs after a normal tidal volume expiration: $FRC = ERV + RV$

Source: Comroe et al., 1962.

Measurements of the static lung volumes in practice are used to reflect the elastic properties of the lungs and thorax. The most useful measurements are the VC, TLC, FRC, and RV. These volumes are reduced by diseases which limit lung expansion (restrictive disorders). In contrast, diseases which cause airway obstruction may cause an increase in the TLC, FRC, and RV as a result of hyperinflation of the lungs.

Dynamic lung volumes and the work of breathing

Much more information can be obtained concerning the ventilatory status if the rate of air movement in and out of the lungs is considered as well as the work of breathing. The following definitions will be useful in the discussion of effective ventilation:

Minute volume, or *minute ventilation* ($\dot{V}_E$) is the volume of air which is breathed in during inspiration or out during expiration during a 1-minute time period. It may be calculated by multiplying the V_T by the respiratory rate. At rest $\dot{V}_E$ is about 6 or 7 liters per minute. The minute volume is measured by collecting the expired air in a large rubber balloon and dividing the volume collected by the number of minutes taken to collect the sample. The small E in the symbol for minute volume means that the measurement is made on the expiratory phase of the tidal volume, and the dot over the V indicates that it is a timed measurement.

Respiratory frequency (f) is the number of breaths taken per minute. At rest the respiratory rate is about 15 breaths per minute.

Tidal volume (V_T) is the amount of air inhaled or exhaled with each breath. The V_T is about 500 ml at rest but may increase to 3000 ml during exercise when deep breaths are taken. It is obtained by dividing the minute volume by the respiratory rate.

Physiologic dead space (V_D) is the volume of inspired air that does not exchange with pulmonary blood; it may be regarded as wasted ventilation. Physiologic dead space is composed of anatomic dead space (the volume of air in the conducting airways, about 1 ml per pound of body weight), alveolar dead space (alveoli being ventilated but not perfused; the alveolar dead space is highly variable), and ventilation in excess of perfusion. In healthy persons, the physiologic dead space is only slightly greater than the anatomic dead space, but it may be increased if ventilated alveoli are underperfused or not perfused at all, as is the case in pulmonary embolism. The ratio of dead space to tidal volume (V_D/V_T) reflects the portion of the tidal volume that does not exchange with pulmonary blood. In other words, it is a measurement of the percentage of the tidal volume that is physiologic dead space. This ratio is calculated from data collected by measuring the P_{CO_2} in the expired air and the P_{CO_2} in the arterial blood. The larger the difference between these two measurements, the greater the physiologic dead space. The V_D/V_T ratio does not exceed 30 to 40 percent in the healthy person. This ratio is frequently used to follow the course of patients receiving mechanical ventilation.

Alveolar ventilation ($\dot{V}_A$) is the volume of fresh air entering the alveoli each minute that exchanges with pulmonary blood; it is the effective ventila-

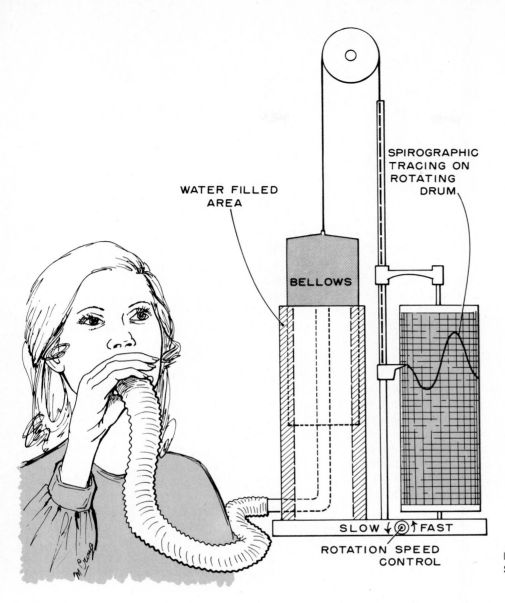

WATER FILLED AREA

SPIROGRAPHIC TRACING ON ROTATING DRUM

BELLOWS

SLOW ↓⊙↑ FAST

ROTATION SPEED CONTROL

FIGURE 32-2
Spirometer.

tion. It is normally about 4.2 liters per minute at rest. Alveolar ventilation is calculated by the formula

$$\dot{V}_A = (V_T - V_D) \times f$$

Alveolar ventilation is a better index of ventilation than minute volume or tidal volume, since it takes into account the volume of air wasted in ventilating the physiologic dead space. The calculations in Table 32.2 illustrate the relation between minute ventilation, breathing pattern, and effective alveolar ventilation. The physiologic dead space for each of the three patients is assumed to be constant at 150 ml, while the rate and depth of breathing vary.

Several deductions can be made from the data in Table 32-2. In each case the total amount of air entering and leaving the lungs is the same (the minute volume),

TABLE 32-2

EFFECTIVE VENTILATION AND RESPIRATORY PATTERN

Patient	V_D (ml)	V_T (ml)	f	$\dot{V}_E$ ($V_T \times f$) (L/min)	$\dot{V}_A$ (($V_T - V_D$) $\times$ f) (L/min)	V_D/V_T (%)
Patient A (rapid, shallow breathing)	150	250	40	10	4	60
Patient B (normal rate and depth)	150	500	20	10	7	30
Patient C (slow, deep breathing)	150	1000	10	10	8½	15

although there is great variation in the percentage of the tidal volume which is physiologic dead space and in the effective ventilation. It is evident that rapid, shallow breathing results in less effective ventilation as more is wasted in dead-space volume. This fact becomes obvious if one considers the formula for the calculation of alveolar ventilation. As tidal volume approaches the physiologic dead-space volume (150 ml), effective ventilation approaches zero regardless of the rapidity of the respiratory rate ($0 \times f = 0$). The percentage of the tidal volume which is physiologic dead space also approaches 100 percent as the tidal volume approaches the dead-space volume. When the fact that total physiologic dead space can vary greatly with disease is also considered, it is obvious that clinical observation of ventilatory adequacy has great limitations, even though some gross qualitative judgments can be made.

In order for air to move in and out of the lungs, the body must work to overcome the combined resistances of the thorax, lungs, and abdomen. The work (in the form of energy expenditure to move the chest bellows) is referred to as the *work of breathing*. The work of breathing can be expressed as the amount of oxygen consumed by the respiratory muscles. In the normal person at rest, this is a small fraction (less than 5 percent) of the total body oxygen consumption, but in disease the proportion may be much greater.

Expenditure of energy is required to overcome two types of resistance: elastic and nonelastic. The *elastic resistance* is the resistance to stretch caused by the elastic properties of the lungs and thorax. The elastic properties of the thorax result from the stretching properties of the tendons, muscles, and connective tissue. The elastic properties of the lungs are produced by the surface tension of fluid lining the alveoli and by the elastic fibers throughout the lung itself. *Nonelastic resistance* is the frictional resistance to airflow in the airways and, to a small degree, resistance resulting from the viscosity of the lung tissues. The work of breathing increases if there is an increase in either the elastic resistance (e.g., "stiff lungs" as in pulmonary fibrosis) or the nonelastic resistance (e.g., turbulent airflow in emphysema as a result of narrowing of the airways).

Compliance (C) is a measure of the elastic properties (distensibility) of the lungs and thorax and is defined as the change in volume per unit change in pressure under static conditions. Total compliance (compliance of the lungs and thorax) or lung compliance alone can be determined. Two manometers are used to measure pressure changes: one is connected to the mouth or nostrils (to measure alveolar pressure or the total pressure exerted by the lung-thorax system) and the other to an esophageal balloon (to measure intrapleural pressure). Volume and pressure changes are then measured under various degrees of lung inflation and breath holding. Compliance is estimated by calculating the slope of the pressure-volume curve which is plotted from the data. Normal lung compliance and thoracic cage compliance over the tidal volume range are each about 0.2 liter per cmH_2O, and total compliance (lungs and thoracic cage) is about 0.1 liter per cmH_2O:

$$C = \frac{\Delta V \text{ (change in lung volume in liters)}}{\Delta P \text{ (change in pressure in centimeters of water)}}$$

Compliance is reduced in restrictive patterns of pulmonary disease which increase the stiffness of the lung or thorax and limit expansion. In these cases, a greater force (ΔP) than normal is required to give the same increase in volume (ΔV), causing the compliance to be smaller. Common causes of decreased lung compliance are atelectasis (collapse of alveoli), pulmonary edema, pneumonia, and pulmonary fibrosis. When pulmonary surfactant is decreased, compliance is also decreased, because the lung becomes stiffer as a result of the increase in surface tension (surfactant normally reduces surface tension). Chest wall compliance is reduced in obesity, abdominal distention, and bony deformities of the chest cage such as kyphoscoliosis.

The *nonelastic airway resistance* (R_{AW}) can be measured by placing the subject in an airtight box (body plethysmograph) and measuring the pressure around the body (which reflects the change in alveolar pressure); at the same time the rate of flow of air at the mouth is measured (see Fig. 32-3). The R_{AW} reflects the nonelastic resistance of the upper airways (first to twelfth generations) and is approximately 1.8 cm H_2O per liter per second of airflow. In patients suffering from obstructive airway disease (e.g., emphysema), R_{AW} is increased and may be greater than 5 cm H_2O per liter per second.

More commonly, however, nonelastic resistance is estimated by measuring forced expiratory volumes and flow rates. This measurement is made on a spirometer or by a portable hand unit which can be used at the bedside. The following volumes of air are measured by the spirometer:

Forced vital capacity (FVC) is the vital capacity measurement performed with expiration as forceful and rapid as possible. This volume of air is normally about the same as the vital capacity but may be significantly reduced in patients with airway obstruction because of premature closure of the small airways and the consequent trapping of air.

Forced expiratory volume (FEV) is the volume of air that can be exhaled in a standard time period during the FVC maneuver. Usually the FEV is

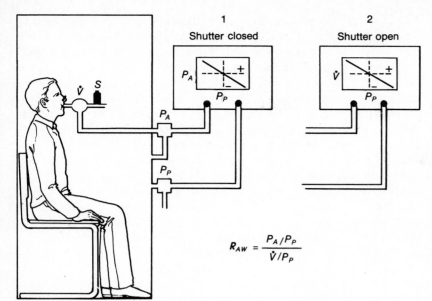

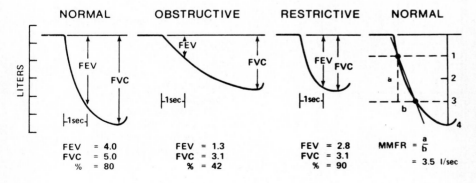

1
Shutter closed

2
Shutter open

$$R_{AW} = \frac{P_A/P_P}{\dot{V}/P_P}$$

FIGURE 32-3

Measurement of airways resistance (R_{AW}) in the body plethysmograph. The ratio between mouth pressure (P_A) (identical to alveolar pressure) and the box pressure (P_P) is determined with the shutter closed. Then the relationship between P_P and airflow ($\dot{V}$) is estimated while the patient pants through the unobstructed pneumotachograph. Now $R_{AW} = P_A/\dot{V}$. (Redrawn from R. M. Cherniack, *Pulmonary Function Testing,* Saunders, Philadelphia, 1977, p. 151.)

measured during the first second of the forced exhalation; this is termed FEV_1. The FEV is a very useful index of the impairment of ventilatory capacity, and values of less than 1 liter during the first second indicate severe impairment of ventilatory function.

The FEV should always be related to the FVC or VC. Normal persons can expire about 80 percent of their vital capacity in 1 second, expressed as the FEV_1/FVC ratio. It makes little difference whether the FVC or VC is used for the ratio; the result is about the same. This ratio is of great value in differentiating between diseases which cause airway obstruction and those that cause restriction of lung expansion. In obstructive diseases such as chronic bronchitis and emphysema, there is a greater reduction in FEV_1 than in the vital capacity (vital capacity may be normal), so that the FEV_1/FVC ratio is less than 80 percent. In a restrictive disease of

the lung parenchyma such as sarcoidosis, both the FEV_1 and the FVC or VC are reduced in about the same proportion and the FEV_1/FVC ratio remains at about 80 percent or more.

The *maximum midexpiratory flow rate* (MMFR) is an important index of airway obstruction which may be derived from a forced expiration. It is the flow rate for the middle two quarters of the forced vital capacity. The MMFR appears to be independent of effort and thus may be a more sensitive index of airway obstruction in early chronic obstructive lung disease than the FEV_1 (Fig. 32-4).

It is important to understand that the routine tests described above can detect only moderate to advanced obstructive disease involving the large airways which account for 80 percent of the resistance. They are not sensitive enough to detect obstruction of the small peripheral airways (bronchioles < 1 mm in diameter), since these airways contribute only a small fraction of

NORMAL	OBSTRUCTIVE	RESTRICTIVE	NORMAL
FEV = 4.0	FEV = 1.3	FEV = 2.8	MMFR = $\frac{a}{b}$
FVC = 5.0	FVC = 3.1	FVC = 3.1	= 3.5 l/sec
% = 80	% = 42	% = 90	

FIGURE 32-4

Measurement of the forced expiratory volume (FEV_1) and maximum midexpiratory flow rate (MMFR). The patient takes a full inspiration and exhales as hard and fast as possible. The pen moves down as the patient exhales. The FEV_1 is the volume exhaled in 1 second. The MMFR is the mean flow rate over the middle half of the FVC. Note the differences between the normal, obstructive, and restrictive patterns. (From J. B. West, in *Harrison's Principles of Internal Medicine,* 10th ed., McGraw-Hill, New York, 1983, p. 1507.)

the resistance (< 20 percent). Obstructive respiratory disease is believed to begin in the peripheral airways. For these reasons new techniques have been devised for detecting early airway dysfunction.

One technique is the *single-breath nitrogen test* to detect uneven distribution of gas in the lung and an increased closing volume. During this test the subject fully exhales, takes a single vital capacity inspiration of 100 percent O_2, and then slowly exhales to the residual volume. During the last expiration, the nitrogen concentration in the expired air (now diluted with inspired O_2) is measured with a rapid nitrogen analyzer and recorded along with the expired volume.

A number of important parameters may be derived from the N_2 curve (Fig. 32-5) including anatomic dead space, residual volume, vital capacity, total lung capacity, closing volume, closing capacity, and the slope of the alveolar plateau. *Closing volume* represents a lung volume at which the small airways in the lowest part of the lung begin to close. It is usually expressed as a percentage of the expired vital capacity (CV/VC). *Closing capacity* consists of the closing volume plus the residual volume and is expressed as a percent of total lung capacity (CC/TLC). The CV/VC ratio is age-dependent and may be as low as 10 percent in young healthy persons and 40 percent at the age of 65 years. An increase in the CV/VC or CC/TLC ratio suggests premature closure of the small peripheral airways due to narrowing or loss of elastic recoil, as in chronic bronchitis and emphysema. An increased CV has been found in apparently healthy cigarette smokers. A rising slope of the alveolar plateau of the N_2 washout curve indicates uneven alveolar gas distribution in the lung and occurs in obstruction of the airways. Excellent and detailed descriptions of these and other pulmonary function tests may be found in Cherniack (1977) and West (1977).

The overall effects on alterations in the elastic and nonelastic properties of the lungs can be assessed by a simple test which measures the *maximum breathing capacity* (MBC), or *maximum voluntary ventilation* (MVV). The MVV (or MBC) can be estimated directly by having the patient breathe as rapidly and deeply as possible for 15 seconds and collecting the expired air in a Douglas bag. This volume is multiplied by 4 to determine the minute volume in liters per minute. This test, used extensively for years, has been largely replaced by the forced expiratory volume (FEV_1) test, which is less demanding and gives essentially the same information. The MBC may be approximated as the product of $FEV_1 \times 30$. The MBC can be affected by changes in compliance because of the increased muscular effort required. It is also affected by changes in airway resistance because of the increased turbulence resulting from airway collapse when breathing at high speeds. The healthy young male adult can move as much as 170 liters of air per minute, compared to a minute volume of about 6 liters per minute at rest. The difference represents the pulmonary reserve, which is very large in the young, healthy adult. The pulmonary reserve is reduced

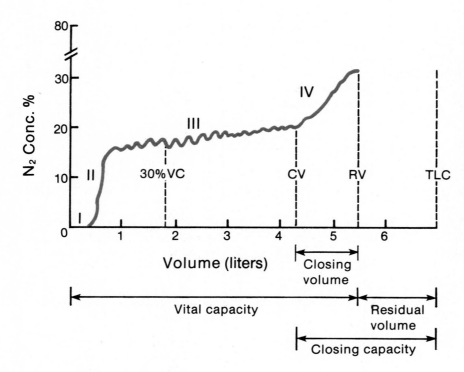

FIGURE 32-5

Measurement of closing volume by the single-breath nitrogen method. If a vital capacity inspiration is followed by slow exhalation to RV, four phases in the N_2 concentration measured at the lips can be recognized. During phase 1 pure oxygen is exhaled from the dead space followed by a rapid rise in N_2 (phase II), representing a mixture of alveolar and dead-space gas and has a nearly horizontal slope when ventilation is even. Near the end of expiration there is an abrupt rise in N_2 concentration (phase IV) signaling closure of the small airways in the dependent zones of the lung. Phase IV represents closing volume, CV. (Redrawn from R. M. Cherniack, *Pulmonary Function Testing*, Saunders, Philadelphia, 1977, p. 158).

in both restrictive and obstructive disease, but much more in the latter.

As already stated, less than 5 percent of the total oxygen consumption is expended for the work of breathing in the normal person at rest. The oxygen cost of breathing is greatly increased in both obstructive and restrictive patterns of pulmonary disease. The patient with emphysema (increased airway resistance) or the person who is very obese (restriction of chest movement) may consume 25 percent or more of the total inspired oxygen for the work of breathing. In severe disease, fatigue may be an important factor in the development of respiratory failure, because of the increased muscular effort required for the work of breathing.

There is also a relation between the mechanical work of breathing and the respiratory pattern (rate and depth of breathing). Respiratory physiologists have demonstrated that for any given alveolar ventilation there is an optimum respiratory rate and tidal volume at which the total work of breathing is minimal. The graphs in Fig. 32-6 show the relation between the me-

chanical work of breathing (including the total work and the elastic and nonelastic work), expressed in kilogram-meters, and the respiratory frequency. The principle illustrated is applied to normal persons as well as to those with pulmonary disease. The total work is the sum of the elastic and nonelastic work. (As you will recall, elastic work is expended to overcome the elastic resistances of the lungs and thorax, and nonelastic work is expended to overcome flow resistance and tissue viscous resistance.) In the normal person at rest, at a particular alveolar ventilation, the total work of breathing is least at about 15 breaths per minute (illustrated by the solid lines in Fig. 32-6). At the same alveolar ventilation, rapid, shallow breathing results in the least amount of work for the patient with a restrictive pulmonary disorder (increased elastic work) such as pneumonia or obesity (long dashed lines in Fig. 32-6). This pattern

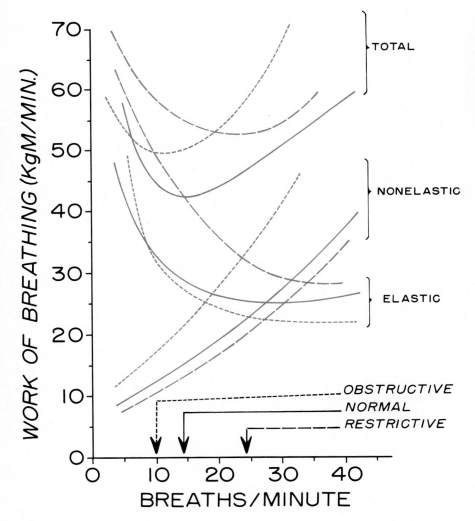

FIGURE 32-6
Relationship between the mechanical work of breathing and the respiratory pattern in health and in pulmonary disease. (Modified from R. M. Cherniack, L. Cherniack, and A. Naimark, *Respiration in Health and Disease*, 3d ed., Saunders, Philadelphia, 1983 p. 17.)

probably occurs because small increments in tidal volume greatly increase the elastic resistance. However, if the pattern of breathing becomes too rapid and shallow, the dead-space volume becomes disproportionately high. On the other hand, the person with an obstructive pulmonary disorder (increased nonelastic work) such as might occur in emphysema adopts a slow, deep pattern of respiration (short dashed lines in Fig. 32-6). This pattern is adopted because a higher flow rate is likely to increase the amount of work needed to overcome resistance to airflow. In fact, if the patient with obstructive disease should voluntarily hyperventilate to blow off more carbon dioxide, the P_{CO_2} might actually rise as a result of its increased production from the increased mechanical work of breathing.

Blood gas analysis

In order to assess respiratory function adequately, it is necessary to look beyond the lung to the volume and distribution of gas transport by the circulatory system. The factors which affect gas transport and removal between the lungs and tissue cells have already been discussed in Chap. 31. In this chapter, the technique used for the collection of blood to measure the blood gases and some general guidelines for the interpretation of measurements are presented.

Usually a sample of arterial blood is used for the blood gas analysis. Figure 32-7 demonstrates the correct technique for drawing a blood sample. The radial artery is often chosen because of its accessibility. The wrist is extended by positioning it over a rolled towel. After the skin has been sterilized, the artery is stabilized with two fingers of one hand while the arterial puncture is made with the other hand using a heparinized syringe. After 5 ml of blood has been drawn into the syringe, air is removed, and the blood is placed on ice and taken immediately to the blood gas laboratory for analysis. This procedure is commonly performed by the intensive care nurse. Table 32-3 lists the normal values for the arterial blood gases.

The Pa_{CO_2} is the best index of alveolar ventilation. When the Pa_{CO_2} rises, the direct cause is always generalized alveolar hypoventilation. Hypoventilation causes respiratory acidosis and a fall in the pH of the blood.

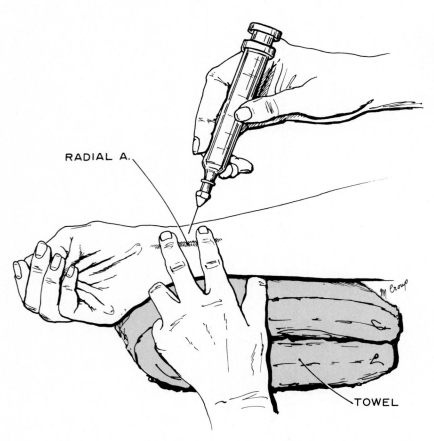

RADIAL A.

TOWEL

FIGURE 32-7
Radial artery punctuate technique for obtaining blood for blood gases.

TABLE 32-3

511

PHYSIOLOGIC METHODS: PULMONARY FUNCTION TESTS

NORMAL VALUES FOR THE ARTERIAL BLOOD GASES

Blood gas measurment	Symbol	Normal value
Carbon dioxide tension	Pa_{CO_2}	36–44 mmHg (average, 40)
Oxygen tension	Pa_{O_2}	80–100 mmHg
Oxygen percent saturation	Sa_{O_2}	97
Hydrogen ion concentration	pH	7.35–7.45
Bicarbonate	HCO_3^-	21–28 meq/L

Alveolar hypoventilation may occur if the tidal volume is decreased (the dead-space effect), as in rapid, shallow breathing. Hypoventilation may also occur if the respiratory rate is decreased as it is in narcotic or barbiturate drug overdose. The Pa_{CO_2} may also rise to compensate for a metabolic alkalosis. Consequently, in order to interpret the Pa_{CO_2} correctly, one must also consider the blood pH and bicarbonate levels to determine whether a change is due to a primary respiratory condition or is compensating for a metabolic condition.

The direct cause of a lowered Pa_{CO_2} is always alveolar hyperventilation. Hyperventilation causes respiratory alkalosis and a rise in the pH of the blood. Hyperventilation is common in asthma and pneumonia and represents an effort to raise the Pa_{CO_2} at the expense of excreting excess CO_2 from the lungs. Hyperventilation may also be caused by brain injury or tumor or by anxiety, or it may be a compensation for metabolic acidosis. Table 32-4 summarizes the acid-base changes in compensated acidosis and alkalosis. The heavy arrows indicate the primary disorder. The change in the bicarbonate level represents the kidneys' attempt to compensate for the respiratory acidosis or alkalosis, while the change in the Pa_{CO_2} in the metabolic disorders represents the lung's role in compensation. The purpose of the compensation is to return the blood pH to normal.

When the Pa_{O_2} falls below the normal value, hypoxemia is the result. Pa_{O_2} levels fall slightly with age, so that it is normal for persons over the age of 60 years

to have a Pa_{O_2} as low as 70 mmHg. In severe respiratory failure, the Pa_{O_2} may fall to 30 to 40 mmHg. Hypoxemia resulting from respiratory disease is caused by one or more of the following mechanisms: (1) ventilation-perfusion imbalance (most common cause), (2) alveolar hypoventilation, (3) impaired diffusion, or (4) intrapulmonary anatomic shunts. Hypoxemia resulting from the first three abnormalities can be corrected by administering oxygen. However, the intrapulmonary anatomic shunt (arteriovenous shunt) cannot be corrected by oxygen therapy.

Changes in the blood gases are critical measurements in the diagnosis of respiratory or ventilatory failure, which may be insidious in onset. Respiratory insufficiency exists when the Pa_{O_2} falls below the normal values, and respiratory failure exists when the Pa_{CO_2} falls to 50 mmHg. The Pa_{CO_2} may be increased or decreased below the normal values in respiratory insufficiency or failure. Respiratory failure is discussed in greater detail in Chap. 37.

Some of the common changes in ventilatory function and blood gases in restrictive and obstructive patterns of pulmonary disease are summarized in Table 32-5.

TABLE 32-4

ACID-BASE CHANGES IN ACIDOSIS AND ALKALOSIS

Acid-base disturbance	pH	HCO_3^-	Pa_{CO_2}
Respiratory acidosis	↓	↑	↑
Respiratory alkalosis	↑	↓	↓
Metabolic acidosis	↓	↓	↓
Metabolic alkalosis	↑	↑	↑

TABLE 32-5

CHANGES IN VENTILATORY FUNCTION AS A RESULT OF PULMONARY DISEASE

Test	Obstructive pattern	Restrictive pattern
RV	↑	↓
FRC	↑	↓
TLC	N or ↑	↓
VC*	N or ↓	↓
FVC	N or ↓	↓
MBC	↓	N or ↓
FEV_1†	↓	N or ↓
FEV_1/FVC	↓ (<80%)	N or ↑ (>80%)
MMFR	↓	N or ↓
CV	↑ for age or > FRC	
C	N or ↑ (slight)	↓
Pa_{O_2}	↓	N (↓↓ exercise)
Pa_{CO_2}	↑	N or ↓
pH	↓ (during exacerbations)	N or ↑

Key: N = normal; ↓ = decreased or tending to decrease; ↑ = increased or tending to increase.
*Useful test to monitor progress of restrictive lung disease.
†Most useful test to monitor progress of obstructive lung disease.
Sources: Crofton and Douglas, 1981; Cherniack, 1977.

Diagnostic procedures in respiratory disease

Directions: Answer the following on a separate sheet of paper.

1. List six radiologic methods commonly used to detect pulmonary disease.

2. List four distinct features that are depicted on a routine chest x-ray.

Directions: Circle the letter which correctly answers the question.

3. Which of the following diagnostic methods is *not* used to detect pulmonary disease and adequacy of pulmonary function?
   a. Blood gas measurements   *b.* Ventilatory function tests   *c.* Intravenous pyelogram   *d.* Fluoroscopy

Directions: Match each of the diagnostic tests in col. A to its description in col. B.

Column A

4. _____ Bronchography
5. _____ Angiography of pulmonary vessels
6. _____ Fluoroscopy
7. _____ Perfusion lung scan
8. _____ Percutaneous needle biopsy of lung
9. _____ Bronchoscopy
10. _____ Sputum studies
11. _____ Tomography
12. _____ Mediastinoscopy

Column B

a. Most accurate method of diagnosing pulmonary embolism

b. Used to obtain information about how various zones of the lung behave during respiratory cycle

c. Reveals the size and appearance of the tracheobronchial tree; useful in confirming the diagnosis of bronchiectasis

d. Closed technique to obtain lung biopsy specimen

e. Useful technique to obtain aspiration of secretions for cytologic examination or biopsy specimen under direct visualization

f. Radiologic technique providing detailed x-rays of "slices of the lung"

g. Technique used to assess spread of lung cancer to hilar lymph nodes

h. Involves the injection into a peripheral vein of albumen microspheres tagged with an isotope

i. Specimen may be obtained by aspiration of gastric contents

Directions: Match each of the diagnostic precedures in col. A to the potential hazards and precautions in col. B. Letters in col. B may be used more than once.

Column A

13. _____ Fluoroscopy
14. _____ Bronchography
15. _____ Bronchoscopic biopsy
16. _____ Perfusion and ventilation scan
17. _____ Pulmonary angiography
18. _____ Lung biopsy by open and closed techniques

Column B

a. Food and fluids are withheld after this examination until the gag reflex returns

b. The major risk during this procedure is development of cardiac arrhythmia

c. Safer procedure for the diagnosis of pulmonary embolism, though less definitive

d. Excess radiation is the chief hazard associated with this procedure

e. Percussion and postural drainage should follow this procedure

f. Pneumothorax and bleeding are possible complications

g. Laryngospasm or edema is a possible complication following this procedure

Directions: Answer the following on a separate sheet of paper.

19. Describe the role of ventilatory function tests and blood gas analysis in the diagnosis and treatment of pulmonary disorders. Are any of these tests specifically diagnostic?

20. Explain why alveolar ventilation is a better index of effective ventilation than minute volume or tidal volume.

21. Describe the procedure for the measurement of compliance of the lungs and thoracic cage. How is compliance calculated from the measurements?

22. List three common causes of decreased lung compliance and three causes of decreased chest wall compliance.

23. Why does a patient with emphysema adopt a slow, deep pattern of respiration?

24. What breathing pattern might a patient with normal airway resistance but very stiff lungs (low compliance) adopt? Why?

25. Describe the correct technique for the collection of blood in the measurement of arterial blood gases.

26. List three causes of alveolar hyperventilation and hypoventilation.

27. List four causes of hypoxemia. Which one is not corrected by oxygen administration?

Directions: Circle T if the statement is true and F if it is false.

28. T   F   Rapid, shallow breathing results in less effective ventilation because the respiratory rate is greater than the normal rate per minute.

29. T   F   The ratio of physiologic dead space to tidal volume does not normally exceed 30 to 40 percent.

30. T   F   Alveolar ventilation in a 120-lb female with a tidal volume of 200 ml and a respiratory rate of 30 breaths per minute is about 6 liters per minute.

31. T   F   The work of breathing refers to the form of energy expenditure required to move the chest bellows (the amount of oxygen consumed by the respiratory muscles).

32. T   F   Elastic properties of the lungs are the result of the surface tension of fluid lining the alveoli and the elastic fibers throughout the lung.

33. T   F   The maximum breathing capacity test is a good test to measure pulmonary reserve.

34. T   F   Nonelastic resistances consist of the frictional resistance to flow in the airways.

Directions: Circle the letter preceding each item below that correctly completes the statement. More than one answer may be correct.

35. The primary lung volume which measures the amount of air inhaled or exhaled with each breath is the:
a. Tidal volume (V_T)   b. Expiratory reserve volume (ERV)   c. Inspiratory reserve volume (IRV)   d. Residual volume (RV)

36. The lung capacity which measures the maximum volume of air that can be expired after a maximum inspiratory effort is the:

a. Total lung capacity (TLC)   b. Vital capacity (VC)   c. Inspiratory capacity (IC)   d. Functional residual capacity (FRC)

37. The spirometer directly measures the combination:
a. V_T, TLC, RV, IC   b. FRC, TLC, ERV, VC
c. V_T, IRV, ERV, VC, IC

38. In healthy young persons, the 1-second forced expiratory volume/forced vital capacity ratio is approximately:
a. 30 percent   b. 50 percent   c. 80 percent
d. 100 percent

39. The normal range for Pa_{CO_2} is:
a. 22–30 mmHg   b. 36–44 mmHg   c. 50–62 mmHg   d. 85–100 mmHg

40. Alveolar hypoventilation can be readily diagnosed by measuring the:
a. Pa_{O_2} b. pH of the arterial blood   c. Respiratory rate   d. Pa_{CO_2} e. Tidal volume

41. Physiologic dead space can be increased by:
a. Enlargement of the anatomic dead space
b. High ventilation/perfusion ratios of pulmonary units   c. Low ventilation/perfusion ratios of pulmonary units

42. Laboratory test results which indicate adequate compensation for a respiratory acidosis are:
a. Increase in pH toward 7.4   b. Decrease in the serum bicarbonate   c. Increase in the serum bicarbonate

Directions: Match each of the pulmonary functions in col. A to its definition in col. B.

Column A
43. ____ FVC
44. ____ FEV₁
45. ____ V_D/V_T
46. ____ $\dot{V}_A$
47. ____ $\dot{V}_E$
48. ____ Pa_{CO_2}
49. ____ MMFR
50. ____ R_{AW}

Column B
a. Carbon dioxide tension in the arterial blood

b. Volume of air exchanged in the airway in 1 minute

c. Volume of air expired during the first second of the forced vital capacity maneuver

d. Proportion of tidal volume that is physiologic dead space

e. Effective ventilation per minute

f. Expiration performed as rapidly and as forcefully as possible following a maximum inspiration

g. Nonelastic resistance of the large airways

h. Maximum flow rate during the middle two quarters of the FVC maneuver

Directions: Answer the following on Table 32-6.

51. Indicate the common changes in ventilatory function and blood gases in restrictive and obstructive patterns of pulmonary disease by filling in the blanks in the table. Use the following key: N = normal, ↓ = decreased, ↑ = increased.

TABLE 32-6

CHANGES IN VENTILATORY FUNCTION AS A RESULT OF PULMONARY DISEASE

Test	Obstructive pattern	Restrictive pattern
Residual volume		
Functional residual capacity		
Total lung capacity		
Vital capacity		
Forced vital capacity		
Maximum breathing capacity		
FEV_1		
FEV_1/FVC		
Compliance		
Pa_{O_2}		
Pa_{CO_2}		
pH		

Directions: Circle the letter preceding the item that best answers the question or completes the statement.

52. Which of the following pulmonary function tests is most sensitive in detecting early obstructive lung disease of the peripheral airways?
    a. MMFR   *b.* R_{AW} *c.* FEV_1/FVC
    d. CV/VC

53. The single-breath nitrogen test can be used to measure:
    a. RV   *b.* V_D *c.* Uneven distribution of alveolar ventilation   *d.* CC/TLC   *e.* All the above

CHAPTER 33

CARDINAL SIGNS AND SYMPTOMS OF RESPIRATORY DISEASE

OBJECTIVES

At the completion of this chapter you should be able to:

1. Describe the following cardinal signs and symptoms of respiratory disease: cough (causes, importance, and types); sputum (cause of excessive secretion, source, color, and consistency); hemoptysis (detection, cause, and importance); dyspnea (causes, classification, and significance); chest pain (type and description); digital clubbing (causes, detection, and significance); cyanosis (types, detection, causes, and importance).

2. Differentiate between hypoxemia and hypoxia.

3. List the laboratory findings associated with hypoxia.

4. List the clinical signs associated with hypoxia in the cardiovascular, respiratory, and central nervous systems.

5. Identify skin changes associated with hypoxia.

6. Differentiate between hypercapnia and hypocapnia.

Pulmonary diseases may give rise to both respiratory and general signs and symptoms. Respiratory signs and symptoms include cough, excessive or abnormal sputum, hemoptysis, dyspnea, and chest pain. General signs and symptoms include cyanosis, digital clubbing, and other manifestations related to inadequate gas exchange. The reader is referred to other textbooks for a discussion of adventitious chest sounds and systematic assessment of the respiratory status.

COUGH

Coughing is a protective reflex caused by irritation of the tracheobronchial tree. The ability to cough is an important mechanism in clearing the lower airways, and many adults normally cough a few times upon first arising to clear the trachea and pharynx of secretions which have accumulated during sleep. Coughing is also the most common symptom of respiratory disease. Any cough persisting for longer than 3 weeks should be investigated to determine the cause.

Stimuli that commonly produce a cough are mechanical, chemical, and inflammatory. Inhalation of smoke, dust, and small foreign bodies is the most common cause of cough. Smokers often have a chronic cough as a result of inhaling foreign bodies (smoke) and chronic inflammation of the airways. Mechanical stimulation from tumors either extrinsic or intrinsic to the airways is another cause of cough (the most common tumor causing cough is bronchogenic carcinoma). Any inflammatory process of the airways, with or without exudate, may produce a cough. Chronic bronchitis, tuberculosis, and pneumonia typically have coughing as a prominent symptom. A cough may be productive, hacking and nonproductive, brassy (as when there is pressure on the trachea), frequent, infrequent, or paroxysmal (intermittent coughing episodes).

SPUTUM

The normal adult produces about 100 ml of mucus in the respiratory tract per day. This mucus is transported to the pharynx by the normal cleansing actions of the cilia that line the airways. When excess mucus is formed, the normal process of removal may be ineffective and may result in the accumulation of mucus. When this occurs, the mucous membrane is stimulated and the mucus is coughed up as sputum. Excess mucus production may be caused by physical, chemical, or infective insults to the mucous membrane.

Whenever a patient produces sputum, it is important to observe its source, color, volume, and consistency. Sputum produced by clearing the throat is most likely to have originated in the sinuses or nasal passages rather than in the lower respiratory tract. Profuse purulent sputum suggests the presence of a suppurative process such as lung abscess, while sputum production which gradually increases over a period of years suggests chronic bronchitis or bronchiectasis.

The color of sputum is also important. Yellow sputum indicates an infection. Green sputum is indicative of stagnant pus. The green color is produced by the presence of verdoperoxidase, which is liberated from polymorphonuclear leukocytes (PMNs) in the sputum. Green sputum is common in bronchiectasis because of the stagnation of sputum in dilated, infected bronchioles. Many patients with lower respiratory tract infection report having green sputum early in the morning, which becomes yellow as the day progresses. This is probably caused by the accumulation of purulent spu-

tum during the night, with the consequent release of verdoperoxidase.

The character and consistency of sputum also yields useful information. Pink, frothy sputum is characteristic of acute pulmonary edema. Sputum may be mucoid, sticky, and grey or white in color in chronic bronchitis. A foul odor to the sputum may indicate a lung abscess or bronchiectasis.

HEMOPTYSIS

Varying amounts of blood may be mixed with sputum, or blood may compose the entire expectoration. *Hemoptysis* is the term applied to the expectoration of both pure blood and blood-streaked sputum. Any process resulting in interruption of the continuity of the pulmonary blood vessels may result in bleeding. The expectoration of pure blood is a serious symptom. It may be the first manifestation of active tuberculosis. Other common causes of hemoptysis are bronchogenic carcinoma, pulmonary infarction, and lung abscess. Blood-streaked sputum (which may be rust-colored) is a common feature of pneumococcal pneumonia. When blood or blood-streaked sputum is expectorated, it is important to determine whether the source is actually the lower respiratory tract rather than the nasal passages or the gastrointestinal tract.

DYSPNEA

Dyspnea is a term used to designate difficulty in breathing and is a cardinal symptom of cardiopulmonary disease. A patient suffering from dyspnea is likely to experience shortness of breath or a sensation of suffocation. Dyspnea is by no means always an indication of disease; the normal person commonly experiences this sensation after varying degrees of physical exertion. The amount of exertion sufficient to induce dyspnea varies with age, sex, altitude, state of physical training, and emotional involvement in the task. Thus it is important to correlate dyspnea in a person with the minimal level of activity sufficient for its induction. Dyspnea may occur (1) after moderate exertion such as climbing a flight of stairs, (2) after a short walk, (3) after light activities such as talking, bathing, or shaving, (4) at rest, and (5) while lying down (orthopnea). The key factor which seems to determine whether or not dyspnea is experienced is whether the level of ventilation or effort is appropriate to the degree of activity. The stimuli, sensory receptors, and nerve pathways by which the appropriateness is recognized have not been established with certainty.

Dyspnea is a prevalent symptom in diseases which affect the tracheobronchial tree, the lung parenchyma, and the pleural space. Dyspnea is commonly associated with pulmonary diseases in which there is increased respiratory work as a result of decreased ventilatory capacity. However, when the work of breathing is increased chronically, the patient may become accustomed to this and not experience dyspnea. Weak respiratory muscles may also result in dyspnea.

CHEST PAIN

There are many causes of chest pain, but the most characteristic pain of lung disease is that resulting from inflammation of the pleura (pleurisy). Only the parietal layer of the pleura is a source of pain, as the visceral pleura and the lung parenchyma are regarded as insensitive organs.

Typical pleurisy may develop gradually but is usually abrupt in onset. The pain occurs at the site of inflammation and is usually well localized. The pain is cutting and sharp in character, aggravated by coughing, sneezing, and deep breathing, so that the patient often adopts a pattern of rapid, shallow breathing and avoids unnecessary movement. The pain may be somewhat relieved by applying pressure (splinting) over the involved area. The most common causes of pleuritic pain are pulmonary infection or infarction, although such conditions may be present without pain.

DIGITAL CLUBBING

Digital clubbing is a peculiar change in the shape of the tips of the fingers and toes, characterized by a bulbous appearance. It is a significant physical sign, since it is associated with a number of serious conditions. Pulmonary disease (such as bronchogenic carcinoma, bronchiectasis, lung abscess, or pulmonary tuberculosis) is the most common cause of digital clubbing (70 to 80 percent of cases). Cardiovascular disease (such as congenital intracardiac shunting or subacute bacterial endocarditis) ranks second (10 to 15 percent of cases); and 5 to 10 percent of the cases of digital clubbing are associated with chronic diseases of the gastrointestinal tract, including the liver. The pathogenesis of digital clubbing is not understood. A popular hypothesis ascribes it to hypoxia, but this does not explain its presence in many entities. Clubbing often develops early in bronchogenic carcinoma and is not associated with arterial desaturation. It is curious that the chronic hypoxia of emphysema rarely seems to be associated with digital clubbing, while the chronic hypoxia of tetralogy of Fallot is often associated with severe clubbing.

It is important to detect clubbing as early as possible because of its diagnostic significance. The earliest sign is a loss of the angle between the nail and the dorsum of the terminal phalanx; this angle is normally 160°. The normal variations, early and advanced clubbing, may be seen in Fig. 33-1. In early clubbing the skin at the base of the nail may have a shiny appearance,

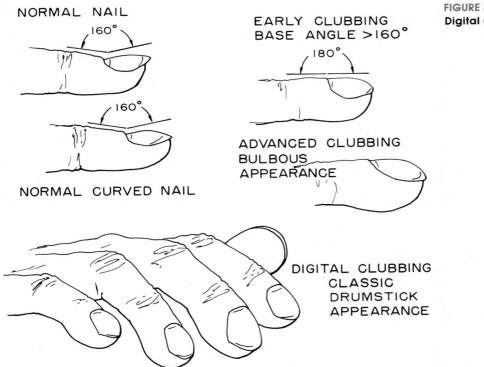

FIGURE 33-1
Digital clubbing.

and gentle pressure on the nail root reveals a spongy feeling (floating nail). Normally the nail plate rests firmly against the bone. Early clubbing must be differentiated from the normal curved nail that is common in blacks. If one views the normal curved nail from the side, the base angle is still about 160°. In early clubbing, the base angle of the nail becomes greater than 160°. As the condition progresses, the tissue at the root of the nail becomes heaped up and the curvature of the nail becomes pronounced, until the soft tissue of the digit tip becomes bulbous, producing the classic drumstick appearance.

SIGNS OF INADEQUATE GAS EXCHANGE

Cyanosis

Cyanosis is a bluish coloration of the skin and mucous membranes which develops as a result of an increase in the absolute amount of reduced hemoglobin (hemoglobin not united with oxygen). It may be a sign of respiratory insufficiency, although this is a highly unreliable indication. There are two types of cyanosis: central and peripheral. Central cyanosis resulting from insufficient oxygenation of hemoglobin in the lungs is most easily observed on the face, lips, and earlobes and under the tongue. Cyanosis is generally not detected until the absolute amount of reduced hemoglobin is 5 g/100 ml or more in a person with normal hemoglobin concentration. The normal amount of reduced hemoglobin in the capillary bed is 2.5 g/100 ml. In the person with a normal hemoglobin concentration, oxygen saturation is about 75 percent and the Pa_{O_2} is 50 mmHg or less when cyanosis is first detected. Anemic patients (low hemoglobin concentration) may never become cyanotic even though they have severe tissue hypoxia, because the absolute amount of reduced hemoglobin is not likely to reach 5 g/100 ml. On the other hand, a person with polycythemia (high hemoglobin concentration) can easily have 5 g/100 ml of reduced hemoglobin when there is only mild hypoxia. Other factors which make cyanosis difficult to recognize are variations in skin thickness, pigmentation, and lighting conditions.

In addition to cyanosis caused by respiratory insufficiency (central cyanosis), peripheral cyanosis occurs when severly reduced blood flow causes a great reduction in the venous saturation, thereby turning an area blue. Peripheral cyanosis may result from cardiac insufficiency, obstruction of blood flow, or vasoconstriction due to cold temperatures.

Cyanosis may also be produced by small amounts of circulating methemoglobin and by even smaller amounts of sulfhemoglobin, although these causes are uncommon. These variations in cause and the difficulty in recognizing cyanosis make it an unreliable sign of respiratory insufficiency.

Hypoxemia and hypoxia

The term *hypoxemia* refers to values of PaO_2 which are abnormally low and is frequently associated with *hypoxia*, or inadequate tissue oxygenation. Hypoxemia is not necessarily accompanied by tissue hypoxia. One can have normal tissue oxygenation with hypoxemia, just as one can have a normal Pa_{O_2} with tissue hypoxia (because of the abnormalities of oxygen delivery and utilization by the cells, discussed in Chap. 31). There is a relation, however, between the Pa_{O_2} and tissue hypoxia, although the precise Pa_{O_2} at which impairment of tissue utilization of oxygen occurs is variable. All things being equal, the more rapid the onset of hypoxemia, the more extensive the tissue abnormalities. In general, Pa_{O_2} values that are persistently less than 50 mmHg are associated with tissue hypoxia and acidosis (caused by anaerobic metabolism). Since hypoxia may exist with both normal and low values of Pa_{O_2}, evaluation of blood gas measurements must always be correlated with clinical observation of the patient. Cyanosis is an unreliable sign of hypoxia, because the oxygen saturation must be below 75 percent in persons with normal hemoglobin before it is detectable. Clinical signs and laboratory findings which indicate hypoxia are listed in Table 33-1.

TABLE 33-1

INDICATORS OF HYPOXIA

Laboratory findings	$Pa_{O_2} < 70$ mmHg $Sa_{O_2} < 90\%$ pH of blood < 7.35 $Pa_{CO_2} < 36$ mmHg if hyperventilation or > 44 mmHg if hypoventilation
Central nervous system	Mental confusion, bizarre behavior Restlessness; agitation Anxious facial expression; sweating Drowsiness progressing to coma when hypoxia severe
Cardiovascular system	Tachycardia early; bradycardia later when heart muscle not receiving adequate oxygen Arrhythmias Rise in blood pressure followed by a drop when hypoxia remains uncorrected
Respiratory system	Increased respiratory rate Dyspnea, yawning Use of accessory respiratory muscles; flared nostrils
Skin	Cyanosis of lips, oral mucosa, and nail beds

Just as ventilation is considered adequate when O_2 supply is matched with O_2 demand, so also must CO_2 elimination through the lungs be matched with CO_2 production for adequate ventilation. Because CO_2 is highly diffusible, the CO_2 tensions are equal in alveolar air and arterial blood; thus Pa_{CO_2} is the direct and immediate reflection of the alveolar ventilation in relation to the metabolic rate. Adequate ventilation maintains the Pa_{CO_2} at about 40 mmHg. *Hypercapnia* is defined as a rise in the Pa_{CO_2} above 44 mmHg; *hypocapnia* occurs when the Pa_{CO_2} is less than 36 mmHg. The direct cause of CO_2 retention is alveolar hypoventilation (ventilation inadequate to cope with CO_2 production). Hypercapnia is always accompanied by some degree of hypoxia when the patient is breathing room air.

The major causes of hypercapnia are obstructive airway disease, respiratory depressant drugs, weakness or paralysis of the respiratory muscles, chest trauma or abdominal surgery causing shallow respirations, and loss of lung tissue. Clinical signs associated with hypercapnia are mental confusion progressing to coma, headache (as a result of cerebral vasodilatation), asterixis or flapping tremor of the outstretched hands, and a pulse of large volume with warm, sweaty extremities (as a result of the peripheral vasodilatation caused by the hypercapnia). In chronic hypercapnia resulting from chronic pulmonary disease, the patient may become abnormally tolerant to the high Pa_{CO_2}, so that the principal drive to respiration is hypoxia. Under these circumstances, if oxygen is administered at a high concentration, respiration is diminished and the hypercapnia is increased.

Excessive loss of CO_2 from the lungs (hypocapnia) occurs when there is hyperventilation (ventilation in excess of metabolic need to remove CO_2). Common causes of hyperventilation, were listed in Chap. 32, and also include excessive mechanical ventilation, anxiety states, cerebral trauma, and compensatory response to hypoxia. Signs and symptoms commonly associated with hypocapnia include frequent sighing and yawning, dizziness, palpitations, tingling and numbness in the extremities, and muscular twitches. Severe hypocapnia ($Pa_{CO_2} < 25$ mmHg) may cause convulsions.

QUESTIONS

Cardinal signs and symptoms of respiratory disease

Directions: Match the signs and symptoms in col. B with the possible causative factors in col. A. Each letter may be used only once.

Column A

1. ____ Interruption in the continuity of the pulmonary blood vessels

2. ____ Inflammation of the pleura

3. ____ Increase in the absolute amount of reduced hemoglobin

4. ____ Physical, chemical, or infectious insults to the mucous membrane of the respiratory tract

Column B

a. Cough

b. Excess sputum production

c. Hemoptysis

d. Dyspnea

e. Digital clubbing

f. Chest pain

g. Cyanosis

5. ____ Protective reflex initiated by irritation of the tracheobronchial tree

6. ____ Pathogenesis unknown; associated with early stage of bronchogenic carcinoma and with certain chronic respiratory, cardiovascular, and gastrointestinal diseases

7. ____ Increased ventilatory work as correlated with the minimum level of activity sufficient for its induction

Directions: Circle T if the statement is true and F if it is false, and correct the false statements.

8. T   F   *Hypoxia* refers to inadequate tissue oxygenation

9. T   F Pa_{O_2} values that are persistently less than 85 mmHg are associated with tissue hypoxia.

10. T   F   Cyanosis is a reliable sign of hypoxia.

11. T   F   Confusion, restlessness, and agitation are clinical signs that may indicate hypoxia.

12. T   F   Anemic patients frequently become cyanotic even with moderate degrees of hypoxemia.

13. T   F   The Pa_{CO_2} is the best index of alveolar ventilation adequacy.

14. T   F   *Hypercapnia* refers to a rise in the Pa_{CO_2} above 44 mmHg.

15. T   F   The direct cause of hypocapnia is alveolar hypoventilation.

16. T   F   Symptoms of headache, drowsiness, and asterixis are associated with hypercapnia.

Directions: Answer the following questions on a separate sheet of paper.

17. What is digital clubbing? Why is it important to detect?

18. How would you detect cyanosis in a black patient?

CHAPTER 34

OBSTRUCTIVE PATTERNS OF RESPIRATORY DISEASE

OBJECTIVES

At the completion of this chapter you should be able to:

1. Describe the pattern of ventilatory dysfunction in chronic obstructive pulmonary disease (COPD).

2. Identify the criteria used to characterize chronic bronchitis, pulmonary emphysema, and asthma.

3. Describe chronic bronchitis, pulmonary emphysema, and asthma, including symptoms, pathologic anatomy, and physiology.

4. Illustrate the interrelation of the disease entities composing COPD.

5. Describe the pathologic changes resulting in airway obstruction found in asthma.

6. Differentiate between the three categories of asthma.

7. Identify the major symptoms, treatment, and complications of an asthmatic attack.

8. Describe the etiology of chronic bronchitis and identify the pathologic changes found.

9. Contrast the two morphologic patterns of emphysema.

10. Identify the process of formation and the significance of blebs and bullae.

11. Outline the objectives of treatment for chronic bronchitis and emphysema.

12. Identify the pathogenesis of COPD and the morphologic types of emphysema which may result.

13. Differentiate between the pure bronchitic (blue bloater) and emphysematous (pink puffer) types of COPD in regard to onset, etiology, sputum, dyspnea, $\dot{V}/\dot{Q}$, body build, polycythemia, blood gases, lung volumes, morphologic type, and tendency to develop cor pulmonale.

14. Describe the clinical course, complications, and treatment of a patient with COPD.

15. Describe the pathologic changes that occur in bronchiectasis.

16. Describe the pathogenesis, clinical features, and treatment of bronchiectasis.

17. Describe the etiology, pathologic features, treatment, and prognosis of cystic fibrosis (mucoviscidosis).

PATTERNS OF RESPIRATORY DISEASE

Respiratory diseases have been classified on the basis of etiology, anatomic site, chronicity, and changes in structure and function. None of these classifications is entirely satisfactory. The etiologic agents are unknown in some cases, while in others the same causal agent may affect different anatomic sites and produce different pathophysiologic effects. In this chapter and the following one, respiratory diseases are classified according to ventilatory dysfunction and are divided into two categories: diseases which primarily produce an obstructive ventilatory disorder and those which produce a restrictive ventilatory disorder. This classification was chosen because spirometric and other tests of ventilatory function are carried out almost routinely, and most respiratory diseases affect ventilation. There are two limitations to this approach. In some respiratory disorders the ventilatory abnormality may produce a mixed pattern (e.g., chronic emphysema with superimposed pneumonia), while in other disorders affecting respiration, ventilatory function may be normal (e.g., anemia or right-to-left shunt). The following pulmonary disorders, which do not readily fit into obstructive or restrictive patterns of disease, are discussed separately: cardiovascular diseases affecting the lung, respiratory insufficiency and failure, pulmonary neoplasms, and tuberculosis. Only those disorders most commonly encountered in hospital practice are considered.

CHRONIC OBSTRUCTIVE PULMONARY DISEASE

Chronic obstructive pulmonary disease (COPD) is a term often applied to a group of pulmonary diseases of long duration which are characterized by increased resistance to airflow as the main pathophysiologic feature. Chronic bronchitis, pulmonary emphysema, and bronchial asthma are the three diseases which make up the entity known as COPD. There appears to be an etiologic and sequential relationship between chronic bronchitis and emphysema which does not seem to exist between these two diseases and asthma. This is particularly true in regard to etiology, pathogenesis, and treatment, as discussed later in this chapter.

Chronic bronchitis is a clinical disorder characterized by excessive production of mucus in the bronchi and is manifested by a chronic cough and production of sputum for a minimum of 3 months a year for at least 2 consecutive years. This definition assumes that diseases such as bronchiectasis and tuberculosis, which also cause chronic cough and sputum production, have been excluded. The sputum produced in chronic bronchitis may be mucoid or mucopurulent.

Pulmonary emphysema is an anatomic alteration of the lung parenchyma characterized by abnormal enlargement of the alveoli and alveolar ducts and destruction of the alveolar walls.

Asthma is a disease characterized by hypersensitivity of the tracheobronchial tree to various stimuli. It is manifested by periodic, reversible airway narrowing caused by bronchospasm.

Note the different bases of the definitions (American Thoracic Society, 1962) of the diseases given above: chronic bronchitis is defined by clinical symptoms, pulmonary emphysema by pathologic anatomy, and asthma by clinical pathologic physiology. Although each disease may exist in its pure form, it is more usual for chronic bronchitis and emphysema to exist together in the same patient. Asthma is more easily separated from chronic bronchitis and emphysema on the basis of a history of paroxysmal attacks of wheezing beginning in childhood and associated with allergies. Occasionally, however, patients with chronic bronchitis have asthmatic features to their disease. The interrelation of chronic bronchitis, asthma, and emphysema are illustrated in Fig. 34-1. The shaded areas represent those persons with features of more than one disease, while the unshaded areas represent each disease in the predominantly pure form. For purposes of clarity, asthma is here considered separately from chronic bronchitis and emphysema, since it is more easily separated from the other two diseases.

Asthma

The term *asthma* comes from the Greek word for "panting" and means attacks of shortness of breath. Although in the past this term has been used for the clinical picture of shortness of breath resulting from any cause, today it is confined to a condition of abnormal responsiveness of the air passages to certain substances.

FIGURE 34-1
Interrelationships between the disease entities composing COPD.

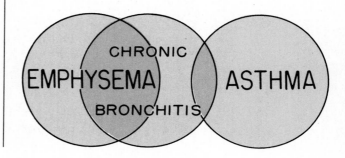

The pathologic changes involved in airway obstruction are found in the medium-sized bronchi and in bronchioles as small as 1 mm in diameter. Airway narrowing is caused by bronchospasm, mucosal edema, and hypersecretion of viscous mucus (see Fig. 34-2).

Asthma can be divided into three categories. *Extrinsic,* or *allergic, asthma,* found in a minority of patients, is clearly caused by a known allergen. This form generally begins in childhood in a member of a family with a history of atopic diseases including hay fever, eczema, and dermatitis as well as asthma. Allergic asthma results from the sensitization of such a person to an allergen, usually a protein, in the form of an inhaled pollen, animal dander, mold spore, feather dust, lint, or, less commonly, to a food such as milk or chocolate. Exposure to the allergen, even in minute quantities, produces an asthmatic attack. *Intrinsic,* or *idiopathic, asthma,* on the other hand, is characterized by the absence of clearly defined precipitating factors. Such nonspecific factors as the common cold, exercise, or emotion may trigger the asthmatic attack. The intrinsic type of asthma is more apt to develop after the age of 40, with the onset of attacks after infections of the nasal sinuses or tracheobronchial tree. The attacks become more frequent and severe as time goes on, and the condition merges into chronic bronchitis and, sometimes, emphysema. *Mixed asthma* is a form of asthma afflicting the majority of patients and is composed of components of both extrinsic and intrinsic types. Often patients with intrinsic asthma later develop the mixed type; children who have the extrinsic type often have complete recovery at adolescence.

The pathogenesis of asthma is discussed in Chap. 10 of this book. The clinical manifestations are easy to recognize. After exposure to the causative allergen or precipitating factor, dyspnea may begin suddenly. Patients feel as if they are suffocating and must stand or sit up and devote all their energy to breathing. On the basis of the anatomic changes which have been described, it is apparent that the major difficulty is with expiration. The tracheobronchial tree widens and lengthens during inspiration, but it is difficult to force air out of the constricted, edematous, mucus-filled bronchioles, which normally contract to a certain degree during expiration. Air is trapped distal to the obstruction, so that there is progressive hyperinflation of the lungs. Prolonged wheezing expirations are thus characteristic as the patient struggles to force the air out. It is usual for an asthmatic attack to last from a few minutes to several hours, followed by a cough which is productive of considerable whitish sputum. Treatment consists in administration of bronchodilator drugs, specific long-term desensitization, avoidance of known allergens, and occasionally corticosteroid drugs. Intervals between attacks are characteristically free from respiratory difficulty. Asthma is distinguished from chronic bronchitis and emphysema by its intermittent nature and the fact that destructive emphysema rarely occurs. An occasional asthmatic attack known as *status asthmaticus,* however, may be sustained for days and be intractable to ordinary methods of treatment. In these cases, ventilatory function may be so impaired as to result in cyanosis and death.

Chronic bronchitis and emphysema

The main pathologic findings in chronic bronchitis are hypertrophy of the bronchial mucosal glands and an increase in the number of goblet cells, accompanied by inflammatory cell infiltration and edema of the bronchial mucosa. The resulting increased production of mucus leads to the characteristic symptoms of cough and expectoration. The chronic cough in the presence of increased bronchial secretions appears to affect the minute bronchioles to the point of destruction and dilatation of their walls. The prime etiologic factors seem to be cigarette smoking and the forms of air pollution common to the industrial environment. Continued air pollution also predisposes to recurrent infections by

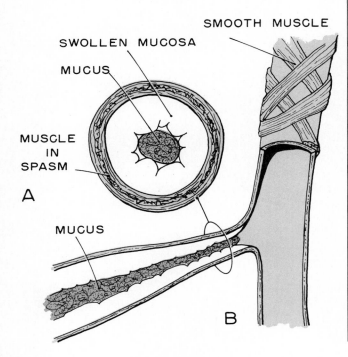

SMOOTH MUSCLE

SWOLLEN MUCOSA

MUCUS

MUSCLE
IN
SPASM

A

MUCUS

B

FIGURE 34-2

Factors causing expiratory obstruction in bronchial asthma. (*A*) Cross section of bronchiole occluded by muscle spasm, swollen mucosa, and mucus in lumen; (*B*) longitudinal section of bronchiole.

slowing down ciliary and phagocytic activity, causing increased mucus accumulation at the same time as defense mechanisms are weakened.

Two types of emphysema are recognized in relation to COPD. *Centrilobular emphysema* (CLE) selectively affects the respiratory bronchioles. Fenestrations develop in the walls, enlarge, become confluent, and tend to form a single space as the walls disintegrate (see Fig. 34-3). Initially, the more distal alveolar ducts and sacs and the alveoli are preserved. This disease commonly affects the upper portions of the lung more severely, but it tends to be unevenly distributed. Centrilobular emphysema is more prevalent in males than in females. It is usually associated with chronic bronchitis and is seldom found in nonsmokers.

Panlobular emphysema (PLE), or *panacinar emphysema*, is a less common morphologic pattern in which there is nearly uniform enlargement and destruction of the alveoli distal to the terminal bronchiole (see Fig. 34-3). As the disease progresses there is gradual loss of all components of the acinus until only a few strands of tissue remain, which are usually blood vessels. PLE

is characteristically uniform in distribution throughout the lung, although the basal sections tend to be more severely affected. PLE, but not CLE, is associated with a small group of patients with primary emphysema. This form of emphysema is characterized by the insidious development of increased airway resistance without evidence of chronic bronchitis. It has an early onset and usually produces symptoms between the ages of 30 and 40 years. In England, less than 6 percent of patients with COPD have primary emphysema, which affects females as often as males. The cause of this form of emphysema is unknown, but a familial kind associated with a deficiency of the enzyme α_1-antitrypsin has been described.

α_1-Antitrypsin is an antiprotease. It has been hypothesized that α_1-antitrypsin is essential in protection against the naturally occurring proteases (Cherniack and Cherniack, 1983, p. 288). Proteases are produced by bacteria, polymorphonuclear leukocytes, monocytes, and macrophages during the phagocytic process (see Chap. 4) and have the ability to break down the elastin and other macromolecules in lung tissue. In the healthy person, lung tissue damage is prevented by the action of antiproteases, which inhibit protease activity. Certain persons may inherit α_1-antitrypsin deficiency as an autosomal recessive trait (Guenter and Buchan, 1977, p. 560). Homozygotes (type ZZ) with two abnormal genes

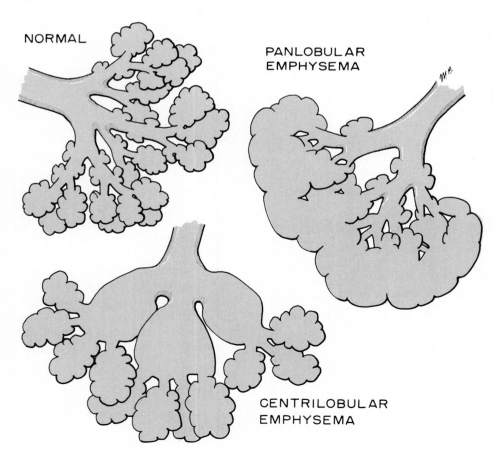

NORMAL

PANLOBULAR EMPHYSEMA

CENTRILOBULAR EMPHYSEMA

FIGURE 34-3

Morphologic types of emphysema: panlobular— entire primary lobule involved, destruction and distention distal to the respiratory bronchioles; centrilobular— destruction is central, primarily involving the respiratory bronchioles.

have less than 10 percent of the normal amount of α_1-antitrypsin and have a 70 to 80 percent chance of developing emphysema of the primary type (panlobular, or emphysematous). Heterozygotes (type MZ) with one abnormal gene have 60 percent of the normal amount of α_1-antitrypsin and are believed to have an increased predisposition to develop emphysema, usually of the bronchitic type (centrilobular). In persons in the latter group, smoking can produce an inflammatory response with the consequent release of proteolytic enzymes (proteases), while at the same time the oxidants in smoke inhibit α_1-antitrypsin (Cherniack and Cherniack, 1983, p. 153).

Panlobular emphysema, although characteristic of primary emphysema, may also be associated with the emphysema of aging and with chronic bronchitis. It is believed that the deterioration of the elastic and reticular fibers of the lung, with the resultant loss of elastic recoil of the lung, leads to progressive generalized distention of the lung in the aging process. Senile emphysema, however, is not true emphysema, since most of these elderly patients do not develop significant impairment of lung function. The panlobular emphysema associated with chronic bronchitis is thought to be an end stage of progressive centrilobular emphysema, since both morphologic patterns may exist in the same lung.

When the thorax of a patient who has emphysema is opened during surgery or at autopsy, the lungs are seen to be grossly enlarged; they remain filled with air and do not collapse. They are whiter than normal and feel downy or billowy. Subpleural air-filled spaces called *blebs* and parenchymal air-filled spaces greater than 1 cm in diameter called *bullae* are commonly seen (see Fig. 34-4). There is also generalized dilatation of the air spaces. Bullae are common in both PLE and CLE but may exist in the absence of either. Bullae generally develop because of a check-valve bronchiolar obstruction (see Fig. 34-5). During inspiration, the bronchiolar lumen widens so that air is able to pass by the obstruction caused by thickening of the mucosa and excess mucus. During expiration, however, when the bronchiolar lumen normally becomes narrowed the obstruction may prevent the egress of air. A loss of elasticity of

FIGURE 34-4
Pulmonary blebs and bullae.

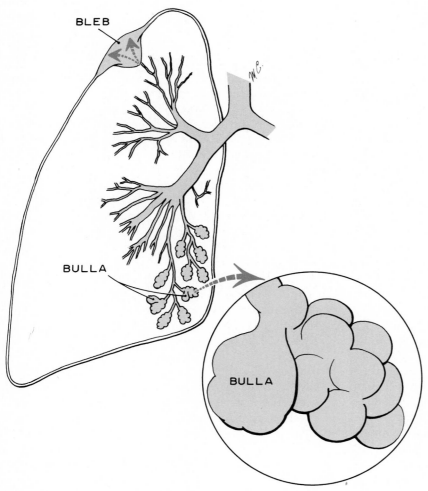

BLEB

BULLA

BULLA

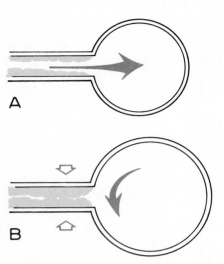

FIGURE 34-5
Check-valve bronchiolar obstruction. (A) During inspiration, lumen widens enough to allow air entry. (B) During expiration, premature collapse and narrowed lumen prevent egress of air which becomes trapped in the alveoli.

the bronchiolar walls in emphysema may also cause premature collapse. Air is thus trapped in the affected pulmonary segment, leading to overdistention and coalescence of several alveoli. This is caused by fragmentation of the interalveolar elastic tissue and subsequent rupture of the attenuated interalveolar septa, resulting in a bulla. In emphysema there may be a single bulla or many, which may or may not communicate with each other. Blebs, which are formed by ruptured alveoli, may rupture into the pleural cavity and cause a spontaneous pneumothorax (collapse of the lung). Other changes commonly seen in the COPD lung are a reduction in the capillary bed and histologic evidence of chronic bronchiolitis (involvement of the minute bronchioles).

The flow diagram in Fig. 34-6 illustrates the pathogenesis of COPD and the morphologic types of emphysema which result. This diagram emphasizes the fact that while a genetic predisposition may be a factor in the development of pulmonary emphysema, and smoking and air pollution are the prime factors in the pathogenesis of the bronchitic type of emphysema, there is an interaction between the two. For example, persons with a genetic predisposition might develop emphysema if exposed to varying degrees of air pollution. Although senile dilatation of the air spaces is not considered true emphysema, it is possible that normal loss of elasticity of the lung parenchyma associated with aging is a factor in the development of true emphysema.

The clinical course of patients with COPD ranges

from what is known as the *pink puffers* to the *blue bloaters*. The clinical hallmark of pink puffers (associated with primary panlobular emphysema) is the development of dyspnea without significant cough and sputum production. Usually the dyspnea begins between the ages of 30 and 40 years and becomes increasingly severe. In advanced disease the patient may be too breathless to eat and characteristically has a thin, wasted appearance. Later on in the course of the disease, the pink puffer may develop secondary chronic bronchitis. The chest of the patient is barrel-shaped; the diaphragm is low and moves poorly. Polycythemia and cyanosis are rare (hence the term *pink*), and cor pulmonale (heart disease resulting from pulmonary hypertension and lung disease) rarely develops until the terminal stage. There is minimal ventilation-perfusion imbalance, so that by hyperventilating, the pink puffer is usually able to keep blood gases within the normal range until late in the course of the disease. The lungs are usually greatly enlarged, so that there is a large increase in total lung capacity and residual volume.

At the other extreme of the COPD range are the blue bloaters (bronchitis with little evidence of obstructive emphysema). These patients usually have a productive cough and frequent respiratory infections which continue for years before there is noticeable functional impairment. Eventually, however, they develop dyspnea on exertion. These patients show a diminished respiratory drive; they hypoventilate and become hypoxic and hypercapnic. There is also a markedly distorted ventilation/perfusion ratio. The chronic hypoxia stimulates the kidney to produce erythropoietin, which in turn stimulates increased production of red blood cells, resulting in secondary polycythemia. Hemoglobin levels may be 20 g per 100 ml or more, and cyanosis is more readily apparent, since there may easily be 5 g per 100 ml of reduced hemoglobin when only a small proportion of the circulating blood hemoglobin is in the reduced form (hence the name *blue bloater*). As these patients are not dyspneic at rest, they appear to be comfortable. There is generally not a great weight loss, and body build is normal. The total lung capacity may be normal, and the diaphragm is in the normal position. Death usually results from cor pulmonale (which develops early) or from respiratory failure. At autopsy, emphysema is often, although not always, seen. The emphysema tends to be of the centrilobular type, although the panlobular type may also be present.

Table 34-1 contrasts the pure bronchitic (blue bloater) and emphysematous (pink puffer) types of COPD. Most patients with COPD lie somewhere between these two extremes.

The typical course of COPD is a long one, beginning in the twenties and thirties with a "cigarette cough" or "morning cough" and the production of a small amount of mucoid sputum. Minor respiratory infections tend to persist longer than usual in these pa-

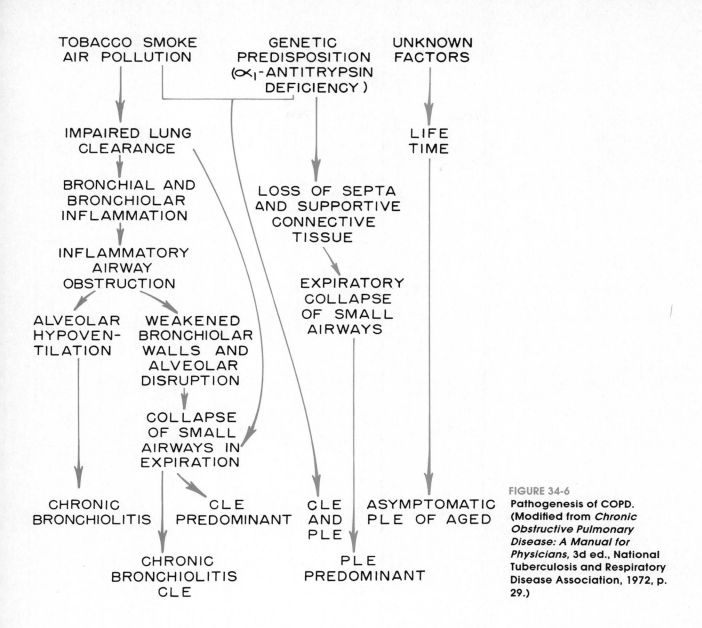

FIGURE 34-6

Pathogenesis of COPD. (Modified from *Chronic Obstructive Pulmonary Disease: A Manual for Physicians*, 3d ed., National Tuberculosis and Respiratory Disease Association, 1972, p. 29.)

tients. Although there may be some decrease in exercise tolerance, it usually goes unnoticed as the patient becomes less energetic with the passage of time. Eventually episodes of acute bronchitis occur more regularly, particularly in the winter, and the patient's working capacity decreases, so that work may have to be given up sometime in the patient's fifties or sixties. In patients of the predominantly emphysematous type, the course appears to be less protracted, with no previous history of a productive cough; severe debilitating dyspnea may develop within a few years. When hypercapnia, hypoxemia, and cor pulmonale develop, the prognosis is poor, and death usually comes within a few years after the onset. A combination of respiratory and heart failure precipitated by pneumonia is the usual cause of death.

Therapy for the patient with chronic bronchitis and obstructive emphysema requires measures to relieve obstruction of the small airways. Although airway collapse secondary to emphysema is irreversible, many patients have some degree of bronchospasm, retention of secretions, and mucosal edema which may be relieved by the appropriate therapy. Of paramount importance is cessation of smoking and avoidance of other forms of air pollution or allergens which may aggravate the symptoms. Often the cessation of smoking alone may bring about a marked relief of symptoms and improvement of ventilation. Infection should be treated promptly, and patients who are particularly susceptible to respiratory infection may be directed to use prophylactic antibiotics. The patient is instructed to seek this medication whenever dyspnea or the amount of sputum production increases. Tetracycline, ampicillin, and penicillin are usually the drugs of choice. All patients should receive influenza vaccine.

Additional measures to relieve airway obstruction include providing adequate hydration to thin bronchial secretions, use of expectorants, and bronchodilator drugs to relieve smooth muscle spasm. Sympathomimetic drugs such as isoproterenol, epinephrine, ephedrine, and xanthines (such as aminophylline) are commonly administered. In patients with copious secretions, percussion and postural drainage are used to assist in the removal of obstructive secretions which may also predispose to infection. Breathing exercises may also be helpful. The patient is taught to use slow, relaxed expiration against pursed lips. This exercise prevents collapse of small bronchioles and reduces the amount of trapped air. A graduated program of physical exercise during the administration of low concentration oxygen may be helpful in improving the patient's sense of well-being. Oxygen, however, must be administered with *caution* in the later stages of the illness when there is hypercapnia and hypoxemia. Respiratory failure may be precipitated, as these patients depend on hypoxia to stimulate breathing. The treatment of cor pulmonale and respiratory failure complications are discussed in Chaps. 36 and 37.

Two other diseases which may result in an obstructive pattern of pulmonary dysfunction deserve mention in this chapter—bronchiectasis and cystic fibrosis.

BRONCHIECTASIS

Bronchiectasis is a condition characterized by chronic dilatation of the medium-sized bronchi and bronchioles (about fourth to ninth generations). Two anatomic types are commonly described. Saccular bronchiectasis consists in rounded cavitylike dilatations, often found in dilated bronchi and typically in adults. Bronchiectasis develops when the bronchial walls are weakened by chronic inflammatory changes involving the mucosa and muscular coat. As seen in Fig. 34-7, purulent materials collect in these dilated areas and lead to persistent infection of the affected segment or lobe. Chronic infection causes further damage to the bronchial walls, and a vicious circle is set up. There is no single, specific cause of bronchiectasis, as it is a disease based on an abnormal anatomic condition. Most commonly, bronchiectasis begins in childhood following a lower respiratory tract infection which develops as a complication of measles, whooping cough, or influenza. Bronchial obstruction resulting from a neoplasm or an aspirated foreign body (especially if it is organic, such as a peanut) may also lead to bronchiectasis and secondary infection

TABLE 34-1

DIFFERENTIATION OF CLINICAL TYPES OF COPD

Feature	Pink puffer (emphysematous)	Blue bloater (bronchitic)
Onset	30–40 years of age	20s and 30s—cigarette cough Disability in middle age
Etiology	Unknown factors Genetic predisposition Smoking Air pollution	Unknown factors Smoking Air pollution Climate
Sputum	Minimal	Copious
Dyspnea	Relatively early	Relatively late
$\dot{V}/\dot{Q}$ ratio	Minimal $\dot{V}/\dot{Q}$ imbalance	Marked $\dot{V}/\dot{Q}$ imbalance
Body build	Thin, asthenic	Well-nourished
AP diameter of chest	Barrel chest common	Not increased
Pathologic lung anatomy	Panlobular emphysema	Centrilobular emphysema predominant
Respiratory pattern	Hyperventilation and marked dyspnea which may occur at rest	Diminished respiratory drive Hypoventilation common, with resultant hypoxia and hypercapnia
Lung volume	Low FEV_1 Increased TLC and RV	Low FEV_1 Normal TLC; moderate increase in RV
Pa_{CO_2}	Normal or low	Elevated
Sa_{O_2}	Normal	Much desaturation due to $\dot{V}/\dot{Q}$ imbalance
Polycythemia	Hemoglobin and hematocrit normal until late	Elevated hemoglobin and hematocrit common
Cyanosis	Rare	Common
Cor pulmonale	Rare except terminally	Frequent, with many episodes

of the distal bronchial tree. Bronchiectasis of the upper lobes may be associated with tuberculosis, although it is frequently asymptomatic because bronchial drainage is achieved by gravity. Cystic fibrosis and Kartagener's syndrome (bronchiectasis associated with sinusitis and displacement of the heart to the right side of the thorax) are examples of congenital diseases associated with bronchiectasis.

The principal clinical feature of bronchiectasis is a chronic, loose cough productive of a large amount of mucopurulent, foul-smelling sputum. Coughing is most severe when the patient changes position. The amount of sputum varies with the stage of the disease but may be 200 ml daily in severe cases. Hemoptysis is common, usually consisting of blood streaks in the sputum. Characteristic features of advanced untreated disease are recurrent pneumonia, malnutrition, digital clubbing, cor pulmonale, and right ventricular failure.

The degree of functional disturbance depends on the extent of involvement of pulmonary tissue. Bronchiectasis localized to one or two segments of the lung may cause little impairment of pulmonary function, while diffuse bronchiectasis may be associated with anastomoses between the bronchial and pulmonary circulation, with resultant right-to-left shunting.

The most important feature of treatment is daily, vigorous bronchial hygiene with postural drainage, which generally must be continued for the rest of the patient's life. Antibiotic therapy for the control of infection is another important aspect of therapy. Before the advent of antibiotics, bronchiectasis was much more common and the prognosis was poor. Patients rarely lived beyond the age of 40 years. Bronchiectasis is much less common today and, except for the congenital forms of the disease, should be regarded as preventable. Timely vaccinations against childhood diseases commonly complicated by pneumonia, vigorous antibiotic and other appropriate treatment of pneumonia, and prompt removal of aspirated foreign bodies are all preventive measures.

CYSTIC FIBROSIS

Cystic fibrosis, or *mucoviscidosis*, is a disease of genetic origin, occurring in about 1 out of 2000 births among whites but rarely seen in blacks. The secretions of the exocrine glands that produce mucus and some other exocrine fluids produce abnormally viscid secretions. (The sweat and saliva are not particularly viscid but do contain abnormal amounts of salt.) The viscid secretions commonly cause obstruction of the pancreatic and hepatic ducts and the bronchioles. The obstruction, in

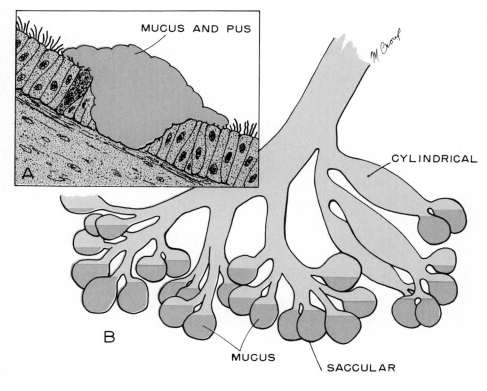

MUCUS AND PUS

A

CYLINDRICAL

B

MUCUS

SACCULAR

FIGURE 34-7
Pathologic changes in bronchiectasis. (A) Longitudinal section of bronchial wall—chronic infection causes damage to the bronchial walls. (B) Collection of purulent material in dilated bronchioles leading to persistent infection.

turn, can lead to fibrotic changes in the involved organs. A few patients may live to be adults, but survival does not generally extend beyond adolescence. Accompanying respiratory disease and complications account for over 90 percent of the deaths from this disease. The sequence of events proceeds from recurrent pulmonary infections that gradually develop into bronchiectasis from retention of thick secretions, to chronic pneumonia, fibrosis, ventilation-perfusion imbalance, chronic hypoxemia, cor pulmonale, and respiratory failure. Since pulmonary dysfunction is the overriding factor in determining survival, the management of this aspect of the disease is crucial, with removal of the obstructing bronchial secretions as the most crucial aspect of treatment. Generally, aerosol therapy is used to liquefy secretions and is followed by percussion and postural drainage. Prevention of infection and its prompt treatment are also important.

QUESTIONS

Obstructive patterns of respiratory disease

Directions: Answer the following questions on a separate sheet of paper.

1. What is the ventilatory functional disorder associated with COPD?

2. Describe the interrelation of chronic bronchitis, pulmonary emphysema, and asthma.

3. Describe the symptoms of an asthmatic attack. How is it treated? What is *status asthmaticus?*

4. Contrast the two morphologic patterns of emphysema according to anatomic changes, distribution in lung, sex prevalence, type of associated COPD, and etiology.

5. What are the objectives of treatment for chronic bronchitis and emphysema?

6. What are the two criteria for establishing a diagnosis of chronic bronchitis? What is the period of time within which these symptoms must be manifested (months per year and consecutive years)?

7. Describe the pathologic anatomic changes in the lung parenchyma in pulmonary emphysema.

8. What are subpleural air-filled spaces called? What is their cause?

9. What are parenchymal air-filled spaces more than 1 cm in diameter called? What generally causes them?

10. How does the tracheobronchial tree of the asthmatic patient respond to various stimuli? How is this manifested?

11. What anatomic changes occur in bronchiectasis? What are some possible precipitating factors, and what features tend to cause persistence and progression of the disease?

12. What are the principal clinical features of bronchiectasis?

13. Identify the mode of treatment for bronchiectasis.

14. What is the most crucial aspect of treatment of cystic fibrosis?

15. Match each of the diseases in col. A with its basis for definition in col. B.

Column A	Column B
____ Chronic bronchitis	a. Pathologic anatomy
	b. Clinical symptoms
____ Pulmonary emphysema	c. Pathophysiology
____ Asthma	

Directions: Circle the letter preceding each item below that correctly completes the statement. More than one item may be correct.

16. The pathologic changes associated with chronic bronchitis include:
a. Hypertrophy of the bronchial mucosal glands *b.* Destruction of alveolar walls *c.* Increase in the number of goblet cells *d.* Edema, scarring, and increased thickness of bronchioles *e.* Decreased production of surfactant

17. In bronchial asthma:
a. Bronchiolar smooth muscle is atrophic *b.* Medium and small-sized bronchi are plugged with viscid mucus *c.* The lungs are pale and emphysematous *d.* The patient is usually free from symptoms between attacks

18. Emphysema is an anatomic entity which:
a. Has one basic morphologic pattern *b.* Causes serious respiratory insufficiency when it develops as a result of the aging process *c.* Is characterized by increased size of the air spaces distal to the terminal bronchioles with associated parenchymal destruction *d.* Is always related to chronic bronchitis

19. The major source of disability and death in pediatric patients with cystic fibrosis is:
    a. Malnutrition   *b.* Recurrent pulmonary infection   *c.* Hyponatremia resulting from the loss of salt in sweat and saliva   *d.* Chronic pancreatitis

20. Centrilobular emphysema:
    a. Is more common than PLE   *b.* Appears to be related to cigarette smoking   *c.* Usually affects the upper lobes more severely   *d.* Is associated with deficiency of α_1-antitrypsin

21. The pathophysiology of asthma is characterized by:
    a. Bronchodilatation   *b.* Alveoli filled with exudate   *c.* Loss of support of bronchiolar walls   *d.* Bronchiolar narrowing

Directions: Circle T if the statement is true and F if it is false in regard to cystic fibrosis. Correct the false statements.

22. T   F   *Mucoviscidosis* is another name for the disease.

23. T   F   It is a disease of genetic origin.

24. T   F   It is more common in blacks than in whites.

25. T   F   Up to 200 ml of mucopurulent, foul-smelling sputum may be produced daily.

26. T   F   The exocrine glands are affected by this disease.

27. T   F   Digital clubbing is a characteristic feature of advanced disease.

28. T   F   The prognosis of cystic fibrosis is generally good.

Directions: Match the pink puffer and blue bloater types of COPD in col. B to their associated features in col. A.

Column A

29. ____ PLE

30. ____ CLE predominant

Column B

a. Pink puffer

b. Blue bloater

31. ____ Genetic predisposition

32. ____ Late onset of dyspnea

33. ____ Minimal sputum

34. ____ Polycythemia common

35. ____ Early cor pulmonale

36. ____ Marked $\dot{V}/\dot{Q}$ imbalance

37. ____ Thin, wasted appearance

38. ____ Hypercapnia (early)

Directions: Match the type of asthmatic condition in col. A with the appropriate descriptive features in col. B. Each item in col. B may be used more than once.

Column A

39. ____ Extrinsic asthma

40. ____ Intrinsic asthma

41. ____ Mixed asthma

Column B

a. Absence of clearly defined precipitating factor

b. Clearly caused by a known allergen; usually develops in early childhood

c. Attacks may be associated with infection of the tracheobronchial tree or of the nasal sinuses

d. Afflicts the majority of patients

e. Exposure to the allergen precipitates an asthmatic attack

CHAPTER
35

RESTRICTIVE PATTERNS OF RESPIRATORY DISEASE

OBJECTIVES

At the completion of this chapter you should be able to:

1. State the physiologic consequences of a restricted pattern of ventilation.
2. Describe at least two extrapulmonary diseases or altered conditions causing alveolar hypoventilation and identify the mechanism responsible for the altered conditions in the following systems or structures: central nervous system, peripheral nervous system, muscular system, and chest cage.
3. List four types of fixed chest wall deformities.
4. Differentiate between kyphosis and scoliosis.
5. Identify the relation of the four types of fixed chest wall deformities to respiratory failure.
6. State the relation between the Pickwickian syndrome and respiratory insufficiency.
7. Describe the effect that multiple rib fractures (flail chest) has on respiration.
8. Define *pleural effusion*.
9. Differentiate between a pleural effusion which is a transudate and one which is an exudate.
10. Define the following terms: *hydrothorax, empyema, hemothorax,* and *chylothorax*.
11. State the possible consequences of inadequately treated empyema.
12. Define *pneumothorax*.
13. List the three classes of pneumothorax according to cause and give examples of each.
14. Differentiate between open, closed, and tension pneumothorax.
15. Describe the complications and treatment of a penetrating chest wound.
16. Explain why pneumothorax occurs.
17. State the most common cause of idiopathic spontaneous pneumothorax in young people.

18. Differentiate between the signs and symptoms of pneumothorax and pleural effusion.

19. Describe the treatment for pneumothorax and pleural effusion.

20. List several conditions that result in damage to lung alveoli and interstitium and identify the specific damage to lung tissue caused by each disorder.

21. Describe two physiologic abnormalities seen in patients with disease of the lung parenchyma.

22. Define *atelectasis*.

23. Differentiate between absorption and compression atelectasis on the basis of cause and mechanism involved.

24. Explain how collateral ventilation prevents absorption atelectasis.

25. Assess the importance of measures used to prevent atelectasis in predisposed persons.

26. List four lung defense mechanisms which play a role in the prevention of atelectasis and factors which interfere with these defense mechanisms.

27. Identify the morbidity and mortality from pneumonia for susceptible population groups.

28. Describe four anatomic patterns of pneumonitis or pneumonia, the micropathologic changes, and the common infecting agent.

29. Identify and describe the four stages in the pathologic response to pneumococcal pneumonia by the name of the stage, the time period, and the lung changes for each stage.

30. Describe the signs, symptoms, physical findings, treatment, and prognosis of pneumococcal pneumonia.

31. List the common complications and prognosis of pneumonias caused by gram-negative or staphylococcus organisms.

32. Describe the symptoms, treatment, complications, and prognosis of pneumonias caused by viruses or *Mycoplasma pneumoniae*.

33. Differentiate between aspiration and hypostatic pneumonia.

34. Name the three most common fungal infections causing lung disease in the United States.

35. Identify the most common causes of diffuse pulmonary fibrosis.

36. List the criteria used to determine whether a particular dust will cause disease of the lung parenchyma.

37. Describe the mechanism causing pulmonary fibrosis; include inorganic and organic dusts and noxious gases.

38. Describe the pulmonary manifestations of diffuse pulmonary fibrosis.

EXTRAPULMONARY DISEASE

A restrictive ventilatory disorder is characterized by increased stiffness of the lungs or thorax or both, resulting from decreased compliance and a reduction in all lung volumes, including the vital capacity. There is an increase in the work of breathing to overcome the elastic forces of the respiratory apparatus, so a pattern of rapid, shallow breathing is adopted. The physiologic consequences of a restricted pattern of ventilation are alveolar hypoventilation and an inability to maintain normal blood gas tensions.

A number of diseases may contribute to pulmonary restriction through varying mechanisms. In this chapter, these diseases are divided into two classes: extrapulmonary disorders, including neurologic, neuromuscular, and thoracic cage disorders, and diseases of the pleura and lung parenchyma.

Neurologic and neuromuscular disorders

In reference to extrapulmonary disorders, the term *extrapulmonary* implies that the lung tissue itself may be quite normal. The common pathophysiologic disturbance in these disorders is alveolar hypoventilation, although this is not entirely true in the case of kyphoscoliosis.

A number of disorders directly affecting the medullary respiratory center may cause alveolar hypoventilation. Carbon dioxide retention from a variety of causes may depress rather than stimulate respiration when the Pa_{CO_2} exceeds about 70 mmHg. A number of drugs are capable of depressing the respiratory center and thereby causing alveolar hypoventilation. For example, narcotic or barbiturate drug overdose is a common cause of death due to respiratory depression and failure. Anatomic damage to the respiratory center re-

sulting from head trauma or cerebral lesions caused by a cerebral vascular accident can also cause respiratory center depression and alveolar hypoventilation. Abnormalities of neural or neuromuscular transmission to the respiratory muscles may result in paresis or paralysis and alveolar hypoventilation. Amyotrophic lateral sclerosis, poliomyelitis, Guillain-Barré syndrome, and myasthenia gravis are all neurologic disorders which may produce ventilatory insufficiency. The muscles themselves are diseased in progressive muscular dystrophy. The severity of the respiratory involvement in any of the above diseases depends on the amount of anatomic involvement: vital capacity is reduced in proportion to the degree of paresis of the respiratory muscles. Although parenchymal lung disease is not primary, secondary infection is frequent because of ineffective coughing and limitation of respiratory excursions. Table 35-1 summarizes the extrapulmonary disorders causing alveolar hypoventilation and the mechanism responsible.

Thoracic cage disorders

Four major types of fixed chest wall deformities may restrict ventilation by interfering with the bellows mechanism: kyphoscoliosis, pectus excavatum, ankylosing spondylitis, and healed thoracoplasty.

Kyphosis is a term which refers to any posterior angulation of the spine (hunchback), and *scoliosis* refers to a lateral displacement of the spine. Kyphoscoliosis is,

TABLE 35-1

EXTRAPULMONARY DISORDERS CAUSING ALVEOLAR HYPOVENTILATION

System or structure	Disease or altered condition	Altered mechanism
Neurologic (central nervous system)	$Pa_{CO_2} > 70$ mmHg	Depression of the respiratory center
	Narcotics and barbiturates	
	Head trauma, CNS lesions	Direct anatomic damage to the respiratory center
	Poliomyelitis	Interruption of nerve transmission to respiratory muscles due to lower motor neuron lesion
	Amyotrophic lateral sclerosis	Interruption of nerve transmission to respiratory muscles due to upper motor neuron lesion
Neurologic (peripheral nervous system)	Guillain-Barré syndrome	Interruption of nerve transmission to respiratory muscles due to inflammation involving ganglion cells and peripheral nerves
	Myasthenia gravis	Interruption of nerve transmission to respiratory muscles due to disease involving the neuromuscular junction
Muscular	Progressive muscular dystrophy	Paresis of the respiratory muscles due to diffuse disease of the skeletal muscles
Chest cage	Kyphoscoliosis	Deformity of the chest cage causing abnormal positioning and functioning of the respiratory muscles and compression of the chest cage contents
	Closed chest wall trauma	Voluntary restriction of ventilation due to pain or paradoxical movement of the chest wall and thoracic contents in flail chest injury
	Pickwickian syndrome (extreme obesity)	Limitation of thoracic movement by accumulated body fat

therefore, characterized by angulation of the spine both posteriorly and laterally. About 80 percent of the cases are idiopathic, while the remaining 20 percent result from the aftereffects of poliomyelitis or tuberculosis of the spine (Pott's disease). Kyphoscoliosis is quite common, with about 1 percent of the American population affected, although the defect is severe enough to produce cardiopulmonary symptoms in only a small proportion of these persons. Severe kyphoscoliosis is associated with marked asymmetry of the chest and leads to abnormal functioning and positioning of the respiratory muscles and to compression of the lungs.

The sequence of events which may lead to both respiratory and cardiac failure in kyphoscoliosis is shown in Fig. 35-1). In these persons, breathing entails a high work and energy cost, so that a rapid, shallow pattern is adopted. This in turn leads to alveolar hypoventilation by preferential ventilation of the anatomic dead space at the expense of alveolar ventilation. In addition, compression of the lungs by the thoracic deformity causes a small lung volume and unequal distribution of ventilation and perfusion, since both alveoli and pulmonary blood vessels are compressed. The consequent physiologic shunting leads to hypoxemia. When alveolar ventilation is also limited, the result is hypoxemia, hypercapnia, and respiratory acidosis. Compression of the pulmonary blood vessels and the acidosis also lead to pulmonary hypertension and cor pulmonale. The common cause of death from this chain of events is a combination of respiratory and heart failure.

Pectus excavatum (funnel chest) is a congenital deformity in which the lower end of the sternum is attached to the thoracic spine by fibromuscular bands, giving the lower sternal area a caved-in appearance. Compare this deformity with kyphoscoliosis in Fig. 35-2. Pectus excavatum, unlike severe kyphoscoliosis, rarely causes more than mild restriction of ventilation.

Thoracoplasty is a surgically induced depression of the thoracic cage which was performed for the treatment of tuberculosis in the past but is no longer common. Since this procedure is performed for an underlying lung disease, the subsequent pulmonary dysfunction is usually more closely related to the original disease than to the induced deformity.

Ankylosing spondylitis is a disease which causes symmetrical reduction in mobility of the bony thorax as a result of the ossification of the vertebral joints and ligaments. Rib fixation and increased stiffness of the chest wall cause mild ventilatory restriction, which is not usually symptomatic.

Closed chest wall injury may also restrict ventilation. The most common chest wall injury is simple rib fracture. As a result of the pain and muscle splinting, there is ventilatory restriction of tidal volume, increase in respiratory rate and frequency, and voluntary inhi-

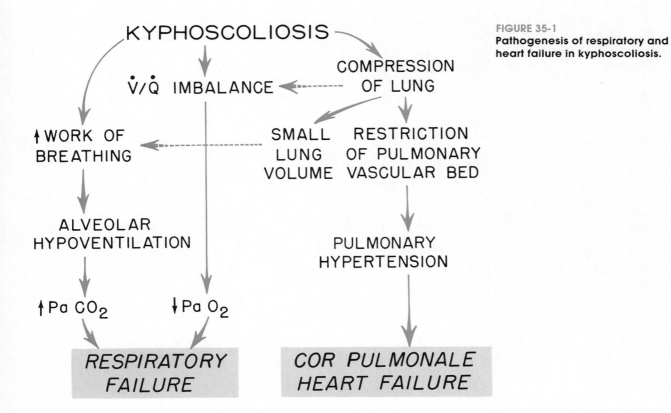

FIGURE 35-1
Pathogenesis of respiratory and heart failure in kyphoscoliosis.

a major defect in chest wall continuity caused by a crushing chest injury (commonly seen in steering wheel injuries in auto accidents) with multiple rib fractures. The resulting instability of the chest wall causes a paradoxical movement of the chest wall accompanied by pendulum movement of the mediastinal contents during the breathing cycle. This condition may cause interference with venous return to the heart and cause dead-space air to be shunted back and forth between the lungs (*pendelluft*), as illustrated in Fig. 35-3. The treatment for flail chest is stabilization of the chest wall and mechanical ventilation.

Pickwickian syndrome is the term used to describe a group of clinical features found in persons who are extremely obese. These features include chronic alveolar hypoventilation, somnolence, polycythemia, hypoxemia, and hypercapnia. (The syndrome was named after the sleepy fat boy in Dickens's *Pickwick Papers*.) The somnolence common to this syndrome can be related to the carbon dioxide retention which depresses the central nervous system; polycythemia is the compensatory response to chronic hypoxia. In persons with the Pickwickian syndrome, the accumulated body fat appears to limit thoracic movement and greatly increases the work of breathing. It is not uncommon for respiratory impairment to progress to the point of cor pulmonale and respiratory failure. It is now known that the Pickwickian syndrome is only one subtype of a group of disorders called *sleep apnea syndromes,* in which elements of upper airway obstruction (which results in snoring) or central hypoventilation or both may be present (Blum, 1983; Fairbanks, 1984). It is also known that nonobese persons may be afflicted. It is important to note also that not all extremely obese persons develop alveolar hypoventilation and blood gas abnormalities. Weight reduction, if successful, seems to be the most effective treatment for the Pickwickian syndrome and may reverse the respiratory insufficiency.

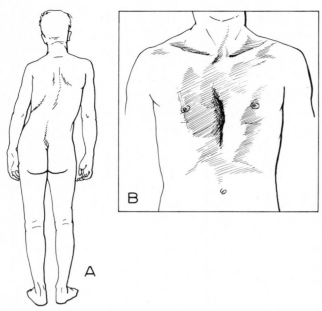
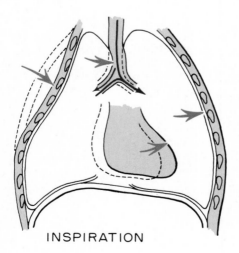

FIGURE 35-2
Thoracic deformities restricting ventilation. (A) Kyphoscoliosis. (B) Pectus excavatum (funnel chest).

bition of the cough reflex. Chest strapping and administration of narcotics further restrict the chest movement and depress the respiratory center and cough reflex, thus compounding the problem. Healthy young persons tend to tolerate these changes well, but in elderly persons, these changes may lead to impaired clearing of secretions, respiratory tract infection, blood gas abnormalities, and even respiratory failure. Flail chest is

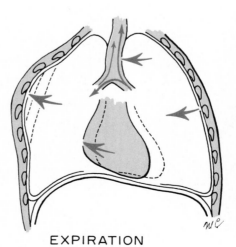

INSPIRATION   EXPIRATION

FIGURE 35-3
Altered cardiopulmonary dynamics in flail chest injury. Arrows indicate the direction of motion; arrows within trachea and bronchi indicate air being shunted back and forth between lungs during respiratory cycle (*pendelluft*). Note the paradoxical motion of the unstable portion of the chest wall on the right side. (After B. Burrows, R. J. Knudson, and L. J. Kettle, *Respiratory Insufficiency*, Year Book, Chicago, 1975, p. 111.)

Pleural disorders

The pleura and pleural space are the site of a number of disorders which may restrict the expansion of the lungs or the alveoli or both. This reaction may result from compression of the lung as a result of the accumulation of air, fluid, blood, or purulent material in the pleural cavity. Pain resulting from inflammation or fibrosis of the pleura may also cause limitation of chest expansion.

Pleural effusion

The parietal and visceral pleura are opposed to each other and are separated by a thin layer of serous fluid. This thin layer of fluid represents a balance between transudation from the pleural capillaries and reabsorption by the visceral and parietal veins and lymphatics as discussed in Chap. 31. *Pleural effusion* is the term applied to a collection of fluid in the pleural cavity (see Fig. 35-4). Pleural effusions may be transudates or exudates. A *transudate* occurs if there is a rise in pulmonary venous pressure, as in congestive heart failure. In these cases the balance of forces favors the passage of fluid out of the vessels. Transudation may also occur if there is hypoproteinemia, as in liver and renal disease, or pressure from a tumor on the venae cavae. The accumulation of transudate in the pleural cavity is called *hydrothorax*. The pleural fluid tends to accumulate at the base of the lungs as a result of the force of gravity. The accumulation of an *exudate* is secondary to involvement of the pleura by inflammation or malignant growth and results from increased capillary permeability or impaired lymphatic absorption. An exudate is differentiated from a transudate by the protein content and specific gravity of the pleural fluid. Transudates have a specific gravity of less than 1.015 and a protein content of less than 3 percent, while exudates have a higher specific gravity and protein content because of their cellular content.

When the pleural effusion contains pus, the condition is termed *empyema*. Empyema is the result of extension of infection from contiguous structures and may be a complication of pneumonia, lung abscess, or perforation of a carcinoma into the pleural cavity. Empyema which is not adequately treated by drainage may have disastrous effects on the thoracic cage. The inflammatory exudate becomes organized, and fibrous adhesions weld the parietal and visceral pleura together. This condition is termed *fibrothorax* (see Fig. 35-4). If the fibrothorax is extensive, it may cause serious mechanical restriction of the underlying tissue. Surgical peeling, called *decortication*, is sometimes necessary to separate the pleural membranes.

The term *hemothorax* is used to designate frank bleeding into the pleural cavity and does not designate a hemorrhagic pleural effusion. Trauma is the most common cause of hemothorax. The trauma may be classified as penetrating (e.g., knife wound) or nonpenetrating (e.g., fractured rib which in turn lacerates the lung or an intercostal blood vessel). The thoracic duct can also drain lymph into the pleural cavity as a result of trauma or malignant tumor; this condition is termed *chylothorax*.

Pneumothorax

The presence of air in the pleural cavity caused by a breach in the pleura is termed *pneumothorax*. A pneu-

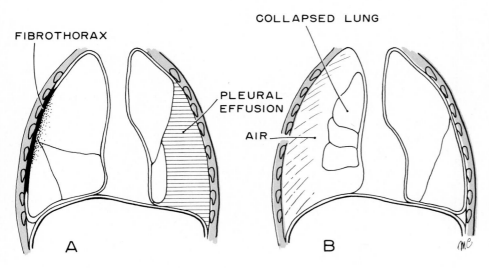

FIBROTHORAX

COLLAPSED LUNG

PLEURAL EFFUSION

AIR

A

B

FIGURE 35-4
Disorders of the pleura: (A) fibrothorax resulting from organization of inflammatory exudate and pleural effusion; (B) collapse of lung due to open pneumothorax.

mothorax may be classified by cause as (1) traumatic, (2) spontaneous, or (3) therapeutic. It may also be classified, according to the sequence of events which follow the breach in the pleura, as open, closed, or tension pneumothorax.

A penetrating wound to the chest is a common cause of *traumatic pneumothorax*. As the air enters the pleural space, which is normally subatmospheric in pressure, the lung collapses to a variable extent. If the communication is *open*, a massive collapse occurs until the pressure in the pleural cavity is equal to that of the atmosphere (open pneumothorax—see Fig. 35-4). The mediastinum is shifted in the direction of the collapsed lung and may shift to and fro during the respiratory cycle as air moves in and out of the pleural cavity. Emergency treatment of a penetrating chest wound consists in application of an airtight seal immediately over the wound. If the defect causing the communication between the pleural space and the atmosphere seals itself off, it is called a *closed* pneumothorax. On the other hand, if the defect remains open during inspiration and closes during expiration (check valve effect), a large volume of air may collect in the pleural space, so that pressure builds up above that of the atmosphere, causing complete collapse of the lung. This is termed *tension* pneumothorax. Tension pneumothorax is a serious emergency which must be treated immediately by aspiration of air from the pleural cavity.

Spontaneous pneumothorax is the term used to designate a sudden, unexpected pneumothorax which may occur with or without underlying pulmonary disease. Common pulmonary diseases which may cause a spontaneous pneumothorax include emphysema (rupture of blebs or bullae), pneumonia, and neoplasms. A pneumothorax occurs when there is communication between a bronchus or alveolus and the pleural cavity, so that air gains access to the pleural cavity through the defect, which may result in an open, closed, or tension pneumothorax. A spontaneous pneumothorax may occur in apparently healthy young persons, usually between the ages of 20 and 40 years, and is termed *idiopathic spontaneous pneumothorax*. The usual cause is rupture of a subpleural bleb at the surface of the lung or localized bullous disease (refer to Fig. 34-4). The cause of such a bleb or bulla in otherwise healthy persons is unknown, but a familial predisposition has sometimes been reported.

A *therapeutic pneumothorax* deserves brief mention for historical reasons. Induced collapse of the lung (therapeutic pneumothorax) was a common treatment for tuberculosis until about 1960, but it is not done today. It was surmised that this procedure inhibited spread of the disease and growth of the bacteria, although there was no definite evidence to support this notion.

Both pleural effusion and pneumothorax limit function by restricting the expansion of the underlying lung. The degree of functional impairment and disability depends on the size and the rapidity of development. If fluid accumulates slowly, as is usually the case in pleural effusion, a large amount of fluid may be accommodated with little apparent distress. On the other hand, rapid decompression of a lung from a massive pneumothorax may be accompanied by rapid development of shock. The signs and symptoms of pleural effusion and pneumothorax are summarized in Table 35-2. The presence of both conditions is confirmed by x-ray.

A first pneumothorax is treated by conservative observation if the collapse is 20 percent or less. The air is gradually absorbed through the pleural surfaces, which act as wet membranes allowing oxygen and carbon dioxide to diffuse through them. If the pneumothorax is large and dyspnea severe, a thoractomy tube attached to water-sealed drainage will be necessary to aid reexpansion of the lung. If bloody effusion is associated with pneumothorax, it must be removed by drainage, because clotting and organization lead to extensive pleural fibrosis. A pleural effusion is treated by needle aspiration (thoracentesis). This is particularly important if the effusion is an exudate, since fibrothorax may result. A small, noninflammatory effusion (transudate) may be resorbed into the capillaries once the cause of the effusion has been reversed.

TABLE 35-2

SIGNS AND SYMPTOMS OF PLEURAL EFFUSION AND PNEUMOTHORAX

Pleural effusion	Pneumothorax
Dyspnea variable	Dyspnea (if large)
Pleuritic pain usually precedes effusion if secondary to pleuritic disease	Pleuritic pain severe
Trachea deviated away from the side of effusion	Trachea deviated away from the side of pneumothorax
Bulging of intercostal spaces (large effusion)	Tachycardia
	Cyanosis (if large)
Diminished and delayed chest movement on the involved side	Diminished and delayed chest movement on the involved side
Flat percussion note over the pleural effusion	Hyperresonant percussion note over pneumothorax
Egophony over compressed lung next to effusion	Flatness to percussion over collapsed lung
Decreased breath sounds over pleural effusion	Decreased or absent breath sounds on affected side
Decreased vocal and tactile fremitus	Decreased vocal and tactile fremitus

Lung parenchymal diseases

A large number of diseases affecting the lung alveoli and/or interstitium either locally or diffusely lead to respiratory impairment of varying degrees. Damage to healthy lung tissue may result from invasion by bacteria, viruses, fungi, or malignant cells and inhalation of irritating dust and fumes. Damage to the alveolar capillary endothelium from a variety of causes leads to interstitial, alveolar wall, and intraalveolar edema. Excess fibrotic tissue may be deposited as a sequela to a variety of diseases, usually inflammatory or allergenic in nature. The result is a reduction in lung compliance (stiff lungs) and interference with the gas diffusion pathway. A deficiency of surfactant, as in respiratory distress syndrome, may also produce the same results.

The physiologic abnormalities seen in patients with disease of the lung parenchyma vary widely and depend, to some degree, on the extent of the pathologic process. A restrictive defect with its concomitant decrease in lung volume and a rapid, shallow breathing pattern is common. Hypoxemia is the most important blood gas abnormality and is commonly caused by a ventilation-perfusion imbalance resulting in excess wasted ventilation or wasted perfusion due to shunting. None of the physiologic abnormalities are specific, but pulmonary function tests are helpful in quantifying the degree of abnormality, guiding therapy, and assessing the results. Only selected, frequently encountered lung parenchymal diseases are discussed in this chapter.

Atelectasis

Atelectasis, although not a disease per se, is a condition which is associated with disease of the lung parenchyma and must be understood in order to prevent its occurrence. *Atelectasis* is a term meaning "imperfect expansion," and it implies that the alveoli in the affected part of the lung have become airless and collapsed. There are two major causes of collapse: absorption atelectasis secondary to bronchial or bronchiolar obstruction and atelectasis caused by compression.

In *absorption atelectasis*, obstruction of the airway prevents air from entering the alveoli distal to the obstruction. The air which is already present in the alveoli is then absorbed gradually into the bloodstream, and the alveoli collapse. (It takes more air pressure and work to reinflate an alveolus from a completely collapsed position, just as one must blow harder at the beginning when blowing up a balloon.) Absorption atelectasis may result from intrinsic or extrinsic bronchial obstruction. Intrinsic bronchial obstruction is most commonly caused by retained secretions or exudate. Extrinsic pressure on a bronchus commonly results from neoplasm, lymph node enlargement, aneurysm, or scar tissue. This discussion is concerned with intrinsic obstruction re-

sulting from retained secretions, since this is more common and is preventable to a large degree.

The physiologic defense mechanisms which act to keep the lower respiratory tract sterile have already been discussed. Some of these mechanisms also act to prevent atelectasis by preventing obstruction. These mechanisms include the combined action of the "ciliary escalator," which may be assisted by cough to move noxious particles and bacteria to the posterior pharynx, where they are swallowed or expectorated. Another mechanism which serves to prevent atelectasis is collateral ventilation. Recent experimental studies of collateral ventilation, a subject of debate for the past 50 years, leave no doubt that air can pass from one lung acinus to another by other than the normal airways. It is now well established that small pores, called the *pores of Kohn* after their discoverer in 1873, between the alveoli provide a path for collateral ventilation.

Figure 35-5 illustrates how collateral ventilation prevents absorption atelectasis in the presence of bronchiolar obstruction by a mucus plug. Also illustrated is one of the causes of ineffective ventilation and its effect. Only deep inspiration is effective in opening up the pores of Kohn and providing collateral ventilation to an adjacent obstructed alveolus. Collapse caused by absorption of gases in the obstructed alveolus is thus prevented. (Normally gas absorption into the blood is favored by the fact that the total partial pressure of the blood gases is slightly less than atmospheric pressure, because more oxygen is absorbed into the tissues than carbon dioxide is excreted.) During expiration the pores of Kohn close, and pressure builds up in the obstructed alveolus, which aids in the expulsion of the mucus plug. Even greater expiratory force may be built up if, after taking a deep breath, the glottis is closed and then suddenly opened as in the normal cough. In contrast, the pores of Kohn remain closed with shallow inspiration, so that there is no collateral ventilation to the obstructed alveolus; pressure adequate to expel the mucus plug is thus not attained. Absorption of alveolar gases into the bloodstream continues, resulting in collapse of the alveolus. As the air leaves the alveolus, it is gradually replaced by edematous fluid.

The purpose of this discussion is to emphasize the importance of coughing and deep breathing exercises and other physical activity to prevent atelectasis in predisposed persons. This is particularly important in postoperative, bedridden, or otherwise debilitated patients, since atelectasis is the prevalent cause of morbidity in this population group. Atelectasis at the lung bases is especially common in patients whose respirations are shallow as a result of pain, weakness, or abdominal distention. Retained secretions may lead to pneumonia and more extensive atelectasis.

Prolonged atelectasis may lead to the replacement of the involved lung tissue with fibrous tissue. Adequate prevention also requires familiarity with factors which interfere with normal lung defense mechanisms. Some of these factors, discussed previously, are listed in Table 35-3 for added emphasis and consideration.

Compression atelectasis results from extrinsic pressure on all or part of the lung, driving the air out and causing collapse. Common causes are pleural effusion, pneumothorax, or abdominal distention elevating the diaphragm. Compression atelectasis is much less common than absorption atelectasis.

Infections of the lung parenchyma: Pneumonias

Acute inflammation of the lung parenchyma, which is usually infectious in origin, is called *pneumonia* or *pneumonitis.* The first term is preferable, since the second term has frequently been used to designate a nonspecific pulmonary inflammation of unknown cause. Pneumonia is a common malady and affects about 1 percent of the American population annually. In spite of antibiotics, it is still a major killer, accounting for 2.7 percent of American deaths in 1977 (*Vital Statistics of the U.S.,* 1977). The infant and young child are particularly susceptible because of poorly developed immune responses. Pneumonia is frequently the terminal event in the elderly and those debilitated by chronic diseases.

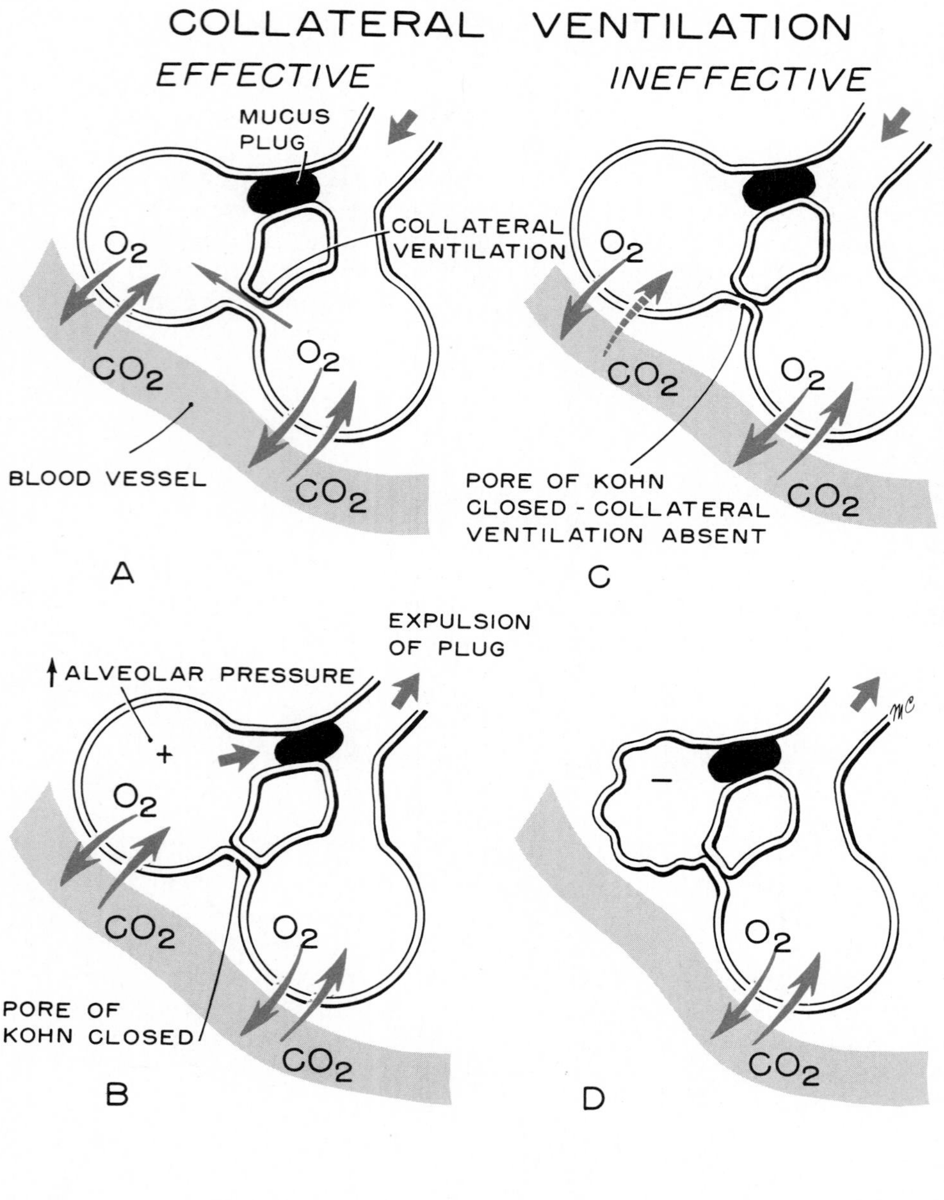

FIGURE 35-5

The role of collateral alveolar ventilation in the prevention of absorption atelectasis. Effective ventilation: (A) during deep inspiration, pores of Kohn open, and air enters adjacent obstructed alveolus; (B) during expiration, the pores of Kohn close; positive pressure builds up in obstructed alveolus and aids in expulsion of mucus plug. Ineffective ventilation: (C) pores of Kohn do not open during shallow inspiration, so that collateral ventilation is not provided to obstructed alveolus; (D) obstructed alveolus collapses as alveolar gases are absorbed into bloodstream. (Modified from Edwin J. Kroeker, "Atelectasis," *Hospital Medicine,* March 1969.)

TABLE 35-3

541

DISEASES OF THE PLEURA AND LUNG PARENCHYMA

LUNG DEFENSE MECHANISMS PREVENTING ATELECTASIS

Protective mechanism	Factors causing interference with mechanism
Mucus and ciliary action	General dehydration causes production of viscous mucus and scant volume Inhalation of dry air increases viscosity of mucus so that crusting occurs Excess mucus production (e.g., chronic bronchitis) overwhelms ciliary escalator Cigarette smoke reduces or paralyzes ciliary action Trauma (suctioning) reduces ciliary action Anesthetics and atropinelike drugs reduce both mucus production and ciliary action
Cough	Pain reduces expiratory force Sedatives and narcotics inhibit cough initiation Airflow rate reduced by COPD
Collateral ventilation	Shallow breathing due to pain or sedation Pulmonary edema from congestion or infection Constant tidal volume respiration on a mechanical respirator Anesthetic gases and oxygen rapidly absorbed, allowing less time for collateral ventilation
Pharyngeal clearing	Unconsciousness; obtundation favors aspiration of gastric contents or upper respiratory tract secretions

Alcoholic and postoperative patients and those with chronic respiratory disease or virus infections are also particularly vulnerable. Infectious agents are most frequently inhaled or are already normal flora of the respiratory tract. Consequently, predisposing factors include any deficiency in the lung's defense mechanisms.

The pathologic picture depends, to some extent, on the etiologic agent. *Bacterial pneumonia* is characterized by an intraalveolar suppurative exudate with consolidation. The infectious process may be classified on an anatomic basis. There is consolidation of an entire lobe in *lobar* pneumonia, while *lobular pneumonia*, or *bronchopneumonia*, refers to a patchy distribution of infectious areas about 3 to 4 cm in diameter surrounding and involving the bronchi. *Virus* or *Mycoplasma pneumoniae* pneumonias are characterized by an interstitial inflammation with accumulation of an infiltrate in the alveolar walls, although the alveolar spaces themselves are free of exudate and there is no consolidation. If the infecting agent is a *fungus* or *Mycobacterium tuberculosis*, the common pathologic pattern is a patchy distribution of granulomas, which may undergo caseous necrosis with the development of cavities (see Fig. 35-6, illustrating the forms of pneumonia and the common etiologic agent).

The pattern of response also depends on the specific etiologic agent. Three organisms most commonly involved in bacterial pneumonia are the pneumococcus, *Streptococcus pneumoniae* (accounting for more than 90 percent of the cases); *Klebsiella*, or Friedländer's bacillus (1 percent); and Staphylococcus (1 to 5 percent). Less commonly, hemolytic streptococci and gram-negative organisms such as *Pseudomonas aeruginosa* and *Escherichia coli* may cause pneumonia.

Among the bacterial pneumonias, the pathogenesis of pneumococcal pneumonia has been the most extensively studied. The current concept is that the pneumococci reach the alveoli in droplets of mucus or saliva. The lower lobes of the lungs are commonly involved because of the effect of gravity. Once established in the alveolus, the pneumococcus elicits a typical pathologic response involving four successive stages:*

1. Engorgement (first 4 to 12 hours)—serous exudate pours into alveloi from the dilated, leaking blood vessels.
2. Red hepatization (next 48 hours)—lung assumes a red, granular appearance (hepatization = liverlike) as red blood cells, fibrin, and polymorphonuclear leukocytes fill the alveoli.
3. Gray hepatization (3 to 8 days)—lung assumes a grayish appearance as the leukocytes and fibrin consolidate in the involved alveoli.
4. Resolution (7 to 11 days)—exudate is lysed and resorbed by macrophages, restoring the tissue to its original structure.

The onset of pneumococcal pneumonia is typically sudden, with chills, fever, pleuritic pain, cough, and rust-colored sputum. Rales and a friction rub may be heard over the involved tissue because of the exudate and fibrin that are in the alveoli and may be deposited on the pleural surface. There is almost always some degree of hypoxemia as a result of the shunting of blood through the nonventilated, consolidated area of lung, and the patient may have a dusky appearance. Chest x-ray, white blood cell count, and sputum examination, including gross appearance, microscopic examination, and culture, may all be helpful in making the diagnosis and following the course of the pneumonia.

The general treatment of patients with pneumonia consists in administration of antibiotic drugs effective

---

*These stages represent the temporal course in untreated pneumococcal pneumonia. With the use of antibiotics the course is now run in about 3 days.

against the specific organism, oxygen therapy for hypoxemia, and treatment of complications. Likely complications and mortality are related to the specific infecting organism. Pneumococcal pneumonia generally runs an uncomplicated course, resulting in restoration of normal tissue structure. The most likely complication is a small pleural effusion. Before the era of antibiotics there was a 20 to 40 percent mortality for pneumococcal pneumonia, but this has now been reduced to 5 to 13 percent. Death is more likely to occur in elderly, chroni-

cally ill persons. The presence of bacteremia also affects the prognosis for pneumonia. The mortality in patients with bacteremia is about double that observed in the absence of bacteremia. Transient bacteremia may occur in all patients with pneumococcal pneumonia. Demonstrable bacteremia suggests ineffective localization of the pulmonary process, and it is not surprising that the mortality is higher in this group. The consequences of bacteremia may be metastatic lesions resulting in such conditions as meningitis, bacterial endocarditis, and peritonitis.

A vaccine for pneumococcal pneumonia is currently available and is 80 to 90 percent effective in adults against the most common pneumococcal serotypes. The vaccine is generally given to persons at high

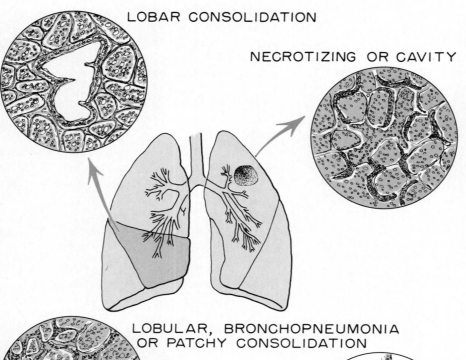

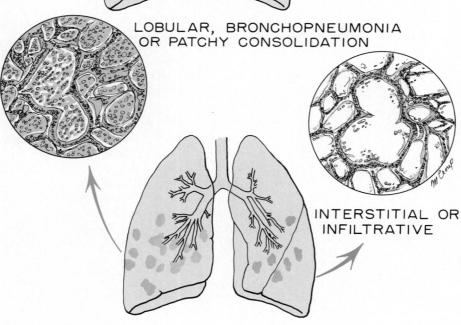

LOBAR CONSOLIDATION

NECROTIZING OR CAVITY

LOBULAR, BRONCHOPNEUMONIA OR PATCHY CONSOLIDATION

INTERSTITIAL OR INFILTRATIVE

FIGURE 35-6

Forms of pneumonia: lobar—entire lobe consolidated, exudate chiefly intra-alveolar (inset), Pneumococcus and *Klebsiella* common infecting organisms; necrotizing—granuloma may undergo caseous necrosis and form cavity, fungi and tubercle bacillus common cause; lobular—patchy distribution, fibrinous exudate chiefly in bronchioles, *Staphylococcus* and *Streptococcus* common infecting organisms; interstitial—perivascular exudate and edema between the alveoli, caused by virus or mycoplasmal infection.

risk of fatal outcome, e.g., those with sickle-cell anemia, multiple myeloma, nephrotic syndrome, or diabetes mellitus.

Pneumonias caused by gram-negative organisms or by staphylococcus frequently have a poor prognosis even with antibiotic therapy. These pneumonias cause extensive damage to the lung parenchyma, and complications such as lung abscess and empyema are common. The mortality is 25 to 50 percent when the infecting organism is *Klebsiella pneumoniae*, 70 percent with *Pseudomonas aeruginosa*, 45 percent with *Escherichia coli*, and 15 to 50 percent with *Staphylococcus aureus*. A large number of patients who survive *Klebsiella* (or Friedländer's) pneumonia develop a chronic pneumonia with severe progressive destruction of lung tissue that ultimately converts the patient into a respiratory cripple. A thick "red currant jelly" sputum is characteristic of this pneumonia. Most cases of *Klebsiella* pneumonia occur in middle-aged or elderly males who are chronic alcoholics or who have some other chronic disease. Pneumonia caused by *Pseudomonas* organisms is most common in hospitalized patients who are terminally ill or who have marked suppression of immunologic body defenses (e.g., a patient with leukemia or a renal transplant who is receiving large doses of immunosuppressive drugs). Other predisposing factors in gram-negative pneumonias include prior antimicrobial therapy which alters the normal resident flora of the respiratory tract and allows overgrowth of certain microorganisms. Contaminated ventilatory equipment is a common source of *Pseudomonas* infection. *Staphylococcus aureus* is commonly a secondary infection in hospitalized, debilitated patients and is most likely to cause a bronchopneumonia.

Viral pneumonias account for about 50 percent of all acute pneumonias and are characterized by symptoms of headache, fever, generalized aching of muscles. extreme fatigue, and a dry cough. Most of these pneumonias are mild, do not require hospitalization, and leave no permanent lung damage. Types A and B influenza virus and adenovirus are common infecting agents. The treatment of viral pneumonia is symptomatic and palliative, since antibiotics are not effective against viruses. Vaccination may give protection for a limited time but does not give protection against the many other types of viruses (some unidentified) which may cause respiratory infections. Viral pneumonia may set the stage for secondary invasion by bacteria, which has already been discussed. More rarely, a fatal patchy or diffuse pneumonitis may be attributed to the virus.

Pneumonia caused by *Mycoplasma pneumoniae* is generally discussed with virus pneumonias even though the infecting organism is a bacterium. The clinical picture of mycoplasmal pneumonia is similar to influenza virus pneumonia with evidence of interstitial pneumonitis. It is highly contagious and, unlike viral pneumonia, responds to tetracycline or erythromycin. My-coplasmal pneumonia is often referred to as *primary atypical pneumonia*.

Aspiration pneumonia refers to a pneumonia caused by the aspiration of gastric contents. The resultant pneumonia is partly chemical as a result of the reaction to the gastric juice and partly bacterial as a result of the organisms which may inhabit the mouth or stomach. Aspiration is most common during or following anesthesia (especially in obstetrical patients and surgical emergencies, because of the lack of surgical preparation), in infants, and in any obtunded patient with depressed cough or gag reflexes. This type of pneumonia may be extremely fulminant and has a high mortality. Massive inhalation of gastric contents may lead to sudden death from obstruction, while aspiration of smaller quantities of gastric contents may lead to widespread pulmonary edema and respiratory failure. The severity of the inflammatory response depends on the pH of the aspirate more than on any other factor. Aspiration pneumonia always results when the pH of the aspirate is 2.5 or less. Abscesses, bronchiectasis, and gangrene are common complications of aspiration pneumonia. It is important to realize that vomiting is not a prerequisite to the entrance of gastric contents into the tracheobronchial tree, as silent regurgitation may occur in obtunded patients. Proper positioning to drain oropharyngeal secretions from the mouth is most important in the care of these patients.

Hypostatic pneumonia is a pneumonia which develops frequently at the lung bases and is caused by shallow breathing and constantly remaining in the same position. Gravity causes blood to become congested in the dependent part of the lung, and infection aids the development of true pneumonia.

Fungi may be the cause of pneumonia, although they are a much less frequent cause than bacteria. A few fungi are capable of producing a chronic granulomatous, suppurative lung disease which is often mistaken for tuberculosis. Many of these fungal infections are endemic to certain geographic regions. The most important fungal infections in the United States are *histoplasmosis* (midwest and east), *coccidioidomycosis* (southwest), and *blastomycosis* (southeast). Spores of these fungi are found in the soil and are inhaled. Spores carried into the smaller divisions of the lung are phagocytized and cause an allergic reaction. After allergy develops, the reaction becomes inflammatory, with tubercle formation, central caseation, scarring, calcification, and even cavity formation. All the pathologic changes resemble tuberculosis so closely that differentiation can only be made by identification and culture of the fungus from lung tissue. Serologic and delayed hypersensitivity skin tests are not positive until a few weeks after the initial infection and may even be negative with severe disease.

It is not unusual for fungal pneumonia to complicate the final stages of terminal diseases such as cancer or leukemia. *Candida albicans*, a yeast frequently found in the sputum of healthy persons, may invade the pulmonary tissue under these conditions. Infection with *Candida* is termed *candidiasis*. Prolonged use of antibiotics may also alter the natural body flora and permit invasion of *Candida*. Amphotericin B is the drug of choice for the pulmonary fungal infections.

Pulmonary fibrosis

Pulmonary fibrosis is not a disease entity but a pathologic term which implies that there is an excessive amount of connective tissue in the lung. Fibrosis results from a method of tissue repair which may follow any disease process of the lung producing inflammation or necrosis. The most common type of pulmonary fibrosis is localized fibrosis, which follows localized damage to the lung parenchyma caused by such conditions as tuberculosis, pulmonary abscess, bronchiectasis, or unresolved pneumonia. Less commonly, pulmonary fibrosis may diffusely involve the lung parenchyma, particularly affecting the interalveolar septa. Unlike localized fibrosis, diffuse pulmonary fibrosis is a disabling and frequently fatal disorder. Diffuse pulmonary fibrosis represents end-stage lung disease from a host of known and unknown causes. A few of the more common causes of diffuse pulmonary fibrosis are listed in Table 35-4.

The *pneumonoconioses* are a group of diseases caused by the inhalation of certain inorganic and organic dusts. Some dusts, when inhaled in sufficient concentration into the lungs, produce a fibrous tissue reaction, while others are quite inert. The dust inhalation diseases are of particular interest, since exposure is usually related to certain occupations, and these diseases are theoretically preventable by the institution of industrial safety standards. Only a few examples of noxious dusts or gases causing pulmonary fibrosis are listed in Table 35-4. Whether a particular dust causes disease depends on (1) the size of the particle—the most dangerous dust particle seems to be 1 to 5 μm, since larger particles never reach the alveoli; (2) the concentration and length of exposure—high concentration is usually required to overcome the action of the ciliary escalator, and long exposure is usually required (e.g., coal miner's pneumoconiosis, or black lung disease, usually requires 20 years of exposure before there is extensive pulmonary fibrosis); and (3) the nature of the dust—certain

materials [particularly the organic dusts such as cotton fiber, which causes bysinosis; sugar cane (bagassosis); and moldy hay (farmer's lung)] have an unusual antigenic effect and cause an allergic alveolitis. The chemical nature of inorganic dusts also influences their capacity to produce disease. Silica dust (commonly inhaled by grinders, sandblasters, and rock quarry workers), which causes silicosis, is particularly harmful. It is thought that these dust particles regularly destroy the macrophages by which they are phagocytized, resulting in the formation of fibrotic nodules. Widespread fibrosis is produced by the coalescence of the fibrotic nodules.

Asbestos is a compound of magnesium and iron silicate. Because of its unique physical characteristics (durability, heat resistance, flexibility) it is widely used in industry (e.g., shipbuilding, car brake and clutch lining, air filters, insulation materials, and roofing). *Asbestosis* is an interstitial process which slowly develops into a diffuse, nonnodular pulmonary fibrosis involving the terminal airways, alveoli, and pleurae. The disease is usually recognized after 10 years of exposure and tends to progress after exposure has ended. The major complications of asbestosis are bronchogenic carcinoma, malignant mesothelioma, and pleural plaques. The risk of bronchogenic carcinoma is largely confined to cigarette smokers, in whom the risk is greater than in smokers without asbestosis (see Chap. 38). Asbestos exposure

TABLE 35-4

COMMON CAUSES OF DIFFUSE PULMONARY FIBROSIS

Diseases of known etiology	Diseases of unknown etiology

1. Pneumoconioses (occupational inhalation of dusts)
  a. Inorganic dusts:
    Silica—silicosis
    Coal—"black lung"
    Iron—siderosis
    Asbestos—asbestosis
    Talc—talcosis
    Beryllium—berylliosis
  b. Organic dusts:
    Cotton—byssinosis
    Sugar cane—bagassosis
    Moldy hay—"farmer's lung"
    Maple bark
2. Noxious gas inhalation—Nitrogen oxides (silo filler), chlorine, sulfur oxides, metal fumes
3. Drug sensitivity to diphenylhydantoin (Dilantin) busulfan (Myleran)
4. Irradiation injury
5. Viral pneumonias
6. Chronic pulmonary edema
	1. Hamman-Rich syndrome
	2. Sarcoidosis
	3. "Collagen diseases"—progressive systemic sclerosis
	4. Chronic interstitial pneumonia
	5. Mucoviscidosis (cystic fibrosis)

occurs not only from mining and the manufacture of asbestos products but from general community air pollution. Asbestos fibers have been found in the autopsied lungs of a high percentage of city dwellers. The potential health hazard of such low concentrations is not clear.

The inhalation of noxious gases may be associated with certain occupations. The result is a chemical pneumonitis. Of particular interest is silo filler's disease, which is not a pneumoconiosis but is caused by the inhalation of nitrogen oxides from fermentation of the vegetation in a freshly filled silo. The severity of reaction to noxious gases depends on the concentration of gas and length of exposure. Viral pneumonias, chronic pulmonary edema, irradiation involving the chest, and certain drugs that produce a hypersensitivity reaction (e.g., diphenylhydantoin and busulfan) are other known causes of diffuse pulmonary fibrosis.

Among diseases of unknown cause leading to diffuse pulmonary fibrosis is the Hamman-Rich syndrome. This is an unusual interstitial pneumonia which may have a rapidly fatal course or a more protracted one, both with the development of severe intraalveolar and interstitial fibrosis. Other chronic interstitial pneumonias also tend to result in progressive pulmonary fibrosis, as do certain systemic diseases such as sarcoidosis, collagen diseases (especially scleroderma), and mucoviscidosis.

The systemic symptoms in the group of diseases causing pulmonary fibrosis vary widely. In the early stages there may be no symptoms at all. The pulmonary symptoms, however, are strikingly similar. The primary symptom seems to be a progressive dyspnea on exertion. The common pathologic denominator is interstitial fibrosis, with the extent of fibrosis determining the effect on pulmonary function. When the fibrosis is extensive, there is a decrease in lung elasticity, total lung capacity, vital capacity, and residual volume, which all indicate restrictive lung disease. The dyspnea reflects the poor compliance and results in a concomitant increase in the work of breathing. With marked destruction of alveoli and pulmonary vessels, hypoxemia, pulmonary hypertension, cor pulmonale, and heart failure may result. In many of the cases, however, the symptoms do not progress beyond mild exertional dyspnea.

QUESTIONS

Restrictive patterns of respiratory disease

Directions: Match each of the extrapulmonary disorders causing alveolar hypoventilation in col. A with its appropriate altered mechanism in col. B.

Column A

1. ____ Kyphoscoliosis

2. ____ Progressive muscular dystrophy

3. ____ Pa_{CO_2} 70 mmHg

4. ____ Myasthenia gravis

5. ____ CNS lesion

6. ____ Amyotrophic lateral sclerosis

Column B

a. Depression of the respiratory center

b. Interruption of nerve transmission to respiratory muscles due to disease involving the neuromuscular junction

c. Interruption of nerve transmission to respiratory muscles due to upper motor neuron lesion

d. Direct anatomic damage to the respiratory center

e. Paresis of the respiratory muscles due to diffuse disease of the skeletal muscles

f. Deformity of the chest cage causing abnormal positioning and functioning of its respiratory muscles

Directions: Circle T if the statement is true and F if it is false. Correct the false statements.

7. T F In kyphoscoliosis, compression of the lungs by the thoracic deformity causes a small lung volume and unequal distribution of ventilation and perfusion.

8. T F *Pectus excavatum* refers to a lateral displacement of the spine.

9. T F Flail chest injury is associated with paradoxical movement of dead-space air between the airways of the right and left lungs during the respiratory cycle.

10. T F Ankylosing spondylitis is a disease which causes asymmetric deformity of the chest cage.

Directions: Circle the letter preceding each item below that correctly completes the statement. Only one answer is correct.

11. The Pickwickian syndrome is characterized by all the following except:

a. Hypoxemia   b. Hypercapnia   c. Increased arterial pH   d. Polycythemia   e. Cor pulmonale

12. Patients with kyphoscoliotic lung disease would be expected to exhibit all the following physiologic abnormalities *except:*
a. Increased nonelastic work of breathing   b. Increased elastic work of breathing   c. Decreased lung compliance   d. Decreased vital capacity

13. Alveolar hypoventilation results in all the following abnormalities of the blood gases *except:*
a. Low Pa_{O_2} b. Low PA_{CO_2} c. High Pa_{CO_2}
d. Low PA_{CO_2}

14. Children with muscular dystrophy are most likely to exhibit the following abnormalities of pulmonary function:
a. Obstructive ventilatory pattern   b. Restrictive ventilatory pattern   c. Pulmonary diffusion block
d. Normal ventilatory function

Directions: Answer the following on a separate sheet of paper.

15. What are two physiologic alterations which occur as a consequence of a restricted pattern of ventilation?

16. List possible causes of the following types of pneumothorax: traumatic, therapeutic, and spontaneous.

17. Describe the emergency treatment of a penetrating chest wound.

18. Why does a pneumothorax occur when there is a communication between a bronchus or alveolus and the pleural cavity?

19. Describe the treatment for a large pneumothorax and a large pleural effusion.

20. What is a collection of fluid in the pleural cavity called?

21. When a transudate occurs, there is a rise in pressure so that the balance of forces favors the passage of fluid out of the vessels. What is this pressure called?

22. What is formed in the pleural cavity as the result of increased capillary permeability or impaired lymphatic absorption?

23. What is pleural fluid called which has a specific gravity of less than 1.015 and a protein content of less than 3 percent?

24. List five general disorders which may cause damage to the lung alveoli and interstitium. State the spe-

cific damage to lung tissue that each disorder causes.

25. Contrast absorption and compression atelectasis with respect to the common cause of each and the mechanism involved.

26. Why are the pores of Kohn important in maintaining collateral ventilation? Illustrate how collateral ventilation prevents absorption atelectasis caused by bronchial obstruction by a mucus plug.

27. List in sequence the four stages describing the pathologic changes in the lung in untreated pneumococcal pneumonia (include name of stage, time period, and description of lung changes).

28. List three principles of treatment for patients with pneumonia.

29. List three criteria used to predict whether a particular dust will cause disease of the lung parenchyma. State the reason why each of these criteria is important.

30. List the three most important fungal infections in the United States causing lung disease.

31. What are two consequences of pulmonary fibrosis?

32. The manifestations of extensive diffuse pulmonary fibrosis are typical of what type of pattern of ventilatory dysfunction?

Directions: Complete the following statements by filling in the blanks.

33. Pulmonary fibrosis is characterized pathologically by _____ fibrosis.

34. Pneumonia caused by gram-negative or staphylococcus organisms causes extensive damage to the lung _____. Common complications include _____ and _____. The prognosis is generally _____.

Directions: Circle T if the statement is true and F if it is false. Correct the false statements.

35. T   F   Patients with Friedländer's pneumonia often develop a chronic pneumonia following the original infection.

36. T   F   Gram-negative pneumonias often occur in hospitalized or debilitated patients.

37. T   F   Viral pneumonia commonly has a poor prognosis.

38. T   F   Viral pneumonia is successfully treated with erythromycin.

39. T F The clinical picture of mycoplasmal pneumonia is similar to that of viral pneumonia.

40. T F Aspiration pneumonia develops at the lung bases and is caused by shallow breathing and constantly remaining in the same position.

41. T F Amphotericin B is the drug of choice for the treatment of candidiasis.

42. T F Fungal pulmonary lesions are often granulomatous and similar to lesions caused by *Mycobacterium tuberculosis*.

Directions: Match the type of pneumothorax in col. A with the correct description in col. B.

Column A
43. ____ Open
44. ____ Closed
45. ____ Tension

Column B
a. Communication between pleural cavity and atmosphere sealed off
b. Communication between pleural cavity and atmosphere open during inspiration and closed during expiration
c. Communication between pleural cavity and atmosphere does not seal off

Directions: Match each of the anatomic patterns of pneumonia in col. A with its pathologic description or common etiologic agent in col. B. More than one letter may be used for each blank in col. A.

Column A
46. ____ Lobar consolidation
47. ____ Lobular consolidation
48. ____ Necrotizing or cavity formation
49. ____ Interstitial

Column B
a. Fungi or *Mycobacterium tuberculosis*
b. Virus or *Mycoplasma* pneumonia
c. Pneumococcus
d. Staphylococcus or streptococcus
e. Perivascular exudate and edema between the alveoli
f. May undergo caseous necrosis
g. Exudate chiefly intraalveolar
h. Fibrinous exudate chiefly in bronchioles

i. Patchy distribution of infection
j. Whole lung lobe infected

Directions: Match each of the protective mechanisms in col. A with the factors causing interference with it in col. B. More than one letter may be used for each blank in col. A.

Column A
50. ____ Cough
51. ____ Mucus and ciliary action
52. ____ Collateral ventilation
53. ____ Pharyngeal clearing

Column B
a. Cigarette smoke
b. General dehydration
c. Pain
d. Shallow breathing
e. Constant tidal volume breathing
f. Sedatives and narcotics
g. Atropinelike drugs
h. Unconsciousness
i. Reduction of airflow rate

Directions: Match each item in col. A with its description or cause in col. B. Items are associated with occupational diseases resulting in diffuse pulmonary fibrosis.

Column A
54. ____ Organic dusts
55. ____ Silica dust
56. ____ Farmer's lung
57. ____ Silo filler's disease
58. ____ Byssinosis
59. ____ Black lung disease

Column B
a. Caused by inhalation of nitrogen oxides
b. Caused by inhalation of cotton dust
c. Mechanism of adverse reaction is allergic alveolitis
d. Caused by moldy hay
e. Mechanism of adverse reaction is production of chemical pneumonitis
f. Mechanism of adverse reaction is destruction of macrophages with formation of fibrotic nodules
g. Common occupational disease among rock quarry workers, grinders, and sandblasters
h. Caused by inhalation of coal dust

Directions: Circle the letter preceding each item below that correctly answers the question. More than one answer may be correct.

60. Which of the following are common causes of diffuse pulmonary fibrosis?
    a. Tuberculosis   *b.* Inhalation of noxious gases   *c.* Inhalation of silica dusts   *d.* Sarcoidosis   *e.* Diphenylhydantoin (Dilantin) therapy

61. Which of the following are *typical* signs, symptoms, and findings associated with pneumococcal pneumonia:
    a. "Red currant jelly" sputum   *b.* "Rusty" sputum   *c.* Dry, nonproductive cough   *d.* Decreased white blood cell count   *e.* Fever, chills, pleuritic pain   *f.* Lobar consolidation evident on chest x-ray

62. What percentage of the American population is affected by pneumonia annually?
    a. 1 percent   *b.* 5 percent   *c.* 10 percent   *d.* 15 percent

63. Which of the following abnormalities are commonly seen in patients with disease of the lung parenchyma?
    a. A restrictive pattern of pulmonary dysfunction   *b.* An obstructive pattern of pulmonary dysfunction   *c.* Rapid, shallow breathing pattern   *d.* Slow, deep breathing pattern   *e.* Decrease in lung volume   *f.* Hypercapnia   *g.* Hypoxemia

Directions: Circle the letter preceding the one best answer to each of the following.

64. Inadequately treated empyema may result in which of the following conditions?
    a. Hydrothorax   *b.* Chylothorax   *c.* Hemothorax   *d.* Fibrothorax

65. Which of the following statements is the best description of a pneumothorax?
    a. Air within the pleural cavity   *b.* Cohesion and positive intrapleural pressure   *c.* A pathologic lesion of the lung   *d.* Accumulation of fluid in the pleural cavity

66. What is the most common cause of idiopathic spontaneous pneumothorax in healthy young adults?
    a. Bulging of the intercostal spaces   *b.* Rupture of a subpleural bleb or localized bullous disease   *c.* Lesions of the parietal pleura   *d.* Diffuse emphysematous disease of the lungs

67. Which of the following signs and symptoms would best differentiate between a pleural effusion and a pneumothorax?
    a. Moderate dyspnea   *b.* Diminished and delayed chest movement on the involved side   *c.* Decreased vocal fremitus over the involved area   *d.* Diminished or absent breath sounds on the affected side   *e.* Egophony over lung above effusion (bleating sound heard by stethoscope when patient speaks)

68. A patient with pneumonia is having severe pain in the right lateral portion of the chest accompanying respiratory movements. Why is this?
    a. Inflamed lung is painful   *b.* Visceral pleura is inflamed and sensitive to pain   *c.* Parietal pleura is inflamed and sensitive to pain   *d.* Patient has an intercostal peripheral neuritis

69. Nosocomial (arising from hospitalization) infections associated with respirators, resuscitation equipment, and humidifiers are especially likely to be caused by:
    a. Klebsiella pneumoniae   *b. Staphylococcus aureus*   *c.* Fungi   *d. Pseudomonas* organisms

70. The normal respiratory tract is sterile:
    a. Below the oropharynx   *b.* Below the larynx   *c.* Below the mainstem bronchi   *d.* Below the terminal bronchioles   *e.* Nowhere

71. The usual course of pneumococcal lobar pneumonia terminates with:
    a. Diffuse pulmonary fibrosis   *b.* Organization of the inflammatory exudate   *c.* Complete resolution of the pulmonary inflammation   *d.* Abscess formation and empyema

CARDIOVASCULAR DISEASE AND THE LUNG

OBJECTIVES

At the completion of this chapter you should be able to:

1. Define *pulmonary embolism*.
2. Identify the morbidity and mortality for pulmonary embolism.
3. List three basic factors related to the development of venous thrombosis and pulmonary embolism.
4. List four diseases and activities that appear to increase the risk of venous thrombosis.
5. State the two most important conditions predisposing to venous thrombosis.
6. Describe the classic syndrome associated with a moderate-sized pulmonary embolus.
7. Describe the signs and symptoms of a massive pulmonary embolus and the signs and symptoms associated with multiple small, recurrent emboli.
8. Identify the physiologic effects of a pulmonary embolism.
9. Identify the most reliable test for the diagnosis of pulmonary embolism.
10. List the objectives of treatment of pulmonary embolism.
11. Compare the preventive treatment for pulmonary embolism accorded to high-risk patients with the treatment accorded to patients with acute pulmonary embolism.
12. Identify four conditions that may precipitate pulmonary embolism.
13. State the most common cause of pulmonary edema.
14. Describe the emergency treatment of acute pulmonary edema.
15. Define *paroxysmal nocturnal dyspnea*.
16. Define *cor pulmonale*.
17. Explain the prerequisite condition for the development of cor pulmonale.
18. List the most common causes of cor pulmonale.
19. Briefly describe the pathophysiologic mechanisms leading to cor pulmonale.
20. State the rational for the treatment of cor pulmonale.
21. Briefly describe a pulmonary infarction and identify the conditions under which it occurs.

Chronic lung disease is an increasingly frequent cause of heart disease, and conversely, heart disease with decompensation or vascular disease may cause changes in the structure and function of the lung. This close interrelation relates to the functional position of the lungs in the circulation (refer to Fig. 31-4). This chapter discusses pulmonary embolism, pulmonary edema, and cor pulmonale, all diseases demonstrating the close relation between the heart and the lungs.

PULMONARY EMBOLISM

Pulmonary embolism occurs when an embolus, usually a blood clot which breaks free from its attachment in a vein of the lower limbs, circulates through the blood vessels and the right side of the heart to become lodged in the main pulmonary artery or one of its branches. *Pulmonary infarction* is the term used to describe a local focus of necrosis resulting from the vascular obstruction (see Figs. 36-1 and 7-9).

The true incidence of pulmonary embolism cannot be determined because of the difficulty of the clinical diagnosis, but it is an important cause of morbidity and mortality in a hospital population and is said to account for 5 percent of sudden deaths. Pulmonary embolism has been described in over 50 percent of consecutive autopsies in some studies, suggesting that many cases are clinically undetected.

Three basic factors are related to the development of venous thrombosis and subsequent pulmonary embolism: (1) venous stasis or slowing of the blood flow, (2) injury to the vein wall, and (3) hypercoagulability. Several diseases and activities seem to increase the risk of forming a thrombus, and patients in these states should be watched closely to detect any evidence of thrombus formation. The risk of thrombus formation is increased by pregnancy, the use of oral contraceptive drugs, obesity, heart failure, varicose veins, abdominal infection, cancer, sickle cell anemia, and any prolonged inactivity such as plane, train, or bus rides. Many of these conditions are common in hospitalized patients. Venous thrombosis and pulmonary embolism occur predominantly in bedridden patients. The single most important condition predisposing to venous thrombosis is congestive heart failure; the postoperative state is next in importance. The most common site for a blood clot to form is in the deep veins of the legs (90 percent), although clots may form in the pelvic veins and in the right side of the heart. Emboli of nonthrombotic origin are uncommon but include obstruction caused by air, fat, malignant cells, amniotic fluid, parasites, vegetations, and foreign material.

The signs and symptoms of a pulmonary embolus are extremely variable, depending on the size of the clot or clots. The clinical picture may range from no signs at all to sudden and almost immediate death caused by

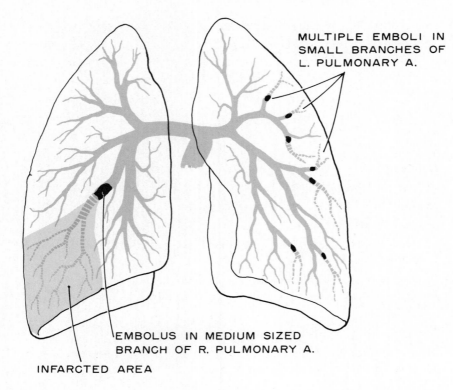

MULTIPLE EMBOLI IN
SMALL BRANCHES OF
L. PULMONARY A.

EMBOLUS IN MEDIUM SIZED
BRANCH OF R. PULMONARY A.

INFARCTED AREA

FIGURE 36-1
Pulmonary embolism and infarction.

a massive saddle embolus at the bifurcation of the main pulmonary artery, resulting in blockage of the entire outflow of the right ventricle. In a patient with the signs of thrombophlebitis in leg veins, the classic syndrome associated with a moderate-sized pulmonary embolus consists in sudden onset of unexplained dyspnea, tachypnea, tachycardia, and restlessness. Pleuritic pain, friction rub, hemoptysis, and fever are not usually present unless infarction has occurred. Massive pulmonary embolism may result in a sudden shocklike state with tachycardia, hypotension, cyanosis, stupor, or syncope. Death usually follows within a few minutes. Frequently, however, the symptoms of pulmonary embolism are subtle, such as unexplained fever or worsening of a preexisting cardiac or cardiopulmonary condition. These subtle symptoms are apt to be associated with recurrent small, multiple pulmonary emboli. They may go unnoticed until right ventricular hypertrophy and failure direct attention to the pulmonary vascular disease.

The effect of pulmonary embolism is to produce an area of lung which is ventilated but underperfused, thus increasing physiologic dead-space ventilation. Reflex bronchoconstriction occurs in the affected area and is thought to result from the release of histamine or serotonin from the clot. Reflex bronchoconstriction is considered to be compensatory in the occluded area, as it reduces the unevenness of ventilation and perfusion. In adjacent areas, however, reflex bronchospasm may result in considerable hypoxemia. If the pulmonary vascular bed is sufficiently reduced by a large embolus or by recurrent multiple emboli, pulmonary hypertension may result. It is estimated that two-thirds of the vascular bed must be obliterated before this happens.

A localized area of ischemic necrosis (infarction) is an uncommon complication of pulmonary embolism because of the lung's dual blood supply. Pulmonary infarction is usually associated with occlusion of a medium-sized lobar or lobular artery and insufficient collateral flow from the bronchial circulation (see Fig. 36-1). A pleural friction rub and a small pleural effusion are common signs.

There are few diagnostic tests which specifically distinguish a pulmonary infarction from a pulmonary infiltrate. Radioactive lung perfusion scans will be abnormal in either case or in the presence of emphysema. The chest x-ray may be normal or a pleural effusion may be present in both cases. Physiologic tests and serum enzymes are likewise of little value in distinguishing an infarction from pneumonia. In addition, the signs and symptoms of pneumonia may be similar to those of pulmonary embolism. The most reliable method of diagnosis is pulmonary angiography.

Treatment of pulmonary embolism is directed to prevention of initial or recurrent embolism, relief of symptoms resulting from the embolus, and surgical removal of a massive embolus. In high-risk patients, the

effectiveness of oral anticoagulants in preventing pulmonary embolism has been clearly shown. Low-dose heparin (3000 to 5000 units every 8 to 12 hours subcutaneously) has also been effective in preliminary studies and may prove to be a valuable prophylactic agent.

The early detection of patients with deep venous thrombosis (and, therefore, at high risk for pulmonary embolism) has been greatly improved by the use of three relatively new noninvasive diagnostic techniques: Doppler ultrasonic examination, impedance plethysmography, and ^{125}I-labeled fibrinogen uptake (see "Venous Disease," Chap. 30). The combined approach of early detection of deep venous thrombosis by these improved techniques and the use of low-dose heparin in persons at high risk of having deep venous thrombosis offers promise for the reduction of pulmonary embolism.

Treatment of an acute pulmonary embolism includes general cardiopulmonary support with oxygen, digitalization, intensive care monitoring, elastic stockings, and the administration of aqueous heparin in full doses of 20,000 to 40,000 units per day by continuous infusion or divided doses. Surgical embolectomy is considered only when the embolus is massive, since the mortality from this kind of surgery is about 50 percent. Other surgical measures to prevent recurrent pulmonary emboli from the lower extremities include ligation of the inferior vena cava and the insertion of a filtering device or screen in the inferior vena cava.

PULMONARY EDEMA

Pulmonary edema is an excessive accumulation of serous or serosanguinous fluid in the interstitial spaces and alveoli of the lungs. If the edema is acute and extensive, death may rapidly ensue. Pulmonary edema may be precipitated by an increase of hydrostatic pressure within the pulmonary capillaries, a decrease in the colloid osmotic pressure as in nephritis, or damage to the capillary walls. Damage to the capillary walls may result from the inhalation of noxious gases, inflammation as in pneumonia, or local interference with oxygenation. The most common cause of pulmonary edema is left ventricular failure resulting from arteriosclerotic heart disease or mitral stenosis (mitral valve obstruction). If the left side of the heart fails while the right side continues to pump blood, the pulmonary capillary pressure rises until pulmonary edema results. There are two stages in the formation of pulmonary edema: the first is interstitial edema characterized by engorgement of the perivascular and peribronchial spaces and increased lymphatic flow; the second is alveolar edema when fluid moves into the alveoli. Blood plasma is poured out into the alveoli faster than coughing or the lymphatics of the lung can clear it. This interferes with diffusion of oxygen, and the consequent tissue hypoxia further increases the tendency to edema. Asphyxia may result unless measures are taken to reverse the pulmonary edema. Emergency treatment for acute pulmonary edema includes measures to reduce pulmonary hydrostatic pressure, such as placing the patient in Fowler's position with the feet dependent; rotating tourniquets; or phlebotomy (removal of about a pint of blood). Other measures include the administration of diuretics, oxygen, and digitalis to improve myocardial contractility.

In the presence of chronic passive congestion of the lungs, structural changes in the lung, namely, pulmonary fibrosis, may result. These changes enable the lung to function for a time with the increased hydrostatic pressure without the development of pulmonary edema. The balance, however, is precarious, and the patient may have attacks of dyspnea at night (paroxysmal noc-

turnal dyspnea) due to the increase in pulmonary hydrostatic pressure which results from a horizontal position.

COR PULMONALE

Cor pulmonale is the condition in which hypertrophy and dilatation of the right ventricle, with or without right ventricular failure, develop as a result of disease affecting the structure or function of the lung or its vasculature. By this definition of the condition, neither disease of the left side of the heart nor congenital heart disease is responsible for its pathogenesis.

The prerequisite for the development of cor pulmonale is pulmonary hypertension. Pulmonary hypertension, in turn, increases the workload of the right ventricle, causing it to hypertrophy and eventually fail. Because the pulmonary circulation is a low-pressure, low-resistance circulation under normal circumstances, cardiac output can increase many times (as happens during exercise) without a significant increase in pulmonary artery pressure. The critical point in the sequence leading to pulmonary hypertension seems to be an increase in pulmonary vascular resistance through the small muscular arteries and arterioles. The increase

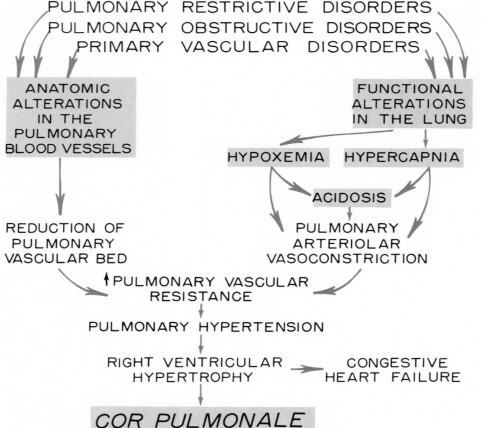

FIGURE 36-2
Etiology and pathogenesis of cor pulmonale.

in vascular resistance may be anatomic or vasomotor in origin. The cross-sectional area of the pulmonary vascular bed may be reduced by a number of pathologic processes. Reduction can occur as a result of a loss of capillaries, as in chronic bronchitis-emphysema; the internal diameter may be occluded by pulmonary emboli; external pressure may reduce the diameter, as in pulmonary fibrosis or high alveolar pressures in obstructive lung diseases; and the various forms of pulmonary fibrosis may reduce the distensibility. When about two-thirds or three-fourths of the vascular bed is destroyed, pulmonary arterial hypertension occurs even at rest.

Anatomic alterations in the pulmonary vascular bed are only one cause of pulmonary hypertension. Another important condition resulting in pulmonary hypertension is pulmonary arteriolar vasoconstriction. Pulmonary vasoconstriction occurs in response to a number of stimuli, but the most important ones are hypoxemia (results in alveolar hypoxia) and hypercapnia (which causes acidosis and evokes pulmonary vasoconstriction). Hypoxemia, hypercapnia, and acidosis, three conditions important in the pathogenesis of pulmonary hypertension and cor pulmonale, are present in a number of different pulmonary diseases as a result of generalized alveolar hypoventilation or as a consequence of ventilation-perfusion abnormalities.

It is evident from the above discussion that any pulmonary disease that affects ventilatory mechanics, gas exchange, or the pulmonary vascular bed may result in cor pulmonale. Since this includes all pulmonary diseases, a list of the causes of cor pulmonale includes all possible types of pulmonary disease. This list also includes extrapulmonary disease such as kyphoscoliosis, the Pickwickian syndrome, and others which affect ventilatory mechanics. The development of cor pulmonale simply means that the primary disease was sufficiently advanced to impair cardiac function. Right ventricular failure is often the terminal event in these diseases. The etiology and pathogenesis of cor pulmonale are illustrated in Fig. 36-2.

The most common cause of cor pulmonale in the United States is chronic obstructive pulmonary disease, which accounts for about 75 percent of the cases. A second important cause is recurrent multiple pulmonary emboli. The exact incidence of cor pulmonale is unknown, but one study in Cleveland during 1941–1947, using the criterion of postmortem ventricular wall thickness, found an incidence of 7.1 percent of all patients with cardiac disease (most patients being over the age of 50).

The treatment of cor pulmonale is directed toward improvement of the underlying pulmonary disorder and correction of the accompanying hypoxemia. In the event of right ventricular failure, digitalis is seldom used, as it may produce toxicity in patients who have fluctuating serum electrolytes and blood gases.

QUESTIONS

Cardiovascular disease and the lung

Directions: Answer the following on a separate sheet of paper.

1. List three factors which directly relate to the development of venous thrombosis.
2. What disease is the most common cause of cor pulmonale in the United States?
3. List four conditions that may precipitate pulmonary edema.
4. What is *paroxysmal nocturnal dyspnea?*
5. Define *cor pulmonale.*
6. What is the relation between left-sided heart failure and pulmonary edema? Is this condition the most frequent cause of pulmonary edema?
7. List three objectives in the treatment of pulmonary embolism.
8. What are the two goals in treatment of cor pulmonale?
9. Describe two mechanisms that can lead to increased pulmonary vascular resistance.

Directions: Circle the letter preceding each item below that correctly answers the question. More than one answer may be correct.

10. The classic signs and symptoms associated with a moderate-sized pulmonary embolism without infarction are:
a. Dyspnea b. Rapid respiratory rate
c. Tachycardia d. Unconsciousness and death within minutes e. Hemoptysis
11. Which of the following types of pulmonary embolism is more frequent?
a. Massive occlusion at bifurcation of main pulmonary artery b. Moderate-sized occlusion of lobar or lobular pulmonary artery c. Occlusion of small pulmonary vessels as a result of recurrent multiple emboli

12. Which of the following are effects of pulmonary embolism?
    a. Pulmonary infarction   b. $\dot{V}/\dot{Q}$ imbalance resulting in increased dead space   c. $\dot{V}/\dot{Q}$ imbalance resulting in increased shunting   d. Reflex bronchoconstriction

13. The most reliable method of diagnosing a pulmonary embolism is:
    a. Chest x-ray   b. Perfusion lung scan with albumin tagged with radioactive isotope   c. Pulmonary angiography   d. Physical examination

14. The usual treatment of an *acute* pulmonary embolism includes:
    a. Oral anticoagulants in low dosage   b. Intensive care monitoring   c. General cardiopulmonary support with oxygen   d. Elastic stockings   e. Surgical embolectomy

15. What is the approximate mortality for surgical removal of a massive pulmonary embolus?
    a. 1 percent   b. 10 percent   c. 50 percent

16. Emergency treatment of acute pulmonary edema might include:
    a. Placing the patient in a high Fowler's position with the feet dependent   b. Placing the patient in a horizontal position with the feet elevated   c. Rotating tourniquets   d. Rapid infusion of intravenous solutions

17. A pulmonary embolism usually occurs when a thrombus from a leg vein breaks off and:
    a. Circulates through the left ventricle and lodges in the main pulmonary artery or its branches   b. Circulates through the right ventricle of the heart and lodges in the pulmonary vein   c. Circulates through the right side of the heart and lodges in the main pulmonary artery or its branches

18. The most likely location for the formation of a blood clot causing a pulmonary embolism is:
    a. A deep vein in the legs   b. The left ventricle   c. An artery in the legs   d. The right ventricle

19. Which of the following conditions is associated with an increased risk of pulmonary embolism?
    a. Carcinoma of the small bowel   b. Postoperative bedridden patient   c. Thrombophlebitis   d. Congestive heart failure

Directions: Determine which are the first and second most important conditions predisposing a patient to venous thrombosis by writing 1 beside the first choice and 2 beside the second.

20. ＿＿ Thrombophlebitis
    ＿＿ Postoperative bedridden patient
    ＿＿ Congestive heart failure
    ＿＿ Carcinoma of the small bowel

Directions: Circle T if the statement is true with respect to pulmonary infarction and F if it is false.

21. T   F   It is a localized area of ischemic necrosis.

22. T   F   It is an infrequent complication of pulmonary embolism as a result of the lung's dual blood supply.

23. T   F   It is frequently associated with a small pleural effusion.

24. T   F   It is easily differentiated from pneumonia by chest x-ray.

Directions: Complete the following statements by filling in the blanks.

25. A freely circulating blood clot which lodges in a blood vessel causing an obstruction is called a(n) ＿＿＿＿＿＿＿＿＿ .

26. Pulmonary embolism is the cause of sudden death in hospitalized patients in at least ＿＿＿＿＿＿ percent of cases.

27. A prerequisite for the development of cor pulmonale is increased pulmonary vascular resistance leading to＿＿＿＿＿＿＿ ＿＿＿＿＿＿＿ .

RESPIRATORY FAILURE

OBJECTIVES

At the completion of this chapter you should be able to:

1. Describe chronic respiratory insufficiency.

2. Define *acute respiratory failure*.

3. List the two broad classes of respiratory failure.

4. Name three examples each of extrinsic and intrinsic lung disorders associated with the two types of respiratory failure.

5. Explain the importance of distinguishing between these two types of respiratory failure.

6. Name nine precipitating factors of respiratory failure in patients with chronic lung disease, two of which are iatrogenic.

7. Describe five pathogenic mechanisms causing hypoxemia and two causing hypercapnia and discuss their relative importance.

8. Explain why hypoventilation causes hypoxemia.

9. Explain why low $\dot{V}/\dot{Q}$ ratios cause hypoxemia but have little effect on increasing the Pa_{CO_2} (use HbO_2 and CO_2 dissociation curves).

10. Explain why respiratory alkalosis may occur in hypoxemic respiratory failure.

11. Differentiate between chronic respiratory insufficiency and acute respiratory failure on the basis of signs and symptoms.

12. Differentiate acute and chronic respiratory acidosis and alkalosis and mixed acid-base disturbances.

13. Explain the significance of the following tests of ventilatory function in the care of a patient in respiratory failure: respiratory rate, tidal volume, minute ventilation, FVC, FEV_1, MIF, VD/VT, Pa_{CO_2}, and arterial blood pH.

14. Calculate the expected value of the Pa_{O_2} with various levels of FI_{O_2}, using the alveolar gas equation.

15. Differentiate between hypoventilation, $\dot{V}/\dot{Q}$ mismatch, and true physiologic shunting using the $P(A-a)O_2$ gradient.

16. Explain the significance of the following tests of oxygenation status in managing a patient in respiratory failure: Pa_{O_2}, $P(A-a)O_2$ gradient, and $\dot{Q}s/\dot{Q}T$.

17. State the primary goal of treatment of respiratory failure.

18. Describe the principles of oxygen therapy for both hypercapnic and hypoxemic respiratory failure.
19. List the priorities and aims of treatment of hypercapnic respiratory failure.
20. Describe adult respiratory distress syndrome (etiology, pathogenesis, clinical features, and treatment).

Respiratory failure is a relatively common problem which is usually, but not always, the end result of chronic disease affecting the respiratory system. Increasingly, this condition is encountered as a complication of acute trauma, septicemia, or shock.

Respiratory failure, like the failure of any other organ system, may be characterized on the basis of clinical features or laboratory tests. However, it must be remembered that the correlation between the clinical features and deviations of laboratory tests from the normal range is far from straightforward in respiratory failure.

Respiratory failure is said to exist when the lung cannot fulfill its primary functions of gaseous exchange, namely, oxygenation of the arterial blood and carbon dioxide elimination. There are various grades of respiratory failure, and the condition may be acute (and possibly remittent) or chronic. *Chronic respiratory insufficiency* or *failure* refers to long-term functional impairment persisting many days or months and represents a compromise between the pathologic processes leading to failure and the compensatory processes stabilizing the situation. Blood gases may be mildly abnormal or within normal limits at rest but markedly abnormal during situations of increased demand such as exercise. Increased work of breathing (and thus decreased respiratory reserve) and reduction of physical activity are the two broad coping mechanisms in chronic respiratory insufficiency.

ACUTE RESPIRATORY FAILURE

Acute or *severe respiratory failure* is numerically defined as respiratory failure having a $Pa_{O_2} \leq 50$ to 60 mmHg with or without a $Pa_{CO_2} \geq 50$ mmHg under resting conditions at sea level. This numerical definition based on blood gases has been established because the line between chronic respiratory insufficiency and respiratory failure is subtle and clinical observations alone are unreliable. On the other hand, it must be understood that the definition based on blood gases is not absolute; the significance of the numbers depends on the

past history of the patient. A previously healthy person who developed this degree of abnormality of blood gases following a near-drowning accident might be expected to be comatose, whereas many patients with COPD can function with some degree of physical activity at the same levels.

Two broad classifications of respiratory failure are based on blood gas pathophysiology: (1) *hypoxemic,* or *normocapnic, respiratory failure* (hypoxemia with normal or low Pa_{CO_2}), and (2) *hypercapnic,* or *ventilatory, failure* (hypoxemia and hypercapnia). This chapter discusses the clinical features, causes, pathogenetic mechanisms, and management of these two types of respiratory failure.

Pathogenesis and etiology

The successful treatment of acute respiratory failure depends not only on its recognition at an early stage but also on identification of the mechanisms at fault. Early recognition may be difficult when the onset is insidious because the clinical signs and symptoms are nonspecific. Although tissue hypoxia cannot be assessed directly, blood gas measurements (one step in the long process which determines tissue oxygenation) can be helpful in drawing inferences about inadequate tissue oxygenation and the faulty mechanisms. Knowledge of the mechanisms at fault provides insight into the pathophysiology of a patient's lung disease, which leads in turn to appropriate treatment.

An important first step in the recognition of impending respiratory failure is awareness of the conditions and settings likely to lead to respiratory failure. Table 37-1 lists some of the common lung disorders causing respiratory failure, classified as extrinsic or intrinsic. Most of these conditions have been discussed in previous chapters. Extrinsic lung disorders (with lungs that are normal or nearly normal) lead to ventilatory, or hypercapnic, respiratory failure through (1) depression of central respiratory drive or (2) interference with the ventilatory response. Narcotic overdose is one of the most common causes of respiratory center depression

TABLE 37-1

CAUSES OF RESPIRATORY FAILURE

A. Extrinsic lung disorders
   1. Respiratory center depression
      a. Drug overdose (sedatives, narcotics)
      b. Cerebral trauma or infarction
      c. Bulbar poliomyelitis
      d. Encephalitis
   2. Neuromuscular disorders
      a. Cervical cord injury
      b. Guillain-Barré syndrome
      c. Amyotrophic lateral sclerosis
      d. Myasthenia gravis
      e. Muscular dystrophy
   3. Pleural and chest wall disorders
      a. Chest injury (flail chest; rib fracture)
      b. Pneumothorax
      c. Pleural effusion
      d. Kyphoscoliosis (abnormal lungs)
      e. Obesity—Pickwickian syndrome
B. Intrinsic lung disorders
   1. Diffuse obstructive disorders
      a. Emphysema, chronic bronchitis (COPD)
      b. Asthma, status asthmaticus
      c. Cystic fibrosis
   2. Diffuse restrictive disorders
      a. Interstitial fibrosis of various causes (e.g., silica, coal dust)
      b. Sarcoidosis
      c. Scleroderma
      d. Pulmonary edema
         (1) Cardiogenic
         (2) Noncardiogenic (ARDS)
      e. Atelectasis
      f. Consolidated pneumonia
   3. Pulmonary vascular disorders
      a. Pulmonary emboli
      b. Severe emphysema

resulting in ventilatory failure. Interference with ventilatory response occurs when there is disease or injury of the neural pathways or ventilatory muscles or mechanical dysfunction of the thoracic bellows due to injury, pain, or deformity. Some of the possible causes of a decreased ventilatory response are listed under neuromuscular and pleural and chest wall disorders.

While extrapulmonary, or extrinsic, lung disorders are important causes of respiratory failure, the pulmonary, or intrinsic, lung disorders are even more important. Chronic obstruction of the airways results in ventilatory failure, with COPD the most common cause. Diffuse restrictive disorders of the lung parenchyma and vasculature generally cause mild hypoxemic respiratory failure. However, acute intrinsic abnormalities of the lung parenchyma such as massive pulmonary edema, atelectasis, extensive consolidated pneumonia, and adult respiratory distress syndrome (ARDS) may cause profound hypoxemia. ARDS accounts for a significant portion of the population of respiratory intensive care units and has a high mortality rate. This condition is

discussed separately from the other causes of respiratory failure later in this chapter.

Finally, it is important to know that a number of precipitating factors can result in acute respiratory failure in persons with chronic lung disease (Table 37-2). Retained secretions, infection, and bronchospasm are the most common precipitating factors in patients with COPD causing *acute-on-chronic respiratory failure*. Important iatrogenic factors include the injudicious administration of narcotics or high fractions of inspired oxygen (FI_{O_2}). Cor pulmonale, pulmonary embolism (especially in patients with polycythemia), and pneumothorax from an emphysematous bleb are other less common precipitating causes of respiratory failure. Some of these precipitating factors cannot be eliminated, but many of them can; this has important implications for patient education and the management of chronic respiratory disease.

Mechanisms of hypoxemia and hypercapnia

By definition, hypoxemia is present in respiratory failure. Hypoxemic respiratory failure is characterized by hypoxemia and either normocapnia or hypocapnia, whereas ventilatory failure is characterized by hypoxemia and hypercapnia. The treatment implications of this distinction will become evident as this discussion proceeds.

Table 37-3 lists the pathogenetic mechanisms involved in hypoxemia and hypercapnia. Only the last three mechanisms shown in the Table (alveolar hypoventilation, low $\dot{V}/\dot{Q}$ ratio, and shunting) are important causes of hypoxemia. The primary cause of hypercapnia is alveolar hypoventilation, but $\dot{V}/\dot{Q}$ inequality generally has a trivial effect on the Pa_{CO_2}. It should be noted that alveolar hypoventilation causes both hypercapnia

TABLE 37-2

PRECIPITATING FACTORS OF RESPIRATORY FAILURE IN CHRONIC LUNG DISEASE

1. Infection of tracheobronchial tree, pneumonia, fever
2. Change in tracheobronchial secretions (increased volume or viscosity)
3. Bronchospasm (inhalation of irritants, allergens)
4. Disturbance in ability to clear secretions
5. Sedatives, narcotics, anesthesia
6. Oxygen therapy (high FI_{O_2})
7. Trauma, including surgery
8. Cardiovascular disorders (heart failure, pulmonary embolism)
9. Pneumothorax

TABLE 37-3

MECHANISMS OF HYPOXEMIA AND HYPERCAPNIA IN RESPIRATORY FAILURE

Hypoxemia	Hypercapnia
1. Low $F_{I_{O_2}}$ (altitude)	1. Alveolar hypoventilation
2. Diffusion impairment	2. $\dot{V}/\dot{Q}$ mismatch (trivial effect as long as overall $\dot{V}/\dot{Q}$ of functional alveoli is adequate)
3. Alveolar hypoventilation	
4. $\dot{V}/\dot{Q}$ mismatch	
a. Low $\dot{V}/\dot{Q}$ ratio (wasted perfusion, physiologic shunting, venous admixture-like perfusion, shunt effect)	
5. Venous to arterial shunt (true venous admixture, right to left shunt)	
a. Anatomic right to left shunt	
(1) Intracardiac	
(2) Intrapulmonary	
b. Alveolar capillary shunt (anatomic-like shunt)	
(1) Atelectasis	
(2) Consolidated pneumonia	
(3) Alveolar edema or exudate	

and hypoxemia, whereas $\dot{V}/\dot{Q}$ mismatch generally causes only hypoxemia.

The determination of the Pa_{CO_2} with respect to the lungs is relatively simple: the Pa_{CO_2} is directly related to CO_2 production and nearly inversely proportional to the alveolar ventilation (West, 1977):

$$Pa_{CO_2} \propto \frac{\dot{V}_{CO_2} \text{ (production of } CO_2)}{\dot{V}_A \text{ (alveolar ventilation)}}$$

Thus if alveolar ventilation is halved, the Pa_{CO_2} will be doubled provided CO_2 production remains constant. Conversely, if alveolar ventilation should double as in hyperventilation, the Pa_{CO_2} would be halved. Ventilatory failure with hypercapnia always involves the mechanism of alveolar hypoventilation. Pure hypoventilation, although relatively infrequent, is associated with the extrapulmonary conditions listed in Table 37-1, in which the lungs are relatively normal (with the exception of kyphoscoliosis). Alveolar hypoventilation develops in these conditions because the minute ventilation falls, as in respiratory center depression from narcotic overdose, or there is a disproportionally high work of

breathing or total body metabolism (increased CO_2 production) for a given alveolar ventilation, as in obesity or chest deformity (Cherniack and Cherniack, 1983). The hypoxemia associated with pure hypoventilation is generally mild (Pa_{O_2} = 50 to 80 mmHg) and is directly caused by the elevation of the alveolar P_{CO_2}. This fact can be explained by recalling that the partial pressure of all the alveolar or all the arterial blood gases must add up to the total (atmospheric) pressure. Thus when Pa_{CO_2} increases the Pa_{O_2} must decrease and vice versa at a constant total atmospheric pressure. The respiratory exchange ratio (R), or ratio of milliliters of CO_2 excreted to milliliters of O_2 absorbed, is 0.8. This means that for every 10 mmHg rise in the Pa_{CO_2}, the Pa_{O_2} will decrease about 12 mmHg.* Thus if the Pa_{CO_2} should increase from a normal 40 to 70 mmHg, the Pa_{O_2} must decrease from, say, a normal 100 to 64 mmHg when there is pure hypoventilation. If the drop in the Pa_{O_2} is greater than expected, other mechanisms causing hypoxemia must also be operating ($\dot{V}/\dot{Q}$ mismatch, shunting). While this degree of hypoxemia in itself is not serious, since oxygen saturation is about 80 percent, this degree of elevation of the Pa_{CO_2} will depress the respiratory center and cause a serious acidosis with an arterial pH of about 7.2.

Ventilation/perfusion ($\dot{V}/\dot{Q}$) inequality or mismatch is by far the most important mechanism causing hypoxemia in persons with chronic airway obstruction and plays a role in most other intrinsic lung disorders. $\dot{V}/\dot{Q}$ inequality, or mismatch, refers to the *regional* imbalance of ventilation and blood flow in the pulmonary gas-exchanging units discussed in Chap. 31. Some pulmonary units have relatively high $\dot{V}/\dot{Q}$ ratios (wasted ventilation or dead-space-like units), while others have low $\dot{V}/\dot{Q}$ ratios (wasted perfusion, physiologic shunt, venous admixture). If some alveoli receive too little ventilation in proportion to perfusion (low $\dot{V}/\dot{Q}$), there is a fall in Pa_{O_2} and a rise in Pa_{CO_2} in the blood leaving these alveoli. In effect, blood is shunted past the alveoli without adequate gas exchange taking place (venous admixture effect). Conversely, alveoli which receive too little perfusion in proportion to ventilation (high $\dot{V}/\dot{Q}$) produce high Pa_{O_2} and low Pa_{CO_2} in the blood flowing from them. Recall that the healthy lung has some $\dot{V}/\dot{Q}$ inequality due to the effects of gravity (see Chap. 31), but this is not significant enough to cause blood gas abnormalities. Low $\dot{V}/\dot{Q}$ ratios can cause significant hypoxemia in lung disease but generally have little effect on the Pa_{CO_2}. The relation between the partial pressures and content of these two gases accounts for the difference.

---

*Equality of alveolar and arterial CO_2 gas tension is assumed as well as equality of alveolar and arterial O_2 gas tension, although this is not strictly accurate. The Pa_{O_2} is about 5 mmHg lower than the PA_{O_2} because of a small $\dot{V}/\dot{Q}$ mismatch and shunt in the normal lung, but the effect on PA_{CO_2} differences is negligible.

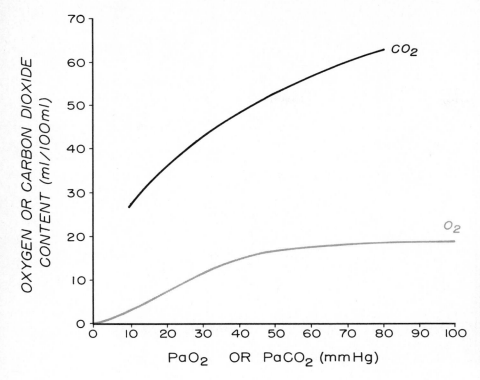

Figure 37-1 illustrates the oxyhemoglobin and carbon dioxide dissociation curves drawn on the same scale for comparative purposes. This figure makes the important point that the oxyhemoglobin curve has a flat portion while the CO_2 curve does not. At a Pa_{O_2} of about 60 (when the curve starts to flatten), the oxygen content of the blood has reached more than 80 percent of the maximum content of about 19.5 volume percent. A large increase in the Pa_{O_2} (e.g., from 60 to 100 mmHg) causes only a small increase in oxygen content. In contrast, CO_2 transport in the blood is much more efficient. Because the CO_2 curve is steep in the physiologic range of the Pa_{CO_2}, a small change (e.g., from 40 to 50) causes a large change in CO_2 content. What this means in terms of $\dot{V}/\dot{Q}$ imbalance is that alveoli with high $\dot{V}/\dot{Q}$ ratios cannot fully compensate for those with low $\dot{V}/\dot{Q}$ ratios with reference to oxygen transport. The hemoglobin from the better ventilated units, when already nearly saturated (flat part of oxyhemoglobin dissociation curve), cannot carry the excess oxygen that would be needed to compensate for the deficit caused by poorly oxygenated blood from the low $\dot{V}/\dot{Q}$ units. Since the CO_2 dissociation curve is more nearly linear in the physiologic range, the hyperventilating units with a high $\dot{V}/\dot{Q}$ ratio can compensate for hypoventilating units with a low $\dot{V}/\dot{Q}$ ratio. The result is that the mixed blood leaving the high and low $\dot{V}/\dot{Q}$ units will have a normal Pa_{CO_2}. However, progressive involvement of more and more of the lung by the disease process will result in more and more alveolar-capillary units with low $\dot{V}/\dot{Q}$ ratios. Eventually a point is reached at which the remaining high $\dot{V}/\dot{Q}$ units cannot compensate for the low units, and hypercapnia ensues. Therefore those diseases characterized by $\dot{V}/\dot{Q}$ abnormalities (most of the intrinsic lung diseases and kyphoscoliosis) demonstrate progression through hypoxemic respiratory insufficiency and failure (which occurs first) to hypercapnic, or ventilatory, failure (which occurs later).

The important principles to remember from this discussion so far are that (1) the factors determining oxygenation and ventilation are different and must be analyzed separately; (2) the Pa_{CO_2} must be regarded as a function of the *overall* ventilation of the entire lung without regard to local inequalities of distribution of ventilation and perfusion; (3) the Pa_{O_2}, on the other hand, depends not only on the amount of alveolar ventilation but also on the matching of ventilation and perfusion; and (4) hypercapnia must be viewed as representing a problem not only with oxygenation but also with ventilation.

The third important mechanism causing hypoxemia is venous to arterial, or right to left, shunting of blood, which bypasses the gas-exchanging units of the lung. A true anatomic right to left shunt may exist in congenital heart disease, as when there is an opening between the right and left chambers of the heart or, rarely, when there is an arteriovenous fistula within the lung (West, 1977). There is a small true shunt in normal lungs (see Fig. 31-12) amounting to about 2.5 percent of pulmonary blood flow. In addition to these rare anatomic vascular abnormalities and the small normal shunt, shunting may also occur when alveolar spaces are nonfunctional, as when the alveoli are collapsed (atelectasis) or filled with edema fluid or with exudate, as in pulmonary edema or pneumonia. This type of shunting may be regarded as an extreme type of $\dot{V}/\dot{Q}$ mismatch in which ventilation of the involved units is zero while perfusion continues. If a large number of gas-exchange units are involved in shunting, the resulting hypoxemia can be severe. However, the Pa_{CO_2} is generally normal or low, since the subject can usually increase ventilation sufficiently in the remaining normal lung to blow off the CO_2 adequately. When overall hyperventilation occurs in response to severe hypoxemia, hypocapnia and respiratory alkalosis may result. Hypoxemic respiratory failure caused primarily by shunting is difficult to treat, since the hypoxemia is not readily correctable by oxygen therapy.

Another type of extreme $\dot{V}/\dot{Q}$ imbalance is that exemplified by a pulmonary unit in which there is ventilation but no perfusion (dead space). The classic example of alveolar dead-space disease is acute pulmonary embolus. Another common cause is acutely decreased pulmonary perfusion due to acutely decreased cardiac output or acute pulmonary hypertension with increased pulmonary vascular resistance (Shapiro, 1982). Destruction of the alveolar septal walls in emphysema, with replacement of several alveoli by large air spaces, results in reducing the surface area for gas exchange. The anatomic dead space can be greatly increased by a rapid, shallow breathing pattern, as illustrated in Table 32-2. The normal physiologic dead space is 30 percent of the tidal volume (V_D/V_T). If dead-space ventilation is increased significantly (wasted ventilation), overall ventilation must increase to maintain effective alveolar ventilation. In advanced disease the work of breathing may be so great as to cause hypercapnia and hypoxemia. When there is both high minute volume and high physiologic dead space, the condition is referred to as *high-output ventilatory failure* (Shapiro, 1982, page 117).

Hypoxemia due to high altitude can generally be ignored in the treatment of respiratory failure, since it is constant for a particular locale. At sea level, barometric pressure (P_B) is 760 mmHg. With increasing altitude the total barometric pressure and the P_{O_2} of inspired air decrease, although the percentage of oxygen in the air remains constant at 20.93 percent. For example, in Boston at sea level the P_B is 760 mmHg and the inspired P_{O_2} is 159 mmHg, while in Denver the P_B is 632.3 mmHg and the inspired P_{O_2} is 132.3 mmHg (Comroe, 1974, page 251).

Most authorities no longer consider diffusion impairment to be a significant factor in producing hypoxemia, although it may play a minor role when there is thickening of the alveolar-capillary membrane, as in pulmonary fibrosis and sarcoidosis. The normal contact time between alveolar gas and pulmonary blood is 0.75 seconds under resting conditions, and equilibration is normally completed in 0.25 second. Thus there is ample diffusion time in reserve (Cherniack and Cherniack, 1983; Shapiro, 1982). When diffusion time is somewhat reduced during exercise, it is possible for diffusion limitation to make a greater contribution to hypoxemia.

In summary, when hypoxemic respiratory failure is present the principal mechanisms involved are low $\dot{V}/\dot{Q}$ ratio or shunting, either alone or in combination. Diffusion impairment may possibly make a minor contribution to the hypoxemia, although this is controversial. Hypoxemic respiratory insufficiency or failure is usually associated with restrictive or vascular diseases of the lung. Even though the work of breathing is increased in these conditions (with consequently increased CO_2 production and O_2 consumption for ventilatory work), the subject has enough strength to increase ventilation sufficiently to maintain a normal Pa_{CO_2}. Any slight rise in the Pa_{CO_2} will stimulate increased ventilation. When the Pa_{O_2} falls to about 50 to 60 mmHg, this also stimulates ventilation. Consequently hyperventilation may result, so that the Pa_{CO_2} is decreased below normal levels (respiratory alkalosis or hypocapnia). Hyperventilation while breathing room air is generally ineffectual in correcting hypoxemia because of the sigmoid shape of the oxyhemoglobin dissociation curve. Oxygen therapy is quite effective in correcting hypoxemia due to $\dot{V}/\dot{Q}$ imbalance or diffusion impairment but ineffective if the cause is shunting.

Hypercapnic, or ventilatory, failure may be caused by hypoventilation alone or in combination with any or all of the other hypoxemic mechanisms–$\dot{V}/\dot{Q}$ imbalance, shunting, or possibly diffusion impairment. Pure ventilatory failure occurs in extrapulmonary disorders involving failure of neural or muscular control of breathing. The classic example of hypercapnic respiratory failure occurs in chronic obstructive pulmonary disease (COPD) and involves $\dot{V}/\dot{Q}$ imbalance and hypoventilation. When respiratory failure is precipitated by retained secretions and pneumonia in such patients, there may also be considerable shunting. Although obstructive disorders of the airways generally result in hypercapnic respiratory failure, reversible airway disease, as in asthma, is an exception to the rule. An acute asthmatic attack is generally characterized by hypoxemia and hypocapnia, since the subjects are usually able to hyperventilate. A rise of the Pa_{CO_2} even to normal levels in a sustained asthmatic attack may be a signal that the functional status is deteriorating (Cherniack and Cherniack, 1983, p. 370). The primary focus in ventilatory failure is on measures to improve ventilation and at the same time prevent serious tissue hypoxia. Methods of differentiating between the mechanisms involved in hypoxemia and hypercapnia are discussed subsequently.

The manifestations of acute respiratory failure represent a combination of the clinical features of the underlying disease, the precipitating factors, and the manifestations of hypoxemia and hypercapnia. Thus the clinical picture may be quite variable, since various factors may precipitate it. The presence or absence of preceding chronic respiratory insufficiency is another factor which modifies the clinical picture.

The signs and symptoms of hypoxemia are a direct result of tissue hypoxia. (These were presented in Chap. 33 but are here reviewed.) The more commonly cited signs and symptoms do not develop until the Pa_{O_2} is in the range of 40 to 50 mmHg. Tissues highly sensitive to oxygen depletion are principally affected, including the brain, heart, and lungs. The most prominent signs and symptoms are neurologic: headache, mental confusion, impairment of judgment, slurring of speech, asterixis, impairment of motor function, agitation, and restlessness which may progress to delirium and unconsciousness. In some cases the neurologic signs and symptoms of hypoxic persons have been misinterpreted as alcoholic inebriation. The initial cardiovascular responses to hypoxemia are tachycardia and increased cardiac output and blood pressure. When the hypoxia persists, bradycardia, hypotension, decreased cardiac output, and arrhythmias may occur. Hypoxemia causes vasoconstriction of the pulmonary blood vessels. The metabolic effect of tissue hypoxia is anaerobic metabolism resulting in metabolic acidosis. Although cyanosis is often regarded as a sign of hypoxia, it is unreliable (see Chap. 33). The classic symptom of dyspnea may also be absent, especially when there is depression of respiratory center drive, as in the respiratory failure of narcotic overdose.

Hypercapnia while breathing room air is always accompanied by hypoxemia. Consequently the signs and symptoms of ventilatory failure represent the effects of both hypercapnia and hypoxemia. The major effect of increases in the Pa_{CO_2} is depression of the central nervous system. It is for this reason that severe hypercapnia is sometimes referred to as *CO$_2$ narcosis*. Hypercapnia results in cerebral vasodilatation, increased cerebral blood flow, and increased intracranial pressure. The resultant headache, worse upon awaking in the morning (since Pa_{CO_2} increases slightly during sleep) is characteristic. Other resultant signs and symptoms include papilledema, neuromuscular irritability (asterixis), fluctuations of mood, and increased drowsiness, which may progress to frank coma. Although an increased Pa_{CO_2} is normally the most powerful stimulus to respiration, it has a depressive effect on respiration at levels above 70 mmHg. In addition, persons with COPD and chronic hypercapnia develop insensitivity to increased Pa_{CO_2} and depend on hypoxic drive. Hypercapnia causes con-

striction of the pulmonary blood vessels, thus aggravating any pulmonary artery hypertension that may be present. When CO_2 retention is severe, decreased myocardial contractility, systemic vasodilatation, heart failure, and hypotension may ensue. Hypercapnia causes respiratory acidosis, which is often combined with metabolic acidosis when there is tissue hypoxia. This combination can cause a serious depression of the blood pH. The renal compensatory response to respiratory acidosis is reabsorption of bicarbonate in order to restore pH to normal. This response takes about 3 days, so respiratory acidosis is much more severe when the onset is rapid.

Diagnosis

There are a number of situations in which anyone can recognize respiratory failure. Examples are cardiac arrest, complete obstruction of the upper airways by, e.g., a piece of meat, head injury serious enough to stop the breathing mechanism, or labored breathing in a person who is cyanotic. However, in many patients the presence of respiratory failure may not be so obvious. The onset of respiratory failure is insidious in many persons with chronic respiratory insufficiency. Signs and symptoms may be nonspecific and correlate poorly with the degree of respiratory impairment until the situation is catastrophic. Great astuteness is needed to recognize every case of respiratory failure. Thus the clinician needs to have a high degree of suspicion and be ready to obtain measurements of arterial blood gases (ABG) when respiratory failure is suspected, since this is the only way a definitive diagnosis can be made. In general, a Pa_{CO_2} of 50 mmHg or more or a Pa_{O_2} of 50 to 60 mmHg or less at sea level is accepted as indicating respiratory failure.

Assessment of respiratory function

Measurement of respiratory function is indispensable in the provision of adequate respiratory care, not only for accurate diagnosis but also for evaluation of response to treatment. Measurement of ABG provides valuable information not only for establishing the degree and type of respiratory failure but also for identifying the mechanisms involved. A number of bedside measurements of ventilatory function are also frequently used to assess ventilatory reserve and the need for mechanical ventilation. The ventilatory status as well as the acid-base status are assessed by examining the arterial P_{CO_2}, HCO_3, and pH.

A normogram may be helpful in determining whether hypercapnic respiratory failure is acute or chronic or whether a mixed acid-base disorder is present. Figure 37-2 shows the relation between the Pa_{CO_2} and pH and the alterations seen in respiratory and metabolic disorders of acid-base balance. Data falling within a particular band usually represent the primary disorder, and data outside the band represent a mixed disorder. The following equivalences need to be emphasized: (1) respiratory acidosis = hypercapnia = alveolar hypoventilation, and (2) respiratory alkalosis = hypocapnia = alveolar hyperventilation. The lettered points on the normogram represent common values in respiratory failure. Any sudden, severe decrease in ventilation resulting in the retention of CO_2 in the blood will produce acute respiratory acidosis (C). This acidosis is frequently aggravated by a coexisting metabolic acidosis due to excess lactic acid produced by the tissue hypoxia that also results from decreased ventilation (B). The renal compensation for a rise in the Pa_{CO_2} is retention of HCO_3^- in order to restore blood pH to normal. This process normally takes about 3 days. Thus point D represents chronic hypercapnia, frequently seen in patients with COPD. Point E could represent partially compensated acute hypercapnia or a mixture of acute and chronic hypercapnia, which might occur when a patient with COPD develops a respiratory infection. Point F represents a mixture of chronic hypercapnia and metabolic alkalosis, which might be caused by rapid correction of the hypercapnia by artificial ventilation. When the Pa_{CO_2} is lowered rapidly in a person with compen-

sated respiratory acidosis (hypercapnia) and consequently with an increased HCO_3^-, there is an excess of base bicarbonate (metabolic alkalosis) until the kidneys can excrete the excess. Point G represents chronic hyperventilation (respiratory alkalosis), which is common in hypoxemic respiratory failure. Point A represents a mild hypercapnia. The acute and the chronic form cannot be distinguished unless the patient's usual Pa_{CO_2} is known.

Evaluation of oxygenation involves examination of several parameters, including Pa_{O_2}, the alveolar-arterial O_2 difference or gradient [the $P(A-a)O_2$ or $A-aDO_2$], cardiac output, and hemoglobin. The Pa_{O_2} should be related to the Pa_{CO_2}, pH, and HCO_3^- in order to determine the type of respiratory failure (hypoxemic versus hypercapnic) and the pathophysiologic mechanism. The inspired oxygen fraction FI_{O_2} must be taken into account when interpreting blood gases. Pure hypoventilation while breathing air ($FI_{O_2} = 0.21$), can be distinguished from the other mechanisms ($\dot{V}/\dot{Q}$ and/or shunt) by calculating the expected value of the Pa_{O_2} for a given change in the Pa_{CO_2}. For example, if the patient's Pa_{CO_2} is 70 mmHg, the expected Pa_{O_2} would be 64 mmHg, since a 10-mmHg change in Pa_{CO_2} causes a 12-mmHg change of Pa_{O_2} in the opposite direction, as explained earlier in this chapter. If the change is greater than expected (e.g., $Pa_{O_2} = 45$ mmHg), $\dot{V}/\dot{Q}$ mismatch and/or shunting must also be involved.

The $P(A-a)O_2$ gradient is even more helpful in distinguishing between the pathophysiologic mechanisms. The normal $P(A-a)O_2$ gradient is about 10 mmHg (because of a small amount of normal shunting). Knowing that high concentrations of inspired oxygen correct hypoventilation and $\dot{V}/\dot{Q}$ imbalance (and diffusion impairment) but not shunting allows one to distinguish between the mechanisms, using the $P(A-a)O_2$ gradient.

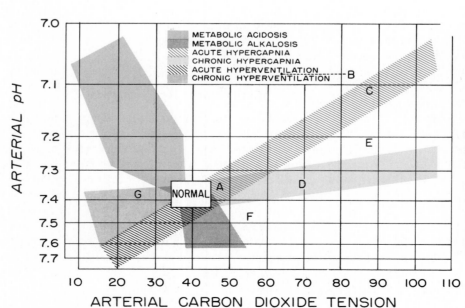

FIGURE 37-2

Normogram for acid-base disturbances. This graph displays the quantity and direction of changes in pH and Pa_{CO_2} in various types of acid-base disturbances. The shaded areas represent the range of variability in persons with pure acid-base disorders. In general, values lying outside the significance bands represent mixed acid-base disorders. See text for explanation of lettered points. (Modified from Burrows, B., Knudson, R. J., and Kettel, L. J., *Respiratory Insufficiency,* Year Book Medical Publishers, Inc., Chicago, 1975, p. 93).

The $P(A-a)O_2$ gradient is normal while breathing air if the cause of the hypoxemia is pure hypoventilation. A $P(A-a)O_2$ gradient of >20 mmHg (25 in older adults) is considered abnormal for clinical purposes when room air is being breathed (Guenter, 1977, page 147). The PA_{O_2} can be calculated by using a simplified version of the alveolar gas equation and then calculating the alveolar-arterial partial pressure difference ($PA_{O_2} - Pa_{O_2}$):

$$PA_{O_2} = PI_{O_2} - \frac{Pa_{CO_2}}{R}$$

where

$$PI_{O_2} = FI_{O_2} \times (PB - PH_2O)$$

Using the figures of 760 mmHg for the barometric pressure (PB at sea level), 47 mmHg for the partial pressure of H_2O at normal body temperature, and 20.93% oxygen for the FI_{O_2}, the PI_{O_2} is seen to be 149.3 mmHg [$0.2093 \times (760 - 47)$].

Making a concrete application of this formula, the following room air (PB = 750 mmHg) blood gas values were obtained on a 30-year-old man during an asthmatic attack: $Pa_{CO_2} = 60$ mmHg and $Pa_{O_2} = 40$ mmHg. Thus, $PI_{O_2} = 0.2093 \times (750 - 47) = 147$, and $P(A-a)O_2 = 147 - (40/0.8) - 60$ mmHg $= 37$ mmHg. Since $P(A-a)O_2$ is greater than 20, alveolar hypoventilation alone does not account for the hypoxemia, and there is either additional $\dot{V}/\dot{Q}$ mismatch or shunting.

$\dot{V}/\dot{Q}$ mismatch may be differentiated from true shunting by determining the $P(A-a)O_2$ after having the patient breathe 100% oxygen (or a lesser concentration) for 15 minutes to wash out the nitrogen gas from the alveoli. Since $FI_{O_2} = 1.0$ when pure oxygen is breathed, the alveolar gas equation simplifies to

$$PA_{O_2} = (PB - 47) - Pa_{CO_2}$$

A healthy person breathing 100% oxygen at sea level would thus have a PA_{O_2} of 673 mmHg ($760 - 47 - 40$). The normal Pa_{O_2} is >500 mmHg and the $P(A-a)O_2$ gradient 30 to 50 mmHg when 100% oxygen is breathed (Bushnell, 1973, page 33). Since $\dot{V}/\dot{Q}$ mismatch is largely corrected by administration of 100% oxygen, a $Pa_{O_2} <500$ mmHg indicates significant shunting (Cherniack and Cherniack, 1983). The $P(A-a)O_2$ gradient is also increased. The calculated PA_{O_2} can also be used to determine the proportion of the cardiac output that is acting like a shunt ($\dot{Q}s/\dot{Q}T$). These calculations are based on equations using arterial and venous oxygen content differences (for formulas, see West, 1977; Cherniack, 1977; and Shapiro, 1982). In practice, the percentage of shunt is often estimated from the Pa_{O_2}. If inhalation of 100% oxygen does not raise the Pa_{O_2} above 100 mmHg, the shunt is 20 percent or greater, indicating significant dysfunction. A 50 percent shunt is compatible with life only if the subject is breathing 100% oxygen (Guenter, 1977). The normal shunt is 2 to 5 percent.

The $P(A-a)O_2$ is a highly sensitive index of oxygen exchange and is not only useful in identifying the mechanism of the hypoxemia but is used regularly by intensive care nurses and physicians to follow the progress of patients in respiratory failure. Table 37-4 lists some of the common measurements used to assess ventilatory function and oxygenation for patients in respiratory failure. The critical values listed are used as criteria of the need for mechanical ventilation. It must be emphasized that these values are only guidelines. Good clinical judgment is based on a thorough understanding of the pathophysiology of respiratory failure and involves integration of qualitative observations of the patient with the quantitative measurements.

Treatment of respiratory failure

The priorities in the management of respiratory failure vary according to the etiology, but the primary aims of treatment are the same in all cases, that is, to treat the cause of the respiratory failure and at the same time ensure adequate ventilation and clear airways.

Since the most life-threatening feature of respiratory failure is the impairment of gas exchange, the first goal of therapy is to ensure that hypoxemia, acidemia, and hypercapnia do not reach hazardous levels. A Pa_{O_2} of 40 mmHg or a pH of 7.2 or less is poorly tolerated by adults and can result in cerebral, kidney, and cardiac impairment and the development of cardiac arrhythmias. A Pa_{CO_2} of 60 mmHg which has developed slowly in a patient with COPD is usually well tolerated, but rapid development to this level is not. A Pa_{CO_2} of 70 mmHg or more is usually poorly tolerated in any patient and causes central nervous system depression and coma.

Oxygen may be delivered at a concentration of 40 to 60 percent to a patient with hypoxemia and a normal or low Pa_{CO_2} (mask or catheter at 8 liters per minute with adequate humidification) in order to achieve a rapid correction of the hypoxemia. However, this concentration should not be continued for more than a few hours, as it has a direct toxic effect on alveolar cells, causing decreased synthesis of surfactant and decreased pulmonary compliance. Prolonged administration of oxygen (more than 24 to 48 hours) at high concentrations ($>50\%$) also causes absorption atelectasis.

Hypoxemia with hypercapnia is always treated with low, graduated oxygen therapy, beginning with a mask which delivers 24% oxygen. The concentration is increased to 28% oxygen if necessary to maintain a

Pa_{O_2} of 50 mmHg or more. Careful monitoring of blood gases is utilized at all times to ensure that the oxygen therapy does not cause a deterioration in the patient's respiratory status: In the patient with COPD, attempts are made to achieve Pa_{O_2} values which are normal for the patient (e.g., 50 to 70 mmHg) and not those normal for the healthy adult (80 to 100 mmHg). When it is not possible to achieve Pa_{O_2} values of 50 mmHg, artificial ventilation with a respirator may be required. See Table 37-4 for critical values indicating need for ventilatory support.

Table 37-5 lists the priorities and aims in the treatment of hypercapnic respiratory failure. The approach to the problem of retained lung secretions includes measures to liquefy and remove them. Liquefaction is best achieved by adequate hydration of the patient. Drugs such as potassium iodide taken orally or aerosol delivery of water may also help in the mobilization of sputum. Secretions are best removed by encouraging the patient to cough or assisting the patient's efforts by percussion, vibration, and postural drainage. When the patient is too depressed or weak to cough, secretions may be removed by aspiration via an endotracheal tube or bron-

TABLE 37-4

MEASUREMENTS OF RESPIRATORY FUNCTION

Test	Significance	Normal value	Critical value
Tests of ventilatory function			
Respiratory rate (f) per minute	Overall indicator of respiratory distress and work of breathing	12–20	>35 or <10
Tidal volume (V_T), ml	Volume of air exchanged during each breath at rest	500–700	<350
Minute ventilation ($\dot{V}_E$), liters	Overall indicator of ventilation	5–10	>10
Forced vital capacity (FVC), ml per kg ideal body weight	Indicates ventilatory reserve; best indicator of need for ventilatory support	65–75	<15
FEV_1, ml/kg	First-second expired volume of FVC; useful in assessing ventilatory reserve in patients with COPD as well as efficacy of measures to overcome airway obstruction	50–60	<10
Maximum inspiratory force (MIF), cmH_2O	Indicates reserve of ventilatory effort	75–100	<25
V_D/V_T	Dead space/tidal volume ratio; allows estimate of ventilation in excess of perfusion; requires collecting sample of expired air to measure PE_{CO_2} and Pa_{CO_2}; $V_D/V_T = Pa_{CO_2} - (PE_{CO_2}/Pa_{CO_2})$	0.25–0.40	>0.60
Pa_{CO_2}, mmHg	Reflects ability of lung to eliminate CO_2; trend should be followed in patient with chronic hypercapnia along with pH of arterial blood; serious acidemia when pH 7.2 or less	35–45	>55
Tests of oxygenation status			
Pa_{O_2} (breathing air), mmHg	Adequacy of oxygen tension in arterial blood; expected Pa_{O_2} can be calculated from alveolar gas equation when patient breathing higher FI_{O_2} than air (O_2 therapy)	80–100	<50–60
$P(A-a)O_2$ or $A-aD_{O_2}$, mmHg (breathing 100% O_2)	Alveolar-arterial oxygen tension difference; indicates oxygenation reserve	30–50	>450
$\dot{Q}s/\dot{Q}T$, %	Proportion of cardiac output shunted past alveoli	<5	>20
Tests of acid-base status			
Pa_{CO_2}, mmHg		36–44	
Arterial blood pH		7.35–7.45	
HCO_3^-, meq/L		24 ± 3	

Values from Cherniack and Cherniack, 1983; Bendixen, 1965.

TABLE 37-5

565

ADULT RESPIRATORY DISTRESS SYNDROME

PRIORITIES AND PRINCIPLES OF THE TREATMENT OF HYPERCAPNIC RESPIRATORY FAILURE

Priority	Problem	Treatment
1	Retained secretions (ineffective cough)	Adequate hydration, expectorants, aerosols Supervised coughing Catheter aspiration (deep suction) Bronchoscopic suction Endotracheal tube aspiration Tracheostomy
2	Hypoxemia	Graduated oxygen therapy with frequent monitoring of blood gases to direct therapy
3	Hypercapnia	Respiratory stimulants (drug overdose) Avoidance of sedation Artificial ventilation via endotracheal tube or tracheostomy
4	Respiratory infection	Antiobiotics
5	Bronchospasm	Bronchodilatory drugs (isoproterenol by inhalation therapy; intravenous, oral, or rectal aminophylline; corticosteroid drugs)
6	Cardiac failure	Diuretics Digoxin (with caution if given at all)

Source: Crofton and Douglas, 1981.

choscopy. If these methods fail, tracheostomy may be necessary.

If bronchospasm is present in respiratory failure, bronchodilatory or corticosteroid drugs may be used. Respiratory infection, which is a common cause of hypoxemic respiratory failure, is treated with the appropriate antibiotics.

Finally, a thorough search is made for other factors which may have induced the respiratory failure, such as pulmonary embolism or left ventricular failure.

A number of excellent books dealing with the management of respiratory failure are suggested in the references for those who wish to gain more extensive knowledge of this subject.

ADULT RESPIRATORY DISTRESS SYNDROME

Adult respiratory distress syndrome (ARDS) is a distinct form of respiratory failure characterized by profound hypoxemia refractory to conventional treatment. It is preceded by a variety of serious illnesses which all result in a characteristic diffuse noncardiogenic pulmonary edema. The term was coined by Petty and Ashbaugh (1971) after observing acute life-threatening respiratory distress in patients with no previous lung disease. Although this syndrome has been called by a variety of other names (*shock lung, wet lung, adult hyaline membrane disease, stiff lung syndrome*) the term *adult respiratory distress syndrome* has been more widely accepted. It has been estimated that 150,000 persons suffer from ARDS each year, and the mortality rate is 50 percent (MacDonnell and Segal, 1977).

Etiology and pathogenesis

ARDS develops when the lung is injured directly or indirectly by various processes. Some of the most common conditions leading to ARDS are listed in Table 37-6.

The mechanism by which such a diversity of insults could produce a common clinical and pathophysiologic syndrome is not clear. The common denominator causing the characteristic alveolar edema seems to involve injury to the alveolar-capillary membrane with the pro-

TABLE 37-6

CAUSES OF ADULT RESPIRATORY DISTRESS SYNDROME

1. Shock from various causes (especially hemorrhagic, hemorrhagic acute pancreatitis, gram-negative sepsis)
2. Sepsis without shock, with or without disseminated intravascular coagulation (DIC)
3. Overwhelming viral pneumonia
4. Critical trauma
   a. Head injury
   b. Direct chest injury
   c. Multiple organ trauma with hemorrhagic shock
   d. Multiple fractures
      (1) Fat embolization (associated with fracture of long bones such as the femur)
5. Aspiration/inhalation injury
   a. Aspiration of gastric contents
   b. Near drowning
   c. Smoke inhalation
   d. Irritant gas inhalation (e.g., chlorine, ammonia, sulfur dioxide)
   e. Prolonged exposure (>48 hours to high concentration of inhaled oxygen (F_{IO_2} >50%))
6. Narcotic overdose
7. Postperfusion cardiopulmonary bypass surgery

duction of a capillary leak. Electron microscopy studies reveal that the air-blood barrier consists of type I pneumocytes (supporting cells) and type II pneumocytes (source of surfactant) along with basement membrane on the alveolar side; these are back to back with capillary basement membrane and endothelial cells. In addition, the alveolus has connective tissue cells that serve as support and regulate volume. The alveolar capillary membrane is normally quite impermeable to particles. However, with injury this permeability is altered, with an influx of fluid, RBCs, WBCs and blood proteins. The fluid first accumulates in the interstitium; when the capacity of the interstitium is exceeded, the fluid accumulates in the alveolus, causing congestive atelectasis. The point of vulnerability seems to be the interdigitations (small spaces about 60 Å wide) between the capillary endothelial cells, which become widened, allowing the influx of small particles, which then cause a shift in oncotic pressure (MacDonnell, 1977). Thus the formation of pulmonary edema depends on the disruption of the normal relations of the Starling forces—hydrostatic pressure, oncotic pressure, and tissue pressure. In addition, alterations in the surfactant system undoubtedly play a role in the diffuse microatelectasis. In fact, light microscopy reveals that the proteinaceous material may be organized into hyaline membranes lining the alveolus. The pathologic picture is similar to that of the respiratory distress syndrome occuring in the infant (Petty, 1978). The consequence of the diffuse edema and atelectasis is marked intrapulmonary shunting, which may affect more than 40 percent of the cardiac output.

The mechanisms of acute lung injury are not known. Bone (1984) has reviewed a number of chemical mediators implicated in the pathogenesis of ARDS. These factors include prostaglandins, histamine, serotonin, bradykinin, fibrin degradation products, and platelet and leukocytic enzymes, which have all been observed in abnormal quantities in blood or secretions or in the lung in animals and humans following insults known to cause ARDS. The relation of these incriminating mediators to the disturbance in capillary permeability is unknown.

Clinical features

The primary features of ARDS include a marked degree of intrapulmonary shunting with hypoxemia, a progressive loss in lung compliance, and extreme dyspnea and tachypnea resulting from both the hypoxemia and the increased work of breathing secondary to the loss of lung compliance. The normal compliance of the lungs and thorax together is about 100 ml/cmH$_2$O. In ARDS compliance may be as low as 15 to 20 ml/cmH$_2$O (Petty, 1978). Functional residual capacity is also reduced. These features are a consequence of the interstitial and alveolar edema. The result is a stiff lung which is difficult to ventilate. It is a hallmark of ARDS that the hypoxemia cannot be relieved by oxygen administration during spontaneous breathing. The full-blown clinical state may become manifest 1 to 2 days following the initiating injury.

The establishment of the correct diagnosis of ARDS largely depends on obtaining an accurate clinical history. The earliest laboratory finding is hypoxemia, so measuring the arterial blood gases in the appropriate clinical setting is important. The Pa$_{CO_2}$ is generally normal or low. Early chest x-ray findings may be normal despite the hypoxemia. Later, as the alveolar and interstitial fluid accumulates and the congestive atelectasis spreads, the chest x-ray shows a diffuse "whiteout" appearance (MacDonnell, 1977). Hence another name for ARDS is *white lung*.

Treatment

The management of ARDS is aimed at correcting the accompanying shock, acidosis, and hypoxemia. Almost all patients require mechanical ventilation and high concentrations of oxygen to avoid serious tissue hypoxia. The use of positive end-expiratory pressure (PEEP) with the volume respirator is a major advance in the treatment of this condition. PEEP helps to correct the respiratory distress syndrome by reexpanding previously atelectatic areas and by reversing the flow of atelectatic edema fluid from capillaries. Another benefit of PEEP is that it allows administration of lower concentrations of F$_{I_{O_2}}$. This is important, since on the one hand a high F$_{I_{O_2}}$ is generally needed to achieve a minimally acceptable Pa$_{O_2}$, and on the other hand high concentrations of oxygen are toxic to the lung and cause ARDS. The net effect of PEEP is to improve arterial oxygen tensions and allow reduction in the F$_{I_{O_2}}$. Potential hazards from the use of PEEP are pneumothorax and interference with cardiac output because of high pressures. Close monitoring and attention is directed toward achieving "best PEEP"—i.e., ventilation at that end-expiratory pressure which results in the best lung compliance and least reduction in the Pa$_{O_2}$ and cardiac output (Petty, 1978).

Since sequestration of fluid in the lung is a problem, restriction of fluids and diuretic therapy are other important measures in the treatment of ARDS. Appropriate antibiotics are given to treat infection. Although the use of corticosteroids is controversial, many centers use them in the treatment of ARDS even though their benefit has not been clearly established.

Respiratory failure

Directions: Answer the following on a separate sheet of paper.

1. What is the relation between respiratory insufficiency and the maintenance of normal arterial blood gases?

2. What is the most common cause of chronic respiratory insufficiency?

3. List the two types of respiratory failure based on blood gas changes.

4. Explain why high concentrations of oxygen must not be administered in hypercapnic respiratory failure.

5. What level of Pa_{O_2} or Pa_{CO_2} would not be well tolerated in most adults?

6. List at least three measures used to treat the problem of retained secretions and pulmonary infection in hypercapnic respiratory failure.

7. What is the primary goal and first priority in the treatment of respiratory failure?

8. What are the three most common precipitating factors of acute-on-chronic respiratory failure in patients with COPD? Name two iatrogenic precipitating factors. Name as many other factors as you can remember.

9. Why is a patient breathing air with a $\dot{V}/\dot{Q}$ mismatch able to maintain a normal Pa_{CO_2} by increasing alveolar ventilation but is unable to achieve a normal Pa_{O_2}? (Explain with respect to the Hb O_2 and CO_2 dissociation curves.)

10. A 25-year-old male heroin addict was admitted to the hospital with severe hypoventilation due to drug overdose. The barometric pressure was 760 mmHg. His body temperature was normal, so the partial pressure of water in his trachea was 47 mmHg. On admission his Pa_{O_2} was 50 mmHg and the Pa_{CO_2} was 80 while breathing air. Is this pure hypoventilation? Calculate the $P(A-a)O_2$ gradient to answer the question. He was given oxygen (FI_{O_2} = 50%). Measurement of blood gases then revealed Pa_{O_2} = 246 mmHg and Pa_{CO_2} = 80 mmHg. What would you expect his Pa_{O_2} to be on 50% oxygen? Do you now think that his hypoxemia was due to pure hypoventilation? [Assume that his respiratory exchange ratio (R) is 0.8.]

11. A 60-year-old man with COPD was admitted to the hospital because of respiratory distress. He reported an increase in sputum production; the sputum was purulent, although his temperature was normal. Measurement of blood gases revealed Pa_{O_2} of 35 mmHg and Pa_{CO_2} of 55 mmHg. Barometric pressure was 747 mmHg. Assume R = 0.8. What was his $P(A-a)O_2$ gradient? Is his hypoxemia due to either hypoventilation or $\dot{V}/\dot{Q}$ imbalance alone or to both these mechanisms? He was given 24% oxygen. Two days later his blood gases were Pa_{O_2} = 50 mmHg, Pa_{CO_2} = 45 mmHg. Is his condition better or worse? Calculate his $P(A-a)O_2$ to answer this question.

Directions: Circle T if the statement is true and F if it is false. Correct false statements.

12. T F The clinical signs of respiratory failure are most easily detected in a patient who has chronic respiratory insufficiency which has progressed to respiratory failure.

13. T F Cyanosis is the most reliable index of respiratory failure.

14. T F Acute respiratory failure may be manifested by cardiovascular and neurologic signs and symptoms.

15. T F Hypoxemia with a normal or low Pa_{CO_2} is associated with conditions affecting the alveolar wall and interstitium of the lung.

16. T F Hypoventilation may cause the Pa_{CO_2} to fall below normal, since CO_2 excretion is directly related to ventilation.

17. T F Hyperventilation when breathing room air fails to correct hypoxemia.

18. T F Cerebral oxygenation may become impaired when significant hypocapnia is combined with hypoxemia.

19. T F Impaired cerebral oxygenation can be explained by the shift of the oxyhemoglobin dissociation curve to the left as a result of respiratory alkalosis.

20. T F When the Pa_{CO_2} rises to 70 mmHg in pure hypoventilation, one expects a normal Pa_{O_2} of 95 mmHg to be decreased to about 45 mmHg.

21. T F Hypoventilation or hyperventilation may be accurately identified at the bedside by observing the respiratory rate and depth.

22. T F A forced vital capacity (FVC) of 700 ml in a 70-kg male of average build indicates a need for ventilatory support.

23. T F A Pa_{O_2} of 80 mmHg with a Pa_{CO_2} of 24 mmHg after breathing 100% oxygen for 15 minutes indicates a serious shunting problem. ($P_B = 747$ mmHg.)

24. T F A person with viral pneumonia and a 50% shunt would be considered as being in good condition.

25. T F Absorption atelectasis is an expected complication with the prolonged administration of 60% oxygen.

26. T F Hypercapnia causes decreased cerebral blood flow and decreased intracranial pressure.

27. T F PEEP is established as the treatment of choice for ARDS.

28. T F Papilledema observed in some persons with acute ventilatory failure is indirectly caused by hypercapnia.

29. T F Alveolar CO_2 tension is inversely related to CO_2 production and directly related to alveolar ventilation.

30. T F Hypoxemic respiratory failure may progress to hypercapnic respiratory failure as the patient tires from the increased work of breathing.

Directions: Circle the letter preceding each item below that correctly answers the question. More than one choice may be correct.

31. Ventilation failure is numerically defined as:
    a. $Pa_{O_2} = 80$ mmHg, $Pa_{CO_2} = 60$ mmHg
    b. $Pa_{O_2} = 70$ mmHg, $Pa_{CO_2} = 35$ mmHg
    c. $Pa_{O_2} \geq 60$ mmHg, $Pa_{CO_2} \geq 40$ mmHg
    d. $Pa_{O_2} \leq 50$ mmHg, $Pa_{CO_2} \leq 50$ mmHg

32. Which of the following best describes the primary causes of respiratory failure?
    a. Hypersensitivity of the tracheobronchial tree to various stimuli   b. Ventilation-perfusion imbalance which increases physiologic shunt or dead space   c. Alveolar hypoventilation associated with obstructive or restrictive disease   d. Impaired diffusion due to alveolar-capillary block

33. The major cause of hypoxemia with hypercapnia is:
    a. Alveolar hypoventilation   b. Alveloar hyperventilation   c. Neither *a* nor *b*   d. Both *a* and *b*

34. Treatment of patients with hypoxemia with hypercapnia includes:
    a. Oxygen delivered at a concentration of 40 to 60 percent in order to achieve a rapid correction of hypoxemia   b. Low graduated oxygen therapy beginning with a mask which delivers 24 percent oxygen concentration   c. Careful monitoring of blood gases   d. Achievement of a Pa_{O_2} of 90 to 100 mmHg for all these patients

35. Tissue hypoxia may occur even when the Pa_{O_2} is normal if:
    a. Severe anemia is present   b. Cardiac output is low   c. The oxyhemoglobin curve is shifted to the left   d. Local vasoconstriction is present

36. Alveolar hypoventilation results in:
    a. Low PA_{CO_2} b. Low Pa_{CO_2} c. High PA_{CO_2} d. High Pa_{CO_2}

37. Which of the following mechanisms can contribute significantly to hypoxemia?
    a. Alveolar hypoventilation   b. Perfusion of underventilated lung units   c. Ventilation of underperfused lung units   d. Diffusion impairment   e. Left to right shunt

38. A low Pa_{O_2} can theoretically be the result of any of the following *except*:
    a. Shunting of arterial blood   b. $\dot{V}/\dot{Q}$ abnormalities   c. Alveolar-capillary diffusion block   d. Alveolar hypoventilation   e. Anemia

39. The predominant cause of hypoxemia in asthma is:
    a. Hypoventilation   b. Diffusion impairment   c. Increased dead-space ventilation   d. Areas of low $\dot{V}/\dot{Q}$ ratio   e. True right to left shunts

40. Decreased pulmonary diffusing capacity plays a role in:
    a. Narcotic overdose   b. Sarcoidosis   c. Myasthenia gravis   d. Asbestosis

41. Even when the Pa_{O_2} is normal, tissue hypoxia can occur if:
    a. Severe anemia is present   b. Cardiac output is low   c. P_{50} is low (oxyhemoglobin curve shifted to the left)   d. Local vasoconstriction is present

42. Hypoxemia can always be significantly improved by administration of oxygen *except* when due to:
    a. Low $\dot{V}/\dot{Q}$ ratio   b. High $\dot{V}/\dot{Q}$ ratio   c. Alveolar hypoventilation   d. True right to left shunt   e. Diffusion defect

43. Which of the following findings is/are compatible with diffusion limitation alone?
    a. Low Pa_{O_2}, high Pa_{CO_2} at rest   b. Normal Pa_{O_2}, normal Pa_{CO_2} at rest   c. Low Pa_{O_2}, high Pa_{CO_2}

during exercise   *d*. Low Pa_{O_2}, normal Pa_{CO_2} during exercise

44. Which of the following findings is compatible with $\dot{V}/\dot{Q}$ mismatch alone?
    a. Low Pa_{O_2}, high Pa_{CO_2} *b*. Low Pa_{O_2}, low Pa_{CO_2} *c*. Low Pa_{O_2}, normal Pa_{CO_2} *d*. Normal Pa_{O_2}, normal Pa_{CO_2}

45. Which of the following findings is compatible with true shunting alone?
    a. Low Pa_{O_2}, high Pa_{CO_2} *b*. Low Pa_{O_2}, low Pa_{CO_2} *c*. Low Pa_{O_2}, normal Pa_{CO_2} *d*. Normal Pa_{O_2}, normal Pa_{CO_2}

46. Some major effects of hypoxemia causing significant tissue hypoxia are:
    a. Vasoconstriction of the pulmonary blood vessels   *b*. Anaerobic metabolism and metabolic acidosis   *c*. Impaired judgment   *d*. Increased or decreased cardiac output   *e*. Cardiac arrhythmias

47. Place the following sequence of events in proper order to explain why a patient with COPD might complain of morning headaches.
    a. Normal hypoventilation during sleep   *b*. Increased cerebral blood flow   *c*. Chronic hypercapnia   *d*. Increase in retained respiratory secretions   *e*. Additional rise of Pa_{CO_2} *f*. Morning headache   *g*. Increased intracranial pressure

48. Which of the following is the best definition of respiratory failure?
    a. Respiratory alkalosis or acidosis   *b*. Any increase or decrease in alveolar ventilation   *c*. CO_2 retention when O_2 is administered   *d*. Inability to maintain normal blood gases   *e*. Hypoxemia at rest

49. High-output ventilatory failure is characterized by:
    a. High effective alveolar ventilation and low dead space   *b*. High tidal volume and high urine output   *c*. High minute ventilation and high physiologic dead space   *d*. High respiratory frequency and low minute ventilation   *e*. High cardiac output and high effective alveolar ventilation

50. Impaired synthesis of surfactant occurs in:
    a. Oxygen toxicity   *b*. Adult respiratory distress syndrome   *c*. Infant respiratory distress syndrome   *d*. Hypercapnia

51. Physiologic correlates of ARDS include:
    a. Severe hypoxemia, usually with hypocapnia   *b*. Increased intrapulmonary shunting   *c*. Increased dead space   *d*. Reduction on FRC   *e*. Increased $P(A-a)O_2$ gradient

52. Pathophysiologic changes in ARDS include:
    a. Low compliance   *b*. Diffuse atelectasis   *c*. Loss of pulmonary surfactant   *d*. Interstitial and alveolar edema and hemorrhage

53. Which of the following test results indicate a need for mechanical ventilation?
    a. Respiratory rate >35 per minute   *b*. VD/VT >0.6   *c*. $P(A-a)O_2$ >450 on 100% oxygen   *d*. FVC <15 ml per kilogram of ideal body weight   *e*. MIF <25 cmH_2O

54. Physiologic effects of PEEP when used to treat ARDS include:
    a. Reduction of $P(A-a)O_2$ gradient   *b*. Increased cardiac output   *c*. Increased functional residual capacity (FRC)   *d*. Improved compliance

55. Complications of PEEP for ARDS include:
    a. Pneumothorax   *b*. Interference with cardiac output   *c*. Infection   *d*. None of the above

56. Oxygen toxicity is associated with:
    a. F_{IO_2} >50% for >48 hours   *b*. Loss of surfactant   *c*. Alveolar collapse   *d*. Reduced lung compliance

57. Satisfactory method(s) of reducing oxygen toxicity are:
    a. Frequent observation for signs of toxicity   *b*. Hyperbaric oxygen treatment   *c*. Limitation of oxygen administration to 48 hours   *d*. Maintenance of the F_{IO_2} at 40% or less   *e*. Intermittent oxygen administration

Directions: Match each type of respiratory disorder in col. B with the type of respiratory failure it is likely to be associated with in col. A.

Column A	*Column B*
58. ____ Hypoxemic respiratory failure	*a*. COPD *b*. Respiratory center depression *c*. Asthmatic attack
59. ____ Hypercapnic respiratory failure	*d*. Bacterial pneumonia *e*. ARDS *f*. Myasthenia gravis *g*. Silicosis

Directions: Match the acid-base status in col. B to the findings it fits best in col. A. (Use the acid-base normogram to check your answers.)

Column A	*Column B*
60. ____ Patient with cystic fibrosis and chronic hypercapnia	*a*. Normal acid-base status *b*. Chronic respiratory alkalosis *c*. Mixed acute and chronic respiratory acidosis

61. ____ Patient with head injury, $Pa_{CO_2} = 40$ mmHg, $HCO_3^- = 24$ meq per liter, pH = 7.41

62. ____ Patient with COPD with respiratory infection, $Pa_{CO_2} = 75$ mmHg, pH = 7.1

63. ____ COPD patient above after being on mechanical ventilator, $Pa_{CO_2} = 55$ mmHg, pH = 7.48, $HCO_3^- = 39$ meq per liter

64. ____ Patient with lobar pneumonia, $Pa_{CO_2} = 24$ mmHg, pH = 7.46, $Pa_{O_2} = 60$

65. ____ Patient who aspirated vomitus during a CVA, 2 days later $Pa_{CO_2} = 20$ mmHg, pH = 7.32, $Pa_{O_2} = 35$ mmHg

d. Mixed respiratory alkalosis and metabolic acidosis

e. Mixed chronic respiratory acidosis and metabolic alkalosis

f. Chronic respiratory acidosis

CHAPTER
38

PULMONARY MALIGNANT NEOPLASMS

OBJECTIVES

At the completion of this chapter you should be able to:

1. List three factors that appear to account for the increase in bronchogenic carcinoma.

2. Describe the relation between cigarette smoking and the development of bronchogenic carcinoma.

3. State one possible reason why bronchogenic carcinoma is more common in the lowest socioeconomic classes.

4. Give at least one example of an important industrial hazard associated with an increased incidence of bronchogenic carcinoma.

5. Describe the four histologic types of bronchogenic carcinoma with respect to anatomic site, frequency, sex, association with smoking, mode of spread, and general prognosis.

6. Define *carcinoid syndrome*.

7. Give one reason why the lung is a common site for cancer metastasis.

8. List the manifestations of bronchogenic carcinoma.

9. Name and describe briefly the diagnostic tests used in the diagnosis of lung cancer and identify the significant findings expected with each technique.

10. State the objectives for the treatment of lung cancer.

11. Describe the TNM staging system for lung cancer.

12. State the general prognosis for patients with lung cancer.

Over 90 percent of primary lung tumors are malignant, and about 95 percent of these malignant tumors are bronchogenic carcinoma. This is the disease that is meant whenever reference is made to lung cancer, since the majority of primary malignant tumors of the lower respiratory tract are epithelial in nature and arise from the mucosa of the bronchial tree.

Although once considered a rare form of malignant growth, the incidence of lung cancer among males in the large cities of the industrialized countries has risen to epidemic proportions in the decades since 1930. Some of the alarming statistics were cited in the introduction to this Part. Although lung cancer is still more common in men than in women (about 5:1), the disease is increasingly rapidly in women. Lung cancer is now the fourth leading cause of cancer death in women. This increase is believed to be related to the increased cigarette smoking by women.

BRONCHOGENIC CARCINOMA

Although the exact cause of bronchogenic carcinoma is unknown, three factors appear to account for the increase in incidence—smoking, industrial hazards, and air pollution. Of these factors, smoking appears to play the major role. Massive statistical evidence indicates that there is a relation between heavy cigarette smoking and the development of lung cancer. Three prospective studies, one involving nearly 200,000 men aged 50 to 69, followed for 44 months revealed that the death rate from cancer of the lung per 100,000 was 3.4 in the male nonsmoker, 59.3 in those who smoked 10 to 20 cigarettes daily, and 217.3 in those who smoked 40 or more cigarettes daily. Those who give up smoking permanently are much less likely to develop carcinoma after an abstinence of 5 years. The risk in pipe smokers or cigar smokers is only slightly greater than that in nonsmokers. Mortality from lung cancer is related to atmospheric pollution, but its effect is small compared to that of cigarette smoking. The death rate from cancer of the lung is twice as high in cities as in rural areas. Statistical evidence also shows that the disease is more common in the lowest socioeconomic classes and decreases in the higher classes. This may be partly explained by the fact that persons in the lowest social classes are more apt to live near their jobs, where the atmosphere may be more polluted. A carcinogen (cancer-producing material) which has been found in polluted air (and also in cigarette smoke) is 3,4-benzpyrene. The nicotine in cigarette smoke is not a carcinogen.

In certain instances, bronchogenic carcinoma appears to be an occupational disease. Of the various industrial hazards, the most important is undoubtedly asbestos, which is widely used in the construction industry. The risk of lung cancer in asbestos workers is about 10 times greater than that in the general population. Local benign or diffuse malignant mesotheliomas of the pleura are rare tumors which have been specifically associated with asbestos exposure (Borow et al., 1967). There is also increased risk in those who work with uranium, chromate, arsenic (insecticide used in agriculture), iron, and iron oxides. The risks of lung cancer from both asbestos and uranium exposure are greatly enhanced in those who also smoke cigarettes.

In many tissues, chronic inflammatory changes are known to precede cancer. Evidence supports the view that chronic inflammation of the bronchial mucosa from inhaled irritants may be of greater importance than the carcinogenic effect of any one substance. Another factor which has not received much attention is the close correspondence between the increase in the number of motor vehicles and the incidence of lung cancer.

These facts suggest that although smoking clearly plays a major part in the increasing incidence of lung cancer, it is by no means the only factor. Chronic infection, air pollution from motor vehicles and industry, occupational exposure to carcinogens, and perhaps other unknown factors may (either alone or in combination) predispose to cancer of the lung.

Primary lung cancer can be classified in terms of its anatomic location and on the basis of histologic type. The approximate anatomic distribution is illustrated in Fig. 38-1. About 50 percent of the lesions arise centrally about the hilus and the first few orders of bronchi; the others have a more peripheral origin in the terminal bronchioles. Bronchogenic carcinoma may be classified in the following histologic types (approximate frequencies are listed in parentheses): (1) squamous cell or epidermoid carcinoma (45 to 60 percent); (2) anaplastic or undifferentiated carcinoma (20 to 30 percent) includes the oat cell, small cell, and large cell varieties; (3) ade-

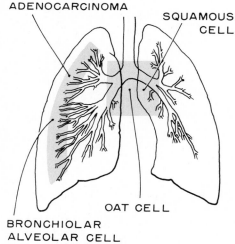

FIGURE 38-1
Anatomic distribution of lung cancer (50 percent is located centrally, while the other 50 percent is peripheral).

nocarcinoma (10 to 15 percent); and (4) bronchiolar-alveolar cell carcinoma (1 to 2 percent).

Squamous cell carcinoma is the most common histologic type of bronchogenic carcinoma and arises from the surface of the bronchial epithelium. Squamous cell carcinoma is usually centrally located about the hilus and is almost always associated with cigarette smoking. The tumor is seldom more than a few centimeters in diameter, and it tends to spread by direct extension to the hilar lymph nodes, chest wall, and mediastinum. Squamous cell carcinoma often presents with manifestations of cough and hemoptysis as a result of irritation or ulceration and pneumonia and abscess formation from the obstruction and secondary infection. The life expectancy in this type of tumor is greater than in the anaplastic variety, since it tends to metastasize only locally and somewhat later.

Anaplastic carcinomas are the second most common histologic type. They are undifferentiated cell types, since no squamous or adenomatous pattern can be defined. Metastasis occurs early, chiefly via the lymphatics, so the prognosis in this type of cancer is very poor. Death usually occurs within a few months after discovery. The oat cell variety of anaplastic carcinoma is the most common; it is generally centrally located about the mainstem bronchi. This type of cancer is also related to heavy cigarette smoking.

Adenocarcinomas, as the name implies, show a cellular organization like that of bronchial glands and may contain mucus. The majority of these tumors arise in the peripheral segmental bronchi and are sometimes associated with focal lung scars and chronic interstitial fibrosis. These lesions often spread via the bloodstream and remain clinically silent until distant hematogenous metastases occur. There is no clear correlation between this type of bronchogenic carcinoma and smoking. Unlike the squamous and oat cell varieties, which are much more common in men, this type affects both sexes about equally.

Bronchiolar-alveolar cell carcinoma is a rare type of malignant lung tumor which arises from the alveolar or possibly the bronchiolar epithelium. This type of lung cancer does not seem to be related to smoking and is equally distributed between the sexes. In contrast to anaplastic and squamous carcinomas, which have a peak incidence between the ages of 50 to 60 and are located centrally, bronchiolar-alveolar cell carcinoma is almost always located in the peripheral portions of the lung and occurs in patients of all ages. The onset is generally insidious, with signs resembling pneumonia. Grossly this neoplasm resembles in some cases the uniform consolidation of lobar pneumonia. Microscopically, groups of alveoli are lined with clear mucus-secreting cells, and there is abundant expectoration of mucoid sputum. The prognosis is poor unless surgical removal of the diseased lobe is performed early.

OTHER FORMS OF LUNG CANCER

Other rare primary lung cancers include sarcomas (accounting for less than 1 percent of lung cancers) and bronchial adenomas. Bronchial adenomas are a group of small malignant neoplasms of low aggressiveness arising in the lower trachea or major bronchi, the most important being the bronchial carcinoid and the rarer cylindroma. Carcinoids affect adults of either sex under the age of 40 years. Some of these tumors secrete serotinin, 5-hydroxy-tryptophan, and other biologically active substances which give rise to a symptom complex known as the *carcinoid syndrome*. Symptoms include hypotension, flushing, bronchoconstriction, cyanosis, anxiety, and tremulousness. Carcinoid tumors follow a relatively benign course, and surgical resection is usually successful.*

Finally, it should be remembered that the lung is affected by metastatic cancer much more often than by a primary malignant neoplasm. The lung is a common site for secondary deposits of cancer cells originating in other organs because bloodborne microscopic tumor emboli are likely to become enmeshed in the pulmonary capillary bed. Lymphborne tumors from the lower half of the body and abdominal cavity may also be arrested as they pass through the thoracic duct. The most common neoplasms giving rise to pulmonary metastasis in descending order of frequency are carcinomas of the breast, gastrointestinal tract, female genital tract, and kidneys; melanomas; and male genital cancer.

MANIFESTATIONS OF BRONCHOGENIC CARCINOMA

Bronchogenic carcinoma imitates a variety of other pulmonary diseases and has no typical mode of onset. It often masquerades as a pneumonitis which fails to resolve. Cough is a common symptom which is often ignored by the patient or attributed to smoking or bronchitis. When bronchial carcinoma develops in a patient with chronic bronchitis, cough often becomes more frequent or the volume of sputum may increase. Hemoptysis is another common sign. Initial symptoms of localized wheeze and mild dyspnea may result from varying degrees of bronchial obstruction. Chest pain may appear in various forms but is commonly experienced as an ache or discomfort caused by neoplastic spread to the

---

*Carcinoid tumors are more common in the gastrointestinal tract than in the lungs. Although usually benign, they can be malignant.

mediastinum. Pleuritic pain may occur when there is secondary involvement of the pleura resulting from neoplastic spread or pneumonia. Rapid development of digital clubbing is an important sign, since it is often associated with bronchogenic carcinoma. General symptoms such as anorexia, fatigue, and weight loss are late symptoms. Symptoms of intrathoracic or extrathoracic spread may also be present when the patient is first seen by the physician. Local extension of the tumor to the mediastinal structures may produce hoarseness as a result of involvement of the recurrent laryngeal nerve, dysphagia from involvement of the esophagus, and paralysis of the hemidiaphragm from involvement of the phrenic nerve. Symptoms of extrathoracic spread depend on the site of metastasis. Structures commonly involved are the scalene lymph nodes (especially in peripheral lung tumors), adrenals (50 percent), liver (30 percent), brain (20 percent), bone (20 percent), and kidneys (15 percent). Oat cell tumors are known to produce virtually any of the polypeptide hormones such as parathormone, ACTH, or ADH, so the patient may show features which resemble hyperparathyroidism, Cushing's syndrome, or fluid retention with hyponatremia.

THE DIAGNOSIS AND TREATMENT OF LUNG CANCER

The main tools in the diagnosis of lung cancer are radiology, bronchoscopy, and cytology. A solitary, circumscribed nodule, or *coin lesion* on the chest x-ray is of particular importance and may be the earliest indication of bronchogenic carcinoma, although it may also occur in many other conditions. Computerized tomography (CT) scan may be of further help in differentiating the suspected lesion. Bronchoscopy with biopsy is the most successful technique in the diagnosis of squamous cell carcinoma, which is generally located centrally. Scalene node biopsy is most successful in the diagnosis of those cancers which are inaccessible to bronchoscopy. Cytologic examination of the sputum, bronchial brushings, and examination of the pleural fluid also play an important role in the diagnosis of lung cancer.

Both the histology and the stage of disease are important in determining prognosis as well as the treatment plan. The TNM staging system for lung cancer formulated by the American Joint Committee for Staging and End Results Reporting is a widely accepted method of determining the extent of disease at the time of diagnosis (see Table 38-1). The TNM system is de-

signed to take into account the size of the tumor, T; the local spread to the hilar and mediastinal lymph nodes, N; and the distant spread, M. Tumor size and histology are determined by the various methods of radiology and of obtaining a tissue specimen described above. Gallium 67 scanning of the lung, mediastinum, and total body is a useful noninvasive method of differentiating benign and malignant primary lung neoplasms and determining whether there is spread to the hilar lymph nodes and distant metastasis. If a single lung lesion seen on x-ray is gallium-positive, there is a 91 percent probability that the lesion is primary lung cancer. If the lesion is gallium-negative, there is a 78 percent probability that it represents a metastatic lesion from another primary or is nonmalignant. If both the lung lesion and an extrathoracic site are gallium-positive, there is a 90 percent chance that the extrathoracic site is a metastasis and should be biopsied (Golomb and DeMeester, 1979). If the mediastinal lymph nodes are gallium-positive, mediastinoscopy and biopsy can confirm the suspected local spread.

The treatment of lung cancer consists in surgical resection and palliation by such methods as chemotherapy, irradiation, and, more recently, immunotherapy using BCG (bacillus Calmette-Guérin) or *Corynebacterium parvum*. If the histologic diagnosis is oat cell carcinoma, the treatment of choice is radiotherapy, since this carcinoma is the most radiosensitive type. Radiotherapy may be integrated with combination chemotherapy, which uses multiple drugs. Most patients with oat cell carcinoma have stage III disease at the time of diagnosis, but regardless of stage the outlook is dismal. Even with treatment it is rare for a patient to survive 5 years, and most are dead within 2 years. In contrast, a patient with well-differentiated squamous cell carcinoma T_1 or T_2 without involvement of nodes or distant metastasis (Stage I) has at least a 50 percent chance of 5-year survival after operation.

One of the primary aims of diagnostic tests and staging is to identify patients who might be helped by surgical resection and to avoid useless thoracotomy on the remainder. Patients with stage I disease receive the maximum benefit from surgery. However, only a small proportion of lung cancer is found at an early stage. Contraindications to surgical resection are evidence of distant metastasis, pleural involvement, mediastinal invasion (i.e., stage III disease), and severe impairment of pulmonary function. Oat cell carcinomas are not generally treated surgically regardless of stage; they may be treated with chemotherapy, radiotherapy, or immunotherapy. Immunotherapy is based on stimulation of the nonspecific immune response, with the resultant killing of tumor cells. This treatment modality holds considerable promise but is yet in the preliminary stages of development. The overall 5-year-survival rate for lung cancer (all stages) is low: 8 percent for men and 12 percent for women (Neptune et al., 1978).

TABLE 38-1

575

QUESTIONS

TNM STAGING SYSTEM FOR LUNG CANCER

	TNM designation	Definition
Primary tumor (T)	T_x	Can be demonstrated only by cytologic study of bronchopulmonary secretions, e.g., malignant cells in sputum but no visualized tumor mass
	T_1	Lesion <3 cm in diameter without extension proximal to a lobar bronchus
	T_2	Lesion >3 cm in diameter or of any size with its associated atelectasis extending to hilum; must be >2 cm from carina and confined to the visceral pleura
	T_3	Lesion of any size within 2 cm of carina or with intrathoracic spread, e.g., the mediastinum, diaphragm, chest wall with pleural effusion
Regional lymph nodes (N)	N_0	Negative hilar or mediastinal nodes
	N_1	Positive ipsilateral hilar nodes
	N_2	Positive nodes in the mediastinum, contralateral hilum, or cervical region
Distant metastasis (M)	M_0	No distant metastasis
	M_1	Systemic metastasis, e.g., contralateral lung, adrenals, bone, brain, liver
Occult	$T_xN_0M_0$	Sputum contains malignant cells, but no other evidence of lung cancer
Stage I	$T_1N_0M_0$ $T_1N_1M_0$ $T_2N_0M_0$	Tumor classified as T_1 with or without involvement of ipsilateral hilar nodes, or T_2 tumor without nodal involvement
Stage II	$T_2N_1M_0$	Tumor classified as T_2 with involvement of ipsilateral hilar nodes
Stage III	T_3 with any N or M N_2 with any T or M M_1 with any T or N	Any tumor more extensive than T_2, or any tumor with involvement of the nodes of the contralateral hilum, mediastinum, or cervical region or evidence of distant metastasis

Source: The American Joint Committee for Cancer Staging and End-Results Reporting: Clinical Staging System for Carcinoma of the Lung, *Cancer*, **24**:87,1974.

On the basis of present knowledge, the only practical means of treating lung cancer is to prevent it by advising people not to smoke cigarettes or live in an atmosphere polluted by industry. Protective measures must also be taken for those who work with asbestos, uranium, chrome, and other carcinogenic materials. Men over the age of 40 should have routine chest x-rays for earlier detection of lung cancer.

QUESTIONS

Pulmonary malignant neoplasms

Directions: Answer the following on a separate sheet of paper.

1. What is the carcinoid syndrome, and what type of tumor causes it?

2. What are some common signs and symptoms of bronchogenic carcinoma, and why is it difficult to diagnose on the basis of these signs and symptoms?

3. List three major diagnostic tools used for the detection of lung cancer and describe the significant findings of each technique.

Directions: Match each histologic type of bronchogenic carcinoma in col. A with its characteristics in col. B.

Column A

4. ____ Squamous or epidermoid

5. ____ Anaplastic (oat cell)

6. ____ Adenocarcinoma

Column B

a. Least common of all types

b. Most common type

c. Spreads chiefly by direct extension to hilar lymph nodes

d. Spreads chiefly via lymphatics

7. ___ Bronchio-
     lar-alveolar cell

e. Spreads chiefly via bloodstream

f. Spreads directly through airways

g. Mucus-producing tumor cells

h. Associated with heavy cigarette smoking

i. Not associated with smoking

j. Located centrally about hilus
   and first few orders of bronchi

k. Located in peripheral part of
   lung

l. Both sexes affected equally

m. Undifferentiated cell type

n. Poorest prognosis

o. May secrete hormones

Directions: Circle T if the statement is true and F if it is false. Correct the false statements.

8. T   F   Three factors which appear to account for the increase in lung cancer
over recent decades are cigarette
smoking, industrial hazards, and air
pollution.

9. T   F   Statistical evidence indicates a negative relationship between heavy cigarette smoking and bronchogenic carcinoma.

10. T   F   Of the industrial hazards, the most
common material responsible for increasing the risk of developing lung
cancer is uranium.

11. T   F   Primary malignant neoplasms of the
lung are more common than second-
ary metastasis to the lung from another primary site.

12. T   F   About 95 percent of primary malignant neoplasms of the lung are bronchogenic carcinoma.

13. T   F   About 50 percent of malignant bronchogenic tumors are centrally located
about the hilus and first few orders of
bronchi.

Directions: Circle the letter preceding each item below that correctly answers the question. More than one choice may be correct.

14. The lung is a common site for secondary metastasis
because:
a. Bloodborne tumor emboli are likely to become
enmeshed in the capillary beds of the lungs   b. It
is anatomically close to the abdominal organs
c. All the lymph of the body passes through the
thoracic duct and may transport lymphborne
tumor cells to the lungs

15. The overall 5-year survival rate for patients with
primary lung cancer is about:
a. 75 percent   b. 50 percent   c. 10 percent
d. 1 percent

16. Methods of treatment of lung cancer include:
a. Irradiation   b. Lung scan   c. Surgical
resection   d. Chemotherapy

17. Of the four patients with the following TNM
stages of lung cancer, which would probably not be
recommended for surgical resection?
a. $T_1N_1M_0$ b. $T_2N_1M_0$ c. $T_2N_2M_1$
d. $T_1N_0M_0$

CHAPTER 39

PULMONARY TUBERCULOSIS

OBJECTIVES

At the completion of this chapter you should be able to:

1. Describe the incidence of and mortality from tuberculosis in the United States.

2. List the characteristics of *Mycobacterium tuberculosis*.

3. Identify the most common mode of transmission and site of implantation of the tubercle bacillus.

4. Describe the inflammatory process at the site of infection (the Ghon complex) that is evoked by the tubercle bacillus.

5. Describe caseous necrosis as to appearance and responses that result from it.

6. Differentiate between the lymphohematogenous and hematogenous dissemination of mycobacterial tuberculosis.

7. Identify the signs and symptoms that are associated with tuberculosis as it develops.

8. List the factors that must be considered for verification of a case of tuberculosis when the *M. tuberculosis* organism has not been identified.

9. Describe a hypersensitivity reaction in the host of the tubercle bacillus.

10. Describe the technique used in tuberculin skin testing with respect to injection site, peak of reaction, interpretation and recording of the result, and significance of the reaction.

11. List the typical pathologic findings of pulmonary tuberculosis on a roentgenographic examination.

12. Evaluate the role of bacillus Calmette-Guérin (BCG) in the control of tuberculosis.

13. Differentiate between the staining and culture methods used to detect the tubercle bacillus.

14. List the antimicrobial drugs used in the treatment and preventive therapy for tuberculosis, with their usual dosage, minimum duration of therapy, adverse side effects, and necessary monitoring.

15. Explain the risk associated with isoniazid therapy.

16. List at least three groups of people who should receive preventive therapy against tuberculosis.

The incidence of and mortality from tuberculosis declined rapidly after the advent of chemotherapy. However, in recent years the decline has reached a plateau and the incidence may increase. Causing this trend are persons with socioeconomic and health-related problems (e.g., alcoholism, poverty, inadequate nutritional intake) and refugees who have entered the United States from areas of high tuberculosis prevalence.

Currently there are approximately 25,000 new tuberculosis cases annually in the United States. There has been an average annual decline in tuberculosis cases in the United States. In 1979–1981, years of a large influx of Indochinese refugees, the average annual decline was 1.4 percent. Whereas, in 1981–1982 the number of cases decreased by 6.8 percent. In 1979–1982, the average annual number of tuberculosis deaths was nearly 2000. Tuberculosis was the leading cause of death among the 38 communicable diseases reported to the Center for Disease Control in 1979, and the number of tuberculosis deaths showed no decline in the 1979–1982 period (Center for Disease Control, 1984).

Tuberculosis is an infectious disease caused by *Mycobacterium tuberculosis*. The aerobic, acid-fast rods include both pathogenic and saprophytic organisms. There are several pathogenic mycobacteria, but only the bovine and human strains are pathogenic to humans. The tubercle bacillus is 0.3×2 to $4 \ \mu m$, which is smaller than a red blood cell.

PATHOGENESIS

The portals of entry for the *M. tuberculosis* organism are the respiratory tract, the gastrointestinal tract, and an open wound in the skin. The majority of tuberculosis infections are contracted by the airborne route through the inhalation of droplet nuclei containing organisms of the tubercle bacillus. The infected particle is usually disseminated from a patient infected with tuberculosis. The gastrointestinal tract is the usual portal of entry for the bovine strain, which is spread by contaminated milk. However, in the United States, with widespread pasteurization of milk and detection of diseased cattle, bovine tuberculosis is rare.

Tuberculosis is a disease that is controlled by a cell-mediated immunity response. The effector cell is the macrophage, and the lymphocyte (usually T cell) is the immunoresponsive cell. This type of immunity is basically a local phenomenon, involving macrophages that are activated at the infection site by lymphocytes and their lymphokines. This response is referred to as a (delayed) *hypersensitivity reaction* (see Chap. 5).

The tubercle bacilli, which are usually inhaled in units of one to three bacilli, reach the alveolar surfaces. Larger clumps of inhaled bacilli tend to impinge on the mucociliary surfaces of the nasal passages and bronchial tree and do not cause disease (Dannenberg, 1982). Once in the alveolar space—commonly in the lower part of the upper lobe or the upper part of the lower lobe—the reaction evoked by the tubercle bacillus is an inflammatory process. Polymorphonuclear leukocytes appear on the scene and phagocytize the bacteria but do not kill the organism. After the first few days, leukocytes are replaced by macrophages. The involved alveoli are consolidated, and acute pneumonia develops. This cellular pneumonia may resolve itself so that no residue remains, or the process may continue, with the bacteria continuing to be phagocytized or to multiply within the cells. There is also lymphatic drainage of the bacilli into the regional lymph nodes. The infiltrating macrophages elongate and partially fuse to form the epithelioid cell tubercle, surrounded by lymphocytes. This reaction usually takes 10 to 20 days.

Necrosis of the central portion of the lesion results in a relatively solid, cheesy appearance called *caseous necrosis*. The area of caseous necrosis and the surrounding granulation tissue of epithelioid cells and fibroblasts evoke different responses. The granulation tissue may become more fibrous, forming collagenous scar tissue which results in a capsule surrounding the tubercle.

The primary lesion in the lung is called the *Ghon focus*, and the combination of regional lymph node involvement and the primary lesion is termed the *Ghon complex*. A calcified Ghon complex may be seen on a routine chest x-ray of healthy persons.

Another response which may occur at the site of the necrotic area is liquefaction, with the liquid material sloughing into a connecting bronchus and producing a cavity. The tubercular material sloughed from the walls of the cavity enters the tracheobronchial tree. The process may be repeated in other parts of the lung, or bacilli may be carried to the larynx, middle ear, or gut.

Even without therapy, small cavities close and leave a fibrous scar. As inflammation subsides, the bronchial lumen may be narrowed and closed by scarring near the junction of the cavity and the bronchus. The caseous material may thicken and be unable to flow through the communicating channel, so that the cavity fills with this material and the lesion becomes similar to the unsloughed encapsulated lesion. It may remain in a quiescent stage for long periods or reestablish its bronchial communication and be the site of active inflammation.

The disease may spread through the lymphatics or blood vessels. The organisms that pass through the lymph nodes reach the bloodstream in small numbers and may initiate occasional lesions in various organs. This dispersal of the organisms, referred to as *lymphohematogenous dissemination*, is usually self-limited. *Hematogenous dissemination*, an acute phenomenon, usually gives rise to miliary tuberculosis; it occurs when a necrotic focus erodes a blood vessel, allowing large numbers of organisms to enter the vascular system and be disseminated to organs in the body.

DIAGNOSIS AND CLINICAL MANIFESTATIONS

In the early stages of tuberculosis there are usually no specific signs or symptoms. Tuberculosis can be diagnosed only by tuberculin testing, roentgenographic examination, and bacteriologic studies.

According to the Center for Disease Control (CDC), a case of tuberculosis is verified by identification of the *M. tuberculosis* organism. When this verification cannot be obtained, reported cases are considered verified if *all* the following factors are present: (1) completed diagnostic procedures; (2) evidence of tuberculosis infection (i.e., positive tuberculin test); (3) abnormal chest x-ray (not stable, i.e., worsening or improving) and/or clinical evidence of current disease; and (4) decision to give a full course of therapy with two or more antituberculosis drugs (April 15, 1980).

As the disease progresses and there is more destruction of lung tissue, sputum production and coughing may increase. Chest pain is usually not a symptom, and hemoptysis is usually associated only with more advanced cases. Some patients present with productive cough, fatigue, weakness, night sweats, and weight loss—similar to the signs and symptoms of acute bronchitis and pneumonia.

HYPERSENSITIVITY REACTION

The pathogenicity of the bacillus does not arise from any intrinsic toxicity but from its capacity to induce a hypersensitive reaction in the host. Tuberculoproteins derived from the bacillus appear to induce this reaction. The tissue responses of inflammation and necrosis are the results of a cellular (delayed) hypersensitivity response of the host to the tubercle bacillus. A tuberculosis hypersensitivity reaction usually develops 3 to 10 weeks from the onset of infection. As stated previously (see Chap. 5), persons who have been exposed to the tubercle bacillus develop sensitized T lymphocytes. If purified protein derivative (PPD) of tuberculin is injected into the skin of a person whose lymphocytes are sensitized to tuberculoprotein, the sensitized lymphocytes interact with the extract and attract macrophages to the area (see Fig. 5-6).

Tuberculin skin testing

Intradermal (Mantoux) tuberculin test

The standard technique (Mantoux Test) is the intradermal injection of 0.1 ml of tuberculin (PPD) containing 5 tuberculin units (TU) into the upper third of the volar aspect of the forearm after the skin has been cleansed with alcohol. A disposable tuberculin syringe with a 26- to 27-gauge needle is usually preferred. The short, bluntly beveled needle is held upward and the tip of the needle inserted beneath the surface of the skin. A wheal 6 to 10 mm in diameter and resembling a mosquito bite should be produced when the prescribed 0.1-ml amount is accurately injected (see Fig. 9-8).

The skin reaction requires 48 to 72 hours to reach its peak after the injection, and the reaction should be read during that time period, in a good light, with the subject's forearm slightly flexed. The reaction must be recorded as the diameter of the induration in millimeters, measured transversely to the long axis of the forearm. Only *induration*, not erythema alone, is significant. Induration may be determined by inspection and by palpation (stroking the area with a finger).

The interpretation of the skin test (see Table 39-1) identifies three types of reactions. An indurated area measuring 10 mm or more is considered a *positive reaction*, reflecting sensitivity resulting from infection with the bacillus. An induration measuring 5 to 9 mm is a *doubtful reaction*; it can result from cross sensitivity to atypical mycobacteria, and the test should be repeated. A 0- to 4-mm area of induration is read as a *negative reaction*; no repetition of the test is usually necessary.

Jet injection tuberculin test

Jet injection is a method of administering large numbers of tuberculin tests rapidly and painlessly. The testing material (5 TU of PPD) is administered intradermally by high pressure. The wheal produced should be 6 to 10 mm in diameter. Reading and interpretation of the test are the same as for the Mantoux.

Multiple-puncture tuberculin tests

Multiple-puncture tests are rapidly administered by devices that pierce the skin at several points simultaneously. For example, the tine test uses four tines pre-dipped in old tuberculin (OT) and pressed into the skin. The test is read within 48 to 72 hours. A positive tine test consists of one or more papules, 2 mm or larger. Multiple puncture tests are less accurate than other techniques, because unknown amounts of tuberculin are administered and the reactions are less precise than with the Mantoux. The Mantoux test is the preferred method and the standard of comparison for other types of tests.

It is important to emphasize that a positive reaction to the tuberculin test indicates the presence of infection but does not necessarily signify clinical disease. However, this test is an important diagnostic tool in the evaluation of an individual patient and is also useful in determining the prevalence of tuberculosis infection in a population.

BCG vaccination

Bacillus Calmette-Guérin (BCG), an attenuated living strain of bovine tubercule bacilli is the most widely used vaccine. In BCG vaccination these organisms are injected into the skin to produce a well-circumscribed, calcified, walled-off primary focus. BCG has retained its capacity to increase the bodily resistance of animals and humans, and primary infection by BCG has the advantage over primary infection by virulent organisms because there is no danger of producing progressive disease in the host (Rosenthal, 1980).

Vaccination with BCG usually leads to the development of tuberculin sensitivity. The degree of sensitivity is variable, depending on the strain of BCG used and the population vaccinated. There is no way of distinguishing tuberculin reactions caused by vaccination with BCG from those caused by natural mycobacterial infections. A 10-mm or 15-mm reaction is considered a significant reaction in BCG-vaccinated persons.

BCG vaccination is mandatory by law in 26 countries and is optional but recommended in 19 others. The World Health Organization and UNICEF have assisted with the establishment of laboratories and with vaccination campaigns in over 45 countries in which over 200 million people have been vaccinated. The worldwide number of vaccinated persons is estimated at 500 million or more (Rosenthal, 1980).

Despite the worldwide acceptance of BCG, vacci-

TABLE 39-1

RECOMMENDED INTERPRETATION OF SKIN TEST REACTIONS

1. Intracutaneous Mantoux and jet injection tests (with standard test dose).
   A. *10 mm or more of induration = positive reaction.* This is interpreted as positive for past or present infection with *Mycobacterium tuberculosis* because reactions this large most likely represent specific sensitivity. The test does not need to be repeated for confirmation in ordinary circumstances, unless there is reason to question the validity of the test.
   B. *5 to 9 mm of induration = doubtful reaction.* Reactions in this size range reflect sensitivity that can result from infection with either atypical mycobacteria or *M. tuberculosis*; hence they are classed as doubtful. However, a person with a doubtful reaction who is known to have been in close contact with an infectious person, i.e., a subject with infectious sputum, or a person having radiographic or clinical evidence of disease compatible with tuberculosis, should be regarded as probably infected with *M. tuberculosis*. For all other persons, if an appropriate antigen for atypical mycobacteria is available, an intracutaneous test with such an antigen may be applied at the same time as a repeat tuberculin test.
   C. *0 to 4 mm of induration = negative reaction.* This reflects either a lack of tuberculin sensitivity or a low-grade sensitivity that most likely is not caused by *M. tuberculosis* infection. No repeat test is necessary unless there is also suggestive clinical evidence of tuberculosis. If the person is in contact with a tuberculosis subject, he or she should be followed up according to the established routine for contacts.
2. Multiple-puncture tests. In determining the size of induration, measure the diameter of the largest single reaction. If the reaction consists of discrete papules, the diameters of separate areas of induration should not be added. For screening tests, the following interpretation is suggested.
   A. *Vesiculation = positive reaction.* If vesiculation is present, the test may be interpreted as positive, in which case the management of the subject is the the same as that for one classified as positive to the Mantoux test.
   B. *2 mm or more of induration = doubtful reaction.* Even though such reactions may be due to *M. tuberculosis*, a significant proportion of them may not be confirmed by a positive standard Mantoux test. This is particularly true of smaller reactions. Therefore, a standard Mantoux test should be done on all subjects in this group, and management should be based on the reaction to the Mantoux test or on the results of dual testing using PPD-tuberculin and PPD-B.
   C. *Less than 2 mm of induration = negative reaction.* There is no need for retesting unless the individual is in contact with a case of tuberculosis or there is clinical evidence suggestive of the disease.

Source: American Lung Association, 1974, pp. 18–19.

nation against tuberculosis in the United States has had only token acceptance. BCG vaccination is about 80 percent effective in preventing tuberculosis infection and nearly 100 percent effective in keeping the infections that do occur from being fatal (Center for Disease Control, 1979). However, most authorities agree that the risk of tuberculosis among nonreactors is too small to justify using BCG vaccine in the general population. BCG is recommended in developed countries such as the United States for high-risk groups, e.g., persons living in communities with high tuberculosis incidence and health personnel or military personnel serving in high-incidence areas.

Sensitivity to tuberculin usually persists throughout life, but it may be altered during certain illnesses or conditions. Immune suppression of cellular (delayed) immunity may be evident in viral infections, in lymphoreticular malignant disease such as Hodgkin's disease and in patients receiving corticosteroid therapy.

Regardless of the factors involved in the initiation of tuberculosis, progressive disease does not tend to maintain an anergy state, whether partial or complete. The tuberculosis infection itself has, or can have, a suppressive effect on cellular immunity and on the ability of the organism to mount an adequate defense to the invading bacilli (Youmans, 1979).

ROENTGENOGRAPHIC EXAMINATION

Roentgenographic examination often suggests the presence of tuberculosis, but it is almost impossible to make a diagnosis on this basis alone, because almost all the manifestations of tuberculosis can be mimicked by other diseases.

Pathologically, the earliest manifestation of tuberculosis involvement of the lung is usually a parenchymal lymph node complex. In adults, the apical and posterior segments of the upper lobe or the superior segments of the lower lobe are the usual sites of lesions, which may appear dense and homogenous. There may also be evidence of cavity formation and scattered disease, which is often bilateral.

BACTERIOLOGIC STUDIES

Stained specimens of sputum, catheterized urine, cerebrospinal fluid, and gastric contents may be microscopically examined, but examination of the sputum is the most important bacteriologic study in the diagnosis of tuberculosis. The Ziehl-Neelsen staining method may be used. The slide is flooded with steaming carbol-fuchsin, then decolorized with acid alcohol. It is then counterstained with methylene blue or brilliant green. The most widely accepted method of staining is the auramine-rhodamine technique of fluorescent staining; the

auramine-rhodamine solution, once attached to the mycobacteria, resists acid-alcohol decolorization. The clinician is provided with an estimate of the number of acid-fast bacilli detected on the slide. A positive specimen gives the clinician a preliminary indication of the diagnosis, but a negative specimen does not rule out infection with the disease.

The most accurate diagnostic method is the culture technique. The mycobacteria are slow-growing and require a complex medium. The microorganism takes 2 or more weeks at 36 to 37°C to grow. Mature colonies are cream-colored or buff, and a warty, cauliflower-like appearance is characteristic. As few as 10 bacteria per milliliter of digested, concentrated material can be detected on the culture medium. The mycobacterial growth that is observed on the culture medium should be quantified as to the number of colonies that are present.

Studies by Harshey and Ramakrishnan (1977) provide evidence that the growth of the tubercle bacilli is slow because the growth rate is limited by their DNA-dependent ribonucleic acid (RNA) polymerase. The *M. tuberculosis* enzyme has structural differences from the corresponding enzyme in *Escherichia coli*. This difference appears to be specific to RNA synthesis rather than to nucleic acid synthesis as a whole. In culture media the rate of RNA chain growth in *M. tuberculosis* is only about one-tenth that seen in *E. coli*, and the ratio of RNA to DNA in *M. tuberculosis* has been demonstrated to be tenfold lower than in *E. coli* on chemical analysis of whole cell abstracts.

Tests are currently available that permit identification of most species of mycobacteria, and computer programs have been developed that aid in the interpretation of data. These programs also suggest additional tests that are needed (Wayne et al., 1980). Currently, these tests have not been adopted for use with inocula measurable in micrograms.

TREATMENT

The treatment of tuberculosis consists primarily in the prolonged administration of antimicrobial drugs. These drugs can also be used to prevent developing clinical disease in an infected person.

Tuberculosis patients with clinical disease should receive a minimum of two drugs to prevent emergence of drug-resistant strains. The drug combination of first choice is isoniazid (isonicotinic acid hydrazide; INH) with ethambutol (EMB) or rifampin (RIF). The usual adult dosage is INH, 5 to 10 mg per kilogram of body weight, or 300 mg daily; EMB, 25 mg/kg for 60 days, then 15 mg/kg; RIF, 600 mg once daily. Side effects of ethambutol include retrobulbar neuritis with a decrease in visual acuity. Monthly tests of visual acuity are recommended in order to detect this condition. Serious side effects of INH are rare. The most serious complication is hepatitis. The risk of hepatitis is low in persons under 20 years of age, reaching a peak among those over 50 years of age. Mild hepatic dysfunction, as evidenced by elevation of serum aminotransferase activity, occurs in 10 to 20 percent of persons taking INH. The minimum duration of the combined therapy is 18 months after sputum conversion to negative cultures, with an additional year of INH alone.

Recently, CDC and the American Thoracic Society (ATS) issued a statement regarding recommendations on short-course chemotherapy for tuberculosis. The recommendations for a treatment duration of 9 months relate to regimens containing *both* INH and RIF (with or without other drugs) and apply *only* to patients with uncomplicated pulmonary tuberculosis, that is, patients without other medical conditions such as diabetes, silicosis, or cancer.

In adults, the usual initial daily therapeutic doses are 300 mg INH and 600 mg RIF. After an initial phase of chemotherapy ranging from 2 weeks to 2 months, the physician may desire to prescribe twice-weekly therapy. The twice-weekly dose of INH would then be 15 mg per kilogram of body weight, with the RIF dosage remaining at 600 mg.

Even though the recommended short-course regimen would be suitable for children, available data concerning the use of RIF in children are limited. Restricting the dose of INH to 10 mg/kg and RIF to 15 mg/kg in children may decrease the likelihood of hepatoxicity. Table 39-2 describes the antimicrobial drugs used in the treatment of tuberculosis.

PRINCIPLES OF CHEMOTHERAPY

In order to be effective in therapy, a drug must interfere with a vital function of the tuberculosis bacillus without harming the host. Stead and Bates (1983, page 1026) emphasize that "the choice of therapy should be guided by several well-established principles" and go on to enlarge on these principles:

1. Drugs should be chosen to which the bacilli are likely to be susceptible. Fortunately, in the United States this presents little difficulty in most newly discovered cases because most strains are suscepti-

ble to the major drugs. If a patient has been treated previously or contracted the infection in an area where drug resistance is common (e.g., Southeast Asia, Philippines, Mexico), it must be assumed that the bacilli will be resistant to isoniazid (INH) and streptomycin (SM); therefore the regimen should include at least two other drugs until the results of susceptibility studies are known.

2. Even in a generally susceptible population of bacilli, a naturally resistant mutant occurs about once in 10^5 to 10^6 organisms. For this reason, at least two effective drugs should always be given to patients with clinical tuberculosis, to avoid multiplication of drug-resistant mutants.

3. Bactericidal drugs are always preferred. Both rifampin and isoniazid are bactericidal for both extra- and intracellular bacilli. Isoniazid is superior to rifampin in producing an early bactericidal effect on actively metabolizing bacteria, but rifampin is superior for sterilizing lesions which contain dormant bacilli that show only rare and short bursts of metabolic activity. For this reason, these two drugs are effective both for immediate reduction in the large extracellular population of bacilli and for ultimate eradication of the smaller intracellular population.

4. When treatment appears to be failing (bacteriology fails to become negative within three to four months), the addition of a single drug is an invitation to disaster. Therapy should always be changed to an entirely new regimen of at least two new drugs, and great care should be taken to ensure that the patient takes the medication regularly.

5. Therapy must be continued long enough to eradicate the bacilli from the body. When two bactericidal drugs are used, this can be accomplished in 9 months, but when one of the drugs is bacteriostatic, a treatment period of 18 to 24 months is required.

6. All medications should be given before breakfast and in a single dose, if possible, in order to achieve a single combined peak concentration for maximum effect on the bacilli.

Treatment of patients who complete a short-course regimen should include (1) interviews for disease symptoms and (2) obtaining of sputum specimens for smear and culture at 3-, 6-, and 12-month intervals after cessation of therapy. Chest x-rays are recommended *only* if the interview and sputum examination suggest the possibility of a recurrence of tuberculosis. Asymptomatic patients with negative sputum can be discharged after the yearly follow-up visit. However, these patients must be instructed to return for follow-up if signs or symptoms of tuberculosis recur.

Isoniazid is also used for preventive therapy in a dosage of 300 mg per day for adults, usually for a 12-month period.

TABLE 39-2

CHEMOTHERAPEUTIC AGENTS FOR TREATMENT OF TUBERCULOSIS

Name	Dosage Daily	Dosage Twice weekly	Common side effects	Monitoring	Remarks
Commonly used medications					
Isoniazid (INH)	300 mg PO or IM (10–20 mg/kg)	15 mg/kg PO or IM	Peripheral neuritis, hypersensitivity, hepatitis	SGOT/SGPT (not as a routine)	For neuritis: pryridoxine, 10 mg as prophylaxis, 50–100 mg for treatment
Rifampin	600 mg PO (10–20 mg/kg)	600 mg PO	GI disturbances (anorexia, nausea vomiting, diarrhea) hepatitis immunosuppression	SGOT/SGPT (not as a routine), alkaline phosphate bilirubin	May necessitate drug adjustments for use with, e.g., oral contraceptives, anticoagulants, corticosteroids
Ethambutol hydrochloride	15–25 mg/kg PO	50 mg/kg PO	Optic neuritis (reversible when drug is discontinued promptly); skin rash	Visual acuity, red-green color discrimination	Not recommended in pregnancy Use with caution in renal insufficiency
Pyrazinamide	2 g PO (20–40 mg/kg)		Hepatotoxicity, hyperuricemia	SGOT/SGPT uric acid	Allopurinol or probenecid to reduce serum uric acid
Streptomycin sulfate	0.75–1 g (15–20 mg/kg) IM	25–30 mg/kg IM	Ototoxicity (8th nerve damage), hypersensitivity, nephrotoxicity—rare	Audiogram, vestibular function, BUN and creatinine	Use with caution in older individual Avoid drug if renal insufficiency
Less commonly used medications					
Capreomycin	1 g IM (15 mg/kg)		Nephrotoxicity, ototoxicity (8th nerve damage), hepatotoxicity	Audiogram, vestibular function, BUN and creatinine	Use with caution in older individual Avoid drug in renal insufficiency
Cycloserine	1 g PO (10–20 mg/kg)		Personality changes, psychoses, convulsions, rash	Psychological testing	Treat neurotoxicity with pyridoxine, 100–200 mg daily; side effects may be blocked by anticonvulsive or ataractic agents
Ethionamide	0.5–1.0 g PO (15–30) mg/kg)		Gastrointestinal intolerance, hepatotoxicity, hypersensitivity	SGOT/SGPT	Divided doses may reduce GI side effects
Kanamycin	1 g IM (15 mg/kg)		Auditory toxicity, nephrotoxicity	Audiograms, vestibular function, BUN and creatinine	Use with caution in older individual Rarely used with renal insufficiency
Para-aminosalicylic acid (PAS; aminosalicylic acid)	12 g PO (200–300 mg/kg)		GI disturbance (nausea, vomiting, diarrhea, abdominal pain), hypersensitivity, hepatotoxicity	SGOT/SGPT	Frequent gastrointestinal disturbances

Source: American Lung Association, 1982.

Priorities must be established for determining which groups should be placed on preventive therapy. The following groups are recommended for preventive therapy:

1. Household members and other close associates of persons who have been recently diagnosed as having tuberculosis.
2. Positive tuberculin skin test reactors with findings on chest x-ray that are consistent with nonprogressive tuberculosis.
3. Newly infected persons. This would apply to persons who have had a tuberculin skin test conversion within the past 2 years.
4. Positive tuberculin reactors in special clinical situations. The following situations increase the risk of developing tuberculosis: (a) therapy with corticosteroids, (b) immunosuppressive therapy, (c) certain hematologic and monocyte-macrophage diseases, (d) diabetes mellitus, and (e) silicosis.
5. Positive tuberculin reactors who are under 35 years of age.

CLASSIFICATION

The classification of tuberculosis is based on broad host-parasite relationships indicated by exposure history, infection, and disease. This classification is divided into six categories (see Table 39-3) applying to both children and adults.

Terms such as *active* and *inactive* that were previously used to describe the status of clinical disease are not included in this classification. Bacteriologic status and chemotherapy status are now used to indicate clinical condition.

EPIDEMIOLOGY

In the United States, it is estimated that 10 percent of the population, or approximately 20 million people, are infected with tuberculosis. An adult tuberculin reactor with an abnormal chest x-ray consistent with tuberculosis has a 5 to 10 percent chance of developing clinical evidence of tuberculosis over the ensuing 10-year period. More than 80 percent of the reported new cases of tuberculosis are in persons over 25 years of age, the majority of whom were infected in the past. In general, 2 or 3 percent of the newly infected population will contract (develop) pulmonary tuberculosis.

When considering a person's susceptibility to tu-

TABLE 39-3

CLASSIFICATION OF TUBERCULOSIS

0. *No tuberculosis exposure, not infected* (no history of exposure, reaction to tuberculin skin test not significant).
1. *Tuberculosis exposure, no evidence of infection* (history of exposure, reaction to tuberculin skin test not significant).
2. *Tuberculosis infection, no disease* (significant reaction to tuberculin skin test, negative bacteriologic studies, if done, no clinical and/or roentgenographic evidence of tuberculosis).
   Chemotherapy status (preventive):
     None
     On chemotherapy since (date)
       Complete (prescribed course of therapy)
       Incomplete
3. *Tuberculosis: current disease* (*M. tuberculosis* cultured, if done; otherwise, *both* a significant reaction to tuberculin skin test *and* clinical and/or roentgenographic evidence of current disease).
   Location of disease:
     Pulmonary
     Pleural
     Lymphatic
     Bone and/or joint
     Genitourinary
     Disseminated (miliary)
     Meningeal
     Peritoneal
     Other
   The predominant site shall be listed. Other sites may also be listed. Anatomic sites may be specified more precisely.
   Bacteriologic status:
     Positive by:
       Microscopy only (date)
       Culture only (date)
       Microscopy and culture (date)
     Negative (date)
     Not done
   Chemotherapy status:
     On chemotherapy since (date)
     Chemotherapy terminated, incomplete (date)
   The following data are necessary in certain circumstances:
   Roentgenogram findings:
     Normal
     Abnormal:
       Cavitary or noncavitary
       Stable or worsening or improving
   Tuberculin skin test reaction:
     Significant
     Not significant
4. *Tuberculosis: no current disease* (history of previous episode(s) of tuberculosis or abnormal stable roentgenographic findings in a person with a significant reaction to tuberculin skin test, negative bacteriologic studies, if done, no clinical and/or roentgenographic evidence of current disease).
   Chemotherapy status:
     None
     On chemotherapy since (date)
     Chemotherapy terminated (date)
       Complete
       Incomplete
5. *Tuberculosis suspect* (diagnosis pending).
   Chemotherapy status:
     None
     On chemotherapy since (date)

Source: American Thoracic Society, 1981.

berculosis, two risk factors must be examined: the risk of acquiring the infection and the risk of developing clinical disease after infection has occurred. The risk of acquiring the infection and of developing clinical disease are dependent on the existence of infection in the population, crowded conditions, socially disadvantaged populations, and inadequacy of medical care. Black and Native American populations have a higher rate of tuberculosis infection than white populations.

PREVENTION AND CONTROL

Public health measures are designed for early detection of cases and sources of infection. Preventive therapy of tuberculosis with antimicrobial drugs is an effective tool in the control of the disease. It is a preventive health measure that benefits not only the infected individual but the community as well. To this end populations that are at risk of developing tuberculosis must be identified, and priorities for setting up treatment programs must take into account the risk of therapy versus the benefit to the individual.

Tuberculosis eradication involves a combination of effective chemotherapy, prompt contact identification and follow-up, and chemoprophylactic therapy of high-risk population groups.

QUESTIONS

Pulmonary tuberculosis

Directions: Answer the following questions on a separate sheet of paper.

1. List four factors that must be considered for verification of a case of tuberculosis when the *Mycobacterium tuberculosis* organism has not been identified.

2. Describe the two risk factors that must be examined when a person's susceptibility to tuberculosis is considered.

3. Explain the rationale for administering bactericidal drugs (rifampin and isoniazid) in the treatment of tuberculosis.

4. What therapeutic regimen should be initiated when treatment for tuberculosis is failing (results of bacteriologic studies fail to become negative within 3 to 4 months)?

5. Evaluate the role of bacillus Calmette-Guérin (BCG) in the control of tuberculosis.

6. What are the primary public health measures for prevention and control of tuberculosis in the United States?

Directions: Circle the letter preceding each item below that correctly completes the statement. More than one answer may be correct.

7. *M. tuberculosis* is described as a(n): *a.* Nonpathogenic organism *b.* Acid-fast rod *c.* Aerobic bacillus

8. The most accurate diagnostic method used for the detection of the tubercle bacilli is:
a. Ziehl-Neelsen method *b.* Auramine-rhodamine technique *c.* Culture technique

9. The portal of entry into the body by the tubercle bacillus which is responsible for the majority of tuberculosis infections in the United States is:
a. Respiratory tract *b.* Lymphoid tissue of the oropharynx *c.* Gut *d.* Open wound in the skin

10. The most common site of implantation of the tubercle bacillus is the alveolar surface of the lung parenchyma in the:
a. Lower part of the upper lobe *b.* Upper part of the lower lobe *c.* Both *a* and *b* *d.* Neither *a* nor *b*

11. The tissue lesion or tubercle produced by the causative agent *M. tuberculosis* usually results in:
a. Hyperplasia of epithelial tissue with many mature cells *b.* Dilatation and erosion of a pulmonary artery *c.* Bacilli surrounded by lymphocytes and fibroblasts *d.* Erosion of the epithelial lining of the mainstem bronchus

12. The earliest reaction to the tubercle bacillus is
a. Cavity *b.* Fibrosis *c.* Calcification *d.* Caseous necrosis

13. The development of caseous necrosis in tuberculosis occurs as a result of:
a. Immunity *b.* Hypersensitivity

14. The period from the onset of infection with tuberculosis bacilli to the development of a tuberculin hypersensitivity reaction is usually:
a. 4 to 6 months *b.* 3 to 10 weeks *c.* 2 to 4 days *d.* 8 to 12 hours

15. A tuberculin skin test detects:
a. A humoral sensitivity reaction to the tubercle bacillus *b.* Tuberculosis infection with disease *c.* Cellular (delayed) immunologic sensitivity to the tubercle bacillus

16. A negative tuberculin skin test usually indicates that a person:
    a. Is immune to tuberculosis   *b.* Has been treated for tuberculosis with drugs   *c.* Has not been exposed to *M. tuberculosis*   *d.* Has not been exposed to the tubercle bacillus or, if recently exposed, has not developed a tuberculin hypersensitivity reaction

17. A positive tuberculin test is indicated by:
    a. Formation of a vesicle followed by a pustule   *b.* A region of 10 mm of erythema around the injection site   *c.* An area of 10 mm of induration   *d.* An area of 5 mm of induration with erythema

18. The signs and symptoms that may be present in the more advanced stages of pulmonary tuberculosis include:
    a. Chest pain   *b.* Hemoptysis   *c.* Increase in sputum production and cough   *d.* Low-grade fever

19. In the treatment of adult pulmonary tuberculosis, the usual daily dosage of INH and of rifampin, respectively (in milligrams per kilogram of body weight), is:
    a. 100; 300   *b.* 200; 400   *c.* 300; 600   *d.* 500; 800

20. Among the groups that should be considered for preventive therapy with isoniazid are:
    a. Positive tuberculin reactors who are receiving adrenocorticoid therapy   *b.* Positive tuberculin reactors over 35 years of age   *c.* Casual contacts of persons who have been recently diagnosed with tuberculosis   *d.* Persons who are newly infected as demonstrated by a tuberculin skin test conversion within the past 2 years

Directions: Circle T if the statement is true and F if it is false. Correct the false statements.

21. T   F   Antimicrobial drugs such as ethambutol and rifampin are usually administered with isoniazid in an attempt to prevent the emergence of drug-resistant strains of *M. tuberculosis.*

22. T   F   The risk of developing hepatitis in persons receiving isoniazid drug therapy is greatest in persons under 20 years of age.

23. T   F   Short-course chemotherapy for tuberculosis may be recommended for uncomplicated pulmonary tuberculosis.

24. T   F   Short-course therapy for tuberculosis refers to treatment duration of 9 months with INH only.

25. T   F   The American Thoracic Society classification system of tuberculosis is based on the status of clinical activity of the disease (i.e., active or inactive).

26. T   F   It is estimated that 10 percent of the population in the United States, or approximately 20 million people, are infected with tuberculosis.

Directions: Match the drug name in Column A with the associated adverse side effect(s) in Column B. Items may be used more than once.

Column A

27. ____ Rifampin
28. ____ Isoniazid (INH)
29. ____ Para-aminosalicylic acid (PAS)
30. ____ Ethambutol hydrochloride
31. ____ Cycloserine
32. ____ Pyazinamide

Column B

a. Peripheral neuritis
b. Hyperuricemia
c. Nausea and vomiting
d. Hepatotoxicity
e. Immunosuppression
f. Personality changes; psychoses
g. Optic neuritis
h. Ototoxicity
i. Nephrotoxicity
j. Hypersensitivity reactions

REFERENCES FOR PART VI

ADLER, R. H.: "Spontaneous Pneumothorax," *Hospital Medicine* 1: 2, May, 1965.

ALBANESE, J. A.: *Nursing Drug Reference,* 2d ed., McGraw-Hill, New York, 1982.

American Cancer Society: *Cancer Facts and Figures,* 1980.

American Joint Committee for Cancer Staging and End Results Reporting: "Clinical Staging for Carcinoma of the Lung," *Cancer,* 24: 87, 1974.

American Lung Association: *Diagnostic Standards and Classification of Tuberculosis and Other Mycobacterial Diseases,* 13th ed., New York, 1974.

————: *Introduction to Lung Diseases,* 5th ed., New York, 1973, pp. 49–58, 87–104.

————: *Tuberculosis: What Every Physician Should Know,* New York, 1982.

AMERICAN THORACIC SOCIETY: "Chronic Bronchitis, Asthma, and Pulmonary Emphysema: A Statement by the Committee on Diagnostic Standards for Nontuberculosis Respiratory Diseases," *American Review of Respiratory Disease,* **85:** 762–768, 1962.

————: *Diagnostic Standards and Classification of Tuberculosis and Other Mycobacterial Diseases,* New York, 1981.

ASHBAUGH, D. G. and T. L. PETTY: "Positive End-expiratory Pressure," *Journal of Thoracic and Cardiovascular Surgery* **65:** 165, 1973.

AUERBACH, O., E. C. HAMMOND, and L. GARFINKEL: "Bronchial Carcinoma in Relation to Smoking," in R. F. Johnston (ed.), *Pulmonary Care,* Grune & Stratton, New York, 1973, pp. 231–242.

AUSTRIAN R.: "Pneumococcal Infections," in R. Petersdorf et al. (eds.), *Harrison's Principles of Internal Medicine,* 10th ed., McGraw-Hill, New York, 1983, pp. 918–922.

BATES, D. V., et al.: *Respiratory Function in Disease,* Saunders, Philadelphia, 1971.

BAUM, G. L.: "Diseases of the Pleura," *Hospital Medicine* **5:** 6, October 1969.

———— and P. B. BARLOW: "Tuberculosis Patients, Old Myths, New Realities," in R. F. Johnston (ed.), *Pulmonary Care,* Grune & Stratton, New York, 1973, pp. 181–193.

BECKLAKE, M. R.: "Asbestos-Related Diseases in Lungs and Other Organs: Their Epidemiology and Implications for Clinical Practice," *American Review of Respiratory Diseases* **114:** 187–220, 1976.

BENDIXIN, H. H., et al.: *Respiratory Care,* Mosby, St. Louis, 1965.

BLUM, J. E.: "Pickwickian Syndrome," *Hospital Medicine* **19**(9): 13–17, 1983.

BONE, R. C.: "The Adult Respiratory Distress Syndrome: Treatment in the Next Decade," *Respiratory Care* **29**(3): 249–262, 1984.

BOROW, M., CONSTON, A., LIVORNESE, L., and SCHALET, N.: "Mesothelioma and Its Association with Asbestos," *JAMA 201:* 92, 1967.

BURNEY, L. E.: "Smoking and Lung Cancer: A Statement on the Public Health Service," *JAMA* **171:** 1829, 1957.

BURROWS, B., R. J. KNUDSON, and L. J. KETTEL: *Respiratory Insufficiency,* Year Book, Chicago, 1975, pp. 25–38, 50–57, 84–96, 110–112, 130–155, 157–158.

BUSHNELL, S. S.: *Respiratory Intensive Care Nursing,* Little, Brown, Boston, 1973.

CATANZARO, A.: "Tuberculosis: Update on Diagnosis and Therapy." *Hospital Medicine* **17**(11): 48E–48M, November 1981.

CHERNIACK, R. M.: *Pulmonary Function Testing,* Saunders, Philadelphia, 1977.

———— and L. CHERNIACK: *Respiration in Health and Disease,* 3d ed., Saunders, Philadelphia, 1983.

COLE, R. B.: *Essentials of Respiratory Diseases,* Medcom, New York, 1975, pp. 103–107, 251–260.

COMROE, J. H., JR.: *Physiology of Respiration,* 2d ed., Year Book, Chicago, 1974.

———— et al.: *The Lung,* 2d ed., Year Book, Chicago, 1962.

CROFTON, J. and A. DOUGLAS: *Respiratory Diseases,* 3d ed., Blackwell, Oxford, 1981.

DANNENBERG, A. M.: "Pathogenesis of Pulmonary Tuberculosis," *American Review of Respiratory Disease* **125**(3): 25–41, March 1982.

DICKIE, H. A.: "Dust Inhalation Diseases," in C. W. Holman and C. Muschenheim (eds.), *Bronchopulmonary Diseases and Related Disorders,* Harper & Row, New York, 1972, vol. 1, pp. 449–467.

FAIRBANKS, D. N. F.: "Snoring: Not Funny, Not Hopeless," *Hospital Medicine* **20**(3): 173–189, 1984.

FISHMAN, F. P.: "Chronic Cor Pulmonale," *Hospital Practice,* May 1971, pp. 101–117.

FITZMAURICE, J. B. and A. A. SASAHARA: "Current Concepts of Pulmonary Embolism: Implications for Nursing Practice," *Heart & Lung* **3:** 209, March-April 1974.

GEIGER, J. R.: "Diagnosis of Chest Injuries," *Hospital Medicine* **7:** 109, October 1971.

GENTON, E. and R. PRYOR: "Acute Pulmonary Embolism," *Hospital Medicine* **9:** 9, April 1973.

GESCHICKTER, C. F.: *The Lung in Health and Disease,* Lippincott, Philadelphia, 1973, pp. 43–62, 99–103, 124–134, 152–159.

GLUCK, L.: "Pulmonary Surfactant and Neonatal Distress," *Hospital Practice,* November 1972, pp. 45–56.

GOLOMB, H. M. and T. R. DeMEESTER: "Lung Cancer: A Combined Modality Approach to Staging and Therapy," *Ca* **29:** 258, 1979.

GRACEY, D. R.: "Adult Respiratory Distress Syndrome:" *Heart & Lung* **4:** 280, March-April 1975.

GUENTER, C. A. and K. A. BUCHAN: "Acute Infectious Respiratory Illness," in C. A. Guenter and M. H. Welch (eds.), *Pulmonary Medicine,* Lippincott, Philadelphia, 1977, pp. 224–307.

HARLAN, D. E. and J. M. MATTLOFF: "Initial Management of Rib Fractures and Their Complications," *Hospital Medicine* **9:** 71, March 1973.

HARSHEY, R. M. and L. RAMAKRISHNAN: "Rate of Ribonucleic Acid Chain Growth in M. tuberculosis," *Journal of Bacteriology* **129:** 612–622, 1977.

HOLLAND, J. and E. FREI: *Cancer Medicine,* Lea & Febiger, Philadelphia, 1982.

HOLMAN, C. W.: "Anatomy," in C. W. Holman and C. Muschenheim (eds.), *Bronchopulmonary Disease and Related Disorders,* Harper & Row, New York, 1972, vol. 1, pp. 3–40.

HOOK, E. W.: "The Pneumonias and Viral Respiratory Infections," in C. W. Holman and C. Muschenheim (eds.), *Bronchopulmonary Disease and Related Disorders,* Harper & Row, New York, 1972, pp. 279–340.

JAWETZ, E., J. MELNICK, and E. ADELBERG: *Review of Medical Microbiology,* 16th ed., Lange, Los Altos, Calif., 1984.

KOOP, C. E.: "Smoking and Cancer," *Hospital Practice* 19(6): 107–132, 1984.

KROEKER, E. J.: "Atelectasis," *Hospital Medicine* 5: 67, March 1969.

LANGLEY, L. L., I. R. TELFORD, and J. B. CHRISTENSEN: *Dynamic Anatomy and Physiology,* 5th ed., McGraw-Hill, New York, 1980.

LIGHT, R. W.: "Postoperative Pleural Effusion: Pathophysiology, Clinical Importance, and Principles of Management," *Respiratory Care* 29(5): 540–549, 1984.

LIPMAN, B. S. and E. MASSIE: "Clubbed Fingers and Hypertrophic Osteo-Arthropathy," in C. M. MacBryde (ed.), *Signs and Symptoms,* 3d ed., Lippincott, Philadelphia, 1957, pp. 258–272.

LONG, M. W., D. E. SNEDER, JR., and L. S. FARER: "U.S. Public Health Service Cooperative Trial of Three Rifampin-Isoniazid Regimens in Treatment of Pulmonary Tuberculosis," *American Review of Respiratory Disease* 119(6): 879–894, June 1979.

LUKAS, D. S. and D. P. BARR: "Dyspnea; Cyanosis," in C. M. MacBryde (ed.), *Signs and Symptoms,* 3d ed., Lippincott, Philadelphia, 1957, pp. 349–375.

MACDONNELL, K. F., and M. S. SEGAL: *Current Respiratory Care,* Little, Brown, Boston, 1977.

Massachusetts Medical Society: "Tuberculosis—United States, 1983," *Morbidity and Mortality Weekly Report* 6(33): 77–78, Feb. 17, 1984.

MINNA, J. D.: "Neoplasms of the Lung," in R. Petersdorf (ed.), *Harrison's Principles of Internal Medicine,* 10th ed., McGraw-Hill, New York, 1983, pp. 1572–1580.

MITCHELL, R. S.: *Synopsis of Clinical Pulmonary Disease,* 3d ed., Mosby, St. Louis, 1983.

MOSER, K. M. "Fiberoptic Bronchoscopy and Other Diagnostic Procedures," in R. Petersdorf et al. (eds.) *Harrison's Principles of Internal Medicine,* 10th ed., McGraw-Hill, New York, 1983.

National Tuberculosis and Respiratory Disease Association: *Chronic Obstructive Pulmonary Disease: A Manual for Physicians,* 3d ed., New York, 1972.

NEPTUNE, W. B., A. J. PIRO, and M. J. STRAUS: "Pri-

mary Cancer of the Lung," in *Cancer: A Manual for Practitioners,* American Cancer Society, Boston, 1978.

NOBLE, J. "Isoniazid Prophylaxis Re-examined," *The New England Journal of Medicine* 285: 687, 1971.

O'DONNEL, W. M., R. H. MANN, and J. L. CROSH: "Asbestos and Extrinsic Factor in the Pathogenesis of Bronchogenic Carcinoma and Mesothelioma." *Cancer (New York)* 19: 1143, 1966.

PETTY, T. L.: "Adult Respiratory Distress Syndrome," in R. S. Mitchell (ed.), *Synopsis of Pulmonary Disease,* 2d ed., Mosby, St. Louis, 1978.

——— and D. G. ASHBAUGH: "The Adult Respiratory Distress Syndrome," *Chest* 60: 233–239, 1971.

POOL, J. L., G. F. GRAY, and C. W. HOLMAN: "Tumors of the Lung and Trachea," in C. W. Holman and C. Muschenheim (eds.), *Bronchopulmonary Diseases and Related Pulmonary Disorders,* Harper & Row, 1972, pp. 785–821.

Public Health Service: "The Health Consequences of Smoking: A Report to the Surgeon General, 1971."

Public Health Service/Center for Disease Control: "Follow-up on Guidelines for Short-Course Tuberculosis Chemotherapy," *Morbidity and Mortality Weekly Report,* 29: 16, 183–189, April 25, 1980.

———: "Tuberculosis—North Dakota," *Morbidity and Mortality Weekly Report,* 27: 52, 523–525, Jan. 5, 1979.

———: *1979 Tuberculosis Statistics: States and Cities,* Atlanta, July 1980, p. 27.

Public Health Service/National Center for Health Research, Statistics, and Technology: "Vital Statistics of the U.S., 1977."

REIMANN, H. A. (ed.): *Acute Respiratory Tract Diseases,* Medcom, New York, 1975.

RELICHEL, J.: "Pulmonary Emphysema," *Hospital Medicine,* February 1980.

ROBBINS, S. and M. ANGELL: *Basic Pathology,* 3d ed., Saunders, Philadelphia, 1981.

ROBIN, E. and R. GAUDIO: "Cor Pulmonale," *Disease-a-Month,* May 1970.

ROBIN, E. D. and L. M. SIMON: "Oxygen Transport and Cellular Respiration," in E. D. Frohlich (ed.), *Pathophysiology: Altered Regulatory Mechanisms in Disease,* 2d ed., Lippincott, Philadelphia, 1976, pp. 167–187.

ROWHEDER, J. J. "Neoplastic Disease in Pulmonary Medicine," in C. A. Guenter and M. H. Welch (eds.), *Pulmonary Medicine,* Lippincott, Philadelphia, 1977, pp. 678–739.

ROSENTHAL, S. R. (ed.): *BCG Vaccine: Tuberculosis—Cancer,* PSB Publishing Company, Littleton, Mass., 1980.

SAID, S. I.: "Metabolid Functions of the Lung," in E. D. Frolich (ed.), *Pathophysiology: Altered Regulatory Mechanisms in Disease,* 2d ed., Lippincott, Philadelphia, 1976, pp. 189–205.

SANDRITTER, W. and W. B. WARTMAN: *Color Atlas and Textbook of Tissue and Cellular Pathology*, 4th ed., Year Book, Chicago, 1973, pp. 74–97.

SCHARER, L.: "Pleurisy, Pleural Effusions, and Empyema," in C. W. Holman and C. Muschenheim (eds.), *Bronchopulmonary Diseases and Related Disorders*, Harper & Row, New York, 1972, vol. 1, pp. 766–783.

SHAPIRO, B. A., R. A. HARRISON, and J. R. WALTON: *Clinical Application of Blood Gases*, 3d ed., Year Book, Chicago, 1982.

SKILLING, D. M.: "Cough; Hemoptysis," in C. M. MacBryde (ed.), *Signs and Symptoms*, 3d ed., Lippincott, Philadelphia, 1957, pp. 321–348.

SPENCER, H.: *Pathology of the Lung*, 3d ed., Pergamon, New York, 1976.

STEAD, W. W. and J. H. BATES: "Tuberculosis," in R. Petersdorf (ed.), *Harrison's Principles of Internal Medicine*, 10th ed., New York, McGraw-Hill, 1983, pp. 1019–1030.

TRAVER, G. A.: *Respiratory Nursing: The Science and Art*, Wiley, New York, 1982.

WAYNE, L. G.: "Pathogenesis of Pulmonary Tuberculosis," *American Review of Respiratory Disease* **125**(3):33–41 March 1982.

WEG, JOHN: *Treatment and Control of Tuberculosis*, American Lung Association, New York, 1972.

WEISS, W.: "Smoking and Pulmonary Disease," in R. F. Johnston (ed.), *Pulmonary Care*, Grune & Stratton, New York, 1973, pp. 221–231.

WELCH, M. H.: "Obstructive Diseases," in C. A. Guenter and M. H. Welch (eds.), *Pulmonary Medicine*, Lippincott, Philadelphia, 1977, pp. 556–677.

WEST, J. B.: *Pulmonary Pathophysiology*, Williams & Wilkins, Baltimore, 1977.

———: *Respiratory Physiology*, 2d ed., Williams & Wilkins, Baltimore, 1979.

WIDMANN, F. K.: *Goodale's Clinical Interpretation of Laboratory Tests*, 9th ed., Davis, Philadelphia, 1983.

WOODBURNE, R. T.: *Essentials of Human Anatomy*, 6th ed., Oxford University Press, New York, 1978, pp. 311–312.

YOUMANS, G. P.: *Tuberculosis*, Saunders, Philadelphia, 1979.

PART VII

LORRAINE M. WILSON

RENAL PATHOPHYSIOLOGY

It has been only within recent years that the role of the kidney as a vital organ has begun to be appreciated and understood. The concept of the kidney as an organ of excretion is no longer adequate. Indeed, the kidney as master chemist of the body has the unique role of regulating the fluid, electrolyte, and acid-base balance of the internal environment. Its excretory function is only incidental to its regulatory function. This new understanding gained from intensive research in normal renal physiology, pathophysiology, and effective methods of treatment has resulted in an appreciation of the impact of renal disease on the health of the nation.

The National Kidney Foundation reports that over 8 million Americans suffer with kidney-related diseases, and these are the fourth greatest health problem in the nation today. The foundation also estimates that 3.3 million persons have unrecognized and undiagnosed infection of the urinary tract. Most of these persons do not develop renal failure, but there is a relation between urinary infection and chronic pyelonephritis, one of the major causes of death due to renal failure. The financial impact of kidney-related diseases on the national economy is in excess of 3.6 billion dollars annually. This figure includes wages lost, medical services, drug costs, and insurance disbursements.*

Deaths directly related to kidney disease have been estimated at about 55,000 annually.† This estimate is conservative, since it does not take into account cases in which renal disease was a contributing cause of death. For example, many patients dying of diabetes, hypertension, or septicemia may have significant renal involvement which is not reported. It should be

*State Health Planning Advisory Council and Office of Health and Medical Affairs: *Management of Renal Disease in Michigan, A Statement of Public Policy,* Lansing, Michigan, November 1973.

†"Report to the Congress, Treatment of Chronic Kidney Failure: Dialysis, Transplant, Costs, and the Need for More Vigorous Efforts," GAO Report no. MWD-75-53, Washington, June 24, 1975.

noted that deaths directly attributed to renal disease exceed those due to diabetes, stroke, rheumatic heart disease, and hypertensive disease through the age of 34 years. In fact, kidney disease continues to be a significant factor throughout the productive years.

Although much more knowledge of the etiology of the major renal diseases (notably chronic glomerulonephritis and pyelonephritis) is needed before effective prevention is possible, much progress has been made in prolonging the lives of persons with end-stage renal failure. These two methods of treatment are chronic dialysis and renal transplantation.

During the past 20 years the numbers of end-stage renal disease (ESRD) patients and treatment facilities have greatly expanded. This expansion has been greatly influenced by public education, better detection, and federal financing of ESRD treatment since 1973. In the United States there are currently about 60,000 patients receiving chronic dialysis treatment in about 1000 facilities and 4000 homes two or three times per week. The number of renal transplants has stabilized at 4700 per year. More than 30,000 renal transplants have been performed in the United States alone, more than 80 percent of them since 1974. About 10,000 newly diagnosed patients with ESRD enter the system annually. The total number of patients has probably reached a plateau. The annual cost of this treatment program was 1.8 billion dollars in 1981 ("End Stage Renal Disease Program," 1982).

This part is concerned with the problem of renal failure. The first three chapters discuss normal kidney structure and function, methods of detecting renal disease, and the etiology and pathophysiology of chronic renal disease. The consequences of renal failure and its treatment are discussed in Chaps. 43 and 44. Acute renal failure is discussed in Chap. 45.

NORMAL RENAL FUNCTION

OBJECTIVES

At the completion of this chapter you should be able to:

1. Identify the anatomic structures of the urinary tract.
2. Describe and recognize the importance of the location of the kidney in relation to other anatomic structures in close proximity.
3. Identify the structures that enter and leave the kidney.
4. Describe the gross anatomy of the kidney.
5. Trace the blood route supplying and draining the kidney.
6. Describe the special features of renal blood flow, including total blood received, its distribution, and autoregulation.
7. Give one example of a possible complication of variations in the renal blood supply.
8. Identify the component parts of the nephron.
9. Name, locate, and describe the function of the various types of cells of the renal corpuscle.
10. Identify and describe the components of the juxtaglomerular apparatus.
11. Describe the function of the juxtaglomerular apparatus in relation to renal blood flow.
12. Describe the renin-angiotensin system.
13. Describe glomerular filtration, including the forces involved, its measurement, and normal values for men and women.
14. Differentiate between *reabsorption* and *secretion* in the nephron.
15. Distinguish two types of transport mechanism in the nephron.
16. Identify three classes of substances and the major components of each which are filtered by the glomerulus.
17. Describe tubular regulation of filtered substances in each component part of the nephron.
18. Describe the role of the kidneys in acid-base regulation.
19. Identify three hormones which influence tubular secretion or reabsorption and the substances influenced.
20. List the major functions of the kidney.
21. Define *osmolality*.

22. Name the single factor that influences osmotic activity.

23. List the four colligative properties of solutions.

24. Illustrate how each of these colligative properties is affected by the addition of particles to water.

25. Differentiate between two methods of measuring the concentration of body fluids (osmometer and urinometer).

26. Write the formula used to calculate the osmotic concentration (osmolality) of a solution and, given appropriate values, calculate the plasma osmolality.

27. Distinguish between *osmolality* and *osmolarity*.

28. Describe reabsorption of glomerular filtrate in the proximal tubule.

29. Differentiate between the cortical and juxtamedullary nephrons (number and anatomic features).

30. Define the *vasa recta*.

31. Explain the two basic processes involved in the countercurrent mechanism.

32. Describe the concentration gradient of the filtrate as it moves from the glomerulus to the end of the collecting duct.

33. Explain the anatomic relations which allow a concentration gradient to become established and maintained in the kidney.

34. Explain how the chloride pump (active chloride transport) is involved in countercurrent multiplication of concentration.

35. Describe how the vasa recta act as a countercurrent exchange system.

36. Describe the effect of antidiuretic hormone (ADH) on the distal tubule, collecting ducts, and vasa recta.

37. Describe the recirculation of urea and its contribution to the osmotic concentration of the interstitial fluid.

38. Explain the role of ADH in maintaining a constant volume and osmolality of the plasma.

ANATOMY OF THE KIDNEYS AND URINARY TRACT

The kidneys perform the vital function of regulating the volume and chemical composition of the blood (and the internal environment) by selective excretion of solutes and water. If both kidneys were to fail to perform this function for any reason, death would follow within three or four weeks. This vital function of the kidney is accomplished within the organ by filtration of the blood plasma through the glomerulus, followed by reabsorption of the appropriate amounts of solute and water along the renal tubules. Excess solutes and water are excreted as urine through the urinary collecting system to the outside of the body. This chapter reviews the gross and microscopic anatomy of the kidney and discusses its physiologic functions.

The urinary tract

The urinary tract consists of the kidneys, which constantly manufacture urine, and the various tubes and reservoirs necessary to carry urine to the outside of the body (Fig. 40-1).

The kidneys are bean-shaped organs situated on either side of the vertebral column. The right kidney is slightly lower than the left because it is pushed down by the liver. Its upper pole lies on the level of the twelfth rib. The upper pole of the left kidney lies at about the level of the eleventh rib.

The two ureters are tubes about 10 to 12 in long extending from the kidneys to the bladder. Their only function is to convey urine to the bladder.

The bladder is a collapsible muscular bag located behind the symphysis pubis. There are three openings in the bladder, two from the ureters and one into the urethra. The bladder has two functions: (1) it serves as a reservoir for urine before it leaves the body, and (2) aided by the urethra, it expels urine from the body.

The urethra is a small dilatable tube leading from the bladder to the outside of the body. It is about 1½ in long in the female and about 8 in long in the male. The opening to the outside of the body is called the *urinary meatus*.

Anatomic relations of the kidney

The kidneys lie at the back of the upper abdomen behind the peritoneum, in front of the last two ribs and three major muscles—the transversus abdominis, quadratus lumborum, and psoas major (Fig. 40-2). They are kept in position by a heavy cushion of fat. The adrenal glands are situated over the upper pole of each kidney.

The kidneys are well protected from direct trauma—posteriorly by the ribs and overlying muscles and anteriorly by a thick cushion of intestines. When they are injured, it is almost always as a result of a force acting upon the twelfth rib, which rotates inward and squeezes the kidney between itself and the bodies of the lumbar vertebrae. This excellent protection from direct injury also accounts for their difficult position for palpation and surgical access. The normal-sized left kidney is not generally palpable on physical examination, be-

cause the upper two-thirds of the anterior surface is overlaid by the spleen. The lower pole of the normal-sized right kidney, however, may be bimanually palpated in many persons. Gross enlargement or displacement of either kidney may be detected by palpation, though this is more easily accomplished on the right.

Gross structure of the kidney

In the adult each kidney is 12 to 13 cm long and 6 cm wide, and weighs from 120 to 150 g. The size does not vary appreciably with body build. Ninety-five percent of the adult population can be expected to have a pole-to-pole kidney length between 11 and 15 cm. A difference of more than 1.5 cm in the length of a particular kidney (compared with its mate) or a change in its shape is significant, since the majority of renal diseases are manifested by structural changes of the organ.

The anterior and posterior surfaces, upper and lower poles, and lateral margin of the kidney have a convex contour, while the medial margin is concave because of the presence of the hilus (Fig. 40-3A). Several structures enter or leave the kidney through the hilus, including the renal artery, renal vein, nerves, and lymphatics. The kidney is encased in a thin, fibrous, glistening capsule, which is loosely adherent to the underlying tissue and can be easily stripped from the surface.

A longitudinal section of the kidney reveals two distinct regions, the outer cortex and inner medulla (Fig. 40-3B). The medulla is divided into triangular wedges called *pyramids*. The pyramids are interspersed with cortical material called the *columns of Bertin*. Pyramids have a striated appearance because they are made up of segments of the tubules and collecting ducts of the nephron. The papilla (apex) of each pyramid forms the papillary ducts of Bellini, which in turn are created by the terminal fusion of many collecting ducts. Each papillary duct is thrust into a cup-shaped terminal extension of the renal pelvis called a *minor calyx* (L. *calix*, cup). Several minor calyces unite to form major calyces, which in turn unite to form the pelvis of the kidney. The renal pelvis is the main reservoir for the renal collecting system. The ureter connects the renal pelvis to the urinary bladder.

Knowledge of renal anatomy is basic to understanding urine formation. Urine formation begins in the cortex and continues as the material flows through the tubules and collecting ducts. The formed urine then flows

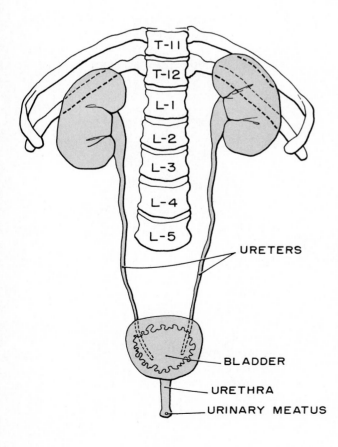

T-11
T-12
L-1
L-2
L-3
L-4
L-5

URETERS

BLADDER

URETHRA

URINARY MEATUS

FIGURE 40-1
The urinary tract, anatomic relations.

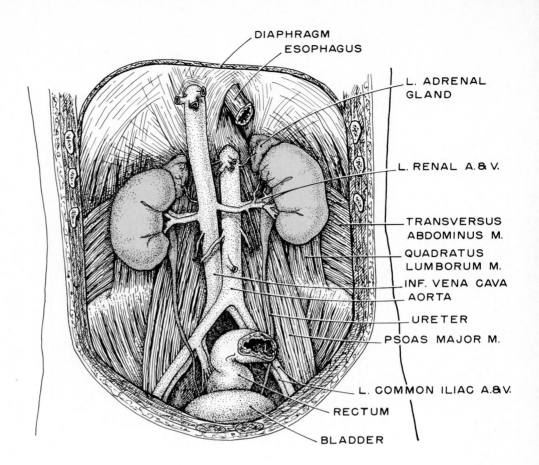

FIGURE 40-2
The kidneys, anatomic relations.

into the papillary ducts of Bellini, enters the minor calyces, major calyces, renal pelvis, and finally exits the kidney via the ureter to the urinary bladder. The walls of the calyces, pelvis, and ureter contain smooth muscle, which contracts rhythmically and helps to propel urine along its course by peristalsis.

Gross vascular supply of the kidney

The renal arteries arise from the abdominal aorta at approximately the level of the second lumbar vertebra. Because the aorta is to the left of the midline, the right renal artery is longer than the left (Fig. 40-2). Each renal artery branches as it enters the hilus of each kidney.

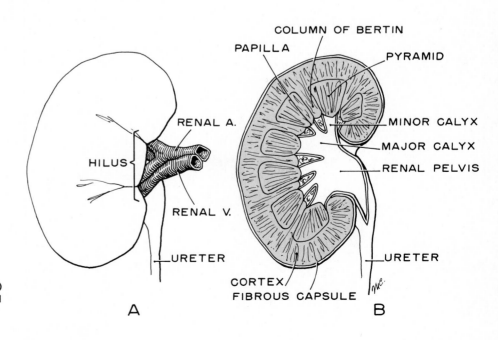

FIGURE 40-3
Gross structure of the kidney. (A) Anterior surface; (B) longitudinal section.

The renal veins which drain each kidney empty into the inferior vena cava, which lies to the right of the midline. Consequently, the left renal vein is about twice as long as the right. Because of these anatomic features, the transplant surgeon generally prefers the left kidney from the donor, which is rotated and placed in the right pelvis of the recipient. Few technical difficulties are encountered with a short renal artery which is anastomosed with the internal iliac (hypogastric) artery. The renal vein, however, must be longer, since it is implanted directly into the external iliac vein (Fig. 44-8).

As the renal artery enters the hilus, it breaks down into the interlobar arteries, which pass between the pyramids to form the arcuate branches, which arch over the bases of the pyramids (Fig. 40-4).

The arcuate arteries give rise to the interlobular arterioles, which form a parallel array in the cortex. These interlobular arterioles give rise to afferent arterioles.

The afferent arterioles terminate in capillary tufts called the *glomeruli*. The glomeruli converge into efferent arterioles, which in turn subdivide into a portal network of capillaries surrounding the tubules, sometimes called the *peritubular capillaries* (not shown). The blood passing through this portal network drains into a venous network to the interlobular, arcuate, interlobar, and renal veins to reach the inferior vena cava.

Special features of renal blood flow

The kidneys are perfused with about 1200 ml of blood per minute—a volume equal to 20 to 25 percent of the cardiac output (5000 ml per minute). This fact is quite remarkable when one considers that the combined weight of the kidneys is less than 1 percent of the total body weight.

More than 90 percent of the blood perfusing the

kidney is distributed to the cortex, while the remainder is distributed to the medulla (the physiologic significance of this for urine concentration is discussed later).

Another special feature of renal blood flow is autoregulation of blood flow through the kidney. The afferent arterioles have an intrinsic capacity to vary their resistance in response to changes in arterial blood pressure thus keeping renal blood flow and glomerular filtration constant. It is effective over an arterial pressure range of 80 to 180 mmHg. The result is the prevention of large changes in solute and water excretion. Autoregulation, however, can be overpowered in certain circumstances even in the autoregulatory range. Renal nerves may cause vasoconstriction in states of emergency and shunt blood away from the kidney to the heart, brain, or skeletal muscles at the expense of the kidney. Disturbances in autoregulation and the distribution of intrarenal blood flow may be important in the pathogenesis of acute oliguric renal failure (see Chap. 45).

Variations in renal vascular supply

There are cases in which multiple arteries or veins supply the kidneys (Fig. 40-5). Anomalies of the renal arteries are far more common than anomalies of the veins. In fact, about 25 percent or more of the population have more than one renal artery supplying a kidney. These additional arteries usually originate as small multiple branches from the aorta and supply the poles of the kidney. An arteriogram of the renal blood supply

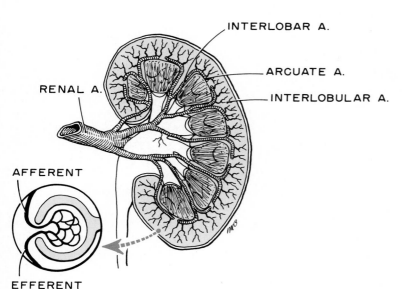

INTERLOBAR A.

ARCUATE A.

INTERLOBULAR A.

RENAL A.

AFFERENT

EFFERENT

FIGURE 40-4
Vascular supply to the kidney. Approximately 90 percent of the blood is distributed to the cortex and 10 percent to the medulla. Inset depicts the glomerular capillary tuft with afferent and efferent arterioles.

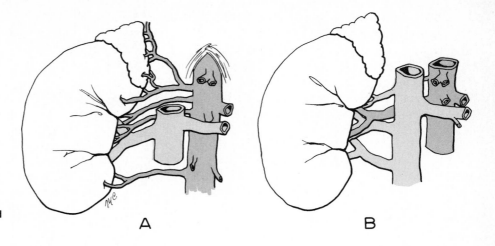

FIGURE 40-5
Anomalies in renal vasculature. About 25 percent of the population have multiple renal arteries supplying a kidney (A); (B) multiple renal veins. (Modified from Netter, 1973.)

A

B

is essential in the donor before kidney transplantation is attempted because of the possibility of these variations, which may present technical difficulties for the surgeon.

Microscopic structure of the kidney

The nephron

The functional work unit of the kidney is called the *nephron*. There are about 1 million nephrons in each kidney, basically similar in structure and function. Thus the work of the kidneys may be considered to be the sum total of the function of all the nephrons put together. Each nephron consists of Bowman's capsule, which surrounds the glomerular capillary tuft, the proximal convoluted tubule, the loop of Henle, and the distal convoluted tubule, which empties into the *collecting ducts* (Fig. 40-6). A normal person can survive, albeit with difficulty, with less than 20,000 nephrons, or 1 percent of the total nephron mass. Thus, it is possible to donate one kidney for transplantation without endangering life.

The renal corpuscle

The renal corpuscle consists of Bowman's capsule and the glomerular capillary tuft. The term *glomerulus* is often used interchangeably with *renal corpuscle*, though it properly refers only to the capillary tuft.

Bowman's capsule is a specialized invagination of the proximal tubule (Fig. 40-7). There is a urine-containing space between the capillary tuft and Bowman's capsule called *Bowman's space*, or the *capsular space*.

Bowman's capsule is lined with epithelial cells. *Parietal epithelial cells* are flat and form the outermost part of the capsule; the much larger *visceral epithelial cells* form the innermost part of the capsule and line the outer side of the capillary tuft. Foot processes, or *podocytes*, form extensions of the visceral epithelial cells which come in contact with the basement membrane at intervals, leaving many areas free of epithelial cell con-

tact. The area between the foot processes, usually referred to as the *slit pore*, has an average width of about 400 Å (angstrom units).

The *basement membrane* forms the middle layer of the capillary wall, sandwiched between the epithelial cells on one side and the endothelial cells on the other. The capillary basement membrane is continuous with that of the tubule. No pores are visible in the basement membrane, although it behaves as if it had pores about 70 to 100 Å in diameter.

Endothelial cells form the innermost layer of the capillary tuft. Unlike the epithelial cells, the endothelial cells are in continuous contact with the basement membrane. However, there are numerous windowlike openings called *fenestrations*, which are about 600 Å in diameter. The endothelial cells are continuous with the endothelial lining of the afferent and efferent arterioles.

The endothelial cells, basement membrane, and visceral epithelial cells are the three layers which make up the glomerular filtration membrane. The function of the glomerular filtration membrane is to allow ultrafiltration of the blood. In separating the formed elements of the blood and the large protein molecules from the rest of the plasma, it delivers the plasma as primary urine to the urinary space of Bowman's capsule. The mechanism involved in the filtration process is not fully understood. Recent evidence seems to indicate that the structural bsasis for the relative impermeability of the glomerular capillary may be the slit pores or the gelatinous basement membrane. A small amount of albumin, molecules of which have a diameter slightly less than that of the smallest pores, enters the filtrate but is reabsorbed in the proximal tubule. Larger protein molecules and blood cells do not normally appear in the filtrate and urine.

The *mesangial cells* are endothelial cells which form a continuous network between the capillary loops of the glomerulus and are thought to function as a supporting network. Mesangial cells are not part of the filtration membrane.

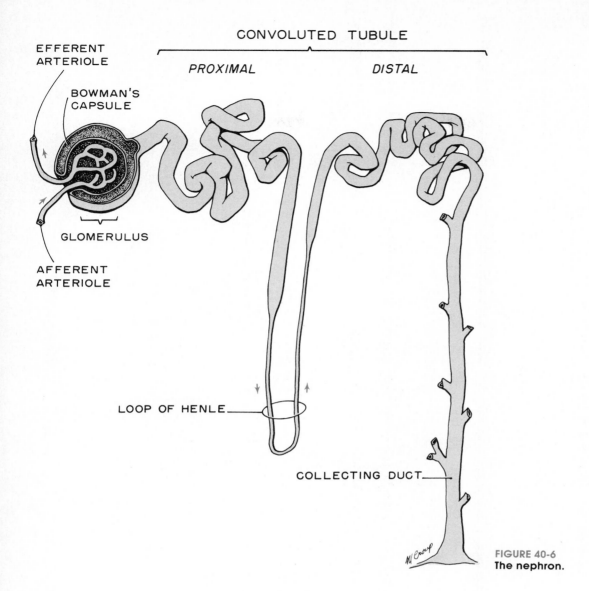

EFFERENT
ARTERIOLE

BOWMAN'S
CAPSULE

GLOMERULUS

AFFERENT
ARTERIOLE

CONVOLUTED TUBULE

PROXIMAL

DISTAL

LOOP OF HENLE

COLLECTING DUCT

FIGURE 40-6
The nephron.

The juxtaglomerular apparatus

In each nephron the first part of the distal tubule rises from the medulla so that it is situated in the angle between the afferent and efferent arteriole of the glomerulus of that nephron (Fig. 40-7). At this point the juxtaglomerular cells within the wall of the afferent arteriole contain secretory granules which are believed to secrete renin. Renin is an enzyme important in the regulation of blood pressure. The distal tubular cells, which come into intimate contact with the granular cells, are called the *macula densa* because of their prominent nuclei. This specialized group of cells (including some connective tissue cells) near the vascular pole of each glomerulus is known as the *juxtaglomerular* (JG) *apparatus* and is believed to regulate renin release.

There are two important theories concerning the regulation of renin release. According to one theory, the juxtaglomerular cells function as baroreceptors (pres-

sure sensors) sensitive to blood flow through the afferent arteriole. A decrease in arterial pressure stimulates increased granularity of the juxtaglomerular cells and increased renin secretion. According to the other theory, the macula densa cells of the distal tubule act as chemoreceptors sensitive to the sodium concentration of the tubular fluid. An increased sodium concentration in the distal tubule influences the juxtaglomerular cells (in close apposition to the macula densa) to increase renin output. A decreased sodium concentration in the distal tubule, however, does not decrease renin release (since sodium concentration in the distal tubule is normally quite low). There is also evidence that the sympathetic nervous system and the catecholamines influence renin secretion. It is probable that both the baroreceptor and macula densa theories are valid, and the juxtaglomerular apparatus may be a site for the integration of several diverse inputs.

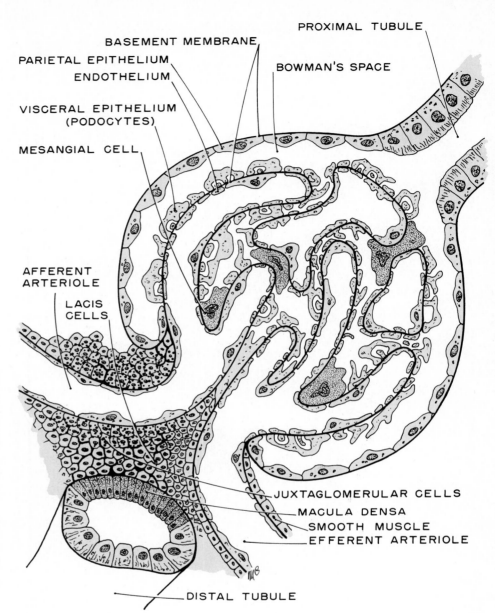

PROXIMAL TUBULE

BASEMENT MEMBRANE

BOWMAN'S SPACE

PARIETAL EPITHELIUM

ENDOTHELIUM

VISCERAL EPITHELIUM
(PODOCYTES)

MESANGIAL CELL

AFFERENT
ARTERIOLE

LACIS
CELLS

JUXTAGLOMERULAR CELLS

MACULA DENSA

SMOOTH MUSCLE

EFFERENT ARTERIOLE

DISTAL TUBULE

FIGURE 40-7
The renal corpuscle. The glomerular capillary filter consists of three layers of cells—the endothelium, basement membrane, and visceral epithelium containing podocytes or foot processes. Mesangial cells (between the capillaries) form a supporting network for the glomerular tuft. The juxtaglomerular apparatus consists of a specialized group of cells (the macula densa and juxtaglomerular cells) near the vascular pole of the glomerulus and is important in the regulation of blood pressure.

The renin-angiotensin system

The release of renin from the kidney results in the conversion of angiotensinogen (a glycoprotein made in the liver) to angiotensin I. Angiotensin I is changed to angiotensin II by a converting enzyme found in the pulmonary capillary bed. Angiotensin II increases blood pressure by causing vasoconstriction of peripheral arterioles and stimulating secretion of aldosterone. Elevated aldosterone levels stimulate sodium reabsorption in the distal tubules and collecting ducts. Increased sodium reabsorption causes increased water reabsorption, and thus plasma volume is increased. This increased plasma volume contributes to blood pressure elevation, which in turn facilitates the reduction of renal ischemia. The schema for the renin-angiotensin mechanism is outlined in Fig. 40-8.

BASIC RENAL PHYSIOLOGY

The primary function of the kidney is to maintain within normal limits the volume and composition of the extracellular fluid. The composition and volume of the extracellular fluid are controlled by glomerular filtration and by tubular reabsorption and secretion, discussed in the following sections. Table 40-1 presents a list of renal functions that may be helpful to review at this point. These functions will be reviewed again at the end of this chapter.

Glomerular ultrafiltration

Urine formation begins with glomerular filtration of plasma. Renal blood flow (RBF) is equal to about 25 percent of the cardiac output, or 1200 ml per minute.

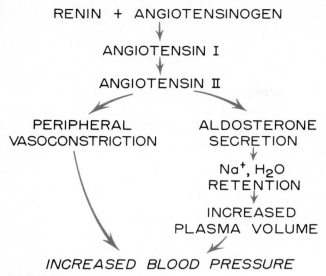

FIGURE 40-8
Schema for the renin-angiotensin system.

Assuming a normal hematocrit of 45 percent, renal plasma flow (RPF) is equal to 660 ml per minute (0.55 × 1200 = 660). Approximately one-fifth of the plasma or 125 ml per minute passes through the glomerulus into Bowman's capsule. This is called the *glomerular filtration rate* (GFR). Filtration at the glomerulus is termed *glomerular ultrafiltration,* because the primary filtrate has the same composition as plasma with the exception of the absence of proteins. Blood cells and large molecules such as proteins are effectively restrained by the filtration membrane "pores," while water and crystalloids (solutes of small molecular dimensions) are readily filtered. Calculation reveals that 173 liters of fluid is filtered through the glomerulus in one day—an astonishing amount in organs whose combined weight is

about 10 oz! As the filtrate travels through the tubules, various substances are added to or subtracted from it so that eventually only about 1.5 liters per day is excreted as urine.

The forces that account for this high glomerular filtration rate are entirely passive, since metabolic energy is not expended by the kidney for the process of filtration. The filtration force is a result of the pressure gradient between the glomerular capillary and Bowman's capsule. The hydrostatic pressure of the blood in the glomerular capillaries favors filtration, and this force is opposed by the hydrostatic pressure of the filtrate in Bowman's capsule and the colloid osmotic pressure (COP) of the blood. The COP in Bowman's capsule is essentially zero. Although never measured in human beings, the glomerular capillary pressure was estimated by R. F. Pitts (1974, p.41) to be about 50 mmHg and intracapsular pressure to be about 10 mmHg. These estimates are based on actual recent measurements in rats. Colloid osmotic pressure of the blood is about 30 mmHg. Net glomerular filtration pressure is thus about 10 mmHg. The glomerular filtration is influenced not ony by these physical forces, but by the permeability of the capillary walls. The balance of forces involved in glomerular ultrafiltration may be summarized as follows:

$$GFR = \begin{matrix} \text{filtration} \\ \text{permeability} \\ \text{factor} \end{matrix}$$

$$\times \left[\begin{matrix} \text{intracapillary} \\ \text{hydrostatic} \\ \text{pressure} \end{matrix} - \left(\begin{matrix} \text{intracapsular} \\ \text{hydrostatic} \\ \text{pressure} \end{matrix} + \begin{matrix} \text{colloid} \\ \text{osmotic} \\ \text{pressure} \end{matrix} \right) \right]$$

$$\text{Net filtration pressure} = 50 - (10 + 30)$$

$$= 10 \text{ mmHg}$$

The most accurate way to measure the GFR is to use a substance such as inulin which is freely filtered at the glomerulus and is neither secreted nor reabsorbed by the tubules. The clearance of a substance is the volume of plasma from which that substance is completely cleared by the kidneys per unit time. The rate of clearance of inulin is exactly equal to the GFR. This is measured by the administration of inulin at a constant IV drip rate to ensure a constant plasma concentration level. Measurement of inulin concentration in plasma (P_{in}) in milligrams per hundred milliliters (mg/100 ml), urine (U_{in}) in milligrams per hundred milliliters, and the volume of urine (V) in milliliters per minute (ml/min) permits calculation of inulin clearance (C_{in}) in milliliters

TABLE 40-1

MAJOR FUNCTIONS OF THE KIDNEY

Excretory functions	Nonexcretory functions
Maintains plasma osmolality near 285 mOsm by varying the excretion of water	Produces renin—important in the regulation of blood pressure
Maintains the plasma concentration of each individual electrolyte within normal range	Produces erythropoietin—important factor in stimulating red blood cell production by the bone marrow
Maintains the plasma pH near 7.4 by eliminating excess H$^+$ and regenerating HCO$_3^-$	Metabolizes vitamin D to its active form
	Degrades insulin
Excretes the nitrogenous end products of protein metabolism, chiefly urea, uric acid, and creatinine	Produces prostaglandin

per minute. The result must be corrected for body surface area, estimated by using a normogram which relates height and weight to body surface area. Example: if a person is passing urine at the rate of 4.2 ml/min, the inulin concentration in the urine specimen is 600 mg/100 ml, and the plasma inulin concentration is constant at 25 mg/100 ml, then

$$\text{GFR} = C_{in} = \frac{(U_{in})\ 600\ \text{mg}/100\ \text{ml} \times (V)\ 4.2\ \text{ml/min}}{(P_{in})\ 25\ \text{mg}/100\ \text{ml}}$$
$$= 100\ \text{ml/min}$$

The calculated GFR of 100 ml/min would then be normalized by correcting it to the standard normal body surface area of 1.73 m². This correction makes it possible to compare function in persons of varying physical stature. The GFR of normal young men averages 125 ± 15 ml/min per 1.73 m², and that of normal young women is 110 ± 15 ml/min per 1.73 m².

Tubular reabsorption and secretion

Three classes of substances are filtered at the glomerulus (Fig. 40-9): electrolytes, nonelectrolytes, and water. Some of the most important electrolytes are sodium (Na^+), potassium (K^+), calcium (Ca^{2+}), magnesium (Mg^{2+}), bicarbonate (HCO_3^-), chloride (Cl^-), and phosphate (HPO_4^{2-}). Important nonelectrolytes are glucose,

FIGURE 40-9

Tubular reabsorption and secretion along the glomerular nephron. Solid arrows indicate active transport, and broken arrows indicate passive transport.

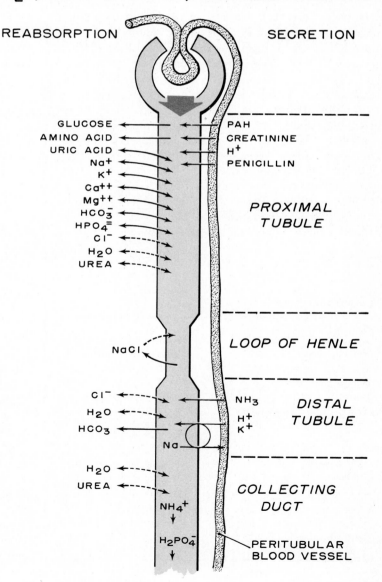

amino acids, and the metabolic end products of protein metabolism: urea, uric acid, and creatinine.

The second step in urine formation after filtration is the selective reabsorption of filtered substances. Most of the substances filtered are reabsorbed through minute "pores" in the tubule, where they pass back into the peritubular capillaries which surround the tubule. In addition, some substances are secreted from the surrounding peritubular blood vessels into the tubule.

Reabsorption and secretion take place by both active and passive transport mechanisms. A mechanism is active if it transports a substance against an electrochemical gradient; i.e., against a gradient of electrical potential, chemical potential, or both. Work is performed directly on the substance reabsorbed or secreted by the tubular cells, and energy is expended in the process. A transport mechanism is passive if the substance being reabsorbed or secreted moves down an electrochemical gradient. No energy is directly expended in moving the substance.

Along the proximal tubule glucose and amino acids are completely reabsorbed by active transport. Almost all the potassium and uric acid is actively reabsorbed, and both are secreted into the distal tubule. At least two-thirds of the filtered sodium is actively reabsorbed in the proximal tubule. Reabsorption of sodium continues in the loop of Henle, distal tubule, and collecting ducts, so that less than 1 percent of the filtered load is excreted in the urine. Most of the calcium and phosphate is reabsorbed in the proximal tubule by active transport. Water, chloride, and urea are reabsorbed in the proximal tubule by passive transport. As large numbers of positively charged sodium ions leave the tubular lumen, negatively charged chloride ions must follow for reasons of electrical neutrality. The exit of a large number of ions and nonelectrolytes from the proximal tubular fluid leaves it osmotically dilute, and as a result, water diffuses out of the tubule into the peritubular blood. Urea then diffuses passively down a concentration gradient established by the reabsorption of water. Hydrogen ion (H^+), organic acids such as para-aminohippurate (PAH) and penicillin, and creatinine (an organic base) are all actively secreted in the proximal tubule. About 90 percent of the bicarbonate is reabsorbed in the proximal tubule indirectly by Na^+–H^+ exchange. When H^+ is secreted into the tubular lumen (in exchange for Na^+), it combines with the HCO_3^- present in the glomerular filtrate to give carbonic acid (H_2CO_3). The H_2CO_3 dissociates to water and carbon dioxide (CO_2). Both CO_2 and H_2O diffuse out of the tubular lumen into the tubular cell. In the tubular cell, carbonic anhydrase catalyzes the reaction of CO_2 and H_2O to form H_2CO_3 once again. The dissociation of H_2CO_3 produces HCO_3^- and H^+. The H^+ is resecreted, and the HCO_3^- passes into the peritubular blood along with Na^+.

In the loop of Henle, Cl^- is actively transported out of the ascending limb, followed passively by Na^+. NaCl then diffuses passively into the descending limb. This process is important for urine concentration and is discussed later in this chapter.

The selective process of secretion and reabsorption is completed in the distal tubule and collecting ducts. Two important functions of the distal tubule are the final regulation of water balance and acid-base balance. If the cells are to function normally, the pH of the extracellular fluid must be maintained within the narrow range of 7.35 to 7.45. Several biological mechanisms working in coordination contribute toward maintaining the pH within normal limits. The principal blood buffer is the bicarbonate-carbonic acid system given by the equation:

$$CO_2 + H_2O \overset{\substack{\text{carbonic} \\ \text{anhydrase}}}{\rightleftharpoons} H_2CO_3 \rightleftharpoons H^+ + HCO_3^-$$

The blood pH is given by the Henderson-Hasselbalch equation:

$$pH = pK + \log \frac{HCO_3^- \text{ (kidneys)}}{H_2CO_3 \text{ (lungs)}}$$

where pK is the dissociation constant of carbonic acid. The lungs eliminate CO_2, which is produced when H^+ is buffered by HCO_3^- (left shift of the reaction above), and thus play an important role in stabilizing the pH. The role of the kidneys in maintaining acid-base balance is the reabsorption of most of the filtered HCO_3^-. When considering disturbances in acid-base balance, it is often helpful to keep in mind that the serum pH is largely a function of the HCO_3^-/H_2CO_3 ratio and that the numerator is largely regulated by renal mechanisms, while pulmonary mechanisms regulate the denominator (through control of CO_2 elimination). A change in the numerator or denominator is followed by a unidirectional change in the other. This change, known as *compensation*, serves to protect the pH.

In addition to reabsorbing and conserving most of the HCO_3^-, the kidneys also eliminate excess H^+. About 60 meq of acids other than H_2CO_3 are produced in the body each day. Since these acids cannot be eliminated by the lungs, they are called *fixed acids*. These acids are eliminated in the tubular fluid, so that it is possible for the urine to achieve a pH as low as 4.5 (a hydrogen ion gradient that is 800 times that in the plasma). All along the tubule, H^+ is secreted into the tubular fluid. The H^+ may then be excreted by combination with filtered dibasic phosphate (HPO_4^{2-}) or with ammonia (NH_3). Thus H^+ is excreted as the titratable monobasic acid salt (NaH_2PO_4) or as ammonium ion (NH_4^+). NH_3 diffuses readily into the tubular lumen, but after combination with H^+ to form the charged particle NH_4^+, it is unable to diffuse back into the tubular cell. Because the minimum urine pH that can be achieved is 4.5, the amount of free H^+ that can be excreted is limited. Therefore the ammonium mechanism (and the phosphate mechanism) is important in eliminating an acid load, since NH_4^+ does not affect the urine pH. The buffering of H^+ by NH_3 or HPO_4^{2-} also has the effect of adding a *new* HCO_3^- to the plasma for every H^+ excreted into the urine. The H^+ that is secreted is derived from H_2CO_3 in the tubular cell leaving HCO_3^- behind in equimolar amounts. In contrast, when HCO_3^- is reabsorbed from the tubular fluid by the mechanism previously described, HCO_3^- is merely conserved, since one H^+ is returned to the plasma for each one that is secreted into the tubular fluid. Therefore the regeneration of HCO_3^- (i.e., the de novo synthesis) by the buffering mechanism is very important in preventing acidosis.

Both uric acid and potassium are secreted into the distal tubule, as already mentioned. Normally about 5 percent of the filtered potassium load is excreted in the urine. Water reabsorption is also completed in the distal tubule and collecting ducts.

Several hormones regulate the tubular reabsorption and secretion of solutes and water. Water reabsorption depends on the presence of antidiuretic hormone (ADH). Aldosterone influences Na^+ reabsorption and K^+ secretion. Increased aldosterone causes increased Na^+ reabsorption and increased K^+ secretion. A decrease in aldosterone has the opposite effect. Parathyroid hormone (PTH) regulates Ca^{2+} and HPO_4^{2-} reabsorption along the tubule. Increased PTH results in increased reabsorption of Ca^{2+} and increased HPO_4^{2-} excretion. A decrease in PTH has the opposite effect.

Figure 40-9 summarizes the major function of each part of the nephron. It is by means of this selective reabsorption and secretion along the tubule that the kidney is able to regulate the internal body environment in a very precise manner. The following discussion examines in greater detail the role of the kidney in water metabolism.

Regulation of water balance

The total solute concentration of body fluids is remarkably constant in the normal person despite wide fluctuation in water and solute intake and excretion. It is through the production of urine much more concentrated or dilute than the plasma from which it is derived that the concentration of the plasma and body fluids is maintained within narrow limits. When a large volume of fluids is ingested, causing dilution of body fluids, the urine becomes dilute and the excess water is rapidly excreted. Conversely, when water deprivation or excess solute intake causes the body fluids to become concentrated, the urine becomes highly concentrated so that solute is lost in excess of water. The water retained tends to return the body fluids to a normal solute concentration.

Before the processes involved in the regulation of body fluid balance can be understood, it is necessary to understand the concept of *osmolality*, a term used to express the concentration of body fluids.

Osmotic concentration

Osmotic concentration (osmolality) refers to the number of particles dissolved in a solution. When a solute is added to water, the effective concentration (activity) of water is lowered relative to that of pure water. Osmotic activity is influenced only by the relative number of solute and solvent particles and is ideally independent of the nature of the solute. Solute particles differing in mass, shape, and charge have the same effect on the osmotic activity of the solvent provided they are equal in number. Thus six sodium and chloride ions which are completely dissociated have the same effect on the osmotic activity as six glucose molecules in 1 kg of water even though they are quite different in mass, shape, and charge (Fig. 40-10).

Colligative properties of solutions

The addition of solute particles to a solvent is manifested as lowering of vapor pressure and freezing point and raising of the boiling point and osmotic pressure of the solvent. These phenomena are referred to as the *colligative properties* of solutions. All these properties depend on osmotic concentration.

Figure 40-11 illustrates the four colligative properties of solutions. The first two colligative properties are vapor pressure lowering and boiling point elevation. When particles are added to water, it is more difficult for the water to escape from the surface, since the effective concentration of water is decreased. Consequently, pure water boils at 100°C, while a solution of glucose and water has a boiling point higher than 100°C.

When solute particles are added to water, the osmotic pressure is increased, which is a third colligative property of a solution. In the diagram in Fig. 40-11, note that there are two glucose molecules in the left compartment and six in the right compartment separated by a semipermeable membrane. The pores in the membrane are too small to allow glucose to diffuse readily. Water, a smaller molecule, diffuses easily from the area of low osmotic concentration in the left-hand compartment to the area of higher osmotic concentration in the right-hand compartment. This process is called *osmosis*. Actually, water is moving from an area of higher water

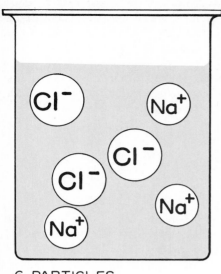

6 PARTICLES
NaCl/KgH₂O

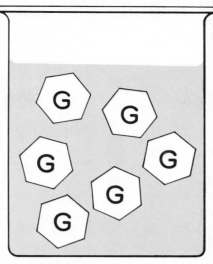

6 PARTICLES
GLUCOSE/KgH₂O

FIGURE 40-10
Osmotic concentration equals the number of particles per kilogram of water. It does not depend on the mass, shape, or charge of the particles in an ideal solution.

concentration (in the left compartment) to an area of lower water concentration (in the right compartment). Osmosis is thus only a special case of diffusion.

The diffusion of water from the left to the right compartment continues until osmotic equilibrium is achieved, with the result that the fluid level is elevated in the right compartment. The force driving the water through the semipermeable membrane is called *osmotic pressure*. To prevent the water from diffusing into the right-hand compartment, it would be necessary to apply

FIGURE 40-11
Colligative properties of solutions.

1. VAPOR PRESSURE LOWERING
2. BOILING POINT ELEVATION
BOILS AT: 100°C   > 100°C

H₂O → G
G
G   G   G
G
G   G

PURE H₂O

GLUCOSE + H₂O

SEMIPERMEABLE MEMBRANE

3. OSMOTIC PRESSURE INCREASE

4. FREEZING POINT DEPRESSION
FREEZES AT: 0°C   < 0°C

PURE H₂O

GLUCOSE + H₂O

physical pressure over the solution in the right-hand compartment which would be equal to the higher potential of water in the left compartment. It is common usage to speak of the osmotic pressure of a solution, though it is virtually never measured. Several other properties of solutions vary in exact proportion to the osmotic pressure and are more easily measured (e.g., depression of the freezing point and vapor pressure lowering). In fact, even the use of the term "osmotic pressure" is rather loose, since it is commonly expressed in terms of concentration rather than pressure (see below).

The principle of osmosis is basic to the movement of water between compartments in the body. This principle is also applied in dialysis by putting high concentrations of glucose in the dialysis bath to facilitate removal of excess fluid from the body which has accumulated while the kidneys were not functioning adequately.

The fourth colligative property of a solution is the freezing point depression. Particles added to water cause the solution to have a lower freezing point than that of pure water, which freezes at 0°C.

Measurement of osmotic concentration

There are two common methods of measuring the osmotic concentration of body fluids. The freezing point depression as measured by the osmometer is a true measure of osmotic concentration, but the measuring procedure is complex and must be carried out in a laboratory.* It is based on the principle that the freezing point of a solution consisting of one gram-molecular weight (mole or mol) of any nondissociated substance dissolved in 1 kg of water will be −1.86°C.† Such a solution is called an *osmolal* solution, and it contains 1 osmol of solute particles (i.e., the number of particles needed to lower the freezing point of water by 1.86°C). The change in temperature is called the *molal freezing point constant* (K_f) and is equal to 1 osmol.

In the absence of dissociation, each molecule of solute behaves as a single particle. Therefore, since molecular size has no effect on colligative properties, 1 gram-mole of albumin (mol wt 70,000) affects the freezing point of water to the same degree as 1 gram-mole of

---

*More recently a device to measure osmotic concentration on the basis of vapor pressure lowering has been used in some laboratories. This method is more rapid and less complicated than the osmometer method.

†One mole of any element or molecular compound contains the same number of particles (Avogadro's number: 6.02×10^{23} molecules/mol) as any other.

glucose (mol wt 180). If dissociation occurs, as with sodium chloride, for example, and two ions are formed, each molecule has the effect of two particles. In this case, then, 1 osmol is one-half the molecular weight.

In order to calculate the osmotic concentration (osmolality) of a solution, it is necessary only to measure the lowering of the freezing point below that of pure water (ΔT). This number is then divided by K_f, the molal freezing point constant:

$$\text{Osmolality} = \frac{\Delta T}{K_f}$$

For example, blood plasma freezes at −0.53°C. When this number is divided by −1.86 (K_f), the calculated concentration is 285 mOsm (1 milliosmol = 0.001 osmol):

$$\text{Plasma concentration} = \frac{-0.53°\text{C}}{-1.86°\text{C})} \times 1000$$
$$= 285 \text{ mOsm}$$

In the healthy person, plasma concentration is 285 ± 10 mOsm/kg H_2O.

The second method of estimating concentration of body fluids is to measure the specific gravity with the urinometer (see photographs of the urinometer and osmometer in Fig. 40-12). Specific gravity is not a true measure of concentration, but because of its simplicity, it is commonly used in the clinical unit. What is actually being measured is the density (which depends on the *weight* of the solute particles) and not the concentration (which depends on the *number* of solute particles). However, estimating the concentration of urine by measuring specific gravity is fairly accurate provided the urine has normal constituents. The correlation between the osmolal and specific gravity measurements are discussed in Chap. 41.

Osmolality vs. osmolarity

In the literature and in practice the term *osmolarity* is frequently used in place of or interchangeably with the term *osmolality* when speaking of the concentrations of intravenous solutions or body fluids. This interchange often causes confusion. *Osmolality* is an expression of concentration *in terms of 1000 g of water*. Accordingly, neither temperature nor space taken up by the solids present in the solution has any bearing on the osmolality figure, and a direct comparison can be made of various body fluids with different water or solids content. On the other hand, such a comparison is not possible when concentration is expressed *in terms of 1 liter of solution* (i.e., *osmolarity*). The amount of water in 1 liter of solution is a function both of its temperature and the space occupied by the solids in solution. Inasmuch as colligative properties are determined only by the

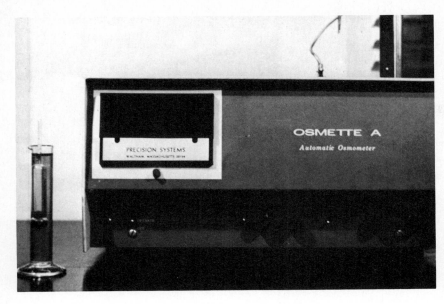

FIGURE 40-12
Osmometer and urinometer. The osmometer measures the freezing point depression of a solution which is used to calculate osmolality. The urinometer (left) does not actually measure osmotic concentration but the density of a solution.

ratio of solute to solvent particles, the osmolarity of various body fluids is not directly comparable. The difference between osmolality and osmolarity is apparent in the diagram in Fig. 40-13. To make up a 1-osmol solution, 1 gram-mole of solute particles is added to a beaker with exactly 1000 g of water. The volume of the solution is thus greater than 1 liter. The one-osmolar solution is made by first adding 1 gram-mole of solute particles to the beaker and then sufficient water to reach the 1-liter mark. Thus the volume of the solute is included in the solution. It is obvious that the concentrations of the two solutions are not equal. The difference between osmolality and osmolarity is negligible in the

range of concentration and temperature of body fluids. It is, however, important to use osmolal units of concentration in the accurate preparation of intravenous solutions.

It is the function of the kidneys to keep the concentration of the body fluids constant at 285 mOsm. How this is accomplished is explored in the following sections.

Isoosmotic reabsorption in the proximal tubule

When the glomerular filtrate first enters the proximal tubule, it has the same concentration as the plasma,

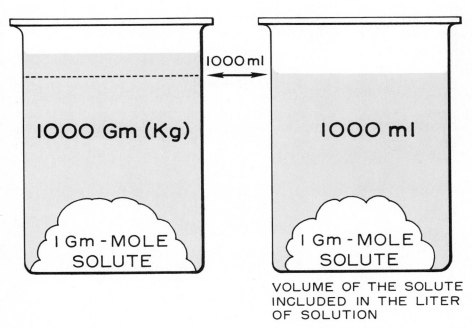

VOLUME OF THE SOLUTE INCLUDED IN THE LITER OF SOLUTION

FIGURE 40-13
Osmolality vs. osmolarity. *Osmolality* is an expression of concentration in terms of 1000 g of water. *Osmolarity* is concentration expressed in terms of 100 ml of solution. Osmolality is approximately equal to osmolarity for dilute solutions when the volume occupied by the solute is very small.

285 mOsm. It is therefore called *isoosmotic*. Along the proximal tubule as much as 80 percent of the filtrate is reabsorbed into the peritubular capillaries.* This reabsorption is isoosmotic, since both water and solutes are reabsorbed in the same proportion as they exist in the filtrate. So at the end of the proximal tubule the concentration of the filtrate is still 285 mOsm, and about 20 percent of the filtrate still remains (Fig. 40-14). Even though the flow has been significantly reduced (from 125 to about 25 ml/min), urine excretion directly out of the proximal tubule would be about 1500 ml/ hour. At this rate of urine excretion, death would occur within a few hours from dehydration, since a loss of 12 to 14 percent of the body weight in water is fatal. The next step in the process of urine formation is to greatly reduce the volume of the filtrate before it is expelled as urine.

Countercurrent mechanism

In the kidney there are two types of nephrons—the cortical and the juxtamedullary (next to the medulla), illustrated in Fig. 40-15. The juxtamedullary nephron has a much longer loop of Henle than the cortical nephron, and its peritubular blood supply is in the form of hairpin loops of vessels which dip down beside the loop of Henle. These blood vessels are called the *vasa recta*. These anatomic features of the juxtamedullary nephrons largely account for the concentration of urine. In fact, the longer the hairpin loop the greater the concentrating ability of an animal. The kangaroo rat, a desert rodent, has unusually long loops and can excrete urine with an osmolality of about 6000 mOsm. In the human, about one out of seven nephrons is juxtamedullary, with long loops, and the maximum concentration of urine is about 1400 mOsm.

*Reported values of filtrate reabsorption in the proximal tubule vary from 66.6 to 87.5 percent, depending on the source (Pitts, 1974, p. 109).

The countercurrent mechanism, which is responsible for the conservation of water by the kidney, actually involves two basic processes: (1) the countercurrent multiplier of concentration in the loop of Henle and (2) the countercurrent exchanger in the vasa recta, which also takes the form of a hairpin loop. The main function of the loop of Henle is to make the interstitial fluid in the medulla hyperosmotic and the tubular fluid which emerges from it into the distal tubule hypoosmotic; these changes permit the concentration of the final urine to be modified over a wide range. The main function of the vasa recta is to prevent the dissipation of the osmotic gradient in the medullary interstitial fluid which has been built up by the loop of Henle. Along the nephron, the fundamental processes involved in the production of a concentrated or dilute urine are the active reabsorption of chloride in the ascending limb of Henle and the variable permeability to the passive diffusion of water and urea along their concentration gradients.

First, let us examine the overall relationships during the production of a concentrated urine (Fig. 40-16). Beginning at the glomerulus, where filtration starts, the filtrate is isoosmotic with the plasma at 285 mOsm. By the end of the proximal tubule, 80 percent of the filtrate has been reabsorbed, although the concentration is still 285 mOsm. As the filtrate moves down the descending limb of Henle, its concentration reaches a maximum at the tip of the loop. Then, as it moves up the ascending limb, the filtrate becomes more and more dilute until it is hypoosmotic at the top of the limb. As it proceeds along the distal tubule it becomes more concentrated, until it is isoosmotic with the blood plasma at the top of the collecting duct. As it moves down the collecting duct, it again becomes increasingly concentrated. At the end of the collecting duct about 99 percent of the water has been reabsorbed and about 1 percent of the filtrate is excreted as urine.

Note on the diagram that there is also a concentration gradient in the interstitial fluid, increasing from the cortex to the medulla. The vasa recta which dip down beside the loop of Henle also have a concentration gradient which increases going down the descending limb and decreases moving up the ascending limb, though the decrease is much less than in the ascending limb of

FIGURE 40-14
Eighty percent isoosmotic reabsorption of the glomerular filtrate in the proximal tubule.

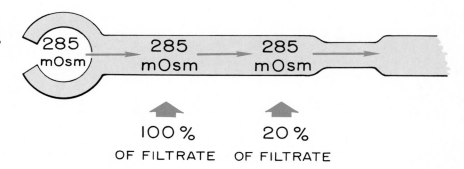

285 mOsm   285 mOsm   285 mOsm

100% OF FILTRATE   20% OF FILTRATE

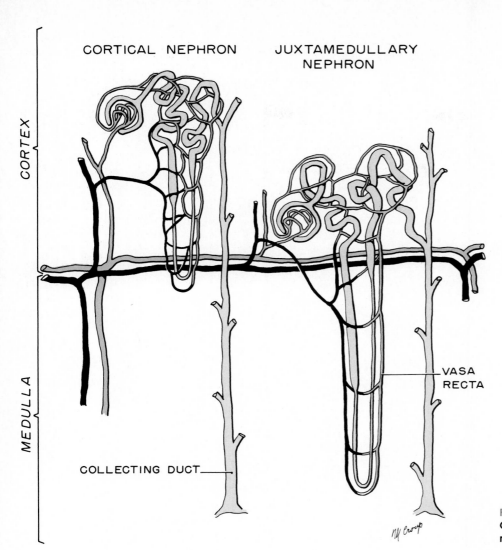

CORTICAL NEPHRON   JUXTAMEDULLARY
                        NEPHRON

CORTEX

MEDULLA

VASA
RECTA

COLLECTING DUCT

FIGURE 40-15
**Cortical and juxtaglomerular
nephrons with vasa recta.**

Henle. Note also that the limbs of the loop of Henle form parallel columns and that the filtrate flow is in opposite directions. This is known as *countercurrent flow* and allows the loop of Henle to function as a countercurrent multiplier building up the concentration gradient in the interstitium. (The principle of countercurrent multiplication is reviewed in Fig. 40-17.) The entire process may now be described in greater detail.

The operation of the countercurrent multiplier in the loop of Henle is initiated by the active transport of chloride out of the ascending limb. This causes sodium to passively follow down the potential gradient created by the active chloride transport. Water, however, cannot passively follow the sodium chloride transport, since the ascending limb is impermeable to water (indicated by the heavy lines in Fig. 40-16). Consequently, the filtrate becomes hypoosmotic as the top of the ascending limb is approached. The interstitial fluid becomes more concentrated, setting up an osmotic gradient between the interstitial fluid and the descending limb of Henle. Water flows out of the descending limb and sodium

chloride passively enters, causing the filtrate to become increasingly concentrated. As this process continues, a concentration gradient increasing from cortex to medulla is established in both the descending limb of Henle and the interstitium until a steady state is reached.

The vasa recta, which dip down beside the loop of Henle, act as a countercurrent exchanger by passive diffusion (active transport is not involved). The blood in the vasa recta is in osmotic equilibrium with the interstitial fluid. As blood flows through the descending limb of the vasa recta, sodium chloride passively moves in and water moves out, causing the blood to become increasingly concentrated as it approaches the tip of the loop. In the ascending limb of the vasa recta, opposite events occur. Sodium passively diffuses out into the interstitium while water is reabsorbed into the blood vessel and returned to the general circulation. The fact that the blood flow through the vasa recta is sluggish allows it to act as an efficient exchanger (recall that the medulla receives only 10 percent of the blood supply to the kid-

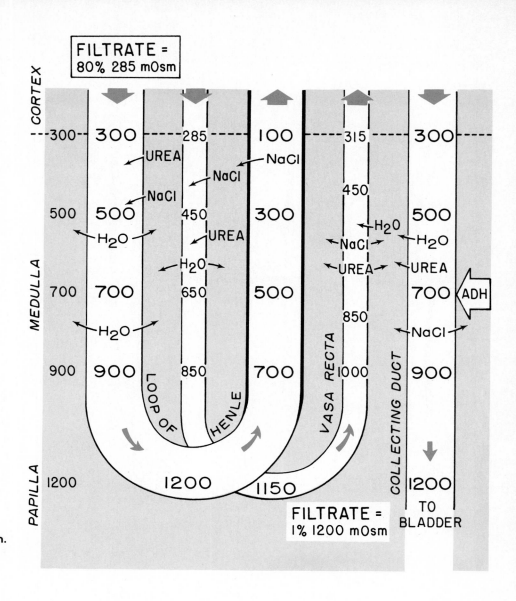

FILTRATE =
80% 285 mOsm

CORTEX

MEDULLA

PAPILLA

LOOP OF HENLE

VASA RECTA

COLLECTING DUCT

ADH

FILTRATE =
1% 1200 mOsm

TO
BLADDER

FIGURE 40-16
The countercurrent mechansim.
See text for explanation.
(Modified from Netter, 1973.)

ney). If the blood flow were very rapid, the sodium chloride which entered the descending limb would be washed away. Thus the vasa recta, acting as a countercurrent exchanger, prevent the dissipation of the concentration gradient in the interstitium built up by the loop of Henle acting as a countercurrent multiplier of concentration.

Along the distal tubule, sodium (chloride) is actively reabsorbed. Under conditions of antidiuresis, the hypoosmotic filtrate at the beginning of the distal tubule becomes isoosmotic by the time it reaches the top of the collecting duct. The final concentration of urine takes place in the distal tubule and collecting ducts under the control of antidiuretic hormone (ADH). The distal tubule and collecting ducts are permeable to water in the presence of ADH. Water diffuses out into the interstitium in response to the osmotic gradient in the medulla, then enters the ascending limb of the vasa recta and is returned to the general circulation. The

final urine produced is low in volume and high in osmotic concentration.

In contrast, under conditions of diuresis and in the absence of ADH, the distal tubule and collecting ducts are virtually impermeable to water. Sodium (chloride) is actively reabsorbed from the distal tubule and collecting ducts, but water does not diffuse out to maintain osmotic equilibrium. Since sodium is reabsorbed and water is left behind, a large volume of dilute urine is produced.

Urea also diffuses out of the collecting ducts into the interstitial fluid, where it contributes to the high osmotic concentration in the medulla. Some of the urea also enters the descending limb of the loop of Henle and the vasa recta and is recirculated. The effect is to trap urea in the medullary interstitium. A person on a low protein diet is unable to concentrate urine as well as a person on a normal or high protein diet, since urea is the end product of protein metabolism.

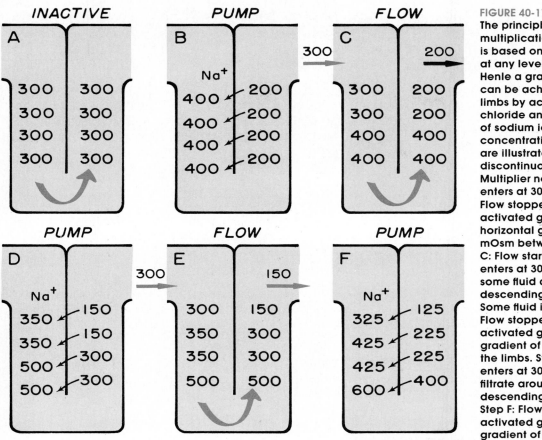

FIGURE 40-17

The principle of countercurrent multiplication of concentration is based on the assumption that at any level along the loop of Henle a gradient of 200 mOsm can be achieved between the limbs by active transport of chloride and passive diffusion of sodium ions. The changes in concentration along the loop are illustrated in a series of discontinuous steps. Step A: Multiplier not active, filtrate enters at 300 mOsm. Step B: Flow stopped, ion pump activated generating a horizontal gradient of 200 mOsm between the limbs. Step C: Flow started, more filtrate enters at 300 mOsm pushing some fluid around the tip from descending to ascending limb. Some fluid is ejected. Step D: Flow stopped, ion pump activated generating another gradient of 200 mOsm between the limbs. Step E: More filtrate enters at 300 mOsm pushing filtrate around the tip from descending to ascending limb. Step F: Flow stopped, ion pump activated generating another gradient of 200 mOsm between the limbs. Note that the concentration of the filtrate at the tip of the loop is now 600 mOsm, and there is a longitudinal gradient of 275 mOsm whereas the ion pump was only able to generate a horizontal gradient of 200 mOsm. Continuation of this process further increases the longitudinal gradient. (Modified from R. F. Pitts, *Physiology of the Kidney and Body Fluids,* 3d ed., Year Book Medical Publishers Inc., Chicago, 1974.)

ADH mechanism for the regulation of plasma osmolality

The ADH mechanism is important in maintaining the volume and osmolality of the extracellular fluid (ECF) at a constant level by controlling the final volume and osmolality of the urine.

Changes in plasma volume or osmolality from the ideal constant of 285 mOsm control the release of ADH. Variations of only 1 to 2 percent from the ideal initiate mechanisms to return the plasma osmolality to normal. ADH is produced in the supraoptic nuclei of the hypothalamus and descends along nerve fibers to the posterior pituitary, where it is stored for subsequent release. ADH release is controlled by a feedback mechanism with two pathways (Fig. 40-18).

ADH release is increased by an increase in the plasma osmolality or a decrease in the plasma volume. Osmo-receptor cells located in the hypothalamus near the supraoptic nuclei are sensitive to the concentration of the circulating blood, and pressure-sensing cells in the left atria are sensitive to blood volume. These sensors stimulate the release of ADH. Increased osmolality and/or decreased volume of the ECF, for example, may be caused by factors such as water deprivation, fluid loss from vomiting, diarrhea, hemorrhage, burns, sweating, or displacement of fluid as in ascites.

The subjective feeling of thirst which drives one to ingest water is also stimulated by a decrease in volume and/or an increase in ECF osmolality, the adaptive significance of both being self-evident in the illustration. The centers which mediate thirst are also located in the hypothalamus, close to those areas which produce ADH. Increased thirst in the person who has suddenly lost 800 ml of blood from hemorrhage (decrease in ECF) or in the person who has just eaten a candy bar (increase in the osmolality of ECF due to more glucose particles in the blood) is explained by this mechanism.

In the kidney, ADH indirectly augments the key events which occur in the loop of Henle by two interrelated mechanisms: (1) blood flow through the vasa recta of the medulla is diminished in the presence of ADH, thus minimizing solute depletion of the interstitium, which in turn becomes more hyperosmotic, and (2) ADH increases the permeability of the collecting ducts and distal tubules, so that more water diffuses out to equilibrate with the hyperosmotic interstitial fluid.

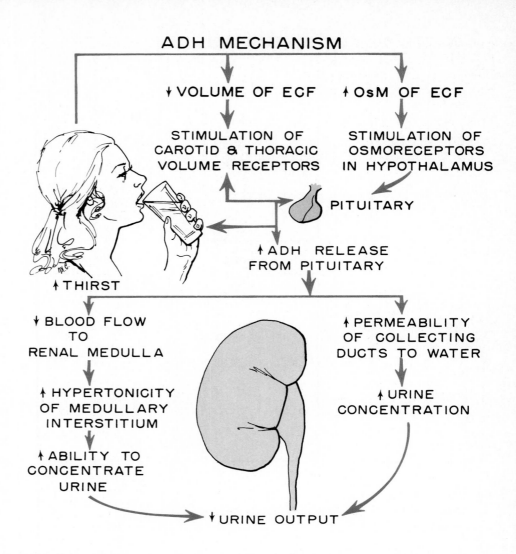

ADH MECHANISM

↓ VOLUME OF ECF   ↑ OsM OF ECF

STIMULATION OF
CAROTID & THORACIC
VOLUME RECEPTORS

STIMULATION OF
OSMORECEPTORS
IN HYPOTHALAMUS

PITUITARY

↑ ADH RELEASE
FROM PITUITARY

↑ THIRST

↓ BLOOD FLOW
TO
RENAL MEDULLA

↑ PERMEABILITY
OF COLLECTING
DUCTS TO WATER

↑ HYPERTONICITY
OF MEDULLARY
INTERSTITIUM

↑ URINE
CONCENTRATION

↑ ABILITY TO
CONCENTRATE
URINE

↓ URINE OUTPUT

FIGURE 40-18
ADH mechanism for the regulation of plasma osmolality.

Both mechanisms operate to produce a concentrated urine and thus reduce the volume of excretion.

Conversely, low plasma osmolality and/or volume expansion from increased water intake inhibits ADH release. The final volume of urine excreted is increased and is more osmotically dilute.

Even in extreme cases of a huge volume of fluid ingestion or of very limited fluid intake, normal human beings have amazing flexibility in maintaining the osmolality of the ECF at a constant 285 mOsm. To accomplish this we are able to excrete urine as dilute as 40 mOsm or as concentrated as 1200 to 1400 mOsm. As will be shown later, the patient with renal insufficiency loses this great flexibility.

Functions of the kidney

The major functions of the kidneys are summarized in Table 40-1, which emphasizes their regulatory role in the body. Vander summarized the function of the kidneys when he said, "This regulatory role is obviously quite different from the popular conception of the kid-

neys as glorified garbage-disposal units which rid the body of assorted wastes and poisons" (Vander, 1975, p. 4). The kidneys do excrete certain foreign chemicals (drugs, etc.), hormones, and other metabolites, but their most important function is maintaining the volume and composition of the ECF within normal limits. This is accomplished, of course, by varying the excretion of water and solutes, and the high filtration rate allows great precision in this function. Renin and erythropoietin production and vitamin D metabolism are all important nonexcretory functions. Excessive renin secretion, which may be important in the etiology of some forms of hypertension, is discussed in Chap. 42. Deficiency of erythropoietin and vitamin D activation, believed to be important in the etiology of anemia and bone disease in uremia, is discussed in Chap. 43.

The kidneys are also importantly concerned with degradation of insulin and production of a group of compounds of possible endocrine significance, the prostaglandins. About 20 percent of the insulin produced by the pancreas is degraded by the renal tubular cells. Consequently, diabetic patients with renal failure may re-

612

quire less insulin. Prostaglandins (PG) are unsaturated fatty acid hormones present in many tissues of the body. The renal medulla produces PGA_2 and PGE_2, which are potent vasodilators. Prostaglandins may play a role in the regulation of renal blood flow, renin release, and Na^+ reabsorption. It is also possible that prostaglandin defiency may contribute to some forms of secondary renal hypertension, although there is insufficient evidence for this at present.

QUESTIONS

Normal renal function

Directions: Label Figs. 40-19 to 40-22 with the appropriate terms from each group.

1. Fig. 40-19: The urinary tract.

Urinary meatus	Ureter
Bladder	Right kidney
Urethra	Left kidney

2. Fig. 40-20: Posterior abdominal wall, vertebrae, and ribs.

Eleventh rib	Psoas major muscle
Twelfth rib	Transversus abdominus muscle

3. Fig. 40-21: Cross section of the kidney.

Pyramid	Minor calyces
Ureter	Major calyx
Renal pelvis	Fibrous capsule
Papilla	Medulla
Cortex	Column of Bertin

4. Fig. 40-22: The nephron.

Proximal convoluted tubule	Bowman's capsule
Distal convoluted tubule	Macula densa
	Juxtaglomerular cells
	Afferent arteriole
Collecting duct	Efferent arteriole
Loop of Henle	Glomerular capillary tuft

5. Draw the kidneys on the diagram in Fig. 40-20 in their correct relation to the ribs and vertebrae.

FIGURE 40-19
The urinary tract.

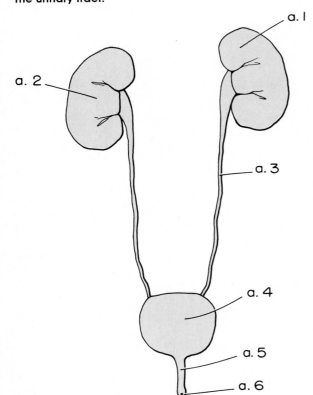

FIGURE 40-20
Posterior abdominal wall, vertebrae, ribs.

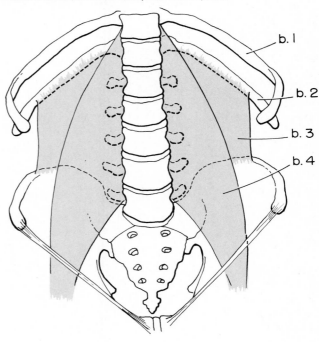

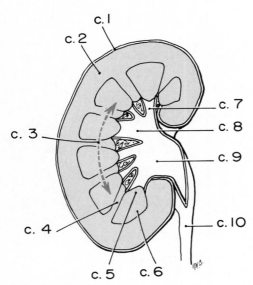

FIGURE 40-21
Cross section of the kidney.

FIGURE 40-22
The nephron.

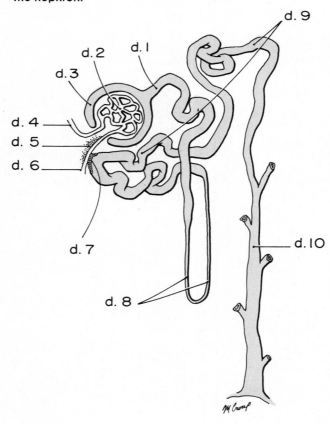

6. Trace the formation and transit of urine from the renal cortex to the bladder by lettering the following structures in sequence.

Ureter
Renal pelvis
Collecting ducts
Bowman's capsule
Proximal convoluted tubule

Bladder
Minor calyces
Distal convoluted tubule
Major calyces
Papillary ducts of Bellini

7. This list contains the names of blood vessels supplying and draining the kidneys. Letter it in the correct sequence beginning with the blood vessel supplying the kidney.

Renal vein
Afferent arterioles
Abdominal aorta
Arcuate arteries
Inferior vena cava
Interlobar veins
Glomerular capillaries
Efferent arterioles

Interlobular arterioles
Interlobar arteries
Arcuate veins
Renal artery
Peritubular capillaries (portal network)
Interlobular veins

Directions: Answer the following questions on a separate sheet of paper.

8. Why is it especially important to obtain a renal arteriogram in a healthy person who is supplying a donor kidney for transplantation?

9. Explain how the juxtaglomerular cells and macula densa cells help to control blood pressure.

10. Why is a heavy blow over the twelfth rib particularly dangerous to the kidney?

Directions: Match the type of renal corpuscular cell in col. A with its proper description in col. B by placing the correct letter in the blank.

Column A

11. ____ Parietal epithelium
12. ____ Visceral epithelium
13. ____ Podocytes
14. ____ Endothelial cells
15. ____ Basement membrane
16. ____ Mesangial cells

Column B

a. Network between capillary loops of the glomerulus

b. Extensions of visceral cells in contact with basement membrane

c. Layer that separates epithelial from endothelial cells

d. Flat cells, outermost part of capsule

e. Innermost layer of capillary tuft containing fenestrations

f. Large cells which line the outside of the capillary tuft

Directions: *Circle the letter preceding each item below that correctly completes the statement. Only one answer is correct.*

615

QUESTIONS

17. The glomerular filtration membrane is composed of all the following cell layers *except:*
    a. Endothelial cells   b. Basement membrane
    c. Visceral epithelium   d. Mesangial cells

18. The structure(s) of the glomerular filtration membrane that is (are) least effective in preventing entry of protein molecules into the filtrate is (are):
    a. Fenestrations in the endothelial cell layer
    b. Slit pores between visceral epithelial cells
    c. Basement membrane   d. Long pores in the mesangial cells

19. Pole-to-pole length of the normal-size kidney is:
    a. 6 to 7 cm   b. 9 to 10 cm   c. 12 to 13 cm
    d. 16 to 19 cm

20. The normal-size kidney that is not generally palpable during physical examination is the:
    a. Right   b. Left

21. The minimal number of nephrons needed to sustain life is about:
    a. 2 million   b. 1 million   c. 200,000
    d. 20,000

22. The substance which *directly* causes peripheral vasoconstriction and increased aldosterone secretion is:
    a. Angiotensinogen   b. Renin
    c. Angiotensin II   d. Angiotensin I

23. The proportion of the cardiac output normally delivered to the kidneys is:
    a. 90 percent   b. 50 percent   c. 25 percent
    d. 10 percent

24. The cortex/medulla ratio of blood distribution in the kidney is normally about:
    a. 9:1   b. 1:9   c. 1:1   d. 1:3

25. The adaptive value of autoregulation of blood flow by the kidney is:
    a. Increase of total renal blood flow in response to hypotensive shock   b. Decrease of cortical blood flow in response to hypotensive shock   c. Increase in sodium and water retention in severe cases of hypertension   d. Increase in medullary blood flow in cases of dehydration shock   e. Prevention of changes in solute and water excretion in response to fluctuations in arterial pressure

Directions: *Answer the following questions on a separate sheet of paper.*

26. Why is glomerular filtration called *ultrafiltration?*

27. How is net filtration pressure derived?

28. Define and give the normal numerical value of the GFR for men and women.

29. What kind of substance must be used to measure the GFR, and why?

30. During an inulin clearance test the following values were obtained from a patient: concentration of inulin in plasma 25 mg/100 ml and in urine 500 mg/100 ml; urine volume 2 ml/min. Calculate this patient's GFR ignoring body surface area. Is it within normal range?

31. What are the two most important functions of the distal tubule and collecting ducts?

32. Explain how the kidneys and lungs work together in the regulation of acid-base balance in the body.

33. How do phosphate excretion and ammonia secretion contribute to the excretion of acid by the kidney?

34. List the major functions of the kidney.

35. How are the four colligative properties of a solution affected by the addition of particles to water?

36. What does the osmometer measure? the urinometer? Which is the most accurate in estimating concentration and why?

37. Write the formula to calculate plasma osmotic concentration from the freezing point. Given that plasma freezes at $-0.53\,°C$, calculate the concentration of plasma in milliosmols.

38. Draw a cortical and juxtamedullary nephron, illustrating their position in relation to the cortex and medulla.

39. What are the vasa recta and what do they do?

40. What is the purpose of the countercurrent mechanism? What are the two basic processes involved?

Directions: *Circle the letter preceding each item below that correctly completes the statement. Only one answer is correct, with exceptions noted.*

41. The forces that determine the glomerular filtrate are:
    a. Hydrostatic pressure of the blood in the glomerulus   b. Plasma protein concentration
    c. Hydrostatic pressure of the fluid in Bowman's capsule   d. All the above.

42. Tubular secretion involves the movement of substances:
    a. From the peritubular capillaries into the tubular lumen   b. From the tubular lumen into the peritubular capillaries   c. From the glomerular capillaries into the tubular lumen   d. From the tubular lumen into the bladder

43. Normal renal plasma flow is about:
    a. 1200 ml/min   b. 660 ml/min   c. 125 ml/min
    d. 1 ml/min

44. The fraction of plasma filtered by the glomerulus
    (filtration fraction) is:
    a. 100 percent   b. 50 percent   c. 20 percent
    d. 1 percent

45. The type of tubular transport involving the move-
    ment of a substance up a chemical or electrical gra-
    dient is called:
    a. Osmosis   b. Passive diffusion   c. Active
    d. Hydrostatic

46. Substances normally filtered by the glomerulus in-
    clude all the following *except*:
    a. Electrolytes   b. Water   c. Nonelectrolytes
    d. Blood cells

47. The proportion of glomerular filtrate reabsorbed in
    the proximal tubule is about:
    a. 20 percent   b. 50 percent   c. 80 percent
    d. 99 percent

48. The osmolality of a solution depends on:
    a. Density of particles   b. Size of particles
    c. Electrical charge of the particles   d. Number
    of particles   e. All of these

49. The ascending limb of the loop of Henle:
    a. Actively transports sodium   b. Is permeable to
    water   c. Is hyperosmotic   d. Actively trans-
    ports chloride   e. Actively transports water

50. The medullary interstitial fluid in health is:
    a. Always hypoosmotic   b. Always hyperosmotic
    c. Hyperosmotic during antidiuresis only   d. Hy-
    posmotic during diuresis and hyperosmotic during
    antidiuresis

51. All the following factors are important in the for-
    mation of a concentrated urine *except*:
    a. Presence of a long loop of Henle   b. Presence
    of ADH   c. Intact chloride pump in the ascend-
    ing limb of Henle   d. Increase in medullary
    blood flow in the vasa recta   e. Diffusion of urea
    into the medullary interstitium

52. ADH release is stimulated by (more than one an-
    swer is correct):
    a. Increase in ECF volume   b. Decrease in ECF
    volume   c. Increase in the osmolality of the ECF
    d. Decrease in the osmolality of the ECF.

53. ADH exerts all the following effects on the kidney
    except (more than one answer is correct):
    a. Increases blood flow in the vasa recta   b. De-
    creases blood flow in the vasa recta   c. Increases

permeability of distal tubule and collecting ducts
to water   d. Decreases isoosmotic reabsorption in
the proximal tubule

54. Under conditions of severe water deprivation in
    human beings, maximum urine osmolality is
    greater than plasma osmolality by a factor of about:
    a. 10   b. 5   c. 3   d. 2

55. The maximum urine dilution ability in human
    beings under conditions of excess water ingestion
    is:
    a. 40 mOsm   b. 100 mOsm   c. 285 mOsm
    d. 1400 mOsm

**Directions: Match the appropriate osmotic
concentration in col. B with each region of the
nephron or interstitium in col. A:**

Column A

56. ____ Bowman's space

57. ____ Ascending limb of Henle

58. ____ Descend-ing limb of Henle

59. ____ Proximal tubule

60. ____ Distal tu-bule

61. ____ Collecting duct

62. ____ Medullary interstitium

63. ____ Cortical interstitium

Column B

a. Hypoosmotic

b. Isoosmotic

c. Hyperosmotic

d. Isoosmotic or hypoosmotic

**Directions: Answer questions 64 to 73 in relation to
the following list of substances.**

a. Sodium   g. Amino acids   m. Ammonia
b. Potassium   h. Creatinine   n. Uric acid
c. Calcium   i. Chloride   o. Hydrogen
d. Phosphate   j. Urea   ion
e. Glucose   k. Bicarbonate   p. Water
f. Urine   l. Renin

64. Which of the substances in this list are filtered by
    the glomerulus?

65. Which two substances are 100 percent reabsorbed
    in the proximal tubule?

66. Which two substances are regulated by parathyroid
    hormone?

67. Which three substances are passively reabsorbed in the proximal tubule?

68. Which substance is actively transported out of the ascending limb of Henle?

69. Which three substances are end products of protein metabolism?

70. Which two substances are regulated by aldosterone?

71. Which two substances are secreted into the distal tubule in exchange for sodium reabsorption?

72. Which substance is secreted into the distal tubule, unites with H^+, and is unable to diffuse out of the tubule?

73. Which substance, when reabsorbed, is most important as a blood buffer?

Directions: Match the correct estimated pressures in col. B to the proper glomerular filtration forces in col. A.

Column A

74. ____ Glomerular hydrostatic pressure

75. ____ Colloid osmotic pressure

Column B

a. 50 mmHg

b. 30 mmHg

c. 10 mmHg

76. ____ Net filtration pressure

77. ____ Hydrostatic pressure in Bowman's capsule

Directions: Circle the letter preceding the item that correctly completes the following statements.

78. The ratio of juxtaglomerular nephrons to cortical nephrons in the human kidney is about:
a. 1:1 b. 1:3 c. 1:7 d. 1:15

79. Osmolality is solute concentration:
a. Per 1000 g (kg) of water b. Per 1000 ml of solution

DIAGNOSTIC PROCEDURES IN RENAL DISEASE

OBJECTIVES

At the completion of this chapter you should be able to:

1. Describe the significance of proteinuria as a pathologic condition.
2. Illustrate some of the advantages and disadvantages of the dipstick test for proteinuria.
3. Describe the diurnal pattern of urine pH.
4. List the points to consider when testing the pH of the urine.
5. Describe the factors contributing to the formation of urinary tract calculi.
6. Discuss the prevention of urinary tract calculi.
7. Explain the significance of hematuria.
8. List the steps for measuring specific gravity with a urinometer.
9. Describe the relation between specific gravity and osmolality of the urine.
10. Describe the creatinine clearance test and its relation to the glomerular filtration rate.
11. State the normal value for serum creatinine and blood urea nitrogen levels and discuss the significance of an elevation of each.
12. Discuss the effects of aging on the glomerular filtration rate.
13. Describe two tests used to estimate renal plasma flow and proximal tubule function.
14. Explain the significance of the concentration and dilution tests as tests of distal tubule function.
15. Describe the test used in the diagnosis of renal tubular acidosis.
16. Discuss the value of a sodium conservation test in renal disease.
17. List four types of morphological renal investigations.
18. List the normal constituents of the urine sediment.
19. List the most common abnormal constituents of the urine and their significance.
20. Describe how casts are formed in the kidney (source of constituents, shape).

21. Differentiate between the various types of casts (hyaline, cellular, granular, fatty, and broad granular).
22. Describe the significance of bacteriuria.
23. Discuss the proper procedure of urine collection for bacteriologic study.
24. Differentiate between an intravenous and a retrograde pyelogram.
25. Describe the procedure, precautions, and indications for a renal arteriogram.
26. Describe the procedure, precautions, and indications for a renal biopsy.

BIOCHEMICAL METHODS

This chapter discusses some of the commonly performed diagnostic tests for the detection of renal disease and evaluation of renal function. These tests are divided into methods which are predominantly biochemical or predominantly morphological. These diagnostic tests are especially important in the detection of renal disease, since many serious renal diseases do not produce symptoms until renal function is significantly impaired.

Chemical examination of the urine

Chemical testing of the urine has been greatly simplified by the introduction of impregnated paper strips which detect substances such as glucose, acetone, bilirubin, protein, and blood. The pH of the urine can also be measured by a dipstick test. Of particular importance in renal disease are the detection of protein or blood in the urine, the measurement of osmolality or specific gravity, and microscopic examination of the urine (considered later in the chapter under "Morphological Methods").

Proteinuria

Normal healthy adults excrete small amounts of protein in the urine—up to 150 mg a day—consisting mainly of albumin and Tamm-Horsfall protein. The latter is secreted by the distal tubule. Proteinuria in amounts greater than 150 mg/day is considered pathologic.

Because it is easy to use, the dipstick test (Albustix, Combistix) is the most commonly used test for proteinuria. The end of the stick is dipped in urine and removed immediately, and the urine is shaken off by tapping the stick on the side of the container. The result is then read by comparison with the color chart on the label. Grading is from 0 to 4+, and the corresponding amounts of protein are trace (less than 30 mg/100 ml urine); 1+ (30 mg/100 ml urine); 2+ (100 mg/100 ml urine); 3+ (300 mg/100 ml urine); and 4+ (1 g/100 ml urine). While the dipstick test is generally accurate, there are a number of pitfalls and difficulties in interpretation. Early morning samples are normally more concentrated and should preferably be tested for protein. A "trace" response found in an early morning specimen is probably within normal limits, less than 150 mg/day. On the other hand, if the urine specimen is collected later in the day and is more dilute (e.g., specific gravity 1.006), a trace response might indicate significant proteinuria. A common cause of a false positive in females is contamination of the urine with vaginal secretions. All routine urine examinations should include a simple test for protein for purposes of screening. More accurate quantitative tests for protein may be carried out in the laboratory on a 24-hour specimen.

Persistent proteinuria almost always indicates renal disease, especially involving the glomerulus. The direct cause of proteinuria is always an increase in glomerular permeability. Recall that the glomerulus is composed of three layers (endothelium, basement membrane, and epithelium) which have a series of pores of varying sizes. Normally, only a small amount of albumin (the smallest protein molecule in the serum) is filtered at the glomerulus, and most of this is reabsorbed in the tubules. Albuminuria is very common in the various types of glomerulonephritis. *Heavy proteinuria* refers to the passage of ≥ 3.5 g/day and is the laboratory definition of the nephrotic syndrome (discussed later). Some patients with the nephrotic syndrome may pass as much as 20 or 30 g of protein per day. *Moderate proteinuria* is associated with a broad spectrum of renal diseases; *minimal proteinuria* (less than 1 g/day) is more apt to be associated with renal diseases such as chronic pyelonephritis, with less glomerular involvement.

Hematuria

The dipstick test for occult blood is an excellent screening test for hematuria. Whenever it is positive, the urine should be examined microscopically. Hematuria is a common finding in a number of renal diseases and pathologic processes in the lower urinary tract, including infections, stones, trauma, and neoplasms. Hematuria is a prominent feature of glomerulonephritis but not of pyelonephritis. The dipstick test can easiily be used by patients to follow the course of hematuria during their treatment.

Hydrogen ion concentration

In the healthy adult, the pH of the urine ranges widely from 4.5 to 8.0, but the average pooled specimen is quite acidic, at 6.0, because of acidic metabolites produced by the normal breakdown of body tissues and nutrients. The usual diurnal pattern consists of a rise in pH after a meal (alkaline tide) followed by a gradual fall until the next meal ingestion, while during normal sleeping hours pH reaches its minimum (nocturnal acid tide due to hypoventilation during sleep). A diet high in animal protein tends to produce an acid urine, while a predominantly vegetable diet tends to produce an alkaline urine.

A persistently acid urine may occur in respiratory or metabolic acidosis and in pyrexia (fever). A persistently alkaline urine is suggestive of urinary tract infection with urea-splitting organisms. For example, in *Proteus* infections, the urine pH is consistently at a pH of 8 or higher. Persistently alkaline urine also occurs in renal tubular acidosis (a renal disease in which there is inability to conserve bicarbonate), in potassium depletion, and in Fanconi syndrome (a renal disease in which ammonia excretion is defective).

Although random pH readings are of little diagnostic value, they are helpful in the management of certain clinical conditions in which the pH of the urine should be kept persistently high or low by diet or drugs. Alkaline urine is desirable in the treatment of patients with calculi which form in acid urine, and acid urine is desirable in patients with calculi which form in alkaline urine or who have urinary tract infections (Table 41-1).

Common stones formed in acid urine are composed of calcium oxalate, uric acid crystals, or cystine. About two-thirds of all urinary calculi are of the calcium oxalate type. Idiopathic hypercalciuria is an important predisposing factor. Thiazide diuretics decrease calcium excretion and are quite effective in preventing recurrence (Coe, 1980). Cystine stones are rare and are re-

TABLE 41-1

FACTORS CONTRIBUTING TO THE FORMATION OF URINARY TRACT CALCULI AND THEIR PREVENTION

Urinary stone content	Predisposing factors	Preventive therapy to achieve desired urine pH*
	Acid urine	Alkaline urine (pH > 6)
Calcium oxalate	Hypercalciuria	Vegetables, milk, fruit (except plums, prunes, cranberries)
Uric acid crystals	Chemotherapy, gout	Sodium bicarbonate or citrate
Cystine	Aminoaciduria	
	Alkaline urine	Acid urine
Triple phosphate	Urinary tract infection	Meat, breads, protein foods, cranberry juice, prunes, plums
Calcium phosphate	Hypercalciuria Prolonged immobility	Mandelamine

*High fluid intake is the most important preventive measure against all calculi.

lated to a hereditary renal tubular transport disorder involving certain amino acids. Cystine, a metabolic product of dietary methionine, is the least soluble of the naturally occurring amino acids. The excess urinary excretion of cystine (cystinuria) in an acid urine results in cystine urolithiasis. Treatment of this disorder is directed toward a reversal of risk factors by forced hydration and bicarbonate or acetazolamide (Diamox) administration to maintain the urine pH above 7.5 (Coe, 1980). Hyperuricemia leading to uric acid crystallization is a particular hazard in patients who are receiving cytotoxic drugs for cancer or leukemia. Uric acid is formed principally as an end product of nucleoprotein metabolism. With increasing proliferation and destruction of cells there is a proportional increase in uric acid because of degradation of cellular nucleoproteins. The physician may order the administration of sodium bicarbonate or citrate to alkalinize the urine. It is important to encourage a high fluid intake in these patients, especially before bedtime, when the urine normally becomes more acid, to prevent crystallization of uric acid in the renal tubules and interstitium and consequent obstruction. Some foods which help alkalinize the urine are milk, vegetables, and fruits (except prunes, plums, and cranberries).

Common stones formed in alkaline urine are composed of calcium phosphate or magnesium ammonium phosphate (triple-phosphate stones). Calcium phosphate or oxalate is often present in triple-phosphate stones. Triple-phosphate stones are often associated with urinary tract infections, especially with urea-splitting organisms. These stones occasionally grow to occupy the entire pelvicalyceal system. Such a stone, referred to as a "staghorn" calculus because of its shape, must be removed surgically. Since 90 percent of all calculi contain calcium, hypercalciuria is an important predisposing cause. Hypercalciuria is associated with hyperparathyroidism, renal tubular acidosis, and prolonged immobilization. All are associated with mobilization of calcium salts from bone. Meat, bread, protein foods, cranberry juice, plums, and prunes tend to produce an acid urine and thus help prevent the formation of these stones. The physician may order a drug such as Mandelamine to acidify the urine for persistent urinary tract infections. Probably the most important factor in the prevention of all stones regardless of composition is a high fluid intake sufficient to produce a urine output of 2½ to 3 liters/day.

The pH of the urine may be tested by using Squibb Nitrazine paper or by a dipstick test. The following points should be kept in mind while performing this test: (1) only fresh urine should be used (when urine is allowed to stand, urea breaks down to ammonia and the pH becomes more alkaline); (2) the test strip should be removed promptly after being dipped in the urine to avoid washing out the test reagent; and (3) the color comparison with the standard should be made immediately in good light (daylight is preferable, and fluorescent light should be avoided).

Specific gravity

Specific gravity is commonly measured in the clinical unit to determine the concentration of urine. It is measured by the flotation of the hydrometer or urinometer in a cylinder of urine (Fig. 41-1). The proper procedure for measuring the specific gravity of urine is as follows:

1. Check the accuracy of the urinometer against distilled water to read 1.000 at its calibration temperature. Most urinometers are calibrated at a temperature of 16°C (60.8°F). This procedure is necessary since the density of water changes with temperature.

2. Fill the cylinder about three-quarters full of well-mixed urine. A uniform solution is necessary, since solute concentration is being measured.

3. Give the urinometer a gentle spin as it is plunged into the urine to avoid errors of surface tension at

the stem and to prevent it from adhering to the sides of the cylinder.

4. Read from top to bottom. The urinometer is calibrated in units of 0.001, starting with 1.000 at the top and progressing downward to 1.060. The correct reading is at the level of the bottom of the meniscus, which should be read at eye level.

5. Correct the specific gravity reading if the temperature of the specimen deviates from the calibration temperature of the urinometer. Use a thermometer to determine the actual temperature of the urine. Add 0.001 to the reading for every 3°C (5.4°F) above the calibration temperature and subtract 0.001 for each 3°C below. For example, if a urinometer calibrated at 16°C is placed in a freshly voided urine specimen with a temperature of 31°C (88°F) and shows a reading of 1.015, then 0.005 is added to the reading

$$31°C - 16°C = 15°C \times \frac{0.001}{3°C} = 0.005$$

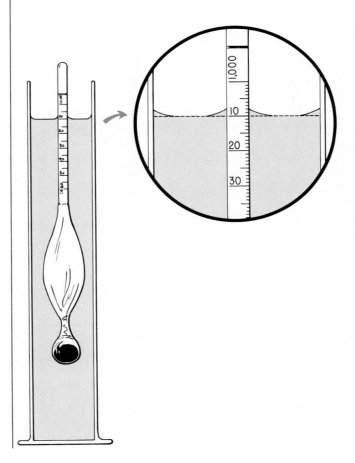

FIGURE 41-1
Urinometer with scale featured.

The true specific gravity corrected for temperature is 1.020.

Although specific gravity measurement is simple and convenient, it is important to realize that density is being measured. The density depends on the weight as well as on the number of the solute particles in solution. The kidney's capacity to concentrate, however, is related to the concentration of particles in solution (i.e., osmolality) and not to their weight. True concentration, osmolality, is measured by freezing point depression or vapor pressure lowering, though this is more expensive and time-consuming to measure.

Fortunately, when urine contains only normal constituents (mainly NaCl), the correlation between specific gravity and osmolality is sufficiently close to use specific gravity as a clinical guide to the osmolality of the urine. The relation between specific gravity and the osmolality of urine is shown in Fig. 41-2. When the urine contains normal constituents (middle line), a specific gravity of 1.010 corresponds to the osmolality of the blood at 285 mOsm. When given large amounts of water, the healthy person can excrete urine with a min-

imum specific gravity of 1.001 (about 40 mOsm). When deprived of fluid, maximum specific gravity is about 1.040 (1300 mOsm). If the urine should contain glucose or protein (dense particles), the specific gravity would be greater at a fixed osmolality than in normal urine (shifted toward the pure glucose curve); and conversely, if the urine contains much urea (a less dense molecule), the specific gravity will be lower. For example, at a concentration of 400 mOsm the specific gravity of urine with normal constituents will be about 1.013. At the same osmolality, if the urine contained a large amount of protein or glucose, the specific gravity would be about 1.030; if it contained a large amount of urea, the specific gravity would be about 1.007. These facts must be taken into consideration when the specific gravity measurement is used to estimate the ability of the kidneys to concentrate urine.

In chronic renal disease, the kidney loses first the ability to concentrate urine. Later, the ability to dilute urine is lost as well, so that the specific gravity of urine becomes fixed near 1.010 (the specific gravity of the plasma). This generally occurs when 80 percent of the nephron mass has been destroyed.

Glomerular filtration rate

One of the most important indices of renal function is the glomerular filtration rate (GFR). The GFR gives in-

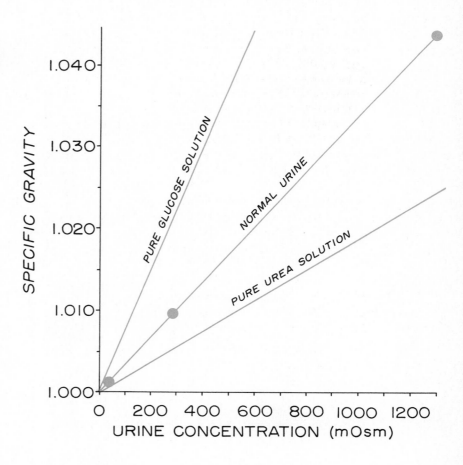

FIGURE 41-2

Relationship between specific gravity and osmolality of the urine. (Modified from H. E. De Wardner, *The Kidney*, 4th ed., Longman, Inc., New York, 1973.)

formation about the amount of functioning renal tissue. As noted previously, the most accurate way to measure GFR is by means of the inulin clearance test. However, this test is infrequently used in the clinical unit because it involves an intravenous infusion at a constant rate and timed collections of urine by catheterization. The endogenous creatinine clearance test is much simpler to carry out.

Creatinine clearance test

Creatinine is an end product of muscle metabolism which is liberated from the muscles at a virtually constant rate and excreted in the urine at the same rate. The plasma (serum) level is therefore nearly constant, ranging from 0.7 to 1.5 mg per 100 ml (higher value in males than in females because of the male's greater muscle mass). Creatinine is excreted in the urine by filtration at the glomerulus, but it is not reabsorbed by the tubules. A small amount, however, is secreted by the tubules, especially when serum creatinine levels are high. In spite of the fact that a small amount is secreted, the creatinine clearance test is a convenient test from which to estimate the GFR in the clinical unit. To perform the creatinine clearance test, it is only necessary to collect a 24-hour urine specimen and a blood specimen during the same 24-hour period (Fig. 41-3). Creatinine clearance (C_{cr}) is then calculated from the clearance formula

$$C_{cr} = \frac{U_{cr}V}{P_{cr}}$$

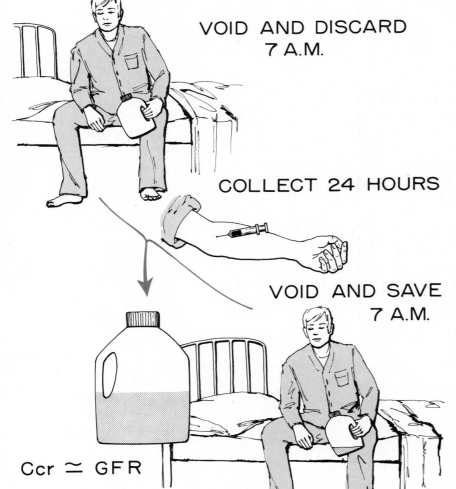

FIGURE 41-3
Creatinine clearance test.

VOID AND DISCARD
7 A.M.

COLLECT 24 HOURS

VOID AND SAVE
7 A.M.

$C_{cr} \simeq GFR$

Creatinine clearance is a fairly good index of GFR, although it is not a true measurement, since creatinine is secreted by the tubules to some extent, and the slight secretion of creatinine tends to cause overestimation of the GFR. Plasma creatinine also may be overestimated because of the difficulties inherent in the laboratory determination. Luckily, these two errors are of nearly the same magnitude and cancel each other out, so that creatinine clearance approximates GFR.

In chronic renal disease the GFR is decreased below the normal value of 125 ml/minute. GFR also decreases with advancing age: after the age of 30, it decreases at the rate of about 1 ml/minute every year.

Plasma creatinine and blood urea nitrogen

The plasma creatinine and blood urea nitrogen (BUN) concentrations are also used as guides to the GFR. The normal BUN concentration is about 10 to 20 mg/100 ml, and plasma creatinine concentration is 0.7 to 1.5 mg/100 ml. Both these substances are nitrogenous end products of protein metabolism normally excreted in the urine. When the GFR decreases, as in renal insufficiency, the plasma levels of creatinine and BUN rise. This condition is called *azotemia* (nitrogenous substances in the blood). The level of plasma creatinine as an index of GFR is more accurate than the BUN, since its production rate is mainly a function of the size of the muscle mass, which changes very little. The BUN, however, is affected by the amount of protein in the diet and the catabolism of body protein. The relation of a rising plasma creatinine and BUN level to a decreasing GFR is discussed in Chap. 42.

Tubular function tests

A number of tests are carried out to evaluate the function and integrity of the renal tubules. The function of the tubules is selective reabsorption of the contents of the tubular fluid and secretion of substances into the tubular lumen which are either circulating in the peritubular capillaries or are formed by the tubular cell. These processes are under the control of a wide variety of hormones, gas pressures, and plasma electrolyte concentrations. Common tests of proximal tubular function include the phenolsulfonphthalein (PSP) and para-aminohippurate (PAH) excretion tests. Distal tubular function tests include tests of concentration, dilution, acidification, and sodium conservation.

PSP excretion test

Phenolsulfonphthalein is a nontoxic dye which is eliminated primarily by secretion into the proximal tubule. Binding of PSP to plasma proteins is so high that only about 4 percent is excreted by glomerular filtration. With the usual 6-mg intravenous dose, the plasma level of the dye is only about one-fifth of the tubular capacity to excrete PSP. The excretion rate of PSP is therefore usually limited by the rate of delivery to the tubules via the renal plasma flow and, in severely impaired kidneys, by proximal tubular function. The 15-minute PSP test is most commonly performed (Fig. 41-4).

Thirty minutes before the PSP dye is given, the patient is asked to drink two or three glasses of water to ensure sufficient bladder urine for urination. Exactly 1 ml (6 mg) of PSP is injected intravenously, using a tuberculin syringe for accuracy. Exactly 15 minutes after the dye is given, the patient is asked to completely empty the bladder. All the urine is then placed in a 1-liter volumetric flask; 5 ml of 10% NaOH is added, and enough water to bring the volume up to 1 liter. A test tube of the pink, diluted specimen is then compared with the appropriate standards visually or by the use of a colorimeter. The person with normal renal function should excrete a minimum of 28 percent of the dye in 15 minutes.

The primary value of the PSP excretion test is in the detection of functional impairment early in the course of renal disease. Many physicians no longer perform this test and consider the creatinine clearance test alone to be an adequate assessment of renal function. The analysis of the PSP test is so simple that it can be performed without the aid of a clinical laboratory, so it might be useful in situations where such a facility is not available.

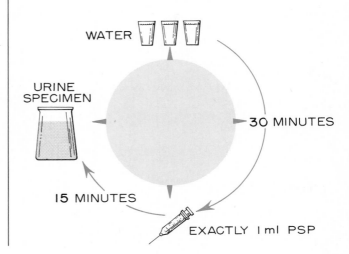

FIGURE 41-4
Fifteen-minute PSP excretion test. Twenty-eight percent or more of the dye is normally excreted in 15 minutes.

PAH excretion test

Para-aminohippurate is a substance which is both filtered by the glomerulus and secreted by the proximal tubule. When given in low concentrations to human subjects, about 92 percent of it is cleared in one circulation through the kidneys. It is, therefore, a fairly accurate measure of renal plasma flow (RPF). In the adult, RPF is approximately 600 ml/minute. If the plasma concentration is further increased until secretory capacity is exceeded, the secretory capacity of the proximal tubule can be calculated from the filtered load and urinary excretion. This test is most commonly used in research.

Concentration and dilution tests

The measurement of urine specific gravity after water restriction is a sensitive measure of the ability of the renal tubules to reabsorb water and produce a concentrated urine. Renal function is considered normal if an early morning urine specimen has a specific gravity of 1.025 or more. When concentrating ability is doubtful, a more elaborate concentration test may be carried out. The Fishberg concentration test is commonly used. To ensure accuracy of results, the patient must be on a normal diet (normal salt, protein, and fluid intake) and must not be taking diuretics prior to the administration of the test. The patient is instructed to eat a normal evening meal at 6 P.M. and not to take food or fluids until the test is completed the next morning. Urine specimens are collected the next morning at 6, 7, and 8 A.M. At least one of these specimens should have a specific gravity of 1.025 (800 mOsm) or more (Fig. 41-5).

The urinary dilution test is performed by having the patient drink 1 liter of water within a 30-minute period. Urine specimens are then collected over the next 3 hours. At least one of these specimens should have a specific gravity of 1.003 (80 mOsm) or less (Fig. 41-5). The urinary dilution test is much less useful than the concentration test, since nonspecific factors such as nausea or emotions may interfere with water diuresis even in normal subjects. Diluting ability may be defective in adrenal insufficiency, hepatic disease, and cardiac failure. The ability to dilute urine is lost late in most renal diseases, while concentrating ability is lost early. Neither the concentration nor the dilution tests should be carried out on azotemic patients, since dehydration and water intoxication could result.

Urine acidification test

The urine acidification test is designed to measure the maximum acid-excreting capacity of the kidney and is specific for the diagnosis of renal tubular acidosis.

In the 5-day test, control urine is collected for 2 days. The patient is then given ammonium chloride (about 12 g/day in the adult) for the next 3 days. The ammonium chloride is metabolized to urea and hydrogen chloride, producing acidosis in the patient. The urinary pH is determined daily, and on the fifth day ammonium and titratable acids are also measured. Normally the kidney excretes the acid load and the urine pH is 5.3 or less (Fig. 41-6). In renal tubular acidosis a hydrogen ion gradient between the tubular lumen and the plasma cannot be maintained, and a low urine pH is not achieved. Many patients with chronic renal failure can achieve a urine pH of 5.3, but excretion of ammonium and titratable acids is impaired.

Sodium conservation test

The healthy person can produce urine that is virtually sodium-free under conditions of dietary restriction of sodium. In renal disease the ability to conserve sodium may be lost, and some patients suffer sodium depletion. If a person is losing more sodium than is ingested, the result is a contraction of the plasma volume, a decrease in the GFR, and an accelerated course toward final renal failure. A salt-losing nephritis is more common in patients who have chronic pyelonephritis or polycystic disease. Both diseases primarily involve the renal tubules. Many patients in renal failure oscillate between states of sodium retention and depletion, so their daily intake of sodium must be defined within very narrow limits.

The sodium conservation test is sometimes used to determine how much sodium is needed in the diet of a patient with a salt-losing nephritis. The patient eats a low sodium diet (10 meq, or 500 mg). Sodium excretion in the urine normally falls to equal sodium intake within a week. In salt-losing nephritis, a large amount of sodium continues to be lost in the urine in spite of the restricted intake. Additional sodium may be added to the diet when the magnitude of the deficit is determined. For example, a patient who is excreting 50 meq of sodium in urine on a 10-meq sodium diet should be allowed an additional 40 meq of sodium in the diet, or 50 meq.

MORPHOLOGICAL METHODS

Diagnostic methods in renal disease which are primarily morphological include microscopic and bacteriologic examination of the urine, renal radiologic examination, and renal biopsy. These methods are discussed briefly.

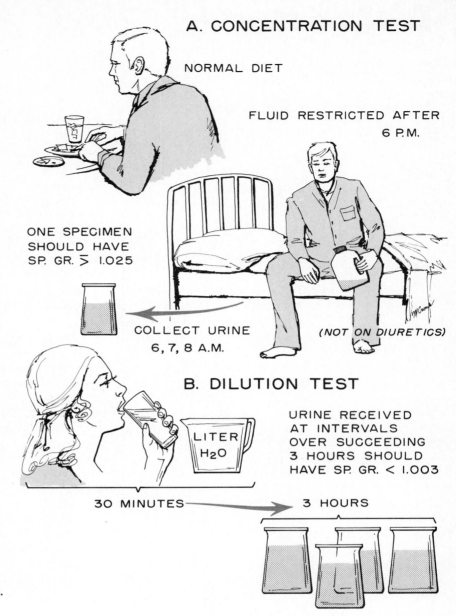

A. CONCENTRATION TEST

NORMAL DIET

FLUID RESTRICTED AFTER 6 P.M.

ONE SPECIMEN SHOULD HAVE SP. GR. ≥ 1.025

COLLECT URINE 6, 7, 8 A.M.

(NOT ON DIURETICS)

B. DILUTION TEST

LITER H₂O

URINE RECEIVED AT INTERVALS OVER SUCCEEDING 3 HOURS SHOULD HAVE SP. GR. < 1.003

30 MINUTES → 3 HOURS

FIGURE 41-5
Urine concentration and dilution tests.
See text for explanation.

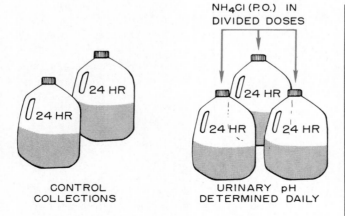

NH₄Cl (P.O.) IN DIVIDED DOSES

24 HR

24 HR

24 HR   24 HR

CONTROL COLLECTIONS

URINARY pH DETERMINED DAILY

pH: NORMAL • 4.5 – 5.3
RENAL TUBULAR ACIDOSIS • > 5.3

Microscopic examination of the urine

Microscopic examination of the urine is carried out on a freshly collected, centrifuged specimen, the deposit from which is suspended in 0.5 ml urine. In health, the urine contains a small number of cells and other elements derived from the entire length of the genitourinary tract—casts, epithelial cells from the lining of the urinary tract and vagina (females), spermatozoa (males), mucus threads, and no more than one or two red blood cells and three or four white blood cells per high-power field.

FIGURE 41-6
Urine acidification test.

The most common abnormal constituents of the urine are red blood cells (RBCs), white blood cells (WBCs), bacteria, and casts. All casts arise in the kidney and are thought to be "moldings" of renal tubules. Thus they indicate conditions exclusively within the kidneys and, for this reason, are of great diagnostic value. Casts consist of a mucoprotein matrix, the Tamm-Horsfall mucoprotein, in which cells or debris are embedded and in which a variety of serum and renal proteins may be absorbed. The Tamm-Horsfall protein is secreted by the distal tubule cells. As it passes down the tubule, it dehydrates and takes on the shape of the tubule. *Hyaline casts* consist of this protein and appear as clear cylinders. Cellular elements may be incorporated into hyaline casts (cellular casts) at the time of their formation. In this way, various types of casts are formed, depending on the cell type embedded in the cast (Fig. 41-7). Normally there is not enough protein in the renal tubules to provide more than an occasional cast. *Cylindruria* (excessive excretion of casts in the urine) usually means increased proteinuria or renal excretion of cells, or both, and indicates renal disease.

Casts are classified according to shape or constituents. Cellular casts may contain RBCs, WBCs, bacteria, or tubular epithelial cells or may be mixed. Red blood cells and *red cell casts* are seen in active glomerulonephritis. *White cell casts* are often seen in pyelonephritis. Oval fat bodies and *fatty casts* are common in the nephrotic syndrome. Oval fat bodies are the remains of degenerated fat-filled tubular cells. *Granular casts* or *waxy casts* represent stages in the degeneration of a cellular cast, and the progression is from coarse to fine and finally to waxy. Broad granular casts are a typical finding in end-stage kidney disease. They are gran-

ular because of dead cells and broad because they are formed in the collecting ducts owing to decreased urinary flow. These broad granular casts are sometimes called *renal failure casts*.

Bacteriologic examination of the urine

Bacterial counts may be carried out by inoculating the surface of a nutrient agar plate, using a calibrated loop which delivers 0.001 ml of urine (Fig. 41-8). The agar plate is then incubated for 24 hours at 37°C, and colonies are counted. Counts of 100 or more colonies (10^5 organisms per milliliter of urine) constitute a significant degree of bacteriuria. The bacteria may be subcultured for identification and for an antibiotic sensitivity test. This procedure is commonly referred to as *C & S*, or *culture and sensitivity*, test. The results of this test are a useful guide in the choice of an antibiotic for the most effective treatment.

In order for a bacteriologic study of the urine to have validity, the specimen must be free of contaminating bacteria from the urethra, external genitalia, and perineum. Proper techniques and precautions are therefore important in the collection of urine specimens. Collection of the urine by catheterization into a sterile container is the best way to ensure that the specimen is uncontaminated. Catheterization, however, is avoided if possible, because of the danger of introducing bacteria into the urinary tract. A "sterile-voided" specimen is

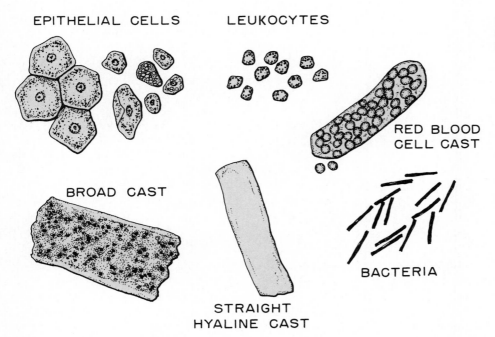

EPITHELIAL CELLS   LEUKOCYTES

RED BLOOD CELL CAST

BROAD CAST

BACTERIA

STRAIGHT HYALINE CAST

FIGURE 41-7
Some formed elements in the urine sediment.

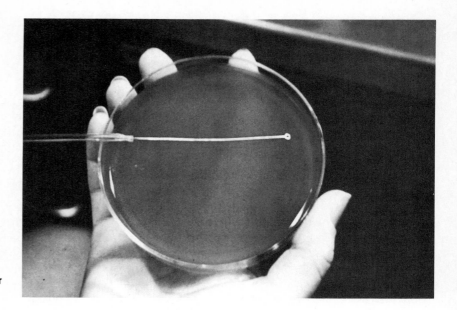

FIGURE 41-8

Inoculation of the surface of a blood agar plate by means of a calibrated loop. The plate is incubated for 24 hours at 37°C. Significant bacteriuria is 10^5 (100,000) or more organisms per milliliter of urine.

generally considered adequate for a bacteriologic study. Men, and particularly women, are instructed to wash the area around the urinary meatus with soap and water. A midstream specimen is then collected in a clean or sterile specimen container. The urine is examined within 30 minutes, or a preservative is added and it is refrigerated at 4°C. Refrigeration prevents the growth of bacteria, and the preservative prevents the deterioration of casts and cells.

Radiologic examinations

A number of radiologic procedures are available to evaluate the urinary system. The excretory urogram or intravenous pyelogram is the most common and important radiologic examination of the kidneys and is usually performed first. Other imaging examinations include ultrasonography, radionuclide (isotopic) imaging, computerized tomography, voiding cystourethrography, and renal angiography.

Intravenous pyelogram (IVP)

The usual procedure for performing the IVP includes a flat plate (plain film) of the abdomen followed by intravenous injection of contrast medium. The contrast medium circulates via the bloodstream and heart to the kidneys, where it is excreted. After injection, a film is taken every minute for the first 5 minutes for the purpose of visualizing the cortex of the kidney. The cortex is thinned in glomerulonephritis and has a moth-eaten appearance in pyelonephritis and ischemia. Adequacy of filling of the calyces is evaluated by examination of the 3- and 5-minute films. Another film is taken at 15 minutes which makes the calyces, pelvis, and ureters visible. Cysts, lesions, and obstructions cause a dis-

tortion of these structures. A final film is taken at 45 minutes which makes the bladder visible. If the patient is severely azotemic (BUN > 70 mg/100 ml) an IVP is not usually done, since this indicates that the GFR is very low. Consequently the dye will not be excreted and the pyelogram will be difficult to visualize.

Sometimes a retrograde pyelogram is done by passing a catheter up the ureter and injecting contrast medium directly into the kidney. The main indications for this procedure are urologic—e.g., further investigation of a nonfunctioning kidney or when visualization of the IVP is not clear. This procedure is avoided if at all possible since it involves anesthesia and there is a very real danger of infection.

The standard IVP serves many purposes. It can establish the presence and position of the kidneys and evaluate their size and shape. The effect of different disease states on the kidney's ability to concentrate and excrete the dye can also be evaluated. The diagram in Fig. 41-9 shows some typical abnormalities revealed by the IVP. The small, atrophic kidney may be due to unilateral renal ischemia or unilateral chronic pyelonephritis (Fig. 41-9A). Bilaterally small kidneys are common findings in chronic nephrosclerosis, pyelonephritis, and glomerulonephritis. Distortion of the renal pelvis with clubbing of the calyces is a common finding in chronic pyelonephritis (Fig. 41-9B). Note also the irregular shape and the greatly thinned cortex.

Renal ultrasonography

High-frequency sound waves (ultrasound) directed at the abdomen are reflected from tissue surfaces of varying density. The reflected waves, or echoes, are used to construct images (sonograms) representing sections of the kidney. Ultrasonography is particularly useful in distinguishing solid tumors from fluid-filled cysts. Since ultrasound evaluation does not depend on renal function, it can be applied to patients in severe renal failure who have kidneys which do not visualize on the IVP. Kidney size can be determined accurately, and an obstruction can be identified. Other applications include evaluation of a unilateral nonvisualizing kidney (often caused by hydronephrosis), evaluation of renal transplants (perirenal abscess or hematoma, for example, can be differentiated from acute rejection), and renal localization for needle placement for percutaneous renal biopsy (see below).

Renal radionuclide imaging

Radionuclide imaging involves the injection of a radioactive material which is subsequently detected externally by a scintillation (gamma) camera which picks up the radioactive emissions. Information is provided for the evaluation of both structure and function. The properties of the compound that bind the radioisotope determine how it is handled by the kidney—whether it is retained within the vascular system, filtered by the glomerulus, or secreted into the tubule. Three main procedures may be performed together or indepen-

dently: *renal scintiangiography* employs serial imaging of the aorta and renal vasculature; *renal scintiscanning* employs imaging of the renal parenchyma using various ^{99m}Tc-labeled compounds, and *renography* is the original technique of radionuclide evaluation of the kidneys using ^{131}I hippuran, which is excreted by tubular secretion. Radionuclide imaging is used for many purposes in renal evaluation but is particularly helpful in renal transplant evaluation. Renal function may be followed, impaired diffusion detected, and acute rejection differentiated from acute tubular necrosis.

Voiding cystourethrogram

The voiding cystourethrogram procedure involves filling the urinary bladder with contrast material via a urinary catheter. Films of the lower urinary tract are taken before, during, and after voiding. Its major diagnostic uses are to investigate abnormalities of the urethra (e.g., stenosis) and to determine whether there is vesicoureteral reflux.

Computerized tomography (CT body scanning)

The application of CT to the abdomen has been a fairly recent development. The x-ray film reveals the anatomy of series of "slices" of the body about 10 mm thick so that abnormalities may be identified. Since CT is more expensive than more conventional x-ray techniques, an important question is what it can show that other investigative methods cannot. One useful application of renal CT is the detection of retroperitoneal masses (e.g., tumor spread) which may be difficult to detect by angiography.

Renal arteriogram

The renal blood vessels may be visualized in an arteriogram. The usual procedure is to introduce a catheter via the femoral artery and abdominal aorta to the level of the renal artery. Contrast medium is injected at this level and then flows into the renal artery and its accessory branches. Additional information often can be obtained by selective renal angiography; the tip of the catheter is maneuvered into a renal artery and more

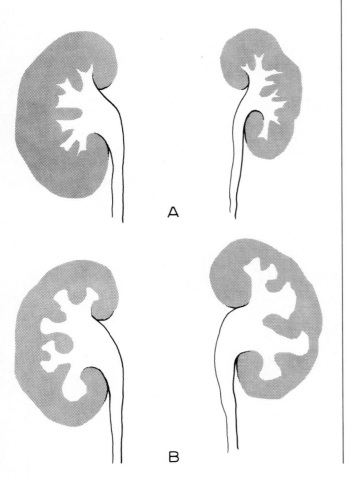

A

B

FIGURE 41-9

Diagram of abnormalities viewed on the intravenous pyelogram (IVP). (A) Small, atrophic kidney due to unilateral renal ischemia. (B) Clubbing of the calyces, irregularity of contour, and thinning of cortical substance may be found in chronic pyelonephritis.

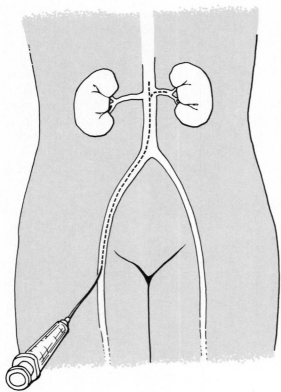

FIGURE 41-10
Transfemoral approach in renal angiography.

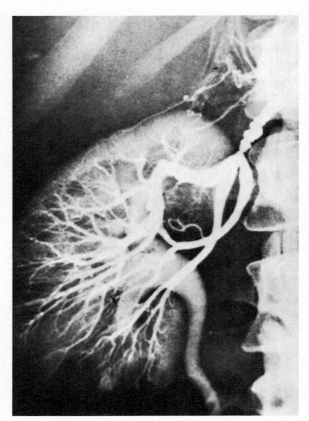

FIGURE 41-11
Renal arteriogram showing stenosis of the right renal artery.

FIGURE 41-12
Percutaneous renal biopsy. Site is located by x-ray reference; patient lies prone with sandbag under abdomen to fix kidney against back. Vital signs are monitored.

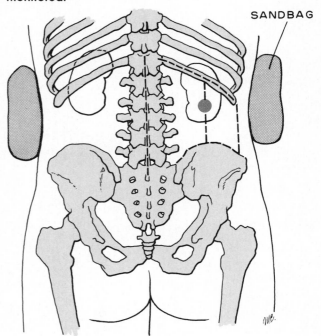

contrast medium is injected (Fig. 41-10). This procedure may be used (1) to visualize renal artery stenosis, which may cause some cases of hypertension; (2) to visualize the blood vessels of a neoplasm; (3) to visualize the blood supply of the cortex, which, for example, may have a patchy appearance in chronic pyelonephritis; and (4) to ascertain the structure of the renal blood supply of a donor before renal transplantation. Figure 41-11 is an arteriogram showing marked narrowing of the right renal artery.

Angiography is not done without discomfort and some hazard. The patient usually experiences an intense burning sensation for a few seconds as the solution enters the blood vessel. Prior to injection the patient is usually tested for iodide sensitivity, to avoid an anaphylactic response. Other complications following arteriogram include thrombus or embolus formation and local inflammation or hematoma at the site of entry. Although these complications are rare, vital signs are checked every 15 minutes until stable and then every 4 hours for 24 hours. Peripheral pulses are also checked for diminished strength to detect occlusion of blood flow due to a thrombus.

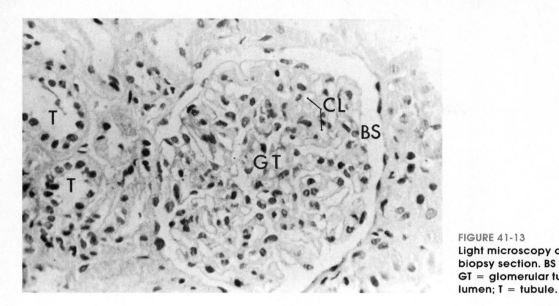

FIGURE 41-13
Light microscopy of normal renal biopsy section. BS = Bowman's space; GT = glomerular tuft; CL = capillary lumen; T = tubule.

Renal biopsy

Renal biopsy is one of the most important diagnostic techniques developed during the past few decades. It has resulted in considerable advancement of knowledge of the natural history of renal disease. Renal biopsy is used chiefly for the diagnosis of diffuse renal disease and for following its progress.

Most commonly the percutaneous, or blind, procedure is used for renal biopsy. The patient lies prone, with sandbags under the abdomen to fix the kidney against the back (Fig. 41-12). Local anesthesia is used. The usual site for the biopsy is over the right renal angle just below the twelfth rib. The site is located by x-ray reference. A biopsy needle is used to obtain a specimen of renal tissue. The tissue is examined, after appropriate preparation, by light microscopy, electron microscopy, and immunofluorescent microscopy. Figure 41-13 illustrates the appearance of a normal renal biopsy by light microscopy.

Renal biopsy should be performed only by a skilled nephrologist. The procedure is dangerous in patients who are uncooperative or who have a coagulative disorder or a solitary kidney. The most common complications are intrarenal and perirenal bleeding. Serious bleeding with gross hematuria occurs in about 5 percent and death in about 0.17 percent. Arteriovenous fistula is the second most common complication.

Immediately after the biopsy, pressure is applied over the biopsy site for 10 minutes with 4- by 4-in sponges, and the patient is kept in a prone position for 30 minutes. A pressure dressing is then applied to the biopsy site. The dressing from above and the sandbag from below provide pressure on the kidney and aid in the prevention of extrarenal bleeding. Lying on the sandbag is usually uncomfortable for the patient but immobilizes the kidney in the anteroposterior plane and is a necessary measure to ensure hemostasis. The patient should be kept in bed and as quiet as possible for the next 24 hours and should be instructed not to cough or sneeze. During this period frequent observations of the vital signs, abdomen, and urine should be made. The patient is kept on bed rest as long as hematuria occurs.

QUESTIONS

Diagnostic procedures in renal disease

Directions: Answer the following questions on a separate sheet of paper.

1. Contrast the amount of protein a healthy adult and a person with nephrotic syndrome might excrete in a day. Explain the significance.
2. What is always the *direct* cause of proteinuria, regardless of the underlying disease process?
3. Explain why only fresh urine should be used for measuring pH.
4. Hyperuricemia leading to uric acid crystallization in the renal tubules is a particular hazard for patients receiving cytotoxic drugs. Why?
5. What are the most common factors predisposing to formation of calculi in alkaline urine? Explain.

6. What is the most important *preventive* measure against all calculi?

7. What are the five important points that must be considered in obtaining an accurate specific gravity measurement with the urinometer?

8. What is creatinine, and what is its normal range of values in the plasma?

9. Why is the creatinine clearance test not a true measure of GFR?

10. What effect does increasing age have on the GFR?

11. What test most accurately measures effective renal plasma flow?

12. Which is the more accurate index of renal fuction, the BUN or the plasma creatinine level? Why? What is *azotemia*?

13. Give two examples of difficulties that may be encountered in the interpretation of the dipstick test for proteinuria.

Directions: Fill in the blanks with the correct words or numbers or circle the appropriate letter to complete the following sentences.

14. Protein excreted in the urine of the healthy adult consists mainly of _____ and _____ _____ protein.

15. The average pooled daily urine specimen has a pH of about _____.

16. After a meal, one expects a (a) rise or (b) fall in the urine pH. This is referred to as the _____ tide.

17. During normal sleeping hours the urine pH reaches its (a) maximum or (b) minimum due to (c) hypoventilation or (d) hyperventilation during sleep. This is referred to as the _____ _____ tide.

18. When the urine contains normal constituents, a specific gravity of 1.010 corresponds to the normal osmolality of the blood at _____ mOsm.

19. When given large amounts of water, the healthy human being can dilute urine to a minimum specific gravity of about _____ (40 mOsm). Under conditions of water deprivation a normal person can excrete a concentrated urine with a maximum specific gravity of about _____ (1300 mOsm). What is the purpose of this great flexibility?

20. In the 15-minute PSP test the kidneys normally excrete _____ percent of the dye in the urine.

21. After about 14 hours of water deprivation, the urine of a person with normally functioning kidneys has a specific gravity of _____ or more. After a water load (1 liter in 30 minutes) the specific gravity should be _____ or less within the next 3 hours.

22. The _____ _____ test is specific for the diagnosis of renal tubular acidosis (RTA). The urine pH should be _____ or less in the 5-day test.

23. The _____ _____ test is used to determine the proper dietary intake of sodium, especially in a patient with "salt-losing" nephritis. A negative sodium balance is most frequently found in patients with renal disorders primarily involving the (a) tubules or (b) glomerulus.

Directions: Circle the letter preceding each item that correctly completes the statement. Only one answer is correct, with exceptions noted.

24. The normal pH range of the urine is:
a. 7.0–14.0 b. 6.0–12.0 c. 4.5–8.0 d. 3.0–6.0

25. The most clinically useful test for the measurement of the glomerular filtration rate is:
a. Urea clearance b. Uric acid clearance
d. Creatinine clearance d. PSP excretion

26. The following foods tend to produce an acidic urine (more than one answer may be correct):
a. Meat b. Vegetables c. Cranberry juice, prunes d. Milk

27. The following data were obtained from a creatinine clearance test on a patient: 24-hour urine volume = 1440 ml; urine creatinine level = 50 mg/100 ml; plasma creatinine level = 2 mg/100 ml. The creatinine clearance (uncorrected for body surface area) is:
a. 100 ml/min b. 1440 ml/min c. 25 ml/min
d. 36,000 ml/min

28. At the usual rate of decrease with aging, the GFR in a 90-year-old man would be about:
a. 25 percent of normal b. 50 percent of normal
c. 75 percent of normal d. 100 percent of normal

Directions: Answer the following questions on a separate sheet of paper.

29. Name the most common abnormal constituents of the urine sediment.

30. When is bacteriuria significant? List proper conditions of urine collection and significant bacterial count.

31. Differentiate between an intravenous pyelogram (IVP) and a retrograde pyelogram. State the purpose of each.

32. List four reasons for performing a renal arteriogram.

33. Why is it not worthwhile to perform an IVP on a patient who is severely azotemic (BUN level greater than 70 mg/100 ml)?

34. Outline a plan of care for a patient after a renal arteriogram.

35. Outline a plan of care for a patient during and after a renal biopsy. What observations should be made?

Directions: Fill in the blanks with the correct words.

36. Four types of morphological renal investigations are:
    a. _____ examination of the urine sediment   b. _____ study of the urine   c. Renal _____, a method which reveals the shape, size, and position of the kidneys   d. Renal _____, a method which reveals the microscopic structure of the kidney

37. Hyaline casts are made up of coagulated _____ protein secreted by the _____ tubule.

38. Excessive excretion of casts in the urine is called _____ and usually means that there is an increased glomerular permeability to _____.

39. A _____ and _____ test is sometimes done to determine the best choice of an antibiotic for treating a urinary tract infection.

40. An abnormality seen on the IVP which is diagnostic of chronic pyelonephritis is _____ of the calyces.

Directions: Circle the letter preceding each item that correctly answers each question or completes the statement. Only one answer is correct.

41. Casts are classified according to:
    a. Number of particles   b. Shape and constituents   c. Number of bacteria

42. Long-standing renal ischemia usually results in which condition of the kidney?
    a. Atrophy   b. Hypertrophy

43. Above what level of RBCs per high-power field would microscopic examination of urine sediment reveal significant hematuria?
    a. 100,000   b. 5000 to 9000   c. 1 to 2

44. Which of these statements with respect to renal biopsy is false?
    a. Death occurs in 1 percent of patients.   b. The procedure is dangerous in patients who are uncooperative.   c. Postbiopsy hematuria occurs in 5 percent of patients.   d. During the procedure the patient lies in a prone position on a sandbag.

Directions: Match the renal disease in col. B to the type of cast most frequently seen in the urine sediment in col. A.

Column A

45. ____ Broad granular casts

46. ____ Red blood cell casts

47. ____ Leukocyte casts

48. ____ Fatty casts and oval fat bodies

Column B

a. Pyelonephritis

b. Nephrotic syndrome

c. Advanced renal disease

d. Active glomerulonephritis

Directions: Match the radiologic technique in col. B to its description or application in col. A.

Column A

49. ____ Used to detect vesicoureteral reflux

50. ____ No radiation hazard involved; fluid-filled cysts can be distinguished from solid tumors

51. ____ Uses radioisotopes; useful for evaluation of renal transplant

52. ____ Image reveals serial "slices" of the body

Column B

a. Computerized tomography

b. Voiding cystourethrogram

c. Ultrasonography

d. Radionuclide imaging

CHRONIC RENAL FAILURE

OBJECTIVES

At the completion of this chapter you should be able to:

1. Differentiate between acute and chronic renal failure.
2. List the three primary structures involved in the kidney in chronic renal disease.
3. Describe the three stages in the natural history of progressive renal failure.
4. Explain why nocturia and polyuria are often early symptoms of chronic renal failure.
5. Describe anatomic changes in chronic renal disease which may alter renal function.
6. Describe the intact nephron hypothesis and give the supporting evidence for this theory.
7. Explain why the original cause of end-stage renal disease may be difficult to determine.
8. List the four leading causes of end-stage renal disease.
9. Name the most common infecting organism in urinary tract infections and explain how it may reach the kidney.
10. Describe the urinary tract defense mechanisms against infection.
11. Describe nine factors which may predispose to urinary tract infection and chronic pyelonephritis.
12. Differentiate between symptomatic and asymptomatic bacteriuria as a cause of chronic pyelonephritis.
13. Compare the sex distribution, clinical features, and gross and microscopic changes in the kidney in acute and chronic pyelonephritis.
14. Explain the principles of treatment of acute pyelonephritis.
15. Delineate controversial issues concerning the etiology of chronic pyelonephritis.
16. Define *glomerulonephritis.*
17. Explain why confusion exists in the classification and separation of the various types of glomerulonephritis.
18. Distinguish between diffuse, focal, and local glomerulonephritis.
19. Discuss the distinguishing features and the natural history of the broad clinical forms of diffuse glomerulonephritis.

20. Describe a classic case of acute poststreptococcal glomerulonephritis (age group commonly affected, specific organisms involved, presenting features, treatment, and prognosis).

21. Describe the sequence of events that results in glomerular injury following an antigen-antibody reaction along the basement membrane.

22. Describe the pathogenesis of the hypertension, edema, hematuria, albuminuria, and urinary casts in acute poststreptococcal glomerulonephritis.

23. Differentiate between the two distinct immune mechanisms involved in diffuse glomerulonephritis.

24. Describe the significance of epithelial crescent formation.

25. Describe the gross and microscopic changes in end-stage kidney disease.

26. Describe four histologic types of glomerulonephritis associated with the nephrotic syndrome (population affected, morphology, treatment, prognosis).

27. Describe the nephrotic syndrome (clinical features, physiologic disturbances, causes, treatment).

28. Describe the relation between hypertension and chronic renal failure.

29. Distinguish between benign and malignant essential hypertension (rate of progress, target organs, clinical signs and symptoms, arterial lesions).

30. Define *nephrosclerosis*.

31. Explain the importance of the early diagnosis of renal artery stenosis.

32. Discuss the relation of connective tissue disorders to renal disease.

33. Relate the histologic changes in lupus nephritis to prognosis and compare the histologic changes with those seen in primary glomerulonephritis.

34. Describe polyarteritis nodosa and scleroderma (pathogenesis, population affected, renal lesions).

35. Compare renal tubular acidosis and polycystic disease of the kidneys (heredity, forms of the disease and population affected, renal lesions or pathophysiology, clinical features, treatment, prognosis).

36. Describe diabetic nephropathy.

37. Explain the importance of gout, hyperparathyroidism, and amyloidosis to renal failure.

38. List three reasons why the kidney is vulnerable to the hazards of drug or chemical toxicity.

39. Describe the characteristic renal changes and presenting clinical features that may result from chronic analgesic abuse with phenacetin.

40. Describe the pathogenesis of lead nephropathy.

The purpose of this chapter is to give an overview of the course of deterioration in progressive renal failure, its general pathophysiology, and its causes.

Renal failure is usually divided into two broad categories—chronic and acute. Chronic renal failure is a progressive, slow development of renal failure, usually over a period of years, as contrasted with acute renal failure, which develops over a period of days or a few weeks. In both cases the kidneys lose their ability to maintain the volume and composition of the body fluids under conditions of normal dietary intake. Although the terminal functional disability is similar in the two types of renal failure, acute renal failure has some unique features and is discussed separately in Chap. 45.

Chronic renal failure follows a great number of conditions which devastate the nephron mass of the kidney. The majority of these conditions involve diffuse, bilateral disease of the renal parenchyma, although obstructive lesions of the urinary tract may also lead to chronic renal failure. In the beginning, some renal diseases primarily involve the glomerulus (glomerulonephritis), while others primarily involve the renal tubules (pyelonephritis or polycystic kidney disease) or may interfere with blood perfusion to the renal parenchyma (nephrosclerosis). In all cases, however, if the disease process is progressive, the entire nephron is destroyed and is replaced by scar tissue. The individual features of the various parenchymal renal diseases are discussed later in this chapter.

Despite the diversity of causes, the clinical features of chronic renal failure are remarkably similar, for progressive renal failure may be explained simply as a deficiency in the total number of functioning nephrons,

and a fairly fixed combination of disturbances is inevitable.

OVERVIEW: CLINICAL COURSE OF CHRONIC RENAL FAILURE

An overview of the general course of chronic renal failure may be obtained by looking at the relation of the creatinine clearance and glomerular filtration rate (GFR), as a percentage of the normal, to the serum creatinine and blood urea nitrogen (BUN) levels as the nephron mass is progressively destroyed by chronic renal disease (Fig. 42-1).

The general course of progressive renal failure may be divided into three stages (designated as I, II, and III in Fig. 42-1). The first stage is called *decreased renal reserve*. During this stage the serum creatinine and BUN levels are normal, and the patient is asymptomatic. Impairment of renal function may be detected only by imposition of severe demands on the kidney, such as a prolonged urine concentration test, or by careful testing of the GFR.

The second stage in the progression is called *renal insufficiency,* when more than 75 percent of the functioning tissue has been destroyed (GFR is 25 percent of normal). At this point the BUN level is just beginning to rise above the normal range. The rise in BUN concentration is variable, depending on the dietary intake of protein (compare the BUN graphs for a low and normal protein intake). Serum creatinine level also begins to rise above normal during this stage. The azotemia is

FIGURE 42-1

The relationship of the blood urea nitrogen (BUN) and serum creatinine levels to the glomerular filtration rate during the three stages of progressive renal failure. Note that a low protein diet delays azotemia.

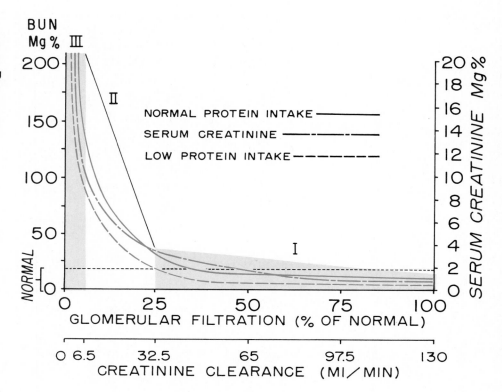

generally mild unless, for example, the patient is stressed by infection, heart failure, or dehydration. It is also during the stage of renal insufficiency that the symptoms of nocturia and polyuria (caused by impaired concentrating ability) begin to appear. These symptoms occur in response to stress and sudden changes in food or fluid intake. The patient usually takes little note of these symptoms, so they may be revealed only by careful questioning. *Nocturia* (urinating at night) is defined as persistent nocturnal output of 700 ml or having to get up more than once to void during the night. Nocturia is due to loss of the normal diurnal pattern of concentrating urine to a greater degree at night. The ratio of day to night urine is normally 3:1 or 4:1. Of course, nocturia may occasionally occur in response to anxiety or to a high fluid intake, especially of tea, coffee, or beer taken just before retiring. *Polyuria* means a persistent increase in the volume of urine. Normal urine output is about 1500 ml a day and varies considerably with fluid intake. The polyuria of renal insufficiency is usually greater in diseases which primarily affect the tubules, though it is generally moderate and rarely exceeds 3 liters a day.

The third and final stage of progressive renal failure is called *end-stage renal failure* or *uremia*. End-stage renal failure occurs when about 90 percent of the nephron mass has been destroyed, or only about 200,000 nephrons remain intact. The GFR is 10 percent of normal, and the creatinine clearance may be 5 to 10 ml a minute or even less. At this point, the serum creatinine and BUN levels rise sharply in response to small decrements in the GFR. During end-stage renal failure the patient begins to suffer severe symptoms as the kidneys are no longer able to maintain fluid and electrolyte homeostasis in the body. The urine becomes isoosmotic with the plasma at a fixed specific gravity of 1.010. The patient usually becomes oliguric (urine output less than 500 ml a day) because of glomerular failure even though the renal tubules may have been initially affected by the disease process. The complex of biochemical changes and symptoms which is called the *uremic syndrome* affects every system in the body and is discussed in detail in Chap. 43. In end-stage renal failure, unless the patient receives treatment in the form of dialysis or renal transplantation, death will surely follow.

Although the clinical course of chronic renal disease has been divided into three stages, in practice there are no sharp divisions between the stages. The hyperbolic shape of the graph of azotemia plotted against GFR reflects this continuous but slowly accelerating course.

General pathophysiology of chronic renal failure

Two theoretical approaches are generally offered to account for the impaired function of the kidneys in chronic renal failure. The traditional point of view is that all the nephron units are diseased to varying degrees and that specific parts of the nephron concerned with particular functions may be destroyed or their structure altered. For example, organic lesions of the medulla disrupting the anatomic arrangement of the loop of Henle and vasa recta or the chloride pump in the ascending limb would interfere with countercurrent multiplication and exchange. The second approach, known as the *Bricker hypothesis* or *intact nephron hypothesis*, maintains that nephrons, when diseased, are totally destroyed. The remaining intact nephrons behave normally. Uremia results when the total number of nephrons is so reduced that fluid and electrolyte balance can no longer be maintained. The intact nephron hypothesis is most useful in explaining the orderly pattern of functional adaptation in progressive renal disease, i.e., the ability to maintain a balance of body water and electrolytes in spite of a marked decrease in the GFR.

The sequence of events in the general pathophysiology of progressive renal failure may be outlined in terms of the intact nephron hypothesis. As chronic renal disease advances, the amount of solute which must be excreted by the kidney in order to maintain body homeostasis does not change, although there is a progressive reduction in the number of nephrons performing this function. Two important adaptations occur in the kidney in response to the threat of fluid and electrolyte imbalance. The remaining nephrons hypertrophy in an attempt to carry the entire workload of the kidneys (Fig. 42-2). There is an increase in filtration rate, solute load, and tubular reabsorption in each individual nephron even though the GFR for the entire nephron mass of the kidneys is decreased below normal. This adaptive mechanism is successful in maintaining body fluid and electrolyte balance down to very low levels of renal function. Finally, when about 75 percent of the nephron mass is destroyed, the filtration rate and solute load per nephron are so high that glomerular-tubular balance (balance between increased filtration and increased tubular reabsorption) can no longer be maintained (note that six out of the eight nephrons are destroyed in Fig. 42-2). There is a loss of flexibility in both the excretion and conservation of individual solutes and water. Modest dietary changes may upset the precarious balance, since the lower the GFR (which means fewer nephrons) the greater must be the change in excretion rate per nephron. Loss of the ability to concentrate or dilute causes the specific gravity of urine to become fixed at 1.010, or 285 mOsm (the concentration of plasma) and accounts for the symptoms of polyuria and nocturia. For example, a person on a normal diet excretes about 600 mOsm of solute each day. If that person is incapable of

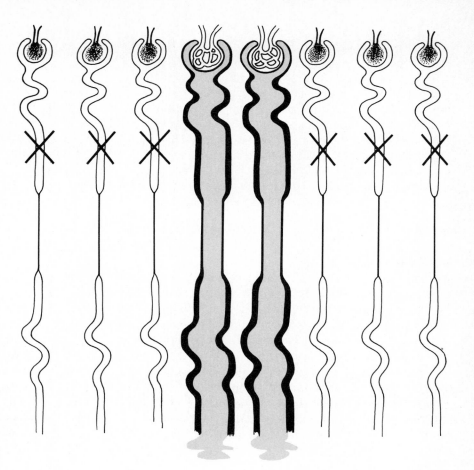

FIGURE 42-2
Diagram illustrating the intact nephron hypothesis. As chronic renal disease advances and nephrons are progressively destroyed, the remaining intact nephrons hypertrophy in an attempt to carry on the entire workload of the kidney. Solute load per nephron is increased, resulting in osmotic diuresis, i.e., rise in urine flow and reduction in concentration. (Modified from Netter.)

concentrating urine from the normal plasma osmolality of 285 mOsm, then there is an obligatory loss of 2 liters of water with the 600 mOsm solute excretion (285 mOsm per liter) regardless of water intake. In response to the same solute load and water deprivation, the normal person could concentrate urine to about four times the plasma concentration and thus excrete a small volume of concentrated urine. As the GFR progresses toward zero, it becomes increasingly important to regulate intake of water and solutes very precisely to accommodate the decreased flexibility in renal function.

The intact nephron hypothesis is supported by several experimental observations. Dr. Neal Bricker and his associates have shown that in patients with naturally occurring pyelonephritis and in dogs with experimental destruction of the kidney, the surviving nephrons hypertrophy and become more active than normal (Bricker, 1969). It is also known that when one kidney is removed in the healthy person, the remaining kidney undergoes hypertrophy and the capacity of this kidney approaches that formerly possessed by both.

It has also been demonstrated that normal kidneys under conditions of increased solute load behave much like the kidney in progressive renal failure, giving further support to the intact nephron hypothesis. The experimental data in Fig. 42-3 illustrate the concept that with progressive increases in solute load, the ability to concentrate the urine under conditions of water deprivation (upper curve) or to dilute the urine under conditions of high water intake (lower curve) is progressively lost. Both curves approach the specific gravity of 1.010 until the urine is isoosmotic with the plasma at 285 mOsm, so that a fixed specific gravity exists.

The above experimental conditions could be induced in a normal person by giving mannitol (an osmotic diuretic). The number 10 on the x axis is arbitrarily chosen to show that the kidneys are excreting 10 times the usual solute load. At this point each normal nephron is undergoing an osmotic diuresis with an obligatory loss of water. The kidney has lost its flexibility to either concentrate or dilute the urine from the plasma osmolality of 285 mOsm.

Similar events probably occur in the patient with progressive renal failure. The patient with 90 percent destruction of nephron mass is at the same point on the graph as the normal person with an induced solute load that is 10 times normal. The remaining 10 percent of the nephrons are forced to excrete 10 times the normal solute load and therefore lose their flexibility; they are unable to compensate properly by the usual changes in tubular reabsorption for excesses or deficiencies of sodium or water.

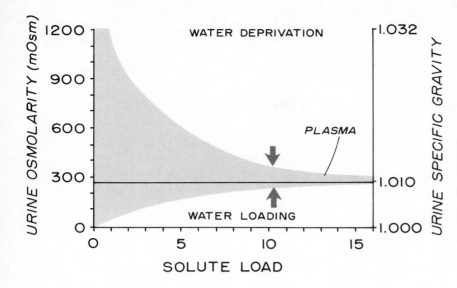

FIGURE 42-3

The response of normal kidneys to an increasing solute load under conditions of water loading and deprivation. Ability to concentrate or dilute the urine is progressively lost as the solute load increases. Urine specific gravity becomes fixed near 1.010 (285 mOsm). (Modified from A. Gordon and M. H. Maxwell, "Reversible Uremia," *Hospital Medicine*, January 1967.)

CAUSES OF CHRONIC RENAL FAILURE

Chronic renal failure is a clinical state of progressive, irreversible renal damage arising from many different causes. The most common causes of chronic renal failure may be divided into the eight classes listed in Table 42-1. No attempt is made to be all-inclusive, and only selected examples are listed under each class. These diseases are discussed in this chapter but not necessarily in

the same order in which they appear in the table. It should be emphasized that while the early stages of renal disease may be quite variable, the end stages are remarkably similar, and in many cases the original cause cannot be identified. According to the 1975 report of the American College of Surgeons/National Institutes of Health, Organ Transplant Registry, the leading causes of end-stage renal disease (in transplant recipients) are glomerulonephritis (56.0 percent), pyelonephritis (13.1 percent), polycystic disease (5.4 percent), and hypertensive nephrosclerosis (4.9 percent).* There is also great variation in the rate of progression of these chronic renal diseases. The course terminating in end-stage renal disease may vary from 2 or 3 months to 30 or 40 years.

Urinary tract infections and pyelonephritis

Urinary tract infection is a common condition and usually implies pyelonephritis or cystitis. *Cystitis* is an infection of the bladder; *pyelonephritis* is an infection involving the renal pelvis and interstitium. Pyelonephritis may be acute or chronic. While both cystitis and acute pyelonephritis are usually benign, they may lead to chronic pyelonephritis and renal failure. Obstruction of the urinary tract is an important predisposing factor in

TABLE 42-1

CLASSIFICATION OF THE CAUSES OF CHRONIC RENAL FAILURE

Disease classifications	Disease
Infections	Chronic pyelonephritis
Inflammatory diseases	Glomerulonephritis
Hypertensive vascular disease	Benign nephrosclerosis Malignant nephrosclerosis Renal artery stenosis
Connective tissue disorders	Systemic lupus erythematosis Polyarteritis nodosa Progressive systemic sclerosis
Congenital and hereditary disorders	Polycystic kidney disease Renal tubular acidosis
Metabolic disorders	Diabetes mellitus Gout Hyperparathyroidism Amyloidosis
Toxic nephropathy	Analgesic abuse Lead nephropathy
Obstructive nephropathy	Upper urinary tract—calculi, neoplasms, retroperitoneal fibrosis Lower urinary tract—prostatic hypertrophy, urethral stricture, congenital anomalies of the bladder neck and urethra

*Figures may overrepresent glomerulonephritis and underrepresent pyelonephritis since patients with pyelonephritis may have been rejected more often as unsuitable for transplant. In the United States in 1964, the Committee on Chronic Dialysis ("Gottschalk Report") reported the following distribution of primary renal diseases: nephritis and nephrosis 45 percent, infections of the kidney 36 percent, and polycystic disease 15 percent. In a 1967 report by Hood in Sweden the diseases responsible for death in uremia were nonobstructive pyelonephritis (includes patients with papillary necrosis in which analgesic abuse may have played a role) 42 percent, chronic glomerulonephritis 21 percent, diabetic renal disease 18 percent, obstructive pyelonephritis 7 percent, polycystic kidney 5 percent, and malignant hypertension 3 percent (Strauss and Welt, 1971, p. 235).

recurrent or chronic infections. Chronic pyelonephritis is the second leading cause of end-stage renal disease and is theoretically preventable by the control of urinary tract infections. Unfortunately, many chronic urinary tract infections involving the kidney may be silent and asymptomatic until irreversible renal damage has occurred.

Etiology and pathogenesis

The most common infecting organism of the urinary tract is *Escherichia coli,* which accounts for more than 80 percent of the cases. *E. coli* is a normal inhabitant of the colon. Other infecting organisms often include the *Proteus, Klebsiella, Pseudomonas,* enterococcus, and *Staphylococcus* groups. In most cases the organisms gain access to the bladder via the urethra. The infection, beginning as cystitis, may remain confined to the bladder or may ascend via the ureter to the kidney. Organisms may also reach the kidney via the bloodstream or lymphatics, but this is believed to be uncommon. The bladder and upper urethra are normally sterile, although bacteria are present in the lower urethra. The normal urinary tract can rid itself of bacteria before they have a chance to invade the mucosa by the flushing action of urine flow. Other defense mechanisms include the antibacterial effect of the urethral mucosa, the bactericidal properties of prostatic fluid in the male, and the phagocytic properties of the bladder epithelium. In spite of these defenses, many urinary infections do occur and are believed to be related to certain predisposing factors listed in Table 42-2.

Obstruction of the urinary outflow proximal to the bladder can result in the accumulation of fluid under pressure in the renal pelvis and ureter. This alone is enough to cause severe atrophy of the renal parenchyma. It is a condition called *hydronephrosis.* In addition, obstruction below the level of the bladder is often associated with vesicoureteral reflux (see later) and infection of the kidney. Common causes of obstruction are renal or ureteral scarring, calculi, neoplasms, prostatic hypertrophy (common in males over 60 years), congenital anomalies of the bladder neck and urethra, and urethral stricture.

Females have a much higher incidence of urinary tract infections and pyelonephritis than males, presumably because of a shorter urethra and its proximity to the anus and consequent fecal contamination. Epidemiologic studies have shown that significant bacteriuria (10^5 organisms per milliliter of urine) exists in 1 to 4 percent of schoolgirls, 5 to 10 percent of women of childbearing age, and about 25 percent of women more than 60 years of age (Papper, 1978, p. 264). Only a few of these persons have clinical symptoms of urinary tract infection, and the relation of significant bacteriuria to the development of chronic pyelonephritis is not known. Infection in the male is rare, and when it occurs, it is usually related to obstruction.

It has been known for some time that hydroureter and hydronephrosis, most marked on the right, always occur during pregnancy and persist for some time afterward. The dilatation is attributed partly to muscular relaxation caused by the high progesterone levels and partly to obstruction of the ureters by the enlarged uterus. About 5 to 7 percent of the women so affected have asymptomatic bacteriuria (Norden and Kass, 1968; Whalley, 1967). In a controlled study, Kass (1960) found that 42 percent of a placebo-treated group of women ($n = 48$) who had asymptomatic bacteriuria during early pregnancy developed pyelonephritis later during the pregnancy or during the first few weeks post partum, while none of the group ($n = 42$) treated with antibiotics for the bacteriuria developed symptomatic infection. Although the issue is not resolved yet, there is evidence suggesting that bacteriuria may also be associated with hypertensive disorders during pregnancy and premature births (Berl and Schrier, 1980).

When the renal pelvis becomes distended with newly formed urine, the smooth muscle contracts, propelling a bolus of urine into the ureter. Dilatation of the ureter then initiates a peristaltic wave which carries the urine into the bladder. Urinary flow is normally unidirectional, from the renal pelvis to the bladder, and reverse flow (reflux) is prevented by the *ureterovesicular valve* (located where the ureter is implanted into the bladder). The action of this one-way valve is vitally important in preventing backflow during the act of micturition when intravesicular pressure rises, since transmission of this pressure can damage the kidney directly. *Vesicoureteral reflux* (VUR) is defined as retrograde flow of urine from the bladder into the ureter, especially during micturition. The presence of VUR may be detected by injecting contrast material into the bladder

TABLE 42-2

PREDISPOSING FACTORS IN THE DEVELOPMENT OF URINARY TRACT INFECTIONS AND CHRONIC PYELONEPHRITIS

Obstruction of urinary outflow

Sex, age

Pregnancy

Vesicoureteral reflux

Instrumentation (especially indwelling catheters)

Neurogenic bladder

Chronic analgesic abuse (phenacetin)

Renal disease

Metabolic disturbances (diabetes, gout, urinary calculi)

through a catheter until the bladder is distended to the point at which the patient has the urge to void. Serial radiographs are taken with the bladder distended and during and after the act of voiding. The entire procedure is known as a *voiding cystourethrography*. VUR has been associated with congenital malformation of the intravesicular ureter, obstruction of the bladder outlet (bladder neck or urethra) and cystitis. Vesicoureteral reflux has been demonstrated in a high proportion of patients, especially children with recurrent urinary tract infections, and appears to be the mechanism by which organisms ascend to the kidney.

Urethral and ureteric catheterization and cystoscopy are common forms of instrumentation by which infection is introduced into the bladder or kidney. About 2 percent of simple, single bladder catheterizations result in infection. There is a 98 percent incidence of infection within 48 hours when an indwelling catheter is placed unless meticulous attention is directed to keeping a closed drainage system. Even when the system is closed, the urine is sterile for only about 5 to 7 days. These facts indicate that catheterization is a procedure to be avoided if possible

The function of the bladder is to serve as a distensible reservoir for urine from which the urine is evacuated at suitable intervals. The innervation of the bladder consists in a reflex arc at the S2 to S4 level of the spinal cord whose function is modified by sensory and motor connections to the higher centers in the brain. The act of micturition (urination) consists in the coordinated contraction of the detrussor muscle (smooth muscle of the bladder wall), abdominal wall, and muscles of the pelvic floor; fixation of the chest and diaphragm; and relaxation of the internal and external sphincter muscles. Accordingly, both autonomic and voluntary activities are involved. Contraction of the detrussor muscle is reflex (stimulated when the bladder contains about 300 ml of urine), and this reflex contraction may be both inhibited and facilitated by supraspinal portions of the nervous system under voluntary control. Interference with efferent or afferent limbs of the reflex arc or with efferent or afferent pathways connecting the sacral spinal cord to the central facilitory or inhibitory mechanisms can disrupt normal micturition; these conditions are referred to as *neurogenic bladder*.

Lapides (1976) identifies five types of neurogenic bladder dysfunction, each associated with a particular neural lesion: (1) uninhibited neurogenic bladder, (2) reflex neurogenic bladder, (3) autonomous neurogenic bladder, (4) sensory paralytic neurogenic bladder, and (5) motor paralytic neurogenic bladder.

Uninhibited neurogenic bladder involves a defect of the corticoregulatory tract. This condition is seen frequently in patients who have lesions involving the cerebral cortex, as in cerebral vascular accidents, or those who have disseminated cord lesions involving the corticoregulatory tracts, as in multiple sclerosis. The un-

inhibited neurogenic bladder resembles that of the infant. The patient is aware of a sudden desire to urinate as the bladder fills but may be unable to inhibit the desire to void even though the situation may not be appropriate. The uninhibited neurogenic bladder dysfunction is the most frequently encounter in clinical practice. In children the upper motor neuron dysfunction is manifested in persistent diurnal and nocturnal diuresis beyond the age of 2 to 3 years. Uninhibited neurogenic bladder dysfunction may be associated with recurrent urinary tract infection, especially in young girls. The patient may be able to suppress urination by voluntarily contracting the striated muscles around the urethra but is unable to control the uninhibited bladder contractions. The resultant rise in intravesicular pressure causes ischemia of the bladder wall and a lowering of local tissue immunity, with consequent infection.

Reflex neurogenic bladder results from disconnection of the sacral reflex arc from higher centers, as in cord injury or transection above the S2 level. All bladder sensation is lost, and emptying occurs reflexly whenever intravesicular pressure rises above a critical level. Emptying of the bladder is incomplete because of the lack of motor input from higher centers, and there is vesicoureteral reflux because of the high intravesicular pressures. Both the VUR and residual urine predispose the patient with spinal cord injury to cystitis and pyelonephritis.

Autonomous neurogenic bladder results from destruction of both limbs of the bladder reflex arc, as by sacral or cauda equina lesions (e.g., gunshot wound, abdominal-perineal resection surgery, neoplasia, and congenital anomalies such as spina bifida and myelomeningocele). Patients with this type of lesion can neither perceive bladder fullness nor initiate urination in the normal fashion. However, they may learn to pass their urine by voluntarily straining and manual pressure over the suprapubic region (Credé's maneuver).

Sensory paralytic neurogenic bladder results from lesions of the sensory limb of the bladder reflex arc, as in diabetic neuropathy or multiple sclerosis. There is a gradual loss of bladder sensation, infrequent urination, and overdistension. Overdistension causes the bladder muscle to lose its tone, so that emptying is incomplete and there is residual urine.

Motor paralytic neurogenic bladder involves interruption of the motor limb of the bladder reflex arc, commonly associated with poliomyelitis, tumor, or trauma. The sensation of bladder fullness is intact, but the patient has either partial or total inability to initiate urination. Painful overdistension may result, requiring catheterization and drainage.

The pathogenic mechanisms predisposing to urinary tract infection in neurogenic bladder dysfunction include ischemia of the bladder wall from overdistention, which lessens resistance to bacterial invasion; residual urine, which provides a medium for bacterial growth; and VUR associated with increased intravesicular pressures. The use of catheters and urinary drainage are additional predisposing factors.

Chronic phenacetin abuse alone may cause chronic interstitial nephritis (see "Analgesic Abuse," later in this chapter), but it also predisposes to chronic pyelonephritis. Various underlying renal diseases increase susceptibility to infection and pyelonephritis. Finally, metabolic disturbances such as diabetes, gout, and renal stones are often complicated by renal infection.

It is not known with certainty what proportion of the cases of chronic bacterial pyelonephritis can be explained on the basis of these predisposing factors. It is clear, however, that infection beginning in the lower urinary tract can ascend to the kidney. Various studies have shown that the renal medulla has unique characteristics which favor the survival of bacteria. This increased susceptibility to infection is apparently due to the high ammonia content and hyperosmolality, which interfere with host defense mechanisms such as leukocyte migration, phagocytosis, and complement activity. In addition, some bacteria when in a hyperosmotic environment enter a spherocyte or protoplast form (bacteria with defective cell walls) in which they become resistant to antibiotics and can revert later to the parent form.

Acute pyelonephritis

The clinical features of acute pyelonephritis are usually quite characteristic. The patient is a woman in about 90 percent of the cases. There is an abrupt onset of fever, chills, malaise, back pain, tenderness to palpation over the costovertebral area, leukocytosis, pyuria, and bacteriuria. These symptoms are often preceded by dysuria, urgency, and frequency, indicating that the infection began in the lower urinary tract. The finding of leukocyte casts indicates that the infection is in the kidney.

Figure 42-4 illustrates the gross and microscopic appearance of the kidney in acute pyelonephritis. The kidney is swollen, with multiple small abscesses on the surface. On cross section, abscesses appear as yellowish gray streaks in the pyramids and cortex. Microscopically, numerous polymorphonuclear leukocytes (PMNs) are found within the tubules (arrow) and in the interstitium surrounding the tubules. Segments of the tubules are destroyed, and this leukocytic material is flushed out into the urine as casts.

E. coli is the most common infecting organism in acute, uncomplicated pyelonephritis. Of patients with this infection, 90 percent respond to antibiotic therapy while the remaining 10 percent may have acute recurrent infections or persistent asymptomatic bacteriuria. When acute pyelonephritis is complicated by obstruction, recurrent or persistent bacteriuria occurs in 50 to 80 percent of patients within 2 years. It is not known with certainty how many of these patients will develop significant renal damage or how long the process might take. Treatment is directed toward appropriate antibacterial therapy, correction of predisposing factors, and careful long-term follow-up, with urine cultures at intervals to ensure that the urine is sterile.

Chronic pyelonephritis

There are many controversial issues among the authorities concerning the causes of chronic pyelonephritis, since about half the patients have no recallable history of urinary tract infection, and more than half of those with established chronic pyelonephritis have negative urine cultures. Nevertheless, many believe that chronic pyelonephritis develops from inadequately treated or recurrent pyelonephritis. Explanations given to account for these facts are that recurrent infection may be subclinical, and bacteria (which can convert to the protoplast form) may be expelled into the urine only intermittently. Evidence against bacterial infection as a cause include the fact that the sex incidence of chronic pyelonephritis is about equal although acute urinary tract infection is probably 10 times more frequent in females. Furthermore, bacterial infection is a common complication of other renal diseases, and nonbacterial agents such as phenacetin produce similar lesions.

In contrast to acute pyelonephritis, the clinical features of chronic pyelonephritis are quite vague. The diagnosis is often made when a patient presents with symptoms of chronic renal insufficiency or hypertension, or proteinuria may be discovered in a routine examination. In some cases there is a documented history of urinary tract infections dating from childhood. In other cases careful questioning may reveal a history of vague symptoms of dysuria, frequency, and sometimes loin pain. Many patients are asymptomatic until the disease is advanced. Typical findings in chronic pyelonephritis include intermittent bacteriuria and white blood cells or white cell casts in the urine. Proteinuria is usually minimal. Because chronic pyelonephritis is chiefly a medullary interstitial disease, the concentrating ability of the kidney is affected early in its course, before there is a significant decrease in the glomerular filtration rate. Consequently polyuria, nocturia, and urine with a low specific gravity are prominent early symptoms. In addition, many patients have a tendency to lose salt in the

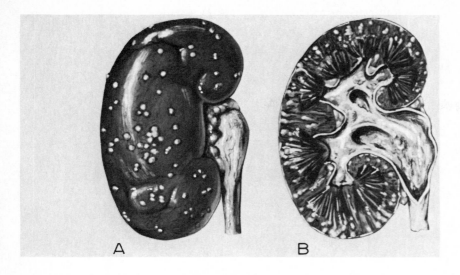

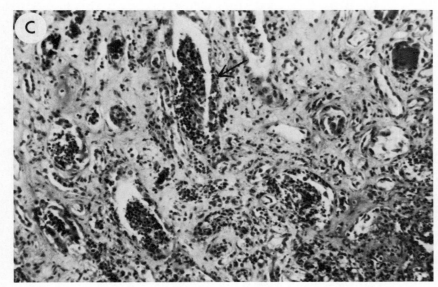

FIGURE 42-4

Gross and microscopic appearance of The kidney in acute pyelonephritis. (A) The kidney is swollen with multiple abscesses on the surface. (B) Abscesses appear as yellowish gray streaks on the cross section. (C) Histologically, many PMNs appear in the interstitium and within the tubules. (Art by Judy Simon, Dept. of Medical and Biological Illustrations, University of Michigan.)

urine. About half the patients may develop hypertension. Azotemia is common in the course of chronic pyelonephritis, but advancement to renal failure is usually only slowly progressive.

The IVP reveals clubbing of the calyces, a thinned cortex, and small, irregular-shaped kidneys which are usually asymmetric (see Fig. 41-9B). Figure 42-5 illustrates the pathologic changes in chronic pyelonephritis. The surface of the kidney is coarsely granular, with U-shaped depressions (Fig. 42-5A), subcapsular scars, and a dilated and fibrosed pelvis; and calyces are seen on the cross section (Fig. 42-5B). Microscopic examination of tissue sections reveals characteristic parenchymal changes: many chronic inflammatory cells consisting of plasma cells and lymphocytes (dark-staining dots) are scattered throughout the interstitium. The three glomeruli are intact but surrounded by many tubules which are small and atrophied or dilated. There is an area of interstitial fibrosis near the glomerulus (arrow,

Fig. 42-5C). Large areas of thyroidization (having the appearance of thyroid gland tissue) are seen, consisting of dilated tubules lined with flattened epithelial cells and filled with glassy-appearing casts (Fig. 42-5D).

Glomerulonephritis

Most deaths from renal failure are due to chronic glomerulonephritis. This disease also accounts for the greatest number of patients who enter chronic dialysis and transplant programs.

Glomerulonephritis is a bilateral inflammatory disease of the kidneys which begins in the glomerulus and is manifested by proteinuria and/or hematuria. Although the lesions are primarily glomerular, entire nephrons may eventually be destroyed, leading to chronic renal failure. The original disease described by Richard Bright in 1827 *(Bright's disease)* is now known to be a collection of many diseases of different causes

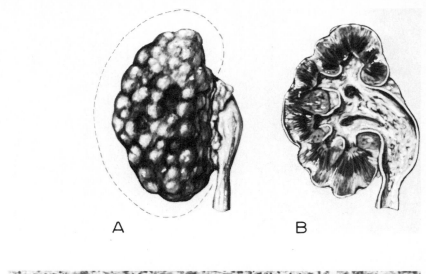

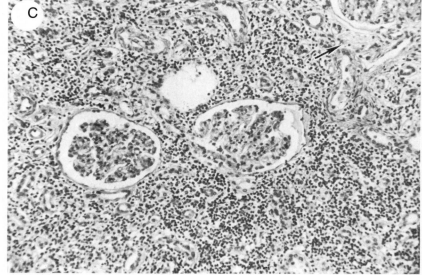

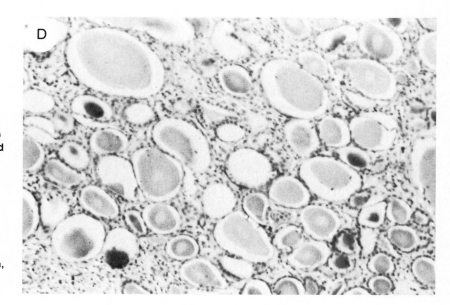

FIGURE 42-5
Gross and microscopic appearance of the kidney in chronic pyelonephritis. (A) Coarsely granular surface with U-shaped depressions. (B) Thinning of the cortex, subcapsular scars, dilated, fibrosed pelvis and calyces. (C) Chronic inflammatory cells throughout interstitium, small, atrophied tubules, and an area of interstitial fibrosis *(arrow).* (D) Thyroid-gland appearance due to dilated tubules containing glassy-looking casts. (Art by Judy Simon, Dept. of Medical and Biological Illustrations, University of Michigan.)

(most of which are unknown), although immune responses seem to be implicated in several forms of glomerulonephritis.

In recent years, knowledge of the pathological changes in renal disease has been greatly expanded by renal biopsy studies using light, immunofluorescent, and electron microscopy. As knowledge has expanded, new categories have emerged based on a greater ability to define the nature of renal lesions. Numerous attempts have been made to separate and classify the various types of glomerulonephritis by relating histologic and clinical features. Unfortunately, the various categories are not exclusive. This overlap is understandable, since the kidney has only a limited number of morphological and functional responses. To add to this confusion, many systemic and metabolic disorders may, when there is renal involvement, have changes in the glomeruli that are indistinguishable from primary glomerulonephritis.

Table 42-3 lists the various ways in which glomerulonephritis is described and classified. This table will serve as a guide for the discussion in the remainder of this chapter and should be read before proceeding. It will be helpful for the reader to remember that the general term *glomerulonephritis* (GN) is commonly used to refer to a number of primary renal diseases predominantly affecting the glomeruli, but it is also used to refer to glomerular lesions which may or may not be the result of primary renal disease. For example, the renal lesion in systemic lupus erythematosis may be referred to as proliferative glomerulonephritis. The following discussion focuses on primary renal diseases which cause glomerulonephritis, although references are made to systemic diseases which cause similar lesions in the kidney. Systemic diseases causing renal injury are considered in more detail later in the chapter.

Acute glomerulonephritis

The classic case of acute glomerulonephritis follows a streptococcal infection of the throat or sometimes of the skin after a latent period of 1 to 2 weeks. The responsible organism is usually a type 12 or 4, group A, β-hemolytic streptococcus, rarely others. However, the streptococcus itself does not cause renal damage by infection. It is believed that antibodies are directed against a specific antigen which is a constituent of the specific streptococcal plasma membrane. An antigen-antibody complex is formed in the blood and circulates to the glomerulus, where it is mechanically trapped in the basement membrane. Complement is fixed, resulting in injury and inflammation which attracts PMNs and platelets to the damaged site. Phagocytosis and release of lysosomal enzymes also damage the endothelium and glomerular basement membrane (GBM). As a response to injury there is proliferation of endothelial

cells, then of mesangial cells, and later epithelial cells may increase as well. The resulting increased porosity of the glomerular capillary permits the escape of proteins and blood cells into the forming urine, causing proteinuria and hematuria. It is presumably these antigen-antibody-complement complexes which appear as subepithelial nodules (or epimembranous humps) on electron microscopy and as a granular, "lumpy-bumpy" pattern on immunofluorescent microscopy; by light microscopy the glomeruli appear swollen and hypercellular, with invasion of PMNs (Fig. 42-6).

Acute poststreptococcal glomerulonephritis (APSGN) most frequently affects children between the ages of 3 and 7 years, though adolescents and young adults are also affected. The ratio of males to females is about 2:1.

The common presenting features of APSGN include hematuria, proteinuria, oliguria, edema, and hypertension. Common symptoms associated with the onset are fatigue, anorexia, and sometimes fever, headache, nausea, and vomiting. Elevation of the antistreptolysin O (ASO) titer may indicate the presence of antibodies to streptococcal organisms. Serum complement levels may be low owing to depletion. This common finding gives further support to the hypothesis that the disease has an immune basis.

The major physiologic disturbances in APSGN are depicted on the diagram in Fig. 42-7. The GFR is usually depressed (though renal plasma flow is generally normal). Consequently the excretion of water, sodium, and nitrogenous substances may be decreased, resulting in edema and azotemia. Increased aldosterone may also play a role in sodium and water retention. Facial edema, particularly periorbital edema, is extremely common in the morning, though it may become more apparent in the lower extremities as the day progresses. The degree of edema usually depends on the severity of the glomerular inflammation, whether there is concomitant congestive heart failure, and how soon dietary salt is restricted.

Hypertension almost always occurs, though the rise in blood pressure may be only moderate. Whether the hypertension results from an expansion of the extracellular fluid (ECF) volume or from vasospasm is not clear.

Damage to the glomerular capillary tuft results in hematuria and albuminuria, as previously described. The urine may be grossly bloody or coffee-colored. Microscopic examination of the sediment reveals cylindruria (many casts), red blood cells (RBCs), and red cell casts. The latter establish the glomerular origin of the bleeding. The loss of protein is usually not great enough

TABLE 42-3

CLASSIFICATIONS OF GLOMERULONEPHRITIS

Classification	Description
1. Distribution	
a. Diffuse	Involves all the glomeruli; most common form results in chronic renal failure
b. Focal	Only a portion of the glomeruli are abnormal
c. Local	Only a part of the glomerular tuft is abnormal, such as a single capillary loop
2. Broad clinical forms of diffuse glomerulonephritis	
a. Acute	Classic, benign disorder which is nearly always preceded by a streptococcal infection and associated with immune-complex deposition in the glomerular basement membrane and proliferative cellular changes
b. Subacute	Rapidly progressive form of glomerulonephritis characterized by intense cellular proliferative changes that destroy the glomeruli and result in death from uremia within a few months from the onset
c. Chronic	Slowly progressive glomerulonephritis leading to sclerosing and obliterative changes in the glomeruli; small, contracted kidneys; and death from uremia. Entire course varies from 2 to 40 years
3. Pathogenetic immune mechanism and immunofluorescent pattern	
a. Immune-complex, granular	Antibody (Ab) to either exogenous or endogenous nonglomerular antigens (Ag) is involved in the formation of circulating Ab-Ag complexes which are passively trapped in the GBM. Complement fixation and the release of immunologic mediators results in glomerular injury; deposit is along epithelial surface and reveals a lumpy or granular pattern on immunofluorescent microscopy; associated with poststreptococcal GN, idiopathic membranous GN, and the GN of serum sickness, subacute bacterial endocarditis, malaria, and anaphylactoid purpura
b. Nephrotoxic (anti-GBM), linear	Antibodies form which react with the patient's own GBM as the antigen (anti-GBM or antikidney antibodies). True autoimmune disease in contrast to immune-complex GN, in which the GBM is like an innocent bystander; immune deposits are subendothelial and result in a ribbonlike linear pattern on immunofluorescence; associated with RPGN and Goodpasture's syndrome
4. Histologic pattern	
a. Minimal change	Also referred to as *lipoid nephrosis* or *foot-process disease*; glomeruli appear normal or nearly normal on light microscopy, while electron microscopy reveals fusion of the foot processes; only major form of GN without evidence of immunopathology; commonly presents as the nephrotic syndrome in children of 1 to 5 years; responds well to corticosteroid therapy; prognosis excellent
b. Proliferative change	Deposition of immunoglobulin, complement, and fibrin leads to proliferation of endothelial, mesangial, and epithelial cells; latter leads to crescent formation which may encircle and obliterate the glomerular tuft—ominous sign, common in RPGN and advanced CGN
c. Membranous change	Epimembranous deposit of immune material along GBM causing the GBM to thicken, but there is little or no inflammation or cellular proliferation, though the capillary lumen may eventually be obliterated; most common lesion in adults with the nephrotic syndrome; responds poorly to corticosteroid and immunosuppressive therapy; generally poor prognosis and slow progression to renal failure; membranous changes are also common in systemic nephritic diseases such as diabetes mellitus and systemic lupus erythematosis (SLE)
d. Membranoproliferative change	Also referred to as *mesangiocapillary, lobular,* or *hypocomplementemic* GN; immune complex material deposited between the GBM and endothelium, causing GBM thickening and proliferation of the mesangial cells and giving the glomerulus a lobular or "wire-loop" appearance on light microscopy; characterized by low serum complement level, hematuria, and the nephrotic syndrome; responds poorly to therapy, generally progresses slowly to renal failure
e. Focal glomerulonephritis	Proliferative or sclerosing lesions which occur at random throughout the kidneys (focal as opposed to diffuse), often affecting only part of the glomerular tuft (local); occurs during at least part of the course of SBE, SLE, polyarteritis nodosa, Goodpasture's syndrome, and purpura; idiopathic focal GN sometimes appears in children; prognosis good

TABLE 42-3 (continued)

Classification	Description
5. Clinical syndromes	
a. Acute nephritic syndrome	Acute nephritis of sudden onset, usually associated with poststreptococcal GN but can occur in many other renal diseases and as an acute exacerbation of CGN
b. Nephrotic syndrome	Clinical complex characterized by massive proteinuria (>3.5 g/day), hypoalbuminemia, edema, and hyperlipidemia. Occurs in many primary renal and systemic diseases; 50 percent of patients with CGN have it at least once
c. Persistent asymptomatic urine abnormalities	"Latent" stage in CGN, characterized by minimal proteinuria and/or hematuria but without symptoms; glomerular function relatively stable or may show slow progression ("silent azotemia")
d. Uremic syndrome	Symptomatic end-stage renal failure

Key: AGN, acute glomerulonephritis; GBM, glomerular basement membrane; GN, glomerulonephritis; CRF, chronic renal failure; CGN, chronic glomerulonephritis; SLE, systemic lupus erythematosis; SBE, subacute bacterial endocarditis; RPGN, rapidly progressive or subacute glomerulonephritis.

to cause hypoalbuminemia, and the nephrotic syndrome rarely occurs in APSGN. The urine specific gravity is usually high despite azotemia, a combination rarely occurring in renal diseases other than APSGN. This finding is explained by the fact that tubular function has been affected very little by the acute disease.

The usual treatment of APSGN is penicillin to eradicate any residual streptococcal infection, bed rest during the acute phase, sodium restriction in the presence of edema or signs of heart failure, and antihypertensive drugs if indicated. Corticosteroid drugs have no known beneficial effect in APSGN. Symptoms usually subside within days, although microscopic hematuria and proteinuria may persist for months. It is estimated that more than 90 percent of children have a complete recovery. The prognosis is less favorable for adults (30 to 50 percent). Death occurs in 2 to 5 percent of all patients during the acute phase. In the remainder of patients, the disease may advance to a rapidly progressive glomerulonephritis (RPGN) or a more slowly progressive chronic glomerulonephritis (CGN). In RPGN, death in uremia usually occurs within a few months, while the entire course may vary from 2 to 40 years in CGN.

The natural history of the various forms of diffuse glomerulonephritis is depicted in the diagram in Fig. 42-8. Contrary to popular belief, only a small percentage of the cases of RPGN and CGN have their origin in APSGN. The precipitating factors are usually unknown.

Although APSGN has been more clearly defined, it should be noted that an acute nephritic syndrome may be associated with many other diseases affecting the kidney [e.g., subacute bacterial endocarditis (SBE), malaria, anaphylactoid purpura, and the collagen diseases]. An acute nephritic syndrome may also occur during the course of CGN (Table 42-3).

Rapidly progressive glomerulonephritis

Rapidly progressive glomerulonephritis (formerly called *subacute*) is a term used to designate a fulminant renal disease with characteristic clinical and morphological features. There is hematuria, proteinuria, and rapidly progressive azotemia resulting in death within 2 years. At autopsy, the salient features are widespread parietal epithelial crescent formation and diffuse glomerular involvement. Goodpasture's syndrome, a rare disease most common in young men, is a good example of this type of disease. The onset may be insidious or acute and is associated with lung hemorrhage and hemoptysis. There is usually no preceding illness to suggest the origin of the autoimmune antibodies against the glomerular basement membrane which develop in the patient's blood. Subendothelial immune complex material is seen with electron microscopy, and a linear pattern of immunofluorescence suggests that a nephrotoxic immune mechanism is involved in the pathogenesis (Fig. 42-9). Immunoglobulin deposits have also been found along the basement membrane in the lung alveoli. There is no known treatment for this condition. The patient may be kept alive by hemodialysis but may die of lung hemorrhage.

Chronic glomerulonephritis

Chronic glomerulonephritis (CGN) is characterized by slow, progressive destruction of the glomeruli from long-standing glomerulonephritis. In most instances, CGN has no known relationship to APSGN and RPGN but appears to represent de novo disease. The onset tends to be insidious, and it is usually discovered late in its course when symptoms of renal insufficiency appear. According to the stage of the disease there may be polyuria or oliguria, proteinuria of varying

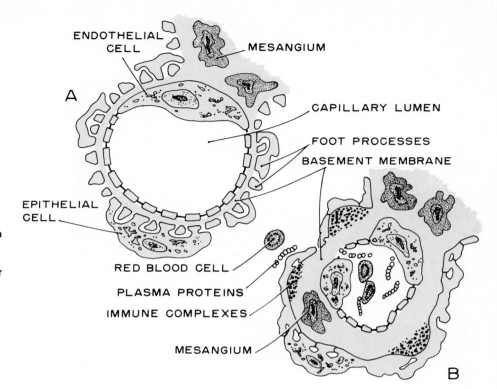

ENDOTHELIAL CELL

MESANGIUM

A

CAPILLARY LUMEN

FOOT PROCESSES
BASEMENT MEMBRANE

EPITHELIAL CELL

RED BLOOD CELL

PLASMA PROTEINS

IMMUNE COMPLEXES

MESANGIUM

B

FIGURE 42-6

Acute poststreptococcal glomerulonephritis. (A) Diagram of electron microscopy (EM) appearance of a single capillary loop of the glomerular tuft. (B) Diagram of EM appearance of subepithelial deposits of immune complex, thickened basement membrane, cellular proliferation, and damage to capillary. (*Continued on next page.*)

degrees, hypertension, progressive azotemia, and death in uremia.

In advanced CGN the kidneys are grossly contracted, sometimes weighing as little as 50 g, and the surface is granular. These changes are due to the loss of nephrons and to ischemia. Microscopically, most of the glomeruli are altered. There may be a mixture of membranous and proliferative changes and epithelial crescent formation. Eventually there is atrophy of the tubules, interstitial fibrosis, and thickening of the arterial walls. When marked damage to all structures has occurred, the organ is called an *end-stage kidney,* and it may be difficult to determine whether the original lesion was glomerular, interstitial and resulting from chronic pyelonephritis, or vascular (Fig. 42-10).

The nephrotic syndrome

Although many patients with CGN have persistent, asymptomatic proteinuria throughout the course of the disease, about 50 percent develop the nephrotic syndrome. The nephrotic syndrome is a clinical state in which there is massive proteinuria (>3.5 g a day), hypoalbuminemia, edema, and hyperlipidemia. Usually the BUN level is normal.

According to Robson's review of over 1400 cases (Robson, 1972), several varieties of primary glomerulonephritis account for 78 percent of the nephrotic syndrome in adults and 93 percent in children. In 22 percent of the adults the condition was due to a systemic disorder (chiefly diabetes, amyloidosis, and renal vein

thrombosis)* in which the kidney was secondarily involved or to an abnormal response to drugs or other allergens.

Four histologic entities found in the nephrotic syndrome are included in the general category of glomerulonephritis. These are minimal change, membranous change, proliferative change, and mixed membranous and proliferative change glomerulonephritis (described in Table 42-3). Focal glomerulonephritis is a less frequent cause of the nephrotic syndrome.

Minimal change glomerulonephritis (GN) is the typical lesion of the nephrotic syndrome in childhood (69 percent) and accounts for 18 percent of adult cases. The older term for this disease is *lipoid nephrosis.* It is also called *foot process disease,* since the normally discrete foot processes (podocytes) of the epithelial cells appear to be fused together on electron microscopy (Fig. 42-11). Minimal change GN is the only major form of glomerulonephritis in which immune pathogenetic mechanisms do not appear to be involved. It is generally treated successfully with corticosteroids. In a minority of patients who do not respond to steroid therapy, the disease can sometimes be suppressed by immunosuppressive drugs such as cyclophosphamide (Cytoxin) or azathioprine (Imuran). The small proportion of patients

*It is unclear whether the renal vein thrombosis is causing the nephrotic syndrome or whether it is a consequence of the hypercoagulable state associated with the nephrotic syndrome (Weller, 1979, p. 157).

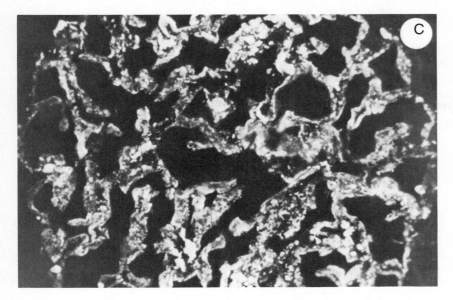

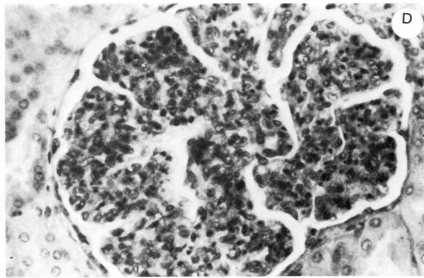

(C) Photomicrograph of immunofluorescent preparation showing lumpy pattern of immunoglobulin and complement deposits along glomerular capillary walls in circulating immune-complex disease. (D) Light microscopy slide from kidney of a patient with APSGN showing infiltration with PMNs and hypercellularity which crowds the glomerulus filling Bowman's space. (Modified Netter, 1973. (Immunoflorescent micrograph courtesy of Michael J. Deegan.)

who do not recover generally follow a long, remitting-relapsing course ending in uremia.

Membranous change GN accounts for 25 percent of the cases of nephrotic syndrome in adults and only 2 percent in children. About 95 percent of these patients develop azotemia and die in uremia in 10 to 20 years. The predominant histologic change is thickening of the basement membrane visible by both electron microscopy and light microscopy.

Proliferative and *membranoproliferative change* GN account for the remaining 35 percent of Robson's adult primary nephrotic syndrome cases and for 22 percent in children. Proliferative change GN is characterized by hypercellularity of the glomerular cells, while there is both hypercellularity and basement membrane thickening in membranoproliferative change GN. Response to therapy is generally poor in these histologic types of GN, and there is progressive renal failure.

The major physiologic disturbances leading to edema in the nephrotic syndrome are depicted in Fig. 42-12. The initial event in most cases is an antigen-antibody reaction at the glomerulus resulting in increased GBM permeability, massive proteinuria, and hypoalbuminemia. Patients with the nephrotic syndrome commonly pass 5 to 15 g protein per 24 hours. Hypoalbuminemia, by decreasing colloid osmotic pressure (COP), favors the transudation of fluid out of the vascular compartment into the interstitium. This serves as a fairly direct mechanism for the production of edema. In addition, the hypovolemia results in a decrease of renal plasma flow (RPF) and GFR, activating the renin-angiotensin mechanism. The hypovolemia also activates volume receptors in the left atria. The result is increased aldosterone and ADH production. Salt and water are retained by the kidneys, further aggravating the edema. By repetition of this chain of events, massive

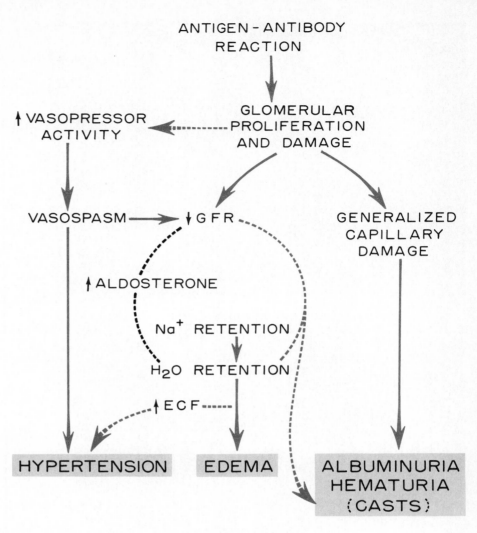

FIGURE 42-7
The major disturbances in acute poststreptococcal glomerulonephritis. (Modified from A. G. White, *Clinical Disturbances of Renal Function,* Saunders, Philadelphia, 1961.)

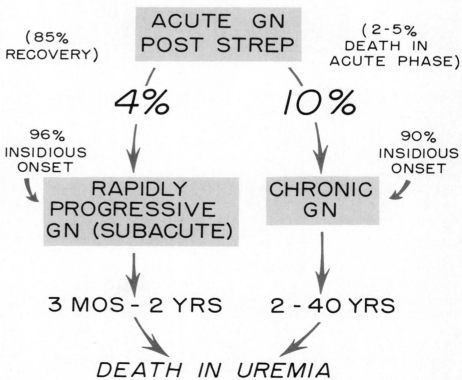

FIGURE 42-8
Natural history of the various forms of diffuse glomerulonephritis.

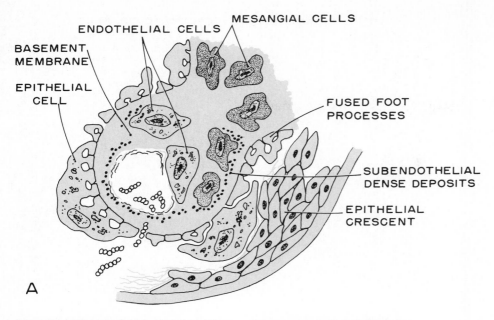

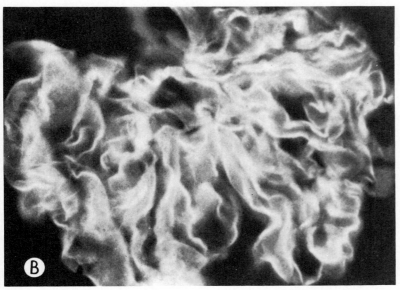

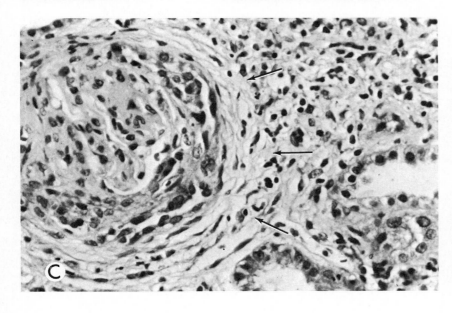

FIGURE 42-9
**Rapidly progressive
glomerulonephritis. (A) Cross section of
a single capillary loop showing
subendothelial dense deposits and
glomerular damage. (B)
Photomicrograph of
immunofluorescent preparation
showing linear pattern of immune
deposit typical of anti-GBM disease.
(C) Light microscopy slide from a
patient with rapidly progressive
glomerulonephritis showing large
fibroepithelial crescent (arrows)
crowding a lobulated glomerular tuft.
(Diagram modified from Netter, 1973.)
(Immunofluorescent slide, from A. J.
Fish, A. F. Michael, and R. A. Good, in
M. B. Strauss and L. G. Welt (eds.),
Diseases of the Kidney, 2d ed., Little,
Brown, Boston, 1971.)**

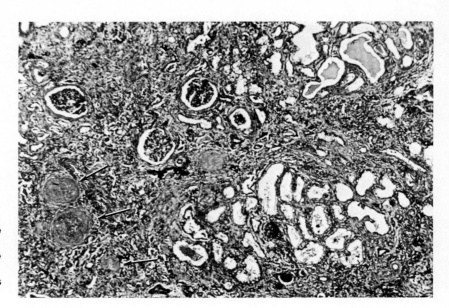

FIGURE 42-10
End-stage kidney (light microscopy) from a patient with chronic pyelonephritis showing marked distortion of the renal architecture. There is interstitial fibrosis, several glomeruli are completely hyalinized (arrows) while three are spared. There is marked tubular distortion and atrophy, and casts appear in several tubules.

edema (anasarca) may occur. The amount of protein lost, however, does not correlate precisely with the severity of the edema, since people vary in the rate of protein synthesis to replace that which is lost. The cause of the hyperlipidemia which often accompanies the nephrotic syndrome is obscure. Serum cholesterol, phospholipids, and triglycerides are all usually increased. Note that the mechanism of nephrotic edema differs from that of APSGN.

Treatment of the nephrotic syndrome consists in corticosteroid and immunosuppressive drugs directed toward the nature of the lesion, high protein and salt-restricted diet, diuretics, sometimes intravenous infusion of albumin, and restricted activity during the acute

phase. It is also important to isolate patients from sources of infection. Patients with the nephrotic syndrome are highly susceptible to infection and in preantibiotic days often died of empyema, pneumonia, or peritonitis. Long-term management is important, since many patients follow a course of repeated exacerbations

FIGURE 42-11
Schema of glomerular loop showing fusion of foot processes in minimal change glomerulonephritis. (Modified from Netter, 1973.)

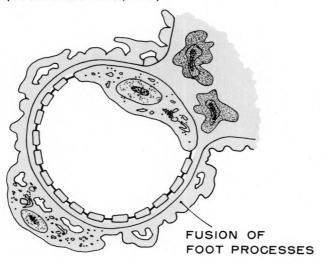

FUSION OF
FOOT PROCESSES

FIGURE 42-12
Pathogenesis of nephrotic edema. (Modified from F. E. Schreiner, "The Nephrotic Syndrome," in M. B. Strauss and L. G. Welt (eds.), *Diseases of the Kidney*, 2d ed., Little, Brown, Boston, 1971.)

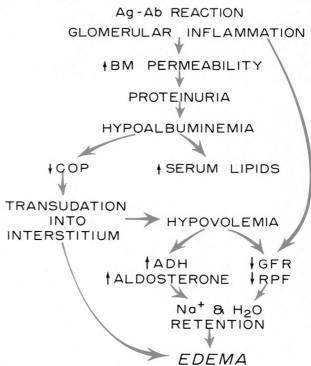

Ag-Ab REACTION
GLOMERULAR INFLAMMATION
↑BM PERMEABILITY
PROTEINURIA
HYPOALBUMINEMIA
↓COP   ↑SERUM LIPIDS
TRANSUDATION INTO INTERSTITIUM → HYPOVOLEMIA
↑ADH   ↓GFR
↑ALDOSTERONE ↓RPF
Na⁺ & H₂O RETENTION
EDEMA

and remissions over a period of years, but with advancing glomerular hyalinization, proteinuria usually diminishes as azotemia progresses.

Hypertensive nephrosclerosis

Hypertension and chronic renal failure are closely related. Hypertension may be the primary disease and cause damage to the kidneys, and conversely, severe chronic renal disease may cause hypertension or contribute to its maintenance through the mechanism of sodium and water retention, the vasopressor effects of the renin-angiotensin system, and possibly prostaglandin deficiency. Sometimes it is difficult for the nephrologist to determine which was primary. Nephrosclerosis (hardening of the kidneys) refers to the pathologic changes in the renal blood vessels as a result of hypertension. It is one of the leading causes of chronic renal failure.

Essential hypertension and the kidneys

Hypertension is defined as a sustained elevation of blood pressure above the accepted normals of 90 mmHg diastolic or 140 mmHg systolic. According to this definition, about 5 percent of the United States population have hypertension. However, as many as 25 percent of individuals may have this disorder by the age of 50 years. The cause of hypertension is unknown in about 90 percent of the cases and is termed *essential hypertension* (unknown etiology and pathogenesis). The onset of essential hypertension is usually between the ages of 20 and 50 years, and it is more frequent in blacks and females. Essential hypertension is classified as benign or malignant. *Benign hypertension* is slowly progressive, while in *malignant hypertension* there is rapid acceleration in the course of the hypertensive disease, resulting in severe organ damage.

The rate of progression of benign essential hypertension is variable, but it generally runs a slowly progressive course over a period of 20 to 30 years. Long-standing hypertension produces structural changes in the arterioles throughout the body characterized by fibrosis and hyalinization (sclerosis) of the blood vessel walls. The chief target organs of this condition are the heart, brain, and kidneys. The usual cause of death is myocardial infarction, congestive heart failure, or cerebral vascular accident. If essential hypertension remains benign, only about 1 percent of patients are likely to suffer renal damage sufficient to die of uremia. Proteinuria and mild azotemia may exist for years without symptoms, and most patients who die of uremia do so as a result of the hypertension entering the malignant phase. This occurs in less than 10 percent of the cases of essential hypertension.

Malignant hypertension implies severe hypertension with diastolic blood pressure greater than 120 to 130 mmHg, grade IV retinopathy,* and renal excretory dysfunction ranging from proteinuria to hematuria to azotemia. Malignant hypertension may occur at any time during the course of benign hypertension but usually occurs after many years. Occasionally it occurs de novo, especially in black males in their third and fourth decades.

In the kidney, renal arteriosclerosis due to longstanding hypertension results in the disorder called *benign nephrosclerosis*. This disorder is the direct result of ischemia due to the narrowed lumen of the intrarenal blood vessels. The kidney may be reduced in size, usually symmetrically, and has a granular, pitted surface. Histologically, the essential lesion is sclerosis of the small arteries and arterioles, which is most marked in the afferent arterioles. The closure of the arteries and arterioles leads to destruction of the glomeruli and atrophy of the tubules, so that entire nephrons are destroyed.

Malignant nephrosclerosis is a term used to designate the structural renal changes often associated with the malignant phase of essential hypertension.† The kidneys may be of normal size, with minimal granularity and some petechiae from rupture of arterioles, or they may be shrunken and scarred. Histologically there are three types of lesions: (1) proliferative endarteritis, (2) fibrinoid necrosis of arteriolar walls, and (3) fibrinoid necrosis of glomerular tufts. At first there is marked thickening of the intima of the interlobular arteries caused by proliferation of the endothelial cells. These changes produce an appearance often referred to as "onion skin." The narrowed lumina produce ischemia of the afferent arterioles and the release of renin, and the blood pressure rises still further. Focal necrosis then occurs in the walls of the afferent arterioles, and as the necrosed areas contain fibrin, the change is called *fibrinoid necrosis*. Fibrinoid necrosis of the glomerular tufts is probably an extension of the fibrinoid necrosis of the feeding afferent arterioles. If the blood pressure remains elevated, these localized changes become widespread, with the formation of thrombi, glomerular hemorrhage, infarction of entire nephrons, and rapid death of all

---

*Grade IV retinopathy refers to the most severe changes in the retina due to hypertension. These changes may be viewed with the ophthalmoscope and consist of vascular sclerosis, exudates, hemorrhages, and papilledema.

†Although these gross and microscopic renal lesions are characteristic of the malignant phase of essential hypertension, they are not specific and may be superimposed upon a variety of diseases associated with hypertension (e.g., chronic pyelonephritis, chronic glomerulonephritis, polyarteritis nodosa).

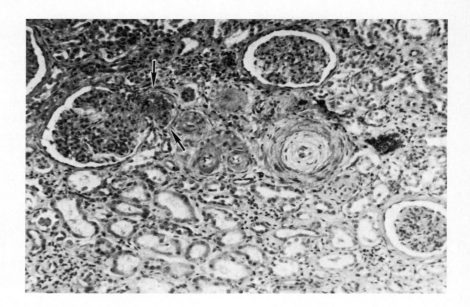

FIGURE 42-13
Malignant nephrosclerosis. Light microscopy slide showing several hyalinized arterioles (center field), dilated tubules with atrophied lining cells (lower center), and an area of fibrinoid necrosis (arrows).

renal cells. Figure 42-13 illustrates some of the above lesions.

Renal artery stenosis

The renal artery may be occluded by atherosclerotic plaques or fibrodysplasia, causing hypertension which is often of the rapidly progressive type. Atherosclerosis is found chiefly in older men and usually involves the proximal one-third of the renal artery near the aorta. Fibrodysplasia is characterized by excesses in fibrous connective tissue within the layers of the blood vessel and is most apt to occur in the middle and distal thirds of the renal artery, sometimes involving segmental branches. There are several histologic types of fibrodysplasia, and the disorder is most common in women between the ages of 20 and 50 years.

Renal artery stenosis may be unilateral or bilateral. If the caliber of the artery is reduced by 70 percent or more, renal ischemia occurs. The renal ischemia activates the renin-angiotensin system, and hypertension follows. Though uncommon (about 5 to 7 percent of hypertension cases), renal artery stenosis is important because surgical correction may alleviate or markedly ameliorate the hypertensive state.

Unilateral renal artery stenosis not only causes ischemic atrophy of the involved kidney but may eventually cause hypertensive nephrosclerosis of the contralateral kidney. The pathogenetic mechanism is depicted in Fig. 42-14. If the contralateral kidney has developed significant nephrosclerosis from the renin-induced hypertension, the function of the ischemic kidney may even be the better of the two, since the stenosed renal artery protects the occluded kidney from the full effects of the systemic hypertension.

Physical findings suggestive of renal artery stenosis include a bruit heard over the epigastrium or the flank and differences in carotid, brachial, or femoral pulses or blood pressure in the extremities (indicative of generalized atherosclerosis).

An intravenous pyelogram suggests unilateral renal artery stenosis when it shows a smaller kidney on the affected side (at least 1.5 cm shorter than the other), when there is delayed appearance of the contrast medium or reduced concentration on the affected side, and when late films show an increased density of contrast material. Selective renal arteriography gives further evidence. An elevated plasma renin measurement implies that a renal artery stenosis is significant. The test can be extended to determine the renin concentration from each renal vein in order to discover the source of an elevated renin level.

Elevated plasma renin levels suggest that surgery would be beneficial. Surgical treatment consists of revascularization of the ischemic kidney, often by means of a saphenous vein bypass graft. The increased perfusion suppresses the increased renin secretion, and the hypertension is cured in more than half the cases. Most of the remaining cases are improved by the surgery, allowing easier medical control of the hypertension.

Connective tissue disorders

The connective tissue diseases (collagen diseases) are systemic diseases whose manifestations are mainly attributable to the soft tissues of the body (see Part XI). They are of particular interest in nephrology because of the high incidence of renal involvement. About two-thirds of patients with systemic lupus erythematosis (SLE) and progressive systemic sclerosis (scleroderma) have clinical evidence of renal involvement. The incidence is about 80 percent for patients with polyarteritis nodosa. Death from renal failure is common in these patients. In addition, death in uremia occurs in one in four patients with rheumatoid arthritis (to be discussed in "Amyloidosis" later).

Systemic lupus erythematosis

Systemic lupus erythematosis is a disease that predominantly affects women, who account for 90 percent of the cases. The age of onset is usually between 20 and

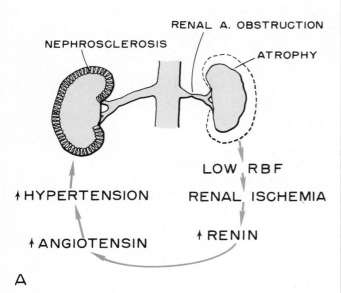

A

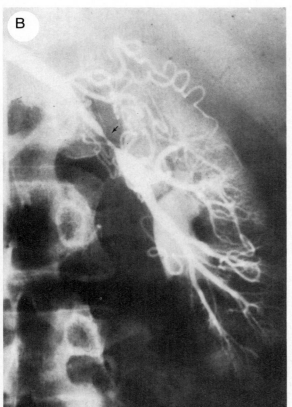

B

40 years. The blood usually gives a positive test for antinuclear factor and LE (lupus erythematosis) cells, especially during the active phase of the disease. Many different tissues and organs may be involved, but renal involvement is the most significant in terms of outcome.

Lupus nephritis is caused by circulating immune complexes which become trapped in the glomerular basement membrane and cause damage. The mechanism is similar to that in APSGN except that the source of the antigen is the body's own DNA rather than the streptococcal plasma membrane. In the case of SLE the body produces antibody against its own DNA. The clinical picture may be one of acute glomerulonephritis or of nephrotic syndrome. Although the basic cause is thought to be the same in both cases, focal, membranous, and proliferative changes in the glomeruli may all be seen. The earliest change often involves only part of the glomerular tuft (local), or only scattered glomeruli may be involved (focal). Focal and local glomerulonephritis respond quite well to corticosteroid drugs, and there may be a complete remission. The prognosis is poor for those who develop diffuse membranous or proliferative changes, and these patients often die of renal failure (Fig. 42-15).

Polyarteritis nodosa

Polyarteritis nodosa is an inflammatory and necrotizing disease involving the medium-sized and small arteries throughout the body. Males are more commonly affected than females, and the peak incidence is in the seventh decade. Although the exact etiology and pathogenesis are unknown, there is evidence to suggest some form of hypersensitivity mechanism. In many cases the onset is associated with a sensitivity reaction to drugs.

Renal lesions are of two types. If the medium-sized vessels within the kidney are affected, areas of renal infarction develop. If the disease is confined to the arterioles, the renal histology is that of severe focal, proliferative glomerulonephritis and fibrinoid necrotic changes with epithelial crescents.

Polyarteritis nodosa is treated with corticosteroid

FIGURE 42-14

(A) Pathogenesis of nephrosclerosis in the contralateral kidney in renal artery stenosis. (B) Renal arteriogram showing renal artery stenosis due to fibrodysplasia. (Arteriogram from James C. Stanley and William F. Fry, "Renovascular Hypertension Secondary to Arterial Fibrodysplasia in Adults," *Archives of Surgery,* **110: 922, 1975. Copyright © 1975, American Medical Association.)**

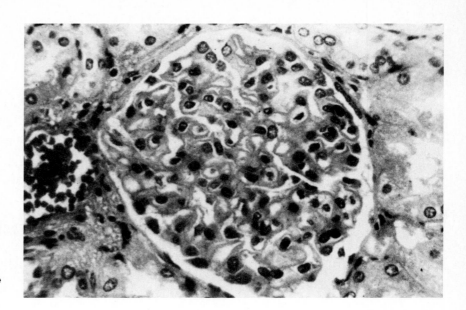

FIGURE 42-15
Glomerulus from a patient with membranous lupus nephritis. Capillary walls (basement membrane) are uniformly thickened, but there is no increase in cellularity. Note the wire-loop appearance. Note the RBCs in the lumen of the tubule (left center).

drugs, which are more effective during the early course of the disease. The prognosis is generally poor. Death results from uremia or hypertension secondary to the arteritis, following a slowly progressive course or one characterized by exacerbations and remissions.

Progressive systemic sclerosis

Progressive systemic sclerosis, or scleroderma, is an uncommon systemic disease characterized by diffuse sclerosis of the skin and other organs. Females are affected more often than males. The onset is usually between the ages of 20 and 50 years. As in SLE, a variety of antibodies may be found in the serum, suggesting that immune mechanisms may be involved in the pathogenesis.

The interlobar arteries typically show changes resembling hypertensive nephrosclerosis. Progressive renal impairment may develop slowly over a period of years. In a few cases, hypertension and uremia may follow a malignant course, with the development of end-stage renal failure within weeks.

Congenital and hereditary disorders

Renal tubular acidosis and polycystic disease of the kidneys are hereditary disorders primarily affecting the renal tubules which may terminate in renal failure, though this is more common in polycystic disease. Both diseases have an infantile and an adult form, whose manifestations may be quite distinct.

Polycystic kidney disease

Polycystic kidney disease (PCKD) is characterized by bilateral multiple, expanding cysts which gradually encroach upon and destroy the normal renal parenchyma by compression. The kidney may be enlarged (sometimes as large as a football) and filled with grape-like clusters of cysts (Fig. 42-16). The cysts are filled with clear or hemorrhagic fluid.

The rare infantile form of the disease appears to be inherited as an autosomal recessive trait. The cysts are closed, blind pouches into which the glomerular filtrate flows. The course of the disease is rapidly progressive, usually resulting in death before the age of 2 years.

In contrast, adult polycystic disease is much more common (about 1 per 500 population); it is an autosomal dominant trait; the cysts communicate with the tubules;

FIGURE 42-16
Polycystic kidney. (Art by Judy Simon, Dept. of Medical and Biological Illustrations, University of Michigan.)

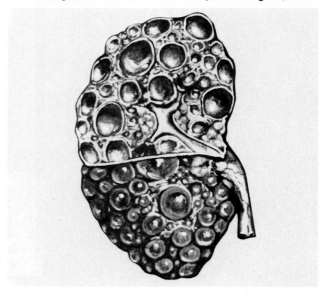

and the course is slowly progressive, with symptoms of renal insufficiency usually occurring during the fourth decade. Flank pain, hematuria, polyuria, proteinuria, and palpably enlarged, "knobby" kidneys are often the presenting signs and symptoms. Hypertension and urinary tract infections are frequent complications. While this disease is ultimately fatal, some persons may complete a normal life span and die of nonrenal causes. Adult PCKD is an important disease because of its frequency (third leading cause of end-stage renal failure) and because it is potentially eradicable by genetic counseling.

Renal tubular acidosis

Primary renal tubular acidosis (RTA) is a clinical disorder in which there is systemic acidosis due to inability to excrete an appropriately acid urine. RTA may stem from disease of the proximal tubule in which there is defective bicarbonate reabsorption or from disease of the distal tubule in which there is a transport defect for hydrogen ion, resulting in an inability to develop an adequate pH gradient between the blood and the urine.

The classic distal RTA in the adult is believed to be transmitted through autosomal dominant heredity. Twice as many females as males are afflicted. The first symptoms generally appear during adolescence or young adulthood. These include bone pain due to osteomalacia, renal colic due to nephrocalcinosis, or calculi, and weakness due to hypokalemia. These changes may be explained as a consequence of the tubular defect. The transport defect of H^+ in the distal tubule results in reduced urine titratable acidity and ammonia. Not all the filtered HCO_3^- is reabsorbed. The missing anion is replaced by Cl^-, giving a hyperchloremic acidosis. There is also increased loss of K^+ and Na^+ in the urine. The sustained acidosis due to H^+ retention (or HCO_3^- loss) results in mobilization of Ca^{2+} salts from the bone and hypercalciuria. Bone resorption is manifested as osteomalacia in adults and as rickets in children. Calcium salts may precipitate diffusely in the renal parenchyma (nephrocalcinosis) or within the collecting system (calculi). Renal failure is secondary to these complications. The condition is diagnosed by the urine acidification test described in Chap. 41. Proximal tubule RTA, however, cannot be diagnosed by this test, since patients with this condition can acidify their urine when given an acid load.

The infantile form of RTA occurs during the first 18 months of life and commonly presents as a failure to thrive. It is not believed to be hereditary. The clinical picture is one of thirst, polyuria, anorexia and vomiting, rickets, and sometimes nephrocalcinosis.

RTA is treated by alkali therapy—sodium bicarbonate or citrate in divided doses. The infant responds well to this therapy, and the condition is usually completely reversed. In some adults the calcium deposits are reabsorbed after prolonged alkali therapy, while in others the nephrocalcinosis is permanent. The prognosis depends on the extent of renal damage prior to treatment.

Metabolic disorders

Metabolic disorders which may lead to chronic renal failure include diabetes mellitus, gout, primary hyperparathyroidism, and amyloidosis.

Diabetes mellitus

Renal involvement is common in diabetes. Approximately 50 percent of juvenile-onset and 6 percent of adult-onset diabetic persons develop renal failure.* The mean duration of the diabetes before uremia develops is 20 years.

Common renal lesions include nephrosclerosis due to lesions of the arterioles, pyelonephritis and necrosis of the renal papilla, and glomerulosclerosis. Glomerulosclerosis is the most characteristic lesion and may be diffuse or nodular. *Nodular glomerulosclerosis,* also known as the *Kimmelstiel-Wilson lesion,* is virtually pathognomonic of diabetes (Fig. 42-17). Both lesions are due to increased deposit of mesangial matrix.† In the diffuse type, the matrix is more diffusely distributed in each glomerulus and is less discrete. There is more thickening of the peripheral basement membrane. In the nodular type the matrix is deposited within the core of the capillary lobule, giving the appearance of a nodule. Initially the capillary lumina are patent, but they are gradually obliterated as the disease progresses.

Diabetic retinopathy, characterized by microaneurysms around the macula, nearly always precedes diabetic glomerulosclerosis. Proteinuria, hypertension, and an increased incidence of pyelonephritis often precede end-stage renal failure.

Gout

Gout is a metabolic disease characterized by hyperuricemia (increased plasma uric acid concentrations). There are two forms of the disease. Primary gout is a hereditary disorder of deranged uric acid metabolism af-

---

*Renal failure is the most common cause of death in juvenile-onset diabetes.

†The mesangial matrix is a spongy network of basement membrane-like trabeculae at the center of the glomerular lobule surrounding the mesangial cells. It merges with the capillary basement membrane.

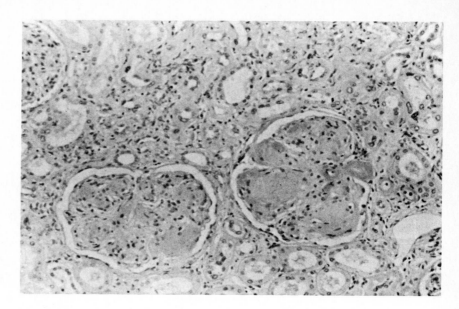

fecting males in 95 percent of the cases. Secondary gout may arise either from increased uric acid production in such conditions as leukemia, polycythemia vera, or multiple myeloma or from decreased uric acid excretion, as in chronic renal failure. The source of the increased uric acid in the myeloproliferative disorders is the massive breakdown of cells (which contain nucleoproteins).

The major lesions of gout are principally due to the deposition and crystallization of urates in the fluids and tissues of the body. The joints and kidneys are the prime targets. In chronic gout, deposit of urate crystals in the renal interstitium causes interstitial nephritis and nephrosclerosis. Approximately 20 percent of the patients eventually develop renal failure. Acute renal failure may develop secondary to complete obstruction of renal tubules by uric acid during cytotoxic drug therapy for malignant disease (discussed in Chap. 41).

Hyperparathyroidism

Primary hyperparathyroidism, resulting in hypersecretion of parathyroid hormone, is a relatively rare disease which can result in nephrocalcinosis and subsequent renal failure. The usual cause is adenoma of the parathyroid glands. Secondary hyperparathyroidism is a common complication of chronic renal failure. Whether the disease is primary or secondary, the manifestations are similar. These are discussed in detail in Chap. 43.

Amyloidosis

Amyloidosis is a metabolic disease in which amyloid, an insoluble, waxy glycoprotein, is deposited in the various soft tissues of the body, where it can produce pressure and cause atrophy of the contiguous cells. In primary or congenital amyloidosis, amyloid is more often found in the tongue, heart, gastrointestinal tract,

and peripheral nerves than in the kidneys. Secondary amyloidosis is frequently associated with chronic infectious disease, such as tuberculosis, chronic rheumatoid arthritis (25 percent), and multiple myeloma (10 to 20 percent), and with paraplegia (40 percent). The kidneys are frequently involved in secondary amyloidosis. The nephrotic syndrome and death from renal failure are common in this condition.

Toxic nephropathy

The kidney is especially vulnerable to the toxic effects of drugs and chemicals for the following reasons: (1) it receives 25 percent of the cardiac output, so it may readily be exposed to large amounts of a chemical; (2) the hyperosmotic interstitium allows chemicals to be concentrated in a relatively hypovascular region; and (3) the kidney is an obligatory excretory route for most drugs, so that renal insufficiency results in drug accumulation and increased concentration in the tubular fluid. The most frequently encountered nephrotoxins result in acute renal failure and are discussed in Chap. 45. Chronic renal failure may result from analgesic abuse and exposure to lead.

Analgesic abuse (phenacetin nephritis)

It is now generally accepted that chronic abuse of analgesics can cause renal injury. The responsible ingredient is believed to be phenacetin, a constituent of the common APC tablet (aspirin, phenacetin, and caffeine) and many other over-the-counter preparations. The American tablet contains 150 mg of phenacetin. The amount sufficient to induce renal failure is not known with certainty. Gault defines *abuse* as the ingestion of five tablets per day for 3 years, the minimum time-dose to induce a nephrotoxic response. The aspirin in the compounds is also believed to contribute to renal injury by uncoupling oxidative phosphorylation in the mitochondria of renal cells and by inhibiting the synthesis of prostaglandins, potent renal vasodilator hormones. Both these effects cause renal hypoxia, making the medulla more susceptible to injury (Brenner et al., 1980). Neurotic persons or those with chronic headaches are the most likely to be analgesic abusers. The highest incidence of this disease is in the Scandinavian countries and in Australia.

The characteristic renal lesion is papillary necrosis and interstitial nephritis. The papillary tips may slough off completely and be excreted in the urine. Since the distal tubule bears the brunt of the disease, urine concentration and acidification tend to be severely impaired, and a salt-losing state may also develop. Common clinical features are hematuria (in cases of papillary necrosis), renal colic (flank pain), and urinary tract infection, including chronic pyelonephritis. Frequently the disease progresses insidiously, so that the patient may have advanced chronic renal failure and hypertension at the time of diagnosis.

Lead nephropathy

Exposure to lead occurs in a number of occupations, and lead may be ingested in illicitly distilled whisky. Lead intoxication is still a problem in the United States, although not as great as when lead-based paints were used. Lead is chiefly incorporated into the bone and gradually released over a period of years; it is also incorporated into renal tubular cells. The basic renal lesion is interstitial nephritis, and there is slowly progressive renal failure.

QUESTIONS

Chronic renal failure

Directions: Answer the following questions on a separate sheet of paper.

1. What is the major difference between acute and chronic renal failure, and what happens to the function of the kidneys in both categories?

2. List the four leading causes of end-stage renal disease and the primary renal structures involved in each.

3. Name in order the three stages in the natural history of progressive renal failure. What percentage of nephrons are destroyed in each?

4. Indicate whether the laboratory values of BUN and plasma creatinine would be normal, rising just above normal, or rising sharply in each of the three stages of renal failure.

5. What happens to the creatinine clearance in progressive renal failure?

6. What is the difference between polyuria and oliguria? Define *nocturia*.

7. Explain why polyuria and oliguria occur as more and more functioning nephrons are destroyed in chronic renal failure. Explain how renal lesions could cause these symptoms.

8. Explain how the normal kidney responds to an increasing solute load, how this condition might be induced, and how the evidence supports the intact nephron hypothesis.

9. What happens to the remaining functioning nephrons in progressive renal failure (size, filtration rate, tubular reabsorption, solute load)?

10. Explain why the original cause of chronic renal failure may be difficult to identify in some cases.

11. Differentiate between symptomatic and asymptomatic bacteriuria as a cause of chronic pyelonephritis.

12. Why is long-term follow-up important in acute pyelonephritis?

13. Why is it often difficult to diagnose chronic pyelonephritis?

14. Give the arguments for and against the bacterial etiology of chronic pyelonephritis.

15. What is the difference between the typical gross appearance of the kidneys in acute and chronic pyelonephritis?

Directions: Circle the letter preceding each item below that correctly answers the question or completes the statement. Only one answer is correct, with exceptions noted.

16. Which of the following best describes nocturia?
    a. A decrease in the volume of urine   *b.* Loss of the normal diurnal pattern of concentrating urine to a greater degree at night   *c.* Both *a* and *b*
    d. Neither *a* nor *b*

17. The earliest symptoms of chronic renal failure are which of the following? (More than one answer is correct.)
    a. Pruritus   *b.* Oliguria   *c.* Polyuria   *d.* Nocturia

18. The most common infecting organism in urinary tract infections is:
    a. Proteus vulgaris   *b. Klebsiella pneumoniae*
    c. Staphylococcus aureus   *d. Escherichia coli*

19. Defense mechanisms present in males but lacking in females which may account for their greater resistance to urinary tract infections include which of the following? (More than one answer may be correct.)
    a. Phagocytic capacity of the bladder epithelium
    b. Bactericidal properties of prostatic fluid
    c. Long entry pathway for bacteria   *d.* Short urethra

20. A simple, single urethral catheterization leads to urinary tract infection in approximately what percentage of cases?
    a. 2 percent   *b.* 20 percent   *c.* 50 percent
    d. 98 percent

21. Conditions interfering with host defense mechanisms in the renal medulla include which of the following? (More than one answer may be correct.)
    a. High ammonia content   *b.* Hypertonicity
    c. Poor blood supply   *d.* High glucose content

22. The salt-losing tendency in early chronic renal failure and especially in chronic pyelonephritis is due to:
    a. Obligatory sodium wastage to preserve acid-base balance   *b.* Defective sodium reabsorption
    c. An osmotic diuresis in each functioning nephron   *d.* Decreased aldosterone production

23. Factors predisposing to urinary tract infection include:
    a. Indwelling catheter drainage   *b.* Urethral stricture   *c.* High progesterone levels in pregnancy   *d.* Vesicoureteral reflux   *e.* All of these

24. The most important cause of chronic renal failure from a preventive or remediable point of view is probably:
    a. Chronic pyelonephritis   *b.* Chronic glomerulonephritis

Directions: Circle T if the statement is true and F if it is false.

25. T   F   Typical findings in chronic pyelonephritis are intermittent bacteriuria or white blood cells or white cell casts in the urine.

26. T   F   Absence of bacteriuria rules out chronic pyelonephritis.

27. T   F   In chronic pyelonephritis, the concentrating ability of the kidney is often diminished before there is a significant decrease in GFR.

Directions: Fill in the blanks with the correct words.

28. In acute pyelonephritis, _____ (inflammatory cells) are usually found throughout the cortex and medulla and segments of the _____ are destroyed, whereas in chronic pyelonephritis, in the interstitium there are many _____ and _____ _____cells.

29. Label Fig. 42-18 by matching the letters with the renal histologic findings from the list below.
    ____ Normal tubule
    ____ Area of interstitial fibrosis
    ____ Hypertrophied tubule with atrophy of epithelial cells

FIGURE 42-18
Histologic findings in chronic pyelonephritis.

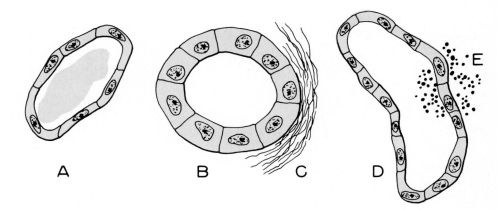

_____ Atrophied tubule containing cast
_____ Inflammatory cells (PMNs)

Directions: Answer the following questions on a separate sheet of paper.

30. Define the term _glomerulonephritis_.

31. Why does confusion exist in the classification and separation of the various types of glomerulonephritis?

32. Name three types of glomerulonephritis based on clinical classification. What is the prognosis of each type, generally speaking? Describe their natural history and relationship.

33. Describe the classic case of acute poststreptococcal glomerulonephritis with respect to common age group affected, causative organisms, signs and symptoms, major physiologic disturbances, pathogenetic mechanisms involved, and treatment.

34. What is the nephrotic syndrome? Why does the patient become edematous? What diseases is it commonly associated with? What are the general principles of treatment?

35. Explain the importance of early diagnosis of unilateral renal artery stenosis. Explain the mechanism resulting in damage to the contralateral kidney (illustrate).

36. List three reasons why the kidney is especially vulnerable to the toxic effect of drugs or chemicals.

Directions: Match the descriptions in col. B to the terms in col. A which refer to the distribution of glomerular lesions.

Column A
37. _____ Diffuse
38. _____ Local
39. _____ Focal

Column B
a. Only a portion of the glomeruli are involved.
b. Part of the glomerulus is involved.
c. All the glomeruli are affected.

Directions: Match the descriptive characteristics in col. B to the appropriate pathogenic immune mechanism in col. A.

Column A
40. _____ Circulating immune complex
41. _____ Anti-GBM

Column B
a. Associated with Goodpasture's syndrome.
b. Associated with APSGN and SLE.
c. Immunoglobulin is deposited subepithelially.
d. Immunoglobulin is deposited subendothelially.

e. Autoimmune mechanism.
f. Linear or ribbonlike pattern of deposit on immunofluorescent biopsy slide.
g. Ag-Ab complexes are mechanically trapped in the filtration membrane.
h. Results in more serious injury to the glomerulus.

Directions: Match the appropriate description in col. B to the histologic type of glomerulonephritis in col. A. Letters may be used more than once.

Column A
42. _____ Minimal change GN
43. _____ Membranous GN
44. _____ Proliferative GN

Column B
a. Primary change in the glomerulus is an increase in endothelial, mesangial, or epithelial cells.
b. Predominant change is thickening of the basement membrane.
c. Only morphological change is fusion of the foot processes.
d. Most common lesion in children associated with the nephrotic syndrome.
e. Nephrotic patients with these lesions often progress to renal failure.

Directions: Match the descriptive phrases in col. B with the terms in col. A to which they apply. Letters may be used more than once.

Column A
45. _____ Polycystic kidney disease (adult form)
46. _____ Polycystic kidney disease (infantile form)
47. _____ RTA (adult form)
48. _____ RTA (child form)
49. _____ Kimmelstiel-Wilson disease

Column B
a. Characteristic lesion of diabetic nephropathy.
b. Hereditary disorder.
c. Commonly presents as failure to thrive.
d. Nephrocalcinosis is a common complication.
e. Deposits in kidney common in rheumatoid arthritis, paraplegia, and multiple myeloma.
f. Cysts communicate with tubules.

50. ____ Gout
51. ____ Hyperparathyroidism
52. ____ Amyloidosis

g. Cysts are closed.
h. Urate crystals may be deposited in the renal tubules or interstitium.
i. Treated with sodium bicarbonate or sodium citrate.
j. Urine acidification test may aid in diagnosis.

Directions: Circle the letter preceding each item below that correctly answers the question. Only one answer is correct, with exceptions noted.

53. Which of the following antibodies is most significant in the pathogenesis of the glomerulonephritis of systemic lupus erythematosis?
    a. Anti-RNA   b. Anti-GBM   c. Anti-DNA
    d. Antikidney

54. Which statement is false with respect to immune-complex glomerulonephritis?
    a. Ag-Ab complexes form in the blood and circulate to the glomerulus.   b. PMNs produce glomerular injury by the release of lysosomal enzymes.   c. Immunofluorescent studies show a pattern of granular deposits.   d. The major glomerular injury is caused by streptococcal renal infection.

55. Which of the following findings is uncommon in APSGN?
    a. Decreased serum complement   b. Ability to produce concentrated urine   c. Massive proteinuria (nephrotic syndrome)   d. Red cell casts

56. Which of the following types of glomerulonephritis (GN) associated with the nephrotic syndrome does *not* show evidence of an immune pathogenetic mechanism?
    a. Idiopathic membranous GN   b. Minimal lesion GN (lipoid nephrosis)   c. Membranoproliferative GN   d. Proliferative GN of systemic lupus erythematosis

57. Death from minimal change GN primarily due to:
    a. Infection   b. Toxic effects of corticosteroid drugs   c. Acute renal failure   d. Chronic renal failure

58. Which of the following statements is false concerning the histologic changes in the end-stage kidney of chronic glomerulonephritis?
    a. Only the glomeruli are involved in the pathologic destruction.   b. Destructive lesions involving the glomeruli, renal tubules, and vasculature are all present.   c. Some glomeruli are completely hyalinized.   d. Epithelial crescents are frequently seen.

59. Which of the following is the characteristic lesion in benign nephrosclerosis?
    a. Fibrinoid necrosis, glomerular hemorrhage   b. Nodular glomerulosclerosis   c. Hyalinized thickening of the arteriolar walls with narrowing of lumina   d. Widespread infarction of entire nephrons

60. What is the leading cause of death in systemic lupus erythematosis?
    a. Infection   b. Renal disease   c. Hemorrhage   d. Neurologic lesions

61. Which of the following commonly precedes diabetic glomerulosclerosis?
    a. Hyperlipidemia   b. Hypertension   c. Retinopathy   d. Increased insulin requirement

62. Which statements are true concerning scleroderma?
    a. Renal changes resemble those of hypertensive nephrosclerosis.   b. Immunopathic mechanisms may be involved in causation.   c. Incidence is higher in females.   d. All are correct.

63. Which statements are true concerning polyarteritis nodosa? (More than one answer may be correct.)
    a. Most frequently affects young adult females.   b. Arterial lesions in the kidney are common.   c. Other renal lesions include proliferative GN and tubular atrophy.

64. Chronic abuse of which of the following drugs may result in papillary necrosis?
    a. Ethyl alcohol   b. Aspirin   c. Phenacetin   d. Caffeine

Directions: Circle T if the statement is true and F if false. Correct the false statements.

65. T   F   Surgical correction of renal artery stenosis or removal of the ischemic kidney always results in cure of the hypertension.

66. T   F   About one-third of all patients with SLE, PN, and scleroderma have clinical evidence of renal disease.

67. T   F   SLE patients with focal and local glomerular lesions respond well to corticosteroid therapy, and the prognosis is good.

68. T   F   The most frequent cause of death in juvenile-onset diabetes is uremia.

69. T   F   Hypoproteinemia is important in the pathogenesis of edema in APSGN.

70. T   F   The kidney is larger than normal,

with multiple petechiae on the surface, in advanced chronic renal failure.

71. T F Polyuria and "salt wasting" are common clinical features of analgesic nephropathy.

72. T F Chronic renal failure may cause hypertension.

73. T F Widespread epithelial crescent formation signifies remission and a good prognosis in chronic renal failure.

74. T F Immunopathic mechanisms are probably involved in the pathogenesis of most of the connective tissue disorders.

75. T F Aspirin inhibits the synthesis of prostaglandins in renal cells, thus favoring medullary hypoxia.

CHAPTER
43

THE UREMIC SYNDROME

OBJECTIVES

At the completion of this chapter you should be able to:

1. Define *uremic syndrome*.
2. Relate the decrease in GFR to the development of the uremic syndrome.
3. Distinguish between two groups of clinical symptoms present in the uremic syndrome.
4. Describe the events that lead to the development of metabolic acidosis in the uremic syndrome.
5. Explain why the total NH_4^+ excretion is decreased in renal failure.
6. Explain why the acidosis of chronic renal failure usually stabilizes at a moderate level.
7. List three symptoms common in the uremic patient which may be associated with renal acidosis.
8. Describe Kussmaul's respiration.
9. Discuss the development of potassium imbalances in chronic renal failure.
10. Explain how systemic acidosis contributes to hyperkalemia.
11. Describe the most serious complication of hyperkalemia.
12. Differentiate between early renal insufficiency and terminal renal failure in relation to the ability of the kidney to regulate sodium.
13. Explain what condition may result in renal failure when magnesium is not excreted.
14. Explain why uremic patients may have attacks of gouty arthritis.
15. Explain the meaning of a constant finding of urine specific gravity at 1.010.
16. Describe how uremia usually affects sexual and reproductive function.
17. Describe cardiovascular, respiratory, and hematologic manifestations of the uremic syndrome.
18. List some of the factors that predispose the uremic patient to infection.
19. Describe changes in skin coloration in the uremic patient for light-skinned and dark-skinned patients.

20. Describe hair and nail changes associated with renal failure.
21. Describe "uremic frost."
22. Explain why the uremic patient often complains of itching.
23. Describe the gastrointestinal manifestations of uremia.
24. Give the rationale for dietary restriction of protein in the uremic patient.
25. Explain how the metabolism of protein, fat, and carbohydrate is altered in the uremic patient.
26. Describe muscular and central nervous system disturbances associated with the uremic syndrome.
27. Describe peripheral neuropathy and the stages in its development.
28. Describe renal osteodystrophy and the types of bone disorders present in this disorder.
29. Discuss the pathogenesis of secondary hyperparathyroidism and the bone disorders associated with terminal renal failure.
30. Explain the significance of the calcium-phosphate cross product.
31. List some common sites of calcium salts deposition in metastatic soft-tissue calcification.
32. Give the etiology of "uremic red-eye."
33. Explain the significance of the middle molecular hypothesis in relation to some of the systemic and metabolic manifestations of the uremic syndrome.

Each of the principal kidney diseases that lead to chronic progressive renal failure has unique features which relate to etiology, pathogenesis, and morphology. These differences were discussed in Chap. 42. It was also pointed out that these diseases produce kidneys which may have many morphological features in common. This is particularly true when the terminal stage of chronic renal disease is reached, when it may be difficult to determine the cause of the chronic renal failure by examination of the end-stage kidney.

As also explained in Chap. 42, from a functional point of view, regardless of cause, there is a common sequence of changes in renal function due to the progressive destruction of nephrons. The rate of destruction can vary greatly, with quiescent periods and exacerbations, and the duration from beginning to end may vary from months to as long as 40 years. However, once the GFR begins to fall and the BUN and creatinine levels rise, there is a tendency toward rapid progression to end-stage renal failure. Because of these common functional patterns, it is possible to consider the events in the pathophysiology of chronic renal failure as a single phenomenon rather than discuss the changes in function on a disease-by-disease basis.

The common sequence of changes has this effect on the patient: When the GFR falls to 5 to 10 percent of normal and progresses toward zero, the patient develops what is called the *uremic syndrome*. The uremic syndrome is a symptom complex that results from or is associated with retention of nitrogenous metabolites because of renal failure. In advanced uremia, some functions of virtually every organ system in the body may become abnormal.

Two groups of clinical symptoms are present in the uremic syndrome. First, symptoms referrable to deranged regulatory and excretory functions are prominent: fluid volume and electrolyte abnormalities, acid-base imbalance, retention of nitrogenous and other metabolites, and anemia due to renal secretory deficiency. A second group of clinical features includes a constellation of cardiovascular, neuromuscular, gastrointestinal, and other abnormalities. Surprisingly little is known about the basis of these multiple-system abnormalities, though diligent research is now being conducted to uncover these mysteries. Table 43-1 lists some of the common manifestations of the uremic syndrome which are discussed in this chapter.

TABLE 43·1

MANIFESTATIONS OF THE UREMIC SYNDROME

Biochemical	Metabolic acidosis (serum HCO_3^- 18–20 meq/L Azotemia ($\downarrow$ GFR $\rightarrow$ $\uparrow$ BUN, $\uparrow$ creatinine) Hyperkalemia Sodium retention or wasting Hypermagnesemia Hyperuricemia	Gastrointestinal	Anorexia, nausea, vomiting $\rightarrow$ weight loss Ammoniacal odor to breath Metallic taste, dry mouth Stomatitis, parotitis Gastritis, enteritis GI bleeding Diarrhea
Genitourinary	Polyuria $\rightarrow$ oliguria $\rightarrow$ anuria Nocturia, reversal of diurnal rhythm Fixed urine sp. gr. 1.010 Proteinuria; casts Loss of libido, amenorrhea, impotence, sterility	Intermediary metabolism	Protein—intolerance, abnormal synthesis Carbohydrate—hyperglycemia, $\downarrow$ insulin need Fat—$\uparrow$ triglycerides

Cardiovascular	Hypertension
	Hypertensive retinopathy, encephalopathy
	
	Circulatory overload
	Edema
	Congestive heart failure
	Pericarditis (friction rub)
	Arrhythmias
		Neuromuscular	Easy fatigability
			Muscle wasting, weakness
			Central nervous system
			  Decreased mental acuity
			  Poor concentration
			  Apathy
			  Lethargy/restlessness, insomnia
			  Mental confusion
			  Coma
			  Muscle twitching, asterixis, convulsions

Respiratory	Kussmaul's breathing, dyspnea
	Pulmonary edema
	Pneumonitis
			Peripheral neuropathy
			  Slowed nerve conduction, "restless leg" syndrome
			  Sensory changes in the extremities—paresthesias

Hematologic	Anemia $\rightarrow$ fatigue Hemolysis Bleeding tendency $\downarrow$ Resistance to infection (urinary tract infection, pneumonia, septicemia)		Motor changes—foot drop $\rightarrow$ paraplegia
		Calcium and skeletal disorders	Hyperphosphatemia, hypocalcemia
Cutaneous	Pallor, pigmentation Hair and nail changes (nails brittle, thin, ridged, alternating red and light bands associated with protein wasting) Pruritus Uremic "frost" Dry skin Bruises		Secondary hyperparathyroidism Renal osteodystrophy Pathologic fractures (demineralization of bones) Calcium salts deposited in soft tissue (around joints, blood vessels, heart, lungs) Conjunctivitis (uremic red eye)

BIOCHEMICAL DISTURBANCES

Metabolic acidosis

Renal failure is characterized by a wide variety of biochemical disturbances. One of the constant abnormalities exhibited by the uremic patient is metabolic acidosis. On a normal diet, the kidney has to excrete daily 40 to 60 meq of H^+ in order to prevent acidosis. In renal failure, impaired ability of the kidney to excrete H^+ results in a systemic acidosis, with a decrease in the plasma pH and HCO_3^- concentration. The HCO_3^- level decreases because it is used up in buffering H^+. NH_4^+ excretion is the kidney's most important mechanism for the excretion of H^+ and the regeneration of HCO_3^- (since it allows de novo addition of new HCO_3^- rather than just reabsorption of the filtered HCO_3^- to the extracellular fluid). Total NH_4^+ excretion is decreased in renal failure because of the diminished number of nephrons. Phosphate excretion provides another mechanism for the excretion of H^+ as titratable acid (i.e., phosphate-buffered H^+). The rate of phosphate excretion, however, is determined by the need to maintain phosphate balance rather than acid-base balance. Phosphate tends to be retained in renal failure because of the diminished nephron mass and factors related to calcium metabolism which are discussed later. The retention of sulfate and other organic anions also contributes to the depletion of HCO_3^-.

The serum bicarbonate level usually stabilizes at about 18 to 20 meq per liter (moderate acidosis) and rarely drops below this level. The most likely explanation for this lack of progression in the presence of a positive hydrogen ion balance is that hydrogen ion is being buffered by calcium carbonate from the bone.

It is possible that the symptoms of anorexia, nausea, and lethargy that are common in the uremic patient may be due in part to the acidosis. One symptom which is undoubtedly due to acidosis is Kussmaul's respiration, though this symptom may be less prominent in chronic acidosis. *Kussmaul's respiration* is the deep, sighing respiration which occurs because of the need to increase carbon dioxide excretion and thus reduce the severity of the acidosis.

Potassium imbalance

Potassium imbalance is one of the serious disturbances which may occur in renal failure, because only a narrow plasma concentration range is compatible with life (normal = 3.5 to 5 meq per liter). About 80 percent of the normal daily intake of 50 to 150 meq is excreted in the urine. Hypokalemia may be associated with the polyuria of early chronic renal failure, particularly in tubular diseases such as chronic pyelonephritis. However, as the patient becomes oliguric in end-stage renal failure, hyperkalemia invariably develops.

The systemic acidosis also contributes to the hyperkalemia by causing K^+ to shift from the cells to the extracellular fluid. The major life-threatening effect of hyperkalemia is its influence on the electrical conduction of the heart. Fatal arrhythmias or cardiac standstill may occur when serum K^+ levels reach 7 to 8 meq per liter.

Sodium imbalance

The average American diet contains 2 to 10 g Na^+ (or 5 to 25 g NaCl) per day. In most normal persons there is great flexibility in the kidney's ability to vary excretion of sodium in response to a variable intake. Salt excretion may vary from nearly zero to more than 20 g daily. Patients with chronic renal failure lose this great flexibility and may be "poised on a razor's edge" with respect to the ability to vary salt output. In early renal insufficiency when there is polyuria, there may be salt wasting because of the increased solute load of each intact nephron. The osmotic diuresis results in obligatory salt losses. This salt-losing tendency is more common in chronic pyelonephritis and polycystic kidneys, which primarily affect the tubules.

When oliguria supervenes in terminal renal failure, the patient is more likely to retain sodium. The retention of sodium and water may result in circulatory overload, edema, hypertension, and congestive heart failure. The development of congestive heart failure secondary to the hypertension and the increased aldosterone levels present in uremic patients may also play a major role in sodium retention.

Hypermagnesemia

Like potassium, magnesium is chiefly an intracellular cation and is excreted chiefly by the kidneys. The normal serum level is 1.5 to 2.3 meq per liter. The ability to excrete magnesium is reduced in the uremic patient. However, hypermagnesemia is generally not a serious problem, since intake of magnesium is usually reduced because of anorexia, reduced protein intake, and decreased absorption from the gastrointestinal tract. A sudden load of magnesium from the ingestion of laxatives such as milk of magnesia or magnesium citrate may cause death.

Azotemia

As previously discussed, a sharp rise in the plasma urea and creatinine levels generally signals the onset of terminal renal failure and accompanies uremic symptoms. There is much evidence, however, that urea itself is not responsible for the symptoms and metabolic defects found in uremia. Some of the substances found in the blood of uremic patients which might act as toxins are the guanidines, phenols, amines, urate, creatinine, aromatic hydroxy acids, and indican. Some of these compounds act as potent enzyme inhibitors. It is likely that a combination of factors such as the acidosis and other electrolyte disturbances, hormonal disturbances, and retained toxins produce the metabolic defects and the multiple-system involvement. Present research postulates that the uremic toxins may lie in the middle molecular range in size (urea is a small molecule), and this has led to the *middle molecular hypothesis* and research into more efficient removal of these molecules. Hemodiafiltration and hemoperfusion are new, experimental types of dialysis now undergoing clinical trials to test the middle molecular hypothesis (see "New Approaches to Solute Removal" in Chap. 44).

Hyperuricemia

The intimate association of gout and the kidney has been alluded to in Chap. 42. A rise in serum uric acid concentration and the formation of obstructive crystals in the kidney can cause chronic or acute renal failure. On the other hand, the serum uric acid level generally rises early in the course of chronic renal failure because of excretory impairment of the kidneys. The kidneys normally account for about 75 percent of the excreted uric acid. A rise in serum uric acid concentration above the normal 4 to 6 mg per 100 ml may or may not be associated with symptoms. It is not uncommon, however, for uremic patients to have attacks of gouty arthritis from the deposition of urate salts in the joints and soft tissues.

GENITOURINARY DISTURBANCES

Urinary symptoms in uremia are intimately associated with water metabolism; these findings have been discussed in previous chapters. Polyuria due to osmotic diuresis gradually gives way to oliguria and even anuria as the nephron mass is gradually destroyed. Nocturia and a reversal of the normal diurnal pattern of urine excretion, resulting in a relatively constant rate of urine formation throughout the day and night, is another important symptom due to the osmotic diuresis. A constant urine specific gravity near 1.010 in the uremic patient reflects loss of the ability to concentrate or dilute the urine from the plasma concentration. These changes make the uremic patient vulnerable to acute changes in water balance. Diarrhea or vomiting may quickly cause dehydration (with subsequent hypovolemia, decreased GFR, and further deterioration of renal function), and excess water intake may cause circulatory overload, edema, and congestive heart failure.

As the nephron mass and the GFR decrease, proteinuria, which may have been prominent earlier in the chronic renal disease, may become insignificant or may disappear altogether. Broad granular casts may occasionally be found in the urine sediment and are characteristic of advanced renal failure.

The young uremic female ceases to menstruate, and the male is generally impotent and sterile when the GFR falls to 5 ml per minute. Both sexes experience a loss of libido as the uremia becomes more severe. Sexual and reproductive function may return after renal transplantation or a regular hemodialysis program. Most physicians, however, advise women not to become pregnant when there is advanced renal insufficiency.

CARDIOVASCULAR ABNORMALITIES

Hypertension and congestive heart failure often accompany the uremic syndrome. About 90 percent of the hypertension is volume-dependent and related to sodium and water retention, while probably less than 10 percent is renin-dependent. The combination of hyperten-

sion, anemia, and circulatory overload due to sodium and water retention all contribute to the increased propensity to congestive heart failure. Other side effects of severe hypertension include retinopathy and encephalopathy. The symptoms of these disorders are the same as in nonuremic patients.

A fibrinous pericarditis is clinically evident in about half the patients presenting with severe uremia. The basis of the problem is unknown. The patient may complain of pain on deep inspiration or when lying down, but about two-thirds of the patients are asymptomatic. A to-and-fro friction rub may be heard over the precordium with auscultation. The chest x-ray may reveal an enlarged cardiac silhouette when there is a pericardial effusion. Occasionally the patient with uremic pericarditis may develop a massive hemorrhagic effusion and cardiac tamponade, especially when anticoagulants are used during hemodialysis. In the event of this emergency, prompt aspiration of the fluid by the physician may be lifesaving.

Finally, it must be remembered that cardiac arrhythmias commonly associated with K^+ imbalance in renal failure are also affected by imbalances in Na^+, H^+, Ca^{2+}, and Mg^{2+}.

RESPIRATORY CHANGES

The deep, sighing (Kussmaul's) respiration of severe acidosis has already been mentioned. However, the patient with moderate acidosis of chronic renal insufficiency is more apt to complain of dyspnea on exertion, and the increased depth of breathing is overlooked except by an experienced observer.

Other respiratory complications of renal failure are the "uremic lung" and pneumonitis. Chest x-ray of the uremic lung reveals a bilateral butterfly-shaped infiltration of the lungs (Fig. 43-1). It is actually pulmonary edema and is inevitably associated with fluid overload due to sodium and water retention and/or left ventricular failure. Why the pulmonary edema takes on this configuration has been an enigma for years. Possibly there is increased permeability of pulmonary capillaries around the hilus of the lung. Bilaterial infection causing a pneumonitis may be superimposed on the chronically wet lung. Pulmonary congestion disappears with the reduction of body fluids by salt restriction and hemodialysis.

HEMATOLOGIC PROBLEMS

A characteristically normochromic, normocytic anemia is an inevitable feature of the uremic syndrome. Usually the hematocrit falls to the 20 to 30 percent range and parallels the degree of azotemia. The primary cause of the anemia is decreased red blood cell (RBC) formation.

Decreased RBC formation is due to deficient production of erythropoietin by the failing kidney. There is also some evidence that uremic toxins may inactivate erythropoietin or suppress the response of the bone marrow to its action (Whitcomb and Bottomley, 1977). A second factor contributing to the anemia is that the life span of the RBC in a patient with renal failure is about half that in the normal person. The increased hemolysis of RBCs appears to be due to the abnormal chemical environment in the plasma and not to a defect in the cells themselves. In addition to the deficient erythropoiesis and hemolytic tendency, blood loss in the gastrointestinal tract may further aggravate the anemia. Other factors contributing to the anemia include iatrogenic blood loss and iron and folic acid deficiency. The blood loss due to frequent sampling for laboratory tests and loss in the hemodialysis tubing may be considerable (average loss is 4.6 liters per year in one study). Iron deficiency may result from blood loss and from poor GI absorption (antacids taken for hyperphosphatemia also bind iron in the gut). Folic acid deficiency is associated with uremia, and if the patient is receiving hemodialysis treatment, water-soluble vitamins are lost through the dialysis membrane. The bleeding tendency of uremia is apparently due to a qualitative defect in the platelets and consequently results in defective adhesion. Inhibition of certain coagulation factors may also play a role.

Pallor due to persistent anemia is characteristic of the anemic patient. The anemia undoubtedly contrib-

utes to the symptoms of fatigue. Dyspnea on exertion may be experienced when the hemoglobin is 8 g per 100 ml or less. Bruising, nosebleeds, and GI bleeding may be manifestations of the coagulation defect.

Infection is a fairly common complication of patients with advanced renal insufficiency. WBC function is apparently normal. Poor nutrition, pulmonary edema, and the use of cannulas and indwelling catheters may be predisposing factors in the increased susceptibility to infection. The use of large doses of corticosteroid and other immunosuppressive drugs following renal transplant to suppress tissue rejection makes these patients unusually susceptible to severe infection which may result in death.

CUTANEOUS CHANGES

The accumulation of urinary pigments (principally urochrome) combined with anemia in advanced renal insufficiency gives the skin of the light-skinned person a peculiar waxy yellow cast. In the brown-skinned person this is observed as a yellowish brown coloration, and in the black-skinned person as an ashen gray color with yellow tones, particularly on the palmar and plantar surfaces. The skin may be dry and scaly, and the hair may be brittle and may change color. The nails may be thin, brittle, and ridged and show alternating light and reddish bands. These nail changes are characteristic of chronic protein wasting (Muehrcke lines). Pruritus is common in the uremic patient and is considered to be a manifestation of increased parathyroid gland function and deposition of calcium in the skin. When the BUN level is very high, fine white crystals of urea may appear on areas of the skin where there is heavy perspiration. This is called *uremic frost.* Multiple bruises caused by minor trauma are often seen on the skin of the uremic patient owing to increased capillary fragility.

GASTROINTESTINAL SIGNS AND SYMPTOMS

The gastrointestinal manifestations of uremia can cause the patient great distress. Anorexia, nausea, and vomiting are common in uremia and are often the first symptoms of disease. They are responsible, in part, for the

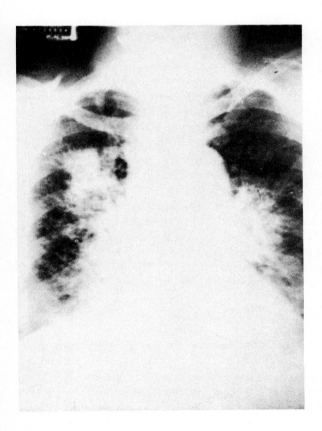

FIGURE 43-1
Uremic lung, showing marked central distribution of pulmonary edema. (From George L. Bailey, *Hemodialysis,* Academic, New York, 1972.)

extensive loss of weight in chronic renal failure. The entire GI tract itself becomes affected in uremia. Patients often complain of a metallic taste in the mouth, and there may be an odor of ammonia to the breath. The mouth may become inflamed and ulcerated (stomatitis), and the tongue may be dry and coated. Occasionally parotitis (inflammation of the parotid gland) occurs. The normal flora of the mouth contains organisms (tooth calculus bacteria) which can split urea in the saliva to produce ammonia. This accounts for the uriniferous odor to the breath and the altered sense of taste and predisposes the tissue to inflammation and infection. Mucosal ulcerations may occur in the stomach and the small or large intestine and may result in profuse bleeding. The effect of GI hemorrhage is extremely serious, as the fall in blood pressure lowers the GFR even further and the digestion of the blood causes a precipitous rise in the BUN level. Diarrhea occurs at times and may cause serious dehydration.

INTERMEDIARY METABOLISM ABNORMALITIES

Abnormalities of intermediary metabolism are characteristic of the uremic syndrome, although the physiologic mechanisms are poorly understood, as are those in other body systems.

Protein

Whatever other elements are responsible for uremic symptoms, the breakdown products of protein metabolism are of prime importance. The dietary restriction of protein generally relieves somewhat the symptoms of lassitude, nausea, and anorexia, though it does not improve the GFR. The patient tends to decrease protein intake voluntarily as azotemia progresses, since the appetite for protein foods generally is lost. Another reason for protein restriction in uremia is that H^+, K^+, and phosphates are derived chiefly from protein foods and must be restricted to prevent their accumulation in the blood. Abnormal protein synthesis in uremia is manifested by elevation or depression of selected amino acids. The significance of this phenomenon is not known.

Carbohydrates and fats

Defective carbohydrate metabolism is commonly associated with uremia. Fasting blood sugar levels are elevated in more than 50 percent of uremic patients, but not usually over 200 mg per 100 ml. Insensitivity of the peripheral tissues to insulin is the possible cause. On the other hand, insulin-dependent diabetics who develop uremia may improve their carbohydrate metabolism and require a lower dosage of insulin, in apparent contradiction to the glucose intolerance of nondiabetics. A possible explanation is an elevated serum insulin level due to a prolonged half-life (the kidney normally inactivates about 15 percent of the insulin) in uremia. Carbohydrate metabolism generally becomes normal with regular hemodialysis.

Abnormal fat metabolism is manifested by high serum triglyceride levels in the uremic patient, even in patients who regularly undergo dialysis. Contributing factors in the elevated triglycerides may include the elevated glucose and insulin levels and the acetate used in the dialysate. The abnormal carbohydrate and fat metabolism undoubtedly contributes to the accelerated atherosclerosis in chronic dialysis patients (Friedman, 1978, p. 225).

NEUROMUSCULAR ABNORMALITIES

Involvement of the neuromuscular system is a nearly universal complication of uremia. Both the central and the peripheral nervous system are involved, with diverse consequences. Muscles may be involved partly because of the peripheral neuropathy and partly because of muscle wasting.

Central nervous system

The degree of cerebral disturbance roughly parallels the degree of azotemia. Early symptoms are decreased mental acuity and ability to concentrate, apathy, and lethargy. The patient complains of feeling weak and tired and may be unable to perform a normal day's work without frequent rest periods. Lethargy may alternate with periods of restlessness and insomnia. The untreated patient will eventually become confused and comatose. If convulsions occur, they are usually associated with hypertensive encephalopathy. Neuromuscular irritability is reflected by involuntary jerking and twitching of muscles. *Asterixis* (flapping tremor of the hands) may sometimes be present and is a manifestation of cerebral toxicity. The physical sign is induced by having the patient raise both arms with forearms fixed and fingers extended; this will result in alterations of flexion and extension at the wrist (flapping tremor).

Peripheral neuropathy

Affliction of the peripheral nervous system follows a characteristic course. The earliest sign of peripheral neuropathy is the slowing of nerve conduction. This is generally tested on the peroneal nerve in the leg. A decreased velocity of nerve conduction may begin before the onset of clinical symptoms. The "restless leg syndrome" may sometimes be an early symptom. The patient may describe this symptom as a peculiar feeling which is relieved by walking or moving the legs. The second stage in the development of peripheral neuropathy is the advent of sensory changes in the extremities. The patient experiences burning pain, numbness, or tingling (paresthesias) of the toes and feet, which progress up the leg in a stockinglike fashion. Later, paresthesias may occur in the fingers and hands. Finally, motor nerves are involved. Motor involvement usually begins as a foot drop and may progress to paraplegia. Pathologically there is a patchy loss of myelin and damage to the peripheral nerves, possibly caused by uremic toxins and electrolyte imbalance.

Hemodialysis may halt the progress of peripheral neuropathy, but once these changes occur they are poorly reversible (sensory) or irreversible (motor). Therefore, hemodialysis (or transplantation preparations) should be started before clinical signs and symptoms occur.

CALCIUM AND SKELETAL DISORDERS (RENAL OSTEODYSTROPHY)

If a patient with chronic renal failure survives long enough, calcium and phosphate imbalances with skeletal involvement are inevitable. The skeletal disorders called *renal osteodystrophy* comprise three lesions.

Osteomalacia is the most common bone disorder and is seen in about 60 percent of all patients with chronic renal failure. It consists of defective mineralization of bone. It is caused by a deficiency of 1,25-dihydroxycholecalciferol [$1,25(OH)_2D_3$], the most active form of vitamin D metabolized by the kidneys. The deficiency of the most active form of vitamin D leads to severely impaired absorption of calcium from the gut. In the bone, osteoblasts continue to manufacture osteoid tissue (the framework on which calcium salts are laid down to produce bone), but the low serum calcium level and ineffective action of vitamin D on the bone do not allow mineralization. Osteoid tissue eventually replaces normal bone, producing osteomalacia in adults and rickets in children. Osteoid is structurally weak and may fracture or deform under stress. On x-ray, osteomalacia presents as a generalized decrease in bone density, especially of the hands, skull, ribs, and spine.

Osteitis fibrosa, occurring in over 30 percent of pa-

tients, is characterized by osteoclastic resorption of bone and replacement by fibrous tissue. The bone demineralization may be localized and may present as cystlike lesions (osteitis fibrosa cystica) or may appear as a generalized decrease in bone density on x-ray. Osteitis fibrosa is caused by the increased levels of parathyroid hormone (PTH) (secondary hyperparathyroidism) in chronic renal failure. The classic x-ray appearance of osteitis fibrosa is often seen in the fingers as subperiosteal bone resorption and in the skull as a patchy loss of bone density (Fig. 43-2).

Osteosclerosis, the third, less common bone disorder, is often manifested as a banded or striped appearance of the vertebrae ("rugger jersey spine") on x-ray

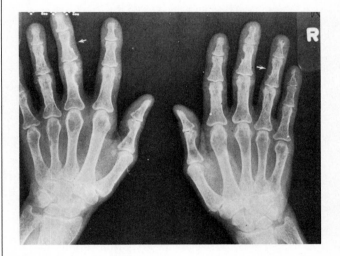

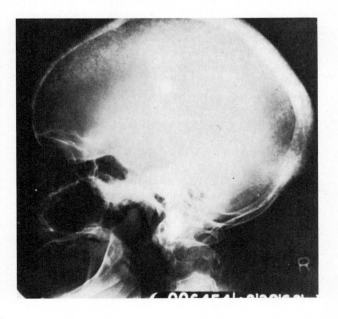

FIGURE 43-2
Renal osteodystrophy. (A) Subperiosteal resorption is present in all phalanges but is seen best on the middle phalanx of both the right and left hands (arrows) producing a jagged appearance. (B) Skull x-ray shows spotty demineralization of bone producing a "moth-eaten" apearance. (Courtesy of D. E. Schteingart.)

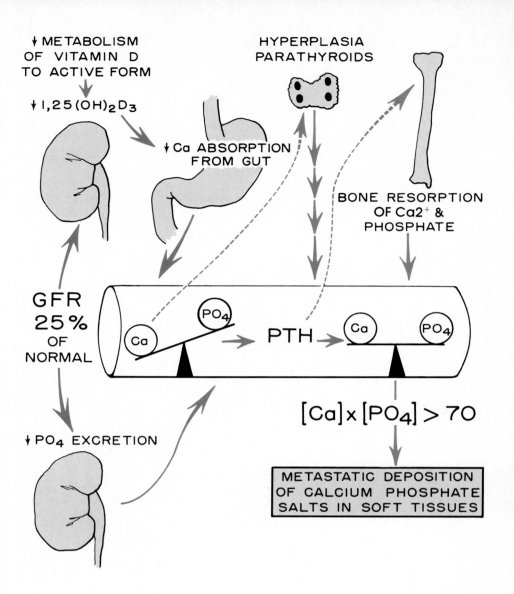

FIGURE 43-3
Pathogenesis of renal osteodystrophy. (See text for explanation.)

due to alternate bands of decreased and increased bone density.

Any of the above lesions may occur alone, but a combination is more common. Hemodialysis alone does not prevent renal osteodystrophy. Only within the past few years has research uncovered some of the complex relationships in the pathogenesis of renal osteodystrophy so that effective treatment is possible. The principal factors are decreased renal function, secondary hyperparathyroidism, and vitamin D deficiency and/or resistance.

Pathogenesis of renal osteodystrophy

The sequence of events leading to secondary hyperparathyroidism and renal osteodystrophy is most easily followed in Fig. 43-3.

Normally the serum calcium and phosphate are in equilibrium with solid-phase calcium and phosphate in the bones. The absorption from the gut, excretion by the kidneys, and deposition and resorption from the bone of these minerals is primarily controlled by PTH and vitamin D. Moreover, serum calcium and phosphate levels have a reciprocal relationship, i.e., when serum calcium levels go up, serum phosphate levels go down and vice versa. This interrelation serves the purpose of keeping the serum calcium-phosphate cross product constant so that calcium phosphate is not precipitated in the vascular system. For example, the normal serum calcium level is 9.0 to 11.0 mg per 100 ml, and the normal phosphate level is 3.0 to 4.5 mg per 100 ml. The normal cross-product value in milligrams per 100 ml of calcium and phosphate is thus 3 to 4.5 × 9 to 11 = 27.0 to 49.5. Precipitation of calcium phosphate salts in the soft tissues is believed to occur when their cross product exceeds 60 to 70 mg per 100 ml.

As renal disease advances, calcium-phosphate interrelations become progressively disrupted. When the GFR falls to about 25 percent of normal, phosphate is retained by the kidneys. Phosphate retention causes the

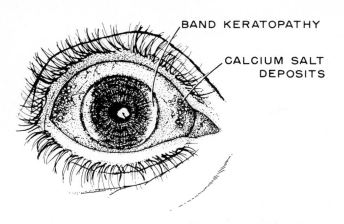

BAND KERATOPATHY

CALCIUM SALT
DEPOSITS

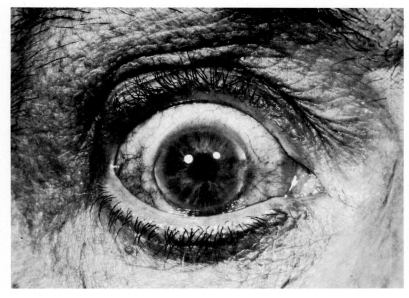

FIGURE 43-4
Band keratopathy due to deposit of calcium salts in the eye. Conjunctival deposits of calcium salts are also present. Diagram of abnormalities seen in photograph. (Photograph from M. H. Maxwell and C. R. Kleeman (eds.), *Clinical Disorders of Fluid and Electrolyte Metabolism,* **2d ed., McGraw-Hill, New York, 1972.)**

depression of serum calcium levels. The azotemic state also interferes with vitamin D activation by the kidney, which is necessary for the absorption of calcium from the gut. Both these factors tend to cause hypocalcemia. Hypocalcemia stimulates the parathyroid glands to put out more PTH, which causes bone resorption of calcium and phosphate, increased excretion of phosphate, and activation of vitamin D by the kidneys. Serum calcium and phosphate levels thus tend to be restored to normal. As the GFR continues to decrease, however, the low serum calcium and high phosphate levels continue to stimulate parathyroid activity more and more. The parathyroid glands may show hyperplasia of the secretory cells, with apparent independence of physiologic controls. The result is increasing demineralization of the bony skeleton. A rise in the serum alkaline phosphatase level is evidence that this process is occurring. The calcium phosphate cross product may become exceedingly high, resulting in the precipitation of calcium phosphate salts in the soft tissues of the body.

Common sites for the deposition of calcium salts are in and around joints, resulting in painful arthritis; in the kidney (nephrocalcinosis), resulting in obstruction; in the blood vessels, which may have the appearance of an arteriogram on the x-ray; in the heart and lung, leading to arrhythmias, cardiomyopathy, and pulmonary fibrosis; and in the eyes. The deposition of calcium salts in the conjunctiva and cornea of the eye is called *band keratopathy*. Band keratopathy appears as grayish or whitish granular opacities in the form of a crescent on the nasal or temporal side of the limbus (where cornea and sclera meet at colored and white part of eye) (Fig. 43-4). Precipitation of calcium phosphate salts occurs on the surface of the eye because here the pH is high and favors precipitation. These depositions can be seen with the naked eye but are most easily outlined by slit lamp examination. The conjunctival deposits sometimes cause intense irritation with redness and watering of the eyes ("uremic red eye").

This completes the description of the syndrome which is called uremia. Not all components are present in every patient, and the dominant features may vary from one patient to another. The prevention and treatment of these complications are considered in Chap. 44.

The uremic syndrome

Directions: Answer the following questions on a separate sheet of paper.

1. What is meant by *uremic syndrome?*

2. What are the two groups of clinical symptoms present in the uremic syndrome? How does the middle molecular hypothesis account for some of these symptoms? What are the implications of this theory?

3. Explain why total NH_4^+ excretion is decreased in renal failure.

4. Why does the acidosis of chronic renal failure generally stabilize at a moderate level when there is a positive H^+ balance? What relation might the acidosis of renal failure have to the bone abnormality?

5. Why is salt wasting associated with polyuria in early renal insufficiency?

6. Name two common laxatives which, if administered to the uremic patient, might result in death.

7. Explain the meaning of a constant finding of urine specific gravity at 1.010.

8. How are sexual and reproductive functions affected in terminal renal failure? (Explain the effects in males and females.)

9. Name four factors which contribute to the development of infection in the uremic patient.

10. Describe skin color changes in uremic patients who are white-skinned, brown-skinned, and black-skinned.

11. Illustrate the mechanisms by which GI bleeding, vomiting, or diarrhea could cause the deterioration of renal function. (Draw flow diagrams.)

12. List several changes you might expect to observe in the mental, emotional, and neuromuscular status and rest pattern of a patient who is developing uremia.

13. List the stages in the development of peripheral neuropathy and the signs and symptoms you would expect to observe in the patient with renal failure.

14. Illustrate the appearance of the phalanges seen on x-ray when there is subperiosteal bone resorption in renal osteodystrophy.

15. Draw a flow diagram of the pathogenesis of secondary hyperparathyroidism and list several examples of the consequences of this condition.

16. A uremic patient has a serum phosphate level of 8 mg per 100 ml and a calcium level of 10 mg per 100 ml. Would you expect metastatic calcification in the soft tissues of the body? Explain.

17. What is *band keratopathy?* Illustrate. What causes "uremic red eye"?

Directions: Circle the letter preceding each item below that correctly answers the question or completes the statement. Only one answer is correct, with exceptions noted.

18. In renal failure there is an impaired ability to excrete H^+. This results in:
    a. Respiratory acidosis *b.* Metabolic acidosis
    c. Respiratory alkalosis *d.* Metabolic alkalosis

19. Which of the following describes the plasma pH and bicarbonate levels in the condition of renal failure?
    a. Increase in pH and decrease in HCO_3^- *b.* Decrease in pH and increase in HCO_3^- *c.* Decrease in both pH and HCO_3^- *d.* Increase in both pH and HCO_3^-

20. Which of the following mechanisms is most important for the excretion of H^+ by the kidney?
    a. Excretion of H^+ as NH_4^+ by combination with NH_3 *b.* Excretion of H^+ as acid phosphate

21. Hypokalemia associated with polyuria is most apt to be associated with:
    a. Acute renal failure *b.* Acute pyelonephritis
    c. Chronic pyelonephritis

22. As the patient becomes oliguric in end-stage renal failure, which of the following K^+ disturbances usually develops?
    a. Hypokalemia *b.* Hyperkalemia

23. Metabolic acidosis contributes to hyperkalemia by which of the following mechanisms?
    a. K^+ (cells) → extracellular fluid *b.* Mg^{2+} (cells) → extracellular fluid *c.* K^+ (extracellular fluid) → cells *d.* Mg^{2+} (extracellular fluid) → cells

24. Fatal arrhythmias and cardiac arrest are most apt to occur when serum K^+ levels reach:
    a. 3.5 to 4.5 meq per liter *b.* 4.5 to 5.5 meq per liter *c.* 6.5 to 7.5 meq per liter

25. When oliguria occurs in terminal renal failure, the patient is likely to do which of the following? (More than one answer may be correct.)
    a. Increase salt-losing tendency *b.* Retain sodium *c.* Increase circulatory overload *d.* Increase aldosterone secretion

26. Symptoms of gouty arthritis experienced by some uremic patients are most likely to be caused by serum elevations of:
    a. Urea *b.* Creatinine *c.* Uric acid *d.* Bicarbonate

27. Which of the following factors contribute to the development of congestive heart failure in uremic patients? (More than one answer may be correct.)
    a. Anemia   b. Hypertension   c. Excess sodium and water intake   d. Circulatory overload

28. Which statements are true in relation to anemia in a uremic patient? (More than one answer may be correct.) Correct the false statements.
    a. Due to excess hemolysis   b. Due to iron deficiency   c. Normochromic, normocytic
    d. Due to excess production of erythropoietin
    e. When severe may cause symptoms of fatigue, dyspnea, and pallor

29. What is the mechanism of the bleeding tendency in uremia? (More than one answer may be correct.)
    a. Defective platelet adhesion   b. Severe thrombocytopenia   c. Inhibition of some of the circulating coagulation factors

30. Symptoms of uremia generally begin when the GFR falls to which of the following ranges of normal?
    a. 80 to 90 percent   b. 50 to 60 percent   c. 30 to 40 percent   d. 4 to 10 percent

Directions: Circle T if the statement is true and F if false. Correct false statements.

31. T   F   Anorexia, nausea, and lethargy are common symptoms in the uremic patient and may be due, in part, to metabolic acidosis.

32. T   F   Kussmaul's respiration is the shallow respiration which occurs because of the need to decrease CO_2 excretion by the lungs.

33. T   F   The symptoms of anorexia, nausea, and lassitude are often relieved by the dietary restriction of protein.

34. T   F   Dietary protein restriction causes a marked improvement of the GFR.

35. T   F   Dietary protein restriction helps reduce K^+, H^+, and phosphate intake.

36. T   F   There is no evidence of abnormal protein synthesis in uremia.

37. T   F   Hypoglycemia is the usual manifestation of abnormal carbohydrate metabolism in uremia.

38. T   F   Insulin-dependent diabetic persons who become uremic often require lower dosages of insulin.

39. T   F   Elevation of serum triglycerides in uremia is related to abnormal fat metabolism in uremia.

Directions: Fill in the blanks with the correct words.

40. Organisms normally in the mouth split _____, producing _____ which contributes to the uriniferous odor to the breath, inflammation and ulceration of the mucous membranes, predisposition to _____, and altered taste sensation common in the uremic patient.

41. Three types of bone lesions seen in renal osteodystrophy are (a) _____ due to hyperparathyroidism; (b) _____ due to vitamin D deficiency; (c) _____ which gives a banded ("rugger jersey") appearance to the spine due to alternating areas of bone demineralization and sclerosis.

Draw arrows from the abnormality found in uremia in col. A to the most likely complication resulting from that abnormality in col. B. More than one arrow from each condition may be drawn from left to right.

Column A

42. ____ Pericarditis

43. ____ Circulatory overload

44. ____ Hypertension

Column B

a. Pneumonia

b. Retinopathy

c. Cardiac tamponade

d. Pulmonary edema

e. Encephalopathy

Directions: Match the following integumentary manifestations of the uremic syndrome in col. B with the probable causative factor in col. A.

Column A

45. ____ Urochrome

46. ____ Anemia

47. ____ Urea

48. ____ Proteinuria

49. ____ Calcium deposits in skin

50. ____ Capillary fragility

Column B

a. Bruises

b. Yellow cast

c. Pruritus

d. Fine white crystal deposits in areas of increased perspiration

e. Brittle, ridged nails with alternating light and red bands

f. Pallor

TREATMENT OF CHRONIC RENAL FAILURE

OBJECTIVES

At the completion of this chapter you should be able to:

1. Describe the two stages in the treatment of chronic renal failure.

2. List four common causes of a sudden deterioration of renal function in chronic renal failure.

3. Describe the principles of dietary regulation in the management of chronic renal failure.

4. Illustrate how fluid allowance is determined in the uremic patient.

5. List common complications encountered in uremia.

6. Describe prevention and treatment measures for the above complications.

7. List two reasons why the treatment of advanced renal insufficiency has been changed in recent years.

8. Describe the modalities of treatment the uremic patient may choose and how they are related to each other.

9. Identify the criteria for transition from conservative methods of treatment of the uremic patient to more definitive therapy.

10. Define *dialysis*.

11. Describe the two major techniques and the basic principles of dialysis (diffusion; osmotic and hydrostatic pressure gradients).

12. Identify the three basic types of hemodialyzers.

13. Describe a hemodialysis system in operation.

14. Differentiate between an external and an internal arteriovenous shunt.

15. Compare the efficiency of hemodialysis and peritoneal dialysis.

16. Name several new, experimental approaches to the removal of uremic solutes.

17. Describe the placement of a transplanted kidney.

18. Identify the two major antigenic groups important in determining histocompatibility in renal transplantation.

19. Differentiate between Class I and Class II HLA antigens (inheritance patterns, methods of assaying, significance, function in rejection).

20. Name four types of test commonly performed before renal transplantation to predict graft survival.
21. Explain the significance of pretransplantation blood transfusions to transplantation outcome.
22. Describe the major complications of renal transplantation and treatment.
23. Compare hemodialysis and renal transplantation as methods of treatment in end-stage renal disease.

The treatment of chronic renal failure may be divided into two stages. The first stage consists of conservative measures which are designed to temper or delay the progressive deterioration of renal function. Conservative measures are begun when the patient becomes azotemic. The physician makes every effort to determine the primary cause of the renal failure and search out any reversible factors such as:

1. ECF volume depletion caused by the overzealous use of diuretics or a salt restriction that is too stringent
2. Urinary tract obstruction from calculi, prostatic enlargement, or retroperitoneal fibrosis
3. Infection, especially of the urinary tract
4. Severe or malignant hypertension

These factors are likely causes of a sudden deterioration of renal function in a patient with chronic renal failure (Schrier, 1976, p. 326). Treatment of reversible factors may stabilize and prevent any further deterioration of renal function.

The second stage of treatment begins when conservative measures are no longer effective. Terminal renal failure exists at this point [glomerular filtration rate (GFR) usually less than 2 ml per minute], and the only effective treatment is either intermittent dialysis or renal transplantation.

CONSERVATIVE MANAGEMENT

The basic principles of conservative management are quite simple and are based on an understanding of the range of excretion that can be achieved by the failing kidney. Dietary regulation of individual solutes and fluid is then adjusted to the limitations. In addition, therapy is directed toward prevention and treatment of complications as they occur.

Dietary regulation of protein, potassium, sodium, and fluids

Dietary regulation is of primary importance in the treatment of chronic renal failure. It is customary to restrict the protein intake of the azotemic patient, though there is controversy about how severe this restriction should be. The restriction of protein not only reduces the BUN level, and perhaps other poorly defined toxic products of protein metabolism, but also reduces the intake of potassium and phosphate and the hydrogen-ion production which stem from protein. Though the GFR is not improved, uremic symptoms such as nausea, vomiting, and fatigue may be ameliorated. One suggested predialysis schedule based on the GFR is as follows:

GFR, ml/min	Protein restriction, g
10	40
5	25 to 30
3 or less	20

Not only is the amount of protein important, but so is its quality. It is possible to maintain nitrogen balance even on a 20-g protein diet, provided the protein is of the highest biological value (i.e., contains all the essential amino acids, as do milk and eggs) and adequate calories are supplied in the form of fats and carbohydrates to prevent the breakdown of body protein to satisfy caloric requirements. However, acceptability may be a problem with a diet of less than 40 g protein per day, and dietary treatment does not seem to be too successful once the GFR has fallen below 4 to 5 ml per minute.

Another approach to protein restriction is to give a diet containing 0.25 g of unrestricted quality protein per kilogram of body weight per day, plus a supplement of essential amino acids or α-keto or α-hydroxy analogues of essential amino acids. This approach allows more variety in the diet and therefore may be more acceptable to some patients. Carbohydrate supplements may be given to ensure adequate calories to prevent breakdown of body protein. Vitamin B complex, pyridoxine, and ascorbic acid supplements should also be given with such regimens (Walser and Mitch, 1977).

The protein allowance is generally liberalized to 60 to 80 g per day (1.0 g/kg daily) when the patient is receiving regular hemodialysis treatment.

Hyperkalemia generally becomes a problem in advanced renal failure, and it becomes necessary also to restrict dietary intake of potassium. The typical dietary allowance is 40 to 80 meq per day. Care must be taken not to administer foods or drugs which are high in potassium. These include salt substitutes (which contain ammonium chloride and potassium chloride), expectorants, potassium citrate, and foods such as soups, dates, bananas, and pure fruit juices. Inadvertent administration of food or drugs high in potassium could cause a serious hyperkalemia.

The dietary regulation of sodium is important in renal failure. The typical sodium allowance is 40 to 90 meq per day (1 to 2 g sodium), but the optimal sodium intake must be determined individually for each patient in order to maintain good hydration. An intake that is too liberal can lead to fluid retention, peripheral edema, pulmonary edema, hypertension, and congestive heart failure. Sodium retention is generally a problem in glomerular disease and in advanced renal failure. On the other hand, if sodium is restricted to the point of negative sodium balance, then hypovolemia, decreased GFR, and a deterioration of renal function will ensue. Sodium depletion is more common in tubular disease and may be precipitated by vomiting or diarrhea. It is therefore important for the physician to determine the optimum sodium intake for each patient. The sodium conservation test and a careful observation of the daily weight, signs of edema, and other complications may all be helpful.

In the sodium conservation test the patient eats a low sodium diet for 5 days (e.g., 10 meq per day). The normal person will conserve sodium and come into balance during this period of time. On the fifth day, 24-hour urine samples are collected and the sodium is measured. The sodium lost in the urine at this time represents an obligatory loss and thus the "sodium floor." For example, a patient on a 10-meq sodium diet who loses 50 meq in the urine on the fifth day has a negative sodium balance of 40 meq (50 − 10 = 40); 40 meq of sodium must be added to the diet. The "sodium ceiling" is determined by observing weight, blood pressure, and

other signs of ECF excess. As stated previously, the range between sodium deficit and sodium excess can be very narrow.

The intake of fluids requires careful regulation in advanced renal failure, as the patient's thirst is an unreliable guide to the state of hydration. Daily weight is the critical parameter to follow, in addition to *accurate* intake and output records. An intake that is too liberal may result in circulatory overload, edema, and water intoxication, and less than optimal intake will result in dehydration, hypotension, and a deterioration in renal function. The general rule for fluid intake is urine output during last 24 hours + 500 ml, the 500 ml representing insensible loss. For example, if the patient's urine output during the past 24 hours was 400 ml, then the total intake per day should be 500 + 400 ml = 900 ml. Anephric patients are allowed 800 ml per day, and patients in dialysis are given sufficient fluid to allow a 2- to 3-pound weight gain between treatments. Obviously, both sodium and fluid intake must be manipulated to achieve fluid balance.

Prevention and treatment of complications

The second category of conservative measures used in the treatment of renal failure comprises those directed toward the prevention and treatment of complications.

Hypertension

It is generally agreed that renal function deteriorates more rapidly if severe hypertension develops. In addition, extrarenal complications such as retinopathy and encephalopathy may develop. Hypertension can usually be controlled effectively by sodium and fluid restriction and by ultrafiltration when the patient is on hemodialysis, since more than 90 percent of hypertension is volume-dependent. In some cases an antihypertensive drug (with or without a diuretic) may be given to achieve blood pressure control. The most common antihypertensive drugs given are alpha-methyldopa (Aldomet), propranolol (Inderal), and clonidine (Catapres), and the most common diuretic is furosemide (Lasix). When the patient is receiving hemodialysis, it is important to withhold the antihypertensive drug before treatment to prevent hypotension and shock that may result as intravascular fluid is removed through ultrafiltration if the normal vascular vasoconstrictive reaction is blocked by the drug. In a small number of cases (<10 percent) the hypertension may be renin-dependent and refractory to sodium-volume control or control with a mild antihypertensive. A more potent antihypertensive drug such as minoxidil (Loniten) can usually bring the blood pressure under control. Bilateral nephrectomy may be considered as a last resort when all other methods have failed. Bilateral nephrectomy causes the anemia to become more severe, since even the end-stage kidney produces some erythropoietin (Epstein, 1977).

Great care is taken to lower the blood pressure gradually so that the patient does not become hypotensive, with consequent lowering of GFR and further deterioration of renal function. Hypertension in the majority of uremic patients is due to fluid overload and is most effectively restored to normal by regulation of sodium and fluid intake and intermittent dialysis.

Hyperkalemia

One of the most serious complications in the uremic patient is the development of hyperkalemia. When serum K^+ reaches a level of about 7 meq per liter, serious arrhythmias and cardiac arrest may occur. In addition, hypocalcemia, hyponatremia, and acidosis intensify the deleterious effects of hyperkalemia. For this reason, the patient may be put on a cardiac monitor to detect the effect of the hyperkalemia (and the effects of all the other ions) on cardiac conduction.

Acute hyperkalemia may be treated by the administration of intravenous glucose and insulin, which drives K^+ into the cells, or by the careful intravenous administration of 10% calcium gluconate, with continuous ECG monitoring if the patient is hypotensive with widening of the QRS complex. The effect of these measures is only temporary, and the hyperkalemia must subsequently be corrected by dialysis. When it is not possible to lower K^+ by dialysis, the cation exchange resin sodium polystyrene sulfonate (Kayexalate) may be used. Each gram of the resin binds 1 meq of K^+. Kayexalate may be given by mouth or by rectal instillation. When given rectally, 50 to 100 g is mixed with 200 to 300 ml of water. To facilitate the K^+ exchange, 25 to 30 ml of 70% sorbitol (a poorly absorbed, osmotically active alcohol which has a laxative effect) is added. Needless to say, orange juice (high K^+ content) should not be given to disguise the taste when Kayexalate is administered orally!

Anemia

The ideal way to treat the anemia of renal failure would be to give erythropoietin, but unfortunately it is not commercially available. However, there are several ways to minimize the severity of the anemia. Iatrogenic blood loss can be reduced by taking the smallest blood sample possible for laboratory tests and by minimizing residual blood left in the tubing in hemodialysis treatment. A multivitamin and a folic acid preparation are commonly given each day since water-soluble vitamins are depleted during dialysis. Oral iron or dextran iron complex (Imferon) may be given parenterally, since iron deficiency may result from blood loss and binding by antacids. Androgens (nandrolone decanoate, or Deca-

Durabolin, for women and depo-testosterone for men) stimulate erythropoietin activity in some patients and are generally more effective in women. However, their masculinizing side effects may be unacceptable to women, and they also tend to cause hyperlipidemia. Patients can usually function quite well and tolerate a hematocrit as low as 18 to 20 percent.

It was formerly believed that blood transfusions should be kept to a minimum, since they would presensitize the host by stimulating antibody formation against leukocyte antigens and thus the chances of graft rejection would theoretically be increased in the event of a subsequent renal transplant. However, recent evidence indicates that cadaver graft survival is greatly enhanced by pretransplant blood transfusions (Opelz and Terasaki, 1978). Thus current practice is more and more to give transfusions to patients on dialysis either for therapeutic reasons or for pretransplant preparation.

Acidosis

The mild chronic metabolic acidosis of the uremic patient usually stabilizes at a plasma bicarbonate level of 16 to 20 meq per liter. It does not usually progress beyond this point, since H^+ production is balanced by bone buffering. The renal acidosis is not usually treated unless the plasma HCO_3^- falls below 15 meq per liter, when symptoms of acidosis may appear. Severe acidosis may be precipitated by the superimposition of an acute acidosis on the mild chronic acidosis. This might occur, for example, in profuse diarrhea with its HCO_3^- loss. When severe acidosis is corrected by the parenteral administration of $NaHCO_3$, it is important to be aware of the hazard involved. Overcorrection of blood pH may precipitate tetany, convulsions, and death. It should be remembered that chronic renal failure patients are usually hypocalcemic. A mild degree of induced alkalosis may reduce the ionized fraction of serum Ca^{2+} (usually in an acidic environment) to the point of severe hypocalcemia. The most logical mode of treatment, finally, is dialysis.

Renal osteodystrophy

One of the most crucial therapeutic measures used to prevent the development of secondary hyperparathyroidism and its consequences is a low phosphate diet along with the administration of gels which bind phosphate in the bowel. The prevention and correction of hyperphosphatemia preclude the sequence of events leading to calcium and bone disorders discussed in

Chap. 43. A low protein diet is also low in phosphate. The treatment should begin early in the course of progressive renal failure, when the GFR is down to one-third of normal. The usual agents chosen as phosphate binders are aluminum antacid gels (Amphojel or Basojel) in tablet or liquid form. *Most other antacids contain magnesium and should not be given.* These antacids form an insoluble aluminum phosphate in the bowel, which is subsequently excreted in the stool. Phosphate-binding gels should be taken *with* meals. The greatest problem is obtaining the cooperation of the patient in carrying out the treatment regimen. Antacids are now available in cookies and in capsule form, which may be more acceptable to some patients.

If severe skeletal involvement occurs for lack of or in spite of preventive therapy with antacid gels, subtotal parathyroidectomy or vitamin D therapy may be indicated. Severe bone demineralization, hypercalcemia, and/or intractable pruritus are considered indications for parathyroidectomy. When the predominant lesion is osteomalacia, the nephrologist may begin vitamin D therapy with great care. This treatment may be quite hazardous. Not only may calcium absorption be increased, but it may in fact lead to progressive soft-tissue calcification when bone resorption and hyperphosphatemia continue unabated.

Other methods used to prevent renal osteodystrophy include increasing calcium intake to 1.2 to 1.5 g daily in the diet or by calcium supplement (only after the serum phosphate level is lowered to normal) and keeping the concentration of calcium in the dialysate between 6.5 and 7.0 meq per liter.

Hyperuricemia

Allopurinol is usually the drug of choice for treating the hyperuricemia of advanced renal disease. This drug reduces uric acid levels by blocking the biosynthesis of some part of the total uric acid produced by the body. Colchicine (anti-inflammatory drug for gout) may be given for the relief of symptoms of gouty arthritis.

Peripheral neuropathy

Usually, symptomatic peripheral neuropathy does not occur until renal failure is far advanced. There is no known treatment for these changes except dialysis, which stops its progression. Therefore the development of sensory neuritis is a signal that dialysis should not be delayed any longer. Motor neuropathy may be irreversible. Nerve conduction velocity tests are commonly performed every 6 months to monitor the progress of peripheral neuropathy.

Prompt treatment of infection

Patients with chronic renal failure have an increased susceptibility to infection, particularly urinary tract infection. Since infection of any sort may accentuate the catabolic process and impair adequate nutrition and fluid and electrolyte balance, infections should be treated promptly to prevent further deterioration of renal function.

Cautious drug administration

Since many drugs are excreted by the kidney, they must be cautiously administered to the uremic patient. The half-life of drugs excreted by the kidney is greatly prolonged in uremia, so toxic serum levels may occur and the dosages of these drugs must therefore be reduced. The nephrologist chooses antibiotics (nonnephrotoxic) and their dosages with these facts in mind. Particular caution is necessary when digitalis drugs are ordered for the treatment of intrinsic cardiac disease in the uremic patient. In fact, *cautious drug administration to the uremic patient should be the rule.*

In progressive renal failure, conservative therapeutic measures finally become inadequate. Hemodialysis and/or renal transplantation are then the only means of preserving life. Continuation of many of the conservative measures may be necessary, particularly with hemodialysis.

DIALYSIS AND RENAL TRANSPLANTATION

The treatment of end-stage renal failure has been transformed by the development of techniques for dialysis and renal transplantation during the past 25 years. In the past, patients with renal failure were doomed to die when all conservative methods failed. Now their lives may be prolonged many years with maintenance dialysis or renal transplantation.

There is an intimate relation between these two techniques, and closely parallel advances in both have been made. For example, the uremic patient may choose to undergo renal transplantation with a related or cadaver donor rather than be maintained on chronic intermittent dialysis. Nevertheless, dialysis will undoubtedly play an important role in the treatment. Dialysis may be used to maintain the patient in an optimum clinical state until the donor kidney is available. In the case of a cadaver renal transplant, the patient may have to wait many months. There are several choices of treatment, depending on the resources available. The initial treatment will be carried out in the medical center hemodialysis unit. The patient may then undergo home dialysis training to permit self-administration of the procedure at home until the donor kidney is available; or more commonly treatment may be given in a satellite (out-of-hospital) or mobile hemodialysis unit near the patient's home. Dialysis may sustain the renal transplant patient through periods of postoperative oliguria, and it provides an alternative if the transplanted kidney should fail because of rejection or other complications. Renal transplantation and chronic maintenance dialysis offer about the same prognosis in regard to longevity. Each mode of treatment has its own unique problems. Renal transplantation, if successful, probably offers a better quality of life because it is less restrictive: there are usually no dietary restrictions, and it is not necessary to commit large blocks of time several times each week for dialysis.

Preparation of the patient

It is important that the patient be prepared for the transition from conservative management to more definitive therapy long before the need arises for maintenance dialysis or renal transplantation. Not only does this give the patient hope, but it also allows time for indoctrination of the patient in preparation for the treatment and makes it possible for the treatment to start at the proper time.

Originally, extremely rigid criteria were used to select patients for either renal transplantation or maintenance dialysis, especially because of limited facilities and the high cost of treatment. The increase in facilities, financial support by the federal government, improvements in techniques, and success in treating some children, older people, diabetic persons, and patients with systemic lupus erythematosis are all factors which have helped to liberalize the criteria so that a greater number of patients can be helped.

When to begin treatment

There are no clear-cut guidelines in terms of measurable blood levels of creatinine or BUN to determine when definitive therapy should begin. Most nephrologists' decisions are based on the well-being of the patient, who is followed closely as an outpatient. Therapy is generally begun when the patient is no longer able to work full-time, develops peripheral neuropathy, or shows other signs of clinical deterioration. The serum creatinine level is generally above 6 mg per 100 ml in males (4 mg per 100 ml in females), and the GFR is below 4 ml per minute. In no case should the patient be allowed to become bedridden or so sick that usual activities are impossible.

Sometimes, in spite of being carefully followed, the patient may deteriorate rapidly over a period of a few days, usually in response to an infectious disease. Sometimes one or two peritoneal dialyses will restabilize the patient. If this is not successful, then intermittent hemodialysis may be initiated. If a decision for a renal transplant has been made, transplantation may be done on an elective basis at a later date.

Dialysis

Dialysis is a process by which solutes and water are diffused through a passive, porous membrane from one fluid compartment to another. Hemodialysis and peritoneal dialysis are the two major techniques used in dialysis, and the basic principles involved are the same for both—diffusion of solutes and water from the plasma to the dialysis solution in response to a concentration or pressure gradient.

Figure 44-1 illustrates the basic principles of diffusion and osmotic and hydrostatic pressure gradients-involved in dialysis. Given a semipermeable membrane with the patient's blood on one side and a solution of known composition on the other side (the *dialysate*, or dialysis bath), substances to which the membrane is permeable will move from where their concentration is high to where it is low. If the blood potassium level is high and the potassium level in the dialysis bath is low (round dots), the net movement of potassium will be out of the blood into the dialysis bath (long arrows indicate direction of net diffusion). The black squares represent solutes which are in higher concentration in the dialysate (e.g., bicarbonate), so that net diffusion is from the bath solution to the blood. Ultrafiltration (water removal) may be achieved by two methods: (1) creating hydrostatic pressure gradient (e.g., by mechanically increasing the positive pressure in the blood compartment) and (2) creating an osmotic pressure gradient by increasing the concentration of glucose in the dialysis bath. The resulting osmotic and hydrostatic pressure gradients cause a net movement of water from the blood to the dialysis bath.* The positive pressure in the blood compartment also speeds up the diffusion of both solutes and water. Ultrafiltration in hemodialysis is primarily achieved by using the first method, whereas peritoneol dialysis uses the second method. Note that protein, blood cells, and bacteria are too large to pass through the pores in the dialysis membrane.

By using a dialysis solution which contains the im-

---

*Some glucose does diffuse from the dialysis bath into the blood, but, since water diffuses much more rapidly than glucose, the major shift will be that of water from blood to bath.

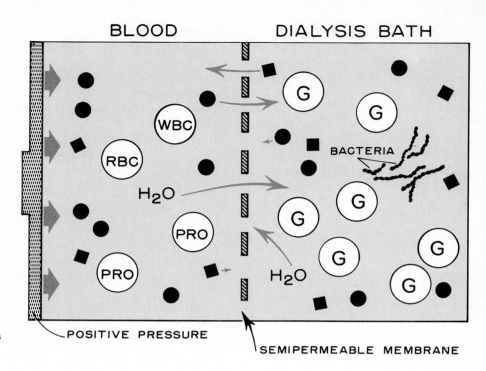

BACTERIA

H₂O

H₂O

POSITIVE PRESSURE

SEMIPERMEABLE MEMBRANE

FIGURE 44-1
Basic principles of diffusion and osmotic and hydrostatic pressures involved in dialysis.

portant electrolytes in concentrations which are normal for healthy persons, the concentration of these electrolytes can be corrected in the blood of the patient with renal failure. The basic practical problem in dialysis is to bring enough blood into contact with enough dialysis solution across a semipermeable membrane of adequate area. This may be accomplished inside the patient's body, using the peritoneum as the semipermeable membrane (peritoneal dialysis), or outside the body, using an "artificial kidney" and cellophane or Cuprophane as the semipermeable membrane (hemodialysis).

Hemodialysis

An artificial kidney machine, or hemodialyzer, consists simply of a semipermeable membrane (cellophane or Cuprophane) with blood on one side and dialysis fluid on the other. Three basic types of dialyzers have been developed. The *coil dialyzer* consists of two cellophane coils arranged in parallel, supported by a rigid mesh screen. Blood is pumped through the inside of the coil, and dialysis fluid is bubbled up around the outside of the coil and recirculated (Fig. 44-2). The *parallel plate dialyzer* consists of two cellophane sheets sandwiched between two rigid supports to form an envelope. Two or more envelopes are arranged in parallel. Blood flows between the membrane layers, and dialysis fluid may flow in the same direction as the blood or in the opposite direction (countercurrent), as shown in Fig. 44-3. The *hollow fiber* or *capillary dialyzer* consists of thousands of tiny capillary fibers arranged in parallel (Fig. 44-4). Each fiber has a wall thickness of 30 μm, an inside diameter of 200 μm, and a length of 21 cm. (For

comparative purposes, a red blood cell has a diameter of 7 μm.) Blood flows down the center of these tiny tubes, and dialysis fluid bathes the outside. The flow of the dialysis fluid is opposite to that of the blood. This dialyzer is very small and compact, because of the large surface area provided by the many capillary tubes. Figure 44-5 is a diagrammatic representation of a hemodialysis system using a hollow fiber dialyzer.

A dialysis system consists of two circuits, one for the blood and one for the dialysis fluid. When the system is in operation, blood flows from the patient through plastic tubing (arterial line), through the hollow fibers of the dialyzer, and back to the patient through the venous line. The dialysis fluid forms the second circuit. Tap water is filtered and heated to body temperature and is then mixed with a concentrate by a proportioning pump to make the dialysate, or bath. The bath is then delivered to the dialyzer, where it flows on the outside of the hollow fibers before exiting to a drain. Equilibrium between the blood and the dialysate takes place across the dialyzing membrane by the processes of diffusion, osmosis, and ultrafiltration described in Fig. 44-1.

The composition of the dialysis bath is designed to approximate the ionic composition of normal blood, modified slightly to correct the common fluid and electrolyte disorders which accompany renal failure. The usual components are Na^+, K^+, Ca^{2+}, Mg^{2+}, Cl^-, acetate, and glucose. Urea, creatinine, uric acid, and phosphate diffuse readily from the blood to the dialysis fluid, since they are not present in the dialysis fluid. Sodium acetate, which is in higher concentration in the dialysis bath, diffuses into the blood. The purpose of adding the

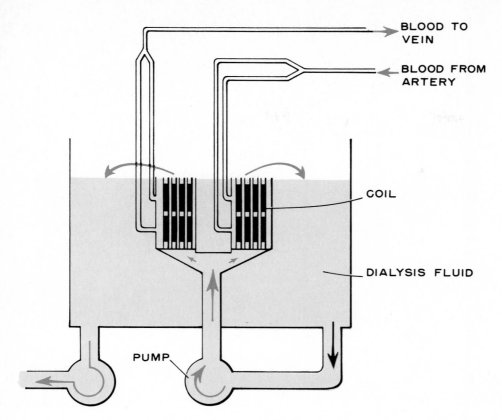

BLOOD TO VEIN

BLOOD FROM ARTERY

COIL

DIALYSIS FLUID

PUMP

FIGURE 44-2
Coil dialyzer.

acetate is to correct the uremic patient's acidosis. Acetate is metabolized into bicarbonate in the patient's body. A low concentration of glucose (200 mg per 100ml) is added to the dialysis bath to prevent glucose diffusion into the dialysis bath with the consequent loss of calories. In hemodialysis, a high concentration of glucose is not necessary since fluid removal may be achieved by effecting a hydrostatic pressure gradient between the blood and dialysis fluid. In hemodialysis, ultrafiltration is achieved mainly by effecting a hydrostatic pressure difference between the blood and dialysis fluid. The hydrostatic pressure gradient is achieved by

increasing the positive pressure within the dialyzer blood compartment by increasing resistance to venous outflow (not shown) or by exerting a vacuum effect in the diaysis fluid compartment by manipulating the negative pressure control. The hydrostatic pressure gradient across the dialyzing membrane also increases the diffusion rate of the solutes.

The blood circuit of the dialysis system is initially primed with saline or blood before connection to the circulation of the patient. The blood pressure of the patient may be adequate to propel the blood through the extracorporeal circuit, or a blood pump may be used to

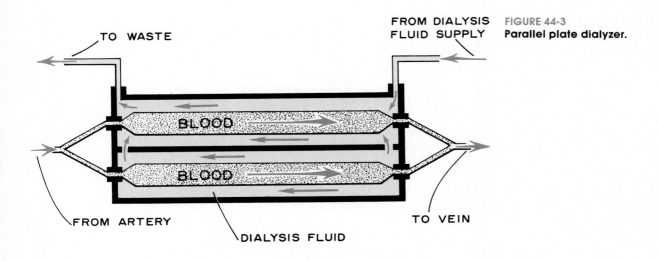

TO WASTE

FROM DIALYSIS FLUID SUPPLY

FIGURE 44-3
Parallel plate dialyzer.

BLOOD

BLOOD

FROM ARTERY

DIALYSIS FLUID

TO VEIN

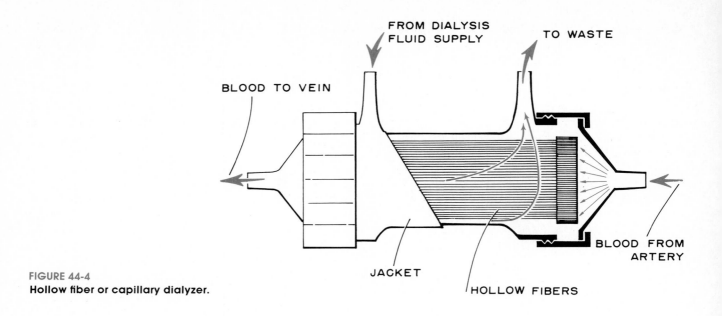

FIGURE 44-4
Hollow fiber or capillary dialyzer.

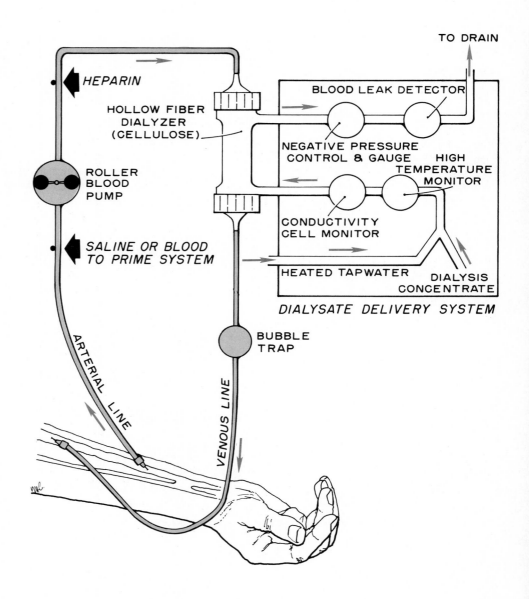

FIGURE 44-5
Diagram of a hemodialysis system using hollow fiber dialyzer.

assist the flow (about 200 ml per minute is a desirable flow rate). Heparin is continuously delivered to the arterial line by a slow infusion pump to prevent clotting. A clot and bubble trap in the venous line prevents air or blood clots from returning to the patient. To ensure patient safety, monitors with alarms for various parameters are included in modern hemodialyzers. A conductivity cell monitors the chemical composition of the dialysis fluid. Dialysis fluid at body temperature increases the rate of diffusion, but a temperature that is too high would cause hemolysis of red blood cells, with possible death to the patient. Any tear in the dialysis membrane causing either a minor or a massive leak is detected by a photocell in the dialysate outflow.

Maintenance hemodialysis is usually performed three times a week, and the length of a single treatment varies from 4 to 6 hours, depending on the type of dialysis system used and the condition of the patient.

Access to the bloodstream

Long-term intermittent dialysis requires reliable access to the circulation. Blood must exit and return to the patient at the rate of about 200 ml per minute. The major access techniques that can provide flow rates of this magnitude are the internal arteriovenous (AV) fistula and the external AV cannula or shunt (Fig. 44-6).

The *external AV shunt* is created by placing Teflon cannula tips in an artery (usually the radial or posterior tibial) and a nearby vein. The cannula tips are then connected by silicone rubber tubing and a Teflon bridge to complete the shunt. At the time of dialysis, the external shunt tubing is separated, and connection is made to the dialyzer. Blood then flows from the arterial line, through the dialyzer, and then back to the vein. The cannula system, devised (Quinton et al., 1960) in 1960, made chronic intermittent dialysis possible for the first time. The main problem with the external shunt is a short life span because of clotting and infection (average life 9 months). The external AV shunt has been supplanted by other methods of angioaccess (see below) and is mainly of historical interest. Occasionally, however, it is used when dialytic therapy is required for short periods of time, as in dialysis for drug overdose or poisoning, acute renal failure, and the initial phase of dialytic treatment for chronic renal failure.

The most popular form of blood access is the *AV fistula*, constructed by anastomosing an artery directly to a vein (usually the radial artery and cephalic vein at the wrist). Blood is shunted from the artery to the vein, causing the vein to enlarge ("ripening") after a few weeks. Venipuncture with large-bore needles becomes easy and gives access to rapidly flowing blood under arterial pressure. Connection with the dialysis system is made by placing one needle distally (arterial line) and the other needle proximally (venous line) in the arterialized vein. The internal fistula circumvents the prob-

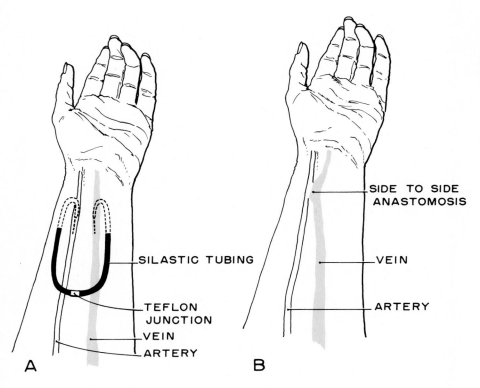

FIGURE 44-6
Access to the circulation. External AV shunt or cannula system (A) and internal AV fistula (B).

SILASTIC TUBING

TEFLON JUNCTION

VEIN

ARTERY

A

SIDE TO SIDE ANASTOMOSIS

VEIN

ARTERY

B

lems of infection, clotting, and possible hemorrhage associated with the cannula. The average life of a fistula is about 4 years. The main problems are painful venipuncture, formation of aneurysms, thrombosis, difficult postdialytic hemostasis, and ischemia of the hand (*steal syndrome*).

Other techniques of angioaccess for hemodialysis include femoral vein cannulation using Shaldon catheters until a more permanent access can be established. A modied internal AV fistula can be constructed, using bovine carotid artery, which is practically nonantigenic. Bovine heterografts have the advantages of providing a large lumen for easy puncture with large-bore needles and of being less susceptible to aneurysms. Disadvantages include increased susceptibility to infection and bleeding from needle puncture sites.

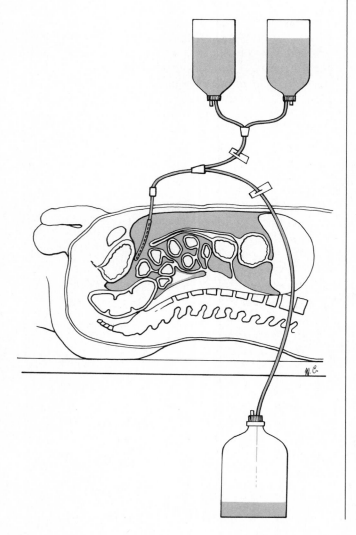

Peritoneal dialysis

Peritoneal dialysis accomplishes the same purposes and operates on the same principles of diffusion and osmosis as hemodialysis. In this instance, however, the peritoneum is the semipermeable membrane. A catheter is placed in the peritoneal cavity by paracentesis (Fig. 44-7). In the adult, 2 liters of sterile dialysis solution is allowed to run into the peritoneal cavity through the catheter (10 to 20 minutes). Equilibrium between the dialysis fluid and the highly vascular semipermeable peritoneal membrane takes place during what is called *dwell time*, generally 30 to 45 minutes. The fluid is then allowed to drain by gravity into a closed, sterile collecting system. The cycle is repeated over a period of 1 to 2 days. The main advantages of this method of dialysis are its simplicity (it does not require highly skilled personnel or sophisticated equipment) and the fact that it does not require access to the bloodstream. On the other hand, peritoneal dialysis requires about six times longer than hemodialysis to achieve the same results. In addition, the procedure is often painful (especially when high glucose concentrations are used to achieve ultrafiltration), and repeated treatments may lead to peritonitis.

New approaches to solute removal

Many patients continue to manifest various disturbed metabolic functions in spite of vigorous hemodialysis through which the concentration of the classic uremic metabolites (e.g., urea, creatinine, uric acid, phosphate) are maintained at near-normal levels. These observations have led investigators to postulate that there is a series of uremic toxins intermediate in molecular weight between the classic small solutes such as urea ($<$ 500 daltons) and the plasma proteins ($>$50,000 daltons) which may partially account for the clinical abnormalities.

Two new experimental primary techniques of solute removal which offer promise of substantially improving future treatment of chronic renal failure are *hemofiltration* (HF), also called *hemodiafiltration*, and *continuous ambulatory peritoneal dialysis* (CAPD). Both methods are based on acceptance of the presence and pathophysiologic significance of middle molecules. The technique of HF is based on the principle of convection rather than diffusion and is more closely analogous to the function of the human glomerulus than is hemodialysis. In HF the standard hemodialysis technique is modified by sequentially prediluting the blood with an electrolyte solution resembling plasma and subsequently ultrafiltering it at high hydraulic pressures. The principal advantage of this technique is more effi-

FIGURE 44-7
Peritoneal dialysis.

cient removal of solutes in the middle molecular range that are inefficiently cleared by hemodialysis. CAPD is a self-dialysis technique using 2-liter exchanges of dialysate every 4 hours on a 24-hour basis. The dialysate is instilled into the peritoneal cavity by gravity from a plastic bag which is rolled and carried in a pouch at the waist during the prolonged 4-hour dwell time. After the dwell time the empty bag is lowered to the floor and allowed to fill by gravity. The cycle is then repeated, using a fresh dialysate bag which is connected to the peritoneal catheter using an aseptic technique. CAPD also results in better removal of middle molecules. Both these techniques are reported to result in an improved sense of well-being, improved hematocrit and blood pressure control, and lower parathyroid hormone levels. Other advantages of CAPD are the absence of the peaks and valleys in blood chemistry levels characteristic of intermittent dialysis, simplicity, ease of learning, independence, and low cost (about one-fifth that of hemodialysis). The primary disadvantage of CAPD is the risk of peritonitis, which occurs on the average about once every 40 patient-weeks.

Additional approaches to solute removal include adjunctive techniques designed to be used with maintenance hemodialysis or in patients with significant residual renal function (GFR equals 5 to 10 ml per minute). All involve the use of sorbents for solute removal. The *Redy system* employs an enzyme-sorbent disposable cartridge for reprocessing dialysate so that a small volume may be used. The sorbent consists of zirconium compounds and carbon. *Hemoperfusion* utilizes activated charcoal, encapsulated in membranes, as the sorbent. Charcoal hemoperfusion systems are efficient in removing middle molecules but do not effectively remove many of the significant uremic solutes, including urea and electrolytes or water. This system must, therefore, be combined with conventional hemodialysis or hemofiltration. There is also serious risk of complications, especially particulate embolization and thrombocytopenia from platelet loss. A third approach to solute removal involves the *oral ingestion of sorbents* such as activated charcoal or oxystarch. The technique of using the GI tract for solute removal is in a primitive state of development, although the use of oral aluminum hydroxides and Kayexalate (orally or by enema) is conventional practice for the control of phosphates and K^+, respectively.

All these primary and adjunctive techniques may be expected to play a role in future treatment of chronic renal failure with the improvement of technology (Friedman, 1978; Moncrief and Popovich, 1979; Henderson and Sanfelippo, 1980).

Renal transplantation

A successful renal transplant is the preferred method of treatment for patients in end-stage renal failure, al-though some patients may elect self-dialysis in their own home after being taught the procedure by a "home-training nurse."

The first successful renal transplant was performed on identical twins in 1954 by Murray, Merrill, and Harrison in Boston. Since that time over 25,000 renal transplants have been performed worldwide, more than 15,000 of them in the United States.

The surgical technique involved in renal transplantation is relatively simple and is generally performed by a surgeon with a background in urologic, vascular, or general surgery. It is standard procedure to rotate the donor kidney and place it in the contralateral iliac fossa of the recipient. The ureter then lies anterior to the renal vessels and is more readily anastomosed or implanted into the recipient bladder. The renal artery is anastomosed end-to-end to the internal iliac artery, while the renal vein is anastomosed to the external or common iliac vein (Fig. 44-8).

The major limiting factor in this procedure is the body's immunologic response that leads to rejection of the transplanted kidney. Rejection may be cell-mediated or humoral. Cell-mediated rejection involves T lymphocytes produced in response to antigens in the donor kidney which are recognized as foreign cells. These lymphocytes invade the foreign donor kidney and contribute to its destruction. Humoral rejection involves the production of antibodies against antigens in the donor kidney which the recipient's plasma cells recognize as foreign. Rejection can occur within hours or several years after a transplantation.

Tissue typing or histocompatibility testing to ensure the closest possible tissue match between donor and recipient and suppression of the immune response with drugs are the two general approaches used to promote successful renal transplant and prevent rejection. Two major antigenic groups have been identified as important in determining histocompatibility: the ABO blood group system and human leukocyte antigens (HLA).

The ABO antigens are present in most tissues of the body as well as on red blood cells. The same rules apply to renal transplants with respect to ABO compatability as to blood transfusions. An O kidney can be transplanted in any recipient, while an A kidney can be given only to an A or AB recipient. Transplantation between ABO-incompatible persons is not done, since it generally leads to immediate hyperacute rejection.

The HLA antigen system is more complex. Histocompatibility appears to be determined by a single autosomal gene complex (called the *MHC*, or *major histocompatibility complex*) on the short arm of the

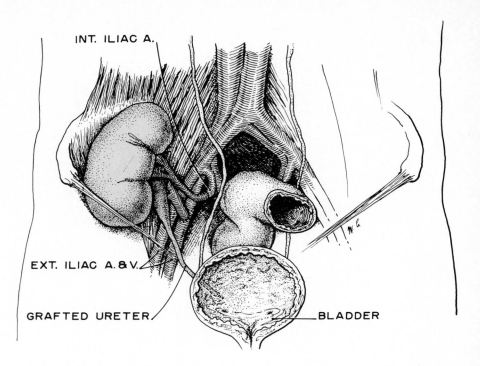

INT. ILIAC A.

EXT. ILIAC A. & V.

GRAFTED URETER

BLADDER

FIGURE 44-8
Renal transplantation.

chromosome 6 (Alfred et al., 1981). Four major HLA sites or loci, designated A, B, C, and D, have been identified in this region. Each sublocus controls a series of antigenic factors, and more than 70 are either known or suspected (Table 44-1). Since chromosomes are paired, a person has a total of eight HLA antigens (two pairs on each of the two chromosomes). Each of these chromosome sets is called a *haplotype*. The genotype of an individual consists of two haplotypes, one from each parent. Within a single family only four genotypes can be present. For example, if the HLA genotype of the mother is AB and that of the father is CD, there are four possible combinations for the children: AC, AD, BC, and BD (Figure 44-9). By the laws of simple Mendelian inheritance, 25 percent of siblings will be HLA-identical, 50 percent will share a haplotype in common, and 25 percent will have a two-haplotype mismatch.

In general, the closer the genetic similarity between donor and recipient the greater the chance of a successful transplant. When the donor and recipient are identical twins or HLA-identical siblings, some 90 percent of the grafts are functioning at the end of 2 years. The next best choices for a donor are a non-identical-HLA sibling, then a parent, and finally an unrelated person (source of cadaver kidneys).

Tissue typing is a technique which has been developed in recent years to predict the outcome of a particular match of antigens between donor and recipient. The HLA antigens are divided into two classes. HLA-A, HLA-B, and HLA-C are *class I antigens*, present on virtually all cells of the body. The Terasaki *microcytotoxicity assay* is used to type class I antigens. Circulating lymphocytes (primarily T lymphocytes) of the po-

tential kidney donor and recipient are exposed to monospecific antiserums. If the serum "recognizes" its HLA antigen on the lymphocyte cell surface, the complement cascade is activated and the cell membrane is lysed, permitting a marker dye to enter the cell (Terasaki et al., 1978).

TABLE 44-1

NOMENCLATURE FOR FACTORS OF THE HLA SYSTEM

Recognized Antigens				
Locus A	Locus B		Locus C	Locus D
A1	BW4	BW41	CW1	DW1
A2	BW6	BW42	CW2	DW2
A3	B5	BW44	CW3	DW3
A9	B7	BW45	CW4	DW4
A10	B8	BW46	CW5	DW5
A11	B12	BW47	CW6	DW6
A25	B13	BW48		DW7
A26	B14	BW49		DW8
A28	B15	BW50		CW9
A29	B17	BW51		DW10
AW19	B18	BW52		DW11
AW23	B27	BW53		
AW24	B37	BW54		*Locus DR**
AW30	B40			DRW1
AW31	BW16			DRW2
AW32	BW21			DRW3
AW33	BW22			DRW4
AW34	BW35			DRW5
AW36	BW38			DRW6
AW43	BW39			DRW7

*B lymphocyte, D-related antigens.
Source: World Health Organization, 1978.

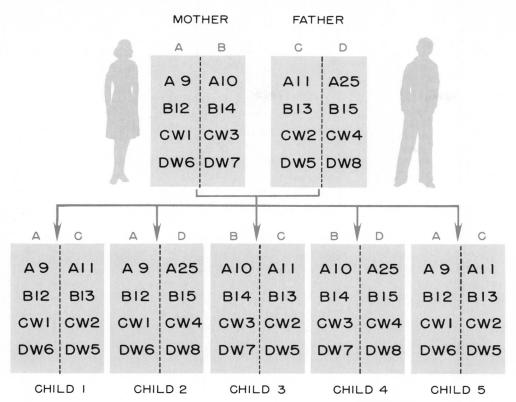

Pattern of inheritance of the HLA antigens. Child 1 and 5 are HLA-identical siblings. All children have a one-haplotype mismatch with each parent and with some their siblings. Some siblings have a two-haplotype mismatch or no antigens in common.

Class II antigens (D and D-related) are determined by the D-locus genes. Class II antigens are found on the surface of B lymphocytes, monocytes, and endothelial cells but only on 2 to 4 percent of T lymphocytes (Alfred et al., 1981). Unlike class I antigens, class II antigens cannot be detected by antiserum tests (since only about 10 percent of B lymphocytes circulate in the blood) but are identified by the *mixed lymphocyte culture* (MLC) test. In the MLC test, lymphoyctes from the donor and recipient are cultured together for 4 or 5 days. Ordinarily both sets of cells would undergo blast transformation in response to antigenic disparity between their cell membrane antigens. However, it is only the antigens present in the donor and lacking in the recipient which are of interest, since they cause the immune response in the transplanted kidney. Thus, to test only the reactivity of the recipient cells, the donor cells are pretreated with irradiation or mitomycin C to inactivate them with respect to capacity to undergo blast transformation without destroying surface antigens. When the two cultures are mixed, only those of the recipient undergo blast transformation. The degree of blast transformation is measured by radioactive tritiated thymidine added to the culture. If the recipient's cells are stimulated by the donor cells, greater quantities of thymidine are taken up for the synthesis of nucleoprotein during blast transformation.

Recently it has been possible to separate the B lymphocytes from the T lymphocytes in blood serum so that class II antigens can be detected serologically. The B-cell antigens detected in this manner are called *D-related*, or *DR*, *antigens*, since they appear to be identical or closely related to the D-locus antigens involved in the MLC test (Alfred et al., 1981).

A mismatch of either class I and class II antigens can lead to rejection of a transplant, although a mismatch of class II antigens may be of greater importance. It has been postulated that class I antigens stimulate the production of both cytotoxic, or "killer," T cells and the antibody-producing B cells which arise in transplant rejection when there is incompatibility of HLA-A, -B, or -C locus antigens. On the other hand, class II antigens stimulate the production of helper T cells which amplify immune response (whether mediated by killer T cells or antibodies) when there is HLA-D or DR incompatibility. The genes that control class I and II antigens are closely linked in the MHC region. Hence among siblings compatibility of class I and class II antigens is positively correlated except in rare cases when a break has occurred during meiosis. That is, when siblings are identical with respect to HLA-A, HLA-B, and HLA-C antigens, the MLC test shows weak stimulation indicating HLA-D antigen compatibility. When there is strong stimulation on the MLC test, the majority of grafts are rejected even when the HLA-A and HLA-B antigens (class I antigens of major importance) are identical (Carpenter and Merrill, 1980). Matching at the HLA-D locus is the most important factor in predicting the success of cadaver transplants. Unfortunately, the MLC test cannot be used prospectively in the case of a cadaver donor, since the length of the test (5 days) exceeds the time the kidney can be preserved (2 to 3 days) before transplantation in the recipient. Typing for HLA-DR antigens offers a rapid method of assessing the D locus of cadaver kidneys, and some studies indicate that DR matching has a significant influence on 1-year graft survival (Morris, 1983; Vanrenterghem et al., 1984).

In addition to pretransplant ABO blood typing and assessing class I and class II antigens, a fourth test routinely performed is the *white cell cross match*. Recipient serum and donor lymphocytes are mixed. If the recipient has preformed antibodies against donor leukocyte antigens from past blood transfusions or pregnancies, these will cause destruction of donor cells (a positive cross match). A negative cross match is essential before proceeding with a transplant, since a positive cross match will result in hyperacute rejection of the donor kidney. As indicated earlier, it was formerly believed that numerous blood transfusions in a patient awaiting transplant would sensitize the patient to a large number of HLA antigens in the general population and decrease the chances of a successful graft. Thus transfusions were kept to a minimum, and only packed washed red blood cells (minus WBCs and platelets) were used. However, recent data show that 1-year cadaver graft survival may be increased by as much as 30 percent (from the usual 45 percent to 75 percent) when 20 or more pretransplant blood transfusions are given (Opelz and Terasaki, 1978). Deliberate donor-specific blood transfusions prior to renal transplantation from living HLA-nonidentical related persons increased graft success to 97 percent compared with an expected succcess rate of 70 percent in another study (Salvatierra et al., 1980). In this study about one-third of the patients became sensitized to donor antigens, as indicated by a positive cross match, and did not receive the intended donor kidney. The other two-thirds were not sensitized to donor antigens and so received the transplant. Apparently this procedure identifies donor-recipient mismatches that are likely to result in unsuccessful transplantation and enhances the success of the procedure in those recipients who do not develop antidonor antibodies. Although the mechanism of the action of blood transfusions in improving graft survival is not well understood, Stuart (1980) has hypothesized that transfusions stimulate enhancing antibodies which inhibit the immune response and prolong graft survival (in contrast to sensitizing antibodies which cause early graft loss).

The nature of the body's immunologic defense against entry of foreign proteins is such that almost all organ transplantation from another person (with the possible exception of an identical twin) is followed by an attempt on the part of the recipient to reject that organ. There are three types of rejection.

Hyperacute rejection occurs within minutes or hours after completion of the transplant and inevitably leads to organ loss. It is caused by ABO incompatibility or previous exposure to transfused WBCs or platelets from another person whose tissues contain the same antigens as the kidney donor. The recipient has preformed circulating antibodies, and such grafts undergo rejection via the humoral immune system, in which the B-cell mechanism predominates. The antibodies are deposited along the kidney vascular endothelium, and complement is activated with consequent tissue damage. The end result is diffuse vascular thrombosis and cortical necrosis (Alfred et al., 1981). Hyperacute rejection can be prevented for the most part by appropriate ABO and lymphocyte cross matching before transplantation.

Acute rejection usually occurs within the first 12 weeks after transplantation. Acute rejection episodes may reoccur at any time after the initial one, but the incidence decreases with time. The greater the HLA antigenic disparity between donor and host (including an unrelated cadaver donor), the greater the likelihood of severe acute rejection episodes. Preformed antidonor antibodies are not present in acute rejection (as in the hyperacute case). Although the cellular immune system is believed to initiate and may predominate in acute rejection, there is also evidence that the humoral immune system plays a synergistic role in the process (Carpenter and Merrill, 1980). Initially, circulating T lymphocytes become sensitized to graft antigens during the induction phase. The sensitized lymphocytes then stop circulating, settle in the thymic regions of secondary lymphoid tissue, and there undergo blast transformation and then an active phase of proliferation and maturation. The first products of this proliferation are large killer T lymphocytes which are strongly cytotoxic and which somehow damage incompatible transplant tissue cells by direct contact. Various lymphokines are also released which amplify the attack on the foreign antigens by converting other T lymphocytes into killer T cells and call macrophages to the site, where they are stimulated to accelerated phagocytosis and degradation of the tissue cells. (See Chap. 5 for a review of cell-mediated immunity.) Histologically there is a perivascular accumulation of monocytes, with varying degrees of vascular injury, and tubular necrosis (Carpenter and Merrill, 1980). There is also evidence that the humoral immune system is involved, since immunofluorescent slides of vascular endothelium show deposition of fibrin, complement, and immunoglobulins (Carpenter and Merrill, 1980).

The first rejection episode commonly occurs about 2 weeks after transplantation and is characterized by renal insufficiency (rising BUN and serum creatinine), oliguria, and sometimes fever and swelling of the graft. A biopsy of the graft may be necessary to make the diagnosis and determine the extent of the lesion. Acute rejection is often reversible with appropriate drug therapy, which is aimed primarily at suppressing T cells (see below). Recovery usually takes 2 to 4 weeks, and during this time the patient requires dialysis.

Chronic rejection occurs months to years after the initial transplant and is characterized by hypertension, proteinuria, and slow loss of renal function. The cause is poorly understood. Histologically the primary changes are in the renal arteries and glomeruli and resemble a reoccurrence of the primary renal disease. Unlike acute rejection, this type of rejection responds poorly to drugs and has a poor prognosis (Alfred et al., 1981).

The survival of the transplanted kidney depends on minimizing the body's defense mechanisms. Common drugs used to suppress the immune response are azathioprine (Imuran) and prednisone. These drugs make the patient more susceptible to infection. Conse-

quently, overwhelming infection is also a major complication in a renal transplant recipient and the principal cause of death. To minimize the danger both of infection and rejection, the general approach is to increase the dosage of corticosteroids for a limited period of time during the initial transplant period and to treat rejection episodes while keeping the maintenance dosage low at other times.

Three new drugs used in some centers to achieve more specific immunosuppression include antilymphocyte globulin (ALG), monoclonal antibodies, and cyclosporin A (Irwin, 1983). ALG is prepared by injecting human lymphoid tissue into an animal, which then makes antibodies against it. These antibodies are then injected into the transplant patient to prevent or treat rejection. The major effect of ALG is to deplete T cells. Monoclonal antibodies are administered intravenously and also act by depleting T cells. This agent is used not only to reverse rejection but also as a research tool to learn more about the lymphocyte subpopulations which trigger rejection reactions (Morris, 1983). Cyclosporin A is the most recent and promising drug added to prevent

TABLE 44-2

COMPARISON OF RENAL TRANSPLANTATION AND HEMODIALYSIS

	Renal transplant	Hemodialysis
One-year survival, %*	90	95
Five-year survival, %*	60	65
One-year graft survival, %†		
Sibling	78.6	
Parent	72.1	
Cadaver	50.8	
Five-year graft survival, %†		
Sibling	68.8	
Parent	57.5	
Cadaver	40.0	
Cost	$10,000–$30,000	$25,000/yr (medical center)
		$20,000/yr (satellite unit)
		$8000–$12,000/yr (home)
Activity restriction	None	Some
General well-being	Complete	Incomplete
Generalized infection	Yes	No
Localized infection	No	Yes
Diet restriction	No	Yes
Renal osteodystrophy	No	Yes
Neuropathy	No	Yes
Rehabilitation	Yes	Yes

*Brundage, 1980.
†Advisory Committee to the Renal Transplant Registry, 1977.

and treat rejection. It is derived from two species of fungus and acts by interfering with the growth and proliferation of helper T cells more than with those of suppressor T cells. In one large European study, cadaver graft survival at 6 months after transplant was increased from 53 percent in those patients receiving conventional azathioprine and prednisone therapy to 75 percent in those patients receiving cyclosporin A (European Multicenter Trial, 1982).

Table 44-2 shows a detailed comparison of hemo-

dialysis and renal transplantation as methods of treatment in end-stage renal failure. A final consideration with respect to treatment is the realization that there is limited choice in opting for renal transplantation as a treatment modality, since there are more than 10,000 newly diagnosed persons with end-stage renal failure each year and a limited supply of good-quality kidneys for transplantation even for ideal recipients. Consequently the overwhelming majority of patients will receive dialysis as a chronic form of treatment. However, the recent significant advances in tissue typing, pretransplant blood transfusions, and improved immunosupression, especially with cyclosporin A, offer hope for greater success in those patients receiving cadaver transplants (the commonest source of organs).

QUESTIONS

The treatment of chronic renal failure

Directions: Answer the following questions on a separate sheet of paper.

1. When are conservative measures of treatment begun for the patient with chronic renal failure? What are the basic principles of conservative treatment? Name four causes of sudden deterioration of renal function in your answer.

2. When conservative therapeutic measures are no longer adequate in the treatment of the uremic patient, what are the alternatives?

3. Describe the principles of dietary regulation of protein, carbohydrate, sodium, and potassium in the treatment of the patient with terminal renal failure.

4. Mr. Walker, who is oliguric and in uremia, has had a total urine output of 500 ml during the past 24 hours. What should his approximate fluid intake be for the next day?

5. What are the two modalities of treatment for the end-stage renal failure patient and how are they related?

6. Define *dialysis*.

7. Differentiate between an external and an internal shunt.

Directions: Match the uremic complications in col. A with the common therapies for the prevention or treatment of the condition in col. B. Conditions may have more than one treatment.

Column A
8. ____ Hyper-
kalemia

Column B
a. Cardiac monitor
b. Kayexalate

9. ____ Hyper-
parathyroidism

10. ____ Hyper-
tension

11. ____ Osteo-
malacia

12. ____ Hyper-
uricemia

13. ____ Peripheral
neuropathy

14. ____ Gouty
arthritis

c. Colchicine
d. IV glucose + insulin
e. Methyldopa
f. Allopurinol
g. Amphojel or Basojel
h. Vitamin D
i. IV calcium gluconate
j. Progress halted only by dialysis
k. Sodium restriction

Directions: Circle the letter preceding each item below that correctly answers the question or completes the sentence. Only one answer is correct, with exceptions noted.

15. Common treatments to ameliorate the anemia of end-stage renal failure are: (More than one answer may be correct.)
a. IV erythropoietin b. Weekly blood transfusions c. Iron and folic acid d. Minimizing blood loss due to hemodialysis and laboratory tests

16. The IV administration of sodium bicarbonate to correct the systemic acidosis in renal failure may result in which of the following complications?
a. Tetany and convulsions b. Hypermagnesemia c. Azotemia d. Renal osteodystrophy

17. Antacids for the uremic patient are properly administered:
a. One hour before meals b. During meals

c. One hour after meals   *d.* Ad lib by patient for gastric distress

18. Which of the following findings in a patient with renal insufficiency would indicate that dialysis treatment should be initiated? (More than one answer may be correct.)
a. BUN 60 mg per 100 ml   *b.* K$^+$ 6.3 meq per liter   *c.* Unable to carry on usual job as telephone operator   *d.* Burning sensation on soles of feet

19. Peritoneal dialysis removes waste products from the blood because of all the following principles except:
a. Water moves across the semipermeable membrane by osmosis.   *b.* The peritoneal surface acts as a semipermeable membrane.   *c.* Red blood cells are removed by ultrafiltration.   *d.* Na$^+$ and K$^+$ are removed by diffusion.

20. The objectives of hemodialysis are all the following except:
a. Removal of excess extracellular and intracellular fluid   *b.* Diffusion of K$^+$ out of the blood   *c.* Stimulation of urine production by the osmotic pressure gradient   *d.* Diffusion of urea out of the blood

21. The most compact of the basic types of hemodialyzer is the:
a. Coil dialyzer   *b.* Parallel plate dialyzer   *c.* Hollow fiber dialyzer

22. All the following substances may leave the blood and enter the dialyzing fluid except:
a. Albumin   *b.* Urea   *c.* Magnesium   *d.* Potassium

23. In hemodialysis, blood is pumped through a _____ tubing bathed in a dialysis fluid which is similar to plasma in composition.
a. Permeable   *b.* Semipermeable   *c.* Osmotic   *d.* Ultrafiltrate

24. The purpose of adding sodium acetate to the dialyzing fluid is to:
a. Correct the hyperuricemia   *b.* Decrease the incidence of peripheral neuropathy   *c.* Alleviate pruritus   *d.* Provide bicarbonate to the body to correct acidosis   *e.* Increase the osmolality of the dialyzing solution to provide for ultrafiltration

25. The flow of blood through an artificially created internal AV fistula causes the vein to enlarge and is referred to as:
a. Fistulation   *b.* Ripening   *c.* Ultrafiltration   *d.* Cannulation

26. Which of the following drugs is used to prevent clotting of blood during extracorporeal circulation?
a. Protamine   *b.* Heparin   *c.* Warfarin sodium (Coumadin)   *d.* Fibrinogen

27. The purpose of histocompatibility testing is:
a. To rule out noncompatible donors   *b.* To demonstrate matching of MHC genes that control synthesis of certain proteins   *c.* To predict the severity of the posttransplant immune response   *d.* None of the above

28. Body cells used in kidney donor and recipient matching include:
a. Endothelial cells of the glomerulus   *b.* Renal tubular cells   *c.* Red blood cells   *d.* White blood cells

29. The probability of HLA-identical siblings in a family is:
a. 10%   *b.* 25%   *c.* 50%   *d.* 75%

30. The most important antigens from the point of view of renal transplant are: (More than one answer may be correct.)
a. ABO blood group   *b.* Leukocytes   *c.* Hemoglobin   *d.* Thrombocytes

31. In general, a donor kidney from which of the following persons would be most likely to be successful?
a. Parent   *b.* Sister   *c.* Cadaver   *d.* Cousin

32. Transplantation should not be carried out with:
a. Cadaver donor with two-antigen HLA matching   *b.* Cadaver donor with two-antigen DR matching   *c.* Related donor with four-antigen matching and different blood group   *d.* Recipient with weak stimulation on the MLC test to related donor   *e.* Recipient with a history of multiple blood transfusions

33. Which of the following statements are true concerning the procedure for renal transplantation? (More than one answer may be correct.)
a. The left kidney of the donor is rotated and placed in the right iliac fossa of the recipient.   *b.* The left kidney of the donor is rotated and placed in the left iliac fossa of the recipient.   *c.* The left kidney of the donor is placed in the left upper abdominal cavity of the recipient, and the renal artery anastomosed to the recipient's renal artery.   *d.* The renal vein is anastomosed to the common iliac vein.   *e.* The renal artery is anastomosed to the internal iliac artery.   *f.* The ureter of the transplanted kidney is implanted into the colon.

34. The immune response to transplantation in acute rejection is mediated by:
a. Humoral antibodies   *b.* T cells   *c.* Complement and humoral antibodies   *d.* Humoral antibodies acting synergistically with T cells

35. The most common cause of failure of a renal transplant is:
    a. Obstruction of the ureterovesicular anastomosis
    b. Infection of the transplanted kidney   c. Immunologic rejection of the transplanted kidney
    d. Recurrence of the patient's original kidney disease

36. The most common cause of death in kidney transplant recipients is:
    a. Surgical complications   b. Hypertension
    c. Viral infections   d. Combined relentless rejection and overwhelming infection

37. The advantage of kidney transplant is:
    a. Generally eliminates the need for dialysis
    b. Side effects easily treated with corticosteroids
    c. No danger to the donor   d. Minimal danger of postoperative infections

Directions: Match the histocompatibility test in col. A with the antigens or antibodies it detects in col. B.

Column A

38. ____ RBC type and cross match

39. ____ Microcytotoxicity assay

40. ____ Mixed lymphocyte culture

Column B

a. Class I antigens
b. ABO antigens
c. Lymphocyte antibodies
d. Class II antigens
e. HLA-DR antigens

41. ____ WBC cross match

Directions: Circle T if the statement is true and F if it is false.

42. T   F   It is only the antigens present in the donor and lacking in the recipient which cause immunologic rejection in a transplanted kidney.

43. T   F   The presence of preformed antibodies against donor ABO antigens or lymphocytes causes hyperacute rejection in the kidney transplant recipient.

44. T   F   Hemodialysis is never needed after a successful renal transplantation.

45. T   F   An immunologic response does not occur when the kidney donor is an HLA-identical sibling.

46. T   F   If acute rejection episodes are untreated, the cells of the transplanted kidney are destroyed.

47. T   F   Most of the immunosuppressive drugs used to prevent or treat transplantation rejection act by depleting T cells.

Directions: Answer the following on a separate sheet of paper.

48. Name three new developments which have potential for greatly increasing survival of cadaver kidney transplants.

49. Name several experimental approaches to the removal of uremic solutes. How are they related to the middle molecular hypothesis?

CHAPTER 45

ACUTE RENAL FAILURE

OBJECTIVES

At the completion of this chapter you should be able to:

1. Define *acute renal failure*.
2. Distinguish between oliguric and nonoliguric acute renal failure.
3. Describe the common clinical situations leading to acute ischemic renal failure.
4. Identify some common causes of postrenal obstructive uropathy.
5. List the two common causes of ATN-type acute renal failure.
6. Discuss five examples of acute nephrotoxic injury to the kidneys.
7. List three causes of acute intrinsic renal failure other than the two major causes.
8. Describe two types of histologic lesion commonly observed in acute tubular necrosis.
9. State the prognosis for each of the two lesions described in Objective 8.
10. Describe the general prognosis, extent of acute damage, and residual effects on the kidney in acute cortical necrosis.
11. Discuss several suggested factors involved in the pathogenesis of acute renal failure.
12. Differentiate between prerenal azotemia, postrenal obstruction, and acute tubular necrosis (etiology, laboratory tests, treatment, prognosis).
13. Describe the clinical course of acute renal failure (three stages and characteristics).
14. Describe the complications of acute tubular necrosis (principles of management, mortality rates).

Acute renal failure (ARF) may be defined as a clinical syndrome resulting from intrinsic metabolic or pathologic damage to the kidney and characterized by a marked and rapid decline of renal function and progressive azotemia (Davidson, 1984, p. 289). ARF is usually associated with oliguria (urine output <400 ml per day). This criterion of oliguria is not arbitrary but is related to the fact that the average American diet contains about 600 mOsm of solute. If the maximum urine-concentrating ability is 1200 mOsm, then there is an obligatory loss of about 500 ml of water in the urine. But, oliguria is not a necessary feature of ARF. Recent evidence suggests that in 30 to 60 percent of the ARF cases, urine output exceeds 400 ml per day and may be as high as 2 liters per day (Anderson et al., 1977). This form of ARF is called *nonoliguric*, or *high-output*, acute renal failure.

The term *acute tubular necrosis* (ATN) is often used interchangeably with the term *acute renal failure* in clinical practice. This usage is not strictly correct, since ATN refers to a renal histologic finding (see below) often present in patients with ARF, although acute renal failure may be present in many patients without tubular necrosis. Despite this fact, the term does serve to distinguish those forms of reversible or potentially reversible ARF attributable to nonrenal causes, i.e., prerenal and postrenal azotemia. It also distinguishes a large spectrum of chronic renal diseases which may be punctuated by episodes of ARF superimposed by generally more reversible factors such as infection and water or salt depletion.

CAUSES OF ACUTE RENAL FAILURE

Acute renal failure is quite common and may result from a wide variety of diseases, drugs, pregnancy-related complications, surgical procedures, and trauma. The causes of ARF are commonly considered under three major diagnostic categories: prerenal, postrenal, and renal (Table 45-1). This classification stresses the fact that only in the third category (renal) is renal parenchymal damage sufficient to cause functional failure in itself. Prerenal and postrenal factors are likely to lead to intrinsic renal failure but with proper diagnosis and treatment are readily reversible. Thus these categories help the clinician to consider a clinical problem involving potential or established acute renal failure in a systematic manner.

The common denominator in all the circumstances leading to prerenal azotemia is renal hypoperfusion.

TABLE 45·1

COMMON CAUSES OF ACUTE RENAL FAILURE

I. Prerenal (circulatory renal failure)
  A. Hypovolemia (hemorrhage, especially postpartum, abruptio placentae, burns, GI losses as in pancreatitis or gastroenteritis, diuretic overuse)
  B. Intravascular pooling (septic shock, anaphylaxis, crush injury)
  C. Decrease in cardiac output (cardiac failure, myocardial infarction, cardiac tamponade, pulmonary embolism)
  D. Increased renal vascular resistance (surgery, anesthesia, hepatorenal syndrome)
  E. Bilateral renal vascular obstruction (embolism, thrombosis)

II. Postrenal (acute obstructive uropathy)
  A. Obstruction to bladder outlet (prostatic hypertrophy, carcinoma)
  B. Bilateral ureteral obstruction (calculi, clots, tumors, retroperitoneal fibrosis, surgical trauma, necrotizing papillitis)
  C. Renal collecting-duct obstruction (uric acid, sulfa drug, Bence Jones protein)

III. Renal (intrinsic renal failure)
  A. Ischemia (all prerenal conditions, postoperative shock)
  B. Nephrotoxins
    1. Organic solvents (carbon tetrachloride, ethylene glycol, methanol)
    2. Heavy metals (bichloride of mercury, arsenic, lead, uranium)
    3. Antibiotics (methicillin, aminoglycosides, tetracyclines, amphotericin, cephalosporins), sulfonamides, phenytoin, phenylbutazone
    4. X-ray contrast media (especially in diabetic persons)
    5. Pigments (intravascular hemolysis due to mismatched blood transfusion, disseminated intravascular coagulopathies; myoglobinuria due to massive crush injuries)
  C. Glomerular-vascular renal disease
    1. Acute poststreptococcal glomerulonephritis
    2. Rapidly progressive glomerulonephritis
    3. Malignant hypertension
  D. Acute interstitial nephritis (overwhelming infection; drug-induced)
  E. Acute-on-chronic renal failure related to salt or water depletion, vomiting, diarrhea, infections

Delay in correcting the perfusion abnormality can lead to true ARF. Postrenal causes of ARF refer to obstruction to the flow of urine at any level of the urinary tract. Obstruction above the bladder, however, must be bilateral unless there is only one functioning kidney. It is important to realize that prolonged obstruction will lead to severe damage to the renal parenchyma and ARF. The remaining causal category of ARF involves intrinsic damage to the renal parenchyma.

The two major causes of acute intrinsic renal failure are (1) renal ischemia (prolonged renal hypoperfusion identified under prerenal conditions) and (2) nephrotoxic injury. Acute tubular necrosis was first identified in relation to ischemic and nephrotoxic acute renal failure and has been extensively studied with animal models. This fact explains the persistent use of the term

ATN, even though it is unsatisfactory in explaining the pathology and pathophysiology of the syndrome of acute renal failure. Ischemic injury is believed to be the most common cause of intrinsic acute renal failure.

Nephrotoxic tubular injury can result from the deliberate or accidental ingestion of bichloride of mercury, ethylene glycol (antifreeze), or carbon tetrachloride. The inhalation of fumes from carbon tetrachloride (CCl_4), a common ingredient of spot remover and other cleaning fluids, accompanied by the ingestion of ethyl alcohol (CH_3CH_2OH), is particularly dangerous because of a chemical reaction between these two compounds, in which a potent toxin is formed which is nephrotoxic. The above set of circumstances (alcohol ingestion at a party and removing a clothing stain with spot remover) has resulted in acute renal failure in a number of unsuspecting persons. For the same reasons, hobbyists using organic solvents and glues should work in well-ventilated rooms and refrain from drinking alcohol at the same time. In the vast majority of cases of nephrotoxic ARF, the agents are iatrogenic, i.e., related to the use of diagnostic or therapeutic agents.

A number of drugs are nephrotoxic. Some may cause an interstitial nephritis, while others are directly nephrotoxic. Antibiotics are the most frequent cause of nephrotoxic acute renal failure, especially in those who are advanced in age or have preexisting renal insufficiency. Often, drug-induced renal failure is nonoliguric. Common nephrotoxic antibiotics include penicillin (especially methicillin), aminoglycosides (neomycin, gentamicin, kanamycin, tobramycin), amphotericin, tetracycline, and the cephalosporins. Other common nephrotoxic drugs include phenytoin, phenylbutazone, and the sulfonamides. A more extended list of nephrotoxic drugs may be found in Papper (1978, p. 561).

X-ray contrast media used in various radiologic studies is a relatively common cause of ARF (Mattern and Finn, 1978). Predisposing factors in the development of radiographic contrast media–induced ARF include (1) juvenile-onset diabetes mellitus with renal insufficiency (creatinine > 5 mg/dl); (2) old age; (3) volume depletion; (4) multiple myeloma; (5) preexisting renal insufficiency, and (6) multiple exposure to contrast agents within a short period of time (Davidson, 1984).

The release of the pigments hemoglobin and myoglobin into the bloodstream may result in ARF. Hemoglobin is normally within red blood cells, and myoglobin normally exists within muscles. Although these agents are included under nephrotoxic causes of ARF, neither are believed to be directly nephrotoxic, and the pathogenetic mechanism of their action is poorly understood. Hemoglobinuria is most commonly associated with mismatched blood transfusions. *Rhabdomyolysis*, or necrosis of skeletal muscle with the release of myoglobin, is often due to trauma and massive crush injuries. However, nontraumatic rhabdomyolysis has re-

cently been recognized as a common cause of ARF. Nontraumatic rhabdomyolysis has been associated with a wide variety of conditions, such as severe exercise accompanied by heat stroke, acute myositis, type A influenza, and alcohol and drug abuse (Mattern and Finn, 1978).

The remaining three categories of intrinsic causes of ARF are glomerular-vascular, interstitial, and acute-on-chronic renal disease. These conditions have been discussed in previous chapters under "Chronic Renal Failure" and are not discussed at length in this chapter. However, they need to be differentiated from nephrotoxic and ischemic causes of ARF.

PATHOLOGY OF ACUTE TUBULAR NECROSIS

The term *acute tubular necrosis* (ATN) is commonly applied to both nephrotoxic and ischemic renal injuries, although it does not reflect the nature and severity of the observed tubular changes. Two types of histologic lesions are commonly observed in ATN: (1) necrosis of the tubular epithelium leaving the basement membrane intact, commonly resulting from the ingestion of nephrotoxic chemicals, and (2) necrosis of the tubular epithelium and the basement membrane, commonly associated with renal ischemia.

The severity of tubular damage in ATN due to nephrotoxins is highly variable, and the prognosis varies accordingly. There may be necrosis of the proximal tubule epithelium with complete healing in three or four weeks. Bichloride of mercury and carbon tetrachloride commonly produce this type of lesion. The prognosis is generally good with conservative management or supportive dialysis. In contrast, other poisons such as glycols may produce irreversible renal failure with infarction of the entire nephron, termed *acute cortical necrosis*. The prognosis in this case is poor. Calcification commonly occurs in the area of cortical necrosis if the patient is fortunate enough to survive.

Tubular damage due to renal ischemic causes is also highly variable. It depends on the extent and duration of the decreased renal blood flow and ischemia. There may be patchy or widespread destruction of the tubular epithelium and basement membrane or cortical necrosis. Many cases of acute cortical necrosis have followed complications of pregnancy, particularly premature separation of the placenta, postpartum hemorrhage, eclampsia, and septic abortion. When the basement membrane is disrupted, epithelial regeneration occurs in a random, haphazard manner, frequently leading to obstruction of the nephron at the site of necrosis. The prognosis depends on the extent of this type of change.

PATHOPHYSIOLOGY OF ACUTE RENAL FAILURE

Although there is now agreement concerning the pathology of the kidney damaged by ATN-type ARF, there is still considerable controversy over the pathogenesis of the suppression of renal function and the usually accompanying oliguria. Most modern concepts concerning possible causative factors are based on studies using animal experimental models in which nephrotoxic acute renal failure is produced by injections of mercuric chloride, uranyl nitrate, or chromate, while ischemic damage is produced by injecting glycerol or clamping the renal arteries, inducing hemorrhagic shock. Several theories have been proposed to explain the moderate reduction in renal blood flow and reduction in GFR observed in both the experimental animals and humans, including (1) tubular obstruction; (2) backleak of tubular fluid; (3) decreased glomerular permeability; (4) vasomotor dysfunction, and (5) tubuloglomerular feedback. None of the proposed mechanisms can account for all the variable aspects of ATN-type ARF. Schrier and Conger (1980) have summarized the supporting and the contradictory evidence for each of the proposed mechanisms.

The tubular obstruction theory proposes that ATN leads to the desquamation of necrotic tubular cells and other proteinaceous materials, which then form casts and occlude the tubule lumina. Cellular swelling as a result of the initial ischemia may also contribute to the obstruction and perpetuate the ischemia. Intratubular pressure increases, so that net glomerular filtration pressure is reduced. Tubular obstruction may be an important factor in ARF due to heavy metals, ethylene glycol, or prolonged ischemia.

The tubular backleak hypothesis proposes that glomerular filtration continues normally but that the tubular fluid "leaks" out of the lumina through the damaged tubular cells into the peritubular circulation. Disruption of the basement membrane may be seen with severe ATN, which provides an anatomic basis for this mechanism.

While the syndrome of ATN implies an abnormality of the renal tubule, recent evidence suggests that in some circumstances the glomerular capillary endothelial cells and/or basement membrane cells undergo changes which reduce permeability or the surface area for filtration. The result is a reduction of glomerular ultrafiltration.

Total renal blood flow (RBF) may be reduced to as low as 30 percent of normal in oliguric ARF (Papper, 1978). This level of RBF could be compatible with a substantial GFR. In fact, RBF in chronic renal failure is often as low as or lower than that found in the acute form, yet reduced but adequate renal function persists. Furthermore, experimental evidence suggests that RBF must be less than 5 percent before renal parenchymal damage occurs (Merrill, 1971, p. 640). Thus it appears that renal hypoperfusion alone cannot account for the degree of reduction in GFR and the tubular lesions found in ARF. However, there is evidence of marked changes in the intrarenal distribution of blood flow from the cortex to the medulla during acute and prolonged hypotension (Merrill, 1971, p. 639). It will be recalled from Chap. 40 that in the normal kidney about 90 percent of the blood is distributed to the cortex (where the glomeruli are located) and 10 percent goes to the medulla. This allows the kidney to concentrate urine and perform its functions. In contrast, in ARF the ratio of renal cortical to medullary blood distribution may be reversed, so that there is relative ischemia of the renal cortex. Constriction of the afferent arterioles provides a vascular basis for the marked reduction in GFR. Renal ischemia would then activate the renin-angiotensin system and perpetuate cortical ischemia after the initiating stimulus has disappeared. The highest concentration of renin is found in the outer cortex of the kidney, the site where ischemia is greatest, in animals and humans with acute renal failure (Schrier and Conger, 1980). Some authors have postulated a role for prostaglandins in the vasomotor dysfunction of ARF (Harter and Martin, 1982). Renal hypoxia normally stimulates the renal synthesis of PGE and PGA (potent vasodilators), causing renal blood flow to be redistributed to the cortex with resulting diuresis (Lee, 1974). It is possible that acute severe or prolonged ischemia may block the synthesis of these renal prostaglandins. Prostaglandin inhibitors such as aspirin are known to reduce RBF in normal persons and potentiate ATN.

The tubuloglomerular theory assumes that the primary injury involves the proximal tubules. The proximal tubules, damaged by ischemia or nephrotoxins, fail to absorb normal quantities of filtered sodium and water. As a result, the macula densa senses the increased sodium concentration in the distal tubular fluid and stimulates increased production of renin from the juxtaglomerular cells. The subsequent activation of angiotensin II results in vasoconstriction of the afferent arterioles, causing reduced renal blood flow and GFR.

Figure 45-1 illustrates a schema in which the various factors involved in the pathogenesis of ARF are combined. The initiating event is generally an ischemic insult and/or a nephrotoxin, which damages the tubules or glomeruli or reduces renal blood flow. Acute renal failure is then maintained through several possible mechanisms which may be present or absent and are a

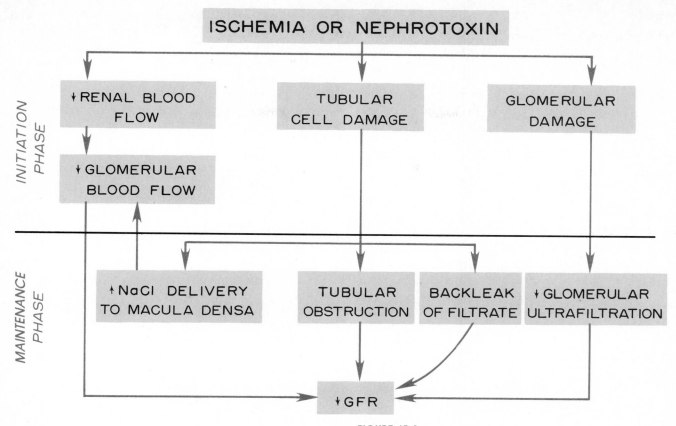

INITIATION PHASE

ISCHEMIA OR NEPHROTOXIN

↓RENAL BLOOD FLOW

↓GLOMERULAR BLOOD FLOW

TUBULAR CELL DAMAGE

GLOMERULAR DAMAGE

MAINTENANCE PHASE

↑NaCl DELIVERY TO MACULA DENSA

TUBULAR OBSTRUCTION

BACKLEAK OF FILTRATE

↓GLOMERULAR ULTRAFILTRATION

↓GFR

FIGURE 45-1

Pathogenesis of actue renal failure. (Redrawn from H. R. Harter and K. J. Martin, "Acute Renal Failure," *Postgraduate Medicine* 72(6): 191, 1982.)

result of the initial injury. Each mechanism differs in the importance of its contribution to the pathogenesis according to the different theories cited. It is likely that the relative importance of these mechanisms varies with the situation and is dependent on the evolution of the disease process as well as the severity of the pathologic damage. The pathophysiology of ARF is far from settled and, much more research is needed to define the relative importance of the various factors.

CLINICAL COURSE OF ACUTE RENAL FAILURE

The clinical course of acute renal failure has been divided traditionally into three stages: oliguria, diuresis, and recovery. This tradition is followed in the discussion below while recognizing that acute renal failure and azotemia may be present with urine output of more than 400 ml per 24 hours. The clinical course of oliguric and of nonoliguric acute renal failure are similar. However, abnormalities of blood chemistry are generally milder and the prognosis for recovery better in cases of nonoliguric acute renal failure.

Oliguric stage

The clinical picture is often dominated by the surgical, medical, or obstetric calamity causing the acute renal

failure. Oliguria is usually present within 24 to 48 hours after the initial injury, though this symptom may not occur until several days after exposure to nephrotoxic chemicals. Azotemia accompanies the oliguria.

It is critically important to recognize the onset of oliguria, determine the cause, and begin treatment of any reversible causes. Acute renal failure of the ATN type must be differentiated from prerenal (hypoperfusion) and postrenal (urinary tract obstruction) failure and other intrarenal disorders (e.g., acute poststreptococcal glomerulonephritis, acute pyelonephritis, acute-on-chronic renal failure). The diagnosis of acute renal failure is made only after the other causes are excluded.

Oliguria due to acute-on-chronic renal failure is usually evident from the history. Since patients with chronic renal failure have a limited ability to adjust fluid and electrolyte balance, they may be easily thrown into acute renal failure by relatively minor upsets. Examples are the patient with chronic glomerulonephritis who has a gastrointestinal upset with vomiting or diarrhea or the patient with chronic pyelonephritis who gets a superimposed acute renal infection. Occasionally, a patient with undiagnosed chronic renal insufficiency may present in acute renal failure. A history of long-standing nocturia, hypertension, systemic diseases such as systemic lupus erythematosis or diabetes mellitus, radiographic evidence of small, contracted kidneys, and signs of long-standing renal disease such as renal osteodystrophy are suggestive of chronic renal insufficiency. The patient can usually be restored to the previous state of health by treatment of the infection, correction of the fluid and electrolyte imbalance, and treatment by peritoneal dialysis if necessary.

Postrenal obstruction must be ruled out, especially if the cause of the renal failure is not apparent. The presence of anuria or of periods of anuria alternating with periods of normal urine flow suggests obstruction. Urethral and bladder neck obstruction can be evaluated by catheterization and determining residual urine in the bladder after an attempt at complete voiding. If outlet obstruction is ruled out but bilateral obstruction proximal to the bladder is suspected, ultrasound or radioisotope renal scan and retrograde pyelography may be performed.

Ultrasonography reveals renal size and may show evidence of obstructing calculi in the renal pelves or ureters. Radioisotope scans may be used to evaluate the integrity of the major renal vessels and is useful when occlusion of the renal artery or vein by an embolus or thrombus is suspected. Retrograde pyelography is used in selected cases of obstructive uropathy and may be therapeutic as well as diagnostic. Potential causes of obstruction are listed in Table 45-1. Prolonged obstruction will lead to intrinsic and often irreversible renal failure. Treatment involves immediate removal of the obstruction. Finally, prerenal oliguria is the most common antecedent situation leading to ARF and must be distinguished from ATN.

Prerenal oliguria versus ATN

Prerenal oliguria and azotemia are physiologic and potentially reversible. They result from shock, decreased plasma volume, and consequent decrease in renal blood flow and GFR. Prerenal oliguria may result from any of the prerenal causes of acute renal failure previously discussed. If left uncorrected, prerenal oliguria may progress to ATN. Serial determinations of the urine output, BUN level, creatinine level, and electrolytes should therefore be made following any major surgery, trauma, serious infection, or obstetric complication.

A few simple tests on the sediment and chemical constituents of the urine are helpful in distinguishing prerenal oliguria or azotemia from true acute renal failure of the ATN type (Table 45-2).

In prerenal oliguria, when there is not yet any damage to the renal parenchyma, the response of the kidney to decreased perfusion is to conserve salt and water. In contrast, intrinsic renal tubular damage is associated with impaired ability to conserve sodium. Consequently, urine sodium concentration in prerenal oliguria is low (<20 meq per liter) and high in ATN (>40 meq per liter).

Water reabsorption by the kidney is assessed by the concentration of a nonreabsorbable solute, such as creatinine, usually expressed as the ratio of the concentration of creatinine in urine to that of plasma (U/P creatinine). A U/P creatinine ratio of 2.0 indicates that 50 percent of the filtered water is reabsorbed, while a U/P creatinine ratio of 100 indicates that 1 percent of the filtered water is reabsorbed. Thus in prerenal azotemia the U/P creatinine ratio is high (>40), while it is low in the presence of intrinsic tubular renal disease (<20).

The U/P urea ratio is >8 in prerenal oliguria and <2 in established ATN. The U/P urea ratio is somewhat lower than the creatinine ratio, since there is some back diffusion of urea but not of creatinine. Thus the U/P creatinine ratio is a truer estimate of water reabsorption across the nephron.

TABLE 45-2

RENAL INDICES IN PRERENAL AZOTEMIA AND ACUTE RENAL FAILURE

Laboratory test	Prerenal azotemia	ATN
Urinary Na concentration	<20 meq/L	>40 meq/L
Urine/plasma creatinine ratio	>40:1	<20:1
Urine/plasma urea ratio	>8:1	<2:1
FE_{Na}, %	<1	>1
BUN/creatinine ratio	>10:1	About 10:1
Urine osmolality	>500 mOsm	Near 287 mOsm (fixed)
Urine/plasma osmolality ratio	>2:1	<1.1:1
Urine specific gravity	>1.015	Near 1.010 (fixed)
Urinary sediment	Normal	Casts, cellular debris

The normal ratio of blood urea nitrogen (BUN) to creatinine is 10:1. In prerenal azotemia this ratio is greater than 10:1 and may be 20:1 or greater. The high ratio of BUN/serum creatinine indicates the disproportionate rise of the blood levels of urea. Blood urea levels rise faster than creatinine because of the greater back reabsorption (its molecule is smaller than that of creatinine) in the situation of reduced renal perfusion. The production of urea may also increase markedly and contribute to the disproportionate increase in the BUN, since a catabolic state is often present in the acute illness and trauma associated with the development of prerenal azotemia.

Urine osmolality, specific gravity, and U/P osmolality ratio are additional indices of water handling by the kidney. In prerenal oliguria, urine osmolaltiy is >500 mOsm (specific gravity > 1.015) but decreases to about 287 mOsm (specific gravity 1.010) in established ATN as ability to concentrate is lost (Coe, 1980). The U/P osmolality progresses toward 1:1 in established ARF, indicating that the urine is isoosmotic with the plasma.

The urinary sodium concentration and U/P creatinine are the most reliable indices in distinguishing prerenal azotemia from ATN. When these indices are combined, the fractional excretion of sodium (FE_{Na}) can be calculated. The fractional excretion of sodium is less than 1 percent in prerenal azotemia and is usually greater than this in established ATN. The FE_{Na} is a very sensitive index in differentiating prerenal azotemia from established acute renal failure. Fractional excretion of sodium is calculated by the following formula (Harter and Martin, 1982):

$$FE_{Na} = \frac{U_{Na}}{P_{Na}} \times \frac{P_{Cr}}{U_{Cr}} \times 100\%$$

where U_{Na} = urinary conc. of sodium in meq/L

P_{Na} = plasma conc. of sodium in meq/L

U_{Cr} = urinary conc. of creatinine in mg/dl

P_{Cr} = plasma conc. of creatinine in mg/dl

Misleading results are occasionally obtained when (1) residual urine which has remained in the bladder for several hours is used; (2) a diuretic has been administered; (3) there is preexisting chonic renal disease, and (4) there is intermittent urinary tract obstruction.

Examination of the urine sediment may also be helpful in the differential diagnosis of ARF. In prerenal azotemia, the urine sediment is essentially normal with a few hyaline casts; brown, granular casts and many epithelial cells are likely to be present in ATN. Prerenal azotemia is fairly easy to exclude on the basis of the clinical setting and the urine chemistry. However, urine chemistry may not be helpful in differentiating postre-

nal obstruction from ATN, and other criteria must be used.

Prevention of ATN in patients at high risk or those with prerenal azotemia or oliguria is an important therapeutic consideration. Correction of circulatory insufficiency and the resulting renal hypoperfusion is important in preventing the progression of prerenal oliguria to ATN. Blood transfusion to replace any losses and hydration with intravenous fluids may be successful in restoring circulation and increased urine output. Mannitol and furosemide have sometimes been successful in inducing diuresis and reducing the risk of oliguric ATN.

Harter and Martin (1982) suggest the following approach. After careful assessment of extracellular fluid (ECF) volume and cardiac function (to exclude ECF volume excess), give 500 ml of intravenous normal saline rapidly to exclude prerenal oliguria. If urine output is unchanged, mannitol 25 g is given slowly IV, followed by furosemide 80 to 320 mg IV. If diuresis occurs (urine output > 40 ml per hour), these doses may be repeated every 3 to 4 hours to maintain high urine flow rates. If this regimen is unsuccessful (urine output still < 30 ml per hour), then established ATN probably exists.

In established ATN the period of oliguria may last no longer than a day or it may last as long as 6 weeks. The average duration of the oliguria is from 7 to 10 days. During the oliguric phase, the usual rise in BUN level is 25 to 30 mg/dl daily, and creatinine rises at the rate of about 2.5 mg/dl daily. The retention of fluids, electrolytes, and nitrogenous substances causes the rapid development of uremic symptoms.

Diuretic stage

The diuretic stage of acute renal failure begins when the urine output increases to more than 400 ml a day. This stage generally lasts two or three weeks. Daily urine output rarely exceeds 4 liters, provided the patient is not overhydrated. The high urine volume of the diuretic phase is due partly to the osmotic diuresis produced by the high blood urea concentration and partly to the impaired ability of the recovering tubules to conserve filtered salts and water. During the diuretic phase patients may develop deficits of potassium, sodium, and water. If the urinary losses are not replaced, death may end the diuresis. During the early diuretic stage the BUN level may continue to rise, largely because urea clearance does not keep up with endogenous urea production. As the diuresis continues, however, the azotemia gradually disappears and there is great clinical improvement.

Recovery stage

The recovery stage of acute renal failure lasts up to a year, during which time the anemia and concentrating ability of the kidneys gradually improve. Some patients, however, are left with a permanent reduction in the GFR.

Even though damage to tubular epithelium is theoretically reversible, ATN is a dangerous condition with a serious prognosis. The mortality rate is still about 50 percent (down from a previous rate of about 90 percent three decades ago) in spite of the most careful management of fluid and electrolyte balance and the aid of dialysis. About two-thirds die during the oliguric stage and about one-third during the diuretic stage. The mortality rate is related to the causal background of the associated illnesses leading up to the acute episode. Mortality is about 60 percent in cases following surgery, crush injuries, and other major trauma, about 25 percent following incompatible blood transfusions and carbon tetrachloride poisoning, and 10 to 15 percent in obstetric cases. In general, patients with nonoliguric ARF have a better prognosis than those with oliguric ARF: only about 25 percent of the former die.

TREATMENT OF ESTABLISHED ACUTE TUBULAR NECROSIS

After ATN is established, the primary consideration in management is the maintenance of fluid and electrolyte balance. The same principles of conservative management which were discussed in the treatment of chronic renal failure also apply to acute renal failure. The early use of hemodialysis to prevent severe fluid and electrolyte imbalance and uremic symptoms has undoubtedly reduced the mortality. Careful attention to fluid and electrolyte balance is necessary not only during the oliguric stage but also during the diuretic stage, when severe sodium and potassium depletion may occur. The most frequent complication in acute renal failure resulting in death is infection. It is the contributing cause of death in about 70 percent of patients and the primary cause in about 30 percent. Not only is the uremic patient more susceptible to infection, but once it is established it is more difficult to control. The presence of infection may go unrecognized because of the lack of the usual symptom of fever, since hypothermia is common in renal failure. Once infection is identified, it should be treated with nonnephrotoxic antibiotics.

QUESTIONS

Acute renal failure

Direcitons: Answer the following questions on a separate sheet of paper.

1. Why is it particularly hazardous to use organic solvents (containing CCl_4) and drink an alcoholic beverage at the same time?

2. List the two major mechanisms of renal injury in acute intrinsic renal failure.

3. What is meant by acute-on-chronic renal failure? What are the precipitating causes?

4. What is the difference between the two types of histologic lesion commonly observed in ATN? What is the common etiology?

5. What is acute cortical necrosis? List the common causes, complications, and prognosis.

6. What is the most common complication resulting in death in acute renal failure?

7. What is the advantage of considering the causes of acute renal failure under the prenatal, postrenal, and renal diagnostic categories?

8. List examples of common conditions causing obstructive uropathy at the level of the bladder outlet, ureters, and kidneys.

9. Name one penicillin and three aminoglycoside antibiotics which are frequently the cause of nephrotoxic acute renal failure. What are the characteristics of patients at high risk?

10. Name and briefly describe five factors suggested as contributing to the pathogenesis of acute renal failure.

11. What is the most sensitive laboratory test in differentiating prerenal azotemia from established acute renal failure? By what formula is it calculated? Name some circumstances which may cause misleading laboratory test results.

12. Name two drugs commonly given in an attempt to correct prerenal oliguria and prevent progression to established acute renal failure.

Directions: Circle the letter preceding each item below that correctly answers the question or completes the statement. Only one answer is correct, with exceptions noted.

703
QUESTIONS

13. Acute renal failure usually refers to the sudden cessation of renal function resulting in urine output of less than:
a. 800 ml per day   b. 1200 ml per day   c. 400 ml per day

14. In ATN, proximal tubular epithelial damage associated with CCl_4 or $HgCl_2$ poisoning (mild exposure) usually results in:
a. Irreversible renal failure with infarction of the entire nephron   b. Complete healing of the lesion in 3 to 4 weeks

15. Acute tubular necrosis may result from: (More than one answer may be correct.)
a. Exposure to nephrotoxic chemicals   b. Obstruction of the ureteropelvic junction   c. Hyperkalemia   d. Massive crush injuries   e. Excessive sodium restriction   f. Prolonged shock

16. Which of the following will *not* cause necrosis of the tubular epithelial cells?
a. CCl_4 b. Severe acute renal ischemia
c. Transfusion reactions   d. Mercuric ions
e. Diodrast (x-ray contrast medium)

17. Which of the following statements is true concerning the treatment and differentiation of prerenal azotemia and established ATN? (More than one answer may be correct.)
a. Oliguric urine is concentrated in established ATN.   b. The urine/plasma osmolality ratio is greater than 2:1 in prerenal azotemia.   c. The urine/plasma urea concentration is less than 1 in established ATN.   d. The correction of circulatory insufficiency by blood and IV administration of fluids may prevent the progress of prerenal azotemia to ATN.   e. The administration of IV mannitol will correct established ATN.

18. The risk of radiographic contrast media–induced acute renal failure is increased by: (More than one answer may be correct.)   a. Age >60 years
b. Dehydration   c. Diabetes mellitus   d. Plasma creatinine >2.0 mg/dl   e. Double dose of medium

19. Sudden deterioration of renal function in a person with diabetes mellitus suggests:
a. Renal calculi   b. Acute poststreptococcal glomerulonephritis   c. Chronic pyelonephritis
d. Papillary necrosis

20. Which of the following conditions is suggested by complete anuria for more than 48 hours?
a. Severe prerenal azotemia   b. Acute-on-chronic renal failure   c. Nephrotoxic antibiotic-induced renal failure   d. Bilateral renal artery or renal vein occlusion

21. Which of the following statements is *incorrect* regarding nonoliguric acute renal failure?
a. Urine volume is >400 ml per day   b. Tubular damage is generally less severe than in oliguric ARF   c. Azotemia is absent   d. Is commonly induced by nephrotoxic antibiotics

22. Mortality is less in nonoliguric than in oliguric ARF but still about:
a. 10 percent   b. 25 percent   c. 35 percent
d. 50 percent

23. Which of the following findings is most consistent with ATN?
a. Urinary Na, 50 meq per liter   b. U/P creatinine ratio, 70   c. Urinary sediment, a few hyaline casts d FE_{Na}, 0.8 percent   d. U/P urea ratio, 10
e. U/P osmolality ratio, 2:1

Directions: Circle T if the statement is true and F if it is false. Give reasons for your answer.

24. T   F   Progressive azotemia is a defining characteristic of nonoliguric acute renal failure.

25. T   F   In acute arterial hypotension, renal cortical blood flow increases from about 10 percent to about 80 to 90 percent while renal medullary blood flow decreases by the same percentage.

26. T   F   Nephrotoxic ARF induced by CCl_4 is potentiated by the ingestion of ethyl alcohol.

27. T   F   Rhabdomyolysis results in the release of large amounts of Tamm-Horsfall protein into the urine, inducing ARF.

28. T   F   Anuria alternating with episodes of polyuria suggests ARF from prerenal causes.

29. T   F   During prerenal oliguria the BUN usually increases faster than serum creatinine because of greater back diffusion and catabolism of body protein.

Directions: Match the stage in the clinical course of acute renal failure in col. B to the statement which best applies to it in col. A.

Column A   Column B
30. ____ Azotemia   a. Oliguric stage

gradually sub-
sides in this
stage.

b. Diuretic stage

c. Recovery stage

31. ____ Concen-
trating ability
of the kidneys
gradually im-
proves during
this stage (may
last up to 1
year).

32. ____ BUN may
rise 25 to 30
mg per 100 ml
daily during
this stage.

33. ____ Average
duration is 7 to
10 days.

34. ____ Most
deaths occur
during this
stage.

35. ____ Most
common com-
plications dur-
ing this stage
are hyperkale-
mia, pulmo-
nary edema,
and cardiac
failure.

36. ____ About
one-third of
the deaths
occur during
this stage.

REFERENCES FOR PART VII

Advisory Committee to the Renal Transplant Registry: "The 13th Report of the Human Renal Transplant Registry," *Transplantation Proceedings* 9: 9–26, 1977.

ALFRED, H. J., L. G. GRAFF, A. J. COHEN, and A. SCHUSTER: "Treatment of Renal Failure," in B. D. Rose (ed.), *Pathophysiology of Renal Disease*, McGraw-Hill, New York, 1981.

ANDERSON, R. J., S. L. LINUS, A. S. BERN, et al.: "Non-oliguric Acute Renal Failure," *New England Journal of Medicine*, 296(20): 1134–1138, 1977.

AVIOLI, P. F.: "Vitamin D Metabolism in Uremia," *The Kidney*, vol. 8, no. 1, 1975.

BAILEY, G. L.: "Uremia as a Total Body Disease," in G. L. Bailey (ed.), *Hemodialysis*, Academic, New York, 1972.

BERL, T. and R. W. SCHRIER: "Renal Function in Pregnancy," in R. W. Schrier (ed.), *Renal and Electrolyte Disorders*, 2d ed., Little, Brown, Boston, 1980, pp. 471–499.

BERLYNE, G. M.: *A Course in Renal Disease*, 3d ed., Blackwell, Oxford, 1971.

————: "Renal Involvement in the Collagen Diseases," in D. A. K. Black (ed.), *Renal Disease*, 4th ed., Blackwell, London, 1979, pp. 653–686.

BRENNER, B. M. and T. H. HOSTETTER, "Toxins" in R. Petersdorf et al. (eds.), *Harrison's Principles of Internal Medicine*, 10th ed., McGraw-Hill, New York, 1983, pp. 1656–1657.

BRICKER, N. S. and L. G. FINE: "The Pathophysiology of Chronic Renal Failure," in M. H. Maxwell and C. R. Kleeman (eds.), *Clinical Disorders of Fluid and Electrolyte Metabolism*, 3d ed., McGraw-Hill, New York, 1980, pp. 799–825.

————: "On the Functional Transformations in the Residual Nephrons with Advancing Disease," *Pediatric Clinics of North America*, 18: 595, 1971.

————: "On the Meaning of the Intact Nephron Hypothesis," *American Journal of Medicine*, 46:1,1969.

————: "Renal Function in Chronic Renal Disease," *Medicine* (Baltimore), 44: 263, 1965.

BROWN, J., et al.: "Diabetes Mellitus: Current Concepts and Vascular Lesions (Renal and Retinal)," *Annals of Internal Medicine*, 68: 643, 1968.

BRUNDAGE, D. J.: *Nursing Management of Renal Problems*, 2d ed., Mosby, St. Louis, 1980.

CAMERON, J. S.: "Natural History of Glomerulonephritis," in D. A. K. Black (ed.), *Renal Disease*, 4th ed., Blackwell, London, 1979, pp. 329–382.

CARPENTER, C. B. and J. P. MERRILL: "Histocompatibility and Transplantation," in K. Isselbacher et al. (eds.), *Harrison's Principles of Internal Medicine*, 9th ed., McGraw-Hill, New York, 1980, p. 360.

CHURG, J. and H. DOLGER: "Diabetic Renal Disease," in M. B. Strauss and L. G. Welt (eds.), *Diseases of the Kidney*, Little, Brown, Boston, 1971, pp. 873–885.

COE, F. L.: "Clinical Stone Disease," in F. L. Coe, B.

M. Brenner, and J. H. Stein (eds.), *Contemporary Issues in Nephrology*, vol. 5, *Nephrolithiasis*, Longmans, New York, 1980, pp. 1–12.

COLTON, R. S. and W. L. EMMERSON: "Uric Acid, Gout, and the Kidney," *Medical Clinics of North America*, **50**: 1031–1041, 1966.

DALGAARD, O. Z.: "Polycystic Disease of the Kidney," in M. B. Strauss and L. G. Welt (eds.), *Diseases of the Kidney*, 2d ed., Little, Brown, Boston, 1971, pp. 1223–1253.

DAVIDSON, W. D.: "Differential Diagnosis and Treatment of Acute Renal Failure," in N. S. Bricker and M. A. Kirschenbaum (eds.), *The Kidney: Diagnosis and Management*, Wiley, New York, 1984.

DE WARDNER, H. E.: *The Kidney*, 4th ed., Longmans, New York, 1973.

DIXON, F. J.: "Glomerulonephritis and Immunopathology," *Hospital Practice*, **2** (11):35–43, 1967.

DOUGLAS, A. P. and D. S. KERR: *A Short Textbook of Kidney Disease*, Pitman, London, 1968, pp. 34–36, 84–86, 156–206.

"End Stage Renal Disease Program," Hearings before the Committee on Government Operations, House of Representatives, 97th Congress, Document 94-793 O, Wahington, 1982.

EPSTEIN, F. H.: "Acute Glomerulonephritis," *Hospital Medicine*, **4** (11): 30–42, 1968.

————: "Signs and Symptoms of Electrolyte Disorders," in M. H. Maxwell and C. R. Kleeman (eds.), *Clinical Disorders of Fluid and Electrolyte Metabolism*, 3d ed., McGraw-Hill, New York, 1980, pp. 499–530.

EPSTEIN, M.: "The Role of Renin Measurements in the Management of Hypertension," *The Kidney*, vol. 10, no. 1, 1977.

European Multicentre Trial: *Lancet*, **2**: 58, 1982.

FINKELBERG, C. and C. M. KUNIN: "Clinical Evaluation of Closed Urinary Drainage Systems," *Journal of the American Medical Association*, **207**: 1657, 1969.

FISH, A. J., A. F. MICHAEL, and R. A. GOOD: "Pathogenesis of Glomerulonephritis," in M. B. Strauss and L. G. Welt (eds.), *Diseases of the Kidney*, 2d ed., Little, Brown, Boston, 1971, pp. 373–395.

FRANKLIN, S. S. and M. H. MAXWELL: "Acute Renal Failure," in M. H. Maxwell and C. R. Kleeman (eds.), *Clinical Disorders of Fluid and Electrolyte Metabolism*, 3d ed., McGraw-Hill, New York, 1980, pp. 745–798.

FREEDMAN, L. R.: "Urinary Tract Infection, Pyelonephritis, and Other Forms of Chronic Interstitial Nephritis," in M. B. Strauss and L. G. Welt (eds.), *Diseases of the Kidney*, 2d ed., Little, Brown, Boston, 1971, pp. 667–713.

FRIEDMAN, E. A.: *Strategy in Renal Failure*, Wiley, New York, 1978, pp. 521–545.

GAULT, M. H., et al.: "Syndrome Associated with the Abuse of Analgesics," *Annals of Internal Medicine*, **68**: 906–925, 1968.

GLASSACK, R. J. and B. M. BRENNER: "The Major Glomerulopathies," in R. Petersdorf (ed.), *Harrison's Principles of Internal Medicine*, 10th ed., McGraw-Hill, New York, 1983, pp. 1632–1649.

GOLDEN, A. and J. F. MAHER: *The Kidney—Structure and Function*, Williams & Wilkins, Baltimore, 1971, pp. 69–87, 145–165, 176–189.

GORDON, A. and M. H. MAXWELL: "Reversible Uremia," in *Hospital Medicine*, January 1969, pp. 11–18.

GUTCH, C. F. and MARTHA STONER: *Review of Hemodialysis for Nurses*, 4th ed., 1983.

HARTER, H. R. and K. J. MARTIN: "Acute Renal Failure," *Postgraduate Medicine*, **72**(6): 175–197, 1982.

HENDERSON, L. W. and M. L. SANFELIPPO: "Newer Approaches to Solute Removal in Chronic Renal Failure," *Advances in Internal Medicine*, **25**: 303–325, 1980.

HEPINSTALL, R. H.: "Pathology of Acute Glomerulonephritis," in M. B. Strauss and L. G. Welt (eds.), *Diseases of the Kidney*, Little, Brown, Boston, 1971, pp. 405–452.

HOOD, B., T. FALKHEDEN, and M. CARLSSON: "Trends and Patterns of Mortality in Chronic Uremia," *Acta Medica Scandanavia*, **181**: 561, 1967.

IRWIN, B. D.: "Renal Transplantation—A Nursing Perspective," *AANNT Journal*, **10**(4): 11–22, 1983.

KASS, E. H.: "Bacteriuria and Pyelonephritis of Pregnancy," *Archives of Internal Medicine*, **105**: 194–1960.

KUNIN, C. M.: *Detection, Prevention, and Management of Urinary Tract Infections*, 2d ed., Lea & Febiger, Philadelphia, 1974.

LAPIDES, J.: *Fundamentals of Urology*, Saunders, Philadelphia, 1976.

LEE, J.: "The Prostaglandins," in R. H. Williams (ed.), *Textbook of Endocrinology*, 5th ed., Saunders, Philadelphia, 1974.

LINDEMAN, R. D.: "Percutaneous Renal Biopsy," *The Kidney*, vol. 7, no. 2, 1974.

MATTERN, W. D. and W. F. FINN: "Changing Perceptions of Acute Renal Failure," *The Kidney*, **11**(6): 25–30, 1978.

MAUDE, D. L.: *Kidney Physiology and Kidney Disease*, Lippincott, Philadelphia, 1978, pp. 123, 171.

MAXWELL, M. and C. R. KLEEMAN: *Clinical Disorders of Fluid and Electrolyte Metabolism*, 3d ed., McGraw-Hill, New York, 1980, pp. 531–589.

MERRILL, J. P.: "Uremia," *New England Journal of Medicine*, **282**: 953–961, 1014–1024, 1968.

———— : "Acute Renal Failure," in M. B. Strauss and L. G. Welt (eds.), *Diseases of the Kidney*, 2d ed., Little, Brown, Boston, 1971

METHANY, N. M., and W. D. SNIVELY: *Nurses' Handbook of Fluid Balance*, 4th ed., Lippincott, Philadelphia, 1983.

MILNE, M. D.: "Renal Tubular Dysfunction," in M. B. Strauss and L. G. Welt (eds.), *Diseases of the Kidney*, 2d ed., Little, Brown, Boston, 1971, pp. 1114–1116, 1071–1127.

MOFFATT, D. B.: "Anatomy of the Human Kidney," in D. A. K. Black (ed.), *Renal Disease*, 3d ed., Blackwell, London, 1979, pp. 3–29.

MONCRIEF, J. W. and R. P. POPOVICH: "Continuous Ambulatory Peritoneal Dialysis," *The Kidney*, vol. 12, no. 3, 1979.

MORRIS, P. J.: "Renal Transplantation—1982," *Transplantation Proceedings*, 15(1): 1033–1038, 1983.

NETTER, F. H.: *Ciba Collection of Medical Illustrations: Kidneys, Ureters, and Urinary Bladder*, Ciba Pharmaceutical Co., Summit, N.J., 1973.

NORDEN, C. W. and E. H. KASS: "Bacteriuria of Pregnancy—A Critical Appraisal," *Annual Review of Medicine*, 19: 431–470, 1968.

OLSSON, O.: "Renal Radiography," in M. B. Strauss and L. G. Welt (eds.), *Diseases of the Kidney*, 2d ed., Little, Brown, Boston, 1971, pp. 139–196.

OPELZ, G. and P. I. TERASAKI: "Improvement of Kidney-graft Survival with Increased Number of Blood Transfusions," *New England Journal of Medicine*, 299: 799, 1978.

PAPPER, S.: *Clinical Nephrology*, 2d ed., Little, Brown, Boston, 1978.

———— and C. A. VAAMONDE: "Nephrosclerosis," in M. B. Strauss and L. G. Welt (eds.), *Diseases of the Kidney*, 2d ed., Little, Brown, Boston, 1971, pp. 735–760.

PAUL, W. E. *Immunogenetics*, Raven Press, New York, 1984.

PICKERING, M. J.: "Treatment of Anemia," *Dialysis & Transplantation*, August 1975, pp. 56–58.

PITTS, R. F.: *Physiology of the Kidney and Body Fluids*, 3d ed., Year Book, Chicago, 1974, pp. 1, 3–10, 40–41, 71–96, 109, 124–168, 198–239.

QUINTON, W., D. DILLARD, and D. H. SCRIBNER: "Cannulation of Blood Vessels for Prolonged Hemodialysis," *Transactions American Society Artificial Internal Organs*, 6: 104–109, 1960.

RAPPAPORT, F. T. and J. DAUSSET (eds.): *Human Transplantation*, Grune & Stratton, New York, 1968.

RELMAN, A. S.: "Pyelonephritis," in D. A. K. Black (ed.), *Renal Disease*, 3d ed., Blackwell, London, 1972, pp. 399–415.

———— and N. G. LEVINSKY: "Clinical Examination of Renal Function," in M. B. Strauss and L. G. Welt (eds.), *Diseases of the Kidney*, 2d ed., Little, Brown, Boston, 1971, pp. 87–96, 116–120, 121–125.

ROBSON, J. S.: "The Nephrotic Syndrome," in D. A. K. Black (ed.), *Renal Disease*, 3d ed., Blackwell, London, 1972, pp. 331–359.

ROSE, B. D.: *Clinical Physiology of Acid-Base Disorders*, McGraw-Hill, New York, 1977, p. 155.

SALVATIERRA, O., JR., F. VINCENT, W. AMEND, et al.: "Deliberate Donor-specific Blood Transfusions Prior to Living Related Renal Transplantation," *Annals of Surgery*, 192: 543, 1980.

SCHREINER, G. E.: "Toxic Nephropathy," *American Journal of Medicine*, 38: 409, 1965.

————: "The Nephrotic Syndrome," in M. B. Strauss and L. G. Welt (eds.), *Diseases of the Kidney*, 2d ed., Little, Brown, Boston, 1971, pp. 503–607.

————: "Renal Biopsy," in M. B. Strauss and L. G. Welt (eds.), *Diseases of the Kidney*, 2d ed., Little, Brown, Boston, 1971, pp. 197–207.

SCHRIER, R. W. and V. D. Conger: "Acute Renal Failure: Diagnosis and Management," in R. W. Schrier (ed.), *Renal and Electrolyte Disorders*, 2d ed., Little, Brown, Boston, 1980, pp. 375–408.

SELDIN, D. W., et al.: "Consequences of Renal Failure and Their Management," in M. B. Strauss and L. G. Welt (eds.), *Diseases of the Kidney*, 2d ed., Little, Brown, Boston, 1971, pp. 211–272.

STABLES, D. P.: "The Scope of Kidney Radiology," *The Kidney*, vol. 10, no. 2, 1977.

STUART, F. P.: "Immunological Enhancement of Allografts: Experimental Basis and Potential Clinical Application," *Dialysis & Transplantation*, 9: 121, 1980.

TERASAKI, P. I., D. BERNOCO, M. S. PARK, et al.: "Microdroplet Testing for HLA-A, -B, -C, and -D Antigens," *American Journal of Clinical Pathology*, 69: 103, 1978.

THEIL, G.: "Membranous Glomerulopathy," *The Kidney*, vol. 5, no. 6, 1972.

THORNBURY, J. R. and J. D. WICKS: "Evaluation of the Kidneys by Imaging Examinations," in J. M. Weller (ed.), *Fundamentals of Nephrology*, Harper & Row, New York, 1979.

VANDER, A. J.: *Renal Physiology*, McGraw-Hill, New York, 1975.

VANRENTERGHEM, Y., L. ROELS, and P. MICHIELSEN: "Prognostic Factors in a Transplantation Center with Good Results," *Clinical Nephrology*, 21(1): 64–71, 1984.

WALSER, M., and M. MITCH: "Dietary Management of Renal Failure," *The Kidney*, vol. 10, no. 3, 1977.

WARHOL, B. A., et al.: "Osmolality," *Archives of Internal Medicine*, 116: 743, 1965.

WELLER, J. M. and J. A. GREENE: *Examination of the Urine*, Meredith, New York, 1966.

WELT, L. G. (ed.): "Symposium on Uremia," *American Journal of Medicine*, **44:** 653–802, 1968.

WHALLEY, P.: "Bacteriuria in Pregnancy," *American Journal of Obstetrics and Gynecology*, **97:** 723–738, 1967.

WHITCOMB, W. H. and S. S. BOTTOMLEY: "Erythropoiesis in Renal Disease," *The Kidney*, vol. 10, no. 4, 1977.

WILSON, L. M. and R. E. EASTERLING: *Fistula or Cannula? Hemodialysis Blood Access Systems*, University of Michigan Renal Disease Control Program, 1975.

WOODS, J. W. and T. F. WILLIAMS: "Hypertension Due to Renal Vascular Disease, Renal Infarction, Renal Cortical Necrosis," in M. B. Strauss and L. G. Welt (eds.), *Diseases of the Kidney*, 2d ed., Little, Brown, Boston, 1971, pp. 772–774.

World Health Organization, Committee on Leukocyte Nomenclature, *WHO Bulletin*, **54:** 461–465, Geneva, 1978.

MARY CARTER LOMBARDO

PART VIII

NEUROLOGIC DISORDERS

More than 200 clinical syndromes associated with dysfunction, disease, and injury of the nervous system are recognized. The clinical manifestations of disease involving the nervous system are perhaps the most complex and intriguing in all of medicine. Signs and symptoms of these diseases vary in type and range from relatively simple, objective, and easily elicited signs to complex and highly individualized signs.

Only a small number of neurologic disorders are presented in this section. Part VIII begins with a concise overview of neuroanatomy, since accurate diagnosis and treatment are most often dependent upon the localization of the disorder within the nervous system. In order for health care professionals to respond to the patient with a neurologic disorder in an intelligent, empathetic, and therapeutic manner, a working knowledge of neuroanatomy is essential.

OBJECTIVES

At the completion of this part you should be able to:

1. Describe the normal structures and functions of the central and peripheral nervous systems and relate these to the elicited signs and symptoms of neurologic disorders.
2. Identify the etiology, pathogenesis, and treatment principles for selected neurologic disorders.

THE NERVOUS SYSTEM*

OBJECTIVES

At the completion of this chapter you should be able to:

1. List three types of neuron according to function.
2. Review the major components of the central and peripheral nervous systems.
3. Name and describe the components of the five major subdivisions of the adult brain.
4. Discuss somatic versus visceral neurons and the structures they innervate.
5. List the general functions of the sympathetic and parasympathetic divisions of the autonomic nervous system.
6. Distinguish between neurons, neuroglia, and Schwann cells.
7. Discuss the functions of microglia, ependyma, astroglia, and oligodendroglia.
8. Discuss the location and function of myelin.
9. Discuss whether nerve cells regenerate.
10. Review the structure of a neuron.
11. List and give examples of three types of neuron classified according to the number and pattern of their processes.
12. Distinguish between Golgi type I and Golgi type II neurons.
13. Discuss the physiology of impulse generation and propagation along the axon of a neuron; between neurons; between a neuron and skeletal muscle.
14. Explain the advantages of convergent and divergent neuronal circuits.
15. Differentiate the structure of a neuron from that of a nerve fiber and a nerve.
16. Identify and describe the protective coverings of the brain and spinal cord.
17. Locate and identify the blood vessels probably involved in the following types of cerebral vascular problem: epidural hematoma, subdural hematoma, subarachnoid hemorrhage, intracranial hemorrhage.

*This chapter was written by A. M. Pizzuti and L. M. Wilson.

18. Explain why laceration of the galea aponeurotica is hazardous.

19. Name and locate the four major sheaths of meningeal dura extending into the cranial cavity.

20. Name the two pairs of arteries supplying the brain.

21. Summarize and diagram the major characteristics of the vascular supply to the brain and spinal cord.

22. Differentiate between conducting and penetrating cerebral arteries.

23. Describe the formation, circulation, and resorption of the cerebrospinal fluid.

24. Discuss the two types of hydrocephalus.

25. Describe the metabolic characteristics of brain tissue.

26. Name the three major subdivisions of the brainstem.

27. Describe the structural and functional characteristics of the following: midbrain, pons, medulla oblongata, cerebellum, diencephalon, limbic system, cerebrum, basal ganglia.

28. Identify functional disabilities associated with lesions of the substantia nigra, red nucleus, subthalamus, pineal body, and hippocampus.

29. Name the three fiber tracts connecting the cerebellum and brainstem.

30. List the major functions of the thalamus and hypothalamus.

31. Identify the lobes of the cerebrum and the major sulci or fissures separating them.

32. Identify three types of cerebral fiber tract and give some examples.

33. State the composition of the internal capsule.

34. Distinguish between the primary and association areas of the cortex as to general functions.

35. Explain what is meant by *contralateral control* with reference to the brain.

36. Identify the voluntary motor and somesthetic areas of the cerebral cortex and describe their somatotopic organization.

37. List the functions associated with each of the lobes of the brain.

38. Identify the likely area of damage to the cerebral cortex associated with the following deficits: socially inappropriate behavior, slovenly dress, alexia, astereognosis, sensory aphasia, motor aphasia, visual field defects.

39. Explain the meaning of the functional specialization of the cerebral hemispheres.

40. State the location and function of the reticular formation.

41. Discuss the role of the CNS monoamines in sleep and emotional behavior.

42. List and describe the functions of the cranial nerves.

43. Describe the components of a typical spinal nerve and how it is connected to the spinal cord.

44. Discuss the number and groupings, major divisions or rami, and sensory distribution of the spinal nerves.

45. Identify the major nerve plexuses and some peripheral nerves arising from each.

46. Identify the vertebral level at which the spinal cord terminates.

47. Describe the structures found in the gray and the white matter of the spinal cord.

The human nervous system is a complex, highly specialized, interconnected network of neural tissue. It coordinates, interprets, and controls the interactions between the individual and the surrounding environment. This important body system is also responsible for the regulation of the activities of most of the other body systems. The body is able to function as a harmonious unit because of the neural regulation of communications between the various systems. The phenomena of consciousness, thought, memory, language, sensation, and movement all originate within this system. Thus the ability to comprehend, learn, and respond to stimuli is a result of the integrated functioning of the nervous system which culminates in the personality and behavior of the individual.

OVERVIEW OF THE HUMAN NERVOUS SYSTEM

The intent of this chapter is to provide a brief overview of selected anatomic and physiologic concepts concerning neural tissue. The constraints and the focus of this textbook do not permit an extensive coverage of this material. Readers are urged to seek out references at the end of this section to review and expand their knowledge of the nervous system.

The nervous system consists of nerve cells (neurons) and supporting cells (neuroglia and Schwann cells) so correlated and integrated that they function as a single unit. *Neurons* are the specialized excitable cells of the nervous system which receive the sensory or afferent input from specialized endings of peripheral nerves or sensory receptor organs and transmit the *motor* or efferent output to muscles and glands, the effector organs. Neurons may transmit neural data to other neurons, in which case they are called *internuncial*, or *association*, *neurons*. *Neuroglia* provide support, protection, and nutrients for the neurons of the brain and spinal cord; *Schwann cells* provide protection and support for the other neurons and neuronal processes outside the central nervous system.

The nervous system is divided into the central nervous system (CNS) and the peripheral nervous system (PNS). The brain and spinal cord constitute the CNS.

The PNS is composed of the afferent and efferent neurons of the somatic nervous system (SNS) and neurons of the autonomic (or visceral) nervous system (ANS).

The CNS is encased by the bones of the skull and vertebral column. It is further protected by suspension in cerebrospinal fluid (CSF), produced within the ventricles (cavities) of the brain, and covered by three layers of tissue collectively referred to as the *meninges* (the dura mater, arachnoid, and pia mater).

The brain has been divided into the forebrain, midbrain, and hindbrain on the basis of embryologic development. These categories have been further subdivided on the basis of anatomic organization of the mature brain (Table 46-1). It is important to note that the mid-

TABLE 46-1

THE FIVE MAJOR SUBDIVISIONS OF THE BRAIN*

I. Telencephalon (endbrain)
  A. Cerebral hemispheres
    1. Cerebral cortex
    2. Rhinencephalon ("nosebrain"); limbic system
    3. Basal ganglia
      a. Caudate
      b. Lenticular (putamen, globus pallidus)
      c. Claustrum
      d. Amygdala
II. Diencephalon (interbrain)
  A. Epithalamus
  B. Thalamus
  C. Subthalamus
  D. Hypothalamus
III. Mesencephalon (midbrain)
  A. Corpus quadrigemina
    1. Superior colliculus
    2. Inferior colliculus
  B. Tegmentum
    1. Red nucleus
    2. Substantia nigra
  C. Cerebral peduncles
IV. Metencephalon (afterbrain)
  A. Pons
  B. Cerebellum
V. Myelencephalon (marrow brain)
  A. Medulla oblongata

*The *prosencephalon* (forebrain) = telencephalon + diencephalon; the *rhombencephalon* (hindbrain) = metencephalon + myelencephalon.

brain, pons, and medulla oblongata together are called the *brainstem.*

The spinal cord is a single continuous structure which extends from the medulla oblongata through the foramen magnum of the skull and down the vertebral column to the lower level of the first lumbar vertebra (L1) in adults. The spinal cord is divided into 31 segments, from which originate the 31 pairs of spinal nerves. These segments are named after the vertebrae corresponding to the exit site for the associated nerve roots, thus giving rise to the cervical, thoracic, lumbar, and sacral divisions of the spinal cord (Fig. 46-1).

The PNS is divided anatomically into the 31 pairs of spinal nerves and the 12 pairs of cranial nerves. A *peripheral nerve* may consist of neurons relaying afferent (sensory) neural messages toward the CNS and/or relaying efferent (motor) neural messages from the

CNS. The spinal nerves carry both afferent and efferent neural messages and are thus called *mixed nerves.* The cranial nerves arise from the surface of the brain; five pairs are motor, three pairs are sensory, and four pairs are mixed nerves. Functionally, the PNS is divided into the somatic nervous system and the autonomic nervous system.

The *somatic nervous system* (SNS) is composed of mixed nerves. The afferents convey conscious and unconscious sensory information (e.g., pain, temperature, touch, conscious and unconscious proprioception, vision, taste, hearing, smell) from the head, body wall, and extremities. The efferents are involved primarily with the skeletal musculature of the body. The SNS is concerned with interaction and response to the external environment.

The *autonomic nervous system* (ANS) is a mixed nervous system. Its afferent fibers carry input from visceral organs (concerning the regulation of heart rate, blood vessel diameter, respiration, digestion, hunger, nausea, elimination, etc.). The motor efferents of the ANS innervate smooth muscle, cardiac muscle, and

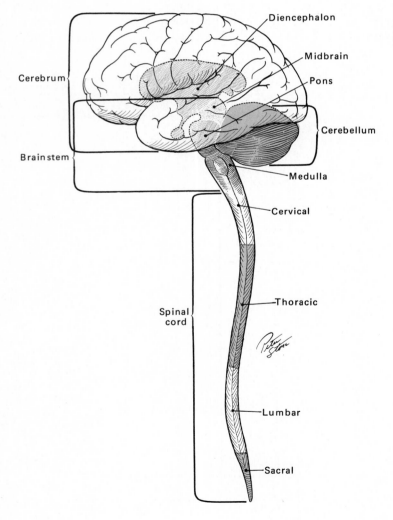

FIGURE 46-1

Lateral view of the central nervous system (From Langley, Telford, and Christensen, 1980, p. 233)

glands of the viscera. The ANS is mainly concerned with the regulation of visceral functions and interactions with the internal environment.

There are two divisions of the autonomic nervous system: the parasympathetic autonomic nervous system (PANS) and the sympathetic autonomic nervous system (SANS). The sympathetic division leaves the CNS from the thoracic and lumbar (thoracolumbar) regions of the spinal cord; the parasympathetic division leaves from the brain (via components of cranial nerves) and the sacral portion (craniosacral) of the spinal cord. Some functions of the sympathetic branch include increase in heart and respiratory rates and decrease in activity of the gastrointestinal tract. Its prime focus is to prepare the body for stress, the so-called fight or flight responses. In contrast, some of the functions of the parasympathetic nervous system are to decrease heart and respiratory rates and to increase gastrointestinal motility as needed for digestion and elimination; it aids in conservation and homeostasis of bodily functions. Table 46-2 lists some of the important functions of the sympathetic and parasympathetic divisions of the ANS.

NEURAL TISSUE

Neuroglia, Schwann cells, and myelin

Neuroglia are the supporting cells for the neurons of the CNS, while *Schwann cells* have this function in the PNS. The neuroglia compose about 40 percent of the volume of the brain and spinal cord. They outnumber the neurons approximately 10:1. Four distinct neuroglia cell types have been identified: microglia, ependyma, astroglia, and oligodendroglia (Fig. 46-2).

TABLE 46-2

AUTONOMIC EFFECTS ON VARIOUS ORGANS OF THE BODY

Effector organ	Effect of sympathetic stimulation	Effect of parasympathetic stimulation
Eye		
Pupil	Dilation (mydriasis)	Contraction (miosis)
Ciliary muscle	Relaxation (far vision)	Contraction (near vision)
Glands of head		
Lacrimal	↓ secretion	Stimulation of secretion
Nasopharyngeal	↓ secretion	Stimulation of secretion
Salivary	Scanty, viscous secretion	Profuse, watery secretion
Heart	↑ rate	↓ rate
	↑ conduction velocity	↓ conduction velocity
	↑ force of beat	↓ force of beat
Blood vessels		
Coronary	Vasodilatation	Minimal
Skeletal muscle	Vasodilatation	Minimal
Abdominal viscera	Vasoconstriction	Minimal
Cutaneous	Vasoconstriction	Minimal
Blood		
Coagulation	Increased	
Glucose	Increased	
Free fatty acids	Increased	
Lungs	Bronchodilatation	Bronchoconstriction
Gut		
Lumen	↓ peristalsis and tone	↑ peristalsis and tone
Sphincters	↑ tone (usually contraction)	↓ tone (usually relaxation)
Secretions	May inhibit	Stimulation of secretions
Liver	Glycogenolysis	
Gallbladder and ducts	Inhibition of contraction	Stimulation of contraction
Adrenal medulla	Secretion of epinephrine and norepinephrine	
Bladder muscle	Relaxation (usually)	Contraction
Sex organs	Ejaculation	Erection
Sweat glands	Stimulation of certain sweat glands	
Pilomotor muscles	Contraction	
Adipose tissue	Lipolysis	

Microglia have phagocytic properties; when nervous tissue is damaged, these cells function to ingest and digest tissue debris. They are found throughout the CNS and are also believed to have a role in fighting infection. These cells have properties similar to those of histiocytes found in peripheral connective tissue and are regarded as belonging to the reticuloendothelial system.

Ependyma are involved in the production of CSF. They are the neuroglia which line the ventricular system of the CNS. These cells provide the epithelial lining of the choroid plexus of the cerebral ventricles.

Astroglia (or astrocytes) are believed to function in providing essential nutrients to neurons and in assisting neurons in maintaining the proper bioelectric potentials for impulse conduction and synaptic transmission. Astroglia have star-shaped cell bodies with multiple processes. Many of the astrocyte processes terminate on blood vessels as perivascular feet or foot processes, and this has implicated them in a system of rapid transport of metabolites. The role of astrocytes in preventing certain substances from passing from the blood vessels to neural tissue, the *blood-brain barrier*, is yet to be determined. It was formerly believed that the foot processes surrounding the capillary wall functioned as the major blood-brain barrier. Most authorities presently believe that the tight junctions between the endothelial cells of the blood capillaries are primarily responsible for the blood-brain barrier. The foot processes of astrocytes also end on ependymal cells in the ventricular system of the CNS and on the pia-covered surface of the brain and spinal cord. Both these structures separate the CSF from nervous tissue.

When there is death of neurons due to injury, astrocytes proliferate and fill in the space formerly occupied by the nerve cell body and its processes, an activity known as *replacement gliosis* (see comments on nerve cell damage below). When there is extensive destruction of CNS tissue, a cavity may be formed which becomes lined with astrocytes.

Oligodendroglia are the glial cells responsible for myelin production within the CNS. Each oligodendroglia surrounds several neurons, and its plasma membrane wraps around the neuronal processes to form the myelin sheath. The Schwann cells form the myelin in the PNS.

Tumors of the neuroglia are referred to as *gliomas* and account for 40 to 50 percent of intracranial tumors (see Chap. 52).

Myelin is a white lipid-protein complex which provides insulation along a nerve process. It prevents the

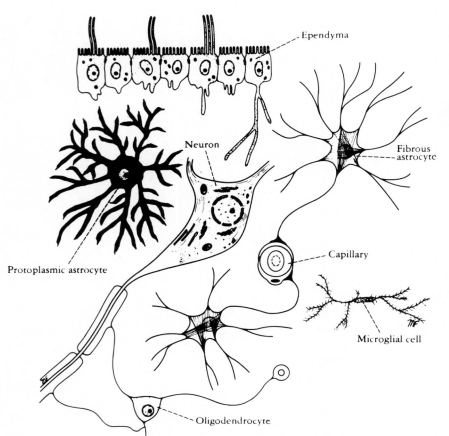

FIGURE 46-2

Diagrammatic representation of the arrangement of different types of neuroglial cell. Note that there are two types of astrocyte. Fibrous astrocytes are found mainly in white matter, while protoplasmic astrocytes are found in gray matter. (From R. S. Snell, *Clinical Neuroanatomy*, Little, Brown, Boston, 1980 p. 74.)

flow of sodium and potassium ions across the neuronal membrane almost completely where it is present. It is not continuous along the nerve processes, and the intervals where it is absent are called the *nodes of Ranvier* (see Fig. 46-3). Nerve processes in the CNS and PNS may or may not be myelinated. Nerve fibers with myelin sheaths are called *myelinated fibers* and within the CNS are called *white matter*. Fibers which have no myelin are called *nonmyelinated fibers* and are present within the *gray matter* of the CNS. Transmission of nerve impulses along myelinated fibers is faster than along nonmyelinated fibers, since the impulses travel, or "jump," from node to node along the myelin sheath; this is known as *saltatory conduction*.

Schwann cells are responsible for forming both the myelin and the neurolemma of peripheral nerves (Fig. 46-3). The plasma membrane of Schwann cells concentrically wraps around nerve processes of the neurons in the PNS to form the myelin sheath. Recall that not all neurons of the PNS are myelinated. The *neurolemma* is a delicate cytoplasmic membrane formed by Schwann cells which wraps around *all* PNS neurons (myelinated and nonmyelinated). The neurolemma provides structural support and protection for the nerve processes.

When there is damage to a nerve cell process in the PNS, there is a potential for regeneration of the nerve fiber. A complex series of degenerative and regenerative changes occurs along the damaged area *as long as the cell body is still viable*. When possible, the neurolemma regenerates along its original course and a new process sprouts and grows within the neurolemma from the cell body of the damaged neuron.

There is no neurolemma in the CNS, hence there is little or no regenerative potential for damaged central neuronal processes. The damaged areas of the CNS neurons are filled with glial cells (primarily astrocytes), a process known as *replacement gliosis*. A gliotic scar following brain injury may result in focal epilepsy (see Chap. 49).

Neurons

A neuron is a nerve cell and is the basic anatomic and functional unit of the nervous system (Fig. 46-3). Each

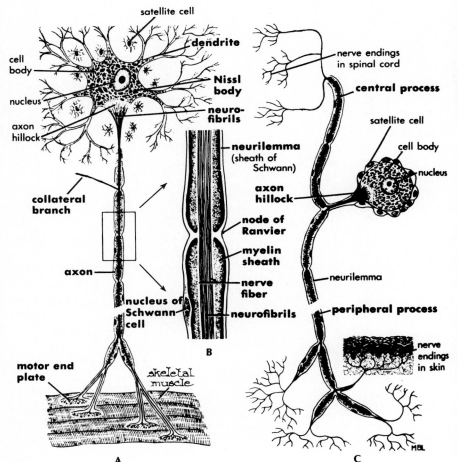

FIGURE 46-3
Motor (panel A) and sensory (panel C) neurons. Panel B shows the structure of a myelinated peripheral nerve. The motor neuron illustrated here is multipolar and the sensory neuron is unipolar. (From J. E. Crouch, *Functional Human Anatomy*, 2d ed., Lea & Febiger, Philadelphia, 1972, p. 480.)

neuron has a cell body which gives rise to one or more processes. *Dendrite* is the name traditionally given to processes which conduct information toward the cell body. The single long process which conducts information away from the cell body is called an *axon*. Dendrites and axons are often referred to, collectively, as *nerve fibers* or *nerve processes*. The ability to receive, convey, and transmit neural messages is a result of the specialized neuronal cell membrane properties of excitability and electrical-chemical conductivity. The human nervous system is composed of approximately 10^{11} neurons, as many (it is estimated) as there are stars in our galaxy. They vary in size, shape, and length of processes. A distinction is also made according to the direction of flow of neural impulses. Thus there are afferent (sensory) neurons, efferent (motor) neurons, and internuncial (associational) neurons.

Neurons are classified as unipolar, bipolar, or multipolar according to the number and pattern of processes arising from the cell body. *Unipolar neurons* have a single process which divides into two branches a short distance from the cell body. One branch is directed toward the periphery, while the other branch travels toward the CNS. An example of a unipolar neuron is the sensory neuron of a spinal nerve (see Fig. 46-3). *Bipolar neurons* have two processes, one axon and one dendrite. Retinal rod and cone cells are bipolar neurons. *Multipolar neurons* have several dendrites and one axon, which may undergo extensive branching. Most neurons of the CNS are multipolar. A notable example of this type of cell is the motor neurons arising in the ventral horn of the spinal cord with their axons extending to skeletal muscle (see Fig. 46-3).

Neurons are also classified by the length of their processes. *Golgi type I* neurons have a long axon which may extend over a meter in length (e.g., motor neuron from the sacral spinal cord to the tips of the toes). The long fiber tracts of the brain and spinal cord and the nerve fibers of the PNS are composed of axons of this type of neuron. *Golgi type II* neurons have short axons which terminate close to the cell body. The dendrites are also short and are clustered around the cell body. Golgi type II neurons are numerous in the brain and spinal cord and are much more common than type I neurons.

A neuron, or nerve cell, shares in the biochemical machinery of all other human living cells and generates chemical energy from the oxidation of nutrients to maintain and repair itself. Neurons primarily use glucose as a source of energy and are, therefore, dependent on oxidative metabolism. In addition, neurons make and

release chemicals called *neurotransmitters*. Nerve cells are metabolically very active.

The majority of the neuronal intracellular organelles are present in the cell body cytoplasm, although some are present within the cell processes. Cellular organelles and inclusions include protein-synthesizing *Nissl substance* (composed of rough endoplasmic reticulum), protein-storing and -processing Golgi bodies, energy-producing mitochondria, neurofibrils, microfilaments, and microtubules involved in intracellular transport. The cell body and dendritic cytoplasm are about equivalent in the types of organelles present, but the axons notably lack Nissl substance. The region of the axon known as the *axon terminal* (see below) is metabolically very active and contains a high concentration of intracellular organelles, especially mitochondria. The nucleus and the prominent nucleolus are located in the cell body. The centrosome may be seen in neurons during prenatal and the first few months of postnatal life, when mitosis is still possible. Centrosomes, however, are generally absent from mature neurons, since these cells are incapable of dividing and increasing their numbers.

Dendrites may be long neuronal processes and branch only at their ends, or they may be short and have multiple branches. Dendrites usually transmit neural impulses toward the cell body and may be considered as extensions of the cell body to increase the receptive area for neural messages. Dendrites undergo terminal branching, and the terminal branches are called *dendritic spines*.

Each neuron has only one axon, which may be short, long, or of an intermediate length, depending on the function of the given neuron. Axons within the human nervous system can be less than 1 mm or more than 1 m in length. Axons usually arise from the cell body in an area called the *axon hillock*. The axon may give rise to a branch along its course called an *axon collateral*. Close to the site of termination, axons branch profusely. The terminal branches, called *telodendria*, are slightly enlarged at their distal ends. These enlargements are called *synaptic boutons* or *knobs*. The diameters of axons vary from neuron to neuron and are related to the function of the neuron: the larger the diameter, the faster the conduction of the impulse. The conduction of a neural impulse along an axon is also affected by whether myelin is present, since conduction along myelinated fibers is faster.

Neurotransmitters are chemicals synthesized in the neurons which are stored in synaptic vesicles in the axon terminals. They are released from the axon terminal by exocytosis and are also reabsorbed and recycled. Neurotransmitters are the method of communication between neurons. Each neuron releases one transmitter. These chemicals cause changes in the cell permeability of a neuron, making it more or less able to conduct an impulse, depending on the neuron and transmitter. There are about thirty known or suspected neurotransmitters. Norepinephrine, acetylcholine, dopamine, serotonin, γ-aminobutyric acid (GABA), and glycine are examples of neurotransmitters.

Neurons conduct neural signals throughout the body. Neuronal impulses are of two types: electrical along the length of a neuron and chemical between neurons. Neurons are not anatomically continuous with one another. The areas where neurons come in contact with other neurons or effector organs are called *synapses*. The synapse is the only location where an impulse can pass from one neuron to another or to an effector. The space between one neuron and the next neuron (or effector organ) is called the *synaptic cleft*. The neuron bringing the nerve impulse toward the synapse is called the *presynaptic neuron;* the one leaving is the *postsynaptic neuron*. It is estimated that there are about 10^{14} synapses in the human nervous system. Synapses can be between an axon and a dendrite *(axondendritic synapse)*, between an axon and a cell body *(axosomatic syn-*

apse), between axons *(axoaxonic synapse)*, and also between dendrites *(dendrodendritic synapse)*. One neuron can make synaptic contact with many neurons *(divergence)* and may receive synaptic contact from many neurons *(convergence)* (see Fig. 46-4).

The electrical component of neural transmission deals with the transmission of the neural impulses along the length of the neuron. Neurons have cell membranes with a variable selective permeability to sodium and potassium ions which is affected by chemical and electrical changes in the neuron (most notably neurotransmitters and receptor organ stimuli, respectively). In the resting state the cell membrane permeability creates a high intracellular potassium concentration and a low intracellular sodium concentration even in the presence of a high extracellular sodium concentration. Electrical im-

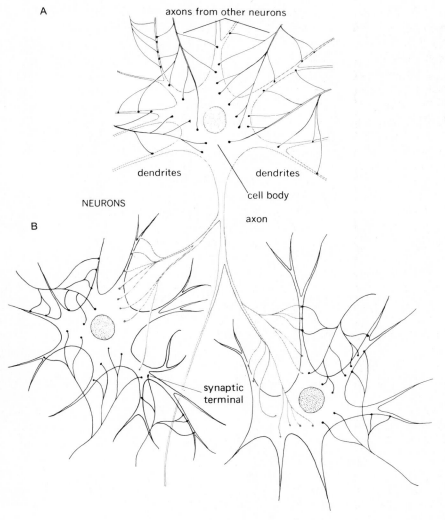

A

axons from other neurons

dendrites

dendrites

cell body

NEURONS

axon

B

synaptic terminal

FIGURE 46-4

(A) Convergence of neural input. (B) Divergence of neural output. Convergence and divergence are important neural mechanisms of processing and integrating information. (From A. J. Vander, J. H. Sherman, and D. S. Luciano, *Human Physiology,* 3d. ed., McGraw-Hill, New York, 1975, p. 168.)

pulses are generated by the separation of charges due to the intracellular and extracellular ion concentration differences across the cell membrane.

If the stimuli causing electrical changes in the neuronal cell membrane cause an increased permeability to potassium ions, the neuron becomes *hyperpolarized* and is in an inhibited state. Hyperpolarized neurons are not able to carry a nerve impulse. When the stimulus causing the electrical changes results in an increased permeability to sodium ions, the neuron is said to be in an excited or *depolarized* state. If the membrane is depolarized to a critical level called the *excitation threshold,* there is a change of membrane permeability with sudden influx of sodium, rapid depolarization, and generation of an action potential at the point of stimulation.

An action potential is transmitted along the axon as an all-or-none phenomenon rather than as a graded response. When the action potential reaches the axon terminal, it causes a release of the neurotransmitter from synaptic vesicles by exocytosis into the synaptic cleft. The transmitter attaches itself to a receptor site on the postsynaptic neuronal or effector membrane and may or may not initiate an action potential in the postsynaptic membrane. Each neuron is covered with a large number of synapses. Whether an action potential will develop or not is determined by the balance of the excitatory and inhibitory impulses the neuron receives at that time from all its synaptic connections. This is another demonstration of the diversity and extensive intercommunication which exist in the human nervous system.

Nerves

A *nerve* is a group or bundle of nerve cell fibers surrounded by a connective tissue sheath *outside* the CNS. (Nerves do not exist in the CNS. The proper term for a group of fibers conducting impulses within the CNS is *fiber tract.*) The peripheral nerves are the cranial and spinal nerves and their branches. Nerves of the autonomic branch of the peripheral nervous system are associated with both cranial and spinal nerves.

A peripheral nerve is composed of a bundle of nerve fibers surrounded by connective tissue layers (Fig. 46-5). Endoneurium surrounds the individual nerve fibers adjacent to the myelin (if present) and the neurolemma. Bundles of nerve fibers (also called a *fasciculus*) are wrapped in perineurium. The epineurium surrounds the various fasciculi of a peripheral nerve. Blood vessels and fat cells are found in this layer. These connective tissue layers are thought to be continuous with the CNS meningeal layers of the pia, arachnoid, and dura, respectively.

THE COVERINGS OF THE BRAIN AND SPINAL CORD

The jellylike tissue of the brain and spinal cord is protected by bone (the skull and vertebral column) and by three connective tissue layers: the pia mater, the arachnoid, and the dura mater. Each is a separate, continuous sheet; there are connections between the pia and arachnoid called *trabeculae.* The dura is also called *pachymeninx;* the pia mater and arachnoid are collectively referred to as the *leptomeninges* (see Fig. 46-6).

The *pia mater* is directly continuous with brain and spinal tissue and follows the contour of their external structure. It is a vascular layer through which blood ves-

FIGURE 46-5

Peripheral nerve in cross section. (From Langley, Telford, and Christensen, *Dynamic Anatomy and Physiology*, 4th ed., McGraw-Hill, New York, 1974 p. 212.)

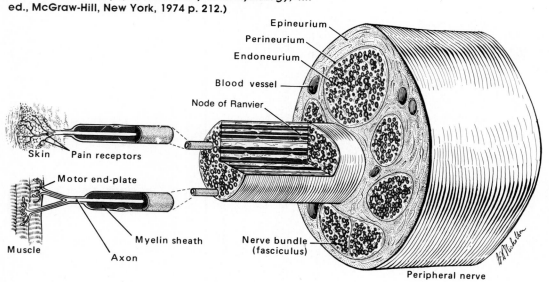

Epineurium
Perineurium
Endoneurium
Blood vessel
Node of Ranvier
Skin   Pain receptors
Motor end-plate
Muscle   Axon   Myelin sheath
Nerve bundle (fasciculus)
Peripheral nerve

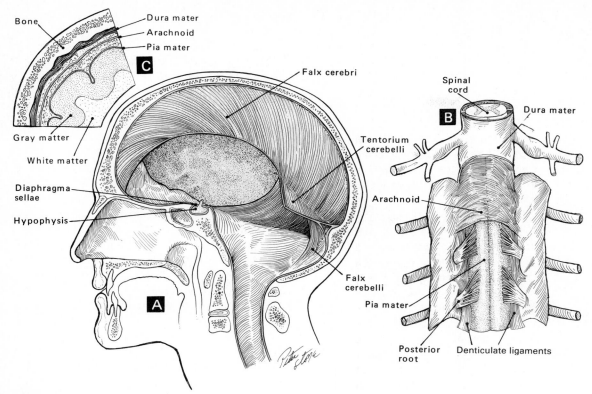

FIGURE 46-6

Meninges. (A) Extensions of the dura mater in the cranial cavity, sagittal view. (B) The dura and arachnoid sheathe the spinal nerves at their origin. The dentate ligament separates dorsal from ventral roots and adheres to the dura. (C) A vertical section through a portion of the calvaria (cranium) and cortex. (From Langley, Telford, and Christensen, 1980, p. 242.)

sels pass to the internal CNS structures to nourish the neural tissue. The pia extends below the spinal cord, which, as previously mentioned, ends at about the lower level of L1. The end of the spinal cord is cone-shaped and is called the *conus medullaris*. A slender filament of pia called the *filum terminale* extends from the conus medullaris.

The *arachnoid* is a thin, fine, fibrous membrane which is avascular. It hugs the brain and spinal cord but does not follow every contour like the pia mater. The area between the arachnoid and pia mater is termed the *subarachnoid space* and contains cerebral arteries, veins, arachnoid trabeculae, and the cerebrospinal fluid that bathes the CNS. There are enlargements in the subarachnoid space called *cisterns*. One notable enlargement is the lumbar cistern in the lumbar region of the vertebral column: The lower lumbar region (usually between L3 and L4 or L4 and L5) is the area where spinal taps are performed to obtain cerebrospinal fluid for examination.

The *dura mater* is a tough, inelastic, leatherlike tissue composed of two layers—the outer endosteal dura and the inner meningeal dura. The endosteal layer

forms the inner periosteum of the skull and is continuous with the periosteal lining of the vertebral canal of the spinal cord. The inner meningeal dura is a thick membrane which covers the brain and dips in between brain tissues to provide support and protection. The layer becomes continuous with the spinal dura mater. The spinal dura continues to the level of the second sacral vertebra, where it fuses with the filum terminale and forms the coccygeal ligament. This extends to the coccyx, where it becomes continuous with the periosteum and serves to anchor the spinal cord in the vertebral canal.

The spinal cord is stabilized along the length of the vertebral canal by a series of 20 to 22 paired longitudinal ligaments referred to as the *dentate* or *denticulate ligaments*. These ligaments, which are attached to the dura at intervals, are lateral extensions of collagenous pial tissue separating the dorsal and ventral roots.

Four major sheaths of the meningeal dura extend into the cranial cavity (Fig. 46-6A). The *falx cerebelli* separate the two cerebellar hemispheres. The left and right cerebral hemispheres are separated along the longitudinal fissure of the *falx cerebri*. The *tentorium cerebelli* separates the cerebrum from the cerebellum. Finally, overlying the pituitary and penetrated by the hypothalamohypophyseal portal system is the *diaphragma sellae*.

The venous sinuses are located between the two layers of dura mater where they separate. Venous sinuses are valveless channels for the drainage of cerebral blood and cerebrospinal fluid. There is no vascular tissue in these sinuses; they are composed of dura mater with an endothelial lining.

When there is damage to the vasculature of the brain, there may be bleeding into the *extradural* or *epidural space* (between the bone of the skull and the endosteal dura), the *subdural space* (between the meningeal dura and the arachnoid), or the *subarachnoid space* (between the arachnoid and pia mater) or beneath the pia mater into the brain itself. The inner table of the skull contains grooves in which lie the anterior, middle, and posterior meningeal arteries. A fracture line running through any of these grooves may damage the contained artery and is the most common cause of extradural or epidural hematoma. A blow to the head over the parietotemporal region damaging the middle meningeal artery is the most frequent cause of extradural hematoma. Subdural hematoma is often caused by damage to the venous vasculature traversing the subdural space. A ruptured aneurysm of the arteries supplying the base of the brain results in subarachnoid hemorrhage. Intracerebral hemorrhage occurs when the vessels that penetrate brain tissue are involved so that blood enters the brain issue itself.

The scalp is an additional structure which must be included in considering the coverings of the CNS. Overlying the skull, to which it is attached by the frontalis and occipitalis muscles, is a freely movable, dense fibrous tissue called the *galea aponeurotica* (Latin *galea*, meaning "helmet"). The galea helps to absorb the force of external trauma, especially glancing blows; without the protection of the scalp the skull would be much more readily fractured. Overlying the galea is a membranous layer containing large blood vessels, a fatty layer, skin, and the hair of the scalp. When severed, the blood vessels constrict poorly and thus may be the cause of severe bleeding, which can, however, be controlled by digital pressure. Between the galea and the outer table of the skull is a potential space called the subaponeurotic space. The *diploic* and *emissary veins* (see Fig. 51-1) penetrate the skull from the dural sinuses into the subaponeurotic space and act as a safety feature (pressure valve) in case of increased intracranial pressure. These veins are also potential access sites for intracranial infection from a pyogenic focus in the scalp or sinuses or in cases of traumatic laceration of the galea. Thus meticulous removal of foreign particles, careful debridement, and flushing with normal saline and sometimes with a bactericidal agent are essential to reduce this hazard whenever the galea has been lacerated.

THE VASCULAR SUPPLY OF THE BRAIN AND SPINAL CORD

The CNS, like all body tissue, is dependent upon an adequate blood supply for its nutrients and for removal of metabolic waste products. The arterial supply of blood to the brain is a branching network of vessels which is highly interconnected to ensure adequate blood supply to the cells. This blood supply is provided via two pairs of arteries, the vertebral arteries and the internal carotid arteries, branches of which anastomose to form the cerebral arterial circle of Willis (see Figs. 46-7 and 46-8).

The venous brain drainage does not closely parallel the arterial supply; it leaves the brain through the large dural sinuses and returns to the general circulation via the internal jugular veins.

The spinal cord arterial and venous systems are quite close parallels of each other and also have extensive branching interconnections to adequately supply the tissue.

Carotid arterial supply

The *internal* and *external carotid arteries* branch from the common carotid arteries at about the level of the thyroid cartilage. The left common carotid stems directly from the aortic arch, but the right common carotid is derived from the innominate or brachiocephalic artery (a 1-inch remnant of the right aortic arch). The external carotids supply the face, thyroid, tongue, and pharynx. A branch from the external carotids, the *middle meningeal artery*, supplies the deep structures of the face and sends a large branch to the dura mater. A slight dilatation in the internal carotids just past the bifurcation is called the *carotid sinus*. Specialized nerve endings within the carotid sinuses respond to changes in arterial blood pressure to reflexly maintain blood supply to the brain and body.

The internal carotids enter the skull and divide, at about the level of the optic chiasm, into the anterior cerebral arteries and the middle cerebral arteries. The middle cerebral arteries are considered to be direct continuations of the internal carotid arteries. Just after entering the subarachnoid space and prior to dividing, the internal carotids give rise to the *ophthalmic arteries*, which enter the orbits and supply the eyes and other orbital contents, portions of the nose, and air sinuses. Occlusion of this branch of the internal carotids (e.g., during a stroke) can result in monocular blindness.

The *anterior cerebral arteries* provide blood supply to such structures as the caudate and putamen nuclei of the basal ganglia, portions of the internal capsule and corpus callosum, and portions (mainly medial) of the frontal and parietal lobes of the cerebrum, including the somesthetic and motor cortices. An occlusion in the

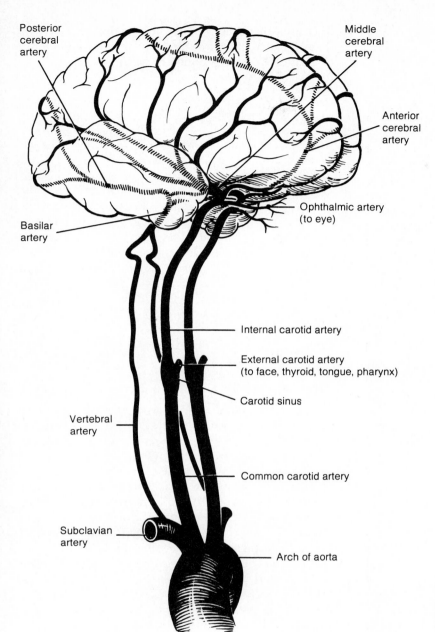

Posterior cerebral artery

Middle cerebral artery

Anterior cerebral artery

Ophthalmic artery (to eye)

Basilar artery

Internal carotid artery

External carotid artery (to face, thyroid, tongue, pharynx)

Carotid sinus

Vertebral artery

Common carotid artery

Subclavian artery

Arch of aorta

FIGURE 46-7

Arterial blood supply to the brain: internal carotids and vertebral-basilar system. Note that the ophthalmic artery is a branch of the internal carotid artery.

main trunk of an anterior cerebral artery results in a contralateral hemiplegia which is greater in the leg than in the arm (lower extremity more involved than upper extremity). Bilateral paralysis and sensory impairment result when there is total occlusion of both anterior cerebral arteries, again more severe in the lower extremities than in the upper.

The *middle cerebral arteries* supply arterial blood to portions of the temporal, parietal, and frontal lobes of the cerebral cortex and form a fanlike distribution over the lateral surfaces. This artery represents the major supply of blood to the precentral and postcentral gyri. Auditory, somesthetic, motor, and premotor cortices are supplied by the artery, as are the association

cortices concerned with higher integrated functions in these central lobes. Occlusion of the middle cerebral artery near the origin of the main cortical branches (in the main trunk of the artery) results in severe aphasia when the language-dominant cerebral hemisphere is involved, contralateral sensory loss of position sense and two-point tactile discrimination, and a severe contralateral hemiplegia predominantly in the upper extremities and the face.

Vertebral-basilar arterial supply

The right and left *vertebral arteries* originate from the subclavian arteries of their respective sides. The right

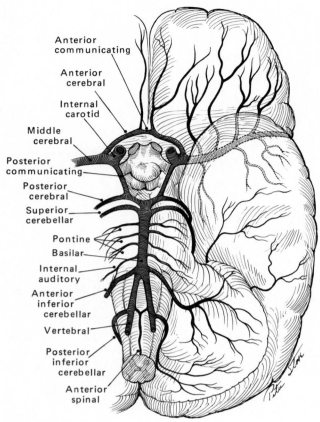

Anterior
communicating

Anterior
cerebral

Internal
carotid

Middle
cerebral

Posterior
communicating

Posterior
cerebral

Superior
cerebellar

Pontine

Basilar

Internal
auditory

Anterior
inferior
cerebellar

Vertebral

Posterior
inferior
cerebellar

Anterior
spinal

FIGURE 46-8
Arteries of the brain, The circle of Willis, at the center, joins branches of the basilar and internal carotid arteries. (From Langley, Telford, and Christensen, 1980, p. 453.)

the result of occlusion of a calcarine artery (see Chap. 52). However, there may be macular sparing as a result of anastomosis of posterior and middle cerebral arteries in the occipital lobe.

Arterial circle of Willis

Although the internal carotids and the vertebral-basilar arteries are two separate arterial systems delivering blood to the brain, they are united by anastomosing vessels to form the cerebral arterial *circle of Willis*. The *posterior cerebral arteries* are connected to the middle cerebral (and anterior cerebral arteries) by the posterior communicating arteries. The *anterior cerebral arteries* are connected by the *anterior communicating arteries* to complete the circle. There is usually only slight blood flow in the communicating arteries under normal conditions; they are a safety feature in case of dramatic changes in arterial blood pressure. The branches of the internal carotid system and of the vertebral-basilar system also have anastomosing vessels.

Conducting and penetrating arteries

In general, cerebral arteries are either conducting or penetrating. The conducting arteries (the internal carotids; anterior, middle, and posterior cerebral arteries; vertebral-basilar arteries; and the main branches from these arteries) form an extensive vascular network over the surface of the brain. The penetrating arteries are nutrient vessels which are derived from branches of the conducting arteries. They enter the brain at right angles and provide blood to the deep cerebral structures, such as the diencephalon, basal ganglia, internal capsule, and parts of the midbrain. For example, the *lenticulostriate (striate) arteries* are penetrating branches of the middle cerebral artery supplying the internal capsule and parts of the basal ganglia (see Figs. 48-1 and 48-3). These small arteries are frequently implicated in the stroke syndrome. Occlusion or rupture of the striate arteries may interrupt the motor pathways of the internal capsule and result in paralysis.

Venous drainage of the brain

The venous drainage for the brainstem and cerebellum closely parallels the arterial vascular distribution in those areas. Most of the venous drainage from the cerebrum occurs via the deep veins draining into superficial venous plexuses and into dural sinuses. The sinuses eventually drain into the internal jugular veins at the base of the skull which rejoin the general circulation. The dural sinuses include the superior and inferior sagittal and the transverse (lateral) sigmoid, straight, and cavernous venous sinuses (Fig. 46-9). When there is a

subclavian is a branch from the innominate artery, while the left subclavian comes directly off the aorta. The vertebrals enter the skull via the foramen magnum, and at the level of the medullary pontine junction of the brainstem (where the medulla oblongata and the pons meet), they fuse to form the basilar artery. The *basilar artery* continues to the level of the midbrain, where it bifurcates to form the paired posterior cerebral arteries. The medulla, pons, cerebellum, midbrain, and part of the diencephalon are supplied by branches from the vertebral-basilar system. The posterior cerebral arteries and their branches supply a portion of the diencephalon, parts of the occipital and temporal lobes, the cochlear apparatus, and the vestibular organs. In the occipital lobe the primary visual cortex is supplied by the calcarine artery, which is a branch of the posterior cerebral artery. A contralateral homonymous hemianopsia is

possibility of a skull fracture, one must consider the possibility of trauma to the cerebral venous sinuses, which may result in a subdural hematoma.

Spinal cord vasculature

The spinal cord receives its supply of nourishing blood via the branches of the vertebral arteries (the anterior and posterior spinal arteries and their branches) and from segmented regional vessels arising from the thoracic and abdominal aorta (the radicular arteries and their branches). From where they branch off the vertebral arteries along the surface of the medulla, the anterior and posterior spinal arteries descend into the spinal cord. The segmental arteries enter the spinal portion of the CNS through intravertebral foramina and divide into anterior and posterior vessels; they encircle the cord, forming an extensive anastomosing vascular plexus on the surface of the cord which also interconnects with the vessels from the vertebral system. Branches from this superficial vascular plexus then penetrate the cord to supply the deep tissue.

The venous drainage follows the arterial distribution for the most part. Some of the spinal cord veins have valves, in contrast to the valveless brain veins and venous sinuses. The vascular system of the spinal cord is directly continuous with the brain venous system. When the venous pressure is increased in the spinal cord, as in coughing or lifting heavy objects, there is an increase in central venous pressure which may temporarily impede brain venous drainage.

THE VENTRICLES AND CEREBROSPINAL FLUID

The ventricles are a series of four interconnected cavities within the brain which are lined with ependyma (a type of epithelial cell which abuts on all cavities of the brain and spinal cord) and contains CSF. There is one lateral ventricle in each cerebral hemisphere (see Fig. 46-10). The third ventricle is in the diencephalon, while the fourth ventricle is in the pons and medulla. The lateral ventricle communicates with the third ventricle via the paired interventricular *foramina of Monro*. The third and fourth ventricles are connected via the narrow *aqueduct of Sylvius* in the midbrain. Three openings extend from the fourth ventricle—the paired lateral *foramina of Luschka* and the single medial *foramen of Magendie*, which are continuous with the subarachnoid space of the brain and spinal cord.

Within each ventricle there is a specialized secretory structure known as the *choroid plexus*. It is composed of a network of blood vessels of the pia mater in

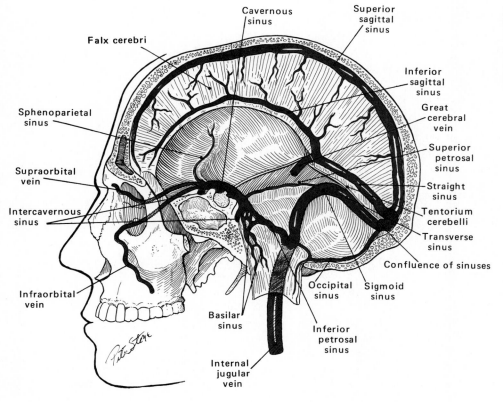

FIGURE 46-9
Venous (dural) sinuses of the head. Superficial veins of the face empty into the cavernous sinus. (From Langley, Telford, and Christensen, 1980, p. 464.)

intimate contact with the ependymal lining. It is the choroid plexus that secretes the clear, colorless CSF which provides a protective fluid cushion around the CNS. The CSF contains water, electrolytes, oxygen and carbon dioxide gases in solution, glucose, a few leuko- cytes (principally lymphocytes), and a slight amount of protein. This fluid differs from other extracellular fluids in that it has higher sodium and chloride concentrations and its glucose and potassium concentrations are lower, indicating that it is a secretion rather than a simple filtrate.

Once in the subarachnoid space, the CSF circulates around the brain and spinal cord and then exits into the vascular system (there is no lymph system in the CNS). Most of the CSF is reabsorbed into the blood through special structures called *arachnoid villi,* or *arachnoid granulations,* which project from the subarachnoid spaces into the superior sagittal venous sinus of the brain. There is constant production and reabsorption of CSF in the CNS. The total volume of CSF in the entire cerebrospinal cavity is about 125 ml, whereas the rate of choroidal secretion is about 500 to 750 ml/day. The CSF pressure is a function of the rate of fluid formation and the resistance to reabsorption of the arachnoid villi.

FIGURE 46-10
Circulation of the CSF. The CSF is formed in the choroid plexuses and circulates within the ventricles and subarachnoid space (gray area). It is reabsorbed by arachnoid villi into the dural sinuses. Direction of circulation (indicated by the arrows) is: lateral ventricles → interventricular foramen (foramen of Monro) → third ventricle → cerebral aqueduct (Sylvius) → fourth ventricle → one foramen of Magendie + two foramina of Luschka → subarachnoid space → arachnoid villi. (From Langley, Telford, and Christensen 1980, p. 244.)

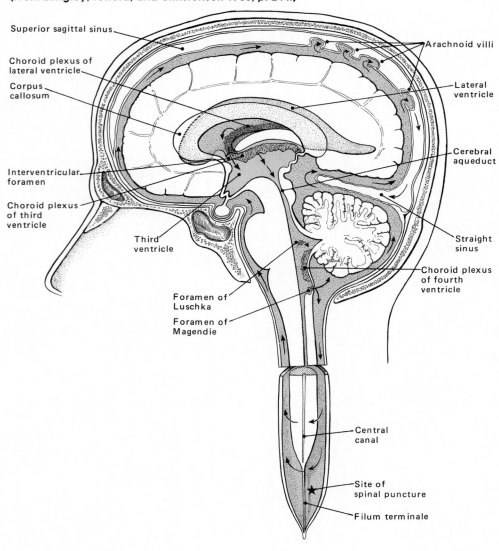

Superior sagittal sinus
Choroid plexus of lateral ventricle
Corpus callosum
Interventricular foramen
Choroid plexus of third ventricle
Third ventricle
Foramen of Luschka
Foramen of Magendie
Arachnoid villi
Lateral ventricle
Cerebral aqueduct
Straight sinus
Choroid plexus of fourth ventricle
Central canal
Site of spinal puncture
Filum terminale

The CSF pressure is commonly measured during a lumbar puncture procedure and normally averages about 130 mmH$_2$O (13 mmHg) in the recumbent position.

Hydrocephalus

Excessive CSF in the cerebrospinal cavity may elevate the pressure sufficiently to damage nervous tissue. This condition is called *hydrocephalus*, a term meaning "excess water in the cranial vault." Hydrocephalus may result from excess formation of fluid by the choroid plexuses, inadequate absorption, or obstruction to flow out of one or more of the ventricles. There are two kinds of hydrocephalus: noncommunicating, in which the flow of fluid from the ventricular system into the subarachnoid space is obstructed, and communicating, in which there is no such obstruction.

Noncommunicating hydrocephalus is the most common pediatric neurosurgical problem and usually has its onset in the immediate postnatal period. It is commonly caused by a congenital narrowing of the aqueduct of Sylvius, so that as fluid is formed by the choroid plexuses of the two lateral and third ventricles, the volumes of these three ventricles increase greatly. This flattens the brain into a thin shell against the skull. The increased pressure also causes the whole head to swell in the newborn. Obstructive hydrocephalus is also frequently associated with *meningomyelocele* (a congenital condition in which there is failure of fusion of the neural tube, so that the spinal cord is open, with cord, nerves, dura, and the more superficial coverings of the cord completely disarranged). Most children with meningomyelocele will develop hydrocephalus, especially after surgical repair of the meningomyelocele. In adults, obstructive hydrocephalus is most commonly due to a posterior fossa tumor with deformity of the aqueduct of Sylvius or fourth ventricle.

Communicating hydrocephalus may be caused by overdevelopment of the choroid plexuses in the newborn infant, so that far more fluid is formed than can be reabsorbed by the arachnoid villi. Fluid therefore collects both inside the ventricles and on the outside of the brain, causing the head to swell tremendously and severely damaging the brain. Communicating hydrocephalus, however, is more commonly caused by interference with reabsorption of the CSF. This situation is usually secondary to meningitis or an irritant that occludes or scars the subarachnoid CSF spaces. This is by far the most common form in the adult. Because of the irritating effect of blood in the subarachnoid space, communicating hydrocephalus can follow subarachnoid hemorrhage by several weeks. A syndrome that often follows communicating hydrocephalus in the adult, especially after subarachnoid hemorrhage, is low-pressure hydrocephalus (or normal-pressure hydrocephalus). The presenting symptoms include difficulty with walking, followed rapidly by dementia, lassitude, and eventual urinary incontinence. It is important to recognize the syndrome of low-pressure hydrocephalus, since it is a treatable form of dementing disease.

All types of hydrocephalus can be treated by shunting the cerebrospinal fluid to the extracranial venous system.

THE BRAIN

The human brain accounts for approximately 2 percent of the total body weight of an adult (about 3 lb). It receives approximately 20 percent of the cardiac output, demands 20 percent of the body's oxygen utilization, and requires about 400 kilocalories of energy daily. The brain is the most energy-consuming tissue in the entire body and is primarily sustained by the oxidative metabolism of glucose. The tissue is fragile, and the demand for oxygen and glucose via the blood supply is constant. *Brain metabolism is steady and continuous, with no rest periods.* Consciousness may be lost in as little as 10 seconds once blood flow has ceased, and a lapse of even a few minutes may cause irreversible damage. Sustained hypoglycemia may also damage brain tissue. The ceaseless activity of the brain is related to its crucial function as an integrative and coordination center between the sense organs and peripheral effector systems of the body, serving to organize incoming information, stored experiences, outgoing impulses, and behavior. The following discussion briefly considers the structure and function of selected parts of the brain.

Brainstem

The brainstem is continuous with the spinal cord caudally and with higher brain centers rostrally. The parts of the brainstem from below upward are the medulla oblongata, pons, and midbrain (see Fig. 46-11). There are many ascending and descending tracts throughout the brainstem. It is an important relay and reflex center of the CNS.

The *medulla oblongata* is an important reflex center for cardiac, vasoconstrictor, respiratory, sneezing, coughing, swallowing, salivation, and vomiting reflexes. All the ascending and descending tracts of the cord are represented here. On its anterior surface are two enlargements called the *pyramids* which contain mainly voluntary motor fibers. Posteriorly, the medulla also has two enlargements which are the fasciculi of the dorsal columns' ascending tracts, the fasciculus gracilis and fasciculus cuneatus. These tracts carry pressure, conscious muscle proprioception, vibratory sensations, and two-

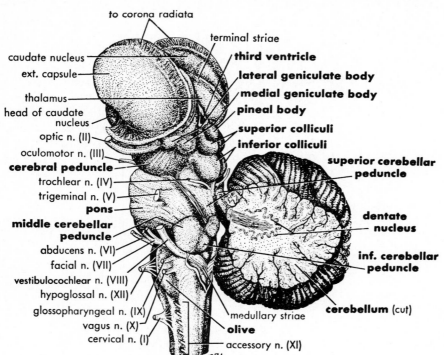

FIGURE 46-11
Diencephalon and brainstem. (From J. E. Crouch, *Functional Human Anatomy*, 2d ed., Lea & Febiger, Philadelphia, 1972, p. 511.)

point tactile discrimination. The medulla contains nuclei of the last four cranial nerves, IX through XII.

The *pons* (Latin for "bridge") consists of a bridge of fibers which connects the halves of the cerebellum and joins the midbrain above with the medulla below. The pons forms an important connecting link in the corticocerebellar path by which the cerebral hemispheres and the cerebellum are united. The lower portion of the pons has a role in respiratory regulation. Nuclei of the Vth to VIIth cranial nerves are located here.

The *midbrain* is the short part of the brainstem which lies above the pons. It consists of a posterior part, the tectum, containing the superior and inferior colliculi, and an anterior part, the cerebral peduncles. The *superior colliculi* are involved in visual reflexes and in the coordination of visual tracking movements. Auditory reflexes, such as turning one's head toward a sound, are mediated through the *inferior colliculi*. The *cerebral peduncles* (or the basis pedunculi) are composed of bundles of descending motor fibers from the cerebrum. The substantia nigra and red nucleus, located in the midbrain, are part of the extrapyramidal or "involuntary" motor pathways. The *substantia nigra* has many connections, including those to the cerebral cortex, basal ganglia, red nucleus, and reticular formation. It is believed to have a complex inhibitory role in the areas to which it has interconnections. Lesions of the substantia nigra produce muscular rigidity, fine tremor at rest, slow and shuffling gait, and a masklike facies. Parkinson's disease is a disease of the substantia nigra and its neurotransmitter, dopamine (see Chap. 50). The *red nu-*

cleus has connections with the cerebellum, cerebral cortex, substantia nigra, basal ganglia, reticular formation, and subthalamic nucleus. It has a role in postural reflexes and righting reflexes dealing with the orientation of the head in space.

Cerebellum

The cerebellum lies in the posterior cranial fossa, covered by the tentlike roof of dura mater, the tentorium, which separates it from the posterior part of the cerebrum. It is composed of a middle portion, the vermis, and two lateral hemispheres. The cerebellum is connected to the brainstem by three bands of fibers called *peduncles*. The *superior cerebellar peduncle* establishes connections with the midbrain; the *middle cerebellar peduncle* connects the two cerebellar hemispheres; and the *inferior cerebellar peduncle* contains fibers of the dorsal spinocerebellar tracts and connects with the medulla. All activities of the cerebellum are below the level of consciousness. Its main function is that of a reflex center through which coordination and refinement of muscular movements are affected and by which changes in tone and strength of contraction are related to maintaining posture and equilibrium.

Diencephalon

Diencephalon is a term used to designate structures surrounding the third ventricle and forming the inner core of the cerebrum. The diencephalon is commonly divided into four areas: thalamus, subthalamus, epithalamus, and hypothalamus. The diencephalon processes sensory stimuli and helps to initiate or modify the body's reaction to those stimuli.

The *thalamus* is composed of two large ovoid structures, each with a complex of nuclei which are interconnected with the ipsilateral cerebral cortex, cerebellum, and many subcortical nuclear complexes such as those in the hypothalamus, brainstem reticular formation, basal ganglia, and possibly substantia nigra. It is an important relay station in the brain and an important subcortical integrator as well. All the main sensory pathways (except the olfactory system) form synapses with thalamic nuclei on their way to the cerebral cortex. Evidence indicates that the thalamus acts as a center of primitive, uncritical sensation through which the individual becomes vaguely conscious of pain, pressure, simple touch, vibratory sense, and extremes of temperature. For example, pain can be felt but it cannot be localized. The finer sensory discriminations require cortical resolution. Emotional responses to the sensory stimuli, however, are possible at the thalamic level of integration. In addition to its role as a primitive sensory center, the thalamus also plays a key role in the integration of motor expressions because of its functional relation to the major motor centers in the cerebral motor cortex, cerebellum, and basal ganglia.

The *hypothalamus* lies beneath the thalamus. It is concerned with the regulation of peripheral autonomic nervous system discharges accompanying behavior and emotional expression. The hypothalamus also plays an important role in hormonal regulation. Antidiuretic hormone and oxytocin are synthesized in nuclei located in the hypothalamus and transported via axons to the posterior pituitary, where they are stored and released. The release of anterior pituitary hormones is also regulated by hypothalamic releasing and inhibiting factors. Regulation of body water and electrolyte composition, body temperature, the endocrine functions of normal sexual and reproductive behavior, and the expression of calm or rage, hunger, and thirst are among the many functions of the hypothalamus.

The *subthalamus* is an important extrapyramidal motor nucleus of the diencephalon. It has connections with the red nucleus, substantia nigra, and globus pallidus of the basal ganglia. Its function is not entirely understood, but a lesion here produces the dramatic dyskinesia known as *hemiballismus*, which is characterized by violent flinging movements of the limbs on one side of the body. The involuntary movement is usually more marked in the arm than in the leg.

The *epithalamus* consists of a narrow band of neural tissue forming the roof portion of the diencephalon. The major structures of this area are the habenular nuclei and commissure, posterior commissure, striae medullaris, and pineal body. The epithalamus has connections with the limbic system and appears to play a role in some of the basic emotional drives. It plays a role in the integration of olfactory information. The pineal body secretes melatonin and is believed to play a role in the regulation of the circadian rhythms of the body and the inhibition of the gonadotropic hormones. In young males, destruction of the pineal gland by a tumor may result in precocious puberty.

The limbic system

The term *limbic* means "border" or "fringe." Thus the limbic system refers to a ring of cortical and subcortical structures that form a border around the corpus callosum (see Fig. 46-12). The principal cortical structures include the cingulate and hippocampal gyri and the hippocampus. Subcortical portions include the amygdala, olfactory bulb and pathway, and septum. Some authors include the hypothalamus and parts of the thalamus in the limbic system because of their close functional relationship. In the lower vertebrates the limbic system is primarily involved with the sense of smell; in humans, its primary function is related to experiences and expressions of mood, feeling, and emotion, especially

FIGURE 46-12
Diagrammatic illustration of the limbic system. The direction in which impulses flow is indicated by the arrows. Its principal function appears to be the arousal of emotions. (From D. B. Stratton, 1981, p. 310.)

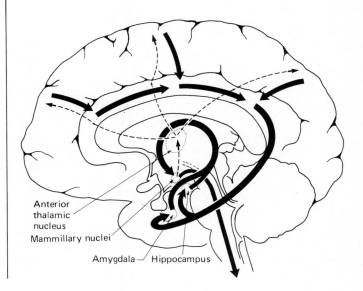

Anterior thalamic nucleus
Mammillary nuclei
Amygdala — Hippocampus

the reactions of fear, rage, and emotions related to sexual behavior. The limbic system is reciprocally connected to numerous central neural structures at several levels of integration, including the neocortex, hypothalamus, and reticular activating system of the brainstem. It is influenced by input from all sensory systems which is integrated and in turn expressed as a behavioral pattern via the hypothalamus, which coordinates the autonomic, somatic, and endocrine responses. The limbic system is also believed to play a role in memory, since lesions of the hippocampus may result in the loss of recent memory. Psychomotor epilepsy begins with and may be confined to the limbic structures that are so involved in the processes of mood, feeling, and emotion. Perceptual distortions, especially memory recall, emotional crises, and alterations in relatedness to other persons and objects characteristic of psychomotor epilepsy, may be accounted for by involvement of limbic structures (see Chap. 49).

Cerebrum

The cerebrum is the largest and most prominent part of the brain. Nerve centers governing all sensory and motor activities as well as reason, memory, and intelligence are located here. The cerebrum is divided into right and left hemispheres by a deep groove or furrow, the great *longitudinal fissure*. The cerebral hemispheres have an outer covering of gray matter called the *cerebral cortex* spread over an inner core of white matter termed the *medullary center*. The two hemispheres are joined by a broad band of fibers called the *corpus callosum*, and gray masses called the *basal ganglia* are embedded in the white matter (see below). Centers for sensory and motor activities are duplicated in each hemisphere and for the most part are associated with the opposite side of the body; i.e., the right cerebral hemisphere controls the left side of the body and the left cerebral hemisphere controls the right side of the body. This functional concept is called *contralateral control*.

The cerebral cortex

The cerebral cortex, or gray mantle, of the cerebrum is thrown into numerous folds called *convolutions* or *gyri* (singular, *gyrus*). Such an arrangement makes it possible for a large surface area (estimated to be about 350 in^2) to be contained within the narrow confines of the cranial vault. Furrows or grooves called *sulci* (singular, *sulcus*) created by the folds divide each hemisphere into distinct areas known as the frontal, parietal, temporal, and occipital lobes (see Fig. 46-13). If the furrow is deep, it may be called a fissure rather than a sulcus. The *central sulcus* (fissure of Rolando) separates frontal and parietal lobes. The *lateral sulcus* (fissure of Sylvius) separates the temporal lobe below from the frontal and parietal lobes. The *parietooccipital sulcus* marks the boundaries of the occipital lobe. An additional subdivision of the cerebrum, the insula, lies within the lateral sulcus and is not visible on the surface.

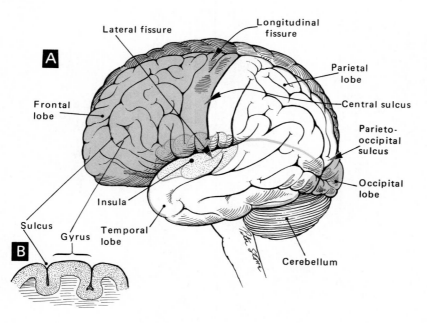

FIGURE 46-13

(A) Lateral view of the cerebrum. Note the line that demarcates the parietal and temporal lobes. (B) A portion of the cortex in cross section. (From Langely, Telford and Christensen, 1980, p. 234.)

Cerebral fiber tracts

The white matter of the cerebrum consists of neuron fiber tracts which may be grouped into three divisions: (1) association tracts, (2) commissural tracts, and (3) projection tracts.

The *association tracts* connect adjacent and distant cortical convolutions of the same hemisphere. *Commissural tracts* link the two hemispheres, the most prominent of which is a broad band of fibers, the corpus callosum. These tracts function to correlate the action of the two halves of the brain as, for example, in coordinating the actions of the two arms and hands in tossing and catching a ball. *Projection tracts* connect the cerebral cortex with other parts of the brain and spinal cord (e.g., basal ganglia, diencephalon, brainstem). The *internal capsule* is a large band of ascending and descending fibers (visible on coronal section as a white irregular mass) bounded by the thalamus and caudate on one side and lenticular nuclei on the other side. The internal capsule is the main pathway for sensory input and motor output between the cerebral cortex and the brainstem. The *corona radiata* is a mass of the fibers which leave the internal capsule in a fanlike radiation to go to various parts of the cerebral cortex.

Functional areas of the cerebral cortex

It has been determined from numerous research investigations that certain areas of the cerebral cortex are primarily concerned with specific functions. Brodmann, a German neuropsychiatrist, in 1909 mapped the cerebral cortex into 47 areas on the basis of cellular structure (cytoarchitecture). Many attempts have been made to ascribe specific functional importance to these areas. In many cases, however, specific functions may overlap several areas. In spite of these limitations, the Brodmann map is a useful general guide for the discussion of cortical functions (Fig. 46-14).

The cerebral cortex can be viewed as having primary and association areas for certain functions. The primary area is that in which the perception or the movement occurs, but the association areas are necessary for integration and higher levels of behavior and intellect. The following discussion considers the highlights of frontal, parietal, temporal, and occipital cortical functions.

The frontal cortex contains the *primary motor area,* Brodmann area 4 (Fig. 46-15), which is responsible for voluntary movements. The primary motor area is located along the *precentral gyrus* (in front of the central sulcus) and is somatotopically organized (see Fig. 46-15). A lesion of area 4 results in a contralateral hemiplegia. The premotor cortex, area 6, is responsible for learned skilled movements such as writing, driving, or typing. A lesion of area 6 on the dominant side may result in loss of the ability to write, or agraphia.

Brodmann area 8 is called the *frontal eye field* and, in conjunction with area 6, is responsible for the voluntary scanning movements of the eyes and conjugate deviation of the eyes and the head. Voluntary eye movements have input from areas 4, 6, 8, 9, and 46.

Brodmann areas 44 and 45 are known as *Broca's motor speech area;* they are responsible for the motor execution of speech. Damage to this area results in difficulty in articulation (motor or expressive aphasia) when the lesion involves the dominant hemisphere. The dominant hemisphere controlling speech is the left in most adults, regardless of whether they are right-handed or left-handed.

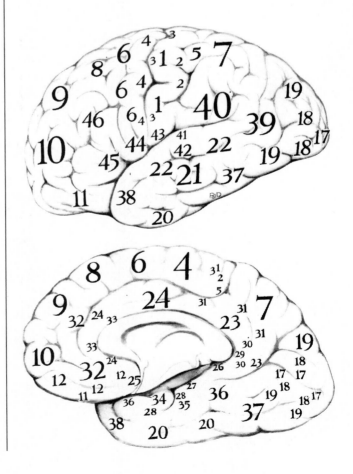

FIGURE 46-14
Cytoarchitectural map of the lateral (top) and medial (bottom) surface of the brain. Numbers represent the Brodmann areas. (From Noback and Demarest, 1981, p. 486.)

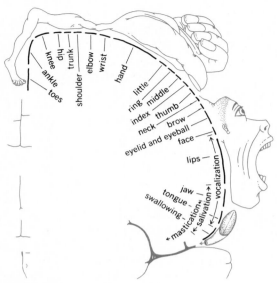

FIGURE 46-15
Motor homunculus, showing the somatotopic organization of the motor cortex along the precentral gyrus. (From A. J. Vander, J. H. Sherman, and D. S. Luciano, *Human Physiology*, 2d ed., McGraw-Hill, New York, 1975, p. 546.)

The *prefrontal cortex*, areas 9 to 12, is associated with the personality of the individual. Complex intellectual activities, some memory functions, sense of responsibility for socially acceptable behavior, ideation, creative thought, judgments, and foresight are all primarily functions of the prefrontal cortex.

The parietal cortex has a major role in the higher level processing and integration of sensory information. The *primary somesthetic area* (areas 1 to 3) is located on the postcentral gyrus parallel to the motor cortex and posterior to the central sulcus. It is also somatotopically organized in a fashion resembling, but not identical to, the primary motor cortex. Sensations from all parts of the body are received in the primary sensory cortex, and it is here that they reach consciousness. These general sensations include pain, temperature, touch, pressure, and proprioception. The fine discrimination and more subtle aspects of sensory awareness are made possible by the primary sensory cortex. A lesion here produces contralateral sensory deficits.

The *somesthetic association area* (Brodmann areas 5 and 7) occupies the superior parietal lobe extending to the medial surface of the hemisphere. It has many connections with other sensory areas of the cortex. The sensory association cortex receives and integrates different sensory modalities, for example, identifying a quarter placed in the hand without looking at it. The qual-

ities of shape, form, texture, weight, and temperature are related to past sensory experiences so that the information may be interpreted and recognition can occur. Awareness of body image, of location of body parts and body posture, and of the self are also functions of this area. Language is a diffuse function which is located throughout many areas of the cortex. A lesion of the *angular gyrus* (area 39) in the dominant hemisphere results in *alexia* (inability to understand written language) and *agraphia* (inability to write) although the individual may be able to speak normally. A lesion of the *supramarginal gyrus* (area 40) of the parietal cortex results in *astereognosis*, the inability to recognize objects by touch. A lesion in this area, such as may occur following a stroke, may also result in a defect in body awareness on the side contralateral to the lesion. For example, the affected person may be unaware of the arm on one side or fail to wash one half of the face.

The temporal lobe is the sensory receptive area for auditory impulses. The *primary auditory cortex* (areas 41 and 42) functions in the reception of sound, while the *auditory association cortex* (primarily area 22, although other parts of the temporal lobe are also included) is necessary for its comprehension. Brodmann area 22 is known as *Wernicke's area*. The temporal lobe (and the nearby hippocampus) also have a role in certain memory processes. The auditory association cortex is essential for the understanding of spoken language, and damage (especially on the dominant side) may result in a severe deficit in which language comprehension, naming objects, and repetition of things heard are severely impaired (*sensory*, or *Wernicke's*, *aphasia*). In Wernicke's aphasia, speech may be grammatically or phonetically correct, but the words chosen are inappropriate or consist of nonsensical syllables. This contrasts with *motor*, or *Broca's*, *aphasia*, in which comprehension may be unimpaired but expression is difficult. Both Wernicke's and Broca's areas (and many other areas of the brain) are necessary for normal speech communication, and these two areas are connected by a bundle of fiber tracts called the *arcuate fasciculus*.

The occipital lobe contains the *primary visual cortex*, area 17, where visual information is received and sense of colors becomes conscious. Damage to area 17 results in visual field defects (see Chap. 52). The primary visual cortex is surrounded by the visual association cortex (areas 18 and 19), where visual information becomes meaningful. This area also has a role in the reflex movement of the eyes when fixing on or following an object. Damage to areas 18 and 19 on the dominant side can result in a lack of recognition of objects and what they are used for even though faces may continue to be recognized. A lesion on the nondominant side may result in a failure to recognize faces (*prosopagnosia*) and to distinguish between forms of life (e.g., cat versus dog). The visual association cortex is adjacent to area 39 of the temporal lobe, and both are related to understanding the symbolism of language. Damage to this area results in sensory alexia, or inability to read with understanding.

Functional specialization of the cerebral hemispheres

A characteristic of the brain with respect to sensation and motor control is that each half of the brain is concerned mainly with the opposite side of the body. Since the brain appears to be bilaterally symmetrical upon first glance, it might also be assumed that the two halves of the brain are functionally equivalent. However, this assumption is false. It has been known for some time that certain learned behaviors such as handedness, language perception, speech performance, and spatial relations are predominantly a function of one or the other hemisphere. About 90 percent of the population is right-handed, a trait which is controlled by the left side of the brain. It has been determined, from observations of patients with strokes and other brain lesions, that linguistic abilities (speech, reading, writing) are predominantly functions of the left side of the brain in about 96 percent of the population. Moreover, recent findings reveal anatomic asymmetry of the hemispheres. The Broca's and Wernicke's speech areas are generally larger in the majority of persons. These observations have led to the concept of cerebral dominance, with the left hemisphere considered dominant over the right.

In recent years the concept of cerebral dominance has been giving way to the newer concept of cerebral specialization and integration of thought processes, since it has become apparent that each hemisphere develops a specialization in many functions. The presence of massive fiber tracts connecting the two halves of the brain suggests that communication and integration of impulses into an overall pattern of action may be an important mode of brain functioning.

The evidence for cerebral specialization has been observed in patients who have undergone a cerebral commissurotomy, a surgical procedure in which the corpus callosum and other commissures joining the two hemispheres are severed for the relief of intractable epileptic seizures. Studies of such split-brain persons have provided increasingly detailed information on the separated hemispheres (see Fig. 46-16). The behavior of such split-brain persons appears normal upon casual observation. However, careful laboratory testing, in which it is possible to ensure that sensory information reaches only one hemisphere at a time and the motor response comes from only one hemisphere, reveals that the two hemispheres are almost completely independent with respect to perception, learning, memory, and ideation. The major hemisphere (usually the left) is specialized in language and mathematical calculation and is limited in spatial tasks. The minor hemisphere (usually the right) is specialized for grasping wholes and perceiving abstract visual patterns, music, and spatial locations but is unable to communicate through verbal language, although communication can take place through gestures and emotional activities. These observations of hemispheric specialization in split-brain persons have led to the notion of two modes of thought—the rational-analytical associated with the left side of the brain and the gestalt-synthetic associated with the right. The former mode of thought is believed to play an essential role in science, while the latter has an essential role in the creative arts such as music, poetry, and imaginative expressions. Supposedly, some persons have left-hemisphere dominance while others are dominated by the right hemisphere. However, the specialization observed in the isolated hemispheres in split-brain experiments should not be overstated. Little is known about how the hemispheres interact in normal behavior, but the presence of the commissures suggests that there must be interaction.

The reticular formation

The *reticular formation* consists of a complex network of cell bodies and interlacing fibers forming the central core of the brainstem. It is continuous with the internuncial cells from the spinal cord below and extends upward into the diencephalon and telencephalon. The chief function of this diffuse reticular system is the integration of a large variety of cortical and subcortical processes, including determination of the state of consciousness and arousal, modulation of the transmission of sensory information to higher centers, modulation of motor activity, control of autonomic responses, and control of the sleep-wake cycle. This system is also the site of origin of most of the monoamines distributed throughout the CNS. The brainstem reticular formation is strategically located in the midst of ascending and descending neural pathways between the brain and spinal cord, enabling it to monitor traffic and participate in all brainstem-hemispheric transactions. It is both diffusely receiving and diffusely projecting. The reticular formation receives input from the cerebral cortex, basal ganglia, hypothalamus and limbic system, cerebellum, spinal cord, and all sensory systems. The efferent fibers of the reticular formation are distributed to the spinal cord, cerebellum, hypothalamus and limbic system, and thalamus (which in turn project to the cerebral cortex and basal ganglia). In addition, an important group of monoamine fibers are distributed widely in ascending paths to subcortical and cortical structures and in descending paths to the spinal cord. There are also a great number of synaptic endings in the brainstem, so that the reticular formation acts upon itself. Thus the reticular formation influences and is influenced by all areas of the CNS.

One of the important functional components of the reticular formation is termed the *reticular activating system* (RAS). The RAS performs a general arousal function in which it activates the cerebral cortex to become receptive to stimuli from other parts of the body. The RAS is essential to maintain the waking state and the waking electroencephalogram. Damage to certain portions of the reticular formation may result in a coma from which the individual cannot be awakened. In addition to controlling the general state of arousal, the RAS performs a screening function with respect to stimuli so that arousal and attention are selective. The reticular system is believed also to play a role in *habituation*, i.e., decreased response to a monotonous stimu-

lus such as the background ticking of a clock. Certain stimuli which are significant to an individual may receive selective attention while others are ignored. This could explain why we notice and pay attention to all restaurant signs when we are driving on the highway and are hungry or why a mother may sleep through a loud thunderstorm yet awaken to the faintest cry of her baby. Input from the cerebral cortex itself to the RAS, which, in turn, projects the impulses back to the cortex, may further increase cortical activity and arousal. This accounts for the fact that such states as a high degree of intellectual activity, worry, or anxiety may increase cortical activity.

Several CNS monoamines, including dopamine, norepinephrine, and serotonin, play an important role in states of sleep and wakefulness. These monoamines are presumably produced in the cell bodies of neurons and distributed in vesicles via axoplasmic flow to nerve terminals. It has been demonstrated by histofluorescent staining techniques that the entire monoamine distribution system in the CNS originates in cell bodies located in the brainstem. Norepinephrine and serotonin

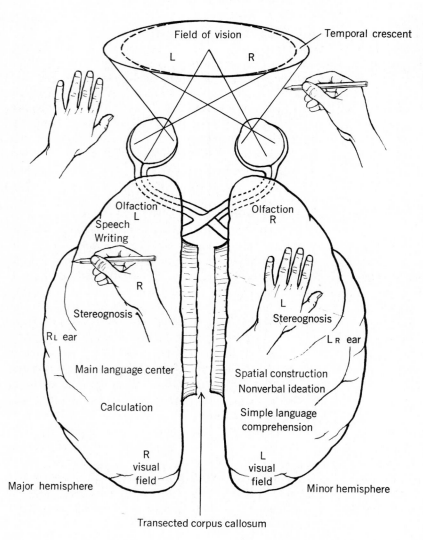

FIGURE 46-16

Some of the specialized functions of the cerebral hemispheres as established by split-brain studies. (From Noback and Demarest, 1981, p. 518.)

pathways project upward to various parts of the brain and downward into the spinal cord, while dopamine pathways project only upward. The norepinephrine pathways as well as those of dopamine are believed to stimulate conscious wakefulness. Norepinephrine tracts are also responsible for rapid eye movement (REM) sleep. Destruction of the locus ceruleus (cell bodies which contain norephinephrine) in the brainstem can suppress REM sleep. Serotonin pathways arising from the raphe nuclei of the brainstem inhibit RAS arousal and promote both REM and non-REM sleep. Destruction of these nuclei produces insomnia. Certain pharmacologic agents which stimulate or inhibit the monoamines can alter sleep and arousal. For example, amphetamine, a drug which stimulates increased synthesis of norepinephrine, decreases total sleep time as well as REM sleep. The administration of p-chlorophenylalanine, a drug which blocks serotonin synthesis, results in insomnia, while the administration of 5-OH-tryptophan (a precursor of serotonin) restores normal sleep.

Another important function of the CNS monoamines is the regulation of emotional behavior through pathways which project to the hypothalamus and limbic system. The mechanisms effecting this control are poorly understood. The major tranquilizing drugs causing alteration in mood are believed to act on CNS monoamine neuronal systems.

CRANIAL NERVES

The cranial nerves arise directly from the brain and exit the skull via openings in the bone called *foramina* (sing. *foramen*). The 12 pairs of cranial nerves, designated by a name or Roman numeral, are olfactory (I), optic (II), oculomotor (III), trochlear (IV), trigeminal (V), abducens (VI), facial (VII), vestibulocochlear (VIII), glossopharyngeal (IX), vagus (X), accessory (XI), and hypoglossal (XII). Cranial nerves I, II, and VIII are purely sensory; III, IV, VI, XI, and XII are mainly motor but do carry proprioceptive fibers from the muscles they innervate; V, VII, IX, and X are mixed. Cranial nerves III, VII, and X also carry some nerve fibers of the parasympathetic branch of the autonomic nervous system. The cranial nerves are discussed at length in Chap. 47. Table 46-3 is a summary of the major functions of the cranial nerves.

SPINAL NERVES

The spinal cord is composed of 31 segments of nervous tissue, each bearing a pair of spinal nerves which emerge from the vertebral canal through the intervertebral foramina (openings in the vertebral bones). The spinal nerves are named according to the intervertebral foramina through which they exit, except for the first cervical nerve pair, which exits between the occipital bone and the first cervical vertebra. Thus there are 8 cervical nerve pairs (and only 7 cervical vertebrae), 12 thoracic nerve pairs, 5 lumbar nerve pairs, 5 sacral nerve pairs, and 1 coccygeal nerve pair (see Fig. 46-17). When localizing a spinal lesion according to cord level rather than vertebral level, it is important to note that the two levels do not correspond. The disparity between the length of the spinal cord and that of the vertebral canal increases the distance between the attachment of the various nerve roots and the intervertebral foramina; therefore the nerve roots arising from the lumbar and sacral segments have to pass for some distance before making their exit.

The spinal nerve is attached to the lateral surface of the spinal cord by two roots, a dorsal, or *posterior (sensory), root* and a ventral, or *anterior (motor), root* (see Fig. 46-18). The dorsal root shows an enlargement, the *dorsal root ganglion*, which is composed of the cell bodies of afferent or sensory neurons. The cell bodies of all afferent neurons of the cord are in these ganglia. The dorsal root fibers are the processes of sensory neurons which are bringing impulses in from the periphery to the cord. The cell bodies of motor or efferent neurons are inside the cord in anterior and lateral columns of gray matter. Their axons form the ventral root fibers which pass to muscles and glands. The two roots emerge from the intervertebral foramen and join beyond it to form the spinal nerve or nerve trunk. Thus all spinal nerves are mixed nerves, i.e., contain both sensory and motor fibers. After a short course the nerve trunk divides into dorsal and ventral divisions, or rami. (There are also two more divisions, a meningeal branch supplying the spinal cord meninges and ligaments and a visceral branch which has two portions, the white and gray rami, and belongs to the autonomic nervous system.)

In general, the dorsal division of the spinal nerves supplies the intrinsic muscles of the back and specific segments of the skin overlying them called *dermatomes* (see below). The ventral division is large and forms the main part of the spinal nerve. The muscles and skin of neck, chest, abdomen, and extremities are supplied by the ventral division.

In all regions except the thoracic, the ventral divisions of the spinal nerves interlace to form networks of nerves called *plexuses*. The plexuses thus formed are the cervical, brachial, lumbar, sacral, and coccygeal. In each instance branches are given off from the plexus to the parts supplied. These branches are the peripheral nerves and have specific names.

The first four cervical nerves (C1 to C4) form the *cervical plexus* which innervates the neck and the back of the head. One very important branch is the phrenic nerve, which supplies the diaphragm.

The *brachial plexus* is formed from C5 through T1 or T2. This plexus supplies the upper extremity. Important branches are the radial, median, and ulnar nerves of the arm.

The thoracic nerves (T3 through T11) do not form a plexus but pass out in the intercostal spaces as the intercostal nerves. They supply intercostal muscles, upper abdominal muscles, and the skin areas of the chest and abdomen.

The *lumbar plexus* is derived from spinal segments T12 through L4, the *sacral plexus* from L4 through S4, and the *coccygeal plexus* from S4 through the coccygeal nerve. L4 and S4 contribute branches to both the lumbar and sacral plexuses. Nerves from the lumbar plexus innervate muscles and skin in the lower trunk and lower extremities. The major nerves from this plexus are the femoral and obturator. The major nerve from the sacral plexus is the sciatic, the largest nerve in the body. The sciatic nerve pierces the buttocks and runs down the back of the thigh. Its many branches supply the posterior thigh muscles, leg and foot muscles, and nearly all the skin of the leg. Nerves from the lower sacral levels and from the coccygeal plexus supply the perineum.

Each of the spinal nerves is distributed to specific segments of the body. The area of skin supplied by the dorsal root of each spinal nerve, and therefore a single segment of the spinal cord, is called a *dermatome*. Although the dermatomes overlap, knowledge of the segmental innervation of the skin makes possible simple

TABLE 46·3

SUMMARY OF CRANIAL NERVE FUNCTIONS

Cranial nerve	Nerve component	Function
I Olfactory	Sensory	Smell
II Optic	Sensory	Vision
III Oculomotor	Motor	Elevation of the upper lid Pupillary constriction Most extraocular movements
IV Trochlear	Motor	Downward inward movement of the eye
VI Abducens	Motor	Lateral deviation of the eye
V Trigeminal	Motor	Temporal and masseter muscles (jaw clenching and chewing); lateral movement of the jaw
	Sensory	Skin of the face, anterior two-thirds of the scalp; mucosa of the eyes; mucosa of the nasal and oral cavity, tongue, and teeth Corneal or blink reflex: sensory limb carried in CN V, motor response in CN VII
VII Facial	Motor	Muscles of facial expression, including those of the forehead and around the eyes and mouth Lacrimation and salivation
	Sensory	Taste on anterior two-thirds of tongue (sweet, sour, salty)
VIII Vestibulocochlear 　Vestibular branch	Sensory	Equilibrium
Cochlear branch	Sensory	Hearing
IX Glossopharyngeal	Motor	Pharynx: swallowing, gag reflex Parotid: salivation
	Sensory	Pharynx, posterior tongue, including taste (bitter)
X Vagus	Motor	Pharynx, larynx: swallowing, gag reflex, phonation; abdominal viscera
	Sensory	Pharynx, larynx: gag reflex; neck, thoracic, and abdominal viscera
XI Accessory	Motor	Sternocleidomastoid and upper portion of trapezius: head and shoulder movements
XII Hypoglossal	Motor	Tongue movements

clinical evaluation, with the help of a pin or wisp of cotton, of the sensory function of a particular segment of the spinal cord or peripheral nerve (see Chap. 47).

The skeletal muscles also receive a segmental innervation from the ventral spinal roots. The segmental innervation of the biceps brachii, triceps, brachioradialis, abdominal muscles, quadriceps femoris, gastrocnemius and soleus, and plantar flexor muscles should be memorized, since it is possible to test them by eliciting simple muscle reflexes using a reflex hammer (see Chap. 47).

THE SPINAL CORD

The spinal cord serves as a center for spinal reflexes and as a conducting pathway for impulses traveling to and from the brain. The spinal cord is composed of *white matter* (myelinated nerve fibers) with an internal core of *gray matter* (unmyelinated neuronal tissue). The white matter serves as a conducting pathway for afferent and efferent impulses traveling between various levels of the spinal cord and the brain. The gray matter is the integrative area for the cord reflexes.

When seen on cross section, the gray matter is in the form of the capital letter H. The two projections of the H which pass toward the front of the body are called *anterior*, or *ventral*, *horns*, and the two projecting backward are the *posterior*, or *dorsal*, *horns* (see Fig. 46-18).

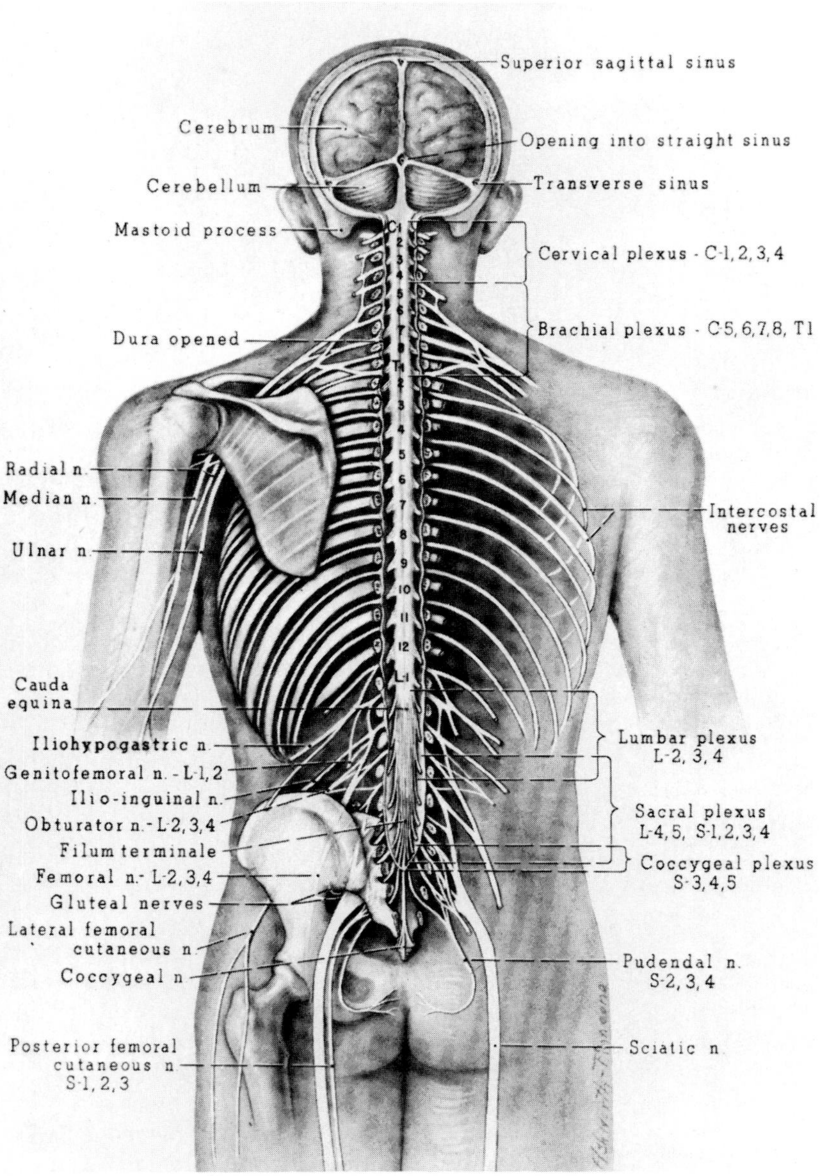

FIGURE 46-17
Spinal nerves and plexuses. (From S. W. Jacob, C. A. Francone, and W. J. Lossow, *Structure and Function in Man*, 4th ed., Saunders, Philadelphia, 1978, p. 256.)

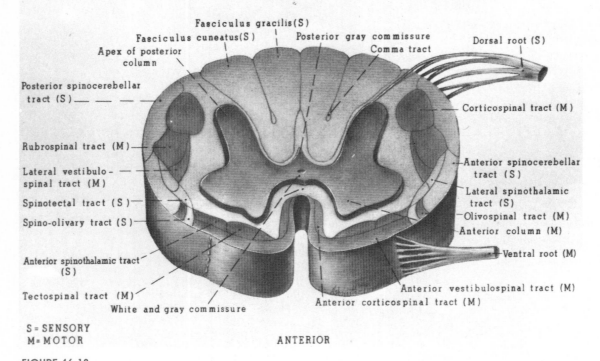

POSTERIOR

Fasciculus gracilis(S)
Fasciculus cuneatus(S)   Posterior gray commissure
Apex of posterior   Comma tract
column   Dorsal root (S)

Posterior spinocerebellar
tract (S)
                                                    Corticospinal tract (M)

Rubrospinal tract (M)

Lateral vestibulo-   Anterior spinocerebellar
spinal tract (M)   tract (S)

Spinotectal tract (S)   Lateral spinothalamic
                                                    tract (S)
Spino-olivary tract (S)   Olivospinal tract (M)
                                                    Anterior column (M)

Anterior spinothalamic tract   Ventral root (M)
(S)

Tectospinal tract (M)   Anterior vestibulospinal tract (M)

White and gray commissure   Anterior corticospinal tract (M)

S = SENSORY
M = MOTOR   ANTERIOR

FIGURE 46-18
Cross section of the spinal cord showing the major ascending and descending tracts. (From S. W. Jacob, C. A. Francone, and W. J. Lossow, *Structure and Function in Man*, 4th ed., Saunders, Philadelphia, 1978, p. 254.)

The ventral horn is composed primarily of cell bodies and dendrites of the multipolar motor efferent neurons of the ventral roots and spinal nerves. The *ventral horn cell*, or *lower motor neuron*, is commonly called the *final common pathway*, since any movement, whether initiated in the cerebral motor cortex, basal ganglia, or reflexly in the sensory receptor, must be translated into action via this structure.

The dorsal horn contains cell bodies and dendrites from which arise sensory fibers which will go to other levels of the CNS after synapsing with sensory fibers from sensory nerves.

The gray matter also contains internuncial, or associational, neurons, autonomic nervous system afferents and efferents, and axons originating at different levels of the CNS. *Internuncial neurons* transmit impulses from one neuron to another within the brain and spinal cord. In the spinal cord, internuncial neurons have many interconnections, and many of them directly innervate the ventral horn cells. Only a few incoming sensory impulses to the spinal cord or motor impulses from the brain terminate directly on the ventral horn cell or lower motor neuron. Instead, most of them are first transmitted through internuncial cells, where they are appropriately processed before stimulating the anterior horn cell. This arrangement allows highly organized patterns of muscle responses.

The reflex arc

The reflex arc is the functional unit of the nervous system. Reduced to its simplest form, it consists of two neurons, a sensory neuron leading from a sensory receptor or ending and a motor neuron which conveys impulses to a muscle or gland. More generally the two neurons are not connected directly but have one or more internuncial neurons interposed between them. Such a mechanism is capable of response quite independent of the higher centers and is sufficient for the performance of such simple acts as withdrawing from painful stimuli. Reflexes may involve only one segmental level of the spinal cord or several levels. The impulses may spread upward or downward from the level at which they enter the cord by passing through internuncial neurons. Because of the multitude of interconnections of neurons within the cord, an almost infinite variety of responses is possible. Knowledge of the segmental levels of the reflexes and of the dermatomes is helpful in localizing lesions of the nervous system (see Chap. 47).

Pathways of selected spinal cord tracts

The white matter of the spinal cord serves as a conducting pathway for the long ascending and descending tracts by which afferent impulses from the spinal nerves reach the brain and those through which efferent impulses pass from motor centers in the brain to ventral horn cells of the cord and thus modify movement. The fibers which make up the white matter of the spinal cord are not scattered in a chaotic fashion but are arranged in bundles which show a functional as well as an anatomic grouping.

Each lateral half of the spinal cord is divided into three longitudinal sections which run the length of the cord, called *dorsal, lateral,* and *ventral columns.* Within each of these divisions are distinct bands of fibers called *tracts* having quite definite locations. A fiber tract is a bundle of fibers all having the same origin, termination, and function. The tracts may be ascending, descending, or associative.

Ascending tracts bring sensory information into the CNS and may travel to parts of the spinal cord and brain. The *lateral spinothalamic tract* is an important ascending tract which carries the fibers for the pain and temperature pathway. The fine touch, conscious proprioception, and vibratory pathways have fibers which compose the *dorsal columns* of the spinal cord white

matter. Impulses from various parts of the brain to the motor neurons of the brainstem and spinal cord are called *descending tracts.* The *lateral* and *ventral corticospinal tracts* represent the voluntary motor pathway in the spinal cord. (See Fig. 46-18 for the location of the tracts of these pathways.) *Associative tracts* are short ascending or descending tracts; for example, they may travel between a few segments of the spinal cord and are thus called *intersegmental tracts.* Table 46-4 lists some of the most important ascending and descending tracts of the spinal cord.

The spinal cord tracts are named to denote the origin and termination of their fibers. *Origin* means the

TABLE 46-4

MAJOR ASCENDING AND DESCENDING TRACTS OF THE SPINAL CORD

Tract	Function
Ascending	
Dorsal (posterior) columns	Fine touch capable of a high degree of localization of the stimulus, fine degree of
Fasciculus cuneatus (T6 and above, upper body)	discrimination of pressure and intensity (two-point discrimination, weight perception)
Fasciculus gracilis (T7 and below, lower body)	Conscious proprioception (position sense)
	Vibration (phasic sensations)
	Rapid transmission of sensory information
Spinothalamic	
Lateral spinothalamic	Pain
	Temperature, including warm and cold sensations
Ventral spinothalamic	Crude touch capable of much less localization of the stimulus and less discrimination of pressure and intensity
	Itching and tickling sensations
	Transmission of sensory information much slower than in dorsal columns
Spinocerebellar	
Dorsal spinocerebellar	Unconscious proprioception (muscle sense)
Ventral spinocerebellar	Coordination of posture and limb movement
	Sensory information transmitted originates almost entirely in the muscle spindles and Golgi tendon apparatus
	Large-tract fibers transmitting impulses faster than any other neurons in the body
Descending	
Corticospinal	
Lateral corticospinal	Pyramidal tract carrying impulses for voluntary control of the muscles of the extremities
Ventral corticospinal	Pyramidal tract carrying impulses for voluntary control of the muscles of the trunk
Rubrospinal	Extrapyramidal tract concerned with unconscious integration and coordination of muscular movement adjusted to proprioceptive input
Tectospinal	Extrapyramidal tract concerned with reflex turning and scanning movements of the head and reflex movements of the arms in response to visual, auditory, or cutaneous sensation
Vestibulospinal	Extrapyramidal tract involved in equilibrium (maintaining balance) and coordination of head and eye movements

location of the cell bodies of the tract, and *termination* refers to the point at which the axon forming the tract ends. Thus it is simple to determine whether a tract is an ascending sensory or descending motor tract by analyzing the name. For example, the rubrospinal tract is a descending motor tract with its cell bodies in the red nucleus of the midbrain and its axon termination in the spinal cord.

Ascending pathways

Sensory information from peripheral receptors is transmitted through the nervous system in a series of neurons organized into an ascending pathway system. The sensory chain consists of three neurons, each having a long axon. The *first-order neuron* has its cell body in a dorsal root ganglion and conducts the impulse from the receptor to the spinal cord. (If the receptors of the first-order neuron lie in the regions supplied by cranial nerves, then its axon enters the brainstem instead of the cord.) The cell body of the *second-order neuron* is located at variable levels of the gray matter of the spinal cord or brainstem and conveys the impulse within the white matter of the cord to the thalamus. The *third-order neuron* conducts impulses from the thalamus to the cerebral cortex, and its cell body lies in the thalamus. In general, the major sensory systems and their pathways are somatotopically organized, and they are crossed pathways. This means that organization according to body surface area is present in the spinal cord and thalamus as well as the primary somesthetic cortex and that each side of the brain registers sensations from the opposite side of the body. It is usually the second-order neuron that crosses at some point on its way to the thalamus. Only two of the ascending pathways are here discussed in detail.

Pain and temperature pathway

The direct neural pathway for the sensations of pain and temperature is the lateral spinothalamic pathway (see Fig. 47-7). The sensory nerve fibers carrying pain or temperature stimuli from receptors enter the dorsal root of the spinal cord, and once in the white matter, they bifurcate and ascend or descend a few segments before synapsing with the second-order neuron in the gray matter of the dorsal horn. The axon of this second-order neuron crosses over to the contralateral side, where it joins the other fibers in the lateral spinothalamic tract. These fibers proceed to the thalamus, where they synapse with a third-order neuron which relays the impulses to the sensory cortex. In the thalamus, the pain and temperature sensations come into con-

sciousness vaguely but are not localized. The full extent of these sensations is consciously perceived and localized as the impulses are received in the primary and secondary somesthetic cortex of the parietal lobe. (Note: There is also an indirect spinoreticular thalamic pathway for pain.)

Fine touch, conscious proprioception, and vibration pathway

The neural pathway for fine (discriminating) touch, conscious proprioception (awareness of body position and movement), and vibratory sense is called the *medial lemniscal system*. This system consists of the tracts that make up the dorsal white columns of the cord (the fasciculi cuneatus and gracilis) plus the medial lemniscus, a flat band of fibers extending through the brainstem.

General mechanoreceptors responsive to fine touch, vibration, body position, and movement conduct impulses into the cord through the dorsal root; they then ascend directly on the same side via the dorsal columns. The dorsal columns are somatotopically organized. Fibers transmitting impulses from the lower part of the body (T7 and below) occupy the medial dorsal column as the *fasciculus gracilis* which terminates the *nucleus gracilis*, the second-order neuron of the medulla. Fibers transmitting impulses from the upper part of the body (T6 and above) occupy the more lateral dorsal column as the *fasciculus cuneatus*, which terminates in the *nucleus cuneatus*, also located in the medulla. The reason for this laminar organization is that the sacral and dorsal column fibers are pushed medially as fibers from higher segments are added. Thus the information for the feet is located in the midline of the cord, while information from the upper extremities is most lateral. (The laminar organization of the spinothalamic tract is opposite to that of the dorsal columns. Fibers from sacral and lumbar segments of the body are pushed laterally by fibers crossing the midline at successively higher levels. Thus the lamination is cervical to sacral segments represented from the medial to more lateral position. Because of this lamination, tumors arising outside the spinal cord first compress the spinothalamic fibers from sacral and lumbar areas, causing the early symptom of a loss of pain in the sacral area.)

Fibers from the second-order neurons cross to the opposite side of the medulla and ascend as a component of a tract called the *medial lemniscus*. The fibers of the medial lemniscus synapse with a third-order neuron in the thalamus which, in turn, sends fibers through the internal capsule to the somesthetic cortex of the parietal lobe. The sensory data reach the conscious level and become localized in the sensory cortex.

Descending pathways

There are two major systems of motor pathways, classified as pyramidal and extrapyramidal. *Pyramidal* tracts (lateral and ventral corticospinal) are those whose fibers come together in the medulla to form the pyramids, hence the name. Most of the descending motor pathways involve two principal neurons, the upper and lower motor neurons. The *upper motor neuron* has its cell body in the cerebral motor cortex or in subcortical areas of the brain and brainstem, and its fibers conduct impulses from the brain to the spinal cord [or from the cerebrum to the brainstem (corticobulbar tract)]. The spinal motor neuron (or cranial motor neuron) which actually innervates the muscle is called the *lower motor neuron*. Thus the upper motor neuron is entirely within the CNS, while the lower motor neuron begins in the CNS (anterior horn of the spinal cord gray matter) and sends its fibers out to innervate muscles. The lower motor neuron is thus a part of the PNS.

Voluntary motor pathway

The lateral and ventral corticospinal tracts are the major voluntary motor tracts of the spinal cord. These tracts are primarily concerned with controlling skilled movements of the extremities. Another important function of the upper motor neuron is to influence reflex movement by sending down facilitating or inhibiting impulses to alpha and gamma motor neurons (see Fig. 47-4).

The upper motor neurons of the corticospinal tracts originate in area 4 of the primary motor cortex, area 6 of the premotor cortex, and various portions of the parietal lobe. From here, fibers descend through the internal capsule to synapse with internuncials at various levels of the spinal cord, which, in turn, synapse with neurons in the ventral horn gray matter. Some fibers, however, may synapse directly with lower motor neurons. It is also true that not all these fibers descend to spinal cord levels, since some may synapse with motor nuclei of cranial nerves (corticobulbar fibers) and in the reticular formation.

Approximately 85 percent of the descending fibers decussate (cross over) in the medulla and extend down the cord on the opposite side as part of the lateral corticospinal tract. The remaining 15 percent of the fibers

remain uncrossed and descend on the same side of the cord as the ventral corticospinal tract. These fibers eventually cross the midline in the ventral gray column of the spinal cord segments (generally in the cervical and upper thoracic regions). Lesions of the corticospinal tracts produce a Babinski sign (see Fig. 47-6) and loss of performance of skilled voluntary movements, especially of the distal segments of the extremities.

THE EXTRAPYRAMIDAL SYSTEM AND BASAL GANGLIA

Precise delineation of the extrapyramidal system (all motor fibers not passing through the pyramids) is difficult anatomically. If the system is considered as an anatomic unit, it is composed of the (1) basal ganglia and their circuits, (2) cortical areas that project to the basal ganglia, (3) cerebellar areas that project to the basal ganglia, (4) parts of the reticular formation that have connections with the basal ganglia and cerebral cortex, and (5) thalamic nuclei which connect the basal ganglia and reticular formation.

The primary function of the extrapyramidal system is to provide coarse control for voluntary muscles. (Fine control is provided by the pyramidal or corticospinal system.) The whole system works as a unit providing for integration on three levels: cortical, striatal, and tegmental. The major effect is inhibition (see Fig. 46-19).

The basal ganglia or basal nuclei are found in each cerebral hemisphere in paired groups and are formed

FIGURE 46-19
Simplified diagram of pyramidal and extrapyramidal systems. Posture and performance of well-coordinated movements result from an integration of information received from both cerebral cortex and extrapyramidal systems. The cortex initiates movement, while the extrapyramidal system provides the facilitation or inhibition needed for production of purposeful, coordinated, controlled movements. Disruption of the extrapyramidal influence results in abnormal, uncontrolled movements. Components of the extrapyramidal system are the reticulospinal, vestibulospinal, tectospinal, and rubrospinal tracts. (Adapted from *Medical Notes on Parkinsonism and Pseudoparkinsonism*, Burroughs Wellcome Co., Research Triangle Park, N. C., 1972.)

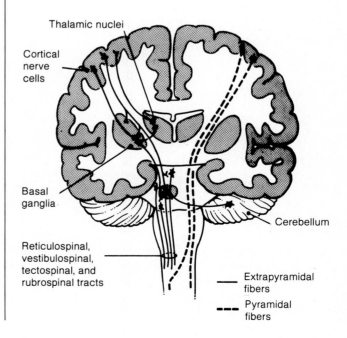

Thalamic nuclei

Cortical nerve cells

Basal ganglia

Reticulospinal, vestibulospinal, tectospinal, and rubrospinal tracts

Cerebellum

——— Extrapyramidal fibers

– – – Pyramidal fibers

from the central gray matter of the telencephalon. They include the claustrum, putamen, globus pallidus, caudate, and amygdala (see Fig. 46-20). The *caudate nucleus*, the most medial of the basal ganglia, is shaped like a comma with an extended tail. The *amygdaloid nucleus* lies as a knob of gray matter at the tip of the tail of the caudate. The putamen and globus pallidus together are called the *lenticular (lens-shaped) nucleus*; it extends from the head of the caudate. The *internal capsule* lies within borders formed by the thalamus, caudate nucleus, and lenticular nucleus. This crucial area is a passageway for all nerve fibers connecting the cerebrum with the rest of the CNS. The caudate and lenticular

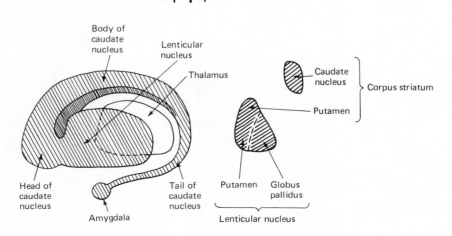

FIGURE 46-20
Illustration of the basal nuclei or ganglia. Upper coronal sections show the basal ganglia in relation to the thalamus, internal capsule, and red nucleus and substantia nigra. The lower illustration shows the caudate nucleus in relation to the lenticular nucleus, amygdala, and thalamus. The nuclei are grouped by commonly used terms. (From Stratton, 1981, pp. 328–329.)

nucleus, along with the adjacent part of the internal capsule, are sometimes referred to as the *corpus striatum.*

Three nuclear masses located in the upper midbrain operate in close association with the basal ganglia and are considered to be part of the extrapyramidal system: the *red nucleus, substantia nigra,* and *subthalamic nucleus,* or *corpus Luysii.*

The basal ganglia have multiple connections with other portions of the CNS, including the cerebral cortex, cerebellum, thalamus, and reticular formation. They are believed to function as important centers of coordination, especially in the control of automatic associated movements. The corpus striatum (caudate nucleus and putamen) is believed to be responsible for the initiation and inhibition of gross intentional body movements that are unconsciously performed in the normal person. They also provide muscle tone so that exact movements can be performed, e.g., fine handwork requiring the coordinated effort of the entire arm and trunk for the hand to be able to perform.

A feedback system seems to operate via circular pathways from the motor cortex to the basal ganglia, thalamus, and motor cortex. Motor signals from the cerebral cortex to the pons and cerebellum are also circuitous, with the return to the cortex being through the ventrolateral nucleus of the thalamus, through which signals from the basal ganglia also pass. Because of the proximity of these circuits, it is hypothesized that basal ganglia and cerebellum feedback signals could be integrated in this area.

Broadly speaking, the basal ganglia are involved in two general activities: control of the body's motor tone and gross intentional movements. The general effect of basal ganglia excitation is of inhibitory signals to the bulboreticular facilitatory areas and of excitatory signals to the bulboreticular inhibitory areas. When the basal ganglia are not functioning adequately, the facilitatory areas become overactive and the inhibitory areas underactive. This results in rigidity throughout the body.

The patient with an extrapyramidal disorder has great difficulty maintaining equilibrium while standing and posture while sitting, changing from a horizontal to a sitting position, rolling from a supine to a prone position, and walking. The righting reflex, the vestibular reflex, and proprioception are all distrubed. If the spinal cord is transected at the level of the mesencephalon, a decerebrate rigidity occurs, indicating that the major effect of the basal ganglia is inhibition. The tremor (abnormal movements) observed in extrapyramidal disorders is a result of excess neural activity in one area of the brain from unopposed activity in another area. This characteristic is called the *release phenomenon* and is common with tissue destruction in the nervous system (a lesion in A removes the regulatory control that A exerted over B, and consequently B becomes overactive).

Both the corpus striatum and the motor cortex are instrumental in the control of gross intentional movements that are normally unconscious. The control is accomplished through two pathways: the globus pallidus through the thalamus to the cortex and downward via corticospinal and extracorticospinal pathways into the spinal cord; and downward through the globus pallidus and substantia nigra to the reticular formation and reticulospinal tracts to the cord. The globus pallidus seems to provide the background muscle tone necessary for performing exacting movements (especially with the hands). Stimulation of the globus pallidus will stop the movement at any point and keep it locked at that point as long as the stimulation is continued.

Parkinson's syndrome and several extrapyramidal disorders of movement which involve the basal ganglia and extrapyramidal system are discussed in Chap. 50.

QUESTIONS

The nervous system

Directions: Circle T if the statement is true and F if it is false. Correct the false statements.

1. T F The nervous system consists of two major cell types: (1) the neurons with their processes and (2) supporting connective tissue.

2. T F The nervous system is a communication system which directs and integrates all bodily activity.

3. T F Dendrites conduct impulses away from the neuronal cell body.

4. T F The central nervous system includes the brain, spinal cord, and cranial nerves.

5. T F All nerve cell bodies are located in the CNS.

6. T F Internuncial neurons relay messages between other neurons in the CNS, and large numbers may be found in the gray matter of the spinal cord forming intersegmental tracts.

7. T F Schwann cells from the myelin for neuronal processes within the CNS.

8. T F Spinal nerve trunks carry both afferent and efferent impulses to the CNS and are thus mixed nerves.

9. T F Nerves of the autonomic nervous system are associated with both cranial and spinal nerves.

10. T F The parasympathetic branch of the ANS forms the thoracolumbar outflow from the spinal cord.

11. T F The autonomic nervous system is primarily concerned with the regulation of visceral functions such as heart rate, blood pressure, and intestinal motility.

12. T F Nerve cells are not mitotic; they do not reproduce.

13. T F The characteristic color of the white matter of the brain and spinal cord is due to the presence of myelin-covered fiber tracts.

14. T F It is possible for a severed nerve fiber in the PNS to regenerate as long as the cell body is still viable.

15. T F Scar tissue in the CNS consists of astrocytes and may result in focal epilepsy.

16. T F Retinal rod and cone cells are examples of multipolar neurons.

17. T F Golgi type II neurons have extremely long axons.

18. T F The direction of a nerve impulse can be reversed.

19. T F Axons lack Nissl substance, and so cannot manufacture protein and must depend on the cell body for such production.

20. T F *Convergence* means that a single neuron receives input from two or more neurons, and the response is the summated effect of all the different types of information.

21. T F Convergence and divergence are important mechanisms enabling the nervous system to perform its integration and control functions.

22. T F The neurilemma is a thin membrane which envelops all nerve fibers.

23. T F A nerve fiber is the axon (or dendrite) of a nerve cell.

24. T F Bundles of nerve fibers found in the CNS are called *cranial nerves*.

25. T F The spinal cord terminates in the vertebral cavity at about L4.

Directions: Circle the letter preceding each item below that correctly answers the question or completes the sentence. More than one answer may be correct.

26. Which of the following structures is *not* included in the CNS?
a. Glia cells b. Cerebellum c. Spinal cord
d. Basal ganglia e. Ganglia of the sympathetic chain

27. Which of the following are characteristic of the ANS?
a. Control of activities which are largely involuntary b. Atrophy of the muscle innervated if the nerve is destroyed. c. Location outside the spinal cord d. Invariable resultant excitation of the effector organ

28. The myelencephalon is composed of the:
a. Medulla oblongata b. Cerebral hemispheres
c. Pons d. Cerebellum

29. Subdivisions of the brain included in the prosencephalon (forebrain) include the:
a. Myelencephalon b. Metencephalon
c. Diencephalon d. Telencephalon

30. Regeneration of nerve fibers will occur if the cell body is intact and the fiber has:
a. A myelin sheath b. An axon c. A dendrite
d. A neurolemma

31. The processes of a neuron are:
a. Cytoplasm b. Axon and one or more dendrites c. Cell body and one or more axons

32. The point at which the electrical activity from one neuron influences the excitability of another neuron is the:
a. Sensory receptor b. Effector c. Synapse
d. Cell

33. The nerve cell has a resting potential because its membrane is selectively permeable to different ions. The most important ion species in the maintenance of resting membrane potential are:
a. Calcium and phosphorus b. Magnesium and calcium c. Phosphorus and sodium d. Potassium and sodium

34. Which of the following statements is *false* concerning the meninges?
a. The denticulate ligaments, located between the

ventral and dorsal roots, are pial tissue which attaches to the dura at intervals.   *b.* The pia mater is the innermost layer.   *c.* The arachnoid is the outermost layer.   *d.* The pia mater and arachnoid are collectively known as the *leptomeninges.*

35. The sheath of meningeal dura separating cerebrum from cerebellum is the:
a. Falx cerebri   *b.* Falx cerebelli
c. Diaphragma sellae   *d.* Tentorium cerebelli

36. An extradural hematoma is most frequently caused by:
a. Rupture of the emissary veins   *b.* Damage to the cerebral venous sinuses   *c.* Laceration of the galea   *d.* Rupture of the middle meningeal artery   *e.* Rupture of the middle cerebral artery

37. The rupture of an aneurysm on the circle of Willis would likely cause bleeding into which of the following spaces?
a. Epidural   *b.* Subdural   *c.* Subarachnoid
d. Subaponeurotic

38. Head injury resulting in laceration of the galea is particularly hazardous and may lead to meningitis or brain abscess, since:
a. The emissary veins provide an access route for infection to enter the skull   *b.* The galea is part of the outer meningeal layer   *c.* The meningeal arteries form a direct conncection between the scalp and dural sinuses through which infection can enter the skull   *d.* The source of infection is via the vertebral and internal carotids, since veins do not penetrate the skull

39. The arterial supply to the brain is provided by the:
a. External carotid arteries   *b.* Internal carotid arteries   *c.* Vertebral arteries   *d.* Jugulars

40. Which of the following arteries is *not* included in the circle of Willis?
a. Anterior communicating   *b.* Posterior communicating   *c.* Internal carotid   *d.* Posterior cerebral   *e.* Vertebral

41. The basilar artery is formed by the:
a. Internal carotid arteries   *b.* Anterior cerebral arteries   *c.* Posterior cerebral arteries   *d.* Vertebral arteries

42. A 65-year-old female with hypertension reports episodes of blindness in the right eye and weakness in the left leg lasting 20 to 30 minutes. An arteriogram revealed atherosclerotic narrowing of an artery supplying the brain. Which artery accounted for the symptoms?
a. Left internal carotid   *b.* Right internal carotid
c. Left posterior cerebral   *d.* Vertebral-basilar

43. The major blood supply to the pre- and postcentral gyrus is provided by the:
a. Middle cerebral artery   *b.* Anterior cerebral

artery   *c.* Posterior cerebral artery   *d.* Anterior communicating artery

44. A compression fracture of the skull from a blow on the crown of the head would be most likely to damage which of the following dural sinuses?
a. Straight sinus   *b.* Superior sagittal sinus
c. Cavernous venous sinus   *d.* Sigmoid sinus

45. Which of the following statements are true concerning the conducting and penetrating arteries of the brain?
a. Conducting arteries form an array over the surface of the brain.   *b.* Penetrating arteries branch off the conducting arteries at right angles to supply the internal capsule and other deep structures.   *c.* Penetrating arteries from the middle cerebral artery are frequently implicated in a stroke syndrome.   *d.* Occlusion of the penetrating blood vessels supplying the internal capsule results in paralysis.

46. Cerebrospinal fluid:
a. Is formed at the rate of about ½ liter per day
b. Provides a protective cushion around the brain and spinal cord   *c.* Is formed in the arachnoid granulations   *d.* Flows out of the third ventricle into the fourth through the foramen of Magendie
e. Has an average pressure of 130 mmH$_2$O when a patient is in the recumbent positon during a spinal tap

47. Noncommunicating hydrocephalus:
a. Is the most common form of hydrocephalus in the adult   *b.* Is a form of low-pressure hydrocephalus   *c.* Is frequently caused by a congenital narrowing of the aqueduct of Sylvius
d. May be treated by shunting CSF to the jugular vein   *e.* Does not usually cause swelling of the head

48. Which of the following does *not* apply to CSF?
a. Clear, colorless   *b.* Higher chloride and sodium content than blood plasma   *c.* Less glucose than plasma   *d.* Absorbed into the arterial system   *e.* Contains little protein

49. Which statement concerning the brain is *not* true?
a. Hypoglycemia can cause brain damage, since the brain is largely dependent on glucose for its energy supply   *b.* Brain tissue may be irreversibly damaged within a few minutes in the event of an untreated cardiac arrest   *c.* Brain metabolism decreases to an almost negligible level during sleep   *d.* The brain uses about 20 percent of the cardiac output   *e.* The brain is the most energy-consuming tissue in the entire body

50. The brainstem includes:
    a. The medulla oblongata b. The pons
    c. The basal ganglia d. The midbrain

51. The following structures are located in the midbrain:
    a. Superior and inferior colliculi b. Hypothalamus c. Red nucleus d. Substantia nigra

52. The superior colliculi are conerned with:
    a. Auditory reflexes b. Visual reflexes
    c. Respiration d. Heart rate

53. An intact medulla is necessary for integration of reflexes involving:
    a. Swallowing b. Vomiting c. Cardiovascular control d. Respiration

54. The thalamus:
    a. Is an important sensory relay center b. Has many interconnections with the cerebral cortex
    c. Is a center of crude sensory awareness d. Relays impulses from the olfactory system e. Is the largest structure of the diencephalon

55. The hypothalamus:
    a. Contains nuclei which produce antidiuretic hormone b. Regulates hormone release by the anterior pituitary c. Is a control center of the ANS d. Contains a center for temperature control

56. Hemiballismus (violent flinging motions of the limbs on one side of the body) may result from a lesion of the:
    a. Pineal body b. Primary motor cortex
    c. Subthalamus d. Hippocampus

57. The limbic system:
    a. Is primarily involved with the expression of primitive emotions b. Is involved in recent memory c. Is believed to be involved in psychomotor epilepsy d. Includes the corpus callosum

58. The two cerebral hemispheres are separated by the:
    a. Central sulcus (fissure of Rolando) b. Great longitudinal fissure c. The fissure of Sylvius
    d. Parietooccipital sulcus

59. Which of the following is *not* visible on the lateral surface of the brain?
    a. Corpus callosum b. Insula c. Precentral gyrus d. Occipital lobe

60. All the following structures are classified as projection tracts *except:*
    a. Corona radiata b. Internal capsule c. Corpus callosum

61. Which sulcus separates the frontal lobe of the brain from the parietal lobe?
    a. Parietooccipital b. Precentral c. Central
    d. Postcentral

62. Projection fibers of the internal capsule are:
    a. Afferent b. Efferent c. Both d. Neither

63. The thin surface of the cerebrum is referred to as the:
    a. Cortex b. Sulcus c. Corona radiata
    d. Midbrain

64. Area 17 of the cerebral cortex is the principal visual cortex and is located in the:
    a. Frontal lobe b. Parietal lobe c. Temporal lobe d. Occipital lobe

65. The somesthetic area of the cortex:
    a. Is located on the postcentral gyrus b. Is located in the frontal lobe c. Receives fibers from the thalamus d. Is represented by areas 3, 1, and 2

66. Wernicke's area (area 22) is important for:
    a. Voluntary scanning movements of the eyes
    b. Comprehension of spoken language c. Ability to recognize objects by touch d. Ability to write e. Comprehension of written language

67. The precentral gyrus is:
    a. Somatotopically arranged with the facial areas in the most medial position b. Areas 3, 1, 2
    c. The motor strip d. Located in the frontal lobe e. Area 4

68. The sensory association areas:
    a. Are necessary for the interpretation and understanding of sensory input to the brain b. Include areas 5 and 7 of the parietal lobe c. Include areas 3, 1, and 2 d. Are involved with awareness of body image

69. A 70-year-old woman, on recovering from a stroke, was found to have difficulty in understanding written speech (alexia) and inability to write (agraphia) but could understand spoken speech. Which area of the cortex was damaged by the stroke?
    a. Broca's area b. The angular gyrus (area 39)
    c. Areas 5 and 7 d. Wernicke's area

70. A young college student was observed to have a marked change of behavior following a tobogganing accident in which he sustained a compression fracture of the skull. His dress became slovenly and he failed to complete his assignments, contrary to his usual behavior. He was sent to the mental health clinic by a professor when he urinated in a wastebasket of the classroom. Which area of his brain was most likely injured and accounted for the behavior change?
    a. Temporal lobe b. Prefrontal cortex c. Area 6 d. Area 40

71. Which of the following functional deficits would be more likely following a stroke involving the left middle cerebral artery?
    a. Failure to recognize faces   b. Aphasia
    c. Loss of topographic memory   d. Left-sided hemiplegia

72. The reticular substance extends through which of the following structures?
    a. Thalamus   b. Midbrain   c. Pons   d. Medulla oblongata   e. Upper spinal cord

73. Some important functions of the reticular formation include:
    a. Screening of sensory stimuli   b. Activation of the cerebral cortex to become sensitive to stimuli
    c. Regulation of the sleep-wakefulness cycle
    d. Modulation of motor activity

74. CNS monoamines produced in nuclei in the brainstem include:
    a. Norepinephrine   b. Epinephrine   c. Dopamine   d. Serotonin

75. The CNS monoamines:
    a. Are involved in the regulation of emotional behavior   b. Are affected by mood-altering drugs such as the tranquilizers   c. Are involved in the regulation of sleep and wakefulness

76. Cranial nerve V:
    a. Is called the facial nerve   b. Is sensory to the face   c. Is motor to the muscles of mastication
    d. Is a purely sensory nerve

77. The hypoglossal nerve:
    a. Carries impulses for taste on the anterior two-thirds of the tongue   b. Supplies the muscles of the tongue   c. Is a purely motor nerve   d. Is cranial nerve XI

78. The cranial nerve concerned with vision is the:
    a. Optic   b. Oculomotor   c. Trochlear
    d. Abducens

79. Which of the following statements are true concerning the spinal nerves?
    a. The dorsal root of a spinal nerve carries both sensory and motor fibers   b. The motor fibers originate in the anterior horn of the spinal cord
    c. There are 31 pairs of spinal nerves   d. Sensory components of the spinal nerves have their origin in the dorsal roof ganglia

80. Spinal nerve roots C5 through T1 or T2 give origin to the:
    a. Brachial plexus   b. Femoral nerve   c. Radial nerve   d. Median nerve   e. Cervical plexus

81. The collection of nerve roots immediately below the spinal cord is called:
    a. Fasciculus gracilis   b. Filum terminale
    c. Cauda equina   d. Posterior columns

82. The simplest reflex arc involves how many neurons?
    a. One   b. Two   c. Three   d. Four or more

83. All the following are ascending tracts in the spinal cord except:
    a. Fasciculus cuneatus   b. Lateral spinothalamic
    c. Ventral spinocerebellar   d. Ventral corticospinal

84. Which of the following sensations is carried by the dorsal columns?
    a. Conscious proprioception   b. Vibration sense
    c. Two-point discrimination   d. Pain
    e. Temperature

85. The lateral spinothalamic tract:
    a. Carries the afferent impulses for fine touch
    b. Is the conscious pathway for pain and temperature   c. Terminates in the fasciculus cuneatus and gracilis   d. Is the motor pathway for voluntary muscle control

86. All the following statements concerning the conscious pathway for pain and temperature are true except:
    a. The cell body for the first-order neuron is located in the ipsilateral dorsal root ganglion.
    b. The cell body for the second-order neuron is located in the ipsilateral dorsal horn, but its axon crosses over to the opposite side of the spinal cord and courses up the contralateral lateral spinothalamic tract.   c. The third-order neuron is located in the nucleus cuneatus.   d. The axon of the third-order neuron terminates in the postcentral gyrus.

87. The lentiform nucleus includes the:
    a. Putamen   b. Globus pallidus   c. Amygdala
    d. Caudate

Directions: Match the numbers in col. B to the appropriate item in col. A.

Column A	Column B
88. ____ Pairs of cranial nerves	a. 7
	b. 3
89. ____ Pairs of spinal nerves	c. 8
90. ____ Number of cervical vertebrae	d. 12
	e. 31

91. ____ Pairs of cervical spinal nerves

92. ____ Oculomotor nerve (cranial nerve number)

Directions: Match the specialized functions in col. B with the cerebral hemisphere they are more likely to be associated with in col. A.

Column A

93. ____ Right hemisphere

94. ____ Left hemisphere

Column B

a. Mathematical calculation

b. Speech

c. Spatial locations

d. Grasping of wholes

e. Music

f. Right-handedness

Directions: Circle the letter preceding each item below that correctly answers the question or completes the statement. Only one answer is correct, with exceptions noted.

95. Which of the following fiber tract impulses are mediated through the ventral horn cell of the final common pathway? (More than one answer may be correct.)
a. Corticospinal   b. Tectospinal   c. Rubrospinal   d. Vestibulospinal

96. The basal ganglia are:
a. Masses of white matter embedded deep inside the cerebrum   b. Paired structures found in each hemisphere   c. Six distinct structures each independent of the others   d. Cortical structures related to vegetative activities and having a steadying influence on muscle

Directions: Answer the following on a separate sheet of paper.

97. Name and outline the components of the extrapyramidal system. What is its function? Name the basal ganglia.

THE NEUROLOGIC EXAMINATION: EVALUATION OF THE NEUROLOGIC PATIENT

OBJECTIVES

At the completion of this chapter you should be able to:

1. List the six major areas of the neurologic examination.

2. Explain the purpose of history taking during a neurologic examination.

3. State the function of the cerebellum.

4. Describe at least one function of each lobe (frontal, parietal, temporal, occipital) of the cerebral cortex.

5. Locate the structures of the brain that regulate vital-organ functions (such as heartbeat and respiration) and other body functions (such as hearing and other sensory impulses).

6. Describe the 12 cranial nerves by identifying their function and explain how to test each one.

7. Differentiate between normal and abnormal responses to each test for the cranial nerves.

8. Describe the neurologic diseases usually associated with cranial nerve responses.

9. Distinguish between upper and lower motor neurons as to origin and their pathways for eliciting a muscle response.

10. Describe a reflex arc.

11. Describe the procedures for eliciting deep tendon and superficial reflexes.

12. Give an example of a deep tendon and a superficial reflex.

13. List four areas that are investigated when examining the sensory nervous system.

14. Describe the effects of a lesion in the lateral spinothalamic tract and the corticospinal tract.

Neurology is a discipline that is concerned with diseases and disorders of the nervous system. This system is a complex and vital network which allows the individual to cope and adapt to environmental stresses. Diseases of the nervous system may develop insidiously, with gradual loss of function (e.g., in multiple sclerosis) or acutely, with sudden interference in normal functioning (e.g., in ruptured aneurysm). Regardless of the cause, the professional health practitioner is dealing with a patient who must adapt to a new method of functioning, whether temporary or permanent.

The clinical examination of the patient with a neurologic disorder yields valuable information. Symptoms presented by patients seeking health care include the ones derived from the primary neurologic disorder as well as those arising from fear, depression, weakness, and other symptoms arising from the individual patient's method of adapting. A logical, systematic, thorough examination of the patient and the presenting complaints can assist the clinician in differentiating and analyzing the complex clinical picture presented by most patients with a neurologic deficit. A good and careful history and physical examination provides the final diagnosis in about 80 percent of cases (Collins, 1982). Despite the advances in diagnostic testing procedures, nothing has been found that can replace the history and physical examination.

In order for the neurologic examination to yield the necessary information, it is important, whenever possible, to gain the patient's cooperation. During the process of examination the patient is often requested to do something that may appear nonsensical or may sound ridiculous. Careful explanation prior to the neurologic examination should allay the patient's anxiety and clarify the importance of the examination to the diagnostic process. Explanation about the length of the examination, the procedure to be followed, and any pain that the patient can expect will help in establishing trust and confidence in the examiner. The patient should be requested to answer all questions as accurately as possible and follow all directions to the best of his or her ability. Time must be allotted for the patient's questions both prior to and following the examination.

THE NEUROLOGIC EXAMINATION

Evaluation of the patient with a neurologic disorder begins by systematically evaluating the patient and the complaints. The history, a summary of the patient's symptoms, and a discussion of similar or related complaints in family members will focus the clinician's thinking, direct the physical examination, and become the keystone for diagnosis of the problem. The close relation between neurologic symptoms and symptoms of other medical disease states (e.g., diabetes mellitus, hypertension, thyroid disorders) necessitates a complete medical evaluation even though the patient's symptoms suggest a neurologic problem. Explanations are especially important to help allay the patient's anxiety, since the neurologic patient, more than any other patients, requires a clinician who sees beyond the symptoms and the disease process to the patient and the family.

The neurologic history focuses on why the patient seeks medical attention. It is important that this information be elicited and recorded in the patient's own words, not in diagnostic terms. A detailed discussion of the neurologic examination is not included here, since it can be found in many standard textbooks on neurology. A brief summary of the examination is included to help review some important points.

Important information to be elicited from the patient and recorded should include past medical history, social history, family history, and onset of the present symptoms. It is important to ask the patient what problems, if any, have been experienced with each major body system and part. The patient is asked specifically about dizziness, headaches, visual disturbances, bowel or bladder dysfunction, weakness, numbness, and pain. While eliciting this information the clinician carefully observes the patient's behavior, attitudes, attention to personal appearance and grooming, ability to answer the questions appropriately, and ability to concentrate. Once this portion of the examination is completed, the clinician can substantiate suspicions and abnormal findings with further examinations and diagnostic tests. In some cases of neurologic disorder (migraine, trigeminal neuralgia) the diagnosis is made purely on the basis of the history, since the physical findings are nil.

Organization of the neurologic examination is very important. Following a particular order allows the clinician to evaluate the information and direct the later segments of the examination. The organization of the examination includes evaluation of (1) mental status/function, (2) level of consciousness, (3) cranial nerve function, (4) motor function, (5) reflexes, (6) coordination and gait, and (7) sensory function. Information from each segment of the examination is correlated with information previously gained, leading to a localization of the disease process.

Examination of mental status

This portion of the examination evaluates the patient's ability to reason, abstract, plan ahead, and make judgments. Changes in behavior and personality may be associated with organic brain dysfunction, and therefore these changes need to be elicited from the patient or the patient's family. In evaluating the patient's mental status the examiner must be cognizant of socioeconomic, ethnic, and educational status. General knowledge and intellect may be evaluated by asking the patient to name five countries or five major rivers. The patient's ability to remember past events may be evaluated by asking the patient questions concerning his or her own past but may be difficult to assess. Recent memory may be assessed by asking the patient to repeat at least six digits. Normal persons have the ability to remember and repeat seven digits forward and four backward. Important information is obtained by evaluating the patient's ability to produce abstract thoughts and generalizations from concrete statements. Asking the patient to interpret a common saying (e.g., "A rolling stone gathers no moss") is a method frequently used.

Level of consciousness

Evaluation of the patient's level of consciousness is an essential component of the neurologic examination. It should be done thoughtfully, with meticulous attention to accuracy. Many tools are available today for catego-

rizing the level of consciousness, using similar terms in different ways. In the use of any tool the most important criterion should be consistency, and a complete understanding of all terminology is essential. It is always better to describe the patient's behavior and responses exactly than to rely on such catch-all terms as *lethargic* or *stuporous*. Table 47-1 lists several terms used in describing levels of consciousness, with descriptions of behavior associated with these terms.

Cerebral Functions

Knowledge of the functions of the cerebral lobes and the subsequently related symptoms associated with deficits of that particular area of the brain assist the clinician in pinpointing the neurologic deficit. Important observations concerning the patient's neurologic problems

TABLE 47-1

LEVELS OF CONSCIOUSNESS

Term	Characteristics
Conscious	1. Freely aware of surroundings; oriented to person, place, and time 2. Cooperative 3. Can repeat several digits a few minutes after being told them
Automatism	1. Relatively normal behavior, e.g., capable of feeding self 2. Speaks in sentences but has difficulty with memory and judgment; no recollection of events prior to period of unconsciousness; may ask the same questions over and over 3. Behaves automatically without immediate or late memory of behavior 4. Obeys simple commands
Confusion	1. Performs purposeful activity (such as feeding) with clumsy movements 2. Disoriented as to time, place, and/or person (acts as if in a daze) 3. Memory impaired, unable to sustain thought or expression 4. Generally difficult to arouse 5. Becomes uncooperative
Delirium	1. Disoriented to time, place, and person 2. Uncooperative 3. Agitated, restless, resistive (may attempt to get out of bed, thrashes around in bed, pulls off dressings, IV, etc.) 4. Difficult to arouse
Stupor	1. Quiet, may appear to be asleep 2. Responds to loud verbal stimuli 3. Annoyed by light 4. Responds appropriately to painful stimuli
Deep stupor	1. Mute 2. Very difficult to arouse (some arousal to painful stimuli) 3. Responds to pain with automatic purposeless movements
Coma	1. Unconscious; body flaccid 2. No response to verbal or painful stimuli 3. Reflexes present; gag, knee jerk, corneal
Irreversible coma and death	1. Reflexes disappear 2. Pupils become fixed and dilated 3. Cessation of respirations and heartbeat

TABLE 47-2

CEREBRAL FUNCTIONS AND DEFICITS

Cerebral lobe	Functions	Deficits
Frontal	Judgment	Impaired judgment
	Personality traits	Impaired grooming and appearance
	Complex mental skills (abstraction, conceptualizing, foresight)	Impaired affect
		Impaired thought process
		Impaired motor functions
Temporal	Auditory memory	Deficits in recent memory
	Recent memory	
	Primary auditory area affecting awareness	Psychomotor seizures
		Deafness
Parietal		
Dominant	Speech	Aphasia
	Calculation (mathematics)	Agraphia
		Acalculia
	Topography of both sides of the body	Agnosia
		Sensory deficits (bilateral)
Nondominant	Sensory awareness	Disorientation
	Synthesis of complex memories	Distortion of concept of space
		Loss of awareness of opposite side
Occipital	Visual memory	Blindness and visual deficits
	Vision	

are made during the neurologic examination. Table 47-2 lists the cerebral lobes and some of their known functions.

Language and speech examination

One of the most important functions of the dominant hemisphere is speech. The left hemisphere is dominant for speech in right-handed persons and in the majority of left-handed persons. There are three speech disorders of neurologic origin—dysarthria, dysphonia, and aphasia.

Dysarthria is a defect in articulation, enumeration, and rhythm of speech related to a weakness in the muscles involved in speech. This abnormality is usually detected in ordinary conversation with the patient but may be confirmed by asking for repetition of a difficult word or phrase, such as "methodist episcopal." The causes for this weakness can be amyotrophic lateral sclerosis, pseudobulbar palsy, or myasthenia gravis.

Dysphonia is a disorder of vocalization giving a hoarse quality to the voice. The disorder can be con-firmed by detecting hoarseness or a rough quality to the voice of a patient responding to a request to say "E" and by indirect laryngoscopy. This problem has many non-neurologic causes; among the neurologic causes are injury to the recurrent laryngeal nerve and tumors of the brainstem.

Aphasia is a general term meaning loss of the ability to comprehend, elaborate, or express speech concepts. Motor aphasia is loss of the ability to express thoughts in speech or writing, and sensory aphasia is loss of the ability to comprehend spoken or written language. For evaluation, the patient may be directed to perform certain tasks by written or verbal orders, such as, "Fold this paper; write your name." The most common cause of aphasia is a cerebrovascular disorder involving the middle cerebral artery, which supplies the speech and language center.

Examination of the cranial nerves

Twelve pairs of cranial nerves arise from the undersurface of the brain through small foramina. They are numbered according to the order in which they emerge, from front to rear (Fig. 47-1).

The cranial nerves are composed of afferent or efferent fibers, and some, referred to as *mixed fibers*, are of both types. The cell bodies of the afferent fibers are located in ganglia outside the brainstem, while the cell bodies of the efferent fibers are located in various nuclei of the brainstem.

The cranial nerves are examined not in sequence but according to function. The method of examination of the cranial nerves and some pathophysiologic implications are discussed in the following sections.

Olfactory nerve (cranial nerve I)

The olfactory nerve conveys smells to the brain for appreciation. With the patient's eyes closed and one nostril occluded at a time, mildly aromatic substances such as vanilla, cologne, and cloves are offered for identification. The patient is requested to indicate the moment of first detection of the odor and, if possible, to identify the substance. Perception of the odor is more important than correct identification of the substance.

Nasal disorders, e.g., sinusitis, allergies, and upper respiratory infections, are the most common causes of loss of smell. A tumor in the olfactory groove (olfactory groove meningioma) is a neurologic cause for the loss of smell.

Anosmia may also occur after meningitis, subarachnoid hemorrhage, or head injury involving the nerve fibers as they pass through the cribriform plate.

Optic nerve (cranial nerve II)

The optic nerve transmits impulses from the retina to the optic chiasm and then through visual pathways

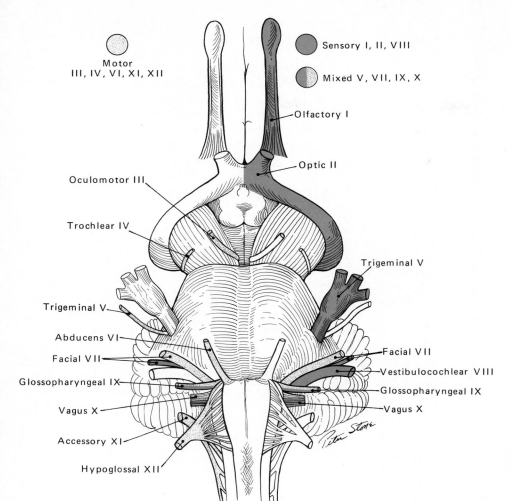

Motor
III, IV, VI, XI, XII

Sensory I, II, VIII

Mixed V, VII, IX, X

Olfactory I

Optic II

Oculomotor III

Trochlear IV

Trigeminal V

Trigeminal V

Abducens VI

Facial VII

Glossopharyngeal IX

Vagus X

Accessory XI

Hypoglossal XII

Facial VII

Vestibulocochlear VIII

Glossopharyngeal IX

Vagus X

FIGURE 47-1

Emergence of the cranial nerves from the ventral surface of the brainstem. (From Langley, Telford, and Christensen, 1980, p. 260.)

to the occipital cortex for recognition and interpretation. Examination of this nerve involves testing visual acuity either by using a Snellen test or, if this is not available, by asking the patient to read various sizes of newspaper print. Reduction of visual acuity is generally caused by diseases involving the eye, the optic nerve, or the optic chiasm. Visual field examinations give the examiner information concerning the optic nerve and visual pathways from the eye to the occipital cortex. For general purposes as part of a neurologic examination, visual fields are examined by confrontation. This is accomplished by asking the patient to cover one eye. The examiner sits directly in front of the patient asking him or her to look straight ahead. A pencil or finger is brought into the field of vision from the four quadrants toward the uncovered eye. The patient is asked to identify when the pencil or finger first enters the visual field. This method provides a gross screening device. For a more thorough evaluation a perimeter and tangent screen are used.

The optic disc is visualized by use of the ophthalmoscope. Neurologically the two most significant findings are papilledema and optic atrophy. Changes in the disc occur with tumors, infections, and trauma. Other changes visualized are exudates, hemorrhages, and arteriovenous abnormalities associated with diabetes and hypertension.

Oculomotor, trochlear, and abducens nerves (cranial nerves III, IV, and VI)

These three nerves are examined together, since they act conjugately to control the extraocular muscles (EOM). In addition, the oculomotor nerve elevates the upper eyelid and innervates the constrictor muscle, which alters the pupil size. The innervation of the EOM is examined by asking the patient to follow a moving finger or pencil with eyes turning upward, downward, medially, and laterally. Weakness in muscles becomes evident when an eye cannot move in a certain direction. Pupils are examined in subdued light and should be round and approximately equal in size, although unequal pupils are found in approximately 20 to 25 percent of the population. However, the difference is rarely greater than 1 mm. Both pupils should react to light directly and consensually.

Pupil Size, mm:

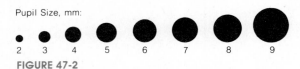

2   3   4   5   6   7   8   9

FIGURE 47-2

**Pupil size reference guide. (From D. A. Jones, C. F.
Dunbar, and M. J. Jirovec,** *Medical-Surgical Nursing,*
McGraw-Hill, New York, 1978, p. 1206.)

In recording the size of the pupils, it is essential to
use millimeters (mm), to ensure accuracy in evaluating
the patient's neurologic status. This practice is particularly important when the practitioner is evaluating a
patient after a head injury. A pupil size reference guide
is given in Fig. 47-2.

The nuclei of the oculomotor nerves and the trochlear nerve are located in the midbrain. The nuclei of the
abducens nerve lies beneath the floor of the fourth ventricle in the lower pons and are close to fibers from the
facial nerve nucleus.

Myasthenia gravis is an important cause of weakness of the extraocular muscles, causing weakness in
more than one muscle and ptosis (see Chap. 50). Horner's syndrome consists of ptosis of the lid, constriction
of the pupil, and absence of sweating on the same side
of the face. This can be due to vascular lesions in the
brainstem, cervical spinal cord injuries and tumors, or
trauma affecting the sympathetic fibers in the neck, or
can be a temporary side effect of cerebral angiography.

Horizontal nystagmus (rapid lateral oscillations of
the eye) is an important neurologic sign. It is seen normally on extreme lateral gaze. Nystagmus can occur in
any direction of gaze and can be unilateral or bilateral.
Neurologic causes include multiple sclerosis, lesions of
one cerebellar hemisphere, and tumor of one side of the
brain. Nonneurologic causes include the use of barbiturates and tranquilizers.

Trigeminal nerve (cranial nerve V)

The trigeminal nerve carries both motor and sensory fibers. It supplies innervation to the temporal and
masseter muscles, which are the muscles of mastication.
The motor division of this nerve is examined by asking
the patient to clench the teeth and move the jaw from
side to side while the examiner palpates the muscles and
judges the strength of contraction.

The sensory fibers of the trigeminal nerve are divided into three main branches—ophthalmic, maxillary,
and mandibular (Fig. 47-3). In order to evaluate areas of
sensory loss, each area is tested by asking the patient to
respond to a touch with a piece of cotton. The corneal

reflex is tested in each eye—a wisp of cotton with a fine
point is touched to the cornea, causing the patient to
blink.

Tumors of the posterior fossa cause loss of corneal
reflex and facial numbness as an early sign. The most
notable disorder affecting the trigeminal nerve is trigeminal neuralgia, or tic douloureux, causing brief, excruciating pain along the maxillary or mandibular divisions of the trigeminal nerve. Myasthenia gravis and
amyotrophic lateral sclerosis cause weakness and fatigue
of the muscles of mastication, causing chewing to be difficult and at times impossible.

Facial nerve (cranial nerve VII)

This nerve has both sensory and motor function. It
carries sensory fibers which mediate taste perception
from the anterior tongue and motor fibers which innervate all the muscles necessary for the varied facial
expressions—smiling, frowning, grimacing, etc.

The motor division of the facial nerve is evaluated
by asking the patient to perform various facial movements and observing the patient talk. Weakness of the
facial muscle may be evidenced by flattening of the nasolabial fold, drooping of one side of the mouth, and sagging of the lower eyelid. The sense of taste is evaluated
by asking the patient to identify sweet, sour, and salty
substances that are applied to the tongue. The ninth
cranial nerve, the glossopharyngeal, carries the sensation of bitterness. It is perceived only on the posterior
segment of the tongue. This is an important point to
remember when testing for the sensation of bitterness.

Since the nucleus of the facial nerve lies in the lateral portion of the lower pons, a lesion in the area of the
brainstem will often cause facial nerve dysfunction.
Since the facial nerve enters the temporal bone and is
in close proximity to the middle ear, it is subject to
trauma from fractures of the base of the skull and the
temporal bone, from surgical procedures, and from diseases of the ear. Other disorders that may result in facial
nerve weakness include myasthenia gravis and Guillain-Barré syndrome. Bell's palsy is the most common type
of nerve paralysis.

Vestibulocochlear nerve (cranial nerve VIII)

The vestibulocochlear nerve functions to maintain
balance and to transmit impulses which allow a person
to hear. Maintenance of balance is the function of the
vestibular division, while the cochlear division mediates
hearing. The cochlear division can be tested by observing the patient's ability to hear a whisper from a distance of 2 ft. Another method of testing involves use of
the tuning fork, which will distinguish between conductive hearing loss and sensorineural loss. People with
normal hearing will hear a tuning fork placed in the
midline of the head or forehead equally well in both

ears. Additionally, they will hear the tuning fork better by air conduction than bone conduction. Normally the tuning fork is heard twice as long by air conduction. The two commonly used tuning fork–hearing tests are the Rinne and Weber tests. In the Rinne test, a vibrating tuning fork is placed on the mastoid process; when the patient indicates that the vibration is no longer audible, the tuning fork is placed next to the ear. If the patient again hears the vibration, then air conduction (AC) is better than bone conduction (BC). This is normal and is arbitrarily called a "positive" Rinne. A "negative" Rinne is indicative of middle ear disease causing conductive hearing loss. In the Weber test, the vibrating tuning fork is placed on the top of the patient's head, in the middle of the forehead, or on the upper front teeth. The patient is asked where the sound is heard the loudest. Normally people hear the sound equally well on both sides. If the sound lateralizes to one side, it may indicate a hearing loss. If the patient has conductive hearing loss, the sound will be heard better in the deafer ear, whereas with sensorineural loss it will

be heard better in the healthy ear. If an abnormality is detected, a complete audiometer evaluation should be done.

Acute dysfunction of the vestibular division of the vestibulocochlear nerve is manifested by vertigo, nausea, vomiting, and ataxia. The cold caloric test is used to screen for problems. It is performed with the patient upright. Ice water (5 ml) is injected into the ear. The normal response to this stimulus is nystagmus of both eyes, vertigo, nausea, and vomiting. Little or no reaction to this stimulus indicates an abnormality of the vestibular nerve. Ménière's disease involves a dilatation of the endolymphatic channels in the cochlea, with eventual atrophy of the hearing mechanism resulting in vertigo, tinnitus, and hearing loss in the affected ear.

The vestibulocochlear nerve leaves the brainstem and travels along a path similar to that of the facial nerve. Like the facial nerve it is subject to damage from fractures of the base of the skull and the temporal bone. Vascular occlusions and tumors of the brainstem are other causes of damage to this nerve.

FIGURE 47-3

(A) Distribution of sensory fibers to the skin by the three branches of the trigeminal nerve. (B) Distribution of the chief motor fibers to muscles of mastication. (C) Distribution of terminal branches. (From Langley, Telford, and Christensen, 1980, p. 263.)

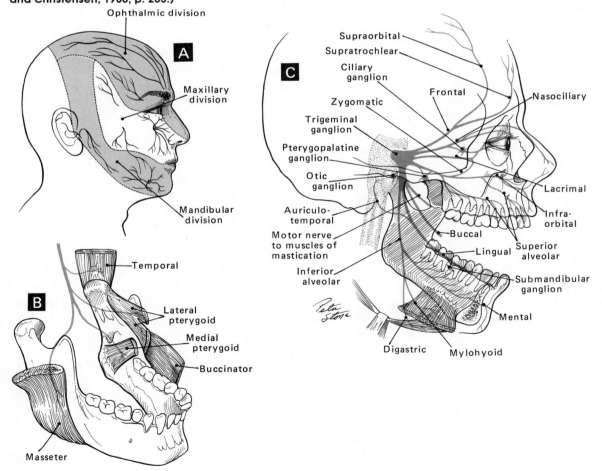

The glossopharyngeal and vagus nerves (cranial nerves IX and X)

These two nerves are closely related anatomically and functionally and are evaluated together. The glossopharyngeal nerve has a sensory division which carries taste from the posterior portion of the tongue, innervates the carotid sinus and the carotid bodies, and supplies sensation to the pharynx. The motor division innervates the posterior wall of the pharynx. The vagus nerve innervates all the thoracic and abdominal viscera and conveys impulses from the walls of the intestines, the heart, and the lungs. It is not possible clinically to examine all these functions; therefore, evaluation of the vagus nerve is directed toward evaluating the motor function of the palate, pharynx, and larynx.

The first step in evaluation of the glossopharyngeal and vagus nerves is inspection of the soft palate. The soft palate should be symmetrical and should not deviate to either side. When the patient says "ah," the soft palate should rise symmetrically. To induce a gag reflex the posterior wall of the pharynx is touched, causing elevation of the palate and constriction of the pharyngeal muscles. The patient's swallowing reflex is tested by observing the reaction to drinking a glass of water. Observations are made of difficulty in swallowing or regurgitation of fluid through the nose, which would indicate weakness of the soft palate and an inability to close off the nasopharynx when swallowing. Indirect laryngoscopy is done when the patient's complaint is a voice disturbance or hoarseness. The vocal cords can be observed for paresis or lesions. Bilateral lesions may cause great difficulty in swallowing and in the ability to mobilize secretions.

The glossopharyngeal and the vagus nerves leave the skull through the jugular foramen with the internal jugular vein. Therefore trauma or a tumor in close proximity to this area would affect these structures. The recurrent laryngeal nerve, a branch of the vagus which supplies the larynx, is susceptible to injury during surgery of the neck because of its close proximity to the thyroid gland. Amyotrophic lateral sclerosis and myasthenia gravis frequently cause weakness in the muscles innervated by the glossopharyngeal and the vagus nerves.

Accessory nerve (cranial nerve XI)

The accessory nerve is a motor nerve innervating the sternocleidomastoid muscle and the upper portion of the trapezius muscle. These muscles act to flex the neck; the sternocleidomastoid muscle acts to rotate the head from side to side, and the trapezius rotates the scapula when the arm is raised.

The function of the accessory nerve is evaluated by observing the sternocleidomastoid and trapezius muscles for atrophy and assessing their strength. In order to test the sternocleidomastoid muscle, the patient is asked to turn the head toward one shoulder and to resist attempts of the examiner to move the head in the opposite direction. This test is repeated on the other side so that both the right and left muscles are evaluated. The trapezius muscle is evaluated by asking the patient to shrug the shoulders while the examiner attempts to push downward. The patient is then asked to elevate both arms to a vertical position. A patient with weakness in the trapezius muscle will not be able to perform this action.

The accessory nerve lies in close proximity to the glossopharyngeal and the vagus nerves. Tumors affecting these nerves frequently affect the accessory nerve. The cell bodies of the accessory nerve lie in the upper part of the spinal cord at levels C1 through C5 and receive innervation from both cerebral hemispheres. A unilateral lesion causes little or no dysfunction in the two muscles innervated by this nerve. The most common cause for accessory nerve dysfunction is neck trauma.

Hypoglossal nerve (cranial nerve XII)

The hypoglossal nerve innervates the musculature of the tongue. Normal functioning of the tongue is essential for normal speech and swallowing. Slight bilateral weakness will be evidenced by difficulty in enunciating consonants and difficulty in swallowing. Severe bilateral weakness causes extreme difficulty with speech and swallowing.

The tongue is examined for asymmetry, deviation to one side, and the presence of fasciculations. This examination is done first inside the mouth with the tongue and rest and then with the tongue protruded. Strength of the muscle is evaluated by asking the patient to push out a cheek with the tongue while the examiner opposes the effort with fingers on the patient's cheek.

The nuclei of the hypoglossal nerves lie within the medulla beneath the floor of the fourth ventricle and receive innervation from both cerebral hemispheres. Injuries to the neck may cause unilateral weakness of the tongue with atrophy and fasciculations. Tumors at the base of the posterior fossa near the foramen magnum may cause ipsilateral paralysis of the tongue. Bilateral weakness can be due to amyotrophic lateral sclerosis and myasthenia gravis.

Examination of motor function

Motor performance is dependent upon an intact muscle, a functioning neuromuscular junction, and intact

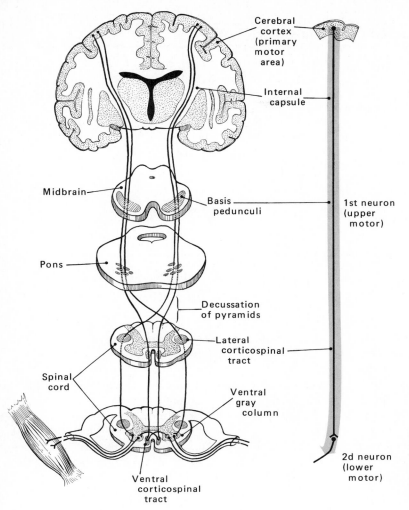

Cerebral cortex (primary motor area)

Internal capsule

Midbrain

Basis pedunculi

1st neuron (upper motor)

Pons

Decussation of pyramids

Lateral corticospinal tract

Spinal cord

Ventral gray column

2d neuron (lower motor)

Ventral corticospinal tract

FIGURE 47-4

Pyramidal motor pathways (corticospinal tracts). The tracts originate in pyramidal cells of the cortex. Fibers that cross at the medulla form the lateral corticospinal tracts, while the remaining fibers form the ventral corticospinal tracts. The basis pedunculi are part of the cerebral peduncles. (From Langley, Telford, and Christensen, 1980, p. 294.)

cranial and spinal nerve tracts. In order to understand how the nervous system functions to coordinate muscle activity, it is important first to be able to distinguish between the upper and the lower motor neuron.

The *upper motor neuron* originates in the cerebral cortex and projects downward, one part (the corticobulbar tract) ending in the brainstem and the other (the corticospinal tract) crossing in the lower medulla and descending into the spinal cord. The cranial nerve nuclei serve as the end point for the corticobulbar tracts. The corticospinal tracts terminate in the region of the anterior horn of the spinal cord from the cervical to the sacral areas. Those corticospinal fibers which travel through the medullary pyramids constitute the pyramidal tracts. Nerve fibers in the corticospinal tract mediate voluntary movement, particularly fine, discrete, conscious movement (Fig. 47-4).

The *lower motor neuron* includes the motor cells of the cranial nerve nuclei and their axons as well as the anterior horn cells of the spinal cord and their axons. The motor fibers leave through the anterior, or motor, root of the spinal column and innervate the muscles.

Lesions involving the upper motor neuron and the lower motor neuron produce characteristic changes in muscle response. Awareness of the differences in muscle weakness will help locate the neurologic lesion. A summary of this information is given in Table 47-3.

Coordination and gait

Coordination is impaired by many disorders at any level of the motor system. Incoordination is a particularly relevant sign, generally indicating problems with cerebellar function and corticospinal tract interruption. Tests revealing a lack of coordination include tandem walking (asking the patient to walk heel to toe); ability of the patient to follow through on simple rapid movements (placing the hand on the knee alternately using the palm and back of the hand); and ability of the patient to place the heel of one foot on the opposite knee and slide it down the front of the leg. Cerebellar disease causes these movements to be slow, nonrhythmic, and inaccurate.

Gait is usually observed by asking the patient to

TABLE 47-3

DIFFERENTIATION BETWEEN UPPER AND LOWER MOTOR NEURON WEAKNESS

	Upper motor neuron*	Lower motor neuron†
Type and distribution of weakness	Lesions in brain—"pyramidal distribution," i.e., distal, especially hand muscles; weaker extensors in arm and weaker flexors in legs Lesions in cord—variable, depending on location	Depends on which lower motor neurons are involved, i.e., which segments, roots, or nerves
Tone	Spasticity—greater in flexors in arms and extensors in legs	Flaccidity
Bulk	Slight atrophy of disuse only	Atrophy—may be marked
Reflexes	Accentuated; Babinski sign present	Decreased or absent; no Babinski sign
Fasciculations	No	Yes
Clonus	Frequently present	Absent

*Synonyms: *pyramidal tract* (referring to fibers in the medullary pyramids), *corticospinal tract, corticobulbar tract.*
†Synonyms: *anterior horn cell, ventral horn cell, somatic motor portions of cranial nerves, final common pathway.*
Source: Simpson and Magee, 1973, p. 60.

walk. Keeping in mind that most people tend to walk slowly and carefully when observed, the examiner looks for lack of arm swing or decreased arm swing, hemiplegia, rigidity, loss of coordinated movement, tremor, and/or apraxia (slow, shuffling steps and difficulty in lifting feet from the ground). Patients with cerebellar disease walk with a wide base of support and have a tendency to stagger laterally. Slow gait, small shuffling steps, and lack of arm swing are characteristics of Parkinson's disease.

Muscle tone and strength

Muscle tone, which is the resistance detected by the examiner when a joint is moved through passive range of motion, is frequently altered in nervous system disorders. Upper motor neuron disorders increase muscle tone, while lower motor neuron disorders decrease muscle tone. Some of the alterations in muscle tone frequently seen in neurologic disorders are listed in Table 47-4.

TABLE 47-4

SOME ALTERATIONS IN MOTOR FUNCTION ASSOCIATED WITH NEUROLOGIC DISORDERS

Muscle disorder	Clinical findings	Neurologic disorder	Muscle disorder	Clinical findings	Neurologic disorder
Dystonia	Persistent abnormal positions of body parts in which there is resistance to passive movement of the part	Extrapyramidal disease Wilson's disease Phenothiazine neuropathy Viral brain infection	Hypotonia	Increased range of motion of joints (overextension and overflexion)	Cerebellar disease
Paratonia (*Gegenhalten*)	Resistance to passive movement throughout the range of motion (somewhat proportional to the amount of force applied)	Frontal lobe disease	Hemiballismus	Unilateral movements, affecting the side opposite to the lesion, involving violent, flinging movements at the proximal joints	Cerebrovascular occlusions involving the subthalamic nucleus
Decerebrate rigidity	Extension and pronation of the upper extremities and extension of the lower extremities	Severe brain injury above the level of the pons	Tremors	Involuntary rhythmic, tremulous movements. Rest tremor: more pronounced at rest. Intention tremor: worse when the patient reaches for an object	Lesions of the cerebellar pathways

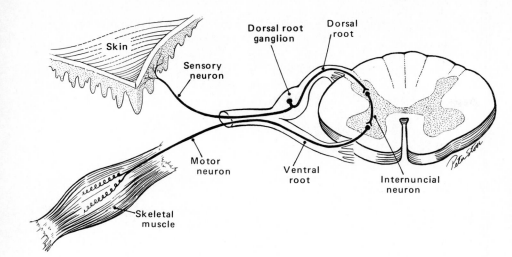

FIGURE 47-5
Components of a simple reflex: a sensory, an internuncial, and a motor neuron. (From Langley, Telford, and Christensen, 1980, p. 287.)

Major muscle groups are observed for evidence of muscle wasting, fasciculations, or contractions. Muscle strength is tested by comparing the strength of the muscles on one side of the body to those on the other side as the patient resists the examiner's counterpressure. Age, sex, and the physical condition of the patient must be considered when evaluating these tests. The patient is observed for any evidence of involuntary movements, including tremors, chorea, hemiballismus, and tic.

Evaluation of reflexes

A deep tendon reflex is elicited by a brisk tap with a reflex hammer over a partially stretched tendon. The impulse then travels along afferent fibers to the spinal cord, where it synapses with a motor, or anterior horn, neuron. After it synapses, the impulse is transmitted down the motor neuron to the anterior nerve root through the spinal nerve and then the peripheral nerve. After it is transmitted across the neuromuscular junction, the muscle is stimulated to contract. In simplest form this is the reflex arc (Fig. 47-5).

The deep tendon reflexes, also known as *muscle stretch reflexes*, commonly tested are the biceps reflex, the triceps reflex, the brachioradialis reflex, the patellar reflex, and the Achilles reflex. The response to reflexes is graded on a scale of 0 to +4 (see Table 47-5, also Table 52-3).

It is important to compare sides when evaluating reflex responses.

Superficial reflexes are tested by stroking the skin with a firm object such as the end of a reflex hammer or applicator, causing the muscles to contract. These reflexes include abdominal, cremasteric, plantar, and gluteal.

Assessment of reflexes gives the examiner information concerning the function of the reflex arc and specific spinal cord segments. Reflexes are altered in disease states involving the upper and lower motor neurons.

Upper motor neuron paralysis is caused by an interruption of the descending motor tracts on one side of a segment of the spinal cord. Immediately after the occurrence of the lesion the deep tendon reflexes are temporarily depressed. This is known as *areflexia*. In addition, the paralyzed muscles are flaccid. Several weeks or months after the lesion occurs, the deep tendon reflexes become hyperactive; the superficial reflexes are lost, and a Babinski reflex (see below) is noted (Noback and Demarest, 1980).

Lower motor neuron paralysis is caused by destruction of the peripheral motor nerves and the anterior horn cells. When this occurs, the muscles become flaccid and hypotonic and the deep tendon reflexes are lost (Adams and Vander Eecken, 1983).

The plantar reflex is elicited by stroking the lateral aspect of the sole from the heel to the ball and curving medially across the ball of the foot. The normal response to this stimulus is flexion of the toes. An abnormal response, dorsiflexion of the great toe with fanning

TABLE 47-5

GRADING OF REFLEXES

Grade	Significance
+4	Very brisk, suggestive of disease of the upper motor neuron, frequently associated with clonus (rhythmic oscillations between flexion and extension)
+3	Brisker than average but not necessarily indicative of disease
+2	Average/normal
+1	Somewhat diminished
0	No response

Source: Modified from Bates, 1983.

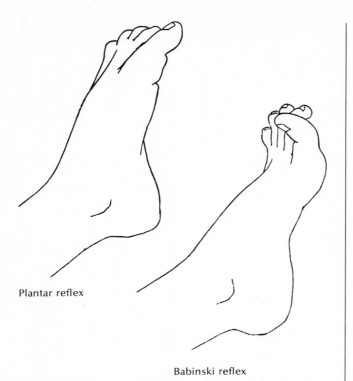

Plantar reflex

Babinski reflex

FIGURE 47-6

The Babinski response. Above, the normal adult response to stimulation of the foot. Below, the normal infant and abnormal adult response. (From Gardner, 1975, p. 215.)

of the other toes, is known as the Babinski reflex and indicates upper motor neuron disease (Fig. 47-6). This reflex is seen in children under the age of 2 years; during periods of deep sleep, general anesthesia, and postictal (after a seizure) depression; and in persons who are drunk or in moderate to severe hypoglycemic shock (Carpenter, 1982).

Sensory evaluation

The sensory system plays a vital role in conveying to the central nervous system information concerning the environment. When examining the sensory system the following four areas are investigated: (1) superficial tactile sensation, including pain, temperature, and touch; (2) proprioceptive sense, which is motion or position sense; (3) vibratory sense; and (4) cortical sensory functions. Patterns of sensory loss may lead to a diagnosis of lesions of the cerebral hemisphere, the brainstem, the spinal cord, the nerve root, and single or multiple peripheral nerves.

Perceptions of pain and temperature are carried by nerve fibers to the dorsal root ganglia where the nuclei of these nerve fibers are located. After synapsing in the dorsal horn they cross over the midline and enter the opposite lateral spinothalamic tract. This tract ascends through the entire length of the spinal cord, medulla,

FIGURE 47-7

The central pathway for impulses perceived as pain (lateral spinothalamic tract). Note that the fibers cross upon entering the spinal cord. (From Langley, Telford, and Christensen, 1980, p. 278.)

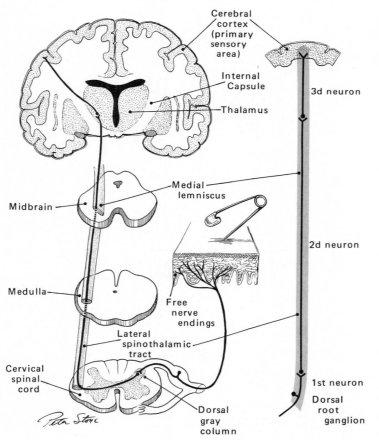

pons, and midbrain and terminates in the thalamus. The thalamus, acting as a relay station, transmits the impulse to the sensory cortex for interpretation. Simple touch sensation is transmitted by the ventral spinothalamic tract. A lesion involving the lateral spinothalamic tract will result in loss of pain and temperature sensation on the opposite side of the body below the level of the lesion. Lesions of the nerve roots and of peripheral nerves impair the perception of touch (Fig. 47-7).

Fibers conducting sensations of position, vibration, and touch requiring a high degree of localization, such as stereognosis, graphesthesia, and two-point discrimination, enter the spinal column and pass into the dorsal column system. Traveling upward to the lower medulla, where they synapse and cross over, the fibers ascend as the medial lemniscus, terminating in the thalamus. The fine distinction and perception of these sensations is carried out in the parietal cortex.

FIGURE 47-8
Arrangement of the dermatomes. Each dorsal (sensory) spinal root innervates one dermatome. The first cervical nerve usually has no cutaneous distribution. The fifth cranial nerve supplies the sensory distribution to the face and anterior aspect of the head. The ophthalmic division is labeled I and VI, the maxillary division is II and V2, and the mandibular division is III and V3 in A and B. (A from Noback and Demarest, 1981, pp. 156–157; B adapted from W. Haymaker, *Bing's Local Diagnosis in Neurological Diseases,* 15th ed., Mosby, St. Louis, 1969.)

The pattern of the dermatomes is shown in Fig. 47-8. Theoretically, a lesion in the dorsal root produces loss of sensation in the area supplied by the root. However, there is considerable overlap of nerve supply, which frequently confuses the clinical picture.

Sensory testing is done with the patient's eyes closed, using a wisp of cotton to test for touch, a safety pin to test for superficial pain, and test tubes filled with hot and cold water to test for temperature.

Proprioception, position, and motion sense are first evaluated in distal joints. If proprioception is normal in the distal joint, then it is not necessary to test the proximal joint. A distal phalanx of one of the patient's fingers is grasped and slowly moved upward or downward and the patient is asked to indicate the movement of the phalanx. The Romberg test evaluates the position sense for the legs and trunk; the normal person should be able to stand with feet together and eyes closed without swaying markedly or losing balance. Frequently patients with abnormality in the proprioceptive pathway can maintain their balance with eyes open, since the visual orientation serves to keep them balanced. The patient with a cerebellar disorder, on the other hand, sways and loses balance with eyes open as well as closed.

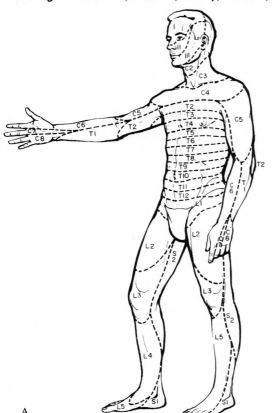

A

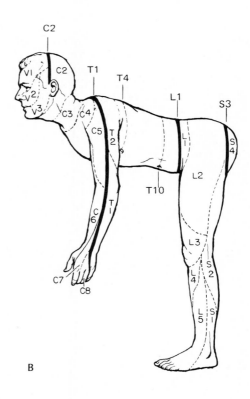

B

The neurologic examination: evaluation of the neurologic patient

Directions: Answer the following questions on a separate sheet of paper.

1. What is the purpose of history taking during a neurologic examination?

2. List the six major areas of the neurologic examination.

Directions: Circle T for true and F for false. Correct the false statements.

3. T F The highest integration and coordination center for perception and interpretation of sensory input is the frontal lobe.

4. T F The neurologic examination of mental status evaluates the patient's ability to reason, think abstractly, plan ahead, and make judgments.

5. T F The right hemisphere is dominant for speech in right-handed persons and in the majority of left-handed persons.

6. T F Dysarthria is a defect in articulation, enunciation, and rhythm of speech related to a weakness in the muscles involved in speech.

Directions: Match the functions in col. B to the location of their cerebral control in col. A.

Column A	Column B
7. ____ Medulla (brainstem)	a. Hearing
8. ____ Frontal lobe	b. Balance, coordination
9. ____ Precentral gyrus of frontal lobe (strip along central fissure in posterior part frontal lobe)	c. Relay center for sensory impulses d. Voluntary muscle movements e. Vital-organ functions—heartbeat, respiration
10. ____ Occipital lobe	f. Reception of fine sensory stimuli
11. ____ Temporal lobe	g. Sight
12. ____ Parietal lobe (strip along central fissure)	h. Intellect, memory, thought

13. ____ Cerebellum

14. ____ Thalamus

Directions: Circle the letter preceding each item below that correctly answers the question or completes the statement. More than one answer may be correct.

15. During a cranial nerve examination, which of the following *may* be abnormal if there is damage to the medulla?
a. Pupillary reflex *b.* Gag reflex *c.* Corneal reflex *d.* Patient's ability to shrug shoulders

16. During a cranial nerve examination, Mr. B. demonstrates the ability to smile without any apparent impairment but indicates that he is unable to chew. Where do you suspect the problem to be?
a. Abducent (VI) *b.* Facial (VII) *c.* Trigeminal (V) *d.* Vestibulocochlear (VIII) *e.* Trochlear (IV)

17. Which of the following cranial nerves is responsible for vision?
a. Olfactory (I) *b.* Optic (II) *c.* Oculomotor (III) *d.* Facial (VII)

18. Mrs. Jones presents with a dilated left pupil, left ptosis (drooping of the eyelid), and inability to look up, down, or medially with her left eye. These signs indicate a problem with:
a. Right optic nerve *b.* Left optic nerve *c.* Left oculomotor nerve *d.* Left trochlear nerve *e.* Left abducent nerve

19. On neurologic examination a Babinski reflex was demonstrated. Which of the following best describes this reflex?
a. Extension of the leg when the patellar tendon is struck *b.* Tremor of the foot following brisk, forcible dorsiflexion *c.* Dorsiflexion of the great toe when the sole is stroked *d.* Flexion of the forearm when the biceps tendon is tapped

20. Mr. J. has an extensive tumor of the cerebellum. In view of the functions of this organ, which symptom would you expect to observe?
a. Absence of the knee jerk and other reflexes *b.* Inability to execute smooth, precise movements *c.* Inability to respond to verbal commands *d.* All the above

21. Reflex activity of the central nervous system:

a. Requires at least two nerve cells b. Is a simple process in higher mammals c. Requires more than three nerve cells to become activated d. Is a mechanical process

22. In the patellar reflex, efferent impulses originate from cell bodies located in the:
a. White matter of the spinal cord b. Ventral gray column of the spinal cord c. Dorsal root spinal ganglion d. Ventral root spinal ganglion

23. A lesion in the corticospinal tract may cause:
a. Problems with visual acuity b. Weakness with decreased reflexes c. Weakness with increased reflexes d. Problems with auditory reflexes

24. A lesion in the lateral spinothalamic tract may cause:
a. Weakness with increased reflexes b. Problems with perception of pain and temperature c. Problems with perception of movement of joint d. Problems with integration of movement

Directions: Match each testing procedure in col. B with the correct cranial nerve in col. A.

Column A
25. ____ Optic (II)
26. ____ Trigeminal (V)
27. ____ Facial (VII)
28. ____ Vestibulocochlear (VIII)
29. ____ Oculomotor (III)
30. ____ Glossopharyngeal (IX)
31. ____ Vagus (X)
32. ____ Accessory (XI)
33. ____ Olfactory (I)

Column B
a. Occlude one nostril with digital compression; have patient indicate when odor is first detected and, if possible, identify substance.
b. Have patient say "ah" in order to note phonation and symmetry of the soft palate.
c. Test positional sense.
d. Cover one of the patient's eyes and bring finger into visual field.
e. Test gag reflex.
f. Have patient raise eyebrows, frown, close eyes, and tightly close eyes; observe symmetry.
g. Test for conductive versus sensorineural hearing loss.
h. Ask patient to shrug shoulders and turn head with and without resistance.
i. Have patient clench teeth; palpate masseters for tension.
j. Check for ptosis of lids and note equality of pupils.

Directions: Match the cranial nerves in col. A with responses indicating abnormality of the respective cranial nerves from col. B.

Column A
34. ____ Trigeminal (V)
35. ____ Glossopharyngeal, vagus (IX, X)
36. ____ Oculomotor (III)
37. ____ Accessory (XI)

Column B
a. Dilatation of the pupil, decreased reaction to light
b. Loss of corneal reflex when cotton wisp is touched to cornea
c. Absence of gag reflex when tongue blade is touched to posterior pharynx
d. Inability to shrug the shoulders
e. Deviation of protruding tongue toward the weak side (muscle atrophy also present on the paralyzed side)

Directions: Answer the following on a separate sheet of paper.

38. List the four areas that are investigated when examining the sensory system.

Directions: Circle the letter preceding each item below that correctly answers the question or completes the statement. More than one answer may be correct.

39. Conductive hearing loss is defined as:
a. Hearing loss of old age b. Person is able to hear better through bone conduction than through air conduction c. Similar to nerve-type hearing loss d. Involves the inner ear

40. When Mrs. T. had her Weber test (a vibrating tuning fork placed at the midpoint of the top of the head), she stated that she heard the sound better in her right ear. Normally, during a Weber test, the patient should hear the sound equally in both ears. Mrs. T.'s abnormal results could be due to a:
a. Sensorineural hearing loss in the left ear
b. Sensorineural hearing loss in the right ear
c. Conductive hearing loss in the right ear
d. Mixed hearing loss in the right ear

41. A Rinne test is then performed on Mrs. T.'s right ear. She hears the tuning fork better when it is

placed on her mastoid bone than when it is placed in front of her pinna. Which type of hearing loss does this suggest?
a. Conductive   b. Sensorineural

Directions: Circle T if the statement is true and F if it is false. Correct the false statements.

42.   T   F   Caloric tests are used in the diagnosis of disorders of the vestibular system.

43.   T   F   A lesion of the lower motor neuron results in a spastic paralysis and hyperactive reflexes.

44.   T   F   When reporting the evaluation of a patient's level of consciousness, one should describe behavior exactly rather than use terms such as *coma* or *stupor*.

Directions: Fill in the blanks with the correct word or words.

45. Interruption of the proprioceptive fibers as in tabes dorsalis (syphilitic infection of the brain and spinal cord) may cause inability to maintain balance when standing with the eyes closed. This is called a positive _____ sign.

46. A right-sided posterolateral herniated intervertebral disc compressing the _____ spinal cord roots might be expected to produce numbness over the lateral aspect of the right foot.

CHAPTER 48

CEREBROVASCULAR DISEASE AND HEADACHE

OBJECTIVES

At the completion of this chapter you should be able to:

1. Explain the importance of vascular disease as compared with other diseases of the nervous system.
2. Describe the historical significance of cerebrovascular disease.
3. State the approximate percentage of the total body weight constituted by the brain and the percentage of the total body oxygen supply utilized by the brain.
4. State how long the brain can survive without oxygen.
5. Describe the arterial blood supply to the brain.
6. Identify the major arteries that form the circle of Willis.
7. Describe the extrinsic (extracranial) factors and the intrinsic (intracranial) factors thought responsible for cerebral circulatory control.
8. Explain the significance of the mortality and morbidity effects of cerebrovascular accidents (strokes) in the United States.
9. List and describe the three types of stroke according to the chronological pattern of their clinical progression and regression of their signs and symptoms.
10. Identify for cerebral arteriosclerosis the characteristic degenerative process, arteries affected, progressive changes, and related diseases and conditions.
11. Describe the association of cerebral thrombosis with atherosclerosis as to etiology, onset, incidence of cerebral vascular accidents, age group most often affected, and prognosis.
12. Describe transient ischemic attacks (TIAs) by identifying the frequency of occurrence, associated symptoms, and prognosis.
13. Identify for cerebral embolism the etiology, incidence, age group most often affected, signs and symptoms, and prognosis.
14. Identify for cerebral hemorrhage the etiology, pathogenesis, incidence of cerebral vascular accidents, onset, neurologic findings, clinical features, age group affected according to vessel involved, and prognosis.
15. Describe for a saccular (berry) aneurysm the most common site of occurrence, signs and symptoms, treatment, and prognosis.

16. Describe the major clinical features associated with arterial insufficiency to the brain from the internal carotid artery; vertebral-basilar system; anterior, middle, and posterior cerebral arteries.

17. Explain the purpose and technique of (1) arteriography, (2) computerized tomography (CT scan), (3) brain scan, and (4) EEG

18. List four critical factors that must be considered in an acute care situation for cerebrovascular accidents (CVAs).

19. Describe the effectiveness of treatment modalities such as vasodilators, anticoagulants, and platelet antiaggregants in the treatment of CVAs.

20. Explain the primary goal of surgical intervention for stroke patients.

21. Describe the procedure and prognosis of these surgical treatments of stroke patients: carotid endarterectomy, revascularization, evacuation of blood clots, and aneurysmal surgery.

22. List the preventive measures (for risk factors associated with the development of a CVA) against cerebral vascular accidents.

23. List several structures and some general mechanisms that seem to be involved in headache.

24. List important points of information to be obtained during the history from a patient with a complaint of headache.

25. Describe the characteristics and treatment of two types of vascular headache: migraine and cluster headaches.

26. Discuss the mechanism, characteristics, and treatment of muscular contraction or tension headache.

27. List several disease conditions or functional abnormalities which may result in traction/inflammatory headache.

Vascular disease of the nervous system is the most commonly occurring neurologic disease. Cerebrovascular disease (or *apoplexy*, as it is called in Europe) was first described pathologically by Morgagni in 1761. The symptoms were assumed to be based on local causes. Not until early in the twentieth century were extracranial factors considered as a significant cause of cerebrovascular disease. Even then, nothing was done with this information until, in 1927, carotid arteriography was introduced by E. Moniz (in Lisbon). In the early 1950s, the importance of internal carotid artery occlusion was recognized as a factor in some cases of cerebral ischemia. Refinement of angiographic techniques and discovery of other valuable diagnostic tools have revolutionized care in certain stroke victims. In the early 1970s, new techniques were developed for the study of fresh cadaver brains. These techniques permitted study of cerebral vessels in extensive detail not possible with earlier methods. Lastly, the use of computed tomography (CT) with contrast media is considered extremely accurate for diagnosis of vascular disease.

The brain accounts for approximately 2 percent of the body's total weight. In a resting state the brain receives one-sixth of the cardiac output; it uses 20 percent of the body's oxygen. When cerebral ischemia occurs, neurons begin to undergo metabolic alterations. Within a period of 3 to 10 minutes the neurons may become totally inactive. Oxygen deprivation leading to loss of function is followed by destruction of the neuron.

When an isolated artery is stenosed, blood flow to the brain continues until the lumen of that vessel is narrowed by 80 percent. Successive stenoses, however, will be significant when the flow is decreased by a lesser amount. For example, if one carotid is occluded, a 50 percent decrease in flow through the other will produce neurologic deficits.

CEREBRAL CIRCULATION

As described in Chap. 46, the arterial blood to the brain is supplied by the two internal carotid arteries (anteriorly) and the two vertebral arteries (posteriorly). They arise from the aortic arch. On the right, the brachiocephalic trunk (innominate) artery divides into the right common carotid, which supplies the head, and the right subclavian artery, which supplies the arm. On the left side, the left common carotid and left subclavian arteries each arise directly from the aortic arch.

In general, the cerebral arteries are either conducting or penetrating. The conducting arteries (carotid and middle and anterior cerebral; vertebral, basilar, and posterior cerebral), and their branches form an extensive network over the surface of the brain. The penetrating arteries are nutrient vessels which are derived from the conducting arteries. These vessels enter the brain at right angles and provide blood to structures below the cortical level (the internal capsule, basal ganglia, etc.) (Fig. 48-1).

Circulation to the two hemispheres is generally symmetrical, with each side retaining its own separate blood supply. However, anomalies of the classic distribution are common and generally insignificant. When a problem arises, these anomalies can cause confusion when an attempt is made to correlate clinical findings with pathophysiologic phenomena.

Collateral circulation may gradually develop when normal flow to a part is decreased. Most cerebral collateral circulation between major arteries is via the circle of Willis. It has been estimated that anomalies in the circle of Willis occur in nearly half of the population. The brain also has collateral circulation sites, such as that between external and internal carotid arteries via the ophthalmic artery, that function only when other routes are impaired. Theoretically, these communicating channels are capable of providing an adequate blood supply to all areas of the brain. Practically, this is often not the case. A major vessel occlusion in one person will produce either no symptoms or a transient neurologic deficit; in another, the same occlusion site may cause a major loss of function. These differences would seem to be related to the state of the individual's collateral circulation.

The normal brain has the ability to regulate its own blood supply. "Normal" needs to be emphasized here, because pathologic states are capable of altering or even abolishing this autoregulatory mechanism. Exactly how this mechanism functions is not entirely clear. McHenry (1976) has arbitrarily divided factors that control cerebral circulation into extrinsic, or extracranial, and intrinsic, or intracranial:

Extrinsic (extracranial) factors	Intrinsic (intracranial) factors
1. Systemic blood pressure	1. Cerebral autoregulatory mechanisms related to cerebral perfusion pressure
2. Cardiovascular function	2. Cerebral blood vessels
3. Blood viscosity	3. Intracranial or cerebrospinal fluid pressure

The extrinsic factors regulating cerebral blood flow (CBF) are related primarily to the cardiovascular system.

If systemic mean blood pressure (BP) drops below 60 mmHg, the brain's autoregulatory mechanism becomes less effectual. The brain will initially attempt to compensate by extracting more oxygen from the available blood, but if the BP continues to drop until CBF is decreased to 30 ml per 100 g of tissue a minute, signs of cerebral ischemia will appear.

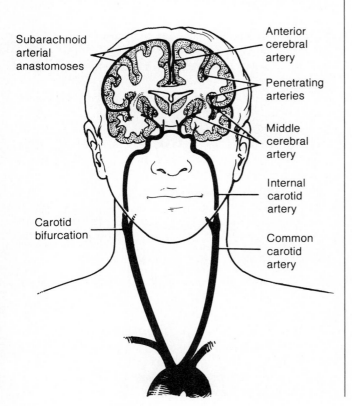

Subarachnoid arterial anastomoses

Anterior cerebral artery

Penetrating arteries

Middle cerebral artery

Internal carotid artery

Carotid bifurcation

Common carotid artery

FIGURE 48-1

Course of the internal carotid artery from the carotid bifurcation to its continuation as the middle cerebral artery. The penetrating lenticulostriate arteries arise from the first portion of the middle cerebral artery to supply the basal ganglia and internal capsule. These arteries are frequently implicated in a stroke syndrome. The middle cerebral artery continues to course over the cerebral hemisphere, sending short and deep penetrating arteries into the brain. The subarachnoid arterial anastomoses, which supply collateral circulation, are shown between the middle and anterior cerebral arteries. (Adapted from Smith, Kline, and French, _Essentials of Stroke and Diagnostic Management_, rev. ed., 1973.)

Cardiac arrythmias can change cardiac output. If cardiac output is decreased by more than one-third, there is often a fall in CBF.

The significance of blood viscosity is demonstrated by the fact that CBF may increase with anemia; in polycythemia it may decrease by 50 percent.

The intrinsic factors, as noted above, are three in number. McHenry calls the cerebral perfusion pressure the "driving force in cerebral circulation." It is the pressure difference between the cerebral arteries and veins. The CBF will remain constant (750 ml per minute) because of autoregulation even when systemic BP fluctuates. The range within which this mechanism can be effective is 150 to 60 mmHg for the systemic BP. When systemic BP falls, there is a compensatory decrease in cerebral vascular resistance. An elevation of BP results in an increase in cerebral vascular resistance.

The cerebral blood vessels are considered the most important factor relating to cerebrovascular resistance.

Recent microcirculatory studies have identified a myogenic response, suggesting that the parenchymal tissue of arterioles releases a vasodilating metabolite in response to their oxygen needs and thereby exerts control on arterial smooth muscle tone:

Decreased → decreased →
perfusion   CBF
pressure

        increased   vasodilatation
        accumulation of → with restora-
           metabolites   tion of blood
                         flow toward
                         normal

The third intrinisic factor regulating CBF is the intracranial pressure (ICP). An increase in ICP will increase cerebrovascular resistance. CBF does not decrease until ICP has increased to 450 mm water (normal range 60 to 180 mm water).

Three metabolic factors considered important (Guyton, 1977) are:

1. *CO_2 concentration.* High CO_2 tension is a potent vasodilator, possibly because of accumulation of CO_2 in vaso-motor centers. In normal subjects CO_2 inhalations have produced up to 75 percent increase in CBF (raising PCO_2 by 9 mmHg will raise CBF by 75 percent).

2. *H^+ concentration.* An increase in H^+ yields an increase in blood flow.

3. *O_2 concentration.* Low O_2 tension is a powerful vasodilator; high O_2 concentration is a moderate vasoconstrictor.

Gradual changes in CBF are resisted by the brain. The brain's ability to adapt and compensate is poorly understood but basic in determining the extent of damage sustained from circulatory disruption. The brain copes most effectively when the changes are gradual.

CEREBRAL VASCULAR ACCIDENTS

Cerebral vascular disease, or stroke, is, in general terms, a disturbance in cerebral circulation. It is a focal neurologic disorder. It may be secondary to a pathologic process within a cerebral blood vessel such as thrombosis, embolus, rupture of a vessel wall, or basic vascular disease such as atherosclerosis, arteritis, trauma, aneurysm, or developmental malformations.

Stroke is responsible for 200,000 deaths in the United States each year. It is the third most frequent cause of death in the country. One-half million Americans each year suffer a new, acute cerebral vascular accident (CVA). There are an estimated 2 million people in the United States today with neurologic deficit that is a result of stroke. About 50 percent of all adult neurologic hospital admissions are due to vascular disease.

The major causes of stroke, in order of importance, are atherosclerosis (thrombosis), embolism, hypertensive intracerebral hemorrhage, and ruptured saccular (berry) aneurysm. Stroke is generally accompanied by one or more associated medical problems such as hypertension, cardiac disease, elevated blood lipids, diabetes mellitus, or peripheral vascular disease.

The severity of the stroke process is variable. Some infarcts are found on autopsy after death from unrelated causes. (Of all adults examined post mortem, 80 to 90 percent have significant atheromatous disease.) In others the stroke is sudden and dramatic, with the patient literally being "struck down." In this latter form, hemiplegia and unconsciousness may both be evident.

Strokes may be categorized according to etiology or on the basis of their course. According to course, or temporal profile (which is defined as the chronological pattern of clinical progression and regression of signs and symptoms), strokes may be divided into three types:

1. *Transient ischemic attacks (TIAs).* These are focal neurologic deficits that develop suddenly and disappear within a few minutes to hours.

2. *Progressive (stroke in evolution).* Evolution of stroke is gradual though acute.

3. *Completed stroke.* Deficits are maximal at onset, with little improvement.

Major clinical features associated with arterial insufficiency to the brain (points of bifurcation or angulation are most vulnerable) may be focal and temporary, or the dysfunction may be permanent, with actual tissue death and neurologic deficit. It is difficult to establish a close correlation between symptoms associated with a particular vessel and actual clinical manifestations in a particular patient because:

1. There is individual variation of collateral circulation with regard to the circle of Willis (Fig. 48-2). Total occlusion of a carotid artery may give no symptoms if the left anterior cerebral and left middle cerebral arteries receive adequate blood from the anterior communicating artery. If this blood supply is not adequate, symptoms may include confusion, contralateral monoparesis or hemiparesis, and incontinence.

2. Leptomeningeal anastomoses are significant over the cerebral cortex between the anterior, middle, and posterior cerebral arteries. There are also anastomoses between the anterior cerebral arteries of the two hemispheres across the corpus callosum.

3. Each of the cerebral arteries has a central area to supply with blood and a peripheral supply area, or border area, which it may share with another artery. Anastomoses exist between external and internal carotid arteries, as around the orbit, with blood from external carotid vessels going to the ophthalmic artery.

4. Various systemic and metabolic factors are of significance in determining the symptoms that a particular pathologic process will produce. A stenosed vessel may produce no symptoms as long as systemic blood pressure is 190/110, but should it be reduced to 120/70, variable symptoms may result depending on the location of the stenotic area. Hyponatremia and hyperthermia are metabolic factors that facilitate development of neurologic deficits in the presence of stenotic blood vessels.

Major clinical features associated with arterial insufficiency to the brain may be associated with the following signs and symptoms:

1. *Vertebral-basilar* (posterior circulation—manifestations usually bilateral)
   a. Weakness in one to four extremities
   b. Increased tendon reflexes
   c. Ataxia

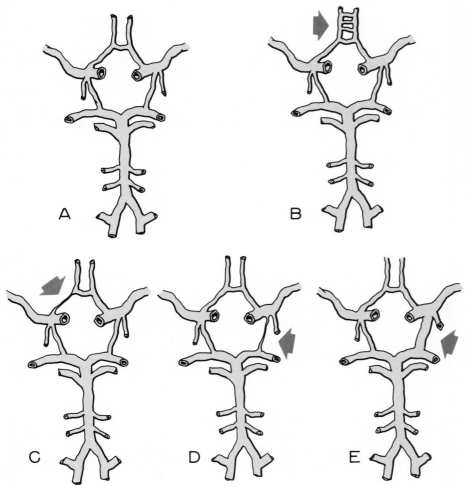

FIGURE 48-2
The circle of Willis and some common anatomic variations. The anomalies are indicated by arrows. (A) Normal circle of Willis. (B) Reduplication of the anterior communicating artery. (C) Stringlike anterior cerebral artery. (D) Stringlike posterior cerebral artery. (E) Embryonic derivation of posterior cerebral artery from the internal carotid artery. (Modified from Alpers et al., 1959.)

    d. Bilateral Babinski sign

    e. Cerebellar signs

    f. Dysphagia

    g. Dysarthria

    h. Syncope, stupor, coma, dizziness, memory disturbances

    i. Visual disturbances (diplopia, nystagmus, ptosis, paralysis of single eye movements)

    j. Numbness of face

2. *Internal carotid artery* (anterior circulation—symptoms usually unilateral). Most common location of lesion is the bifurcation of the common carotid into the internal and external carotid. Branches of the internal carotid are the ophthalmic, posterior communicating, anterior choroidal, anterior cerebral, and middle cerebral. Variable syndromes may develop. The pattern depends on the amount of collateral circulation

    a. *Monocular blindness*, episodic and called *amaurosis fugax*, on the side of involved carotid; it is due to retinal artery insufficiency. Sensory and motor symptoms involve contralateral extremities because of middle cerebral artery insufficiency.

    b. Lesion in the area between the anterior and middle cerebral arteries or the middle cerebral artery: symptoms will initially develop in upper extremities (weak, numb hand), and may involve the face—supranuclear-type weakness. If the lesion is in the dominant hemisphere, expressive aphasia occurs (because of the involvement of Broca's motor-speech area).

3. *Anterior cerebral artery* (confusion is the primary symptom)

    a. Contralateral weakness greater in leg. Proximal arm may also be involved. Voluntary movement of that leg impaired

    b. Contralateral sensory deficits

    c. Dementia, grasp, pathologic reflexes (frontal lobe dysfunction)

4. *Posterior cerebral artery* (in lobe of midbrain or thalamus)

    a. Coma

    b. Contralateral hemiparesis

    c. Visual aphasia or word blindness (alexia)

    d. Third cranial nerve palsy—hemianopsia, choreoathetosis

5. *Middle cerebral artery*

    a. Contralateral monoparesis or hemiparesis (usually affecting arm)

    b. Occasional contralateral hemianopsia (blindness)

    c. Global aphasia (if *dominant* hemisphere is involved)—disturbance of all functions involving speech and communication

    d. Dysphasia

Etiology

Thrombosis

Thrombosis (thrombocclusive disease) is the most common cause of stroke. It accounts for about 40 percent of all pathologically verified strokes. It is usually associated with local damage to the blood vessel wall caused by atherosclerosis.

The *atherosclerotic process* is characterized by fatty plaques which involve the intima of large arteries. The intima of the cerebral artery becomes thin and fibrous, with loss of muscle cells. The internal elastic lamina is split and frayed, and sclerotic material partly fills the lumen of the vessel.

The plaques show a tendency to form at branchings and curves. Thrombi are also associated with these specific sites. The blood vessels at risk, in decreasing order, are the internal carotid, upper vertebral, and lower basilar. The connective tissue is exposed from loss of the intima. Platelets adhere to this exposed, roughened surface. They release an enzyme, adenosine diphosphate, which initiates the coagulation mechanism. This fibrinoplatelet plug may break off and embolize, or it may remain in place and eventually cause complete occlusion of the artery (Fig. 48-3).

Cerebral thrombosis is a disease of older age groups; the peak age of occurrence is 60 to 69 years. In addition to atherosclerosis, hypertension appears to be an important underlying factor (Mancall, 1975).

The onset of progression of symptoms tends to occur during sleep or soon after arising. Maximum intensity is generally realized within 48 hours. Progression is generally stepwise (a series of sudden changes) rather than smooth. Postural hypotension is more common in patients with cerebrovascular disease than in normal controls, possibly because of interference with the baroreceptor reflex. The pressor response to the Valsalva maneuver is often absent in the aged with atherosclerosis. Recumbency even for a night's rest can decrease sympathetic activity and lower blood pressure in the elderly. Additional factors, such as sedation or prolonged rest, can seriously compromise their precarious position.

Transient ischemic attacks (TIAs) are episodes of neurologic dysfunction that are usually of short duration (a few minutes) but may persist for 24 hours. TIAs involving the carotid arterial system last on the average about 14 minutes. Those involving the basilar-vertebral system last for about 7 minutes. TIAs are reversible, and the symptom pattern is the same with each attack, because the same vessel is involved. This is an important observation in terms of differential diagnosis, since small emboli from diseased heart valves might give similar symptoms but there would be no consistent pattern, because different blood vessels might be involved each time. Other problems, besides cardiac emboli, that may initially be misdiagnosed as TIA include small strokes, seizures, migraine syndromes, postural hypotension, and Stokes-Adams syndrome.

Some TIAs seem to be related to vascular stenosis due to atherosclerosis of the large arteries of the neck and less often the intracranial arteries. TIAs are more frequent in males than in females (2:1). They are less common in blacks than in whites (although completed strokes are more common in blacks).

Additional research is necessary to establish the relation between TIAs and strokes. In the recent past this relationship seemed to be clear-cut, with 30 to 70 percent of patients reporting a history of TIAs prior to stroke. The validity of these data is now being questioned, and there is diverse opinion concerning the risk of cerebrovascular accident when there is a history of TIAs.

Anoxic encephalopathy may occur with cerebral thrombosis. Symptoms and the clinical picture are dependent on the location. The brain distal to the clot becomes swollen. There may be discoloration, with the appearance being muddy-looking. There is a loss of demarcation between the gray and white matter. As time passes, nerve cells disintegrate and are replaced by glia.

Pathologically, these infarcts may be classified as bland or ischemic, because the infarct is arterial and does not have blood flowing into it (see Fig. 3-6).

Embolism

Cerebral embolism is the second most common cause of stroke. The patients are younger than those with thrombosis. Most cerebral emboli originate from a thrombus in the heart, so this problem is essentially a manifestation of heart disease. Less frequently the embolus originates from an atheromatous plaque in the carotid sinus or internal carotid artery. Any area of the brain may be involved, but generally the embolus will lodge at a narrow area. The middle cerebral artery, especially the upper division, is the most frequent site of cerebral emboli.

Symptoms may occur at any time, and they are rapidly progressive. Symptoms of small emboli differ from those of TIAs in that the latter tend to recur with the same clinical picture each time (same vessel or vessels involved). With numerous small emboli (as from a chronic atrial fibrillation), the pattern varies with each episode, depending upon the vessels involved.

In general, there is a greater amount of tissue death with emboli than with more gradually occurring situations, because anastomotic vessels do not have time to dilate and thus compensate.

Cerebral hemorrhage

Cerebral hemorrhage is the third most frequent cause of CVA, accounting for one-tenth of all cases. Ruptured cerebral arteries are the usual source of intracranial bleeding. Extravasation of blood occurs in the brain and/or subarachnoid space. Adjacent tissue may be displaced and compressed. Blood is particularly irritating to brain tissue, causing vasospasm in arteries adjacent to the bleeding site. This spasm may spread to the entire hemisphere and circle of Willis. The clot,

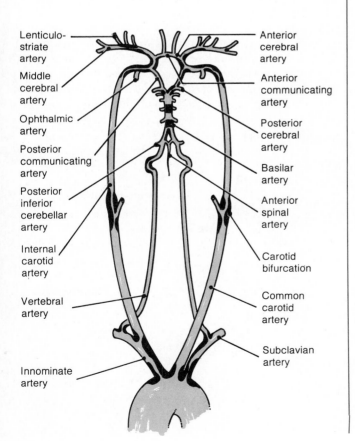

Lenticulo-
striate
artery

Middle
cerebral
artery

Ophthalmic
artery

Posterior
communicating
artery

Posterior
inferior
cerebellar
artery

Internal
carotid
artery

Vertebral
artery

Innominate
artery

Anterior
cerebral
artery

Anterior
communicating
artery

Posterior
cerebral
artery

Basilar
artery

Anterior
spinal
artery

Carotid
bifurcation

Common
carotid
artery

Subclavian
artery

FIGURE 48-3

Extracranial and intracranial arteries supplying blood to the brain. The circle of Willis and its principal branches are also shown. The sites of atherosclerosis of the cerebral blood vessels are designated, the main locations being the carotid bifurcation and the takeoff of the branches from the aorta, innominate, and subclavian arteries. These are the sites that are amenable to surgery. (Redrawn from Smith, Kline, and French, *Essentials of Stroke and Diagnostic Management*, rev. ed., 1973.)

which is originally soft and resembles red currant jelly, eventually resolves and decreases in size. Histologically, the brain adjacent to the clot may be swollen and necrotic. Through enzymatic action, liquefaction occurs and a cavity forms. Over a period of several months all necrotic tissue is replaced. Astrocytes and new capillaries form a weavelike pattern in the cavity. Eventually, astroglial fibers proliferate and fill in the cavity.

Subarachnoid hemorrhage is often associated with a rupture of an aneurysm. The majority of aneurysms involve a vessel in the circle of Willis. Hypertension or a bleeding disorder may contribute to the occurrence of rupture. Often, more than one aneurysm is present.

Neurologic findings are dependent upon the site and severity of the hemorrhage. The vessel involved is usually a penetrating artery such as one of the lenticulostriate branches of the middle cerebral artery which supply some of the basal ganglia and most of the internal capsule.

The onset is abrupt and evolution rapid and steady, lasting minutes, hours, and occasionally days.

Frequently the clinical features include severe headache, nuchal rigidity, vomiting, stupor, coma, and convulsions. Cerebrospinal fluid is bloody in 90 percent of patients (when hemorrhage is small and away from the ventricles, it may be clear). Of these patients, 70 to 75 percent die in 1 to 30 days, generally from hemorrhage extending into the ventricular system, temporal lobe herniation and midbrain compression, or seepage into vital centers.

Cerebrovascular hemorrhage patients may do well if a vital center is not involved. An area in the cerebral hemisphere may tolerate a relatively large accumulation of blood (100 ml) with no significant clinical manifestations, while a 5-ml clot in the brainstem may be lethal (see Fig. 7-3).

When cerebral hemorrhage occurs because of a ruptured aneurysm, the patients are generally young, and 20 percent have more than one aneurysm. As noted earlier, most cerebral aneurysms are located in the circle of Willis.

Saccular (or berry) aneurysms can be smaller than a pinhead or 2 to 3 cm in diameter. They are frequently the size of a pea and arise at or close to points of divisions of an artery. These aneurysms are thin-walled (covered only by intima) blisters protruding from the artery at a point where a local weakness exists. They gradually enlarge, and rupture can occur. Often they are asymptomatic until they rupture. Generally, rupture occurs during activity. The usual clinical pictures include sudden violent headache, "like something snapped in my head"; collapse; brief unconsciousness and confusion; no warning symptoms; and few, if any, lateralizing signs. An outstanding feature of aneurysms is their tendency to rebleed (Fig. 48-4).

Diagnosis

A thorough history and physical examination should be carried out on all patients with cerebrovascular disease. An inadequate history may result in diagnostic error. Neither the patient nor the family may be able to recall when the initial symptoms started. The specific type of stroke should be determined. Contributory diseases need to be identified and treated.

Two significant phenomena that are characteristic of all varieties of stroke are (1) the temporal profile: suddenness of evolution, especially, marks the event as vascular, along with the finding of some degree of improvement following stabilization; and (2) focal or lateralizing neurologic signs. Hemiplegia is the classic sign of stroke and is found in lesions involving the cerebral hemispheres or brainstem.

Angiography

With the clinical diagnosis of cerebrovascular disease, arteriography is essential to demonstrate the cause and site. Practically all intracranial vascular areas, from the aorta on up, may be visualized. Special magnification and stereoscopic techniques have increased the diagnostic and localizing capabilities of these studies. The medium used is less toxic and irritating than in the past.

Direct punctures into the carotid artery are avoided whenever possible, as they may result in a disruption of

FIGURE 48-4

The common sites of saccular (berry) aneurysms. Each is drawn in direct proportion to the frequency at that site. (From F. McDowell, in Beeson and McDermott, 1979, p. 795.)

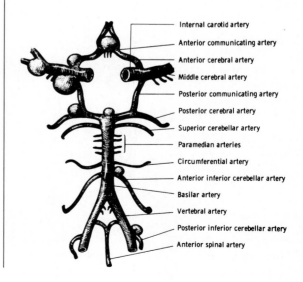

Internal carotid artery
Anterior communicating artery
Anterior cerebral artery
Middle cerebral artery
Posterior communicating artery
Posterior cerebral artery
Superior cerebellar artery
Paramedian arteries
Circumferential artery
Anterior inferior cerebellar artery
Basilar artery
Vertebral artery
Posterior inferior cerebellar artery
Anterior spinal artery

plaque formation and consequent emboli. Extravasation in this area can also result in respiratory difficulty. Instead, the femoral arteries are used. Typically, a catheter is threaded, under fluoroscopy, from the femoral artery in the groin to the appropriate artery (carotid), and dye is then injected.

Computerized tomography (CT scan) is a valuable diagnostic tool for demonstrating hematomas, infarcts, and hemorrhage. It is totally reliable in diagnosing lesions 1.5 cm or more in diameter. It is completely non-invasive if done without contrast media. The device consists of a rotating x-ray tube with a recorder, a digital readout system, and an oscilloscope with a Polaroid camera. CT scan depends on the difference in densities between x-rays absorbed by normal and by damaged tissue. It is safe and rapid and seems accurate.

Brain scans are good as a screening device, and if the lesion has damaged the blood-brain barrier, the isotope may localize in the area. It is best for lesions near the surface. Scans are safe and can be repeated as desired.

Electroencephalograms (EEG) may assist in localization. The delta waves are slower over the affected area.

Treatment

In the acute care situation the critical factors to be considered are:

1. Stabilization of vital signs, which entails (a) maintaining a patent airway (frequent and deep suctioning, O₂, tracheotomy, respiratory assistance if brainstem is involved), and (b) blood pressure control on an individualized basis. This entails correcting hypotension as well as hypertension.

2. Detection and correction of cardiac arrhythmias.

3. Bladder care. When feasible, indwelling catheters are avoided. They have been replaced by in-out catheterizations every 4 to 6 hours.

4. Proper positioning is stressed immediately. The patient should be turned every hour and passive range of motion (ROM) exercises instituted every 2 hours. Within a few days full ROM to a total of 50 times per day is recommended. This is necessary to avoid pressure areas and contractures (especially at shoulder, elbow, and ankle).

No single method of treatment is consistently useful. Several modes of therapy seem useful, but mortality rates have not improved.

FIGURE 48-5
Diagram of a carotid endarterectomy, A bypass tube is used during the removal of an atherosclerotic lesion at the carotid bifurcation. (From Smith, Kline, and French, *Essentials of Stroke and Diagnostic Management,* **rev. ed., 1973.)**

Conservative Treatment

Vasodilators have increased cerebral blood flow (CBF) experimentally but have not proved beneficial in human strokes. Effective dilators of vessels in other areas of the body have little or no effect on cerebral vessels, especially when used orally (nicotinic acid, tolazoline, papaverine, etc.). On the basis of a few clinical trials the following have been suggested as useful: histamine, aminophylline, acetazolamide, intraarterial papaverine.

The use of vasodilators may also exert an adverse effect on CBF by lowering systemic BP and thereby decreasing intracerebral anastomotic flow.

Platelet antiaggregants such as aspirin are used to inhibit the platelet aggregation-release reaction which occurs after ulceration of an atheroma. Many patients and people at risk for developing clots are currently taking 10 gr of aspirin once or twice a day (in some cases once every other day) for prophylaxis against platelet aggregation.

Surgical therapy

Several surgical procedures are now being utilized in stroke clients. The proper selection of the individual who will most benefit from surgery remains a most difficult task. Improving cerebral blood flow is the primary goal of surgical intervention.

Carotid endarterectomy is done to improve cerebral circulation (Fig. 48-5). Patients undergoing this pro-

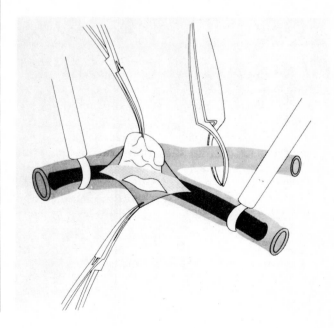

cedure frequently have other complicating problems such as hypertension, diabetes, and widespread cardiovascular disease. The procedure is done under general anesthesia so that good airway and ventilatory control can be maintained. A temporary shunt is used in order to minimize ischemia to the brain. It is essential to maintain a normal or slightly high arterial blood pressure in order to maintain adequate cerebral circulation, since regional blood flow in these patients is directly proportional to the systemic arterial pressure.

In the 1960s, with the use of stereoscopic microscopes and microsuturing techniques, patent anastomoses were successfully performed through the revascularization procedure. Revascularization procedures are being done to increase regional blood flow to areas where circulation is being compromised. Various vessels can be utilized. Commonly, the superficial temporal artery is anastomosed to a superficial cortical artery. In another procedure (the subclavian–external carotid bypass graft), a segment of the saphenous vein is anastomosed to the subclavian artery and the proximal end of the external carotid. Revascularization is primarily a prophylactic procedure and is most likely to benefit clients with TIAs or those who are at an early stage in the course of a thrombosis-in-evolution. Patients manifesting fixed neurologic deficits can expect no benefit from these procedures and are not considered appropriate candidates.

Evacuation of blood clots is seldom beneficial in the acute stage of stroke. Exceptions to this are surface lesions where the client is conscious and some cerebellar hemorrhages where surgical evacuation of the clot has led to improvement.

Surgical intervention in the case of aneurysms is directed toward prevention of a recurrence of the hemorrhage. Ligation of the common carotid artery in the neck is the most conservative treatment of aneurysm.

Intracranial procedures such as clipping or ligating the neck of the aneurysm necessitate major neurosurgical intervention. Aneurysms can also be painted with a physiologic glue which provides an elastic cap and keeps them from rupturing. Before surgery can be undertaken, arteriograms are necessary. Arteriograms are a serious threat to the patient because, first, the dye, like the original free blood, can cause vasospasm due to irritation. Second, the pressure necessary to insert the dye may cause rebleeding in the newly ruptured area. The patient must be stabilized before surgery. The vasospasm must be resolved or minimal. Toward this end, the patient is placed on an aneurysm protocol which may include the following precautions adapted to the individual patient:

Darkened room. No rectal temperatures (may stimulate vagus and elevate blood pressure).

Phenobarbital 30 mg IV every 6 hours to decrease possibility of seizures.

Dexamethasone (Decadron) 20 mg IV every 6 hours for its diuretic effect. It seems to protect the brain by stabilizing cerebral membranes and decreasing cerebral edema.

Cimetidine (Tagamet) 300 mg IV every 6 hours to prevent the gastrointestinal irritation which may be a side effect of dexamethasone administration.

Aminocaproic acid (Amicar) 2 g IV every 6 hours to prevent lysis of the clot. Amicar levels, streptokinase levels, and clot lysis times are monitored daily with this medicine.

Hydralazine hydrochloride (Apresoline) 5 mg every 3 hours if blood pressure is more than 140 mmHG systolic.

Fluid restriction based on serum osmolality; may be as severe as 800 to 1200 ml per 24 hours.

Various shunt procedures may be done (ventriculoatrial shunt) if obstructive hydrocephalus is an overriding concern. Free blood in the subarachnoid space may obstruct cerebrospinal fluid circulation and cause acute hydrocephalus. Shunts are done more frequently than in the past and have all but replaced the decompression craniotomies that were formerly done to reduce the symptoms of increased intracranial pressure.

Preventive measures

In a 24-year follow-up study by the American Heart Association involving 5184 men and women (ages 30 to 62 years at entry into the study), 345 had suffered strokes; 60 percent of these had suffered thrombosis (called *atherothrombotic brain infarction,* or ABI, in this work). Unlike other manifestations of atherosclerosis, ABI occurs equally among men and women. The most important risk factor identified was hypertension, which was even more dangerous when coupled with other factors such as diabetes, left ventricular hypertrophy identified by ECG, elevated blood cholesterol level, cigarette smoking, and cardiac impairments. This study cites the control of blood pressure as the key to ABI prevention (American Heart Association, 1977).

Several other general preventive measures can be identified:

1. Decrease in salt intake—beginning in early life with salt-free or low salt baby food.
2. Especially with the elderly, extreme care to maintain blood pressure during surgical procedures; avoid oversedation and prolonged bed rest.
3. Increased activity—daily walking as part of a fitness program.

4. Decrease in weight if overweight.
5. Discontinuance of cigarette smoking.
6. Discontinuance of oral contraceptive use by women who smoke, since the risk of cerebrovascular problems in a woman who smokes and takes an oral contraceptive is increased 16 times over that of a woman who does neither.

HEADACHE (CEPHALGIA)

Headache is a common symptom that nearly all people experience, at least episodically, during their lifespan. Headache may be part of a sequela related to increased intracranial pressure, head injury, brain tumor, eyestrain, sinusitis, changes in atmosphere, food allergies, etc. The list of possible etiologic factors is inexhaustible. Three basic types of headache are discussed here: (1) vascular (migraine and cluster headache), (2) muscular contraction (also called *psychogenic* or *tension headache*), and (3) traction inflammatory headache (usually secondary to an organic disease process).

General considerations

Pain-sensitive cranial structures which may be involved in headache include all the extracranial tissues, among them skin, scalp, muscles, arteries, and periosteum of the skull; cranial sinuses; intracranial venous sinuses and their tributary veins; parts of the dura at the base of the brain and the arteries within the dura; and the trigeminal, facial, vagus, and glossopharyngeal cranial nerves and the cervical nerves (C2 and C3). The brain parenchyma, much of the meningeal tissue, and the skull (except for the periosteum) are insensitive to pain. Periosteal stretch may cause local pain.

The tentorium is a sheet of dura that serves as a line of demarcation and point of reference within the cranium. It separates the posterior fossa (brainstem and cerebellum) from the anterior cerebrum (see Fig. 46-6). The posterior area (about one-third of the cranial cavity) is referred to as *infratentorial,* and the anterior area (two-thirds of the cranial cavity) is referred to as *supratentorial.*

When head pain involves structures in the infratentorial area, it is referred to the occipital area of the head and neck by the upper cervical nerve roots. Supratentorial pain occurs in the anterior portion of the head (frontal, temporal, and parietal areas) and is mediated largely by the trigeminal nerve.

Some general mechanisms that seem to be responsible for evoking headache include:

Distention or displacement of blood vessels: intra- or extracranial

Traction of blood vessels

Contraction of head and neck muscles (muscular overaction)

Stretching of periosteum (local pain)

Degeneration of the upper cervical spine with compression of cervical nerve roots (e.g., arthritis of the cervical vertebrae)

Deficiency of enkephalins (opiate-like brain peptides; active ingredient of endorphins; (Lance, 1978, p. 6)

The sympathetic nervous system is basically responsible for neural control of the cranial and extracranial blood vessels.

A thorough assessment of the patient with a complaint of headache necessitates compiling a history which should include the following points:

1. What, if anything, brings on the headache (precipitating factors)?
2. When was the onset (number of years, medical conditions, past head injury)?
3. Any early warnings (prodromal symptoms)?
4. Headache alone or associated features such as nausea, vomiting, dizziness, photophobia, blurred vision?
5. Subjective description of headache (quality, location, frequency, time of day, duration, precipitating factors, relieving factors).
6. Does anyone else in the family have headache or similar symptoms?

Thus, in a majority of patients, a clinical pattern may be established.

Vascular headache

Vascular headaches include the migraine, cluster, toxic vascular, and hypertensive varieties. Because of their vascular origin, they tend to throb with the pulse.

Migraine headache is the prototype, a throbbing vascular headache involving vasodilatation and probably a localized inflammation which sensitizes the arteries to pain. Cerebral blood flow is decreased during the period prior to the onset and increased during the actual headache.

A current hypothesis postulates that the early vasoconstriction and subsequent vasodilatation are induced by a release of biogenic amines such as serotonin, norepinephrine, and epinephrine in persons with a genetic predisposition to vascular hypersensitivity. There is an increased excretion of the degradation products of these amines during a migraine headache in some patients. A corresponding decrease in the blood serotonin levels has also been found. Since these amines are powerful vasoconstrictors, they may be responsible for the prodromal vasoconstriction. After their release, degradation, and depletion, a reactive hyperemia could account for the vasodilatation during the migraine attack. This hypothesis is supported by the fact that (1) the administration of reserpine, a drug which depletes serotonin levels in brain tissue and platelets, may induce a migraine attack; (2) the injection of serotonin may relieve migraine headache; and (3) the administration of methysergide, a serotonin antagonist, may prevent migraine in many instances.

Another vasoactive substance which has been implicated in migraine is *neurokinin*, a polypeptide similar to bradykinin. Neurokinin has been found in the fluid which collects around the involved cranial artery during a migraine attack and may be responsible for the inflammatory response.

There are two types of migraine headache. The *classic migraine* has a preheadache or prodromal phase associated with neurologic symptoms such as visual disturbances, paresthesias or paresis on one side of the body, or a slight speech disturbance. These symptoms are believed to be caused by intense vasoconstriction. In about 15 minutes the prodromal phase is followed by the onset of a unilateral headache and sometimes nausea and vomiting. The *common migraine* does not have a prodromal or vasoconstrictive phase prior to the onset.

Migraine headache is more common in women and most often begins before age 40. Seventy percent of patients have a positive family history. Attacks are more likely to occur when the patient becomes overly tired and fatigued. The majority of women have their attacks at some time related to menstruation (prior to, during, or at the end). During pregnancy most are without headache by the third month. A small number experience their initial attack during a pregnancy. Oral contraceptives usually increase the problem, as does hormone therapy in the postmenopausal patient.

The majority of patients experience a unilateral headache that is initially a dull ache and finally a throbbing or pulsating pain which may become bilateral. The frontal and temporal areas are the most frequently involved sites. However, the pain may occur behind the eye and in other regions of the face and neck. Two to four attacks per month, usually lasting 1 or 2 days, are most common.

Manifestations frequently accompanying migraines include photophobia, increased sensitivity to noise, vascular changes (cold hands and feet, pale skin), increased weight, and hyperesthesia of the scalp.

Treatment of migraine has traditionally been by use of vasoconstrictor substances, specifically ergot alkaloids (ergotamine tartrate). Cafergot, a combination of caffeine and ergotamine, is also used. Other vasoconstrictors used in an attempt to prevent headaches or lessen the number a patient may be experiencing are methysergide (Sansert) and cyproheptadine (Periactin). Propranolol (Inderal), a beta-adrenergic blocking agent, is now being used experimentally to decrease the vasodilatory response. Another beta blocker, cimetidine (Tagamet), is also under investigation for use with migraine.

The other important vascular headache, although far less common than migraine, is the *cluster headache* (other synonyms include *migrainous headache, histamine headache, Horton's headache,* and *paroxysmal nocturnal neuralgia*). It is so named because it tends to occur nightly for a few weeks or months (clusters), then not to occur for a period of years.

Cluster headaches occur much more frequently in men than in women. The characteristic pain is constant, severe, nonthrobbing, and unilateral and is often localized to the eye or side of the face. The onset is characteristically two or three hours after falling asleep and is apparently associated with REM sleep. It lasts from minutes to hours and is associated with conjunctival injection, lacrimation, blocked nostril, and sometimes flushing of the cheek on the affected side. Alcohol is often mentioned as a precipitating factor if drinking occurs during a headache-prone period. The ophthalmic and extracranial arteries and the facial and scalp capillaries are usually dilated, while the internal carotid is narrowed.

At the peak of the headache, the pain is intolerable and incapacitating. In contrast to the person with migraine, the cluster headache victim paces the floor restlessly and is unable to lie down or sit still. Many persons have even contemplated suicide. Ergotamine tartrate and methylsergide are both used for treatment. Prednisone and lithium carbonate have also been used successfully in the treatment of cluster headaches. Generally, however, the condition is difficult to treat.

Muscular contraction headache (tension headache)

Muscular contraction, or tension, headache produces pain by a sustained contraction of the scalp, forehead, and neck muscles that is accompanied by extracranial vasoconstriction. The pain is characterized by a band-like tightness around the head and tenderness of the occipitocervical area. This type of headache is very common. The acute form is associated with conditions of temporary stress, anxiety, and/or fatigue generally lasting a day or two. The chronic tension headache is more common in women and is typically bilateral, unremitting (occurring during both day and night and lasting from months to years), dull, nonpulsating, and often associated with anxiety, depression, and repressed feelings.

Ideally medications should not be prescribed for the person with chronic tension headache. Analgesics may be abused and may lead to tolerance (renal failure occurs in some persons who abuse phenacetin; see Chap. 42). Tranquilizers are probably not beneficial and may actually increase the depression. In patients who are tense and anxious, diazepam (Valium) 5 mg tid for 1 month may be effective. If the patient is also depressed, the tricyclic antidepressant drug amitryptyline (Elavil) 25 mg tid is added. In some headache treatment centers, tricyclic antidepressants are being used alone and are effective in increasing cerebral norepinephrine. Biofeedback, relaxation, self-hypnosis, and other conditioning techniques have been beneficial to some patients with headache and are expected to play an increasing role in therapy in the near future.

Traction inflammatory headache

Traction inflammatory headache is usually secondary to organic disease. Masses of any origin (tumor, blood clot, abscess, etc.) may cause traction and displacement of pain-sensitive structures. Headache is the outstanding symptom of a brain tumor (primary or metastatic), and as the tumor grows the pain becomes more frequent and severe. Headache, vertigo, and other localizing neurologic signs are the usual manifestation of chronic subdural hematoma. A rapidly expanding intracranial mass causing increased intracranial pressure may displace cerebral structures, resulting in headache.

Headache is a symptom associated with many inflammatory processes. Meningitis, encephalitis, infection of the sinuses, teeth, nose, and eyes frequently present with the symptom of headache. Traction on the attached parts of the brain and especially traction on the trigeminal and hypoglossal nerves are likely to cause headache. Headache is also a symptom in particular immunologic disorders, especially periarteritis nodosa and giant cell arteritis.

Headache following a lumbar puncture occurs in one out of four patients. The headache occurs when the patient is in an upright position and is decreased or eliminated by lying down. This headache is thought to be caused by the persistent leakage of CSF through the needle puncture site.

A complete diagnostic workup is warranted when an organic condition is believed to be the cause of the headache. Treatment of the underlying problem is then the proper approach.

QUESTIONS

Cerebrovascular disease and headache

Directions: Circle the letter preceding each item below that correctly answers the question or completes the statement. More than one answer may be correct.

1. Which of the following is the most commonly occurring neurologic disease?
   a. Tumors of the nervous system   *b.* Vascular disorders of the nervous system   *c.* Spinal cord diseases   *d.* Epilepsy

2. Which of the following statements is (are) true concerning the pathogenesis of cerebrovascular disease as it has historically been defined?
   a. Early investigators considered extracranial factors significant in the causation of cerebrovascular disease.   *b.* Symptoms were assumed to develop from local causes.   *c.* Internal carotid occlusion was identified as a cause of cerebral ischemia in the eighteenth century.

3. Death of brain cells from a lack of oxygen occurs in approximately:

   a. 15 minutes   *b.* 10 minutes   *c.* 4 minutes
   d. 1 minute

4. The major arterial blood vessels that supply blood to the circle of Willis are:
   a. External carotid   *b.* Internal carotid
   c. Ophthalmic   *d.* Basilar-vertebral system

Directions: Answer the following on a separate sheet of paper.

5. Describe the arterial blood supply to the brain.

6. Briefly describe the three extrinsic (extracranial) factors and the three intrinsic (intracranial) factors which are thought responsible for cerebral circulatory control.

7. Cerebrovascular accident (stroke) is responsible for how many deaths in the United States each year? Approximately how many people in the United States have a neurologic deficit that is a result of a stroke?

8. List and describe the three types of stroke according to the chronological pattern of clinical progression and regression of signs and symptoms.

Directions: Circle the letter preceding each item below that correctly answers the question or completes the statement. More than one answer may be correct.

9. Which of the following cerebral arteries are most likely to form fatty plaques, in order of occurrence?
a. Ophthalmic   *b.* Basilar   *c.* Carotids
d. Vertebral

10. Cerebral emboli can be composed of:
a. Blood clot (especially with underlying heart or vascular disease)   *b.* Fatty tissue   *c.* Tumor cells   *d.* Bacterial clumps (often from heart disease)

11. Major sites of origin of cerebral emboli causing a stroke include all the following except:
a. Mural thrombi in the left atrium associated with atrial fibrillation   *b.* Mural thrombi overlying ventricular infarcts   *c.* Thrombi formed in rheumatic valve disease   *d.* Thrombi formed on arteriosclerotic plaques in the aortic arch and carotid arteries   *e.* Thrombi formed in the deep leg veins

Directions: Circle T for true and F for false. Correct the false statements.

12.   T   F   Cerebral thrombosis usually has a gradual onset, whereas cerebral embolism usually has a sudden onset.

13.   T   F   In cerebral vascular disorders the signs and symptoms the patient experiences depend upon which vessel is involved and the amount of collateral circulation in the affected area.

14.   T   F   In order for a cerebral vascular disorder to be referred to as a *transient ischemic attack* there must be evidence of cerebral tissue necrosis.

15.   T   F   Cerebral thrombosis is a disease of the older age groups.

Directions: Circle the letter preceding each item below that correctly answers the question or completes the statement. More than one answer may be correct.

16. Mr. B., a 60-year-old male, was admitted to the general hospital. On admission his vital signs were: temperature 99.8°F, pulse 90, respirations 20 per minute, and blood pressure 250/140 mmHg. Lumbar puncture disclosed that the spinal fluid contained red blood cells and was under increased pressure. Shortly after admission he became comatose. He was diagnosed as having a cerebral hemorrhage. Which of the following symptoms would probably indicate a hemorrhage in the area of the brain involving the posterior cerebral artery and the thalamus?
a. Contralateral hemiplegia or hemiparesis
b. Ipsilateral numbness and sensory loss on the face   *c.* Dementia   *d.* Tremor

17. The predisposing factors that probably contributed to Mr. B.'s intracerebral hemorrhage include all the following *except:*
a. History of preexisting hypertension   *b.* Weakness of the vascular wall   *c.* Sudden rise in blood pressure   *d.* History of episodic hypotension

18. Miss K., a 32-year-old woman with a history of rheumatic heart disease complicated by mitral stenosis and atrial fibrillation, was admitted to the hospital with a high fever, changing heart murmurs, large tender spleen, and *abrupt* onset of a right hemiplegia and aphasia which persisted for 48 hours. The *most likely* type of neurologic deficit is:
a. Embolism   *b.* Transient ischemic attacks
c. Thrombosis   *d.* None of the above

19. Mr. G., aged 67, was referred to the neurologist by the public health nurse after he had experienced several transient ischemic attacks. Symptoms experienced during these attacks included falling because of weakness of extremities, dizziness, and loss of equilibrium; double vision; and difficulty with speech. The most likely site of arterial occlusion is:
a. Internal carotid artery   *b.* Basilar-vertebral arteries   *c.* Radial artery   *d.* Anterior cerebral artery

20. Mr. K., a 75-year-old man with a history of mild diabetes mellitus and a previous myocardial infarction, was admitted to the hospital with a mild left hemiparesis which evolved slowly over several hours with no other neurologic deficit. This deficit improved slightly after several days in the hospital but did not entirely clear. The most likely diagnosis is:
a. Subarachnoid hemorrhage   *b.* Wallenberg's syndrome (lateral medullary syndrome) on the right side of the medulla   *c.* Transient ischemic attack involving the right middle cerebral artery
d. Cerebral thrombosis involving the right middle cerebral artery

21. A subarachnoid hemorrhage is most frequently associated with:
a. Mycotic aneurysms   *b.* Severe hypertension
c. Berry aneurysms   *d.* Atherosclerotic aneurysms

22. Characteristics of transient ischemic attacks include which one of the following?
    a. Lasting damage to the brain after an attack
    b. Similarity to epileptic attacks in the duration of neurologic dysfunction   c. Return to "normal" after an attack   d. Hemiparesis

23. Mr. O., a 50-year-old male, was admitted to a local general hospital convulsing and unconscious. His temperature was 99°F rectally, pulse rate 98 beats per minute, respirations 20 per minute, and blood pressure 240/140 mmHg. Twenty-four hours after admission, Mr. O. regained consciousness. His right arm and right leg were paralyzed, and he was unable to speak. The hemorrhage responsible for his symptoms probably occurred from rupture of a branch of the:
    a. Anterior cerebellar artery   b. Posterior cerebral artery   c. Middle cerebral artery   d. Vertebral artery

24. Berry aneurysms:
    a. Occur most often at the bifurcation of arteries
    b. Commonly occur on or near the circle of Willis   c. Are usually not discovered until they bleed   d. Cause subdural hemorrhage when they rupture

25. A cerebral infarction in the distribution of the middle cerebral artery would be likely to cause all the following symptoms except:
    a. Contralateral hemiplegia   b. Aphasia
    c. Cerebellar signs   d. Homonymous hemianopsia (loss of vision in half of the visual field)

26. A patient is admitted to the hospital with a diagnosis of mild CVA. The patient demonstrated left-sided weakness of upper and lower extremities. The patient probably has a lesion located in the:
    a. Left cerebral hemisphere   b. Right cerebral hemisphere   c. Brainstem   d. Medulla

27. Which of the following diagnostic studies are used to visualize the intracranial vascular areas?
    a. Brain scan   b. Arteriography   c. Tomography (CT scan)

28. Which of the following diagnostic procedures is able to demonstrate hematomas, infarcts, and hemorrhage?
    a. Brain scan   b. Arteriography   c. Tomography (CT scan)

Directions: Answer the following on a separate sheet of paper.

29. For the acute period of a stroke, describe four critical factors in the patient's treatment.

30. Describe the effectiveness of vasodilators and platelet antiaggregants in the treatment of CVA.

31. State the primary goal of surgical intervention for stroke patients.

32. Describe a surgical procedure used to increase collateral blood flow to the brain.

33. What is the major purpose of clipping the neck of a berry aneurysm located on the anterior communicating artery of the brain?

34. What are the principles of prevention and therapy after neurologic deficit?

Directions: Circle the letter preceding each item below that correctly completes each statement. More than one answer may be correct.

35. The most common type(s) of headache is (are):
    a. Classic migraine   b. Cluster headache
    c. Tension headache   d. Inflammatory headache

36. All the following are postulated mechanisms of headache except:
    a. Dysfunction of the extracranial arteries
    b. Traction of intracranial blood vessels
    c. Compression of the cervical nerve roots
    d. Pressure on the cranial nerves   e. Pressure on the brain parenchyma

37. Pain-sensitive structures of the head include:
    a. All extracranial tissues, especially the arteries
    b. Intracranial venous sinuses and their tributary veins   c. Cranial nerves V, VII, IX, X plus the upper cervical nerves   d. Brain parenchyma
    e. Some basal dural and basal arteries

38. Migraine headache:
    a. Is more common in men   b. May be induced by reserpine, a drug which depletes serotonin
    c. May be heralded by visual disturbances
    d. May be continuous, lasting for weeks   e. May be aggravated by oral contraceptives

39. In migraine:
    a. During the attack, there is increased excretion of the metabolites of the biogenic amines   b. Reserpine may cause a drop in the level of serum serotonin   c. Neurokinin may be found in the fluid surrounding the involved blood vessel
    d. During the attack, there is intense vasoconstriction   e. Methysergide, a serotonin antagonist, may prevent attacks

40. In cluster headache:
    a. The onset typically occurs at night during REM sleep   b. The attacks last 1 to 2 days, then promptly subside   c. The facial skin becomes pale   d. The pain is unilateral and nonthrobbing
    e. There may be conjunctival injection and tearing of the eye on the involved side

41. In headache presumed to be caused by muscle contraction:

a. The patient often complains of a bandlike tightness around the head   b. The headache may last for years   c. The headache is often thought to have psychogenic causes   d. There is commonly tenderness to palpation   e. This type of headache is sometimes treated successfully with tricyclic antidepressants

Directions: Circle T if the statement is true and F if it is false. Correct the false statements.

42. T   F   The common migraine headache is characterized by a vasoconstrictive prodromal phase associated with neurologic disturbances.

43. T   F   Postlumbar puncture headache can often be avoided by using a small needle.

44. T   F   Horton's headache is a synonym for cluster headache.

45. T   F   Alcohol may induce attacks of cluster headache.

46. T   F   The pain in tension headache is often described as dull and nonpulsating.

47. T   F   Headache associated with an expanding intracranial mass such as a tumor generally becomes more severe as the mass enlarges.

Directions: Fill in the blanks with the appropriate words

48. Headache involving supratentorial structures is referred to the _____ two-thirds of the head, and the pain pathway involves the _____ nerve.

49. Headache involving infratentorial structures is referred to the _____ area and _____ and is conveyed by the _____ nerves.

Directions: Match the headache characteristics in col. B to the three categories of headache in col. A. Letters may be used more than once.

Column A
50. ____ Classic migraine headache
51. ____ Cluster headache
52. ____ Tension headache

Column B
a. Flushed skin
b. Pale skin
c. Generally unilateral
d. Generally bilateral
e. Throbbing quality
f. Dull ache, constant day and night
g. Precipitated by stress, fatigue
h. Precipitated by alcohol
i. Genetic predisposition
j. Vasodilatation during headache
k. Mechanism involves sustained contraction of head and neck muscles

Directions: Answer the following on a separate sheet of paper.

53. List several questions you would ask a client with a complaint of chronic headache during history taking.

CHAPTER 49

EPILEPSY

OBJECTIVES

At the completion of this chapter you should be able to:

1. Define *epilepsy*.
2. Compare the incidence of epilepsy in the general population and in the offspring of epileptic persons.
3. List at least three conditions that may cause seizures.
4. Name the areas of the brain associated with lesions that are likely to epileptogenic.
5. Describe the factors that may play an instrumental role in precipitating seizures.
6. Describe the metabolic changes that can occur during and immediately following a seizure.
7. Differentiate between the expected clinical manifestations in tonic-clonic, absence, and partial seizures with both elementary and complex symptoms.
8. Define *status epilepticus*.
9. Identify on an electroencephalogram the changes associated with activity and the layers of the brain responsible for electrical activity, and give an interpretation of the tracing.
10. Identify the drugs used to control tonic-clonic, absence, and partial seizures with elementary and complex symptoms.
11. Discuss the medical and surgical treatment modalities for epilepsy.

Epilepsy is a relatively common neurologic problem. It is a multifarious disorder which is chronic and characterized by recurrent seizure activity. The seizure, which is the chief symptom or manifestation of epilepsy, can be any abnormal dysfunction (motor, sensory, or psychic) that is brief, uncontrolled, and episodic and which interrupts the patient's ongoing behavior. It is associated with excessive local discharge by cerebral neurons. The terms *epilepsy* and *seizure* are often used interchangeably.

Epilepsy was identified as a problem related to the brain by Hippocrates. It can affect any age group; it occurs in all races throughout the world. Some people seem constitutionally more prone to develop seizures than others. In most cases there is probably interaction between an inherited predisposition and environmental factors. The incidence of epilepsy is higher in the off-spring of persons with epilepsy compared with the general population. Relatives of patients exhibit abnormal brain waves more frequently than do control groups.

The true incidence of epilepsy is not known. The commonly cited figure is 0.5 percent of the population. This estimate is considered too conservative by many in the field. There is a reluctance to report the problem on the part of the patient and physician, along with confusion as to when the problem of seizures constitutes epilepsy. Many patients do not reveal their condition because of society's negative view of epilepsy. Learning to cope with occupational, educational, and social discrimination may be more difficult than dealing with the epilepsy per se.

Although epilepsy may occur at any age, the incidence is highest during childhood: 75 percent of cases occur before the age of 20 years. When the first seizure occurs after the age of 25 years, epilepsy is usually secondary.

Epilepsy may be classified as idiopathic or symptomatic. In the *idiopathic,* or *essential,* category, no known cerebral lesion can be demonstrated. In *symptomatic,* or *secondary,* epilepsy there is cerebral abnormality that is promoting seizure response. Among the many conditions that may be responsible for secondary seizures are head injury (including that before or during birth), metabolic and nutritional disorders (e.g., hypoglycemia, PKU, vitamin B_6 deficiency), toxic factors (alcohol withdrawal, uremia), encephalitis, anoxia, circulatory disturbances, and neoplasms.

PATHOLOGY

Seizure activity may follow insults to the brain, depending partly on the severity and location of the lesion. Lesions in the midbrain, thalamus, and cerebral cortex are most likely to be epileptogenic, whereas lesions in the cerebellum and brainstem do not generally evoke seizures.

At the cell membrane level, certain biochemical phenomena characterize the epileptic neuron. These include:

1. Instability of the nerve cell membrane, allowing the cell to be more susceptible to activation.

2. Hypersensitive neurons with lowered thresholds for firing and firing excessively.

3. Possibly polarization abnormalities (excessive polarization, hypopolarization, or lapses in repolarization).

4. Ionic imbalances that alter the chemical environment of the neuron. During a seizure the electrolyte balance at the neuronal level is altered. The imbalance causes the neuronal membrane to depolarize.

Metabolic changes occur during and immediately following a seizure. They are, in part, due to increased energy needs from the neuronal hyperactivity. Metabolic needs are drastically increased during convulsions; the electrical discharges of motor nerve cells may be increased to 1000 per second. Cerebral blood flow is increased, as is tissue respiration and glycolysis. Acetylcholine appears in cerebral spinal fluid (CSF) during and following seizures. Glutamic acid may be depleted during seizure activity.

There is generally no gross change found at autopsy. Histopathologic evidence supports the hypothesis that the lesion is neurochemical rather than structural. No consistent pathologic factor has been identified. Focal abnormalities in the metabolism of potassium and acetylcholine are found to be present between seizures. Seizure foci seem especially sensitive to acetylcholine, a facilitatory transmitter; they are slow to bind and remove the acetylcholine.

SEIZURES

Each major clinical center for epilepsy uses the classification that works best for its purposes. Table 49-1 shows the classification (modified) adopted by the International League Against Epilepsy. Electroencephalographic study, clinical assessment, and history are utilized to identify the type of seizure.

The two major classes of epilepsy are *partial,* or *focal, seizures,* which begin in a specific area of the brain, usually the cerebral cortex; and *generalized seizures,* presumably involving the entire cerebral cortex and diencephalon. The generalized type of seizure is the more common.

Partial seizures may present with elementary or complex symptoms. Partial seizures with elementary symptoms are focal attacks which involve motor or sensory symptoms. Jacksonian epilepsy is the most common form of this type of epilepsy, and generally the focus is located in the sensory or motor cortex. Psychomotor, or temporal lobe, epilepsy is an example of partial seizures with complex symptoms. Complex partial seizures involve disturbances in higher level cerebral functions such as memory and thought processes, as well as complex motor behavior which is automatic. The epileptic focus for this type of epilepsy is often the temporal lobe. Both types of partial seizure may spread and become generalized (major motor) seizures.

TABLE 49·1

INTERNATIONAL CLASSIFICATION OF EPILEPTIC SEIZURES

International classification	Traditional name	Characteristics
1. Partial seizures		Consciousness not generally impaired.
a. Elementary symptoms (motor, sensory, or autonomic)	Jacksonian, or focal, epilepsy	Focal onset—usually unilateral spasm or twitching of the fingers or face which may spread in a progressive march to involve the entire side
		Similar pattern when the symptoms are sensory
b. Complex symptoms	Psychomotor, or temporal lobe, epilepsy	Patient usually conscious during attack but does not recall what happened
		Transient mental disturbances, automatic purposeless movements (clapping hands, smacking lips)
		Sudden recollection of past events, visual or auditory hallucinations, personality changes, antisocial behavior, inappropriate moodiness
		Precipitated by music, blinking lights, and other stimuli
2 Generalized seizures		Bilateral, symmetrical, and without local onset
a. Absence	Petit mal	Short lapses of consciousness lasting a few seconds indicated by a brief pause in conversation, a vacant stare, or rapid blinking of the eyes
		Almost exclusively in children; may disappear at puberty or be replaced by tonic-clonic epilepsy
b. Tonic-clonic	Grand mal	Classic seizure of epilepsy
		Generally preceded by an aura
		Loss of consciousness
		Generalized tonic and clonic spasms of the muscles
		Tongue may be bitten
		Bladder and/or bowel incontinence
		Mental confusion and amnesia for seizure event
3. Unilateral seizures		
4. Unclassified seizures		

Source: Modified from Gastaut, 1970.

Jacksonian motor seizures are characterized by a focal onset thought to be caused by a lesion in the contralateral cortex. The seizure generally starts with either a tonic spasm or a clonic rhythmic twitching of the fingers of one hand, face on one side, etc. This disorder then spreads in a progressive march, for example, from face to neck, hand, forearm, arm, trunk, and leg, all on one side of the body. In some instances there is progression to the opposite hemisphere with a loss of consciousness. It is extremely important to observe where the seizure begins, as this may offer a clue to location of the lesion.

Jacksonian seizures may also be sensory. The patient complains of transient abnormal sensations (e.g., numbness, crawling sensation, pins and needles) that begin as focal phenomena and then progressively march to involve one side of the body. Usually some clonic movements are associated with the sensory seizure, since there is some motor representation in the sensory cortex.

Psychomotor (temporal lobe) *seizures* are characterized by transient mental disturbances and automatic, purposeless movements (clapping hands, smacking lips, chewing motions). Patients may have a clouded, "dreamy" feeling of unreality.

The patient is usually conscious during the attack but generally does not recall what has happened. Other behavior associated with this form of epilepsy includes sudden recollection of past events, hallucinations (visual or olfactory are common), forgetfulness, word-finding difficulty, personality change, antisocial behavior, and inappropriate moodiness. In the postictal (postseizure) period the patient may enter a fugue state in which complex and organized activities may be performed which are not remembered (amnesia).

These attacks may be precipitated by music, blinking lights, and other stimuli. They may occur at any age but primarily occur in adults. Psychomotor seizures are often associated with small focal lesions in the anterior temporal lobe, especially in the hippocampal (uncinate) gyrus. They may also involve lesions outside the temporal lobe (in the insula, orbital cortex, anterior olfactory centers, and diencephalon). The involvement of these structures accounts for the fact that when an *aura* (warning symptoms of an impending seizure) occurs in psychomotor epilepsy, it often takes the form of a perceptual illusion such as an unpleasant taste or smell.

Generalized seizures are characterized by the onset of bilateral, symmetrical epileptic activity (not local).

They include absences, or petit mal seizures and the tonic-clonic, or grand mal, seizure.

Absence, or *petit mal*, epilepsy is characterized by short lapses of consciousness, rarely lasting more than a few seconds. For example, there may be a brief pause in conversation, a vacant look, or a rapid blinking of the eyes. The patient may have one or two seizures a month or several a day. Absence seizures occur almost exclusively in children; the onset is rarely after 20 years of age. It may disappear after puberty or be replaced by other seizures, especially tonic-clonic.

Tonic-clonic, or *grand mal*, is the classic seizure of epilepsy. It may be characterized by an aura followed by a loss of consciousness and tonic-clonic spasms. The aura is a sensory indication of an impending seizure; it may consist of a momentary visual or auditory sensation.

The seizure starts with a rapid loss of consciousness. A cry may be uttered, from the forced expiration caused by thoracic or abnormal spasms. There is loss of upright position, tonic then clonic movements, and bladder and/or bowel incontinence, along with other autonomic dysfunctions. In the tonic phase, muscles contract and body position may be distorted. This phase lasts for a few seconds. The clonic phase involves opposing muscle groups contracting and relaxing, giving a jerking movement. The contractions gradually decrease in number but not in strength. The tongue may be bitten; this occurs in approximately half the cases (spasms of the jaw and tongue). The entire seizure lasts from 3 to 5 minutes and is followed by a period of unconsciousness which may last from a few minutes to as much as a half hour. The patient regaining consciousness may appear confused, stuporous, or dull. Generally there is no recollection of the seizure.

In addition to the common types of generalized seizure just discussed, other forms included in this category are epileptic myoclonus, infantile spasms, clonic seizures, tonic seizures, atonic seizures, and akinetic seizures.

STATUS EPILEPTICUS

Status epilepticus refers to a state in which there is a succession of seizures with no recovery between them. Two types are possible: (1) major motor status, in which one tonic-clonic seizure follows another, and (2) absence continuing, involving a series of absence seizures. Status epilepticus is not a common phenomenon.

Major motor status epilepticus is an emergency which may be fatal if unrelieved. Several medications may be given to relieve this condition. Diphenylhydan-

toin (Dilantin) may be given intravenously and has the advantage of not altering neurologic signs and not depressing the patient. If this treatment is not successful in stopping the seizures, phenobarbital or diazepam (Valium) may be given IV. These drugs are more apt to cause cardiac or respiratory depression.

Status epilepticus often causes elevation of the blood pressure and temperature, respiratory difficulty, and other systemic changes. Proper ventilation is crucial, and cardiopulmonary support systems may be warranted. Care must be taken to avoid aspiration of vomitus and saliva. Fluid and electrolyte balance must be maintained. Exhaustion and acidosis may cause death. Once the patient is under control, causes of the episode should be explored. Abruptly stopping antiepileptic medications may be a precipitating factor, as may alcohol withdrawal.

ELECTROENCEPHALOGRAM

The electrical activity of the cortex is of very low voltage. It is amplified and recorded by an electroencephalograph. The record is called an *electroencephalogram* (EEG).

Brain waves are individualized and vary with activity (e.g., intense mental activity = low amplitude, high frequency; slow-wave sleep = low frequency, amplitude increased). Spikes indicate an irritative focus. Brain waves are slowed with hypoxia, anesthesia, sedatives, low CO_2, deep sleep, and relaxation; they are accelerated with increased CO_2 levels, sensory stimulation, light anesthesia, and drugs such as methylprednisolone (Medrol).

The superficial layers of cortex are responsible for the electrical activity recorded on EEGs. Masses of dendrites forming a dense network are thought to be the source. The cerebellum has a similar network, and a similar pattern can be recorded from that area.

EEGs should be used in conjunction with careful clinical evaluations. The EEG is a physiologic recording and does not distinguish one entity from another (for example, a tumor cannot be distinguished from a thrombosis by EEG). Ten percent of patients with seizures have normal EEGs. Also, an abnormal record does not mean a person has epilepsy. In fact, even in cases of diagnosed epilepsy, most seizure activity is nonclinical.

The EEG is one test, not a conclusive diagnostic determination. Caution should be employed in the interpretation of EEG tracings. For example, scalp electrodes frequently may not perceive the electrical activity from the inferior aspect of the frontal and temporal and occipital lobes.

Certain activating techniques such as hyperventilation, sleep, and visual stimulation are used to initiate abnormal electrical patterns in some patients.

In tonic-clonic seizures, EEG abnormalities are dependent on the frequency and duration of the seizures. EEG abnormalities are more common in patients with frequent seizures than those with infrequent seizures. A normal EEG, however, is common in children with tonic-clonic seizures.

In some centers (such as the Neuropsychiatric Institute at the University of California at Los Angeles), patients can be monitored on a 24-hour basis with radiotelemetry. Electrodes are implanted and attached to a telemetry pack which is secured to the patient's head. The EEG recordings along with a video camera are used to identify specific areas of the brain involved in abnormal discharges.

TREATMENT

The primary mode of management for the epileptic patient is drug therapy to prevent the occurrence of seizures or to reduce their frequency, so that the patient can lead an essentially normal life. Approximately 70 to 80 percent of patients benefit from anticonvulsant

drugs. The drug selected is determined by the type of seizure, and dosages are individualized. Table 49-2 lists some of the common drugs used for epilepsy and their side effects.

Historically, a combination of drugs has been used, on the premise that lower dosages were thus possible and fewer side effects would occur. It was also believed that the drugs would potentiate one another. The current trend, however, is to use a monopharmaceutical approach and minimize, as much as possible, the total number of drugs used.

Careful clinical assessment is the most important factor in drug management for the majority of patients. However, the ability to determine anticonvulsant medication serum levels by gas-liquid chromatography techniques has enhanced the ability to control the seizures of some patients who might otherwise have had their

TABLE 49-2

ANTICONVULSANT DRUGS

Drug	Therapeutic uses (type of seizure)	Effective blood level	Side effects
Phenobarbital	First choice for major motor seizures Used prophylactically with absence to avoid developing tonic-clonic epilepsy; if no seizures occur by age 14, it is gradually withdrawn over a 1-year period	10 to 30 μg/ml	Drowsiness, usually dose-related Hyperactivity, especially in children, not dose-related
Primidone (Mysoline)	Partial seizures, especially complex partial Generalized tonic-clonic	5 μg/ml	Drowsiness, dizziness, diplopia, ataxia Metabolized to phenobarbital and phenylethylmalonamide
Phenytoin (Dilantin)	First choice for tonic-clonic seizures, especially in adults Partial seizures May increase frequency of absence seizures	10 to 20 μg/ml 15 to 25 μg/ml in many	Hypertrophic gums, gastric irritation Diplopia, nystagmus, blurred vision Dizziness, hirsutism Anemia, especially with long-term use, owing to blocking of folic acid synthesis in susceptible persons Serum levels 40 μg/ml are associated with phenytoin encephalopathy
Ethosuximide (Zarontin)	Drug of choice for absence seizures	40 to 90 μg/ml	Nausea, vomiting, weight loss Drowsiness, headache, dizziness Neurologic and psychologic reactions, sleep disturbances Blood dyscrasias
Carbamazepine (Tegretol)	Drug of choice for complex partial seizures	None definite 4 to 8 μg/ml used by some	Bone marrow depression, nausea and vomiting Drowsiness, blurred vision Skin rash
Valproic acid (Depakene)	Tonic-clonic and absence seizures Partial seizures that are refractory	50 to 100 μg/ml	Nausea, hepatotoxicity, pancreatitis Temporary hair loss, lens opacities Tremor
Diazepam (Valium)	Given IV in the treatment of status epilepticus (Dilantin and phenobarbital IV may also be used)		Sedation, cardiovascular and respiratory depression

medications changed or additional medications added. Monitoring blood levels of the drugs gives assurance that the serum level is within the usual therapeutic range. Patient compliance can be assessed, and patients may be confronted with the fact that they are not taking their medication if this is the case. It is important to look at the total person in these cases and attempt to explore with him or her the possible reasons for noncompliance. Some patients may not absorb the drug adequately, may lack enzyme systems necessary to metabolize the drug properly, or may metabolize the drug more rapidly than normal. It is important to be aware of the normal serum levels of the common anticonvulsant drugs in the laboratory with which one is dealing.

Other forms of treatment for epilepsy include diet and surgery. The original ketogenic diet for epilepsy was popular in the 1920s. It is still used occasionally, especially for minor motor (myoclonic) seizures in children when there is resistance to anticonvulsant drugs. A variation of the ketogenic diet, the medium-chain triglyceride diet, was introduced in the early 1970s. The diet is high in fat and low in carbohydrate. Apparently it alters body chemistry by producing ketones. The urine is monitored for ketones during the dietary regimen to ascertain their presence. The acidotic state seems to have an anticonvulsive effect in some of these children.

When acetazolamide (Diamox) is used in conjunction with anticonvulsant drugs, it produces a relative acidosis similar to a ketogenic diet. Again, this state seems to create a climate less likely to produce seizure activity. Dehydrated states also seem to decrease seizure activity, as does physical exercise (possibly because of the production of lactic acid).

Surgical treatment by excision of cortical scars is debatable issue. It is restricted to focal epilepsy if the area is not indispensable (as the speech center is). It is considered only after drug therapy has proved ineffective. Indications for surgery include:

1. Focal lesion identified by EEG and compatible with clinical manifestations
2. Area accessible and dispensable
3. Patient a good candidate for rehabilitation (normal IQ, motivated)

When a person is having a seizure, the two major concerns are maintaining a patent airway and protecting the head. The airway is best maintained by rolling the person onto the side. The tongue will gravitate forward. If regurgitation has occurred, it is important to prevent aspiration of stomach contents. Anything in the mouth that could cause occlusion should be removed.

If the seizure has occurred on a hard surface such as a gymnasium floor, the head may be cradled in the lap of an assistant, or padding, if available, can be placed under the head. The aim is to protect the head, eyes, and ears from injury. Obviously, sharp objects would be removed from the vicinity.

The importance of a holistic approach in the management of the person with epilepsy cannot be overstated. As with any chronic problem, many psychosocial problems can develop. Patients need help in learning to cope not only with the epilepsy itself but also with the public's attitudes toward it. It is important for them to be able to see themselves as persons with epilepsy rather than as epileptics.

QUESTIONS

Epilepsy

Directions: Answer the following on a separate sheet of paper.

1. Define *epilepsy*.
2. (a) What is the incidence of epilepsy in the general population of the United States? (b) For the offspring of epileptic persons?
3. What conditions may cause seizures?
4. List the areas of the brain associated with lesions that are likely to be epleptogenic.
5. Describe the factors that may play an instrumental role in precipitating seizures.
6. Describe the metabolic changes that can occur during and immediately following a seizure.
7. Define *status epilepticus*.

Directions: Circle the letter preceding each item below that correctly answers the question or completes the sentence. More than one answer may be correct.

8. Which of the following statements concerning epilepsy are true?
   a. The single most important factor in diagnosing epilepsy is careful observation and reporting of a seizure.   b. The majority of patients can be brought under reasonable control   c. There are characteristic disease inheritance patterns.
   d. Epileptic persons may have difficulty in obtaining employment.

9. Complex partial seizures are usually characterized by:

a. Inappropriate behavior *b.* A disturbance in the temporal lobe *c.* Most common occurrence in children *d.* Temporary loss of consciousness

10. Uncontrollable tonic, then clonic, muscular spasms with loss of consciousness are characteristic of the following types of seizure:
a. Elementary partial *b.* Absence *c.* Tonic-clonic *d.* Complex partial

11. A seizure involving a momentary loss of consciousness and often characterized by a blank stare and a facial twitch is referred to as:
a. Elementary partial *b.* Tonic-clonic *c.* Complex partial *d.* Absence

12. Which of the following interventions are of primary importance when one encounters a patient having a seizure?
a. Insertion of a tongue blade *b.* Observation of the seizure to determine progression of muscular involvement *c.* Restraint of the patient to limit outward movement of the arms and legs *d.* Establishment of an open airway by maintaining the patient in a side-lying position

13. Which of the following are likely indications for the surgical treatment of an epileptic patient?
a. Focal lesion identified by EEG and compatible with clinical manifestations *b.* Area accessible and dispensable *c.* Drug therapy not effective

d. High motivation for a rehabilitation program

Directions: Match the type of drug in col. A with the associated therapeutic uses and side effects in col. B.

Column A

14. ____ Phenytoin
15. ____ Ethosuximide
16. ____ Valproic acid
17. ____ Carbamazepine
18. ____ Diazepam
19. ____ Primidone

Column B

a. Hepatic damage, lens opacities, hair loss

b. Drug of choice for tonic-clonic, elementary, and complex partial seizures

c. Primary drug for absence seizures

d. Sedation, vertigo, ataxia, diplopia, nystagmus (drug metabolized to phenobarbital)

e. Drug of choice for complex partial seizures

f. Given IV to treat status epilepticus

CHAPTER
50

DEGENERATIVE AND OTHER DISORDERS OF THE NERVOUS SYSTEM

OBJECTIVES

At the completion of this chapter you should be able to:

1. Identify the three current theories of the etiology of amyotrophic lateral sclerosis.

2. Define Wernicke-Korsakoff syndrome and discuss the treatment of choice.

3. Define the following disorders of movement: *tremor, chorea, athetosis, dystonia, hemiballismus.*

4. Define *Parkinson's syndrome,* discussing the various types and their frequency.

5. Identify two classes of drugs which may induce parkinsonlike symptoms.

6. Discuss the role of hydrogen peroxide in parkinsonism.

7. Describe the signs and symptoms of Parkinson's syndrome.

8. Define: *"lead-pipe"* and *"cogwheel" rigidity, resting tremor, bradykinesia, akinesia, micrographia, festinating gait.*

9. Explain how the glabellar reflex is tested and briefly describe the sign.

10. Explain the basis for the resting tremor in Parkinson's syndrome.

11. Name the site in the brain affected in Parkinson's syndrome, the type of nerve tract involved, and the chemical substance believed to be involved.

12. Explain why the administration of L-dopa or Sinemet as a dopamine replacement is effective in the treatment of Parkinson's syndrome; describe precautions necessary in its administration.

13. Describe acute disseminated encephalomyelitis (etiology, pathology, mortality, and prevention).

14. Describe multiple sclerosis (pathology, clinical features, etiology, diagnosis, prognosis, and treatment).

15. Explain the anatomic basis for the various signs and symptoms in multiple sclerosis.

16. Describe the structure and function of the neuromuscular junction and the pathophysiology in myasthenia gravis.

17. Describe the clinical types of myasthenia gravis and its diagnosis, prognosis, and treatment.
18. Differentiate between a myasthenic and a cholinergic crisis.
19. Discuss the three current theories of the etiology of Alzheimer's disease.
20. Describe Alzheimer's disease, including the natural history, treatment, and management.
21. List five possible causes of dementia.
22. Discuss the signs and symptoms of viral central nervous system infections.
23. List four viruses known to cause meningitis and encephalitis.
24. Describe the common presenting signs and symptoms of viral meningitis.
25. Describe the pathophysiology seen in Reye's syndrome.
26. Discuss the ways infection may invade the brain.
27. Discuss the signs and symptoms of brain abscess.

Diseases of the nervous system with a progressively downhill course have been traditionally referred to as *degenerative*. Pathologic processes of the nervous system are generally classified by their effects on a person's functioning rather than their causes, since for many the cause is under investigation or as yet undiscovered. The effects of a degenerative neurologic disease tend to be long-lasting or permanent, requiring the patient to seek new methods of adapting. Families are also affected by the long-term nature of these neurologic disorders.

Degenerative diseases affecting the nervous system are of many types. Three particular types are discussed here: inherited, nutritional, and demyelinating. Each of these diseases produces characteristic changes in nerve cells; the symptoms can and do overlap, making diagnosis difficult, particularly in the early stages of the disease.

INHERITED DEGENERATIVE DISEASES

Amyotrophic lateral sclerosis (ALS) is a progressive neurologic disease affecting persons in the fourth through seventh decades of life. The precise cause is as yet unknown, although current research has provided several clues. It has been suggested that the disease may be the result of (1) genetic predisposition, (2) a slow latent viral infection (e.g., mutated poliovirus), or (3) an autoimmune disorder.

Pathologic changes involve the anterior horn cells of the spinal cord and lower brainstem and the motor neurons of the cerebral cortex that give rise to the corticospinal tract. As a result of the deterioration of these neurons, the musculature innervated by these neurons undergoes neurogenic atrophy. Symptoms of this neurogenic atrophy are muscle weakness and muscle atrophy. These symptoms can occur rapidly or slowly, following a distal to proximal pattern. Fasciculations occur with acute and widespread denervation of entire motor neuron units. In addition, patients experience muscle cramps. As the disease progresses, symptoms demonstrating the involvement of the lower motor neurons develop. Intellectually the patients remain normal, although they demonstrate emotional lability. ALS can be differentiated from other diseases by its painless, neurogenic muscle impairment, with spasticity but no sensory changes. Treatment is directed toward supportive and symptomatic care of the patient and family.

NUTRITIONAL DEGENERATIVE DISEASE

Lack or deficiency of particular nutrients are known to have a deleterious effect on the brain. Several vitamins in particular are known to be essential for normal brain metabolism. Deficiencies of the B vitamins B_1, B_6, B_{12}, niacin, and pantothenic acid are associated with various neurologic disorders. Despite continued research, much is yet unknown about the role of nutrition on the development of the nervous system and its healthy maintenance.

Alcoholism is a major problem in the United States.

The alcoholic person is frequently the victim of severe nutritional deficiencies caused by decreased appetite, abusive drinking, and the presence of chronic illnesses, untreated infections, and anemia.

Wernicke-Korsakoff syndrome is a disease associated with extensive alcohol abuse and nutritional deprivation (as in gastric carcinoma, thyrotoxicosis, and hyperemesis gravidarum). The term *cerebral beriberi* is used in reference to this disease. Pathologic changes involve necrosis of nerve cells and myelinated structures. Symptoms are related to the brain structures involved. Paralysis of gaze, nystagmus, and ataxia are caused by lesions in the midbrain, the cerebellar vermis, and the floor of the fourth ventricle. The psychological symptoms, dull mentation, impairment of recent memory, and amnesia are generally due to lesions of the thalamic nuclei and the hypothalamus. In addition, these patients suffer from postural hypotension, dyspnea, tachycardia, cirrhosis of the liver, and anemia.

Thiamine is now accepted as the therapy of choice for patients suffering from Wernicke-Korsakoff syndrome. Improvement of symptoms varies, the disorders of mentation (apathy, inattentiveness, and listlessness) improving rapidly, while ataxia and nystagmus demonstrate slow but gradual improvement. Unfortunately, not much change is seen in the amnesia.

EXTRAPYRAMIDAL SYNDROMES

Extrapyramidal syndromes are disorders concerned with movement which result from lesions involving those parts of the brain other than the corticospinal pathways, principally the basal ganglia (see Chap. 46). More data are available on the clinical aspects of extrapyramidal dysfunction than on its pathophysiologic basis. Neurochemical changes seem to be involved in some cases.

Tremor

The tremor is an involuntary movement which results from an excess of neuronal activity in one area that is a result of unopposed activity in another area. The tremor is most marked peripherally. It may be suppressed by will or with vigorous activity. In general, there are alternating contractions of the flexor and extensor muscle groups, so that movement is at right angles to the axis of the limb. The tremor of parkinsonism occurs at rest and temporarily disappears during voluntary activity. In contrast, a tremor due to cerebellar deficiency is an intention tremor and is increased with purposeful activity.

Chorea

Chorea is a term referring to movements which are sudden, random, and involuntary. Fragments of purposive movement are apparent, but there is a lack of normal progression and the movements are disorganized. Chorea may be generalized or lateralized.

A generalized form is *Huntington's chorea*, a progressive disease involving the extrapyramidal system (along with cortical degeneration). The caudate nucleus, putamen, and frontal lobes of the cortex seem to be particularly affected. This disease is inherited as an autosomal dominant disorder which becomes manifest at about the age of 35 years.

A lateralized chorea is seen with lesions in the ventrolateral thalamus or subthalamic nucleus. Occlusion of a penetrating branch of the posterior cerebral artery results in an infarct of the thalamic area and is often the basis of the hemichorea.

Chorea may involve proximal or distal extremities, face, head, and trunk. In some cases, speech and mastication are affected. The involuntary movements in the limbs may make walking and purposeful movement of the hands difficult. Movements and environmental stimuli aggravate the symptoms, while the movements may disappear during sleep.

The pathology in chorea involves extensive areas of the nervous system, most notably, degeneration of the corpus striatum and the cerebral cortex. The pathophysiology in chorea may be related to an increased (or altered) response of striatal dopamine receptors. This hypersensitivity hypothesis is supported by biochemical and pharmacological data. L-Dopa can cause an increase or exacerbation of chorea; neuroleptic drugs can decrease or ameliorate the abnormal movements, supposedly by competing with dopamine at the receptor sites.

Athetosis

Athetosis is marked by involuntary movements combined with instability of posture. It is evidenced by slow, rhythmic, writhing, wormlike movements that usually occur in the peripheral parts of the upper extremities (especially the fingers and hands). The face, neck, tongue, lips, and lower extremities may be affected. An attempt to perform a voluntary activity and emotional stimuli cause an exaggeration of the abnormal movements. Coordinated activity is not possible in the affected muscle groups.

The globus pallidus, putamen, and possibly the corpus striatum are involved in the pathology of athetosis. Hypoxia at birth is a causative factor in some cases; others are related to kernicterus, in which the unconjugated bilirubin is taken up by lipid-rich brain tissue (especially the basal ganglia, thalamus, cerebellum, and cerebral gray matter) and causes damage (see Chap. 23). Four types of cerebral palsy (a popular term referring to a motor dysfunction that is congenital or acquired during infancy) are identified: cerebral spastic diplegia (legs affected more than arms), the hemiplegic variety, double athetosis (choreoathetosis), and ataxic. Clinical manifestations often overlap. Cerebral palsy may be but is not always associated with mental retardation, disorders of perception and higher sensory function, and seizure disorders.

Dystonia

Dystonia is closely related to athetosis, differing only in that the larger axial muscles rather than the appendicular muscles are involved. Bizarre or grotesque postures of the limbs or trunk from excessive muscular tone are noted. Voluntary movement is seriously impaired, and sometimes the entire musculature of the body may be thrown into spasm by an effort to move an arm or leg or to speak. The pathology seems to involve the putamen and thalamus. Surgical lesions made in the ventrolateral thalamus may result in improvement.

Hemiballismus

Hemiballismus is the involuntary, violent movement of a large body area (entire leg, shoulder, pelvic girdle). It usually involves only one side of the body. Attempting a normal activity may invoke a ballistic movement instead. This syndrome is believed to be due to extensive lesions of the subthalamic nuclei usually secondary to hemorrhage or, less commonly, infarct or tumor. Death occurs in 4 to 6 weeks in 60 percent of patients and is generally the result of exhaustion, pneumonia, or congestive heart failure. The recent use of neuroleptics (dopamine antagonists) such as haloperidol and chlorpromazine has improved the survival rate.

Parkinsonism

Parkinsonism, or Parkinson's syndrome, is a clinical syndrome characterized by rhythmic tremors, bradykinesia, rigidity of muscles, and loss of postural reflexes. Of all diseases involving the basal ganglia, Parkinson's syndrome is the most common (see Chap. 46). It affects over 1 million Americans and is a major cause of disability. There are several different causes of parkinsonism. The idiopathic type (paralysis agitans) is the most common, affecting persons between the ages of 50 and 60. Postencephalitic parkinsonism was a common sequela of an encephalitis (Economo's disease) that occurred between 1918 and 1925; studies indicate that an influenza A virus may have been responsible. Drug-induced parkinsonism is sometimes a side effect of drug therapy with the phenothiazines, haloperidol and other butyrophenones, and *Rauwolfia* agents. Symptoms generally disappear within days of the cessation of drug therapy, but some patients have been known to remain symptomatic for weeks, months, or even years. In addition, parkinsonism may be seen with heavy metal (lead, manganese, mercury) poisoning and also with hypoparathyroidism.

The cause of parkinsonism is essentially unknown. Research has uncovered several promising leads. Evidence exists which links the problem to the enzymes involved in catecholamine metabolism. The by-product of catecholamine metabolism is hydrogen peroxide. Hydrogen peroxide is removed by two enzymes: peroxidase and catalase. These enzymes are found in large quantities in the substantia nigra. In parkinsonism patients the level of these enzymes is significantly reduced, causing a buildup of hydrogen peroxide which in turn causes destruction of the nigral cells and loss of the enzyme tyrosine hydroxylase. Tyrosine hydroxylase is responsible for the production of dopamine.

Clinical manifestations

The cardinal signs of Parkinson's syndrome are rigidity, tremor (especially with rest), and akinesia or bradykinesia. The dysfunction is chronic and progressive but varies with each individual.

Rigidity may be isolated to one muscle group and may primarily involve one side, or it may be widespread and bilateral. It decreases muscle strength and speed and is a major factor in the deformities associated with parkinsonism. Passive movement of the involved limbs or trunk meets with a taffylike resistance that is relatively constant throughout the range of motion. It has been compared with bending a lead pipe and is sometimes called *lead-pipe rigidity*. Often there are "catches" during passive movement, giving a cogwheel or rachetlike character to the rigidity called *cogwheel rigidity*. Both flexor and extensor muscles are tightly contracted (increased tonus), indicating impairment of reciprocal inhibitory muscle groups. The rigidity of parkinsonism is different from the spasticity associated with pyramidal tract disorder (upper motor neuron). With the latter, additional force will cause a sudden loss of resistance. Decerebrate rigidity is due to hyperactivity of the muscle spindle system.

When the rigidity involves the trunk, it is responsible, in large measure, for the gait and postural problems associated with parkinsonism.

The tremor associated with parkinsonism occurs at rest and is called a *rest tremor*. When muscles are tensed to perform a purposeful activity, the tremor usually stops. (About one-third of patients have an intention tremor along with the rest tremor, but intention tremors are generally associated with cerebellar dysfunction.) Tremors involving the hands are described as *pill-rolling* and are the result of rhythmic movement of the thumb and first two fingers. Tremors are the result of regular alternating contractions (four to six cycles per second) of antagonistic muscles. Tremors are likely to be worse when the pateint is tired, under emotional stress, or focusing attention on the tremor. The basis for the tremor is not clear. Degeneration of the basal ganglia results in loss of inhibitory influence, and the increased feedback in various circuits may result in oscillation. Not every patient has an obvious tremor. If hemiplegia should incidentally occur, the tremor disappears on the paralyzed side.

Akinesia is a freezing or absence of movement. The patient has a decrease in spontaneous movement and difficulty in initiating new movements. *Bradykinesia* refers to an abnormal slowness in deliberate movement. Either symptom is very disabling and obvious when the patient attempts any voluntary activity such as walking, talking, or writing. Loss of associated movements is noted—e.g., the patient does not swing the arms while walking. The face is expressionless and the voice low and monotonous. Writing becomes progressively cramped and may reflect the tremor. *Micrographia* is the small handwriting that eventually trails off and cannot be deciphered. When automatic movement (normally unconscious) is performed consciously, much more energy and effort are necessary. It is more work for the patient to lift an arm than it would be for a normal person. The patient is fatigued and complains of muscle pain.

Secondary signs include gait disturbances, postural problems, and autonomic nervous system disorders. Gait disturbances reflect increasing impairment of postural and righting reflexes. The patient cannot stop and turn quickly but turns *en bloc* rather than sequentially as a normal person would. The gait is slow and shuffling, with short steps and hastening gait *(festinating)*. The posture is stooped, and balance is poor. To remain upright, patients hurry along trying to keep up with the center of gravity. They have difficulty in making adjustments to changes in position and have a tendency to fall.

Among the autonomic manifestations seen with Parkinson's disease are sweating, oily skin with a tendency toward seborrheic dermatitis, swallowing difficulties, constipation, and bladder problems which are aggravated by anticholinergic drugs and prostatic hypertrophy. Additional features include:

Oculomotor disorders such as blurring convergence resulting from inability to sustain contraction of the ocular muscles. *Oculogyric crisis* was associated with the postencephalitic type of parkinsonism (1917 to 1925). Spasms of the conjugate eye muscles occurred and the eyes were fixed, usually upward, for minutes to hours. It is rarely encountered today, because there are fewer patients with this type of parkinsonism still living.

Extreme fatigue and muscle pain. The muscles are exhausted by rigidity.

Postural hypotension. Some feel this is due to medications, but as patients are living longer, it may be a part of the natural history of the disease.

Respiratory difficulties. Many are secondary to hypoventilation and inactivity.

Diagnosis

No specific laboratory data are significant, so the diagnosis of Parkinson's syndrome is based on clinical findings. The major neurologic findings are listed in Table 50-1.

Treatment

Pharmacotherapy of Parkinson's disease attempts to restore the balance between dopamine and acetylcholine by the use of dopaminergic drugs. Dopamine does not cross the blood-brain barrier. Levodopa (L-dopa) is a metabolic precursor of dopamine that will cross the blood-brain barrier. However, levodopa is largely decarboxylated in the periphery (stomach, liver,

TABLE 50-1

MAJOR NEUROLOGIC FINDINGS IN PARKINSON'S SYNDROME

Neurologic finding	Comment
Rest tremor	Pill-rolling movement of fingers characteristic. Tremor decreased with voluntary movement and during sleep.
Masklike facies	Wide-eyed, unblinking, staring expression. Blinks two or three times per minute. Normal blinking, 12 to 20 times per minute.
Cogwheel rigidity	Motion interrupted by "catches." Resistance relatively constant throughout range of motion.
Postural and gait abnormalities	Stooped, shuffling, festinating gait; unable to turn quickly, turns *en bloc*.
Micrographia	Small handwriting that trails off; tremor may be obvious when drawing concentric circles.
Monotone	Expressionless speech.
Hyperactive glabellar (blink) reflex	Exaggerated sensitivity to finger tapping over glabella (between eyebrows) causes the patient to blink with each tap. It takes effort for a normal person to blink. Early sign of Parkinson's syndrome.

kidneys, and heart), and only small amounts reach the basal ganglia. Large doses are necessary to achieve results. The key was to improve the efficiency of L-dopa. This was achieved by combining L-dopa with a decarboxylase inhibitor that will not cross the blood-brain barrier. There is less breakdown of the drug in peripheral tissues, so that more is available to the brain and side effects are greatly reduced. Sinemet (carbidopa and levodopa), released in 1974, is available in two sizes, but the ratio is always 1:10—10 mg carbidopa and 100 mg levodopa or 25 mg carbidopa and 250 mg levodopa. Therapy with L-dopa or Sinemet is begun with small doses, which are gradually increased until symptoms disappear or improve or drug side effects appear. All patients on these drugs have side effects to some degree. These include gastrointestinal effects such as nausea and vomiting; 80 to 90 percent lose weight. The drug should be given after meals to decrease this effect. Cardiac arrhythmias, postural hypotension, and CNS symptoms (nightmares, confusion, insomnia, hallucinations, and depression) may also occur. Abnormal involuntary movements (dyskinesias) are bothersome and increase with long-term use of these drugs, especially Sinemet. These are dose-related, but decreasing the dose often results in return of the symptoms of parkinsonism.

Despite progression of the disease, these drugs have maintained improvement in patients for 6 to 8 years. Before their discovery the average patient was totally disabled in 9 years.

Other drugs used in the treatment of Parkinson's disease include anticholinergics, antihistamines (which also have anticholinergic action), and amantadine, a synthetic antiviral compound used in the prevention of Asian influenza. (The use of amantadine for parkinsonism is based on the discovery that symptoms were greatly reduced in a patient taking the drug for influenza prevention.) These drugs may be given alone or in combination with Sinemet. The belladonna alkaloids atropine and scopolamine were the first centrally active anticholinergics used to treat parkinsonism but have been largely supplanted by synthetic anticholinergics such as trihexyphenidyl (Artane) and benztropine (Cogentin). The use of diphenhydramine (Benadryl) and other antihistamines in parkinsonism is based on their central cholinergic blocking action.

Surgical lesions (using stereotaxic techniques) made in the globus pallidus or ventrolateral thalamus may be a successful treatment in selected patients with parkinsonism. Rigidity may improve, but there is no effect on the akinesia. Many patients will not be benefited by surgery. Surgical treatment is best reserved for those who do not respond to drug treatment, who have unilateral involvement and normal blood pressure, and who are relatively young.

Physical therapy, occupational therapy, and a positive attitude of encouragement are important adjuncts to treatment.

DEMYELINATING DISEASES

A large number of neurologic disorders are termed *demyelinating diseases* because their common pathologic feature is focal areas of destruction involving the myelin sheath of nerve fibers in the central nervous system. The axon often suffers damage as well, but destruction of myelin is the primary change. Multiple sclerosis is the primary demyelinating disease and is the focus of the discussion.

Acute disseminated encephalomyelitis

Acute disseminated encephalomyelitis (postvaccinial or postinfectious), although rare, is a demyelinating disorder that deserves mention because it is essentially preventable. This is an acute encephalitic or myelitic process of variable course characterized by symptoms indicating damage to the white matter of the brain or spinal cord. The pathologic findings consist of numerous circumscribed areas of perivascular demyelinization. About 1 week following measles and 10 days to 2 weeks following vaccination for rabies or smallpox, there is rapid development of neurologic symptoms consisting of headache, drowsiness, stupor, ocular palsies, and often a flaccid paralysis of all four limbs caused by a transverse cord lesion. Variations in severity are common.

Postvaccination encephalomyelitis may occur following rabies vaccination, presumably from sensitization to a vaccine containing brain tissue. This is essentiall an allergic encephalitis and does not occur with the use of the newer duck embryo vaccines free of nerve tissue. Encephalomyelitis may also follow smallpox vaccination, especially the primary vaccination, but the source of the material used for the vaccination seems to have little bearing on its occurrence. The incidence is estimated to be 1 in 5000 vaccinations. The recent decision not to include smallpox vaccination as part of the routine pediatric immunization program in the United States should decrease the incidence of this complication.

Postinfectious encephalomyelitis following a viral infection, especially measles, occurs in about 1 in 1000 cases. The mortality rate is 10 to 20 percent, and about 50 percent of those who survive are left with some neurologic damage. The use of measles vaccine in the United States has greatly reduced the occurrence of encephalomyelitis. There is some evidence that the measles virus may play a role in the etiology of multiple sclerosis (see below).

Multiple sclerosis

Multiple sclerosis is one of the most common neurologic disorders affecting young people. It is slightly more common in females. The mean age of occurrence is 30 years, with a range between 18 and 40 in the majority of cases. It is characterized by the widespread occurrence of patches of myelin destruction followed by gliosis in the white matter of the nervous system. The hard yellow plaques found on autopsy are responsible for its being so named. The characteristic course of the disease consists of a series of isolated attacks affecting different parts of the central nervous system. Each attack subsequently shows some degree of remission, but the overall picture is one of deterioration.

Etiology and pathology

The fundamental nature of the disturbance which leads to multiple sclerosis is unknown and is consequently the subject of much speculation. The illness is more common in temperate climates (northern Europe and northern United States), with an incidence of 30 to 80 per 100,000 population, and it is rare in the tropics; but in Japan multiple sclerosis is uncommon at any latitude. There is also a slightly higher familial incidence of the disease: it is about eight times more common in close relatives. There is a question as to whether this increased familial occurrence is due to a genetic predisposition (a hereditary pattern does not exist) or whether there is common exposure to an infectious agent (probably viral) during childhood which in some way may lead to multiple sclerosis during early adulthood. Migration studies reveal that if adults move from a high- to a low-risk area they retain the high risk for developing multiple sclerosis. However, a person who emigrates before the age of 15 years acquires the low risk of the second residence. These data are consistent with a possible viral cause with a long latent period between initial exposure and clinical onset of the disease. The mechanism of action may be that of an autoimmune reaction attacking myelin.

A number of viruses have been proposed as possible causative agents in multiple sclerosis. The measles (rubeola) virus is suspected by some investigators. Various measles antibodies have been found in the serum and CSF of patients with multiple sclerosis, and there is evidence that these antibodies are produced in the brain. If the measles virus is involved, it probably invades the subject in early life, lies dormant for a number of years, and then stimulates an autoimmune response. Another line of inquiry suggests that certain genetic factors render some people more susceptible to CNS invasion by various "slow" viruses. Slow viruses have long incubation periods and possibly develop only in conjunction with an abnormal or deficient immune status. Certain histocompatibility antigens (HLA-A3 and HLA-A7) have been found to be more common in multiple sclerosis patients than in controls. The presence of these antigens may possibly be related to a deficient immunologic defense against viral infection. Other researchers are attempting to find a relationship between multiple sclerosis in humans and distemper in dogs and cats. In one dramatic case, a family dog with the neurologic disease distemper recovered, but later three family members began to exhibit symptoms of multiple sclerosis. Such supposed precipitating situations are viewed by many as having occurred by pure chance.

Several events are generally considered to be precipitating factors, among them pregnancy, infection (especially with fever), emotional stress, and injury. Complete recovery is usual following the first attack. Remission usually occurs within 1 to 3 months with successive attacks. Eventually, however, recovery is not complete and patients are left with additional permanent damage after each bout.

The lesions of multiple sclerosis occur only in the white matter of the CNS. Autopsy examination shows that the lesions are most prominent in the pyramidal tracts and posterior columns of the cord, around the ventricles of the brain; in the optic nerve and its tract, brainstem, and cerebellar peduncles; and around large veins. In the acute phase the involved area is edematous, inflamed, and pinkish in color. The size may vary from a few millimeters to several centimeters in diameter. Macrophages remove the areas of degenerating myelin, and as the acute phase subsides, there is a reactive gliosis. The end result is a shrunken area of demyelination called a *plaque*. The axon cylinders and cell bodies are not destroyed, although the scar is capable of damaging the underlying axon fiber so that nerve fiber conduction is disrupted. The symptoms of multiple sclerosis due to the demyelinization become irreversible as the condition progresses.

Clinical features

The location of the lesions determines the clinical manifestations. Any combination of the following signs and symptoms may coexist:

1. *Sensory disorders.* Paresthesias (numbness, tingling, "dead" feeling, "pins and needles") may vary in degree from one day to the next. If there is a lesion of the posterior columns of the cervical cord, flexion of the neck causes shocklike sensations to run down the cord (*Lhermitt's sign*). Proprioceptive disorders often give rise to sensory ataxia and incoordination of the arms. Vibration sense is often

diminished. Since sensory disorders cannot be demonstrated objectively, these symptoms may be thought hysterical.

2. *Visual complaints.* A large number of patients experience visual problems as an initial symptom. Blurred vision, abnormal visual fields with blind spots (scotomas), and diplopia are reported in one or both eyes. Vision may be totally lost in one eye for a period of several hours to days. An optic neuritis is the basis for these visual disturbances. Diplopia as a result of brainstem lesions affecting the nuclei or fiber tracts of the extraocular muscles and nystagmus are other common complaints.

3. *Spastic weakness of the limbs.* Weakness of a limb on one side of the body or an asymmetric distribution in all four limbs is a common complaint. The patient may complain of tiredness and heaviness in one leg and noticeably drags that foot and has poor control. The patient may complain that the leg jumps spontaneously, especially when in bed. More profound spasticity is accompanied by painful spasm of the muscles. The tendon reflexes may be hyperactive and abdominal reflexes absent; the plantar responses are extensor (Babinski sign). These signs indicate involvement of the corticospinal pathways.

4. *Cerebellar signs.* Nystagmus (rapid oscillation of the eyeball horizontally or vertically) and cerebellar ataxia are other common symptoms and indicate involvement of the cerebellar and corticospinal tracts. Cerebellar ataxia is manifested by uncoordinated voluntary movements, intention tremors, balance disturbances, and dysarthria (scanning speech with words broken into syllables and pauses between syllables).

5. *Bladder dysfunction.* Lesions in the corticospinal tracts often cause disorders of sphincter control; hesitancy, urgency, and frequency are common and indicate a reduced-capacity spastic bladder. Acute retention and incontinence also occur.

6. *Disorders of mood.* Many patients develop *euphoria,* an unrealistic feeling of well-being. This is believed to be due to involvement of the white matter of the frontal lobes. Other signs of cerebral impairment may include loss of memory and dementia.

Diagnosis, prognosis, and treatment

The diagnosis is usually made on a clear history of relapses and remissions and signs of multiple lesions in the central nervous system. Many times it is impossible to confirm the diagnosis until the patient is followed for several years. The colloidal gold test on the cerebrospinal fluid is positive (in the absence of a positive serologic test) in many cases and is supportive evidence. In about 60 percent of cases of established multiple sclerosis the gamma globulin level in the cerebrospinal fluid is elevated, but this test is not helpful in establishing an early diagnosis. One test which is helpful in determining the presence of active demyelination is the basic protein assay (BPA) of the spinal fluid. The level of the BPA drops rapidly once the acute exacerbation is over (Antel and Arnason, 1983).

The progression of multiple sclerosis is extremely variable. The classic picture is one of intermittent relapses followed by more or less complete remissions. The remissions are usually less complete with each ensuing attack, so that within 10 to 20 years the patient is physically disabled; in a few cases the patient may become severely disabled within a couple of years.

The treatment of multiple sclerosis is symptomatic. During an acute relapse the patient should rest in bed, although prolonged bed rest is to be avoided. During acute relapses, vitamin B_{12} and corticosteroid drugs may be given, but evaluation of this treatment is difficult because of the episodic nature of the disease. Courses of ACTH are given IM or IV. This medication has been tested and used extensively in multiple sclerosis therapy and has been shown to result in earlier and greater improvement when compared with placebos, especially if given soon after an attack. Dexamethasone (Decadron) is given IV to relieve symptoms that are life-threatening, such as inability to swallow or breathe. The beneficial effects of either of these drugs are probably nonspecific or are based on their anti-inflammatory action. They do not prevent progression of the disease. Diazepam (Valium) or baclofen (Lioresal) are used to reduce muscle spasticity if this is a problem. Physical therapy is valuable; it tends to increase the patient's comfort and build morale. Gait retraining, muscle stretching, and muscle strengthening may all be necessary.

MYASTHENIA GRAVIS

The name *myasthenia gravis* means grave muscle weakness. It is the only neuromuscular disease that incorporates both rapid fatigue of voluntary muscle and prolonged recovery time (recovery may actually take 10 to 20 times longer than normal). Mortality rates in the past have been as high as 90 percent. The death rate has been drastically reduced since medications and respiratory care units have become available.

The clinical syndrome was first described in 1600. In the late 1800s myasthenia gravis was distinguished from muscle weakness due to true bulbar palsy. In the 1920s a physician with myasthenia gravis noticed an improvement after taking ephedrine for menstrual cramps. Finally, in 1934, another physician from England (Mary Walker) noted the similarity of symptoms in myasthenia gravis and curare poisoning. She used the curare antagonist physostigmine for myasthenia gravis and observed marked improvement.

The incidence of myasthenia gravis in the United States is often cited as 1 in 10,000. Some experts in the field think that this figure is low and that many cases are never diagnosed. The peak age of onset is 20 years, with a ratio of 3:1 favoring females. A second peak (though lower than the first) occurs in the older adult male.

Pathophysiology

Skeletal or striated muscles are innervated by large myelinated nerves that originate in the anterior horn cells of the spinal cord and the brainstem. They send their axons out in the spinal or cranial nerves to the periphery. Individual nerves branch many times and are capable of stimulating up to 2000 skeletal muscle fibers. The combination of the motor nerve and the muscle fibers it innervates is called a *motor unit*. Although each motor neuron innervates many muscle fibers, each muscle fiber is innervated by a single motor neuron.

The area of specialized contact between the motor nerve and the muscle fiber is called the *neuromuscular synapse* or *junction* (see Fig. 50-1). The neuromuscular junction is a chemical synapse between a nerve and muscle consisting of three basic components: a presynaptic element, a postsynaptic element, and a synaptic cleft about 200 Å wide between two elements. The presynaptic element consists of the axon terminal, which contains synaptic vesicles filled with the neurotransmitter acetylcholine. Acetylcholine is synthesized and stored in the axon terminal (bouton). The plasma membrane of the axon terminal is called the *presynaptic membrane*. The postsynaptic element consists of the *postsynaptic membrane* (postjunctional membrane), or *motor end plate*, of the muscle fiber. The postsynaptic membrane is formed by an invagination, called the *synaptic gutter* or *trough*, of the muscle membrane or sarcolemma into which the axon terminal protrudes. It has many folds (subneural clefts), which greatly increase the surface area. The postsynaptic membrane contains acetylcholine receptors and is capable of generating an end-plate potential which in turn can generate a muscle action potential. Acetylcholinesterase, an enzyme which destroys acetylcholine, is also located in the postsynaptic membrane. The *synaptic cleft* refers to the space be-

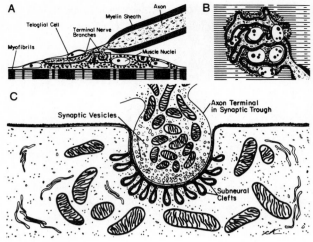

FIGURE 50-1

Muscle and neuromuscular junction. Schematic representations of the motor end plate as seen by light and electron microscopy. (A) End plate as seen in histologic sections in the long axis of the muscle fiber. (B) As seen in surface view with the light microscope. (C) As seen in an electron micrograph of an area such as that in the rectangle in (A). (From Curtis, Jacobson, and Marcus, 1972, p. 115.)

tween the pre- and postsynaptic membranes. The space is filled with a gelatinous material through which extracellular fluid may diffuse.

When a nerve impulse reaches the neuromuscular junction, the presynaptic axon terminal membrane is depolarized, causing the release of acetylcholine into the synaptic cleft. The acetylcholine diffuses across the synaptic gap and unites with the acetylcholine receptor sites in the postsynaptic membrane. This combination causes a change in permeability to both sodium and potassium in the postsynaptic membrane. The sudden influx of sodium ions and efflux of potassium ions lead to depolarization of the end plate known as the *end-plate potential* (EPP). When the EPP reaches threshold, it generates an action potential in the nonjunctional muscle membrane, which is propagated along the sarcolemma. This action potential sets off a series of reactions resulting in the contraction of the muscle fiber. Once transmission across the neuromuscular junction has occurred, acetylcholine is destroyed by the enzyme acetylcholinesterase. In normal persons, the amount of acetylcholine released is more than sufficient to result in an action potential.

In myasthenia gravis, neuromuscular conduction is impaired. The number of normal acetylcholine receptors is reduced as a consequence of an autoimmune injury. Antibodies to the acetylcholine receptor protein have been found in the serum of many myasthenia gravis patients. Determination of whether this is a primary or secondary consequence of receptor damage

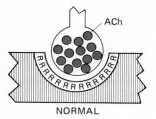
ACh

NORMAL

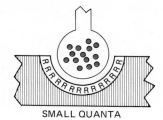
SMALL QUANTA

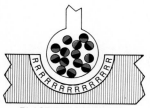
FLASE TRANSMITTER

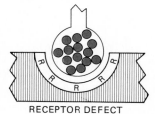
RECEPTOR DEFECT

FIGURE 50-2

Possible defects in myasthenia gravis. Schematic representations of neuromuscular junctions. Circles within nerve endings indicate ACh-containing vesicles; R represents ACh receptors. (From Drachman, Kao, Pesbronk, et al., 1976.)

caused by an unknown primary agent will be of great value in determining the exact pathogenesis of myasthenia gravis. Figure 50-2 illustrates some possible defects in myasthenia gravis.

In patients with myasthenia gravis, the muscles appear normal macroscopically. If atrophy is present, it is on the basis of disuse. Microscopically, in some cases lymphocytic infiltrates may be found within the muscle and other organs, but no consistent abnormality is found in the skeletal muscle.

Clinical manifestations

As mentioned previously, it is currently hypothesized that myasthenia gravis is an autoimmune disorder that impairs acetylcholine receptor functioning and decreases the efficiency of the neuromuscular junction. It most frequently presents as an insidious, progressive disease. However, it may remain localized to a specific group of muscles. Because the course is so variable from one patient to another, it is difficult to determine the prognosis. Table 50-2 divides myasthenia gravis patients into two groups—those with ocular myasthenia and those with generalized myasthenia. Generalized myasthenia may be mild, moderate, or severe, and the onset may be slow or rapid.

In 90 percent of patients the initial symptoms involve the ocular muscles, causing ptosis and diplopia. The diagnosis can be established by attention to the levator palpebrae muscles of the eyelids. If the disease

remains confined to the eye muscles, the course is very mild, and there is no mortality.

The facial, laryngeal, and pharyngeal muscles are also frequently involved in myasthenia gravis. This may result in regurgitation through the nose when swallowing is attempted (palatal muscles); abnormal, nasal speech; and failure of the mouth to close—called the *hanging jaw* sign.

Respiratory muscle involvement is evidenced by a weak cough, eventual attacks of dyspnea, and inability to clear the tracheobronchial tree of mucus. The shoulder and pelvic girdles may become involved in advanced cases; there may be generalized weakness of any of the skeletal muscles.

Generally, symptoms of myasthenia gravis are relieved by rest and anticholinesterase agents. Symptoms are aggravated or exacerbated by (1) alterations in hormonal balance, as during pregnancy, fluctuations in the

TABLE 50-2

CLINICAL CLASSIFICATION OF MYASTHENIA GRAVIS

Group I Ocular myasthenia
Involvement of ocular muscles only, with ptosis and diplopia. Very mild, no mortality

Group II Generalized myasthenia

A Mild generalized
Slow onset, frequently ocular, gradually spreading to skeletal and bulbar muscles. Respiratory system not involved. Response to drug therapy good. Low mortality rate.

B Moderate generalized
Gradual onset with frequent ocular presentation, progressing to more severe generalized involvement of the skeletal and bulbar muscles. Dysarthria, dysphagia, and poor mastication more prevalent than in mild, generalized myasthenia gravis. Respiratory muscles not involved. Response to drug therapy less satisfactory and the patient's activities restricted, but mortality rate low.

C Severe generalized
1 Acute fulminating
  Rapid onset of severe bulbar and skeletal muscle weakness with early involvement of respiratory muscles. Progression of disease usually complete within 6 months. Percentage of thymomas highest in this group. Response to drugs poor, incidence of myasthenic, cholinergic, and mixed crises high. Mortality rate high.
2 Late severe
  Severe myasthenia gravis develops at least 2 years after onset of group I or group II symptoms. Progression of myasthenia gravis may be either gradual or sudden. Second highest percentage of thymomas. Response to drug therapy and prognosis poor.

Source: Professional Information Committee of the National Medical Advisory Board: *Myasthenia Gravis: A Manual for Nurses,* Myasthenia Gravis Foundation, Inc., New York, 1975.

menstrual cycle, or disturbances in thyroid function; (2) concurrent illness, especially upper respiratory tract infections and those associated with diarrhea or fever; (3) emotional upsets—most patients experience more muscular weakness when they are upset; and (4) alcohol (especially with tonic water, which contains quinine, a drug promoting muscle weakness) and other drugs.

Diagnosis

A diagnosis can be made by a suspicious clinician on the basis of the patient's history and the physical examination. One must keep in mind that there *is* such a disease, affecting a small number of people. Many patients have been bluntly told to see a psychiatrist. Asking the subject to perform a repetitive action until tiredness is evident can help establish a diagnosis. The diagnosis is confirmed by the *Tensilon test*. Endrophonium chloride (Tensilon), a cholinesterase inhibitor drug, is given intravenously. In myasthenia patients, there is a marked improvement of muscle strength within 30 seconds. When a positive result is obtained, it is important to make a differential diagnosis between true myasthenia gravis and myasthenic syndrome. Patients with myasthenic syndrome have the same symptoms as those with true myasthenia gravis, but the cause is related to other pathologic processes such as diabetes, thyroid abnormalities, and widespread malignancy. The age at onset of the two conditions is an important distinguishing factor. Patients with true myasthenia are usually young; those with myasthenic syndrome are generally older. Symptoms in the myasthenic syndrome usually disappear if the basic disease can be controlled.

Abnormalities of the thymus gland occur in myasthenia gravis. Even when too small to be radiologically observable, the thymus glands of the majority of patients are histiligically abnormal. The tendency is for younger females to have thymic hyperplasia while older males have thymic neoplasms. Electomyography reveals a characteristic falling off in the amplitude of motor unit potential with continued use.

Treatment

If the patient survives for 10 years, the disease usually remains benign, and death from myasthenia gravis itself would be rare. These patients must learn to live within the limits prescribed by their disease. They need 10 hours of sleep at night to awaken refreshed, and they need to alternate work and rest periods. They must avoid precipitating factors and must take their medications on time.

Medical treatment with anticholinesterase drugs is the treatment of choice. Neostigmine inactivates or destroys cholinesterase, so the acetylcholine is not destroyed immediately. The effect is restoration to almost normal muscular activity, at least 80 to 90 percent of former strength and endurance. Besides neostigmine (Prostigmin), pyridostigmine (Mestinon), and ambenonium (Mytelase), there are other synthetic analogues of the drug originally used, physostigmine (Eserine). Disagreeable side effects in the gastrointestinal tract (cramping, diarrhea) are called *muscarinic side effects*. It is important that the patient realize that these symptoms can mean there has been too much medication on a particular day and that the next dose must be decreased accordingly to avoid a cholinergic crisis (see below). Since neostigmine is the most apt to cause muscarinic effects, it may be prescribed initially so that the patient is made aware of exactly what this side effect is like.

Pyridostigmine is available in a time span form and is often used at bedtime so the patient can sleep through the night without having to awaken to take medication.

The routine use of belladonna or atropine to neutralize muscarinic side effects is not recommended and could result in a dangerous overdose. Prednisone has been used since the 1960s. Many patients who were lost because they did not respond to Mestinon will do well on a regimen that combines prednisone and Mestinon.

Thymectomy in selected patients seems to bring about an earlier and more complete remission than might otherwise be expected. Young women with increasing disability and within the first 5 years after onset and patients who do not respond to the Mestinon and prednisone combination seem to get the most benefit from this procedure.

Crisis in myasthenia gravis

When unable to swallow, clear secretions, or breathe adequately without artificial assistance, the myasthenic patient is in crisis. There are two types of crisis: (1) *myasthenic crisis*, a condition in which there is a need for more anticholinesterase drugs; (2) *cholinergic crisis*, a condition due to an excess of anticholinesterase drugs. In either situation, artificial respiration and an adequate airway must be maintained. Tensilon (2 to 5 mg) is given intravenously as a test to differentiate between the types of crisis. The drug produces a temporary improvement in myasthenic crisis and no improvement or worsening of symptoms in cholinergic crisis.

If in myasthenic crisis, the patient is maintained on the respirator. Anticholinesterase drugs are withheld, since they increase respiratory secretions and may precipitate a cholinergic crisis. Medicines are restarted gradually, and often the dosage can be lowered following a crisis.

In a cholinergic crisis the patient may have taken

an excess of medication by mistake or the dosage may have been excessive because of a spontaneous remission. Many who develop this type of crisis are called *brittle myasthenics*. They are difficult to control with medication and have a narrowed therapeutic range between underdose and overdose. Their response to drugs is often only partial. In cholinergic crisis the patient is maintained on artificial ventilation, anticholinergic drugs are withheld, and 1 mg of atropine may be given intravenously and repeated if necessary. When atropine is given the patient must be carefully observed, since respiratory secretions can thicken, making suctioning difficult, or a mucus plug can occlude a bronchus, causing atelectasis.

ALZHEIMER'S DISEASE

Alzheimer's disease is the most disabling disease of the population over the age of 65. It affects approximately 15 percent of the population over the age of 65 and is severe in about 5 percent, affecting 1,200,000 persons in the United States. With the elderly population of the United States growing, the problem can be expected to get worse.

Pathologically the patient with Alzheimer's disease experiences a severe loss of hippocampal and cortical neurons with no loss of brain parenchyma. In addition, there are diffuse neurofibrillary tangles and senile plaques (the larger the number of senile plaques the worse the symptoms). These last two pathologic changes are not unique to Alzheimer's disease but are also found in patients suffering from lead encephalopathy and Down's syndrome. The latest research findings indicate that problems with neurotransmitters and the enzymes associated with their metabolism are involved. It appears that choline acetyltransferase (the enzyme that synthesizes acetylcholine) is decreased. Its decrease is particularly remarkable in the cerebral cortex, the hippocampus, and the amygdala. Another area under investigation by researchers is peptide neurotransmitters, since somatostatin is decreased in the brain of those suffering from Alzheimer's disease. An additional factor undergoing investigation is aluminum neurotoxicity. Crapper (1979) is the major proponent of a theory in which the membrane transport system fails in patients with Alzheimer's disease, allowing an interaction between aluminum and chromatin that causes the pathologic changes in protein synthesis and neurofibrillary changes.

No one etiologic factor has been identified at present but there are three major theories: (1) slow viruses, (2) an autoimmune process, and (3) aluminum toxicity. Currently the most popular theory (although still unproven) is that of slow viruses. These viruses have an incubation period of 2 to 30 years; therefore transmission is difficult to prove. Certain varieties of viral en-

cephalopathy (kuru, Creutzfeldt-Jakob disease) are characterized by pathologic changes that resemble the senile plaques seen in Alzheimer's disease.

The autoimmune theory is based on the presence of increased levels of brain-reactive antibodies in Alzheimer's disease. There are two types of amygdaloid (a protein complex with starchlike characteristics that is produced and deposited in certain pathologic states), one composed of IgG chains and the other of unknown composition. The theory suggests that the antigen-antibody complexes are catabolized by phagocytes and the immunoglobulin fragments degraded in lysosomes, leading to extracellular amygdaloid deposits.

Aluminum toxicity theory is based on the fact that aluminum is neurotoxic and can induce neurofibrillary changes in the brain. However, certain of the pathologic changes seen in Alzheimer's disease are not seen in aluminum toxicity. In addition, the serum aluminum levels in patients with Alzheimer's disease are normal, and there is no history of environmental exposure to aluminum.

The diagnosis of Alzheimer's disease is complicated by the fact that no test truly identifies the disease; the diagnosis is based on clinical observations and the family's description of the patient's behavior. The patient presenting with dementia should be evaluated to eliminate other causes of dementia, listed in Table 50-3.

Clinically the patient presents with disturbances of problem-solving capacity, forgetfulness, inability to cope with complex situations and think abstractly, emotional lability, apathy, and loss of recent and then of remote memory. As the disease progresses patients be-

TABLE 50-3

CAUSES OF DEMENTIA

Infections	Toxic substances
Neurosyphilis	Drugs
Tuberculosis	Alcohol
Viral diseases	Arsenic
Metabolic disorders	Vascular disorders
Hypothyroidism	Cerebral embolus
Electrolyte imbalance	Cerebral vasculitis
Nutritional deficiencies	Miscellaneous
Vitamin B_{12} deficiency	Parkinson's disease
Niacin deficiency	Wilson's disease
Korsakoff's deficiency	Huntington's disease
(thiamine)	Depression
Space-occupying lesions	
Subdural hematoma	
Tumor	
Abscess	

come totally dependent, unable to care for even their basic needs. Generally patients die of malnutrition and/or infection.

Patients seen for diagnostic evaluation of Alzheimer's disease should undergo a complete physical examination, including blood studies for syphilis, vitamin B_{12} level, and thyroid function; and, in particular, x-rays, electrocardiogram, CT scan, lumbar puncture, and electroencephalogram. In addition, extensive evaluation of cognitive skills as part of the neurologic examination is indicated. It is essential that other treatable causes for the symptoms be evaluated and eliminated, since several of the causes of dementia are treatable, whereas Alzheimer's disease is at this time untreatable.

Management of the patient involves both the patient and his or her family. Tranquilizers and antidepressants may be useful in managing the patient's behavior. Family support groups are essential. Some communities have day care programs available, giving the family a respite from the 24-hour-a-day care. Visiting nurses are helpful, especially as the patient's condition deteriorates and total care is needed.

INFECTIONS OF THE NERVOUS SYSTEM

Infections of the central nervous system constitute a serious medical problem requiring immediate recognition and treatment if serious neurologic sequelae are to be minimized and the patient is to survive.

Infection of the central nervous system by viruses is relatively uncommon but can be serious. Generally viruses invade the central nervous system via the blood, although certain infections such as rabies and varicella-zoster invade the central nervous system via the peripheral nerves.

Signs and symptoms of viral central nervous system infections vary greatly according to the susceptibility of the different nervous system cells to the virus. Infections limited to the meninges give symptoms suggestive of meningitis (nuchal rigidity, headache, fever), whereas if the brain parenchyma is involved the patient shows a decreased level of consciousness, seizures, focal neurologic deficits, and increased intracranial pressure.

Viral meningitis and encephalitis

Viral meningitis is an infection involving the meninges; it tends to be benign and self-limiting. Viral encephalitis involves the brain parenchyma and is more serious.

Various viruses are known to cause meningitis and encephalitis (see Table 50-4).

Viruses generally replicate themselves at the original site of infection—e.g., nasopharyngeal or gastrointestinal systems—and then spread to the central nervous system via the vascular system. Contrary to previous thought, the blood-brain barrier does not provide complete protection against the invasion of viruses. Encephalitis involves an inflammatory reaction of the brain parenchyma, causing degeneration and phagocytosis of neural cells.

With viral meningitis, the patient presents with abrupt onset of headache, fever, and nuchal rigidity; the patient may also experience malaise, sore throat, nausea, vomiting, and abdominal pain. In addition, viral meningitis caused by the enteroviruses is associated with rashes; mumps meningitis is associated with parotitis as well as oophoritis and pancreatitis. Type 2 herpes simplex may coincide with eruption of herpes lesions on the genitals.

In addition to the meningeal signs, viral encephalitis presents with decreasing levels of consciousness, seizures, and focal symptoms, depending on the area of brain involved. Patients with herpes simplex encephalitis may show bizarre behavior and hallucinations.

In evaluating the patient presenting with the signs and symptoms of viral meningitis and encephalitis, it is important to differentiate these diseases from other more treatable infections such as subacute bacterial endocarditis or brain abscess. Cerebrospinal fluid pressure may be normal or elevated and may contain protein in small or large quantities; the electroencephalogram may show changes, especially in encephalitis. Virologic studies can specifically identify the virus; this has become more important, because herpes simplex encephalitis is currently treated with adenine arabinoside.

Other specific antiviral agents are not currently used, and patients are treated supportively as their condition dictates. The prognosis is good for patients with meningitis but poorer for patients with encephalitis.

TABLE 50-4

VIRUSES CAUSING CENTRAL NERVOUS SYSTEM INFECTIONS

Enteroviruses
  Poliovirus
  Coxsackie virus types A, B
  ECHO virus
Herpesviruses
  Herpes simplex virus types 1 and 2
  Cytomegalic virus
Myxoviruses
  Measles virus
  Mumps virus
  Influenza virus

Mortality rates vary from 50 percent in herpes simplex encephalitis to less than 1 percent in specific types of arbovirus encephalitis. Sequelae such as seizures, hydrocephalus, and other neurologic deficits are common.

Reye's syndrome

Reye's syndrome is a rare, acute encephalitis and liver dysfunction seen in children and young adolescents after common viral infections. The children have a history of previous infection with influenza, varicella, adenovirus, Coxsackie virus, ECHO virus, or parainfluenza virus, with apparent recovery from the original viral infection. The asymptomatic or recovery period in postviral infection varies from hours to days. Vomiting and convulsions, then delirium and coma follow this apparent recovery.

Pathologically, the brain swells with injury to the neuronal mitochondria. Fatty infiltration of the liver occurs, spreading rapidly through the parenchyma. Fat deposits can also be found in the myocardium and in the renal tubules. The relation between the viral infection and the encephalopathy and liver damage is unknown.

Coma and decerebrate posturing due to increased intracranial pressure are often seen. Electrolyte imbalances, especially hyponatremia and hypokalemia, are a serious problem. Treatment is nonspecific and is directed toward reducing intracranial pressure and correcting metabolic and electrolyte abnormalities.

Measures to control or reduce cerebral edema include hyperventilation and corticosteroids. Elevation of the head of the bed to approximately 30°, hypothermia, and administration of intravenous mannitol are other means of reducing cerebral edema.

Correction of electrolyte imbalances and clotting factor deficiencies is accomplished with neomycin and low protein intake. In cases with refractory metabolic abnormalities, peritoneal dialysis and exchange transfusions may be used.

Hypertonic glucose solutions are used for hydration to maintain a blood sugar of 200 to 300 mg/dl, since low blood sugar leads to increased production of ammonia and fatty acids.

Some children who recover have residual neurologic deficits including impaired mental capacity, seizures, and hemiplegia. Mortality ranges from 25 to 50 percent, depending on such factors as age, severity of symptoms, and how early the condition is diagnosed and treated.

Bacterial infections

Bacterial infections of the central nervous system present a challenging problem. A variety of bacteria infect the meninges and brain parenchyma. The most common infecting bacteria are *Staphylococcus aureus*, *Streptococcus pneumoniae*, and *Haemophilus influenzae*. Isolation of the specific agent involved is essential in the treatment of bacterial central nervous system infections.

Bacteria enter the central nervous system by several different routes. The ears, sinus, mastoid, and face are the most common sites of the original infection. Bacteria are able to travel from the site of origin to the central nervous system because of the high vascularity of the face and neck and the anatomic structuring of the venous sinuses within the brain. Early and conscientious treatment of these primary infections significantly reduces the incidence of secondary central nervous system infections.

Brain abscess

Brain abscess is an infective process involving the brain parenchyma. It is primarily caused by the spread of an infection from adjacent foci or through the vascular system. A previous history of otitis media, mastoiditis, suppurative sinusitis, or infection of the face, scalp, or skull is common. Bronchiectasis, lung abscess, empyema, and bacterial endocarditis are also known to lead to brain abscess.

Infection may invade the brain several different ways. In otitis media the infection may extend through the tympanic cavity or through the mastoid and meninges to reach the brain tissue. The infection extends via the veins of the inner ear, causing the veins to thrombose. This thrombosis impairs cerebral circulation, leading to ischemia and infarction, which facilitate the development of a local infection. Any tear in the dura caused by trauma is a potential source of infection of the brain.

Generally, abscesses are localized near to the original site of infection. However, those resulting from retrograde venous propagation are located at some distance from the primary site in the distribution of the nearest venous sinus. Metastatic abscesses are generally located along the middle cerebral artery. Early in the course of the disease, the infected tissue is edematous and infiltrated with leukocytes. Gradually, the outer portion becomes thickened because of the presence of collagen forming the abscess wall. In the center of the abscess liquefaction necrosis occurs. Abscess cavities can spread through the white matter, penetrating the walls of the ventricles into the meninges.

Brain abscess most frequently occurs between the ages of 20 and 50 but has been found in all age groups. The patient presents with headache and focal neurologic signs varying with the location of the abscess (see Table 50-5). Signs of increased intracranial pressure (especially nausea, vomiting, and decreasing level of consciousness) are the most common findings.

Generally a CT scan identifies and localizes the abscess as well as surrounding smaller abscesses. Lumbar puncture is generally avoided when the signs point to a large mass. Early diagnosis and prompt antibiotic therapy are essential if the patient is to survive. Residual neurologic deficits, especially convulsions, are common.

TABLE 50-5

FOCAL SYMPTOMS SEEN IN BRAIN ABSCESS

Lobe	Symptoms
Frontal	Drowsiness, inattentiveness, disturbed judgment, impaired intelligence, occasionally convulsions
Temporal	Inability to name objects; inability to read, write, or understand spoken words; hemianopia
Parietal	Impaired position sense and stereognostic perception, focal seizures, homonymous hemianopia, dysphasia, acalculia, agraphia
Cerebellar	Suboccipital headache, stiff neck, impaired coordination, nystagmus, impaired gait, intention tremor

QUESTIONS

Degenerative diseases of the nervous system

Directions: Answer the following on a separate sheet of paper.

1. Name the sites in the brain that are affected in Parkinson's disease. How are these areas of the brain affected? Where are these areas located in the brain?

2. Name the type of fiber tract that is involved in Parkinson's disease. What is the general function of this fiber tract?

3. Define *Parkinson's syndrome* and name three types of the disease.

4. Discuss the role of hydrogen peroxide and dopamine in parkinsonism.

5. Name and briefly describe five movement disorders of the extrapyramidal motor tracts.

6. Name two drugs known to cause extrapyramidal dysfunction and parkinsonian signs and symptoms.

7. Name several neurologic findings (include one reflex) common in patients with Parkinson's disease.

8. What serious demyelinating disorder may follow measles or vaccination for rabies? How can this be prevented?

9. Describe the pathology in multiple sclerosis. What are the most likely symptoms which would cause you to suspect this disease in a patient?

10. List the major theories of the etiologic factors in Alzheimer's disease.

Directions: Circle the letter preceding each item below that correctly answers the question or completes the statement. Only one answer is correct, with exceptions noted.

11. Which of the following are degenerative diseases of the nervous system? (More than one answer may be correct.)
a. Brain abscess   b. Multiple sclerosis   c. Amyotrophic lateral sclerosis   d. Viral meningitis
e. Wernicke-Korsakoff syndrome

12. The chief symptom complex of Parkinson's disease is:
a. Rigidity, aphasia, and oculogyric crisis
b. hemiplegia, drooling, and tremor   c. Tremor, rigidity, and weakness   d. All the above

13. The preferred treatment for Parkinson's disease is:
a. Medical treatment with L-dopa   b. Surgical treatment of the older patient with bilateral disease   c. Anticholinergic drugs   d. Medical treatment with dopamine

14. Symptoms of Parkinson's disease include: (More than one answer may be correct.)
a. Masklike face   b. Intention tremor
c. Bradykinesia   d. Choreiform movements

15. The probable site of abnormality in athetosis is the:
a. Neuromuscular junction   b. Fifth cranial nerve   c. Globus pallidus   d. Motor cortex

16. In multiple sclerosis:
a. Convulsions occur in about half the cases.
b. Visual loss is generally unilateral.   c. Headaches and aphasia are not unusual.   d. Euphoria is an uncommon disturbance.

17. A patient who receives L-dopa with a decarboxylase inhibitor should avoid taking large doses of:
a. Thiamine (B_1)   b. Pyridoxine (B_6)   c. Cyanocobalamin (B_{12})   d. Any of the B vitamins

18. Multiple sclerosis is:
a. Usually inherited   b. Most common in tropical areas   c. Often a familial disease   d. Most common in the 20- to 40-year age group

19. Which of the following statements is true about myasthenia gravis?
a. Ptosis of the eyelids is an uncommon symptom.
b. By nature it is an acute disease common in cold climates.   c. It is characterized by acetylcholine receptor deficiency at the junction of a motor nerve and skeletal muscle.   d. There is experimental evidence that the parathyroid glands are involved in some way.

20. The only manifestations of myasthenia gravis are:
a. Rigidity and tremor   b. Flaccid and/or spastic paralysis of voluntary muscle   c. Rapid fatigue of skeletal muscle and prolonged time for recovery of power   d. Rapid fatigue of smooth muscle and prolonged time for recovery of power

21. Myasthenia gravis is often associated with disorders of the:
a. Heart   b. Thyroid   c. Thymus   d. Liver

22. Your client has demonstrated a positive Tensilon test. Which of the following symptoms would indicate this result?
a. Muscarinic effect on smooth muscle   b. Immediate decrease in muscle strength   c. Difficulty in keeping eyes open (ptosis)   d. Immediate increase in muscle strength

23. Anticholinesterase drugs are used to treat myasthenia gravis. The most common side effects of these medications involve the:
a. Central nervous system   b. Skeletal muscle
c. GI tract   d. Respiratory system

24. Which of the following is *not* used in the treatment of myasthenia gravis?
a. Neostigmine   b. Pyridostigmine
c. Ambenonium   d. Endrophonium

25. When a patient with myasthenia gravis is in crisis, the first consideration is to:
a. Identify the type of crisis (cholinergic versus myasthenic)   b Control the hemorrhage   c Establish an adequate airway   d Restore electrolyte balance

26. Signs and symptoms of Wernicke-Korsakoff syndrome include: (More than one answer may be correct.)
a. Impairment of recent memory   b. Postural hypotension   c. Amnesia   d. Anemia

27. Signs and symptoms of Alzheimer's disease include: (More than one answer may be correct.)
a. Forgetfulness   b. Cognitive rigidity
c. Inability to cope with complex situations
d. Bradykinesia   e. Emotional lability

28. Which of the following are routes of entry of bacteria into the central nervous system?
a. Ears   b. Eyes   c. Nasal sinuses   d. Vascular system   e. All the above

29. Which of the following is common in the previous history of patients with a brain abscess?
a. Otitis media   b. Face or scalp infection
c. Mastoiditis   d. Suppurative sinusitis   e. All the above

Directions: Circle T if the statement is true and F if it is false. Correct the false statements.

30.   T   F   Alzheimer's disease affects approximately 15 percent of the population over the age of 65.

31.   T   F   Neurofibrillary tangles and senile plaques are unique to Alzheimer's disease.

32.   T   F   Mangement of Alzheimer's disease involves the patient's family as well as the patient.

33.   T   F   Metastatic brain abscesses are generally located along the middle cerebral artery.

34.   T   F   Amyotrophic lateral sclerosis (ALS) has been conclusively linked to arsenic toxicity.

35.   T   F   Deficiencies of the B vitamins B_1, B_6, B_{12}, niacin, and pantothenic acid are associated with various neurologic disorders.

36.   T   F   Niacin is accepted as the therapy of choice for patients suffering from Wernicke-Korsakoff syndrome.

37. T   F   Viral meningitis is a viral infection involving the meninges; it tends to be benign and self-limiting.

38. T   F   Viral encephalitis involves the brain parenchyma and is potentially not a serious condition.

39. T   F   The blood-brain barrier provides complete protection against invasion by viruses.

40. T   F   Reye's syndrome is a rare acute encephalitis and liver dysfunction seen in children and young adolescents following common viral infections.

41. T   F   Fatty infiltration involves the liver, myocardium, and renal tubules in Reye's syndrome.

CHAPTER 51

CENTRAL NERVOUS SYSTEM INJURY

OBJECTIVES

At the completion of this chapter you should be able to:

1. State the normal levels of intracranial pressure and several causes of increased intracranial pressure.
2. Explain how the body compensates for increased intracranial pressure.
3. Differentiate the early signs and symptoms of increased intracranial pressure from the later signs and symptoms.
4. Identify and describe the layers of tissue which protect the brain from external trauma.
5. Explain how infection may enter the brain when the galea is torn.
6. Locate and describe the function of the three tissue layers which make up the meninges.
7. Describe the two general mechanisms which account for brain damage in head trauma.
8. Describe a *contrecoup* injury.
9. Explain why fracture of the temporal bone of the skull is most likely to result in an epidural hematoma.
10. Differentiate between subdural and epidural hematoma with respect to blood vessels involved, common site, type of trauma, early findings, signs and symptoms, clinical course, and treatment.
11. Differentiate between acute, subacute, and chronic subdural hematoma according to symptoms, causes, treatment, and prognosis.
12. Describe the characteristic changes in the contents of a subdural hematoma.
13. List the early and late signs and symptoms of increased intracranial pressure and explain their pathogenesis.
14. List the three most common sites of spinal cord injury, the types of physical forces generally involved, the type of injury that may result, and the immediate consequences.
15. Define *spinal shock* (pathogenesis, duration, effect on body functions).
16. Describe spinal cord injury at various levels, including the common cause, expected neurologic deficit, type of paralysis, course, and prognosis.

17. Describe the emergency and long-term treatment of spinal cord injuries.
18. Describe the structure and function of an intervertebral disc.
19. Discuss the pathophysiology, signs and symptoms, diagnosis, and treatment of herniated intervertebral disc disease.

INCREASED INTRACRANIAL PRESSURE

Increased intracranial pressure is defined as an increase in the pressure exerted within the cranial cavity. Normally the cranial cavity is occupied by brain tissue, blood, and cerebrospinal fluid. Each portion occupies a specific volume giving a normal intracranial pressure of 50 to 200 mm water or 4 to 15 mmHg. Intracranial pressure is normally influenced by everyday activities and rises temporarily to levels much higher than normal. A few of these activities are deep abdominal breathing, coughing, and straining. Temporary increases in intracranial pressure present no difficulty, but sustained pressure has a detrimental effect on living brain tissue.

The cranial cavity is a rigid compartment filled to capacity with incompressible substances—the brain (weighing 1400 g), the cerebral spinal fluid (approximately 75 ml), and the blood (approximately 75 ml). An increase in the volume of any of these three major substances results in encroachment on the space occupied by the others and increased intracranial pressure. Increased intracranial pressure is not only seen after head injury but has many additional causes.

A brain tumor is an added mass of tissue occupying the cranial cavity. Any blockage to the flow of cerebrospinal fluid would allow a backup to occur in the ventricles, increasing the space occupied by the cerebrospinal fluid and decreasing the space available for brain tissue and blood. A tumor that obstructs the jugular vein and, therefore, venous drainage from the cranial cavity would lead to increased intracranial pressure.

Cerebral edema, perhaps the most common cause of increased intracranial pressure, itself has many causes. These include an increase in intracellular fluid, hypoxia, fluid and electrolyte imbalances, cerebral ischemia, meningitis, and, of course, injury. Regardless of the cause, the effects are basically the same.

Intracranial pressure generally increases gradually. After head injury edema formation may take 36 to 48 hours to reach its maximum (Schwartz, 1984, p. 1790). A rise in intracranial pressure to 33 mmHg (450 mm H_2O) significantly reduces cerebral blood flow. The ischemia that results stimulates the vasomotor centers, and the systemic blood pressure rises. Stimulation of the cardioinhibitory center produces bradycardia, and respiration is slowed. This compensatory mechanism, known as the *Cushing reflex*, helps to maintain cerebral blood flow. (The decreasing respiration, however, leads to CO_2 retention and resultant cerebral vasodilatation, which contributes to increasing intracranial pressure.) Systemic blood pressure will continue to rise proportionately to the increasing intracranial pressure, although eventually a point is reached when the intracranial pressure exceeds the arterial pressure and cerebral circulation ceases, with resultant brain death. Generally, this event is heralded by a rapidly decreasing arterial blood pressure (Escourolle and Porrier, 1978; Ganong, 1977).

Additional compensatory mechanisms include a slight shifting of volumes within the cranial cavity. Intracranial cerebrospinal fluid is shunted to the spinal subarachnoid space. There is also a slight decrease in cerebral blood flow in an attempt to decrease the rising intracranial pressure. These compensatory mechanisms are ineffective in dealing with serious and sustained intracranial pressure.

The clinical manifestations of increased intracranial pressure are many and varied and are subtle in their appearance. Alteration in the patient's level of consciousness (LOC) is the most sensitive indicator of all the signs of increased intracranial pressure (see discussion in Chap. 47). The classic triad of symptoms is headache due to stretching of the dura and blood vessels, papilledema due to pressure on and swelling of the optic nerve, and vomiting—frequently projectile. The presence of widened pulse pressure and decreased pulse and respiratory rates signals brain decompensation and impending death. Other signs of increased intracranial pressure include hyperthermia, motor and sensory changes, altered speech, and seizures.

HEAD INJURY

Introduction

The brain is protected from injury by the hair, skin, and bones that surround it. Without this protection the delicate brain which makes us what we are would be very susceptible to injury and destruction. Moreover, a neuron once destroyed does not regenerate. Head injury can have catastrophic implications for a person. Some problems are caused directly by the injury, many others are secondary to the injury. It is these effects that the medical team works to prevent and to detect early in order to avoid the sequence of events that leads to mental and physical deficit and even death.

Just above the skull lies the *galea aponeurotica*, a freely moveable, dense, fibrous tissue which aids in absorbing the force from external trauma. Between the galea and the skin is a fatty layer and a deep membranous layer which contains large vessels. Awareness of this fact is important, because when severed, these vessels constrict poorly and may cause significant blood loss in a patient with a scalp laceration. Directly beneath the galea is the subaponeurotic space, in which are found the *emissary* and *diploic veins*. These vessels may carry infection from the scalp to deep within the skull, which underscores the extreme importance of thorough cleansing and debridement of the scalp whenever the galea has been torn (Schwartz, 1984).

In the adult, the skull is a rigid compartment allowing for no expansion of intracranial contents. The bone is actually composed of two walls or tables which are separated by cancellous bone. The outer wall is called the *outer table*, and the inner wall is called the *inner table*. This structure provides for greater strength and insulation with less weight. The inner table contains grooves in which lie the anterior, middle, and posterior meningeal arteries. When fracture of the skull involves tearing of one of these arteries, the resultant arterial bleeding, which accumulates in the epidural space, may lead to a fatal outcome unless it is detected and treated immediately. This constitutes one of the true neurosurgical emergencies, demanding immediate surgical intervention (Schwartz, 1984).

Covering the brain for added protection are the meninges. The three layers of the meninges are the dura mater, the arachnoid, and the pia mater. Each has a separate function and differs from the other two in structure (Fig. 51-1). (See also Chap. 46.)

The *dura* is the tough, semitranslucent, inelastic outer membrane. It functions to (1) protect the brain, (2) enclose the venous sinuses (which are composed of dura mater and endothelial lining only—no vascular tissue), and (3) form the periosteum of the inner table. It is closely attached to the interior surface of the skull. In view of the problems that arise when a tear in the dura is not completely repaired and made airtight, its most important function is perhaps protection. There may be expansion of the fracture instead of healing and a chronic leakage of cerebrospinal fluid which may lead to the development of meningocerebral cicatrix, causing focal epilepsy. However, there are instances when the dura is not closed but instead is left open. These situations include: cerebral edema (to allow for decompression of the bulging brain), drainage of cerebrospinal fluid, or after exploratory trepanning (to allow for inspection and evacuation of clots).

FIGURE 51-1
Meninges in greater detail. Coronal section through the superior sagittal sinus. Emissary vein shown connecting scalp with superior sagittal sinus. The subarachnoid space is filled with cerebrospinal fluid. It enters the sinus through the arachnoid villi. (From Langley, Telford, and Christensen, 1980, p. 245.)

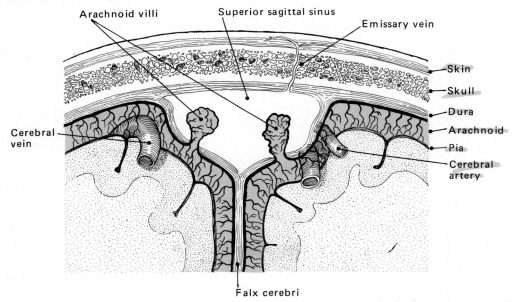

The dura has a rich blood supply. The middle and posterior areas are supplied by the middle meningeal artery, which branches off the internal carotid and vertebral arteries. The anterior and ethmoid vessels are also branches of the internal carotid and supply the anterior fossa. A branch of the occipital artery, the posterior meningeal, supplies blood to the posterior fossa.

Lying close to the dura but not attached to it is the fine, fibrous, elastic membrane known as the *arachnoid*. This membrane is not attached to the dura mater. However, the space between the two membranes—the subdural space— is a potential space. Bleeding between the dura and the arachnoid spreads freely, limited only by the barriers of the falx cerebri and tentorium. The cerebral veins passing through this space have little support except that provided by the dura and the arachnoid and are therefore susceptible to injury and rupture in head (cerebral) trauma.

Between the arachnoid and the pia mater (which lies directly beneath the arachnoid) is the *subarachnoid space*. This space widens and deepens in places and allows for the circulation of cerebrospinal fluid. In the superior sagittal and transverse sinuses, the arachnoid forms villous projections (the Pacchionian bodies) which serve as a pathway for the emptying of cerebrospinal fluid into the venous system.

The *pia mater* is a delicate membrane which is richly supplied with minute blood vessels. The pia dips into all the sulci and blankets the ridges of the gyri. It is the only meningeal layer to do this; the other two meningeal layers bridge the sulci. In some of the fissures and sulci on the medial side of the hemispheres, the pia forms a barrier between the ventricles of the brain and the sulcus or fissure. This barrier provides a structural support for the choroid plexus of each of the ventricles.

The brain damage seen in head trauma can be caused in two different ways: (1) by the immediate effects of the trauma on the functioning brain and (2) by the later effects of the brain cells' response to the trauma.

Immediate neurologic damage is caused by the penetration and laceration of brain tissue by an object or piece of bone, by the effects of force or energy transmitted to the brain, and, lastly, by the effects of acceleration-deceleration on the brain, which is confined in a rigid compartment.

The degree of damage caused by these problems can be dependent upon the force applied—the greater the force, the greater the damage. Two kinds of force are applied in two ways, causing two different effects. First, there is local injury caused by a sharp object with low velocity and little force. Disruption of neurologic

functioning occurs in a localized area and is caused by penetration of the dura at the point of impact by the object or fragments of bone. Second, there is generalized injury, which is more commonly seen in blunt trauma to the head and after automobile accidents. The damage occurs as the energy or force is transmitted to the brain. Much of the energy or force is absorbed by the protective layers of hair, scalp, and skull, but with violent trauma these are not enough to protect the brain. The remaining energy is transmitted to the brain as this energy passes through the brain tissue, causing damage and disruption along the way as delicate tissues are subjected to the force (Schwartz, 1984). If the head is moving and is suddenly and violently stopped, as in an automobile accident, damage is caused not only by local injury to tissue but also by acceleration and deceleration (Schwartz, 1984). The force of acceleration and deceleration causes the contents within the rigid skull to move, thereby forcing the brain against the inner surface of the skull on the side opposite the impact. This is also called *contrecoup* injury. As has been noted before, some areas within the cranial vault are rough, and as the brain moves across these areas (e.g., the sphenoid ridge), they tear and lacerate the tissues. The damage is intensified when trauma also causes rotation of the skull. The areas of the brain likely to receive the greatest amount of damage include the anterior portion of the frontal and temporal lobes, the posterior sections of the occipital lobes, and the upper portion of the midbrain (Schwartz, 1984).

The secondary effects of the trauma, which cause severe neurologic alterations, are due to the tissue response to the injury. Whenever tissue is injured, it responds in a predictable way—there is alteration in intracellular and extracellular fluid content, extravasation of blood, increased blood supply to the area, and mobilization of cells to repair damage and remove cellular debris.

The neurons, the functional cells within the brain, are dependent from minute to minute on a constant supply of nutrients in the form of glucose and oxygen and are very susceptible to metabolic injury when supplies are cut off. As a result of injury the cerebral circulation may lose its ability to regulate the available circulating blood volume, causing ischemia of certain areas within the brain.

Epidural hematoma

Epidural hematoma is a serious sequela to head injury and carries a mortality rate of approximately 50 percent (Schwartz, 1984). Epidural hematoma occurs most frequently in the parietotemporal area from a tear in the middle meningeal artery (Fig. 51-2). In the frontal and occipital areas hematomas are frequently not suspected and produce poorly localizing signs (Beeson and McDermott, 1979). When epidural hematoma is not associated with additional brain injuries, early treatment is generally followed by recovery with little or no neurologic deficit.

The typical patient with epidural hematoma gives a history of head injury followed by a short period of unconsciousness. After this short period of unconsciousness a lucid period follows. It is important to note, however, that this lucid interval is not reliably diagnostic of epidural hematoma. First, the lucid interval may go unobserved, especially if it is short in duration. Second, the patient with additional serious brain injury may remain stuporous (Beeson and McDermott, 1979).

An expanding hematoma in the temporal area causes the temporal lobe to be forced downward and inward. This pressure causes the medial portion of the lobe (the uncus and part of the hippocampal gyrus) to herniate under the edge of the tentorium, causing the neurologic signs observed by the medical team (Fig. 51-3).

The pressure of the herniation of the uncus on the arterial circulation to the reticular formation of the medulla causes unconsciousness. Also located in this area are the nuclei to the third cranial nerve (oculomotor). Compression of this nerve produces dilatation of the pupil and ptosis of the eyelid. Compression of the corticospinal pathways ascending in this area causes weakness in motor responses contralaterally (i.e., side opposite the hematoma), brisk or hyperactive reflexes, and a Babinski sign.

As the developing hematoma enlarges, it pushes the entire brain toward the opposite side, causing severe intracranial pressure. Late signs of increased intracranial pressure develop, including decerebrate rigidity and disturbances in vital signs and respiratory functioning.

Epidural hemorrhage is diagnosed from clinical signs and symptoms as well as by carotid arteriogram and echoencephalogram. Treatment is surgical evacuation of the hematoma and control of the bleeding from the lacerated middle meningeal artery. Surgical intervention must take place early, before serious compression of brain tissue causes brain damage. Mortality re-

mains high even when the condition is diagnosed and treated early because of the associated severe brain trauma and sequelae (Cohen et al., 1983).

Subdural hematoma

While an epidural hematoma is generally arterial in origin, a subdural hematoma is venous (Fig. 51-2). It is caused by rupture of the veins in the subdural space. Subdural hematomas are divided into types which differ in symptoms and prognosis: acute, subacute, and chronic.

Acute subdural hematoma

Acute subdural hematomas are those which cause serious and significant neurologic symptoms within 24 to 48 hours after injury. Frequently associated with serious brain trauma, these hematomas are also associated with a high mortality rate (Schwartz, 1984).

Progressive neurologic deficit is due to the compression of brain tissue with herniation of the brainstem into the foramen magnum, leading to compression of the brainstem. This quickly leads to cessation of respiration and loss of control of pulse and blood pressure.

Diagnosis is made by carotid arteriogram and echoencephalogram or computed tomography (CT scan). Acute subdural hematoma should always be considered a possibility in patients who have suffered severe neurologic trauma and show signs of deteriorating neurologic status. Since more than half of these hematomas are bilateral, it is extremely important to consider the type of injury incurred and to use appropriate diagnostic measures (e.g., bilateral arteriograms) to rule out the possibility of bilateral hematomas (Schwartz, 1984; Cohen et al., 1983).

Treatment consists mainly of removal of the he-

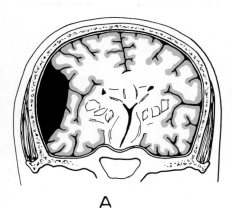
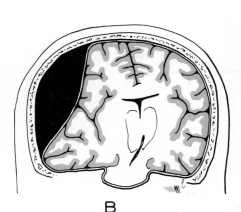

A   B

FIGURE 51-2

(A) Subdural hematoma, usually a result of laceration of the subdural veins. (B) Epidural hematoma in the temporal fossa, usually a result of laceration of the middle meningeal artery.

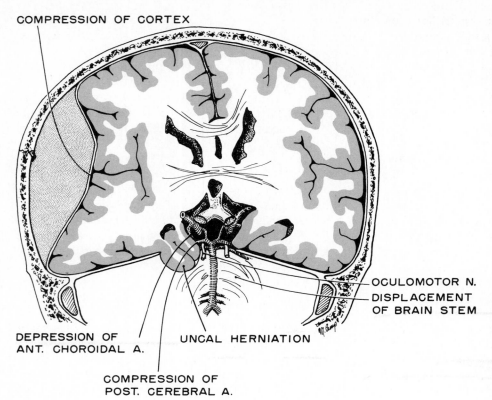

COMPRESSION OF CORTEX

DEPRESSION OF
ANT. CHOROIDAL A.

UNCAL HERNIATION

COMPRESSION OF
POST. CEREBRAL A.

OCULOMOTOR N.
DISPLACEMENT
OF BRAIN STEM

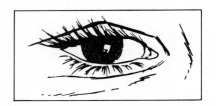

FIGURE 51-3
Mechanisms of signs and symptoms of an expanding intracranial hematoma over the parietotemporal region. The expanding hematoma compresses the cortex, pushing the brain to the opposite side and displacing the brainstem, cranial nerves, and vessels. The extreme medial portion of the temporal lobe (uncus) becomes herniated under the edge of the tentorium cerebelli. Compression of the oculomotor nerve by the herniated uncus may lead to ipsilateral pupil dilation, ptosis, and eventual pupil fixation. Compression of the cerebral cortex and/or distortion of the brainstem will result in depression of consciousness. In the brainstem the reticular activating system is involved. The arterial supply and venous return to the brainstem may be compromised by pressure. Interference with the cardiorespiratory centers will be evidenced by irregularity or slowing of the pulse, elevation of the blood pressure, and abnormalities of respiratory rate, depth, and rhythm. Pressure on the corticospinal and associated pathways may result in a contralateral Babinski sign and contralateral weakness or paralysis.

matoma, decompression by removal of areas of skull and portions of the frontal or temporal lobes if necessary, and relaxation of the compressing dura. Even with prompt diagnosis and surgical intervention, mortality rates are 80 to 90 percent, most related to the severe brain trauma and major organ failure that accompanies severe trauma (Beeson and McDermott, 1979.)

Subacute subdural hematoma

Subacute subdural hematoma is that which causes significant neurologic deficit more than 48 hours but less than 2 weeks after injury (Schwartz, 1984). Like the acute subdural hematoma, it is caused by venous bleeding into the subdural space.

The typical clinical history of a patient with a subacute subdural hematoma shows head trauma causing unconsciousness with subsequent gradual improvement in neurologic status. After a period of time the patient demonstrates signs of deteriorating neurologic status. The level of consciousness begins to decrease gradually over a period of hours. As the intracranial pressure in-

creases from the accumulating hematoma, the patient may become difficult to arouse and nonresponsive to verbal and painful stimuli. As with acute subdural hematoma, the shift of intracranial contents and the increasing intracranial pressure due to the accumulation of blood will lead to herniation of the uncus. This will give rise to third nerve compression and its associated clinical signs—ptosis of the eyelid and dilatation of the pupil.

Treatment, like the treatment of acute subdural hematoma, is early and prompt removal of the clot. This can be accomplished by various means, according to the clinical condition of the patient. Since many of these clots are bilateral, as with the acute subdural hematomas, measures should be taken to ensure that both subdural spaces have been evaluated and, if indicated, surgically explored (Schwartz, 1984).

Chronic subdural hematoma

Chronic subdural hematoma presents an interesting clinical history. The cerebral trauma responsible for

810

it may be trivial or even nonexistent or forgotten. The onset of symptoms is usually delayed for weeks, months, and possibly years after the initial injury.

The initial trauma ruptures one of the veins traversing the subdural space. Slow bleeding thus occurs into the subdural space. Within 7 to 10 days after bleeding has occurred, the blood is surrounded by a fibrous membrane. Breakdown of blood cells within the hematoma occurs as an osmotic pressure gradient is built up, pulling fluid into the hematoma. It is this increase in the size of the hematoma that may cause further bleeding by tearing the surrounding membrane or vessels, increasing the size and pressure of the hematoma (Schwartz, 1984). If allowed to follow its natural course, the contents of the subdural hematoma undergo characteristic changes (see Table 51-1).

Chronic subdural hematoma has frequently been nicknamed "the imitator" because the signs and symptoms are generally nonspecific and nonlocalizing and could be caused by many different disease processes. Some patients complain of a headache. The most typical signs and symptoms include progressive alteration in level of consciousness, including apathy, lethargy, and decreased attention span, and decreased ability to use higher cognitive skills. Hemianopsia, hemiparesis, and pupillary abnormalities are observed in less than 50 percent of cases. The spinal fluid is rarely helpful in confirming a diagnosis and may be nonspecifically abnormal, with increased protein content and xanthochromia, or may contain a few red blood cells; the pressure is generally normal. When aphasia is present, it is usually an anomic type (a fluent aphasia with repetition and comprehension) (Schwartz, 1984; Beeson and McDermott, 1979; Cohen et al., 1983).

Diagnosis is best made by arteriography. CT scan may demonstrate a hematoma, thereby avoiding the necessity of an arteriogram, but a negative CT scan does not necessarily rule out a diagnosis of subdural hematoma.

TABLE 51-1

STAGES IN THE NATURAL HISTORY OF NONLETHAL SUBDURAL HEMATOMA

Stage	Description
Stage I	Dark blood spreads widely over the brain surface beneath the dura.
Stage II	Blood congeals; becomes darker, thicker, and "jellylike" (2 to 4 days).
Stage III	Clot breaks down and after about 2 weeks has color and consistency of crankcase oil.
Stage IV	Organization begins with formation of encasing membranes: an outer thick, tough one derived from dura and a thin inner one from arachnoid. The contained fluid becomes xanthochromic.
Stage V	Organization is completed. Clot may become calcified or even ossified (or may resorb).

Source: Modified from Jackson, 1966.

Small hematomas resolve spontaneously if allowed to follow their natural course. In patients with small hematomas with no neurologic signs who can be closely followed, this is probably the best medical course. But for the patient with progressive neurologic deficit and debilitating symptoms, the best course of treatment is surgical removal, since the greatest danger in chronic subdural hematoma is that in acting like an enlarging mass, it may cause herniation of the temporal uncus and death (Schwartz, 1984; Cohen et al., 1983).

SPINAL CORD INJURY

Most spinal cord injuries occur during sports activities such as diving and skiing and in automobile accidents. Many of those affected are young males under the age of 30. The common mechanism of cord injury is flexion-extension and rotation.

The vertebral column is constructed with a circumferential bony ring which provides ideal protection for low-velocity penetrating injuries and contusions, but the intervertebral articulations are weak points for flexion, extension, or rotational stress. According to Schwartz (1984), dislocations and fractures that do not break the vertebral ring allow the vertebrae above and below the area of injury to act as fulcrums for other vertebrae and their attached soft tissue to undergo concussion, stretching, and contusion and disrupt the spinal cord.

The stresses of flexion, extension, and rotation, along with the relative weakness of the articulations of the vertebrae, cause fractures and dislocations to occur most commonly at points where a relatively mobile portion of the vertebral column meets a relatively fixed segment, namely, between the lower cervical area and the upper thoracic segment; between the lower thoracic and upper lumbar segments; and between the lower lumbar segment and the sacrum (Schwartz, 1984).

Most of the damage in spinal cord injury occurs at the time of injury. Secondary cord injury occurs from movement of the unstable vertebral column; the injury that occurs is a movement of the spinal cord against sharp fragments of bone projecting into the canal and continued compression of the spinal cord.

The primary changes occurring after spinal cord injury include small hemorrhages in the gray matter that occur as spinal cord blood flow falls and hypoxia ensues, followed by edema. Hypoxia of the gray matter stimulates the release of catecholamines which contribute to the hemorrhage and necrosis and cause further spinal cord dysfunction. This mechanism is still under investigation but has stimulated researchers to suggest cooling of the injured segment, norepinephrine blocking agents, and steroids as possible therapeutic measures to prevent additional damage (Beeson and McDermott, 1979; Schwartz, 1984).

When the spinal cord is completely severed, two functional disasters are immediately evident: (1) all voluntary activity in the body parts innervated by the spinal segments is permanently lost, and (2) all sensation, which depends upon the integrity of the ascending spinal pathways, is lost. A third occurrence is immediate spinal areflexia, frequently called *spinal shock*.

Spinal shock

Spinal shock is a temporary condition of decreased excitability of neurons above the level of the transection. Spinal shock may extend over a period of many months. Under normal conditions axons descending from the supraspinal portions of the nervous system deliver low-frequency impulses to the neurons. This serves to maintain the neuron in a state of excitability, ready to respond to a higher frequency impulse. When this "background tone" (Mountcastle, 1980) is removed by transection, the resting excitability of the spinal cord is greatly reduced, resulting in spinal shock.

Spinal shock is not due to any form of irritation at the site of the transection nor is it due to the drop in blood pressure that follows transection. The phenomenon of spinal shock is confined to the region above the level of the transection.

Spinal shock may occur in partial transection of the cord. Studies reported by Mountcastle (1980) have shown that it is the reticulospinal and vestibulospinal tracts whose severance produces the phenomenon of spinal shock.

Transection of the spinal cord produces widespread alterations in visceral functions. Immediately after transection of the spinal cord there is complete atony of the smooth muscle of the bladder wall. At the same time there is an increase in constrictor tone of the sphincter muscle, probably due to loss of an inhibitory influence. With recovery of somatic reflexes, which may occur in 25 to 30 days after cord section, tone returns to the bladder muscles and reflex emptying of the bladder occurs. This is produced by simultaneous contraction of the smooth muscle walls and, to a certain extent, relaxation of the tone of the sphincter. After reflex emptying of the bladder, a considerable residual volume is left. Cutaneous stimulation to the abdomen, perineum, or lower extremities greatly facilitates reflex emptying.

In the intestinal tract it appears as if digestion and absorption proceed normally. Great difficulty is encoun-

tered in the evacuation of feces from the lower bowel and rectum. Normally the presence of fecal matter in the lower bowel and rectum passively stretching the walls produces active contraction and peristalsis; this, combined with inhibitory relaxation of the sphincter, causes defecation. This mechanism is depressed during spinal shock. The sphincter ani muscles relax only slightly in response to passive dilatation; therefore retention of fecal material occurs. With the recovery of reflex excitability there is reflex evacuation of the bowel. It is facilitated by tactile stimulus of the skin areas of the sacral segments and/or by manual dilation of the sphincter ani muscle.

Reflex actions upon the peripheral vessels and organs innervated by the autonomic nervous system are profoundly affected by spinal shock. Transection of the spinal cord causes an immediate and profound fall in arterial pressure. This is the result of elimination of the bulbar vasoconstrictor mechanism; when spinal nerves are separated from the medullary centers, the important coordination between the state of the blood vessels and subsidiary centers in the spinal cord is lacking. In the person with an intact spinal cord, the spinal centers are regarded as subordinated to the higher vasoconstrictor center in the medulla. The hypotension persists for some time after transection. Spinal neurons innervating peripheral effectors concerned with body temperature control are permanently severed from the descending influences of the thermoregulatory center.

The duration of spinal shock varies greatly from one patient to another. In general the reappearance of any reflex which has been completely abolished by cord injury is a sign of recovery from spinal shock and cord activity (Mountcastle, 1980; Frohlich, 1984).

Cervical spine injury

Forced flexion injury to the cervical spine compresses the vertebral bodies, dislocates a vertebra forward on the one below, and interlocks the articular facets. Compression of the spinal cord is caused by displaced fragments of bone or a prolapsed intervertebral disc. In a flexion injury a prolapsed intervertebral disc does not occur except in conjunction with a fracture dislocation.

Direct pressure or injury to the anterior spinal artery or injury to the radicular or vertebral artery in the intravertebral foramen occludes circulation through these arteries, leading to ischemic injury.

Hyperextension injuries to the cervical spine buckle the ligamentum flavum forward, pinching the cord. Such injury can damage several centimeters of the cord. The effects of such an injury leave the upper limbs weaker than the lower limbs and cause variable loss of sensation, with sparing of touch, position, and vibration sense. Hematomyelia (bleeding into the central cord) may complicate the injury.

Cervical spinal cord injuries above the level of C3

are usually fatal. Injuries at C4 may be fatal and are usually associated with respiratory embarrassment due to lack of innervation to the diaphragm and the respiratory muscles. As a general rule, cervical spinal cord injury causes quadriplegia; patients with a C5 injury may have partial function of shoulder and elbow; with a C6 injury, partial function of the wrist in addition to the shoulder and elbow may return; in C7 and C8 injury, shoulder, wrist, elbow, and hand function may return, with some weakness in the hand.

Thoracic-lumbar spinal cord injury

The usual mechanism for thoracic-lumbar spinal cord injury is hyperextension. A hyperextension injury causes compression of one or more of the vertebral bodies, generally in the region of T12 and L3. A heavy, direct blow is needed to fracture the midthoracic vertebral bodies unless they have been previously softened by osteoporosis or neoplasm.

Damage to the cord in the thoracic-lumbar region generally causes paraplegia. Initially the paralysis is a flaccid one, usually followed by spastic paralysis (Schwartz, 1984; Beeson and McDermott, 1979).

Treatment of spinal cord injuries

The first and foremost rule in treatment of spinal cord injury is stabilization of the vertebral column. The presence of foreign bodies adjacent to or in the spinal cord allows for additional damage from body movements. Therefore patients with spinal cord injuries are moved carefully, with the body kept in alignment.

The primary treatment for cervical injury is reduction and stabilization of the fracture, most effectively achieved by skeletal traction with tongs or wires inserted in the skull to achieve and maintain reduction. Stabilization is achieved by anatomic reduction and by tension of the spinal ligaments and soft tissue of the cervical area. Slight extension of the neck gives tension to the anterior spinal ligament.

Reduction of fracture dislocations of the thoracic and lumbar spines is no longer recommended. At present, treatment consists of bed rest until pain subsides. Single compression fractures of the body of a vertebra, with flexion angulation of the spine without spinal cord deficit, may be treated by positioning on a Bradford frame (also called a Foster frame), utilizing extension to stretch the anterior spinal ligament and expand the vertebral body.

A controversial therapy is decompression of the spinal cord. There are two schools of thought on early surgical decompression. Some neurosurgeons believe that severe injury to the cord can rarely be reversed; that the damage that occurs in spinal cord injury occurs early in the injury, and surgical intervention at this time seriously jeopardizes the patient's life with little or no chance of improving postoperative functioning; and that, since function returns gradually over a period of up to 2 years, the risk of surgery is not warranted. Another school of thought believes that the postinjury edema and swelling of the spinal cord increase the neurologic deficit, therefore laminectomy with decompression always has some potential value. All surgeons agree that patients showing progressive deficit in neurologic function and those with open fractures benefit from surgical decompression.

HERNIATED INTERVERTEBRAL DISC DISEASE

One of the most common causes of back pain in the adult is herniated nucleus pulposus (herniated disc). Although more common in adults, there are cases of disc disease in children and teenagers.

The vertebral column consists of a series of joints between the bodies of the adjacent vertebrae, the joints of the vertebral arches, the costovertebral joints, and the sacroiliac joints.

Longitudinal ligaments and the intervertebral discs join the bodies of adjacent vertebrae. The *anterior longitudinal ligament*, a broad, thick band, runs longitudinally on the front of the vertebral bodies and intervertebral discs and fuses with the periosteum and annulus fibrosus. Lying within the vertebral canal on the posterior aspects of the vertebral bodies and intervertebral discs is the *posterior longitudinal ligament*.

Between the vertebral bodies from the second cervical vertebra down to the sacral vertebrae are the *intervertebral discs*. These discs form a resilient fibrocartilaginous joint between the vertebral bodies. The intervertebral disc consists of two basic parts: the nucleus pulposus at the center and the annulus fibrosus surrounding it. The disc is separated from the bone above and below it by two thin hyaline cartilage plates (see Fig. 51-4).

The *nucleus pulposus* is the semigelatinous central portion of the disc. It contains bundles of collagenous fibers, connective tissue cells, and cartilage cells. This material functions as a shock absorber between adjacent vertebral bodies. It also plays an important role in the exchange of fluid between the disc and the capillaries (Ganong, 1977).

The *annulus fibrosus* consists of concentric fibrous rings which surround the nucleus pulposus. The functions of the annulus fibrosus are to permit motion between the vertebral bodies (by reason of the spiral structure of the fibers), to retain the nucleus pulposus, and to function as a shock absorber. Thus, the annulus func-

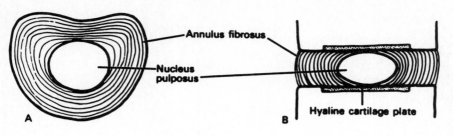

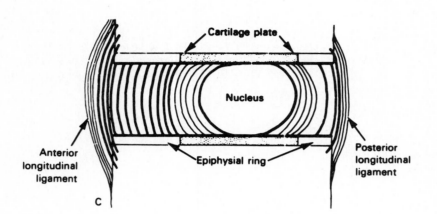

FIGURE 51-4

(A) Annulus fibrosus is composed of concentric fibrous rings which surround the nucleus pulposus. (B) Nucleus pulposus abuts on the hyaline cartilage plate. (C) Annulus fibers form three groups, innermost fibers passing from one cartilage plate to the next, middle fibers passing between the epiphyseal rings of the vertebral bodies, and outermost fibers attaching between the vertebral bodies and the undersurface of the epiphyseal ring. The anterior fibers are more numerous and are supported by the powerful anterior longitudinal ligament, while the posterior longitudinal ligament gives only weak reinforcement to the less numerous posterior fibers. (From MacNab, 1977, p. 3.)

tions like the hoops around a water barrel or like a coiled spring pulling the vertebral bodies together against the elastic resistance of the nucleus pulposus, while the nucleus pulposus acts like a ball bearing between the vertebral bodies (see Fig. 51-5).

Intervertebral discs account for approximately one-fourth of the length of the vertebral column. The thinnest discs are in the thoracic region, while the thickest ones are in the lumbar region. With increasing age the water content of the discs is reduced and they become thinner (Schwartz, 1984).

Pathophysiology

The lumbar region is the most common area for herniation of the nucleus pulposus. The water content of the disc decreases with increasing age (from 90 percent in infancy to 70 percent in old age; Schwartz, 1984). In ad-

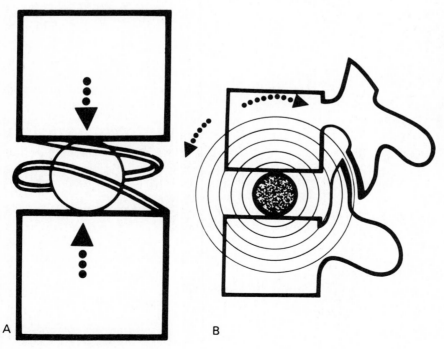

FIGURE 51-5

(A) Annulus acts like a coiled spring, pulling the vertebral bodies together against the elastic resistance of the nucleus pulposus. (B) Nucleus pulposus acts as a ball bearing, with the vertebral bodies rolling over the incompressible gel in flexion and extension while the posterior vertebral joints guide and steady the movement. (From MacNab, 1977, p. 7.)

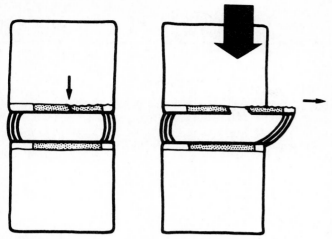

FIGURE 51-6
The first morphologic change to occur in a disc rupture is a separation of the cartilage plate from the adjacent vertebral body. When a vertical compression force is then applied, the detached portion of the cartilage plate is displaced posteriorly and the nucleus pulposus exudes through the torn fibers of the annulus. (From MacNab, 1977, p. 5.)

dition, the fibers become coarsened and hyalinized, and this contributes to the changes that lead to herniation of the nucleus pulposus through the annulus with compression of the spinal nerve roots (see Fig. 51-6). As a general rule, herniation is most likely to occur in regions of the vertebral column where there is a transition from a more mobile segment to a less mobile one (lumbosacral and cervicothoracic junctions).

The vast majority of disc herniations occur in the lumbar area at the L4 to L5 or L5 to S1 interspace (Keim and Kirkaldy-Willis, 1980). The most common direction of herniation of the nuclear material is posterolateral. Because the nerve roots at the lumbar area slant in a downward direction as they exit through the neural foramina, a disc herniation between L5 and S1

affects the S1 nerve root rather than L5 as might be expected. A herniation of the disc between L4 and L5 compresses the L5 nerve root (Fig. 51-7).

Cervical disc herniations, although less common than lumbar disc herniations, usually involve one of the three lower cervical roots. A cervical disc herniation is potentially serious, since spinal cord compression is possible, depending on the direction of protrusion. A lateral herniation of a cervical disc generally compresses the root below the disc level. Thus a C5 to C6 disc compresses the C6 nerve root, and a C6 to C7 disc involves the C7 root (Schwartz, 1984).

The patient generally gives a history of transient episodes of pain and gradual loss of spinal mobility. Although the patient tends to associate the problem with a particular incident of lifting or bending, herniation is a gradual process marked by periods of nerve root compression (causing many symptoms and periods of anatomic readjustment).

The clinical symptoms depend upon the location of the herniation and variation in the individual anatomy. A summary of the most common signs and symptoms can be found in Table 51-2.

The diagnosis of herniated intervertebral disc is often made from the history alone and can be confirmed during physical examination. Such maneuvers as leg raising and having the patient walk on the toes or heels are also helpful in making the diagnosis. X-rays may be normal or may show evidence of distorted spinal alignment (generally caused by muscle spasm). It is impossible to diagnose a herniated disc by x-ray alone. X-rays are helpful in ruling out other causes of back pain such as spondylolisthesis (forward slippage of the anterior portion of a vertebral segment over a lower segment,

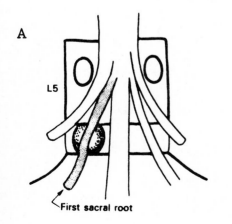

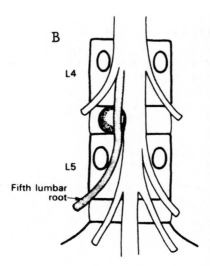

FIGURE 51-7
(A) Posterolateral herniation of the L5 to S1 disc generally compresses the S1 nerve root. (B) Herniation of the L4 to L5 disc compresses the L5 root. (From MacNab, 1977, pp. 95–96.)

TABLE 51-2

SIGNS AND SYMPTOMS OF HERNIATED DISC DISEASE

Location of herniation	Nerve root involved	Pain	Weakness	Paresthesia	Atrophy	Reflexes
L4–L5	L5	Over sacroiliac joint, hip, lateral aspect of thigh and calf, medial aspect of foot. (The pain which radiates down the hip and leg is called *sciatica*)	May produce foot drop and difficulty in dorsiflexion of foot and/or great toe; difficulty walking on heels	Lateral leg, distal portion of foot, and between great and second toes (see dermatome map, Fig. 47-8)	Unremarkable	Usually unremarkable; knee or ankle reflexes may be diminished
L5–S1	S1	Over sacroiliac joint, posterior portion of entire leg to heel, lateral aspect of foot	May produce weakness of plantar flexion, abduction of toes and hamstring muscles; difficulty walking on toes	Midcalf and lateral aspect of foot, including fourth and fifth toes (see dermatome map, Fig. 47-8)	Gastrocnemius	Ankle reflex may be absent or diminished
C5–C6	C6	Neck pain radiating to shoulder, arm, and forearm	Biceps	Radial aspect of forearm, thumb, and index finger	Unremarkable	Biceps reflex diminished or absent

usually at L4 or L5), spinal cord tumors, or bony spurs. Myelograms, electromyography, and nerve conduction studies are used for final verification of the diagnosis and are particularly helpful in diagnosing the rare thoracic herniation.

Conservative treatment is effective for most patients: 1 to 2 weeks of bed rest on a firm mattress, application of moist heat, and analgesics. Traction is useful in the care of patients with cervical herniations. Once the pain has subsided, the patient is started on a program of graded exercise to strengthen the back and abdominal muscles. It is important that the patient limit lifting and use the proper body mechanics whenever lifting. Proper technique involves keeping the spine straight, bending the knees, and keeping the weight close to the body in order to use the powerful leg muscles and avoid using the back muscles. Surgery is generally reserved for patients who experience persistent intractable pain or frequent attacks of pain, symptoms involving both sides, or the presence of a major neurologic deficit such as bowel and bladder incontinence or foot drop. Surgery, if and when performed, relieves the symptoms of nerve root compression but may not relieve the back pain.

QUESTIONS

Central nervous system injury

Directions: Answer the following on a separate sheet of paper.

1. What is normal intracranial pressure, in mmHg? What causes increased intracranial pressure and why is it dangerous?

2. Explain the mechanisms which account for the following signs and symptoms of intracranial hematoma: hemiparesis, seizures, mental dysfunction, depression of consciousness, changes in vital signs (increased systolic blood pressure, bradycardia), decerebrate rigidity, dilated ipsilateral pupil.

3. What are the two general mechanisms which account for brain damage in head trauma?

4. What is a *contrecoup* injury? What areas of the

brain are most likely to be injured in a deceleration automobile accident?

5. List the three most common sites of spinal cord injury.

6. What is the first and foremost rule in the treatment of spinal cord injury?

7. Contrast the mechanisms for posttraumatic epidural and subdural hematomas.

Directions: Circle the letter preceding each item below that correctly answers the question or completes the statement. Only one answer is correct, with exceptions noted.

8. Infection from a scalp wound may be transmitted to the brain tissue via the:
a. Emissary and diploic veins   *b.* Middle meningeal artery   *c.* Cerebral veins of the subdural space   *d.* Carotid artery

9. Brain injury can cause: (More than one answer may be correct.)
a. Increased intracranial pressure   *b.* Hypoxia
c. Hypercarbia   *d.* Hyperthermia

10. Billy, a 10-year-old boy, was hit by a baseball over the temporal area while playing sandlot baseball in the afternoon. Because of a short period of "dizziness," Billy sat on the bench for the next inning and then resumed playing the game. Following dinner at 6 P.M., Billy vomited, complained of a headache, lay down on the sofa, and appeared to be slightly confused. His mother took him to the emergency room of the local hospital. Which of the following types of brain hemorrhage might one suspect?
a. Subdural   *b.* Subarachnoid   *c.* Subperiosteal
d. Epidural

11. If the diagnosis suspected in question 10 is correct, which other of the following neurologic signs and symptoms would Billy be expected to develop if his case is untreated? (More than one answer may be correct.)
a. Ptosis of the contralateral eyelid   *b.* Dilatation of the ipsilateral pupil   *c.* Positive Babinski sign
d. Ipsilateral hemiparesis   *e.* Decrease in blood pressure

12. If the suspected diagnosis in question 10 is correct, therapy should consist of:
a. Conservative observation for the next 24 hours prior to craniotomy   *b.* A spinal tap with the removal of cerebrospinal fluid to relieve the increased intracranial pressure   *c.* Immediate surgical removal of the hematoma and interruption of the arterial bleeding   *d.* Administration of a stimulant to improve mental alertness   *e.* Administration of hypertonic urea to relieve cerebral edema, with craniotomy planned within the next 3 days

13. Following a motorcycle accident, which of the following changes in the neurologic status of a patient would be most significant in indicating damage involving the central nervous system?
a. Localization of headaches   *b.* Change from alertness to increasing lethargy   *c.* Pain and edema located near the eye   *d.* Increase in pulse and respiratory rate

14. Which of the following statements are true concerning chronic subdural hematoma? (More than one answer may be correct.)
a. Usually a result of trivial injury   *b.* Develops very slowly   *c.* Can be diagnosed by arteriogram
d. Develops very rapidly

15. Which of the following mechanisms best explains the sign of ipsilateral pupil dilatation in intracranial hematoma? (More than one answer may be correct.)
a. Hemorrhage from the anterior cerebral artery
b. Herniation of the uncus into the tentorial ring, compressing the third cranial nerve.   *c.* Hemorrhage from the middle cerebral artery   *d.* Traction of the oculomotor nerve against the posterior cerebral artery

16. A young male with a head injury shows a rise in temperature together with a slowing of the pulse and respirations. Which of the following would probably be responsible for his symptoms?
a. Injury to the cortical motor speech area
b. Organization of the clot   *c.* Injury to the vital centers within the medulla   *d.* Lesion in the occipital lobe

17. A subdural hematoma which causes the development of significant signs and symptoms within 24 to 48 hours is classified as:
a. Acute   *b.* Subacute   *c.* Chronic

18. An injury causing unilateral transection of the spinal cord causes which of the following changes below the level of the injury?
a. Contralateral loss of vibration sense and ipsilateral loss of tactile sensation   *b.* Contralateral loss of vibration sense and tactile discrimination and a contralateral increase in touch threshold   *c.* An ipsilateral loss of the vibration sense and tactile discrimination and a contralateral increase in the touch threshold   *d.* An ipsilateral loss of the vibration sense and tactile discrimination and an ipsilateral increase in the touch threshold

19. Which of the following changes is expected immediately following transection of the spinal cord? (More than one answer may be correct.)

a. A general increase in skeletal muscle tone
b. A period of spinal shock lasting approximately
2 days   c. Retention of urine and feces   d. Hypotension

Directions: Match each meningeal structure in col. A with the appropriate statements from col. B.

Column A

20. ___ Dura mater

21. ___ Arachnoid

22. ___ Pia mater

Column B

a. Fine, fibrous middle layer of the meninges

b. Inner meningeal layer closely applied to the brain and spinal cord

c. Encloses the venous sinuses and separates the brain into compartments

d. Circulation of cerebrospinal fluid in a space directly under this layer

e. Middle and posterior portions supplied by the middle meningeal artery

Directions: Circle T if the statement is true and F if it is false. Correct the false statements.

23.   T   F   An epidural hematoma is a hemorrhage between the dura and the arachnoid.

24.   T   F   Paraplegia may be caused by a bilateral lesion at C5.

25.   T   F   A bilateral lesion in the middle or lower thoracic cord causes paraplegia.

26.   T   F   Cervical spinal cord injuries above the level of C3 are generally fatal.

27.   T   F   A quadraplegic with a C6 injury might be expected to have partial function of the shoulder, elbow, and wrist.

28.   T   F   The initial treatment of all serious spinal cord injuries consists of laminectomy with decompression.

29.   T   F   An ipsilateral lesion of the spinal cord at C5 would cause hemiplegia.

30.   T   F   Spinal shock is a temporary condition of decreased excitability of neurons above the level of the cord transection and may last up to 2 years.

Directions: Fill in the blanks with the correct words.

31. The semigelatinous central portion of the intevertebral disc which acts as a ball bearing and shock absorber is called the _____
_____.

32. The _____ _____ functions in a manner similar to a barrel hoop in the intervertebral disc.

33. The direction of herniation of the nucleus pulposus is frequently posterolateral, since the _____ fibers are fewer in this area and the _____ _____ ligament offers weak reinforcement.

Directions: Circle the letter preceding each item below that correctly answers the question or completes the sentence. Only one answer is correct.

34. A herniated intervertebral disc:
a. Is most common between L3 and L4   b. Usually involves the nerve root of the interspace below the site of herniation in the lumbar area
c. Involving S1 root compression may cause numbness of the web of the great toe   d. Can easily be diagnosed by x-ray alone

35. A herniated nucleus pulposus involving the L4 to L5 interspace may cause:
a. Compression of the L5 nerve root   b. Weakness of the dorsiflexors of the ankle   c. Loss of sensation in the medial aspect of the foot
d. Sciatica   e. All the above

36. Herniated cervical discs may cause:
a. Symptoms in the lower extremities   b. Pain in the neck which radiates down the arms
c. Weakness of the arm muscles and diminished biceps or triceps reflexes   d. All the above

37. Which of the following statements are true of suspected herniated lumbar discs?
a. Immediate surgery is advisable to prevent complications   b. Most patients recover completely without surgery   c. The pain may last for years   d. All the above

CHAPTER

52

CENTRAL NERVOUS SYSTEM TUMORS

OBJECTIVES

At the completion of this chapter you should be able to:

1. Explain why the diagnosis of brain tumors may be difficult.

2. Identify the most common brain tumors in adults and children.

3. Identify three types of glial cells and describe their functions.

4. Identify the characteristics of astrocytomas and glioblastomas (common locations, prognosis).

5. Discuss the pathology, growth characteristics, common symptoms, and treatment of meningiomas.

6. Identify three types of pituitary tumor and the characteristics of each.

7. Describe neurilemmomas (pathology, symptoms, treatment, and sequelae).

8. Identify the two most common locations of the primary site of metastatic brain tumors.

9. Identify three types of cerebral blood vessel tumor and their common locations.

10. Identify several brain tumors of congenital origin and their common locations.

11. Describe the effects of adnexal tumors.

12. Describe the pathophysiology of focal disturbances and increased intracranial pressure in brain tumors.

13. Describe the mechanism causing cerebral edema.

14. Explain how the body compensates for increased intracranial pressure, and describe the effects of untreated intracranial pressure.

15. Identify three of the classic clinical manifestations of brain tumor (pathogenesis, significance).

16. Define *papilledema, amaurosis fugax, hemianopsia, quadrantanopsia, hypotonia.*

17. Describe some localizing symptoms for tumors of the frontal, occipital, temporal, and parietal lobes, the cerebellum, ventricles, and hypothalamus.

18. Describe noninvasive and invasive techniques for the diagnosis of brain tumors.

19. Compare brain and spinal cord tumors with respect to frequency and malignancy.
20. List the common locations of spinal cord tumors and common lesions associated with each.
21. List several disorders of movement seen in cerebellar tumors.
22. Describe the signs and symptoms of spinal cord compression at various levels.

BRAIN TUMORS

Intracranial tumors include space-occupying lesions, both benign and malignant, that develop in the brain, meninges, and skull. Because brain tumors present with diverse and confusing symptoms, diagnosis can be difficult. Brain tumors can occur at any age; they are not uncommon in children under 10 but are most commonly found in adults during the fifth and sixth decade.

There are many classifications of brain tumors. Perhaps the one easiest to understand is the Kernahan and Sayre classification, in which the tumor is named for the cells present in the adult nervous system, in vascular tissue, and in developmental defects and the degree of malignancy is graded I to IV (IV being the most malignant; see Table 52-1).

Certain tumors occur more frequently in a particular age group. During infancy and childhood, posterior fossa tumors are far more frequent than supratentorial lesions (middle or anterior fossa), which are more common in adults. The brain tumor of a child is likely to be a malignant astrocytoma of the cerebellum of grade I or II. In the middle-aged or elderly person the most common brain tumor is a glioblastoma multiforme—this is the most malignant glioma, characterized by a rapid growth rate.

Gliomas

Gliomas account for approximately 40 to 50 percent of brain tumors. Gliomas are classified on the basis of embryological origin. In the adult the neuroglia of the central nervous system provide for the repair, support, and protection of the delicate nerve cells. Gliomas consist of connective tissue and supporting cells. The neuroglia possess the potential to continue to divide throughout life. Glial cells congregate to form dense cicatricial scars in regions of brain where neurons disappear because of injury or disease (Snell, 1980).

There are three types of glial cell—microglia, oligodendroglia, and astrocytes. The microglia are of mesodermal embryological origin and therefore are generally not classified as true glial cells. The microglia enter the nervous system through the vascular system and function as phagocytes—clearing away the debris and combating infection.

The oligodendroglia and the astrocytes are true neuroglia and, like neurons, arise from the ectoderm. Oligodendroglia are involved in myelin formation. The function of astrocytes is still under investigation; evidence shows that they may play some role in impulse

TABLE 52-1

BRAIN TUMORS

Tumor	Percent of all brain tumors
Gliomas	40–50
Astrocytoma grade I	5–10
Astrocytoma grade II	2–5
Astrocytoma grades III and IV (glioblastoma multiforme)	20–30
Medulloblastoma	3–5
Oligodendroglioma	1–4
Ependymoma grades I–IV	1–3
Meningioma	12–20
Pituitary tumors	5–15
Neurilemmomas (mainly cranial nerve VIII)	3–10
Metastatic tumors	5–10
Blood vessel tumors	
Arteriovenous malformations, hemangioblastomas, endotheliomas	0.5–1
Tumors of developmental defects	2–3
Dermoids, epidermoids, teratomas, chordomas, paraphyseal cysts	
Craniopharyngiomas	3–8
Pinealomas	0.5–0.8
Miscellaneous	
Sarcomas, papillomas of the choroid plexus, lipomas, unclassified, etc.	1–3

Source: Schwartz, 1984, p. 1800.

conduction and synaptic transmission of neurons and may serve as conduits between blood vessels and neurons (Mountcastle, 1980).

Astrocytomas infiltrate the brain and are frequently associated with cysts of various sizes. Although they infiltrate the brain tissue, the effect on brain functioning is minimal early in the illness. Generally, astrocytomas are nonmalignant, although they may undergo a malignant change to a glioblastoma—a highly malignant astrocytoma. These tumors are generally slow-growing. Because of this the patient frequently does not seek medical attention for several years, until debilitating symptoms occur—for instance, epileptic seizures or headaches. At the time of surgery complete excision is generally not possible because of the invasive nature of the tumor.

The glioblastoma multiforme is the most malignant of the gliomas. This tumor has a rapid growth rate, and complete surgical excision is impossible. Life expectancy is usually about 12 months. The tumor may occur anywhere but most commonly involves the cerebral hemisphere and often spreads to the opposite side via the corpus callosum.

The oligodendroglioma is similar to the astrocytoma but is composed of oligodendroglial cells. It is relatively avascular and is prone to calcification.

Ependymoma is a malignant tumor arising from within the walls of the ventricle. In children the most common site is the fourth ventricle. This tumor invades the surrounding tissue and obstructs the ventricles. Death usually occurs in 3 years or less.

Meningeal tumors

The meningioma is the most important tumor arising from the meninges, the mesothelial lining cells, and the connective tissue cells of the arachnoid and the dura. The majority of meningeal tumors are benign and encapsulated and do not infiltrate adjacent tissue but rather compress the underlying structures. These tumors are often quite vascular and will therefore take up radioactive isotopes during a brain scan. Complete surgical excision is possible, especially if the tumor is not in a critical area and diagnosis is made early. Because of the slow growth of this tumor, symptoms may be overlooked and the diagnosis missed completely. Symptoms include idiopathic epilepsy, hemiparesis, and aphasia.

Pituitary tumors

Pituitary tumors arise from the chromophobe, eosinophil, or basophil cells of the anterior pituitary. These tumors cause headache, bitemporal hemianopsia (due to pressure on the optic chiasm), and signs of abnormal secretion of hormones from the anterior pituitary. Figure 52-1 illustrates the various visual field defects common when lesions involve the optic tract.

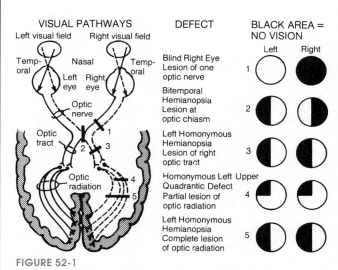

FIGURE 52-1
Visual field defects produced by selected lesions in the visual pathways. (Adapted from *Programmed Practice in Anatomy and Physiology of the Nervous System*, Prentice-Hall, Washington, 1972, p. 49.)

Chromophobe tumors are nonsecretory tumors which compress the pituitary gland, the optic chiasm, and the hypothalamus. Symptoms of this brain tumor include depression of sexual function, secondary hypothyroidism, and adrenal hypofunction (amenorrhea, impotence, loss of hair, weakness, hypotension, low basal metabolism, hypoglycemia, and electrolyte disturbances).

Eosinophilic adenoma is generally a smaller and slower-growing tumor than the chromophobe tumor. The symptoms include acromegaly in adults and gigantism in children, headache, sweating disturbance, paresthesias, muscular pain, and loss of libido. Disturbances in visual fields (bitemporal hemianopsia) are rare.

Basophil adenomas are generally small. These tumors are associated with the symptoms of Cushing's syndrome (obesity, muscle wasting, skin atrophy, osteoporosis, plethora, hypertension, salt and water retention, hypertrichosis, and diabetes mellitus).

Neurilemmoma (auditory nerve tumor)

Auditory nerve tumors constitute 3 to 10 percent of intracranial tumors. They probably arise from the Schwann cells of the nerve sheath. The nerve fibers in the eighth cranial nerve are eventually destroyed. Bilateral auditory neurilemmoma may occur in von Recklinghausen's disease. Generally benign, these tumors occasionally undergo malignant change.

Symptoms of auditory neurilemmoma include first deafness, tinnitus, loss of caloric vestibular reactivity, and vertigo, followed by suboccipital discomfort, staggering gait, involvement of adjacent cranial nerves, and signs of increased intracranial pressure. Nystagmus, especially horizontal, is usually present. Treatment consists in complete removal of the tumor, if possible, since incomplete removal is generally accompanied by recurrence of the tumor. Surgery leaves the patient with facial paralysis and deafness.

Metastatic tumors

Metastatic lesions, which account for approximately 5 to 10 percent of brain tumors, may originate from any primary site. The most common primary tumors are those of the lung and breast, but neoplasms from the genitourinary tract, gastrointestinal tract, bone, and thyroid may also metastasize to the brain. The metastatic lesion may be single or multiple and may be a late stage in the metastatic process or the first sign of a previously unrecognized primary tumor.

Blood vessel tumors

These tumors include the angiomas, the hemangioblastomas, and the endotheliomas and make up a small percentage of brain tumors. *Angiomas* are congenital arteriovenous malformations, present from birth, which slowly enlarge. They may compress surrounding brain tissue and bleed intracerebrally or into the subarachnoid space. *Hemangioblastomas* are neoplasms composed of embryological vascular elements most commonly found in the cerebellum. The von Hippel-Lindau syndrome is a combination of cerebellar hemangioblastoma, angiomatosis of the retina, and cysts of the kidney and pancreas.

Tumors of developmental defects (congenital)

Rare congenital tumors include chordomas, which are composed of cells derived from the embryonic notochord remnants and are found at the base of the skull. They grow slowly but are highly invasive, making complete surgical removal impossible. Dermoids and teratomas may occur anywhere in the central nervous system. Teratomas frequently occur in the ventricular system and obstruct the third ventricle, the aqueduct, or the fourth ventricle. Craniopharyngiomas arise from remnants of the embryonic craniopharyngeal duct (Rathke's pouch) and are usually located posterior to the sella turcica. Symptoms of congenital tumors generally manifest themselves early in a child's life but may be silent for many years. The symptoms include defects in visual fields, generally irregular, and hypothalamic and pituitary dysfunctions.

Pinealomas (adnexal tumors)

Pinealomas account for a very small number of intracranial lesions and include tumors that originate within the pineal body (pinealoma) as well as those from the surrounding choroid plexus (choroid papilloma). Pinealomas compress the aqueduct, causing obstructive hydrocephalus, as well as the hypothalamus, giving rise to precocious puberty and diabetes insipidus. Choroid papilloma causes intraventricular bleeding and also obstructs the ventricular system.

Pathophysiology of brain tumors

Brain tumors give rise to progressive neurologic deficit. The symptoms occur on a continuum. This underscores the importance of the history when examining the patient. Symptoms should be discussed within a time perspective. When did the symptom develop? Was it associated with anything? How long have you had this?

The neurologic deficit in brain tumors is generally thought to be caused by two factors: the focal disturbances caused by the tumor and the increased intracranial pressure.

Focal disturbances occur when there is compression of brain tissue and infiltration or direct invasion of brain parenchyma with destruction of neural tissue. Dysfunction, of course, is greatest with the fastest-growing infiltrating tumors (e.g., glioblastoma multiforme).

Alteration in blood supply because of compression due to the growing tumor causes necrosis of brain tissue. Interference with arterial blood supply is usually manifested by an acute loss of function and may be confused with primary cerebrovascular disorders.

Seizures as a manifestation of altered neuronal excitability are related to the compression, invasion, and alteration in the blood supply to the brain tissue. Some tumors form cysts, which also compress the surrounding brain parenchyma, increasing the focal neurologic deficit.

The increased intracranial pressure may be due to several factors: an increase in the mass within the skull, edema formation around the tumor, and alteration in cerebrospinal fluid circulation. The tumor's growth causes an increase in mass, because it occupies space within the relatively fixed volume of the rigid compartment of the skull. Malignant tumors produce edema in the surrounding brain tissue. The mechanism is not completely understood, but it is thought that an osmotic gradient causes absorption of fluid by the tumor. Some tumors may cause hemorrhage. Venous obstruction and edema due to breakdown of the blood-brain barrier cause an increase in intracranial volume and in intracranial pressure.

Obstruction of cerebrospinal fluid circulation from the lateral ventricles to the subarachnoid space causes hydrocephalus.

Increased intracranial pressure becomes life-threatening when any of the previously discussed causes develops rapidly. Compensatory mechanisms require days or months to be effective and are therefore not useful when intracranial pressure develops rapidly. Compensatory mechanisms include decreased intracranial blood volume, decreased cerebrospinal fluid volume, decreased intracellular fluid contents, and decreased parenchymal cell numbers (Schwartz, 1984). Untreated increased pressure causes herniation of the uncus or the cerebellum. Uncal herniation is caused when the medial gyrus of the temporal lobe is displaced inferiorly through the tentorial notch by a mass in the cerebral hemisphere. This compresses the midbrain, causing loss of consciousness and compression of the third cranial nerve. The cerebellar tonsils are displaced downward through the foramen magnum by a posterior mass in cerebellar herniation. Compression of the medulla and respiratory arrest rapidly ensue. Other physiologic changes that occur with rapidly developing increased intracranial pressure include progressive bradycardia, systemic hypertension (widening pulse pressure), and respiratory failure (Beeson and McDermott, 1979).

Clinical manifestations

The classic triad of symptoms in brain tumor consists of headache, vomiting, and papilledema. But there is great variety in symptoms, depending upon the site of the lesion and the rapidity of growth.

Headache

Headache is perhaps the most common symptom found in patients with brain tumors. The pain may be describe as deep, aching, steady, dull, and sometimes agonizingly severe. It is most severe in the morning and is aggravated by activities that normally increase intracranial pressure, such as stooping, coughing, or straining at stool. The headache is somewhat relieved by aspirin and application of cold packs to the site.

The headache associated with brain tumor is caused by traction and displacement of pain-sensitive structures within the intracranial cavity. These pain-sensitive structures include the arteries, veins, venous sinuses, and cranial nerves.

The headache has a localizing value in that one-third of headaches overlie the tumor site and the other two-thirds are near or above the tumor. Occipital headache is the first symptom in tumors of the posterior fossa. Approximately one-third of supratentorial lesions give rise to a frontal headache. A complaint of a generalized headache has little localizing value and usually indicates extensive displacement of intracranial contents with increased intracranial pressure (Beeson and McDermott, 1979).

Nausea and vomiting

Nausea and vomiting occur as a result of stimulation of the emetic center in the medulla. Vomiting is most frequent in children and in association with increased intracranial pressure with brainstem displacement. The vomiting may occur without preceding nausea and may be projectile.

Papilledema

Papilledema is caused by venous stasis, which leads to engorgement and swelling of the optic disc. When seen by fundoscopy, it suggests increased intracranial pressure. It is often difficult to use this sign as diagnostic of brain tumor, since the fundi in some persons may not show papilledema even with very high intracranial pressure.

In association with the papilledema, some disturbances in vision may occur. These include enlargement of the blind spot and *amaurosis fugax* (fleeting moments of dimmed vision).

Localizing symptoms

Other signs and symptoms of brain tumor occur which tend to have a greater localizing value.

Tumors of the frontal lobe give symptoms of mental changes, hemiparesis, ataxia, and disturbances of speech. Mental changes are manifested by subtle changes in personality. Some patents experience periods of depression, confusion, or bizarre behavior. The most common changes involve higher level reasoning and judgment skills. Hemiparesis is caused by pressure on the neighboring motor areas and pathways. If the motor area is involved, jacksonian seizures and obvious motor weakness may occur. Tumors involving the lower end of the precentral cortex cause weakness of the face, tongue, and thumb, whereas tumors of the paracentral lobule produce weakness in the foot and lower extremity. Tumors of the frontal lobe may cause unsteadiness in the gait, often imitating cerebellar ataxia. When the left or dominant frontal lobe is affected, aphasia and apraxia may be evident.

Tumors of the occipital lobe may give rise to convulsive seizures preceded by an aura. With involvement of the occipital cortex, contralateral homonymous hemianopsia occurs (Fig. 52-1). There may be visual agnosia, difficulty in judging distances, and a tendency to get lost in familiar surroundings.

Temporal lobe tumors cause tinnitus and auditory hallucinations, probably from irritation of the temporal auditory receptive or adjacent cortex. Varying degrees of sensory aphasia, beginning with difficulty in naming objects, appear when the temporal lobe of the dominant hemisphere becomes involved. Mental symptoms similar to whose which occur with frontal lobe tumors are not uncommon. Pressure from a growing tumor on the frontal cortex may result in facial weaknesses. Lesions of the anterior temporal pole cause a superior quadrantanopia, which may progress to a complete hemianopsia.

Tumors in the parietal lobe of the parietal sensory cortex cause loss of cortical sensory function and impairment of sensory localization, two-point discrimination, graphesthesia, position sense, and stereognosis. Visual defects from parietal or parietooccipital tumors ordinarily involve inferior homonymous quadrants.

Cerebellar tumors cause early papilledema and frequently produce nuchal headache. Cerebellar lesions also cause disorders of movement, varying according to the size and specific location of the tumor within the cerebellum. The most common of these disorders are listed in Table 52-2. Less conspicuous but equally characteristic of cerebellar tumor is hypotonia (absence of normal resistance to stretch or to displacement of a limb from a given posture) and hyperextensibility of joints. In speech there is a tendency to decompose words into separate syllables pronounced in a staccato rhythm—this is also called *scanning speech*.

Tumors of the ventricles and hypothalamus produce varied deficits. Invasive lesions of the third ventricle and the hypothalamus produce somnolence, diabetes insipidus, obesity, and disturbances of temperature regulation. A small tumor in the third ventricle, on the other hand, causes steady headache and papilledema with few localizing signs. Tumors involving the fourth ventricle give rise to rapid development of increased intracranial pressure with papilledema and cerebellar symptoms.

Diagnosis

Any patient suspected of having an intracranial lesion should undergo a complete medical evaluation with special attention to the neurologic examination. Specific diagnostic studies are done after the neurologic examination and proceed from the noninvasive procedures that

TABLE 52-2

DISORDERS OF MOVEMENT SEEN IN CEREBELLAR TUMORS

Disorder	Description
Intention tremor	Oscillating tremor most marked at the end of fine movements.
Asynergia	Lack of cooperation between muscles, e.g., failure of the wrist extensors during flexion of the fingers, allowing the wrist to flex.
Decomposition of movement	Performance of actions in successive parts rather than as a whole, e.g., touching the nose by first flexing the forearm, then the arm, and lastly adjusting the wrist and forearm.
Dysmetria	Errors in the range of movement, e.g., in touching a point, stopping the action before reaching the point or moving past it.
Deviation from line of movement	Example: carrying food to the ear instead of the mouth.
Adiadochokinesis	Inability to perform alternating movements, e.g., tapping quickly and smoothly.
Nystagmus	Rapid oscillation of the eyes while fixing the gaze on region and object.

cause the least risk to those which use more dangerous, invasive techniques.

Skull x-rays give valuable information concerning bone structure, thickening, and calcifications; the position of the calcified pineal gland; and the position of the sella turcica. The electroencephalogram gives information concerning the altered excitability of the neurons. A shift of intracerebral contents can be seen on the echoencephalogram. A radioactive brain scan will show areas of abnormal accumulation of radioactive substances. Brain tumors as well as vascular occlusion, infection, and trauma bring about breakdown of the blood-brain barrier, causing an abnormal accumulation of the radioactive substance.

Pneumoencephalography and cerebral angiography are two invasive procedures which aid in the final diagnosis and help the physician decide what treatment measures are to be carried out.

SPINAL CORD TUMORS

Spinal tumors are those which develop in the spine or its contents and generally produce symptoms by involvement of the spinal cord or nerve roots. Primary cord tumors are about one-sixth as common as brain tumors and have a better prognosis, since about 60 percent are benign. The spinal cord suffers not only from actual tumor growth but also from compression caused by an encroaching tumor.

Spinal tumors occur in all age groups but are rarely encountered before the age of 10.

Spinal tumors are classified according to the location of the tumor in relation to the dura and the spinal cord. The major classification divides tumors into extradural and intradural. Intradural tumors are then subdivided into extramedullary and intramedullary.

Extradural tumors generally arise from the bone of the spinal column or within the extradural space. Ninety percent of extradural tumors are malignant. The most common tumor affecting the spinal vertebral column is a metastatic carcinoma. Extradural neoplasms within the extradural space are commonly metastatic carcinomas and lymphomas.

Intradural extramedullary tumors lie between the dura mater and the spinal cord (Fig. 52-2). The most common tumors in this area are benign neurofibromas and meningiomas. These tumors compress the spinal cord and can be surgically removed.

Intradural intramedullary tumors arise from within the spinal cord itself. The same tumors that affect the brain also affect the spinal cord. Ependymomas are the most common, followed by astrocytomas, glioblastomas, and oligodendrogliomas.

The spinal cord accommodates to compression that occurs slowly, as seen in meningiomas, and neurofibromas, producing few signs and symptoms, especially in the early stages. Acute compression of the cord such as that which occurs with metastatic lesions causes rapid, progressive neurologic deficit. Resulting symptoms depend largely upon the area affected as well as the location of the lesion within the spinal column.

Because of the anatomic organization within the cord, compression from lesions outside the cord generally produces symptoms well below the site of the lesion, the level of sensory impairment gradually ascending as the compression increases and affects areas deeper within the cord. Lesions located deep within the cord may spare superficially arranged fibers and give rise to sensory dissociation, with loss of pain and temperature senses and preservation of the sense of touch. By disturbing position sense, cord compression may also result in ataxia.

Spinal cord compression at different levels

Tumors of the foramen magnum

Tumors of the foramen magnum are most commonly meningiomas. Symptoms of spinal cord compression at this level are due to compression of the spinal cord, nerve roots, and intracranial contents. Suboccipital pain is perhaps the earliest symptom. This pain is aggravated by nodding. Nerve root compression causes sensory and motor weakness in the occipital region (C2 dermatome) and the neck (C3 dermatome). Extension of the tumor into the intracranial cavity causes increased intracranial pressure, cerebellar dysfunction, nystagmus, and compression of cranial nerve nuclei, with trigeminal sensory loss and atrophy of the tongue.

Tumors of the cervical region

Cervical lesions produce radicularlike motor and sensory signs that involve the shoulders and arms and may involve the hands. Involvement of the hands from an upper cervical lesion (i.e., above C4) is thought to be due to compression of the descending blood supply to the anterior horns via the anterior spinal artery. There is generally weakness and atrophy involving the shoulder girdle and arms. Lower cervical tumors (C5, C6, C7)

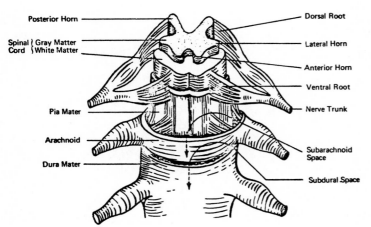

Posterior Horn
Spinal Cord { Gray Matter / White Matter
Pia Mater
Arachnoid
Dura Mater
Dorsal Root
Lateral Horn
Anterior Horn
Ventral Root
Nerve Trunk
Subarachnoid Space
Subdural Space

FIGURE 52-2
Structure of the spinal cord. (From *Programmed Practice in Anatomy and Physiology of the Nervous System,* Prentice-Hall, Washington, 1972.)

may cause the loss of upper extremity tendon reflexes (biceps, brachioradialis, and triceps). Sensory loss extends along the radial border of the forearm and thumb in a C6 compression and involves the middle and index fingers in lesions at C7; C7 lesions cause sensory loss of the index and middle fingers (see Table 52-3).

Tumors of the thoracic region

Lesions of the thoracic area often present with insidiously developing spastic weakness in the lower extremities and later development of paresthesia. Patients may complain of pain and a tight, binding feeling across the chest and abdomen that may be confused with pain from intrathoracic and intraabdominal disorders. In lower thoracic lesions there may be loss of lower abdominal reflexes and Beevor's sign (the umbilicus elevates when the patient, in the supine position, raises the head against resistance).

Tumors of the lumbar-sacral region

A complex diagnostic situation exists in the case of a tumor involving the lumbar and sacral regions because of the close proximity of the lower lumbar and sacral segments and the descending nerve roots from higher levels of the cord. Upper lumbar cord compression spares the abdominal reflexes, abolishes the cremasteric reflexes, and may produce weakness of hip flexion and spasticity of the lower legs. There is loss of the knee jerk

reflex with brisk ankle reflexes and bilateral Babinski signs. Pain is usually referred to the groin. Lesions involving the lower lumbar and upper sacral segments cause weakness and atrophy of perineal, calf, and foot muscles and loss of the ankle jerk reflex. Loss of sensation in the perianal and genital area with impairment of bowel and bladder control are characteristic signs of lesions involving the lower sacral area.

Tumors of the cauda equina

Lesions of the cauda equina cause early sphincteric symptoms and impotence. Other characteristic signs include dull, aching pain in the sacrum or perineum, sometimes radiating to the legs. Flaccid paralysis corresponds to the nerve roots involved and is sometimes asymmetrical.

Symptoms are produced not only by the anatomic location of the spinal cord but by its position within the spinal canal. The pathology of extradural and intradural tumors is discussed below.

Extradural tumors

Extradural tumors are primarily metastases from a primary lesion in the breast, prostate, thyroid, lungs, kidney, or stomach. Pain is generally the first symptom. It is described as being dull, constant, and localized over the area of the tumor, followed by pain radiating along the dermatome pattern. The localized pain is most severe at night and is aggravated by movements of the spine and bed rest. The radicular pain is intensified by coughing and straining. Pain may be present for weeks or months prior to spinal cord involvement.

TABLE 52-3

SYMPTOMS AND SIGNS OF COMMON ROOT LESIONS

Root	Location of pain	Sensory loss	Reflex loss	Weakness and atrophy
C5	Lower neck, tip of shoulder, arm	Deltoid area (inconsistent)	Biceps	Shoulder abductors, biceps
C6	Lower neck, medial scapula, arm, radial side of forearm	Radial side of hand, thumb, index finger	Biceps	Biceps
C7	Lower neck, medial scapula, precordium, arm, forearm	Index finger, middle finger	Triceps	Triceps
C8	Lower neck; medial arm and forearm, ulnar side of hand; fourth and fifth fingers	Ulnar side of hand, fourth and fifth fingers		Intrinsic hand muscles
L4	Low back, anterior and medial thigh	Anterior thigh	Quadriceps	Quadriceps
L5	Low back, lateral thigh, lateral leg, dorsum of foot, great toe	Great toe, medial side of dorsum of foot, lateral leg and thigh		Toe extensors, ankle dorsiflexors and evertors
S1	Low back, posterior thigh, posterior leg, lateral side of foot, heel	Lateral foot, heel, posterior leg	Achilles	Ankle dorsiflexion and plantar flexion

Source: Simpson and Magee, 1973, p. 114.

The common clinical course of extradural tumors is rapid compression of the spinal cord from encroachment of the tumor on the cord, collapse of the vertebral column, or hemorrhage from within the metastasis. Once symptoms of spinal cord compression develop, they rapdily cause total loss of spinal cord function. Spastic weakness and loss of vibration and joint position senses below the level of the lesion are the first signs of cord compression. Without prompt surgical decompression, paresthesia and sensory loss progress quickly to irreversible paraplegia.

Extradural spinal cord tumors can be diagnosed by x-rays of the spine. Most patients with tumors will demonstrate osteoporosis or obvious bone destruction of the vertebral body and pedicles. A myelogram definitely localizes the tumor. The cerebrospinal fluid will show elevated protein and normal glucose levels.

Surgical decompression with laminectomy is the treatment of choice when symptoms of cord compression are present. Used as adjunctive measures are hormones, radiation, and chemotherapy.

Intradural tumors

Intradural tumors, in contrast to the extradural, are generally benign. The clinical course is much slower and may extend over a period of months to years. Intradural tumors are divided into two types—extramedullary and intramedullary.

Extramedullary

Approximately 65 percent of all intradural tumors are extramedullary. They may be either neurofibromas or meningiomas.

Neurofibromas arise from the dorsal nerve roots. They sometimes form a dumbbell-like or hourglasslike growth extending into the extradural space. A small percentage of neurofibromas undergo sarcomatous changes and become invasive or metastasize.

Meningiomas are usually loosely attached to the dura, arising probably from the arachnoid membrane, and approximately 90 percent are found in the thoracic region. These tumors are more frequent in middle-aged females. The posterolateral aspect of the cord is the most common site for these tumors.

Extramedullary cord lesions cause compression of the spinal cord and the nerve roots at the affected segment. The Brown-Séquard syndrome may result from lateral compression of the cord. This syndrome, caused by damage to one-half of the cord, is characterized by ipsilateral signs of dysfunction of the corticospinal tract and the posterior column below the level of the lesion and contralateral reduction in pain and temperature perception below the level of the lesion. The patient complains of pain, first in the back and then along the spinal roots. As with extradural tumors, pain is aggravated by movement, coughing, sneezing, or straining and is most severe at night. The nocturnal aggravation of pain is caused by traction on the diseased nerve roots when the spine elongates with removal of the shortening effect of gravity. The sensory loss is at first vague and located below the level of the lesion (because of dermatome overlap). It gradually rises to below the segmented spinal cord level. Tumors of the posterior aspect may be manifested by paresthesia and, later, proprioceptive sensory loss, adding ataxia to the weakness. Anteriorly situated tumors may cause little sensory loss but severe motor disability.

With extramedullary tumors cerebrospinal fluid protein is almost always elevated. Spine x-rays may show enlargement of a foramen and thinning of the adjacent pedicle. As with extradural tumors, myelogram is essential for precise localization. Early surgical removal is essential for a complete recovery.

Intramedullary

The histologic structure of intramedullary tumors is essentially the same as that of intracranial tumors. Over 95 percent of these tumors are gliomas. In contrast to intracranial tumors they tend to be more benign histologically and have a more benign course. Approximately 50 percent of intramedullary tumors are ependymomas, 45 percent are astrocytomas, and the rest are oligodendrogliomas and hemangioblastomas.

Ependymomas arise at all levels of the spinal cord but are found most commonly in the conus medullaris of the cauda equina. All other intramedullary tumors occur equally frequently in all areas of the spinal cord.

Intramedullary tumors grow into the central part of the spinal cord and destroy crossing fibers and neurons of the gray matter. The destruction of crossing fibers results in bilateral sensory loss of pain and temperature sense extending throughout the segments involved in the lesion, leading to damage to peripheral skin areas. The senses of touch, motion, position, and vibration are usually preserved unless the lesion is large. The loss of pain and temperature sensation with preservation of the other senses is known as *dissociated sensory loss*. Alteration in the function of muscle stretch reflexes results from damage to the anterior horn cells. Weakness, with atrophy and fasciculations, is due to involvement of the lower motor neurons.

Intramedullary tumors may extend through several segments of the spinal cord. As the lesion progresses, involvement of the corticospinal and spinothalamic tracts causes loss of pain and temperature sense, and upper motor neuron signs extend below the level of the lesion. See Table 47-3, which lists some differentiating features between upper and lower motor neuron lesions.

Other signs and symptoms include dull, aching pain localized to the level of the lesion, impotence in males, and sphincter disturbances in both sexes.

X-rays will show visible widening of the spinal canal and erosion of the pedicles. On myelogram the spinal cord appears enlarged.

Surgical removal is sometimes possible with intramedullary tumors, especially ependymomas and hemangioblastomas, but recurrences are not uncommon. Again, early diagnosis is imperative to ensure a good prognosis.

QUESTIONS

Central nervous system tumors

Directions: Answer the following question on a separate sheet of paper.

1. What makes the diagnosis of a brain tumor so difficult? What are the most common general signs and symptoms?

Directions: Match the type of glioma in col. A with its characteristic in col. B.

Column A	Column B
2. ___ Glioblastoma multiforme	a. Often contains calcium
3. ___ Medulloblastoma	b. Most malignant
4. ___ Oligodendroglioma	c. Commonly arises in the fourth ventricle in children
5. ___ Ependymoma	d. Radiosensitive posterior fossa tumor of childhood

Directions: Match the brain tumors in col. A to the statements in col B.

Column A	Column B
6. ___ Chromophobe adenoma	a. Arises from remnants of Rathke's pouch; predominantly a tumor of childhood.
7. ___ Basophilic adenoma	b. Associated with acromegaly; does not cause chiasmal compression.
8. ___ Eosinophilic adenoma	c. Symptoms include tinnitus, deafness, vertigo, and caloric vestibular reactivity.
9. ___ Craniopharyngioma	d. Associated with Cushing's syndrome.
10. ___ Neurilemmoma	

11. ___ Hemangioblastoma

12. ___ Pinealoma

e. Symptoms include those of hypopituitarism, hypothyroidism, hypoadrenalism, and often visual field defects.

f. Often compresses the aqueduct, causing obstructive hydrocephalus, and the hypothalamus, causing precocious puberty and diabetes insipidus.

g. Often bleeds intracerebrally or into the subarachnoid space; most common in cerebellum.

Directions: Match the localizing symptoms of brain tumors in col. A with their probable location in col. B.

Column A	Column B
13. ___ Homonymous hemianopsia	a. Frontal lobe
14. ___ Impairment of sensory localization, two-point discrimination	b. Temporal lobe
	c. Occipital lobe
	d. Parietal lobe
15. ___ Superior quadrantanopsia progressing to hemianopsia	e. Hypothalamus
16. ___ Disturbances of judgment; jacksonian seizures; ataxia and tremor	

17. ____ Obesity and disturbance of temperature regulation

Directions: Match the disorders of movement seen in cerebellar tumors in col. A with the proper descriptive statement in col. B.

Column A

18. ____ Nystagmus
19. ____ Dysmetria
20. ____ Asynergia
21. ____ Intention tremor
22. ____ Deviation from line of movement
23. ____ Adiadochokinesis

Column B

a. Error in range of movement: carrying food to ear instead of mouth
b. Inability to perform tapping movement smoothly and quickly
c. Quick oscillation of eyes while fixing gaze on an object
d. Lack of cooperation between muscles, e.g., failure of wrist extensors during flexion of the finger, allowing the wrist to flex
e. Oscillation tremor most marked at the end of fine movements
f. Inability to arrest a movement at a given point and difficulty in performing successive movements

Directions: Circle the letter preceding each item below that correctly answers the question or completes the sentence. Only one answer is correct, with exceptions noted.

24. All the following statements concerning brain tumors are true except:
a. A glioblastoma is the most malignant form of brain tumor. b. Brain tumors in children occur most often in the posterior fossa. c. Astrocytomas are generally nonmalignant. d. Glioblastomas are generally cured by surgical excision.
e. Meningiomas are benign tumors of perineural tissue.

25. The two most common sources of metastasis to the brain are the:
a. Lung and colon b. Colon and rectum
c. Lung and breast d. Uterus in women and prostate in men

26. Which of the following statements concerning chordomas is true?
a. They are highly invasive, making complete surgical excision impossible b. They arise at the base of the skull c. They grow slowly d. All the above

27. Compensatory mechanisms for increased intracranial pressure include all the following *except:*
a. A decrease in the systemic blood pressure
b. A decrease in intracerebral blood volume
c. A decrease in the volume of CSF d. A decrease in the number of parenchymal cells

28. Noninvasive techniques helpful in the diagnosis of brain tumors include: (More than one answer may be correct.)
a. History and neurologic examination b. Pneumoencephalogram c. Electroencephalogram
d. Arteriogram e. Echoencephalogram

29. The most common cause of extradural extramedullary cord compression is:
a. Metastatic disease b. Glioma c. Astrocytoma d. Ependymoma

30. The most common types of intradural extramedullary spinal lesions are:
a. Gliomas and angiomas b. Meningiomas and neurofibromas c. Sarcomas and lymphomas
d. Gliomas and herniated nucleus pulposus

31. A spinal cord tumor which caused weakness and atrophy of the intrinsic hand muscles, sensory loss in the ulnar side of the hand, and Horner's syndrome, together with a "claw hand" would most likely be:
a. Intramedullary at C6 b. Extramedullary at C6 c. Extramedullary at C7 d. Intramedullary at C8

32. One of the most important tests in the diagnosis of spinal cord compression is:
a. Ultrasound b. Myelography c. Spinal x-ray

33. All the following are characteristics of lower motor neuron lesions except:
a. Fasciculations b. Depressed reflexes below level of lesion c. Spastic paralysis below level of lesion d. Marked atrophy of muscle innervated below level of lesion

Directions: Circle T if the statement is true and F if it is false. Correct the false statements.

34. T F An osmotic gradient causing absorption of fluid into a malignant brain tumor is the most likely mechanism of cerebral edema.

35. T F Hypotonia is an absence of normal resistance to stretch and is seen in cerebellar tumors.

36. T F Astrocytes function as cerebral phagocytes.

37. T F Oligodendroglia are involved in myelin formation.

38. T F Ependymoma is the most common type of intradural intramedullary spinal cord tumor.

39. T F Meningiomas of the spinal cord tend to be located in the cauda equina.

40. T F Papilledema is enlargement of the blind spot in the eye.

Directions: Match the site of spinal cord pathology in col. A with the signs and symptoms in col. B. (Letters may be used more than once.)

Column A

41. ____ Pain increased by coughing or sneezing

42. ____ Loss of vibratory and position sense

43. ____ Babinski reflex

44. ____ Fasciculations

45. ____ Spasticity

46. ____ Ataxia

Column B

a. Posterior (dorsal) root

b. Posterior column (major ascending tract)

c. Corticospinal tract (major descending tract)

d. Anterior horn cells

REFERENCES FOR PART VIII

ADAMS, R. D. and H. VANDER EECKEN: "Motor Paralysis," in R. Petersdorf et al. (eds.), *Harrison's Principles of Internal Medicine*, 10th ed., McGraw-Hill, New York, 1983, pp. 86–92.

ALPERS, B. J. and E. I. MANCALL: *Essentials of the Neurological Examination*, Davis, Philadelphia, 1971.

————et al.: "Anatomical Studies of the Circle of Willis in Normal Brain," *Archives of Neurology and Psychiatry* 81: 409, 1959.

American Heart Association: *Stroke*, 8: 1, 1977.

American Society of Hospital Pharmacists, *American Hospital Formulary Service, Drug Information*, 1985.

————: *Sourcebook on Clinical Pharmacy*, 2d ed., 1980.

ANTEL, J. P. and B. G. ARNASON: "Multiple Sclerosis and other Demyelinating Diseases," in R. Petersdorf et al. (eds.), *Harrison's Principles of Internal Medicine*, 10th ed., McGraw-Hill, New York, 1983, pp. 2098–2104.

APPENZELLER, O: *Autonomic Nervous System*, 3d ed., Elsevier, New York, 1982.

————(ed.): *Pathogenesis and Treatment of Headache*, Spectrum, New York, 1976.

BATES, B.: *A Guide to Physical Examination*, 3d ed., Philadelphia, Lippincott, 1983.

BEESON, P. B. and W. McDERMOTT (eds.): *Cecil and Loeb Textbook of Medicine*, 15th ed., Saunders, Philadelphia, 1979.

BERK, J., J. SAMPLENER, J. S. ARTZ, and B. VINOCUR: *Handbook of Critical Care*, 2d ed., Little, Brown, Boston, 1982.

BLOOM, W. and D. FAWCETT: *Textbook of Histology*, 10th ed., Saunders, Philadelphia, 1975.

BROBECK, J.: *Best and Taylor's Physiologic Basis of Medical Practice*, 10th ed., Williams & Wilkins, Baltimore, 1979, pp. 9-3 to 9-145.

BURCH, G. E. and N. P. DePASQUALE: "Axioms on Cerebrovascular Disease," *Hospital Medicine*, 11(6): 8–21, 1975.

CARINI, E. and G. OWENS: *Neurological and Neurosurgical Nursing*, 8th ed., Mosby, St. Louis, 1982.

CARPENTER, M. B.: *Core Text of Neuroanatomy*, 2d ed., Williams & Wilkins, Baltimore, 1978.

————: *Human Neuroanatomy*, 8th ed., Williams & Wilkins, Baltimore, 1982.

CHEE, C.: "Seizure Disorders," *Nursing Clinics of North America*, 15(1): 71–82, 1980.

COHEN, A., R. FREIDAN, and M. SAMUELS: *Medical Emergencies*, 2d ed., Little, Brown, Boston, 1983.

COLLINS, D. R.: *Illustrated Manual of Neurological Diagnosis*, Lippincott, Philadelphia, 1982.

CRAPPER, D. R., S. QUITTKAT, and U. DeBON: "Altered Chromatin Formation in Alzheimer's Disease," *Brain*, 102: 483–495, 1979.

CURTIS, B., S. JACOBSON, and E. MARCUS: *An Introduction to the Neurosciences*, Saunders, Philadelphia, 1972.

DeVIVO, D. C. and J. P. KEATINE: "Reye's Syndrome," *Advanced Pediatrics* 22: 175–229, 1980.

DIAMOND, S. and D. J. DALESSIO: *The Practicing Physician's Approach to Headache*, 3d ed., Williams & Wilkins, Baltimore, 1982.

DiPALMA, J. (ed.): *Basic Pharmacology in Medicine*, 2d ed., McGraw-Hill, New York, 1981.

DRACHMAN, D. B., I. KAO, A. PESBRONK, et al.: "Myasthenia Gravis as a Receptor Disorder," *Annals of the New York Academy of Sciences,* **274:** 226–234, 1976.

DUVOISIN, R.: "Parkinsonism," *Ciba Clinical Symposia,* **28:** 1, 1976.

Editorial, *Archives of Neurology,* **33:** 395, 1976.

ELLIOTT, F. F.: *Clinical Neurology,* 2d ed., Saunders, Philadelphia, 1971, p. 383.

ESCOUROLLE, R. and J. PORRIER: *Manual of Basic Neuropathology,* 2d ed., Saunders, Philadelphia, 1978.

FIELDS, W.: "Aortocranial Occlusive Vascular Disease," *Ciba Clinical Symposia,* vol. 26, no. 4, 1974.

FISHER, M.: "Occlusion of the Internal Carotid Artery," *Archives of Neurologic Psychiatry,* **65:** 346–377, 1951.

FROHLICH, E. (ed.): *Pathophysiology: Altered Regulatory Mechanisms in Disease,* 4th ed., Lippincott, Philadelphia, 1984.

GANONG, W. F.: *Review of Medical Physiology,* Lange, Los Altos, Calif., 1977.

GARDNER, E.: *Fundamentals of Neurology,* 6th ed., Saunders, Philadelphia, 1975.

GASTAUT, H. (Secretary General): "International Clinical and Electroencaphalographic Classification of Epileptic Seizures," *Epilepsia,* **11:** 102–113, 1970.

———: *Dictionary of Epilepsy: Part I. Definitions,* World Health Organization, Geneva, 1973.

GESCHWIND, N.: "Specialization of the Human Brain," *Scientific American,* **241**(3): 180–199, 1979.

GILROY, J. and J. MEYER: *Medical Neurology,* 3d ed., Macmillan, New York, 1979.

GLASER, G.: "Are the Benefits of Steroid Therapy in Myasthenia Gravis Worth the Risk?" *Modern Medicine,* May 15, 1976, pp. 61–72.

GOODMAN, L. S. and A. GILMAN: *The Pharmacological Basis of Therapeutics,* 6th ed., Macmillan, New York, 1980.

GOSS, C. M. (ed.): *Gray's Anatomy of the Human Body,* 29th ed., Lea & Febiger, Philadelphia, 1973.

GUYTON, A.: *Textbook of Medical Physiology,* 6th ed., Saunders, Philadelphia, 1977.

HARVEY, A., R. JOHNS, A. OWENS, and R. ROSS: *The Principles and Practice of Medicine,* 20th ed., Appleton-Century-Crofts, New York, 1980.

HAWKINS, M. and J. OZUNA: "Practical Aspects of Anticonvulsant Therapy," *American Journal of Nursing* 79(6): 1062–1068, 1979.

HOUSE, E. L., B. PANSKY, AND A. SIEGEL: *A Systematic Approach to Neuroscience,* 3d ed., McGraw-Hill, New York, 1979.

HOWE, J. R. and G. KINDT: "Cerebral Protection during Carotid Endarterectomy," *Stroke,* **5:** 340, 1974.

HUBEL, D. H.: "The Brain," *Scientific American,* **241** (3): 45–53, 1979.

JACKSON, F. E.: "The Pathophysiology of Head Injuries," *Ciba Clinical Symposia,* vol. 18, no. 3, 1966.

JENNETT, B., et al.: "Severe Head Injuries in Three Countries," *Journal of Neurology, Neurosurgery, and Psychiatry,* **40:** 291, 1977.

KEIM, H. A. and W. H. KIRKALDY-WILLIS: "Low Back Pain," *Ciba Clinical Symposia,* **32**(6): 2–35, 1980.

LANCE, J. W.: *Mechanism and Management of Headache,* 3d ed., Butterworth, London, 1978.

LANGLEY, L. L., J. R. TELFORD, and J. B. CHRISTENSEN: *Dynamic Anatomy and Physiology,* 5th ed., McGraw-Hill, New York, 1980.

LIVINGSTON, S.: "Medical Treatment of Epilepsy: Part I," *Southern Medical Journal,* 71(3): 298–310, 1978.

———et al.: "Maintenance of Drug Therapy," *Pediatric Annals* 8(4): 47–84, April 1979.

LUCIANO, D., A. VANDER, and J. SHERMAN: *Human Anatomy and Physiology,* 2d ed., McGraw-Hill, New York, 1983.

MACNAB, I.: *Backache,* Williams & Wilkins, Baltimore, 1977.

MANCALL, E.: "The Stroke: A Review of Current Diagnostic and Therapeutic Considerations," *Hospital Medicine,* 11(4): 8–25, 1975.

MCHENRY, L. C.: "Cerebral Blood Flow Measurement and Regulation in Man: Part II," *Current Concepts of Cerebrovascular Disease—Stroke,* 11(2): 5–8, 1976.

MCLAURIN, R.: "Answers to Questions on Head Injuries," *Hospital Medicine,* 5(1): 54–69, 1969.

MONTOURIS, G. D.: "The Pregnant Epileptic: A Review and Recommendations," *Archives of Neurology,* **36:** 601–603, 1979.

MOUNTCASTLE, V. B.: *Medical Physiology,* 14th ed., Mosby, St. Louis, 1980.

NOBACK, C. R. and R. J. DEMAREST: *The Human Nervous System,* 3d ed., McGraw-Hill, New York, 1981.

NORMAN, R., W. BLACKWOOD, and J. CORSELLEYN: *Greenfield's Neuropathology,* 2d ed., Arnold, London, 1963.

PERRY, T. M. and F. N. MILLER, JR.: *Pathology,* 3d ed., Little, Brown, Boston, 1978.

PETERSDORF, R. G., et al. (eds.): "Alterations in Nervous System Function," in *Harrison's Principles of Internal Medicine,* 10th ed., McGraw-Hill, New York, 1983, sec. 3, pp. 66–155.

PRIOR, J. and J. SILBERSTEIN: *Physical Diagnosis,* 15th ed., Mosby, St. Louis, 1979.

ROBBINS, S. L., R. S. COTRAN, and V. KUMARV: *Pathologic Basis of Disease,* 3d ed., Saunders, Philadelphia, 1984.

Roche Handbook of Differential Diagnosis: Signs and Symptoms of the Nervous System, Coma II, Hoffman-LaRoche, Inc., 1979.

RUBIO, R. and R. BERNE: "Intrinsic Factors in the Control of the Cerebral Circulation," *Current Concepts of Cerebrovascular Disease—Stroke,* 11(5): 21–25, 1976.

SANDS, H. and F. MASTERS: *The Epilepsy Fact Book,* Scribner, New York, 1979.

SCHWARTZ, S. I. (ed.): *Principles of Surgery,* 4th ed., McGraw-Hill, New York, 1984.

SIMPSON, J. and K. MAGEE: *Clinical Evaluation of the Nervous System,* Little, Brown, Boston, 1973.

SNELL, R. S.: *Clinical Neuroanatomy,* Little, Brown, Boston, 1980.

STEVENS, C. F.: "The Neuron," *Scientific American,* **241**(3): 54–65, 1979.

STRATTON, D. B.: *Neurophysiology,* McGraw-Hill, New York, 1981.

SUNDT, T. M.: "Bypass Surgery for Vascular Disease of the Carotid System," *Mayo Clinic Proceedings,* vol. 51, November 1981.

THOMAS, J. and G. MALNER: "The Unconscious Patient," *Hospital Medicine,* 4(11), 6, 1978.

WALLE, J., H. NAUTA, and M. FEIRTAG: "The Organization of the Brain," *Scientific American,* **241**(3): 88–111, 1979.

WEINER, H. and L. LEVITT: *Neurology,* 2d ed., Williams & Wilkins, Baltimore, 1978.

PART IX

DAVID E. SCHTEINGART

ENDOCRINE AND METABOLIC DISORDERS

This part deals with basic concepts in endocrinology and metabolism. These concepts should help you acquire an understanding of clinical problems associated with endocrine diseases. The part examines general physiological concepts, including structure and mechanism of action of hormones, principles of neurohypothalamic control of pituitary function, circadian rhythms, feedback control of endocrine function, and mechanisms which control blood glucose.

The following clinical entities have been selected for discussion: Cushing's syndrome, Addison's disease, primary and secondary aldosteronism, hirsutism, hyperparathyroidism, hypoparathyroidism, panhypopituitarism, acromegaly, diabetes mellitus, hyperthyroidism, hypothyroidism, goiter, carcinoma of the thyroid, and disorders of the reproductive cycle.

OBJECTIVES

At the completion of this part you should be able to:

1. Enumerate basic concepts concerning the endocrine system and the structure of hormones, their mechanisms of action, and the regulation of their secretion.
2. Identify the etiology, pathogenesis, and clinical expression of selected endocrine diseases.
3. Explain the rationale for the treatment of these diseases.
4. Describe the regulation of blood glucose.
5. Give a definition of diabetes mellitus and describe its prevalence, possible etiology, clinical presentation, biochemical diagnosis, treatment, and complications.

PRINCIPLES OF ENDOCRINE AND METABOLIC CONTROL MECHANISMS

OBJECTIVES

At the completion of this chapter you should be able to:

1. Explain the mechanism by which the central nervous system and the endocrine system are integrated.

2. Describe the five vital functions of the endocrine system.

3. Explain the three mechanisms by which hormones work on their target tissues.

4. Differentiate between the two types of hormones as to their chemical structure and sites of production. Give two examples of each type.

5. Describe the characteristics of hormone receptors, including location and degree of specificity.

6. Describe how the tropic hormone angiotensin II is synthesized in the blood and stimulates a peripheral gland.

7. Describe positive and negative feedback control systems of hormonal secretion regulation.

8. Identify at least two examples each of diseases caused by hormonal deficit and hormonal excess.

9. Describe the function of the hypothalamic-hypophyseal portal system.

10. Give an example of the way a feedback control mechanism regulates hormone secretion.

11. Explain a circadian rhythm by describing changes in adrenocorticotropic hormone (ACTH) levels (high or low) and the time of day each level occurs.

12. Describe the cyclic pattern of gonadotropin secretion.

13. Explain the way the central nervous system controls pituitary function through the hypothalamus.

14. Describe the process by which corticotropin-releasing hormone (CRH) influences ACTH.

15. Explain the feedback control of follicle-stimulating hormone (FSH) and thyroid-stimulating or thyrotropic hormone (TSH).
16. Describe the two postulated mechanisms for endocrine disturbances.
17. State the general principles of treatment of diseases caused by hormonal deficit or excess.

As living organisms develop complex structure and function, integration of their various components becomes essential to their survival. This integration is effected by two systems: (1) the central nervous system and (2) the endocrine system. These two systems are related from the embryologic, anatomical, and functional standpoints. For example, many of the endocrine glands originate from the neuroectoderm, an embryonic layer which also gives origin to the central nervous system. In addition, there are anatomical connections between the developed central nervous system and the endocrine system, primarily through the hypothalamus. As a consequence, stimuli which disturb the central nervous system frequently also alter the function of the endocrine system. The integrated operation of the nervous and endocrine systems helps to maximize the response of the organism to stressful stimuli.

FUNCTIONS OF THE ENDOCRINE SYSTEM

The endocrine system helps maintain and regulate vital functions such as (1) response to stress and injury, (2) growth and development, (3) reproduction, (4) ionic homeostasis, and (5) energy metabolism.

When injury or stress occurs, the endocrine system triggers a series of responses aimed at maintaining blood pressure and preserving life. The hypothalamic-pituitary-adrenal axis is chiefly involved in this response.

Without the endocrine system there is failure to grow and reach maturity; infertility also occurs. The hypothalamic-pituitary-gonadal axis is chiefly involved in this function.

The endocrine system is important in maintenance of ionic homeostasis. Mammalian organisms live in an external environment which changes constantly. However, tissues and cells live in an internal environment which must remain constant. The endocrine system participates in the regulation of this internal environment through maintenance of sodium, potassium, water, and acid-base balance. Aldosterone and antidiuretic hormone are responsible for this function. The calcium concentration is also controlled by endocrine

function. Calcium is required for regulation of many biochemical reactions in living cells and for normal neural activation of muscle cell function. The parathyroid glands regulate calcium homeostasis.

Finally, the endocrine system acts as a regulator of energy metabolism. The basal metabolic rate is increased by thyroid hormone, and energy is made available to cells through the integrated action of gastrointestinal and pancreatic hormones.

HORMONES

The endocrine system is made up of glands which synthesize and secrete substances called *hormones*. Hormones cause the physiological and biochemical changes which mediate the types of regulation described above. Once they are released into the bloodstream, hormones are transported to target tissues where they exert their effects. These effects frequently involve the regulation of ongoing enzymatic reactions. Hormones are generally secreted in very low concentrations. For instance, hormones are present in blood at a concentration of 10^{-6} to 10^{-12} molar. In contrast, another blood component, sodium, is usually present at a concentration of 10^{-1} molar. Despite these low concentrations, hormones exert marked metabolic and biochemical effects on their target tissues.

Hormones fall into two main classes: (1) steroids and thyronines, which are lipid-soluble, and (2) polypeptides and catecholamines, which are water-soluble. In addition, some hormones are in the category of glycoprotein, a combination of a sugar moiety and a protein. The main characteristic of steroid hormones is the presence of a multicyclic structure, the cycloperhydrophenanthrene nucleus (see Fig. 53-1). Examples of steroid hormones are the adrenocortical hormones and the hormones produced by the gonads. The molecular structure of insulin, a polypeptide hormone, is illustrated in Fig. 53-2. In addition to insulin, other polypeptide hormones are parathyroid or parathormone hormone (PTH), the tropic hormones of the pituitary gland [with the exception of thyroid-stimulating or thyrotropic hor-

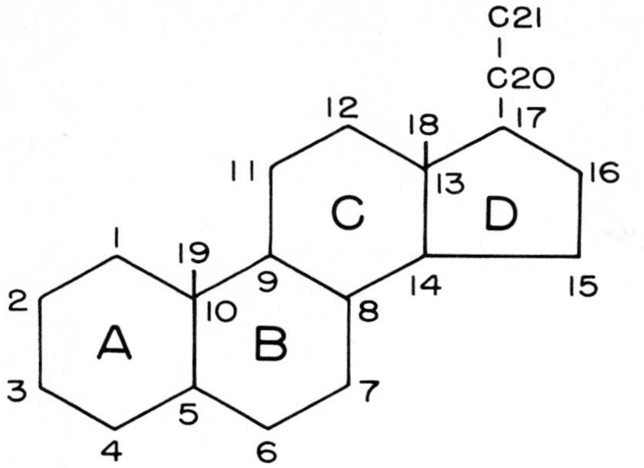

FIGURE 53-1
A steroid nucleus. It has four rings: A, B, C, and D. The numbers designate the carbons within the molecule. Groups attached to different carbons are recognized by the respective numbers. For example, 17-hydroxy steroids have a hydroxyl group attached to the carbon in the 17 position.

mone (TSH) and gonadotropins], pitressin, and glucagon. Examples of glycoprotein hormones are TSH and gonadotropins. Most hormones are synthesized as larger-molecular-weight precursors and are designated in their initial stages as preprohormones, prohormones, or larger-molecular-weight precursors. For example, insulin is synthesized as proinsulin, a continuous peptide which—after losing a portion of the molecule, the C peptide—becomes a two-chain structure. ACTH is derived from proopiomel anocortin (POMC), a 31,000-molecular-weight glycoprotein, which by sequential enzyme catalyzation cleavages generates a series of peptides, including opiates and the 39-amino-acid peptide ACTH.

In addition to the classical hormones, which are produced by specific endocrine glands and act on specific target organs, there are a number of substances generated by hormone action which act directly on cells and promote growth. Some of these substances have insulinlike activity, while others mediate the action of hormones, like growth hormone. Somatomedin C is a well-recognized growth factor, generated in tissues under the effect of growth hormone, which is capable of promoting tissue growth. There are also compounds

which are hormonelike in their mechanism of action but are produced in the blood itself. An example is angiotensin II, a polypeptide hormone which stimulates the adrenal cortex to secrete aldosterone. Angiotensin I is synthesized in the blood from renin substrate (a hepatic protein) under the catalytic effect of renin, an enzyme secreted by renal cells.

While most hormones are synthesized by distinct endocrine glands, there are organs not classically considered endocrine glands which contain groups of cells capable of synthesizing hormones. Many of these cells are derived from the neural crest and have the capacity to take up amine precursors and decarboxylate them for synthesis of hormones. These cells have been described as being part of the APUD (Amine Precursor Uptake and Decarboxylation) system. Tumors derived from these cells may acquire the capacity to secrete hormones which, because of their origin in cells outside the classical endocrine glands, are called ectopic hormones.

Much is known about the way hormones work on their target tissues or cells. Hormones influence cellular metabolic processes either directly or indirectly by first interacting with specific cell receptors. The combination of the hormone with its receptor may bring about changes within the cell by one of two mechanisms: (1) generation of a second messenger within the cell or (2) translocation of the hormone-receptor complex into the nucleus, where the complex induces new protein synthesis by the cell. Polypeptide hormones and catecholamines appear to act via a second messenger mechanism, whereas steroid hormones are freely permeable to the cell membrane and exert their effects directly on the cell nucleus. More specifically, polypeptide hormones act by first interacting with a specific cell membrane receptor, and as a result of this interaction, a membrane-

FIGURE 53-2
Molecular structure of insulin, a polypeptide hormone. The hormone has two chains, A and B. The A chain has 21 amino acids, and the B chain has 30 amino acids. The two chains are linked to each other by disulfide linkages.

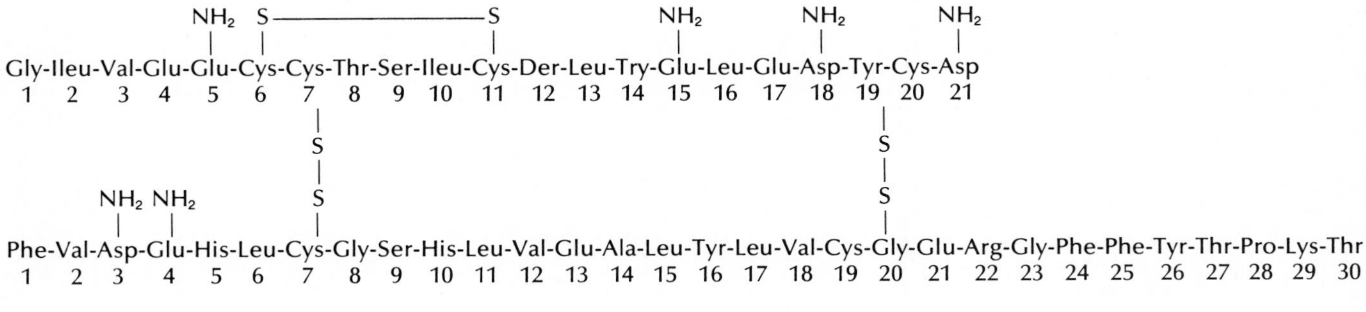

bound enzyme, adenylate cyclase, is activated and adenosine triphosphate (ATP) is converted to adenosine 3′,5′-monophosphate (cyclic AMP). The latter then binds to the regulatory subunit of a protein kinase, thereby liberating a catalytic subunit of this enzyme. This in turn initiates the phosphorylation of certain key enzymes that specifically either activate or inactivate the biological potency of these enzymes (see Fig. 53-3). Different polypeptide hormones activate different specific enzyme mechanisms, which mediate hormone action. For example, glucagon activates the enzyme phosphorylase by the process described, which brings about the enzymatic cleavage of glycogen to glucose 1-phosphate. ACTH increases steroidogenesis by activating one or several enzymes of the steroidogenic pathway. In contrast, other peptide hormones, such as insulin, may not have cyclic AMP as a secondary messenger. Instead, by binding to its receptor, insulin causes a small polypeptide fragment to be cleaved off the cell membrane. This fragment is then responsible for both the membrane effect and the intracellular metabolic effects of insulin. These effects may include enhancement of glucose transport, changes in the flux of certain ions, and other actions not well defined. In contrast to the way peptide hormones exert their effects, steroid hormones work directly inside the cell by entering the cell across the cell membrane and binding to cytosol receptor proteins. The steroid-receptor complex then is translocated to the nucleus of the cell, where it binds specifically to its locus on the chromatin, activing ribonucleic acid (RNA) polymerase and ultimately causing synthesis of one or several specific messenger RNAs. These products leave the nucleus and travel to the ribosome, where they direct the synthesis of proteins. By changing messenger RNA, steroids can modify the way protein is synthesized (see Fig. 53-4).

In summary, hormonal action involves the combination of the hormone with its specific receptors in cells which are the targets of hormone action. The physiological action of the hormone and the specificity of such action are intimately linked to the interaction of the hormone with its specific receptor.

PHYSIOLOGY OF THE ENDOCRINE SYSTEM

The central nervous system is connected to the pituitary through the hypothalamus; this is the most clearly established link between the central nervous system and the endocrine system. The two systems are interrelated by both neural and vascular connections.

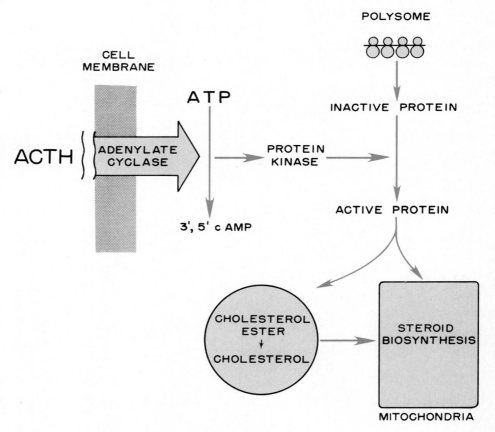

FIGURE 53-3
Mechanism of action of ACTH, a protein hormone. ACTH activates adenyl cyclase, increasing the synthesis of 3′,5′-cyclic AMP. In turn, cyclic AMP stimulates a protein kinase which activates rapid turnover protein. This protein causes (1) increased release of cholesterol for use in steroid biosynthesis and (2) stimulation of conversion of cholesterol to pregnenolone in the cell mitochondria.

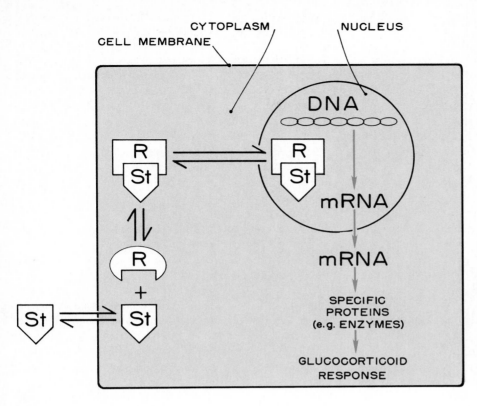

CELL MEMBRANE — CYTOPLASM — NUCLEUS

DNA

R
St

R
St

mRNA

mRNA

R

+

St

St

SPECIFIC
PROTEINS
(e.g. ENZYMES)

GLUCOCORTICOID
RESPONSE

FIGURE 53-4

Mechanism of action of steroid hormones. These hormones bind to intracellular receptor proteins, which subsequently carry the steroid molecule to the cell nucleus. In the nucleus the steroid modifies the formation of messenger RNA and protein synthesis.

As demonstrated in Fig. 53-5, the pituitary is divided into an anterior, a posterior, and an intermediate lobe. Blood vessels link the hypothalamus with the cells of the anterior pituitary gland. These blood vessels end in capillaries at both ends and, for this reason, are known as a *portal system*. In this particular case, the system connects the hypothalamus with the pituitary gland (hypophysis) and is called the *hypothalamic-hypophyseal* portal system. The portal system is an important vascular channel, since it allows for the movement of releasing hormones from the hypothalamus to the pituitary gland, enabling the hypothalamus to modulate

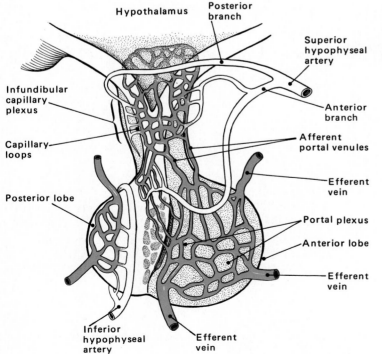

Hypothalamus

Posterior branch

Superior hypophyseal artery

Infundibular capillary plexus

Anterior branch

Capillary loops

Afferent portal venules

Posterior lobe

Efferent vein

Portal plexus

Anterior lobe

Efferent vein

Inferior hypophyseal artery

Efferent vein

FIGURE 53-5

Hypothalamic-hypophyseal portal system. (From L. L. Langley, J. R. Telford, and J. B. Christensen, *Dynamic Anatomy and Physiology*, 4th ed., McGraw-Hill, New York, 1980, p. 689.)

pituitary function. Stimuli originating in the brain activate neurons in the hypothalamic nuclei, which synthesize and secrete low-molecular-weight proteins. These proteins, or neurohormones, are known as *releasing hormones*. They are discharged into the blood vessels of the portal system, through which they reach cells in the pituitary gland. The pituitary gland responds to these releasing hormones by discharging pituitary tropic hormones. In this chain of events, the hormones which are released by the pituitary gland travel with the blood and stimulate other glands, causing the release of target gland hormones. The target gland hormones, in turn, act upon the neuromechanism or the pituitary cells and modify hormone secretion (see Fig. 53-6).

Figure 53-7 illustrates a modality of feedback control in which the hormonal product of the target gland inhibits the release of the corresponding pituitary tropic hormone. This type of regulation of hormone secretion is known as a negative feedback control system. In the hypothalamic-pituitary-adrenal system (Fig. 53-7A), corticotropin-releasing hormone (CRH) causes the pituitary to release ACTH. Then ACTH stimulates the adrenal cortex to secrete cortisol. Cortisol, in turn, feeds back on the hypothalamic-pituitary axis and inhibits the production of CRH-ACTH. The system fluctuates,

varying with the physiological requirements for cortisol. If the system produces too much ACTH and, therefore, too much cortisol, the cortisol feeds back and inhibits the production of ACTH. This is a sensitive system, since an excessive production of cortisol or the administration of cortisol or other synthetic glucocorticoids can quickly inhibit the hypothalamic-pituitary axis and shut off the production of ACTH. The concept of feedback control has practical implications in patients on chronic corticosteroid therapy. These patients have suppressed ACTH release. If steroids are suddenly withdrawn, patients may develop adrenal insufficiency.

Another example of feedback control (Fig. 53-7B) is the action of gonadotropin-releasing hormone (GnRH), which stimulates the pituitary to secrete follicle-stimulating hormone (FSH) and luteinizing hormone (LH). In the female, estrogens are initially produced by the ovary in small amounts; the estrogens feed back on the hypothalamus, stimulating the secretion of GnRH. This, in turn, triggers FSH and LH release, ovulation, and secretion of estrogen and progesterone. The action of estrogens is an example of positive feedback control. A third example (Fig. 53-7C) of feedback control is release of TSH-releasing hormone (TRH), which is secreted by the hypothalamus and causes the pituitary to secrete TSH. In turn, TSH stimulates the thyroid to secrete thyroxine. Thyroxine then feeds back on the pituitary and inhibits production of TSH.

While the interaction between pituitary hormones and the target gland hormones occurs through systemic circulation (the long-loop system), other interactions occur between pituitary hormones and their releasing factors (the short-loop system).

There are other systems which regulate hormone production independently of the hypothalamic-pituitary axis. One example is the renin-angiotensin-aldosterone system. As illustrated in Fig. 53-8, the kidney has juxtaglomerular (JG) cells, which are located in the wall of the afferent arteriole of the glomerulus. These cells secrete the enzyme renin. The production of renin is influenced by the perfusion pressure in the renal arteriole. Changes in the pressure of blood flowing through the afferent arteriole into the glomerulus are sensed by stretch receptors near the JG cells. This causes changes in the secretion of renin, which in turn activates angiotensin II. Angiotensin II stimulates the production of aldosterone by the adrenal cortex. Aldosterone promotes renal tubular reabsorption of sodium. As sodium is reabsorbed, volume is expanded, the pressure rises in the afferent arteriole, and renin production is shut off. Thus, renin, angiotensin, and aldosterone release are deter-

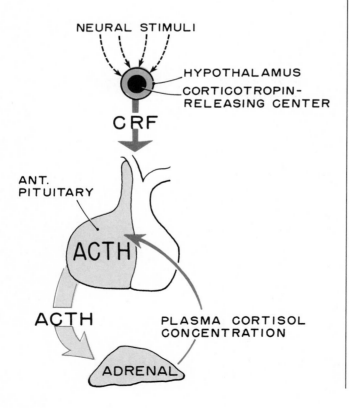

FIGURE 53-6

Feedback regulation of adrenocortical function and ACTH release.

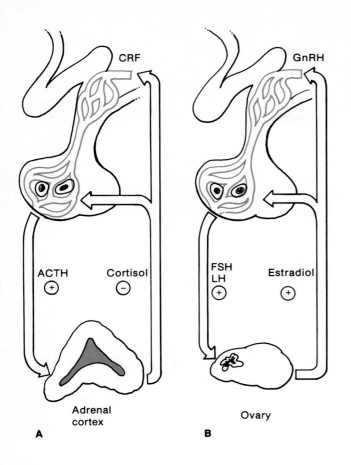

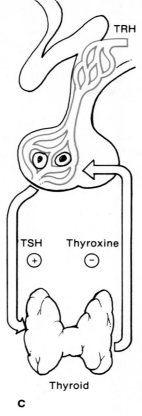

FIGURE 53-7

Diagrammatic representations of feedback-regulating systems where the target gland hormone feeds back to the hypothalamus. Pituitary release of the tropic hormone follows.

mined by volume and pressure changes affecting the JG cells.

Figure 53-9 illustrates another modality of feedback control, in which the metabolic substance controlled by the hormone acts directly upon its release. In example A, insulin and glucose are depicted. Insulin responds to changes in the level of glucose in blood. When glucose levels increase, insulin is secreted. When glucose levels decrease, insulin is shut off. Although some of the pi-

tuitary hormones may indirectly influence insulin release, there is no clear evidence that the pituitary gland directly and specifically controls insulin secretion.

PTH and calcium constitute another unique control system (Fig. 53-9B). A drop in calcium level stimulates PTH secretion. Conversely, an increase in calcium shuts off PTH production.

Another physiological characteristic of the hypothalamic-pituitary axis is the presence of rhythms.

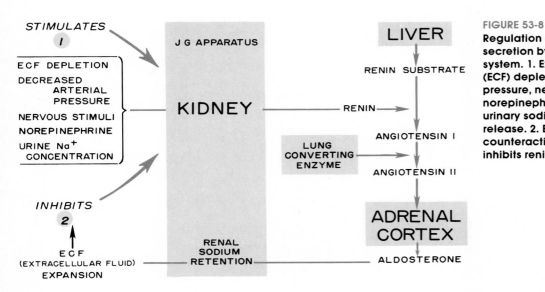

FIGURE 53-8

Regulation of aldosterone secretion by the renin-angiotensin system. 1. Extracellular fluid space (ECF) depletion, decreased arterial pressure, nervous stimuli, norepinephrine, and increased urinary sodium stimulate renin release. 2. ECF expansion, by counteracting these factors, inhibits renin release.

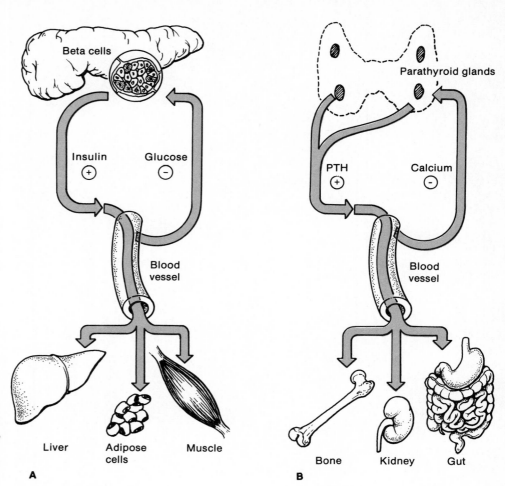

FIGURE 53-9
Diagrammatic representation of feedback-regulating systems where the metabolic substrate of hormone action controls the release of the hormone.

A

B

Rhythms are a common feature of the production of many hormones, and they originate in brain structures. ACTH provides an excellent example of rhythmic, or cyclic, hormone release. When ACTH and cortisol levels are measured on an hourly basis for 24 hours, the levels are seen to rise early in the day, decline later, and rise again during the night to reach a peak by the next morning (see Fig. 53-10). This type of rhythm is referred to as a *diurnal*, or *circadian*, *rhythm*. Since hormonal release by the pituitary gland occurs in short spurts, it is also said that there is *episodic hormonal release*.

Gonadotropins, the tropic hormones of the pituitary gland which control gonadal function, are involved in a different kind of cycle or rhythm. In the female, the release of gonadotropins is cyclic and occurs on a monthly basis rather than on a diurnal basis (see Fig. 53-

FIGURE 53-10
Circadian rhythm of cortisol secretion.

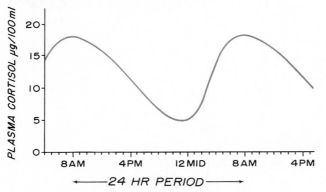

FIGURE 53-11
Monthly cyclic release of gonadotropins in normally menstruating women. Depicted is the midcycle surge of FSH and LH.

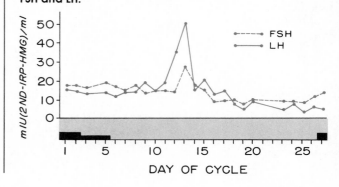

11). The presence of the normal cyclic release of gonadotropins is specific and characteristic of female reproductive endocrine function. In the male, on the other hand, the release of the same gonadotropins does not have this cyclic character, and it occurs at a constant rate. If the cyclic release of gonadotropins in the female is abolished, there is cessation of normal menstrual cycles, disappearance of ovulation, and infertility.

There are other hormones which are not released with a spontaneous rhythm, but are released in response to a stimulus. For example, insulin and growth hormone are released in response to food intake.

DISEASES OF THE ENDOCRINE SYSTEM

Hormones do not act directly on cells or tissues, but they must first bind to specific receptors in the cell membrane or in the cytosol of the cell. For a metabolic event to occur, the metabolic steps distal to the interaction of the hormone and the receptor must all be intact. It thus appears that not only is the hormone concentration important for the final strength of the signal which turns on the cellular machinery, but the number and affinity of the receptors for the hormone are also critically important. As a consequence, two mechanisms for endocrine disease can be postulated: (1) disturbances in which primarily the hormone concentrations are changed and (2) disturbances in which primarily the receptors are defective. Most endocrine diseases can be understood conceptually in terms of the metabolic actions of the hormones involved. They result from either excessive or deficient hormone production or action. Thus, knowledge of the metabolic consequence of the excessive or deficient hormone secretion will help to identify the clinical picture emerging from these disturbances. For example, if there is an excessive production of thyroxine, the thyroid hormone, one can predict an increase in the basal metabolic rate and in heat production. In effect, patients with hyperthyroidism demonstrate a high metabolic rate, increased heat sensitivity, and weight loss. Conversely, lack of thyroxine results in the opposite metabolic effects, such as low basal metabolic rate and increased sensitivity to cold temperature. Primary disturbances at the receptor level have been described in patients with familial homozygous hypercholesterolemia. In this disorder, there is a lack of the low-density lipoprotein (LDL) receptor, which results in an inability of cells throughout the body to take up cholesterol, a lipid normally circulating in plasma and associated with the LDL lipoprotein fraction. A second type of disorder with a disturbance at the receptor level is Graves' disease, where through an autoimmune process, antibodies against the TSH receptor are formed and stimulation of thyroid function results from this receptor abnormality. Some forms of diabetes mellitus, such as is seen in patients with non-insulin-dependent

diabetes, are a consequence of a decreased sensitivity of peripheral tissues to the action of insulin, probably as a result of a decrease in the number or affinity of insulin receptors.

Treatment of endocrine diseases

The treatment of endocrine disease is based on the change in hormone production underlying the specific disease. In simple terms, patients who have a disease caused by a deficit of hormone secretion are treated by replacement of these hormones. Consider the example of a diabetic who is not making enough insulin. Treatment for the metabolic consequence of insulin insufficiency is the administration of insulin. Similarly, a patient who is not making enough thyroid hormone and becomes hypothyroid is treated with replacement amounts of thyroxine.

The treatment of diseases of hormone excess is more complex, since several therapeutic alternatives are usually available. Removal of the whole gland or part of the gland which produces the hormone in excess is one such alternative. The removal of the entire gland, however, results in total deficit of hormone, necessitating hormonal replacement to restore levels to normal. In contrast, removal of part of a gland can eliminate the hormone excess, leaving only enough hormone production to maintain normal function.

The pituitary gland provides an example of the consequence of total glandular removal. Since it is a gland with multiple functions—the anterior lobe secretes tropic hormones, and the posterior lobe antidiuretic hormone, among others—its removal leads to cessation of secretion of many hormones, or panhypopituitarism. Modern surgical techniques allow for removal of only the part of the gland that is abnormal. These techniques are used when a small tumor of the pituitary gland causes excessive hormone production. The tumor can be resected under microscopic view without removal of the rest of the pituitary gland. In other cases, removal of only a part of a gland is not possible. For example, if the adrenal glands are removed, both the adrenal cortex and the adrenal medulla must be removed. Although the body can function well without the adrenal medulla, the capacity of the body to secrete catecholamines may be impaired.

Another alternative for dealing with hormone excess is the administration of drugs which interefere with hormone production by either blocking or destroying the tissue that makes the hormone. For example, a patient who has an overactive thyroid can be given radioactive iodine in large concentrations. The radioactive iodine concentrates in the thyroid gland and destroys the cells that make thyroxine, causing remission of the disease. Another example is adrenal hyperfunction, in which the glands can be blocked by drugs which interfere with the biosynthesis of adrenal cortical hormones.

Suppression of hormone production is also illustrated by oral contraceptives. Estrogens and progestogens are given to inhibit pituitary release of gonadotropins; this, in turn, suppresses normal ovarian function and ovulation.

Another method of controlling excessive hormone effects is by hormone antagonism. An excess production of female hormone can be counteracted by administration of male hormone, or vice versa. Thus, the metabolic effects of a hormone are opposed by the metabolic effects of an opposite hormone, causing cancellation of the effects of the first one. A hormone can also antagonize the effect of another hormone by blocking binding of the latter to its receptors in its target cells.

Another example of treatment of endocrine abnormalities at the receptor level is the administration of sulfonylureas for the treatment of insulin resistance in non-insulin-dependent diabetes mellitus. Sulfonylureas appear to increase the interaction between insulin and its receptors and, therefore, improve the action of insulin.

In summary, endocrine diseases are those of either hormone deficit or hormone excess; the deficit state is treated by replacing the deficient hormone, while the excessive state can be treated either by surgically removing the whole gland or part of the gland that is working excessively or by giving drugs that block or destroy the tissues making the hormone.

QUESTIONS

Principles of endocrine and metabolic control mechanisms

Directions: Answer the following questions on a separate sheet of paper.

1. List in any order the five vital functions of the endocrine system.

2. Cite two mechanisms by which hormones can work on their target cells.

3. In Table 53-1 list the two types of hormones which are differentiated by their chemical structure. State two examples of each type, and identify the location of production for each example.

4. Write a brief description of the way angiotensin II is synthesized in the blood and stimulates a peripheral gland.

5. Identify the role played by the hypothalamus in the hypothalamic-pituitary system.

6. What is the function of the hypothalamic-hypophyseal portal system?

7. Give an example of the way the feedback control mechanism operates to regulate endocrine hormone secretion.

8. Define *circadian rhythm* by identifying the hormonal levels (high or low) of ACTH and the time of day each level occurs.

9. Cite the two postulated mechanisms for endocrine disturbances.

10. State the rationale for providing hormone replacement or suppression as treatment for endocrine diseases caused by hormonal deficit or excess.

TABLE 53-1

TYPE OF HORMONE, LOCATION OF PRODUCTION, AND EXAMPLES OF EACH TYPE

Type of hormone	Location of production	Examples
a	1	1
	2	2
b	1	1
	2	2

Directions: Complete the following statements by filling the blanks with the appropriate words.

11. An overproduction of thyroxine may cause a condition known as _____.

12. The system that connects the hypothalamus with the pituitary gland is called the _____.

13. Thyrotropin-releasing hormone (TRH) secreted by the hypothalamus causes release of _____.

Directions: Circle T if the statement is true, F if the statement is false. Correct any false statements.

14. T   F   Receptors for polypeptide hormone action are located in the membrane of the cell.

15. T   F   Receptors for hormone action are usually not specific for a particular hormone.

CHAPTER 54

DISORDERS OF THE PITUITARY GLAND

OBJECTIVES

At the completion of this chapter you should be able to:

1. Locate the pituitary gland and describe its structure, embryologic origin, and anatomical relations with the hypothalamus.

2. Describe the origin, chemistry, control, and function of growth hormone, prolactin, melanocyte-stimulating hormone (MSH), adrenocorticotropic hormone (ACTH), follicle-stimulating hormone (FSH), luteinizing hormone (LH), thyroid-stimulating hormone (TSH), and antidiuretic hormone (ADH).

3. Identify the etiology, pathogenesis, characteristic manifestations in children and adults, and treatment of panhypopituitarism.

4. Describe the etiology, characteristic manifestations in children and adults, and treatment of excessive secretion of growth hormone.

GENERAL CONCEPTS

The pituitary gland is a complex structure at the base of the brain lying within a bony wall cavity, the sella turcica, in the sphenoid bone at the base of the skull. It is formed early in embryonic development from the fusion of two ectodermal hollow processes. An invagination from the roof of the primitive oral region, Rathke's pouch, extends upward toward the base of the brain and is met by an outpouching of the floor of the third ventricle, destined to become the neurohypophysis. The developed human pituitary gland is thus formed by a posterior lobe, or neurohypophysis, in continuity with the hypothalamus and an anterior lobe, or adenohypophysis, connected to the hypothalamus through the pituitary stalk. A vascular structure—the hypothalamic-hypophyseal portal system—also connects the hypothalamus with the anterior pituitary gland. It is through this system that releasing hormones from the hypothalamus reach the cells of the pituitary gland to promote hormone release.

The posterior lobe of the pituitary gland, or neurohypophysis, is concerned mainly with the regulation of fluid balance. Antidiuretic hormone is synthesized primarily in the supraoptic and paraventricular nuclei of the hypothalamus and stored in the neurohypophysis. The anterior pituitary gland has multiple functions, and because of its ability to regulate the function of other endocrine glands, it is also known as the master gland. The anterior pituitary cells are specialized to secrete specific hormones. Seven such hormones have been well identified, and their physiological metabolic roles defined. These are ACTH, MSH, TSH, FSH, LH, growth hormone, and prolactin. Some of these hormones (ACTH, MSH, growth hormone, and prolactin) are polypeptides, while others (TSH, FSH, and LH) are glycoproteins. Morphologic studies indicate that each hormone is synthesized by a specific cell type. In a sense, the anterior pituitary gland is a conglomeration of independent glands, all of which are under hypothalamic control.

PHYSIOLOGICAL AND METABOLIC ROLES OF ANTERIOR PITUITARY HORMONES

Growth hormone, prolactin, and MSH have direct metabolic effects on target tissues. In contrast, ACTH, TSH, FSH, and LH exert their main effects through the regulation of secretion of other endocrine glands and are, therefore, known as *tropic* hormones.

Growth hormone, or somatotropin, has major metabolic effects in both children and adults. In children, growth hormone is required for somatic growth. In adults, it may preserve normal adult organ size, and it participates in the regulation of protein synthesis and nutrient disposal. The growth-promoting effect of growth hormone appears to be mediated through the production by growth hormone of somatomedin. It is likely that without somatomedin, growth hormone cannot promote growth. Secretion of growth hormone is regulated by a growth hormone–releasing hormone from the hypothalamus and by somatostatin, an inhibiting hormone. The release of growth hormone is stimulated by hypoglycemia and by amino acids such as arginine.

MSH is similar in structure to a portion of the ACTH molecule. It appears to increase skin pigmentation by stimulating the dispersion of melanin granules in melanocytes. It is likely that its secretion is regulated by a corticotropin-releasing hormone (CRH) and that it may be inhibited by a rise in cortisol. In fact, deficient secretion of cortisol can stimulate MSH release, while high cortisol levels suppress its secretion.

Prolactin has similarity in its molecular structure with growth hormone and some overlap with some of its biological properties. Prolactin is one of a group of hormones necessary for breast development and milk secretion. The release of prolactin is under tonic inhibition by a hypothalamic inhibitory factor (PIF) and by dopamine, a brain neurotransmitter. In their absence increased prolactin secretion and lactation may occur.

ACTH regulates the growth and function of the adrenal cortex and is especially important in the control of the production and release of cortisol. By itself, ACTH does not appear to have significant extra-adrenal effects.

TSH stimulates the growth and function of the thyroid gland. TSH causes thyroxine and triiodothyronine release, and these in turn regulate the secretion of TSH.

FSH and LH are also known as gonadotropins. In the male, FSH maintains and stimulates spermatogenesis, and LH the secretion of testosterone by the Leydig, or interstitial, cells of the testes. FSH and LH are secreted in the male in a continuous or tonic fashion. In contrast, in the female, FSH stimulates follicular development and the secretion of estrogens by the follicular cells. LH maintains and stimulates the secretion of progesterone by the corpus luteum, which develops from the follicle after ovulation has occurred. The release of FSH and LH in the female follows a cyclic pattern such that the levels of these two hormones rise at midcycle, triggering ovulation, and slowly decline toward the end of the cycle, when menstruation occurs.

The clinical consequences of deficiencies in ACTH and TSH release are adrenal insufficiency and hypothyroidism, respectively. Absence of gonadotropin release leads to hypogonadism. Conversely, excessive secretion of ACTH leads to adrenocortical hyperfunction, or Cushing's syndrome. Syndromes of excessive TSH or gonadotropin release are more rare.

Clinical disorders of the pituitary gland

Clinical syndromes associated with abnormal function of the pituitary gland include diseases of hormone deficit and of hormone excess.

Pituitary insufficiency commonly affects all the hormones normally secreted by the anterior pituitary gland. The clinical manifestations of panhypopituitarism are, therefore, a composite of the metabolic effects caused by the deficient secretion of each one of the pituitary hormones.

Several pathological processes may result in pituitary insufficiency: (1) pituitary tumor which destroys normal pituitary cells, (2) vascular thrombosis leading to necrosis of the normal pituitary gland, (3) infiltrative granulomatous diseases which destroy the pituitary, and (4) idiopathic or possible autoimmune destruction of pituitary cells.

The clinical syndrome resulting from panhypopituitarism differs in children and in adults. In children, there is interference with somatic growth caused by deficiency of growth hormone release. Pituitary dwarfism develops as a consequence of this deficiency. As the child reaches adolescence, there is absence of development of secondary sexual characteristics and of the external genitalia (see Fig. 54-1). In addition, patients may present with various degrees of adrenal insufficiency

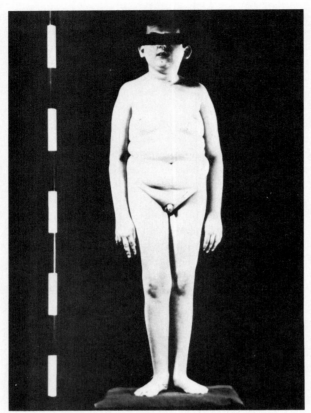

FIGURE 54-1
Short stature and absence of secondary sexual characteristics in a patient with panhypopituitarism developing during childhood.

and hypothyroidism. They may have difficulty in school and exhibit slow intellectual development. Their skin is usually pale because of the absence of MSH.

When hypopituitarism develops in adults, loss of pituitary function frequently has the following chronology: loss of growth hormone, hypogonadism, hypothyroidism, and adrenal insufficiency. Since the adult has already completed somatic growth, adult patients with hypopituitarism are of normal height. Manifestations of growth hormone deficiency may be expressed by unusual sensitivity to insulin and by fasting hypoglycemia. With the development of hypogonadism, male adults exhibit a decrease in libido, impotence, and a progressive decrease in body hair growth, beard, and muscular development (see Fig. 54-2). In women, cessation of menstrual periods, or amenorrhea, is one of the early manifestations of pituitary failure. This is accompanied by atrophy of the breasts and of the external genitalia. Both men and women show various degrees of hypothyroidism (see Chap. 55) and adrenal insufficiency (see

Chap. 58). Deficiency of MSH causes a sallow or pale appearance in these patients.

Occasionally, patients exhibit isolated pituitary hormone failure. Under these circumstances the cause of the deficiency is likely to be in the hypothalamus and involve the corresponding releasing factor.

GIANTISM AND ACROMEGALY

Giantism and acromegaly are caused by excessive secretion of growth hormone. This can result from a pituitary tumor which secretes growth hormone or from a hypothalamic abnormality involving growth hormone release. There are also patients who develop acromegaly in response to extrapituitary neoplasia which secrete growth hormone–releasing hormone (GHRH) ectopically. In these cases there is hyperplasia of pituitary somatotropes and hypersecretion of growth hormone. When growth hormone excess occurs during childhood and adolescence, the patient experiences rapid longitudinal growth and becomes a giant. After somatic growth is completed, growth hormone hypersecretion will cause not giantism but thickening of bones and soft tissue. This condition is termed *acromegaly*, meaning

FIGURE 54-2
Panhypopituitarism in the adult. There is a loss of body hair growth and pallor.

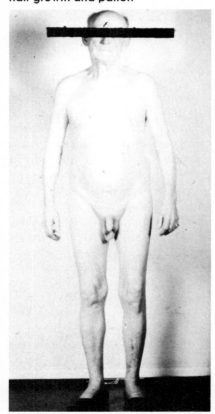

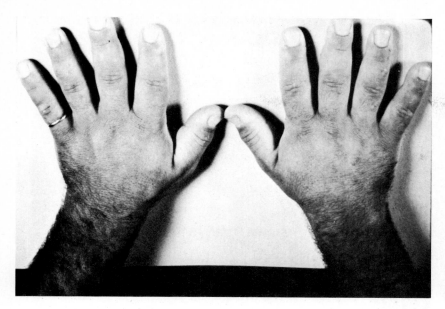

FIGURE 54-3
Hands of a patient with acromegaly.

large hands and feet. Patients with acromegaly exhibit enlargement of hands and feet. Hands become not only larger but also more square (spadelike), and the fingers become more round and stubby (see Fig. 54-3). Patients may relate the need for larger glove size. The feet also become larger and wider, and patients describe changes in shoe size (see Fig. 54-4). The enlargement is usually caused by growth and thickening of bones and by increased growth of soft tissue (see Fig. 54-5). In addition, there are changes in facial features which help diagnose the condition on simple observation. Facial features become coarse, and there is enlargement of the paranasal and frontal sinuses. There are frontal bossing, prominence of the supraorbital ridges, and deformity of the mandible with development of prognathism and under-

bite (see Fig. 54-6). Enlargement of the mandible causes the teeth to spread apart. There is enlargement of the tongue, which causes difficulty with speech (see Fig. 54-7). The voice becomes deeper as a result of thickening of the vocal chords. Deformities of the spine, caused by overgrowth of bone, lead to back pain and changes in the physiological curvature of the spine. The x-ray examination of the skull in acromegaly shows typical changes, including enlargement of paranasal sinuses, thickening of the calvaria, deformity of the mandible which resembles a boomerang, and, most important, enlargement and destruction of the sella turcica suggesting a pituitary tumor (see Fig. 54-8).

When acromegaly is associated with a pituitary tumor, the patients may exhibit bitemporal headaches

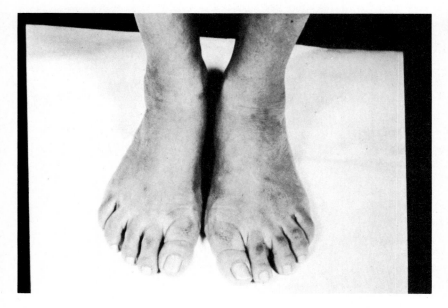

FIGURE 54-4
Feet of a patient with acromegaly.

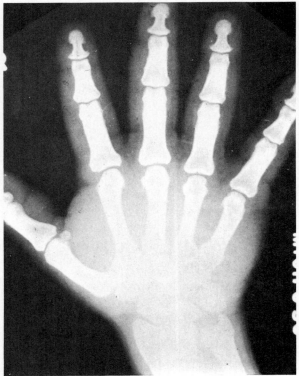

FIGURE 54-5
Radiographic appearance of the hand of an acromegalic patient. There are increases in soft tissues and in density of the bones, squaring of the phalanges, and increased tufting of the terminal phalanges.

and visual disturbance with bitemporal hemianopsia resulting from suprasellar extension of the tumor and compression of the optic chiasma.

EVALUATION OF PATIENTS WITH PITUITARY DISEASE

A clinical diagnosis of a pituitary disorder requires biochemical confirmation by specific tests that reveal the abnormality of pituitary function characteristic of the suspected condition. The pituitary hormones described, ACTH, MSH, TSH, FSH, LH, growth hormone, and prolactin, can all be measured by radioimmunoassay in serum or plasma.

In patients with panhypopituitarism, the baseline level of these hormones is low, as is the level of hormones produced by the target glands controlled by these hormones. In contrast, patients with giantism and acromegaly exhibit high basal growth hormone levels.

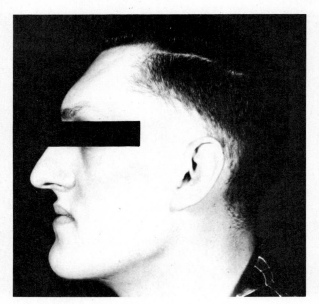

FIGURE 54-6
Profile of a patient with acromegaly. There is prominence of the supraorbital ridges and of the nose (prognathism) and coarsening of facial features.

Patients with hypopituitarism have, in addition to low basal hormone levels, a blunted or absent response to the administration of hormone secretagogues. Combined pituitary function tests can be performed on these patients by injecting (1) insulin in order to produce hypoglycemia, (2) thyrotropin-releasing hormone (TRH), and (3) gonadotropin-releasing hormone (GnRH). Hypoglycemia, with a serum glucose level of less than 40

FIGURE 54-7
Enlargement of the tongue in a patient with acromegaly. Note also a typical acromegalic hand.

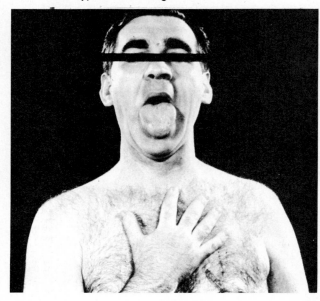

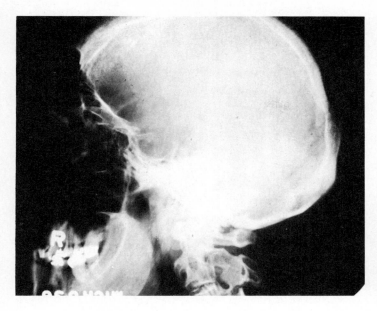

FIGURE 54-8
Radiographic appearance of the skull of a patient with acromegaly. There is marked enlargement and destruction of the sella turcica and suggestion of intrasellar calcification. The calvaria is thick, and there is marked prominence of the frontal and paranasal sinuses. The angle of the mandible is rounded. There is also evidence of underbite.

mg/dl, normally causes the release of growth hormone, ACTH, and cortisol; TRH stimulates TSH and prolactin release, and GnRH stimulates the release of FSH and LH. Following the administration of these three secretagogues, patients with panhypopituitarism fail to respond. Patients with giantism or acromegaly with elevated basal levels of growth hormone can be tested further by the administration of oral glucose. In normal subjects, the induction of hyperglycemia by oral glucose suppresses growth hormone levels. In contrast, patients with giantism or acromegaly fail to suppress. In addition to the biochemical studies, radiographic examination of the pituitary gland is mandatory in patients with suspected pituitary disease, since pituitary tumors are a common cause of these disorders. A plain radiograph of the skull, coned-down on the sella turcica, demonstrates significant changes, including enlargement, demineralization, or erosion in patients with pituitary tumors which exceed 10 mm in diameter. Computerized axial tomography (CAT) scanning of the sella turcica demonstrates pituitary microadenomas as well as macroadenomas with extracellular extension involving the suprasellar cistern, the parasellar regions, or the sphenoid sinus (see Fig. 54-9).

The treatment of hypopituitarism is simple. It consists of replacement of the deficient hormones. Human growth hormone, the only one effective in humans, is available in small quantities for experimental studies. When administered to patients with pituitary dwarfism, it may cause significant increase in height. All the pituitary hormones can be administered only by injection. Thus, for long-term, daily replacement therapy, the hormones of the target glands affected by the pituitary deficiency are administered instead. For example, treatment of adrenal insufficiency caused by deficiency of

ACTH secretion consists of the administration of hydrocortisone orally. Treatment of hypothyroidism caused by TSH deficiency consists of the administration of thyroxine orally. Gonadotropin deficiency can be treated by administering androgens and estrogens. However, induction of ovulation necessitates the administration of gonadotropins.

Treatment of acromegaly or giantism is rather complex. Pituitary irradiation, surgery to the pituitary gland in order to resect a pituitary tumor, or combinations of these procedures may result in amelioration or remission of the disease.

PROLACTIN–SECRETING PITUITARY TUMORS

The combination of persistent milk discharge and absent menses—galactorrhea-amenorrhea—is a relatively common endocrine syndrome in women. It is associated with increased prolactin secretion.

The presence of galactorrhea is usually demonstrated by manual expression of the nipple, although it may occur spontaneously and range from mild to severe. The associated amenorrhea is probably caused by the elevated prolactin levels. Prolactin is believed to inhibit the secretion of gonadotropic hormones by interfering with the hypothalamic secretion of GnRH. In addition, prolactin may block the effect of gonadotropins on the gonad.

Approximately 20 percent of patients with galactorrhea exhibit a prolactin-secreting pituitary adenoma. In many instances, the adenoma is small and barely detectable by radiographic visualization of the sella turcica. In other instances, larger pituitary adenomas have been described. Normal prolactin levels range from 2 to

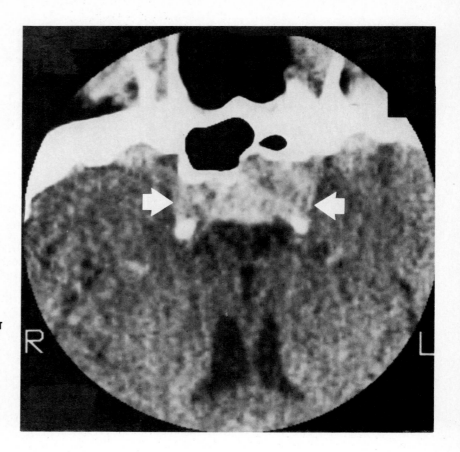

FIGURE 54-9
Coronal cut of the sella turcica by a CAT scan of a patient with a large prolactin-secreting macroadenoma. The enhancing intrasellar mass extends superiorly and laterally beyond the confines of the sella turcica. Also, there is destruction of the floor of the sella, which, instead of a straight horizontal contour, has an irregular appearance.

25 ng/ml. In patients with prolactin-secreting pituitary adenomas, levels may range from 100 ng/ml for small tumors to greater than 1000 ng/ml for large pituitary tumors.

Other patients may have galactorrhea and elevated prolactin levels without detectable pituitary adenomas. They may have undergone interruption of the normal tonic inhibition of prolactin release by the hypothalamus. Galactorrhea can be observed with (1) hypothalamic lesions which interrupt the release of prolactin-inhibiting factor (PIF), (2) drugs with effects on the central nervous system (phenothiazines, antidepressants, haloperidol, alpha-methyldopa), (3) oral contraceptives and estrogens, (4) endocrine disorders such as hypo- and hyperthyroidism, (5) local neurogenic factors, (6) breast stimulation, (7) chest wall injury, and (8) spinal cord lesions.

In the presence of the galactorrhea-amenorrhea syndrome, it is necessary to obtain a basal serum prolactin level. If the prolactin level is elevated above normal, radiographic examination of the sella turcica, including polytomography and computerized axial tomography with coronal cuts of the pituitary gland, should be performed. These studies may demonstrate the presence of abnormalities suggestive of a pituitary microadenoma.

When the diagnosis of a prolactin-secreting pituitary tumor is confirmed, two forms of treatment are usually available: (1) transsphenoidal resection of the prolactin-secreting pituitary tumor and (2) suppression of prolactin secretion by the administration of bromocriptine, an ergot alkaloid derivative which acts as a dopamine agonist. Treatment of hyperprolactinemia by the methods described frequently leads to disappearance of galactorrhea and restoration of normal menstrual cycles and fertility.

Prolactin-secreting pituitary tumors also occur in males, in whom the hyperprolactinemia is associated with hypogonadism and oligospermia. These tumors are frequently large and extend beyond the confines of the sella turcica. The management of prolactin-secreting pituitary microadenomas in the male is similar to that which has been described for the female patient. In patients with large prolactin-secreting macroadenomas, bromocriptine may result in rapid and dramatic decrease in tumor size, without the need for surgical resection.

Disorders of the pituitary gland

Directions: Match the statements in col. A with the structures of the pituitary gland in col. B.

Column A

1. ____ Derived from neural cells of the developing third ventricle

2. ____ Derived from Rathke's pouch

3. ____ Connected to the hypothalamus by the hypothalamic-hypophyseal portal system

4. ____ Confined within the sella turcica of the sphenoid bone

Column B

a. Adenohypophysis

b. Neurohypophysis

c. Both of the above

Directions: Match the hormones in col. A with one of the functions in col. B.

Column A

5. ____ Adrenocorticotropic hormone

6. ____ Growth hormone

7. ____ Luteinizing hormone

8. ____ Follicle-stimulating hormone

9. ____ Prolactin

10. ____ Thyrotropin

11. ____ Melanocyte-stimulating hormone

12. ____ Antidiuretic hormone

Column B

a. Stimulates spermatogenesis in the male

b. Stimulates the formation and release of thyroid hormones

c. Initiates milk secretion after delivery

d. Stimulates the secretory activity of the adrenal cortex

e. Stimulates somatomedin

f. Decreases free water clearance

g. Stimulates the corpus luteum to secrete progesterone and estrogens in human females

h. Increases pigmentation of the skin

Directions: Circle the letter preceding each item below that correctly answers the question. More than one answer may be correct.

13. The hypothalamus secretes neurohormones which:
a. Facilitate the formation of a corpus luteum in the ovary   b. Inhibit the release of prolactin from the pituitary   c. Increase the synthesis of hydrocortisone by the adrenal cortex   d. Facilitate thyroid growth   e. Increase the release of parathormone by the parathyroid glands

14. Antidiuretic hormone is:
a. Synthesized in the neurophypophysis   b. Secreted by the adenohypophysis   c. Synthesized in the supraoptic and paraventricular nuclei in the hypothalamus   d. Stored and released from the neurohypophysis

15. MSH secretion is:
a. Inhibited by high serum levels of cortisol
b. Depressed in Cushing's disease caused by pituitary ACTH excess   c. Greatly increased in Addison's disease   d. Probably controlled by a releasing hormone

16. Which of the following statements about growth hormone is false?
a. It is released in response to hypoglycemia.   b. Its release is controlled by a hypothalamic releasing factor and somatostatin.   c. Its release is inhibited by administration of arginine.   d. Its anabolic effect is mediated through somatomedin.

17. Prepubertal panhypopituitarism may be manifested by:
a. Acromegaly   b. Retardation of growth
c. Pale, dry skin   d. Precocious sexual development   e. Slow intellectual development

18. A 35-year-old multiparous female seeks medical help because of vague symptoms of lethargy, lack of energy, and intolerance to cold. The history reveals that her menstrual periods ceased 1 year earlier following the birth of her last child, which was complicated by postpartum hemorrhage. She is concerned that she is losing her sexual attractiveness. Physical examination reveals an asthenic female with thin hair, atrophied breasts, and thin pubic hair. Blood pressure is 94/60, TPR 97-54-16. Laboratory findings include low thyroidal radioiodine uptake; normal serum cholesterol; depressed serum levels of ACTH; depressed urinary levels of

paranasal and frontal sinuses   c. Increased length and thickness of the mandible   d. Enlargement of the sella turcica

17-ketosteroids, 17-hydroxysteriods, and gonadotropins. The above data are suggestive of:

a. Primary hypothyroidism   b. Premature menopause in an otherwise healthy female   c. Galactorrhea-amenorrhea   d. Primary adrenal insufficiency   e. Panhypopituitarism

19. A possible explanation for this patient's condition is:

a. A congenital disorder   b. Postpartum necrosis of the pituitary   c. Adrenal carcinoma   d. A prolactin-secreting pituitary adenoma

20. Acromegaly results from:

a. Hypersecretion of growth hormone in a child   b. Extrapituitary neoplasia which causes secretion of GHRH ectopically   c. Hypersecretion of growth hormone in an adult   d. Parathormone hypersecretion   e. Pituitary insufficiency

21. Physical signs of acromegaly include:

a. Frontal bossing   b. Prominence of the supraorbital ridges   c. Broad, greatly enlarged, spade-shaped hands   d. Prognathism

22. Patients with acromegaly often experience:

a. Slurred speech   b. Weight loss   c. Hypoglycemia   d. Headaches

23. Common radiologic signs in acromegaly include:

a. Thickened calvaria   b. Enlargement of the

Directions: Circle T if the statement is true and F if it is false. Correct any false statements.

24. T   F   Gondotropin deficiency in hypopituitarism may be treated by the administration of androgens and estrogens.

25. T   F   Growth hormone for treatment of hypopituitary dwarfs is obtained by extraction of the hormone from the pituitary glands of cattle and swine.

26. T   F   Giantism and acromegaly are caused by excessive secretion of somatotropin.

27. T   F   Patients with suspected pituitary disease require only biochemical confirmation by specific tests that reveal abnormality of pituitary function characteristic of the suspected condition.

28. T   F   Computerized axial tomography (CAT) scanning of the sella turcica demonstrates pituitary microadenomas and macroadenomas with extrasellar extension involving the suprasellar cistern, the parasellar regions, or the sphenoid sinus.

CHAPTER 55

DISEASES OF THE THYROID GLAND

OBJECTIVES

At the completion of this chapter you should be able to:

1. Locate the thyroid gland and describe its structure, embryologic origin, and function.

2. Describe the sequential steps in the biosynthesis of thyroid hormones.

3. Differentiate between thyroxine (T_4) and triiodothyronine (T_3) in terms of structure, function, and potency.

4. Explain the physiological effects of thyroid hormones.

5. Describe tests of thyroid function.

6. Give a classification of thyroid diseases on the basis of disturbances in thyroid function.

7. Identify the etiology and major signs and symptoms associated with Graves' disease and toxic nodular goiter. Describe the thyroidal and extrathyroidal manifestations.

8. Define hyperthyroidism.

9. Identify three types of approaches that may be used for the treatment of hyperthyroidism.

10. Differentiate between primary and secondary hypothyroidism.

11. Differentiate between cretinism, juvenile hypothyroidism, and adult hypothyroidism according to age group affected, signs and symptoms, reversible changes, and treatment.

12. Indicate the rationale for measuring thyroid-stimulating or thyrotropic hormone (TSH) levels in the diagnosis of hypothyroidism.

13. Describe the risk factors, clinical features, and diagnostic studies which may help distinguish benign from malignant thyroid nodules.

GENERAL CONSIDERATIONS

The thyroid is a gland with two lobes joined by a thin isthmus located below the cricoid cartilage in the neck. Embryologically the thyroid gland originates from an evagination of the pharyngeal epithelium which carries with it cells from the lateral pharyngeal pouches. This evagination descends from the base of the tongue into the neck until it reaches its final anatomical location. Some thyroid tissue may occasionally be left along this track, giving rise to thyroglossal cysts, nodules, or a pyramidal thyroid lobe. The thyroid gland normally weighs between 10 and 20 g in adults. Histologically, the gland is made up of nodules composed of tiny follicles, which are separated from each other by connective tissue (see Fig. 55-1). The thyroid follicles are lined by cuboidal epithelium, and their lumen is filled with colloid. The follicular epithelial cells initiate the synthesis of thyroid hormones and activate their release into the circulation. The colloidal material, thyroglobulin, is the site where thyroid hormone is synthesized and eventually stored. The two principal thyroid hormones produced by the follicles are thyroxine and triiodothyronine. Another hormone-secreting cell present within the thyroid gland

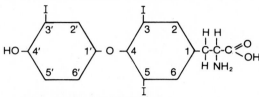

3 - MONO IODOTYROSINE

3, 5, 3', 5'-TETRAIODOTHYRONINE (Thyroxine; T₄)

3, 5 , 3'-TRIIODOTHYRONINE (T₃)

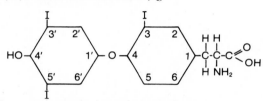

3, 3', 5'-TRIIODOTHYRONINE (reverse T₃; RT₃)

FIGURE 55-2
Chemical structures of thyroid hormones.

FIGURE 55-1
Histology of the thyroid gland. Note colloid of filled follicles. (Courtesy of Dr. Ronald Nishiyama, Pathology Department, University of Michigan.)

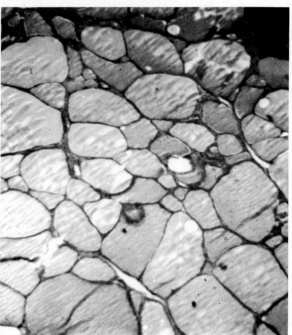

is the parafollicular cell, or C cell, found in the basal portion of the follicle in contact with the follicular membrane. These cells originate in the embryologic ultimobranchial body. They secrete calcitonin, a hormone which lowers serum calcium levels, and thus contribute to the regulation of calcium homeostasis. The follicular thyroid hormones are derived from the iodination of tyrosyl residues in thyroglobulin. Thyroxine contains four iodine atoms (T_4), and triiodothyronine three iodine atoms (T_3) (see Fig. 55-2). Thyroxine is secreted in larger quantities than triiodothyronine, but when compared on a milligram per milligram basis, triiodothyronine is the more active of the two hormones.

Biosynthesis and metabolism of thyroid hormones

The biosynthesis of thyroid hormones involves a sequence of steps which are regulated by specific enzymes. These steps are (1) trapping of iodide, (2) oxidation of iodide to iodine, (3) organification of iodine into mono- and diiodotyrosine, (4) coupling of iodinated precursors, (5) storage, and (6) hormone release (see Fig. 55-3). The trapping of iodide by the thyroid follicular cells is an active, energy-requiring process. This energy is derived from oxidative metabolism within the gland. Iodide is available to the thyroid from that which is ingested in food or water or released by deiodination of thyroid hormones or iodinated agents. The thyroid takes up and concentrates large amounts of iodide from the circulating iodide pool. The thyroid/plasma gradient is 20 to 30:1 at a wide range of plasma inorganic iodide concentrations. Iodide is converted to iodine, catalyzed by an iodide peroxidase enzyme. Iodine is then

FIGURE 55-3
Synthesis and secretion of thyroid hormones. The box indicates steps which occur within the thyroid gland. Thyroid function is regulated by the hypothalamic-pituitary axis. (Adapted from C. Ezrin et al. (eds.), *Systematic Endocrinology*, Harper & Row, New York, 1973.)

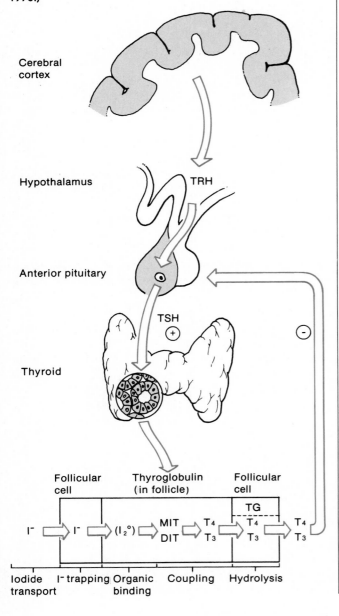

incorporated into a tyrosine molecule, a process described as organification of iodine. This process takes place at the cell-colloid interphase. The resulting compounds, monoiodotyrosine and diiodotyrosine, are then coupled as follows: two molecules of diiodotyrosine make T_4, and one molecule of diiodotyrosine and one molecule of monoiodotyrosine make T_3. The coupling of these compounds and the storage of the resulting hormones take place within thyroglobulin. Hormone release from storage occurs by incorporation of colloid droplets into the follicular cells by a process called *pinocytosis*. Within these cells, thyroglobulin is hydrolyzed and the hormones are released into the circulation. The various steps described are stimulated by thyrotropin (TSH).

Thyroid hormones circulate in plasma bound to plasma proteins: (1) thyroxine-binding globulin (TBG), (2) thyroxine-binding prealbumin (TBPA), and (3) thyroxine-binding albumin (TBA). Most of the circulating hormone is bound to these proteins, and a very small proportion (less than 0.05 percent) is free. The bound and free hormones are in a state of reversible equilibrium. The free hormone is the fraction which is metabolically active, while the larger, protein-bound fraction is not readily accessible to target tissues. Of the three binding proteins, TBG binds thyroxine most specifically. In addition, thyroxine has greater affinity than triiodothyronine for these binding proteins. As a consequence, triiodothyronine is transferred more readily to its target tissues, a factor which accounts for its greater metabolic activity.

Thyroid hormones are chemically altered before excretion. An important alteration is deiodination, which accounts for the disposal of 70 percent of the secreted hormone. Another 30 percent is lost in the stool through biliary excretion as glucuronide or sulfate conjugates. As a result of deiodination, 80 percent of T_4 may be converted into 3,5,3'-triiodothyronine, while the remaining 20 percent is converted to reverse 3,3',5'-triiodothyronine (RT_3), a metabolically inactive hormone.

Thyroid function is controlled by the pituitary glycoprotein hormone TSH, which in turn is regulated by thyrotropin-releasing hormone (TRH), a hypothalamic neurohormone. Thyroxine exerts negative feedback regulation of TSH secretion by acting directly upon the pituitary thyrotropes.

Several drugs and conditions can alter the synthesis, release, and metabolism of thyroid hormones. Drugs like perchlorate and thiocyanate are capable of inhibiting thyroxine synthesis. As a result, they cause a decrease in thyroxine levels and, through negative feedback stimulation, increased release of TSH by the pituitary gland. This condition leads to enlargement of the thyroid gland and the development of a goiter. These drugs are, therefore, called *goitrogens*. Other drugs, such as thiourea derivatives and mercaptoimidazoles, can be used as antithyroid drugs because they inhibit the initial oxidation of iodide, the conversion of monoiodotyrosine to diiodotyrosine, or the coupling of iodotyrosine to produce iodothyronine. These drugs are useful in the treatment of conditions caused by excessive thyroid hormone secretion. Iodine, when given acutely and in large doses, is capable of blocking the organic binding and coupling reactions. The continued administration of large doses of iodine may lead to goiter development and a hyperthyroid state. Finally, drugs like lithium carbonate and glucocorticoids inhibit thyroid hormone release.

Changes in the concentration of TBG can also cause changes in the level of total circulating thyroxine. Increases in TBG, as seen in pregnancy, with birth control pills, and in chronic liver disease, may lead to increased levels of protein-bound thyroxine. Conversely, decreases in TBG, as seen with chronic liver disease, severe systemic illness, nephrotic syndrome, and large doses of glucocorticoids, will cause a decrease in circulating protein-bound thyroxine.

Nutritional changes such as observed during fasting or carbohydrate- and protein-deprived diets can decrease the proportion of thyroxine deiodinated to T_3 and increase the proportion of thyroxine converted into the less metabolically active RT_3. This alteration in the deiodination of thyroxine appears to be a mechanism for fuel conservation in states of food deprivation.

Action of thyroid hormones

The physiological effects of thyroid hormones involve increased transcription of messenger RNA and protein synthesis. This step appears to be necessary for the subsequent stimulation of cell respiration. Specifically, both thyroxine and triiodothyronine stimulate energy-producing electron transfer processes in the respiratory enzyme system of the cell mitochondria. The stimulation by thyroid hormones of oxidative processes leads to stimulation of thermogenesis. In addition to these thermogenic effects, thyroxine and triiodothyronine potentiate the action of epinephrine by increasing the sensitivity of β receptors to catecholamines. Thyroid hormones also stimulate somatic growth and are involved in the normal development of the central nervous system. In their absence, mental retardation and delayed neurological maturation may be present at birth and in infancy.

Tests of thyroid function

The functional status of the thyroid gland can be ascertained by means of thyroid function tests. The following tests are presently used in the diagnosis of thyroid disease: (1) radioactive iodine (RAI) uptake, (2) serum thyroxine and triiodothyronine, (3) T_3 resin uptake, and (4) serum TSH levels. These tests assess the physiological steps described above. For example, the radioactive iodine (^{131}I) uptake test measures the ability of the thyroid gland to trap iodide. The measurement of the serum level of thyroxine gives a good estimation of the circulating level of this hormone, and the T_3 resin uptake test measures the saturation of plasma-binding proteins by thyroxine. When the RAI uptake test is performed, the patient receives a tracer dose of ^{131}I, which the thyroid traps and concentrates over a 24-hour period. By measuring the radioactivity present over the thyroid, it is possible to calculate the percentage of tracer which has been taken up by the thyroid over that period of time. Normally, the RAI uptake ranges from 10 to 35 percent of the administered dose. Values are high in hyperthyroidism and low in hypothyroidism.

The serum thyroxine and triiodothyronine levels can be measured by radioligand assays. Normal levels for thyroxine are 4 to 11 $\mu g/100$ ml; for triiodothyronine they are 80 to 160 ng/100 ml. The T_3 resin uptake test measures the saturation of thyroxine-binding protein by thyroxine and indirectly the level of thyroid hormone. When this test is performed, the patient's plasma is placed in a test tube together with radioactive T_3 and a resin. The radioactive T_3 binds to both the plasma and the resin. Normally 25 to 35 percent of the added T_3 is taken up by the resin. This result can also be expressed as a percent of normal values. A normal T_3 resin uptake ranges between 86 and 110 percent of normal. When the plasma level of thyroxine is high and the protein is completely saturated by thyroid hormone, more of the T_3 will be bound by the resin and less by the protein. The T_3 resin uptake will be high. Conversely, when the thyroxine level is low and the binding proteins are at a low level of saturation, more of the T_3 will bind to the protein and less to the resin. The T_3 resin uptake will be low. Thus, one can assess indirectly the level of thyroxine by the degree of the saturation of the binding protein. By combining the values of the serum thyroxine level and T_3 resin uptake, it is possible to estimate the level of the metabolically active circulating free thyroxine. The free thyroxine index (FTI) is an expression of this value and results from multiplying serum T_4 by T_3 resin uptake. Plasma TSH levels can be measured by radioimmunoassay. Normal values range from 0 to 10 $\mu U/ml$. The plasma TSH level measures the state of homeostatic control of thyroid function by the pituitary gland. Values are high in patients with primary hypothyroidism, in whom the low thyroxine levels are associated with a feedback increase in pituitary TSH release. Some tests are also available that measure the metabolic response to circulating thyroid hormone levels. These tests include the basal metabolic rate (BMR), which measures the oxygen consumption in the resting state; the serum cholesterol level; and the characteristics of response of the Achilles tendon reflex. In patients with hypothyroidism, the BMR is decreased and the serum cholesterol level is high. The Achilles tendon reflex shows slow relaxation. Opposite findings are seen in patients with hyperthyroidism.

At the present time, there is no single thyroid function test which consistently provides all the answers in any given patient with suspected thyroid disease. Therefore, a combination of tests is frequently necessary in order to diagnose the nature of the patient's thyroid problem. Hyper- and hypothyroidism are the two major functional abnormalities for which one needs reliable laboratory tools. Very few supportive laboratory investigations may be required in severe cases. However, reliable tests are essential in the diagnosis of mild cases of thyroid dysfunction. Table 55-1 summarizes the changes in thyroid function tests observed in patients with hypo- and hyperthyroidism.

DISEASES OF THE THYROID GLAND

As with other endocrine diseases, those of the thyroid gland may involve (1) excessive thyroid hormone production—hyperthyroidism, (2) deficient hormone production—hypothyroidism, or (3) thyroid enlargement—goiter—without evidence of abnormal thyroid hormone production.

Hyperthyroidism

Also known as thyrotoxicosis, hyperthyroidism may be defined as the response of body tissues to the metabolic effects of excessive amounts of thyroid hormone. The condition may develop spontaneously or may result from the intake of excessive amounts of thyroid hormone. Occasionally, the therapeutic misuse of thyroid hormone leads to clinical manifestations of hyperthyroidism. Some patients with psychiatric illness may take large amounts of thyroxine or triiodothyronine and be-

come thyrotoxic. These patients frequently deny taking thyroid hormones and pose a real challenge to the medical personnel attempting to establish the proper diagnosis. This form of thyrotoxicosis is called *thyrotoxicosis factitia*. Characteristic of it is the presence of high thyroxine levels and T_3 resin uptake with low RAI uptake and TSH levels.

There are two types of spontaneous hyperthyroidism: (1) Graves' disease and (2) toxic nodular goiter. Graves' disease is the more common.

Graves' disease usually occurs in the third and fourth decades of life and more frequently in females than males. There is a familial predisposition to Graves' disease and frequent association with other forms of autoimmune endocrinopathy. In Graves' disease, there are two major groups of features, thyroidal and extrathyroidal, either of which may be absent. The thyroidal features include a goiter, caused by hyperplasia of the thyroid gland, and hyperthyroidism, which results from excessive thyroid hormone secretion. Symptoms of hyperthyroidism include manifestations of hypermetabolism and of sympathetic overactivity. Patients complain of fatigue; tremor; heat intolerance; increased sweating with warm, moist skin; weight loss, often with increased appetite; palpitations and tachycardia; diarrhea; and muscle weakness and atrophy. The extrathyroidal manifestations include ophthalmopathy and localized skin infiltrations, usually confined to the lower legs. The ophthalmopathy present in 50 to 80 percent of these patients is characterized by stare, widening of the palpebral fissures, decreased blinking, lid lag, and failure of convergence. The lid lag is manifested by a slower movement of the eyelid relative to the eyeball when patients are asked to slowly lower their gaze. Infiltration of the orbital tissues and ocular muscles with lymphocytes, mast cells, and plasma cells leads to exophthalmos (proptosis of the eyeballs), congestive oculopathy, and weakness of extraocular movements (see Fig. 55-4A and B). The ophthalmopathy can be quite severe, and in extreme cases vision may be threatened. Graves' disease appears to develop as a manifestation of an autoimmune disorder. An immunoglobulin (IgG) antibody is present in the serum of these patients. This antibody appears to react with the TSH receptor or the thyroid plasma membrane. As a result of this interaction, the antibody is capable of stimulating thyroid function independently of pituitary TSH, leading to hyperthyroidism. This antibody may result from an inherited abnormality of immune surveillance which permits a particular clone of lymphocytes to survive, proliferate, and secrete stimulatory immunoglobulins in response to some precipitating factor. A similar immune response appears to be re-

TABLE 55-1

Thyroid Function Tests

Test	Hyperthyroidism	Hypothyroidism
RAI uptake	↑	↓
Serum thyroxine	↑	↓
T_3 resin uptake	↑	↓
Serum TSH	↓	↑

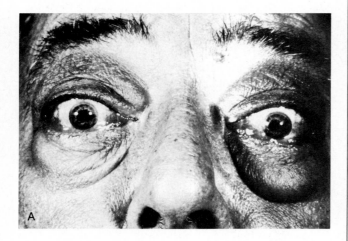

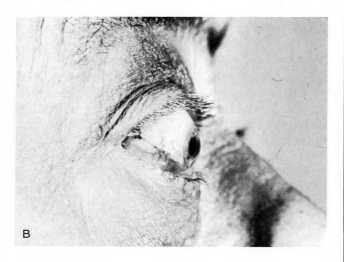

FIGURE 55-4
Exophthalmos with periorbital edema in a patient with Graves' ophthalmopathy. (A) Frontal view. (B) Lateral view. (Courtesy of Dr. James C. Sisson, Department of Internal Medicine, University of Michigan.)

membrane. As a result of this interaction, the antibody is capable of stimulating thyroid function independently of pituitary TSH, leading to hyperthyroidism. This antibody may result from an inherited abnormality of immune surveillance which permits a particular clone of lymphocytes to survive, proliferate, and secrete stimulatory immunoglobulins in response to some precipitating factor. A similar immune response appears to be responsible for the ophthalmopathy observed in these patients.

Toxic nodular goiter develops most frequently in elderly patients as a complication of chronic nodular goiter. The onset of hyperthyroidism in these patients is insidious and the clinical manifestations of hyperthyroidism less severe than in Graves' disease. Patients may present with arrhythmias and heart failure which are resistant to digitalis therapy. Patients may also show evidence of weight loss, weakness, and muscle wasting. The multinodular goiter usually present in these patients contrasts with the diffuse thyroid enlargement seen in patients with Graves' disease. Patients with toxic nodular goiter may show eye signs (stare, widening of palpebral fissure, decreased blinking) resulting from sympathetic overactivity. However, they lack the more dramatic manifestations of infiltrative ophthalmopathy seen in Graves' disease.

Patients with severe manifestations of hyperthyroidism may develop thyroid crisis or storm. In these cases, there is a general worsening of the clinical manifestations described above, to the point where they become life-threatening. Fever is almost always present and may be an important clue to the onset of serious complications. Crisis can be precipitated by minor trauma and stress.

In the presence of clinical manifestations of hyperthyroidism, laboratory tests show a high serum thyroxine and triiodothyronine (T_3) resin uptake. RAI uptake by the thyroid is increased and serum TSH levels are low. In addition, TSH fails to respond to stimulation by TRH, the hypothalmic thyroid-releasing hormone.

Management of hyperthyroidism includes one or several of the following procedures: (1) Prolonged treatment with antithyroid drugs such as propylthiouracil or methimazole, given for at least 1 year. These drugs block thyrozine synthesis and release. (2) Surgical subtotal thyroidectomy after preoperative drug therapy with proplythiouracil. (3) Treatment with radioactive iodine.

Treatment with radioactive iodine is used in the majority of adult patients with Graves' disease. It is usually contraindicated in children and pregnant women. In patients with toxic nodular goiter, antithyroid drugs and ablative therapy with radioactive iodine can also be used. However, if the goiter is very large and there is no contraindication for surgery, surgical resection of the goiter should be considered. Treatment of the ophthalmopathy of Graves' disease involves correction of hyperthyroidism and prevention of hypothyroidism which may develop following surgical or radiation ablative therapy. In many patients, the ophthalmopathy follows a self-limiting course and no further treatment is necessary. However, in severe cases in which vision is threatened, treatment with large doses of glucocorticoids and orbital decompression procedures may be necessary to salvage the eye. Hypothyroidism may develop in patients with hyperthyroidism receiving surgical or radioactive iodine therapy. Of patients treated with radioactive iodine, 40 to 70 percent may go on to develop hypothyroidism over the following 10 years.

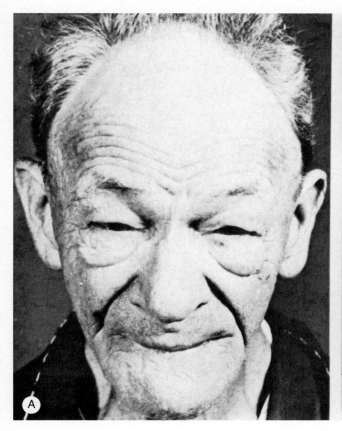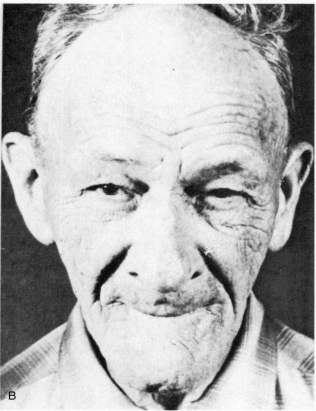

Hypothyroidism

There are several types of hypothyroidism. Depending on the location of the initiating problem, the disease can be classified as (1) primary, resulting from a pathological process which destroys the thyroid gland, or (2) secondary, caused by deficiency of pituitary TSH secretion. Depending on the age of onset of the hypothyroid state, the disease can be classified as (1) adult hypothyroidism, or myxedema, (2) juvenile hypothyroidism (onset after age 1 to 2 years), or (3) congenital hypothyroidism, or cretinism, caused by lack of thyroid hormone before or shortly after birth.

Some patients with hypothyroidism have an atrophic or absent thyroid gland. This results from surgical or radioisotopic ablation of the gland or from its destruction by circulating autoimmune antibodies. Congenital developmental defects may also account for the absence of thyroid gland in patients with congenital hypothyroidism. Other patients with hypothyroidism exhibit a goiter. This is frequently observed in patients with hereditary defects in thyroid hormone biosynthesis, where the concomitant increase in TSH release causes thyroid enlargement, and in patients with Hashimoto's thyroiditis. The latter is an autoimmune disease as a result of which lymphocytic infiltration and destruction of the thyroid gland supervene in association with antithyroglobulin or antithyroid cell microsomal antibodies. Patients with secondary hypothyroidism may exhibit pituitary tumors and deficiency of other pituitary trophic hormones.

The clinical manifestations of hypothyroidism in the adult and juvenile forms include fatigue; hoarseness; cold intolerance; decreased sweating; cool, dry skin; facial puffiness; and slow movements (Fig. 55-5). There is slowing of intellectual and motor activity and slow relaxation of deep tendon reflexes. Women with hypothyroidism frequently complain of hypermenorrhea.

Congenital hypothyroidism, or cretinism, may be present at birth or become evident within the first several months of life. Early manifestations of cretinism include persistent physiological jaundice, hoarse cry, constipation, somnolence, and feeding problems. Subsequently, the child shows delay in reaching the normal milestones of development. The child with congenital hypothyroidism exhibits short stature; coarse features; a protruding tongue; broad, flat nose; widely set eyes; sparse hair; dry skin; a protuberant abdomen; and umbilical hernia. Radiographic examination of the skeleton shows retarded bone age, epiphyseal dysgenesis, and delayed dental development. A major complication of unrecognized and untreated hypothyroidism in a child is mental retardation. This development can be prevented by early correction of hypothyroidism. It is, therefore, mandatory that the medical personnel attending newborn and small infants be aware of this condition.

Laboratory tests used to confirm the presence of hypothyroidism include low serum thyroxine and triiodothyronine levels, low BMR, and elevated serum cholesterol. Serum TSH levels may be high or low, depending on the type of hypothyroidism. In primary hypothyroidism, serum TSH levels are high, together with low thyroxine and T_3 resin uptake. In contrast, all three measurements are low in patients with secondary hypothyroidism.

Treatment of hypothyroidism includes the administration of thyroxine, which is usually instituted at low dose levels of 50 μg per day and gradually increased over days to weeks to a full maintenance dose of 200 μg per day. The measurement of serum thyroxine levels and T_3 resin uptake as well as TSH levels in patients with primary hypothyroidism may be used to determine the adequacy of the replacement therapy.

Nontoxic goiters

Nontoxic diffuse colloid goiters and colloid nodular goiters are very common disorders which affect 16 percent of women and 4 percent of men age 20 to 60, as demonstrated in a survey of Tecumseh, a community in Michigan. Usually there are no symptoms other than the cosmetic appearance, but occasional complications may occur. The thyroid may be diffusely enlarged and/or contain nodules.

The etiology of nontoxic goiter includes iodine deficiency or an intrathyroidal chemical defect caused by a variety of factors. As a result of this defect, the thyroid gland has an impaired capacity to secrete thyroxine, leading to an increase in TSH levels and hyperplasia and hypertrophy of the thyroid follicles. The enlargement of the thyroid gland in patients with nontoxic goiter frequently follows a course of exacerbations and remissions with hyperevolution and involution of areas of the thyroid gland. Fibrosis may alternate with hyperplasia, and nodules containing thyroid follicles may develop.

Clinically, patients may demonstrate a protruberance in the lower third of the neck. With large goiters, mechanical compression problems may develop, including displacement of the trachea and esophagus and symptoms of obstruction.

If the impairment of thyroid function is severe, the goiter may be accompanied by hypothyroidism. In order to ascertain the functional status of the goiter, measurements of serum T_4 and T_3 resin uptake may be neces-

sary. In addition, radioactive iodine scintiscan with technetium pertechnate shows whether the nodules are "cold" or "hot." Cold nodules may represent carcinoma, while hot nodules are nearly always benign. Ultrasound scanning of the thyroid gland may be used to detect cystic changes in thyroid nodules. Cystic nodules are almost never cancerous.

Therapy of goiter involves suppression of TSH by thyroid hormone. Prolonged treatment with thyroxine results in suppression of pituitary TSH and inhibition of thyroid function with atrophy of the thyroid gland. Surgery may be indicated for large goiters, in order to remove the mechanical and cosmetic problems they cause. In communities where goiters develop as a consequence of iodide deficiency, the addition of iodide to table salt should be instituted.

Thyroid neoplasms

Thyroid neoplasms frequently present as discrete enlargements of the thyroid gland. At times, they may resemble a benign nodular goiter. Thyroid nodules are clinically palpable in approximately 5 to 10 percent of adults in the United States. The majority of these nodules are benign, but some nodular goiters are carcinomatous. To determine whether a thyroid nodule is benign or malignant, known risk factors and the clinical characteristics of the mass should be assessed and certain laboratory studies should be made.

Risk factors

The risk of a carcinoma in a thyroid nodule is high, approximately 50 percent, in a child under 14 years of age. In contrast, the risk is less than 10 percent in adults. Men have a higher incidence of carcinomatous thyroid nodules than women. The recent appearance of a nodule or rapid enlargement of a preexisting nodule should raise a suspicion that the nodule is malignant. A previous exposure to therapeutic radiation to the head and neck regions may also increase the risk to patients of developing thyroid carcinoma in the future. The incidence of radiation exposure during childhood in patients under age 15 years with thyroid carcinomas has been reported to be as high as 50 percent; for patients under 30 years of age, 20 percent. Certain types of thyroid cancer such as medullary thyroid carcinoma may occur with familial incidence. The discovery of a goiter in a patient with a positive family history for this type of carcinoma is, therefore, significant for the diagnosis of a thyroid malignancy.

Clinical characteristics

A thyroid carcinoma should be suspected on clinical grounds if the nodule is single, hard on palpation, fixed to overlying tissue, and associated with satellite lymphadenopathy.

Laboratory studies

Thyroid carcinomas usually take up less radioactive iodine than the surrounding normal thyroid gland. When a thyroid scintiscan is performed, the nodule therefore appears as an area of decreased uptake, a cold lesion. Another diagnostic technique that can be used in the differential diagnosis of a thyroid nodule is thyroid echography. This test is based on an analysis of echoes produced by an ultrasonic beam directed into the thyroid nodule. This technique permits accurate differentiation between cystic and solid masses. Thyroid carcinomas are generally solid, while cystic masses usually represent benign cysts.

It is generally agreed that thyroid cancer can be subdivided clinically into a large group of well-differentiated neoplasms of slow growth and high curability and a smaller group of highly anaplastic tumors with a uniformly fatal outlook. There are four main types of thyroid cancer according to morphology and biological behavior: (1) papillary, (2) follicular, (3) medullary, and (4) anaplastic.

Papillary carcinoma is the most common type of thyroid cancer and accounts for 80 percent of malignant thyroid tumors in children and in adults less than 40 years of age. It is approximately twice as common in females as in males. These neoplasms grow slowly and spread via lymphatics to regional nodes in approximately 50 percent of the cases. Treatment is surgical excision of the local lesion together with removal of regional lymph nodes if they are suspected of being involved.

Follicular carcinoma composes approximately 20 percent of all thyroid cancers. The sex and age distributions are similar to those of the papillary cancer, although the incidence is somewhat higher later in life. In its most indolent form, the tumor closely resembles normal thyroid, although at times it may be rapidly progressive, spreading rapidly to distant sites. These tumors not only resemble thyroid follicles histologically, but also are capable of taking up radioactive iodine. The mode of metastasis is via the bloodstream to distant sites such as lung and bone. Like papillary tumors, the growth of this type of cancer is slow, the disease evolving over many years. The treatment is also local surgical excision of the lesion, and if the metastases are capable of taking up radioactive iodine, ablation of the metastases with large doses of radioactive iodine can be carried out.

Medullary thyroid carcinoma is rather uncommon, composing 5 to 10 percent of all cases. The cell of origin of this neoplasm is the parafollicular, or C, cell. Like its precursor cell, the tumor is capable of secreting calcitonin. Medullary thyroid carcinoma has been described in members of families with multiple endocrine neoplasia. Its progression and clinical course can frequently be followed by measurements of serum calcitonin levels. Although the tumor apparently grows slowly, it tends to metastasize to local lymph nodes at an early stage. Later, it spreads by the bloodstream to lungs, liver, bone, and other organs. Because of the tendency to early metastases, these types of cancer are treated with total thyroidectomy.

Anaplastic carcinomas of the thyroid are histologically undifferentiated and extremely malignant, often progressing to death in weeks or months. They show evidence of early local invasion of structures surrounding the thyroid and of metastases, via both the lymphatics and bloodstream. At the present time, the outcome of this type of carcinoma is uniformly fatal regardless of the mode of treatment. Surgical resection should be attempted, followed by radiation therapy and chemotherapy.

Patients who have had resection of either papillary or follicular thyroid carcinomas should be followed for many years for evidence of recurrence or metastases. Following thyroidectomy for papillary or follicular carcinoma, patients are placed on suppressive doses of levothyroxine. Periodically, patients are taken off thyroid replacement and stimulated with TSH. A large dose of radioactive iodine is administered, and the neck as well as the rest of the body is scanned for areas of radioactive uptake. If metastases are detected in this manner, large ablative doses of radioactive iodine can be administered.

QUESTIONS

Diseases of the thyroid gland

Directions: Circle the letter preceding each item below that correctly answers the question. More than one answer may be correct.

1. Which of the following are characteristics of T_3 as compared with T_4?

a. Has a greater affinity for binding proteins, which results in a more potent effect on body tissues in regulating general metabolic rate
b. Configuration consists of two molecules of diiodotyrosine   c. Both a and b   d. Neither a nor b

2. Which of the following levels of TSH indicate primary hypothyroidism (hypothyroidism of thyroidal origin)?
   a. Above-normal serum TSH levels   b. Normal TSH levels   c. Undetectable TSH levels

3. Parafollicular, or C, cells within the thyroid gland secrete:
   a. Tyroxine   b. Triiodothyronine   c. Calcitonin   d. Renin

4. Which of the following are characteristic signs and symptoms of Graves' disease?
   a. Weight gain   b. Diffuse hyperplasia of the thyroid gland   c. Muscle fatigue   d. Bradycradia

5. Mr. B., 40 years of age, was found to have Graves' disease. Which of the following treatment programs may be prescribed?
   a. Long-term administration of propylthiouracil   b. Subtotal thyroidectomy following short-term administration of antithyroid drugs and ^{131}I treatment   c. Total thyroidectomy   d. Administration of 50 mg per day of thyroxine

6. A nurse in the newborn nursery observes a newborn baby boy who is very lethargic and has an umbilical hernia and dry skin. His respirations are noisy, and he has an abnormally hoarse cry. These signs suggest:
   a. Hyperthyroidism   b. Cretinism   c. Colloid goiter   d. Euthyroidism

7. Which of the following signs and symptoms is characteristic of hypothyroidism?
   a. Weight loss   b. Mental, physical slowness   c. Cold intolerance   d. Moist skin

8. Which of the following is characteristic of nontoxic goiters?
   a. Increase in TSH levels   b. Hyperplasia and hypertrophy of the thyroid follicles   c. IgG autoantibodies always present in the serum

9. Which of the following is not characteristic of a malignant thyroid nodule?
   a. It usually presents as a hot nodule   b. It usually appears as a single, firm, fixed nodule   c. It is functioning   d. Prognosis following early detection and treatment is excellent

10. The most likely mechanism by which goitrogens inhibit thyroxine synthesis is to:
    a. Decrease thyroxine levels   b. Increase release of TSH by the pituitary gland   c. Convert monoiodotyrosine to diiodotyrosine   d. Inhibit the initial oxidation of iodide

Directions: Circle T if the statement is true and F if it is false. Correct the false statements.

11. T   F   The T_3 resin test measures the saturation of thyroxine-binding protein and indirectly the level of thyroid hormone.

12. T   F   The most common form of hypothyroidism is caused by a lesion in the pituitary gland.

13. T   F   Hypothyroidism of all forms is best treated with thyroxine.

14. T   F   The process referred to as deiodination converts 80 percent of T_4 into $3,5,3'$-T_3, while the remaining 20 percent is converted to RT_3.

15. T   F   Thyroid function is controlled by the hypothalamic glycoprotein hormone TSH and is regulated by thyrotropin-releasing hormone (TRH), a pituitary neurohormone.

16. T   F   Iodine is an essential element for the production of thyroxine.

Directions: Answer the following questions on a separate sheet of paper.

17. Describe the location and function of the follicular epithelial cells in the thyroid gland.

18. List the steps and describe the process of biosynthesis of thyroid hormones.

Directions: Fill in the blanks with the appropriate word.

19. Normal levels of thyroxine are _____ μg/100 ml; for triiodothyronine, _____ ng/100 ml.

20. Two types of spontaneous hyperthyroidism are _____ and _____ .

CHAPTER 56

DISORDERS OF CALCIUM METABOLISM

GENERAL CONCEPTS

Calcium plays an important role in biological processes. It is an important constituent of biological membranes, affecting their permeability and electrical properties. For example, a lowering of the concentration of calcium outside the cell causes an increase in permeability and excitability of the cell membrane. Calcium also has an effect on neuromuscular activity. A decrease in calcium concentration increases the excitability of nerve tissue and can stimulate muscle contraction. In fact, calcium acts as a coupling factor between muscle excitation and contraction of actomyosin. Calcium is involved in the release of preformed hormones by endocrine cells and in the secretion of transmitter substances at synaptic junctions. It also participates in the mechanism of action of hormones within the cells. For example, it may be an important component in the action of cyclic adenosine monophosphate (AMP), the secondary intracellular messenger. Calcium is important in the property of ad-hesiveness that binds cells together, in enzyme activity, and in blood coagulation.

The maintenance of normal serum calcium levels depends on the balance between calcium input and output from the bloodstream. The main sources of calcium are the diet and the skeleton, with its large pool of calcium salts. The average adult intake of calcium in the North American diet is 600 to 1000 mg per day. This calcium is absorbed widely from the gastrointestinal tract. Calcium output is through the kidney and bone; 98 percent of the filtered calcium load is reabsorbed by the renal tubule by a process similar to that which regulates sodium excretion. Gastrointestinal losses, deposition of calcium into the bone mineral, and urinary clearance of calcium are the major mechanisms of calcium loss (see Fig. 56-1).

Several factors regulate or alter the movement of calcium in the bloodstream. Parathyroid hormone, calcitonin, and vitamin D are the three major factors concerned with this regulation.

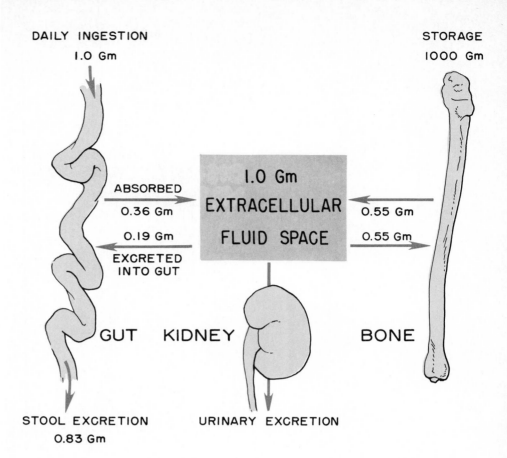

DAILY INGESTION
1.0 Gm

STORAGE
1000 Gm

ABSORBED
0.36 Gm

1.0 Gm
EXTRACELLULAR
FLUID SPACE

0.55 Gm

0.19 Gm

0.55 Gm

EXCRETED
INTO GUT

GUT   KIDNEY

BONE

STOOL EXCRETION
0.83 Gm

URINARY EXCRETION

FIGURE 56-1
**Outline of calcium intake,
absorption, excretion, and
storage in human beings.**

Parathyroid hormone or parathormone (PTH) is a polypeptide secreted by the parathyroid glands, which are located in the neck behind the lobes of the thyroid gland. There are four parathyroid glands, two right and two left, two superior and two inferior. Release of PTH varies with the concentration of calcium perfusing the parathyroid glands. For example, PTH release occurs in response to hypocalcemia, while secretion is suppressed by hypercalcemia. PTH acts on the gastrointestinal tract, bone, and kidney. It stimulates calcium absorption through the intestinal mucosa, it stimulates bone reabsorption by enhancing osteoclastic activity, and it increases the renal clearance of phosphorus by diminishing its tubular reabsorption (see Fig. 56-2). Excessive PTH secretion results in hypercalcemia and hypophosphatemia, while deficiency of PTH secretion leads to hypocalcemia and hyperphosphatemia.

Calcitonin is a hormone produced by the C cells, or parafollicular cells, of the thyroid gland. Calcitonin is released in response to hypercalcemia. It lowers serum calcium levels by inhibiting bone reabsorption. The actual physiological role of calcitonin in the minute-to-minute regulation of calcium levels has not yet been clarified.

Vitamin D works in concert with parathyroid hormone in the regulation of calcium levels. Vitamin D_3, or cholecalciferol, is either ingested with the diet or synthesized through activation of 7-dehydrocholesterol in the skin by ultraviolet radiation from sunlight. Vitamin

D_3 is absorbed in the jejunum and ileum and subsequently metabolized into an active form, first in the liver and ultimately in the kidney. The metabolism of vitamin D_3 involves sequential hydroxylations. In the liver it is converted to 25-hydroxycholecalciferol, and in the kidney to 1,25-dihydroxycholecalciferol (see Fig. 56-3). Vitamin D_3 in its active form acts on the intestine and the bone. In the intestine it promotes absorption of calcium, while in the bone it stimulates bone reabsorption. Vitamin D_3 is an essential cofactor for PTH in both bone and kidney. In its absence, hypocalcemia and disturbances in bone mineralization may occur.

The total serum calcium concentration reflects the concentration of calcium present in several physical chemical states. As indicated in Table 56-1, slightly less than 50 percent of the circulating calcium is present in a form bound to protein. The rest is non-protein-bound, of which the major portion is ionized and freely diffusible. It is this fraction which exerts biological effects and best correlates with the physiological actions of calcium in body fluids and systems perfused by them. The normal total serum calcium level is 9 to 10.5 mg/100 ml.

HYPERCALCEMIA

Hypercalcemia is defined as a calcium level above 10.5 mg/100 ml. Many conditions may lead to hypercalcemia, but PTH excess is by far the most common

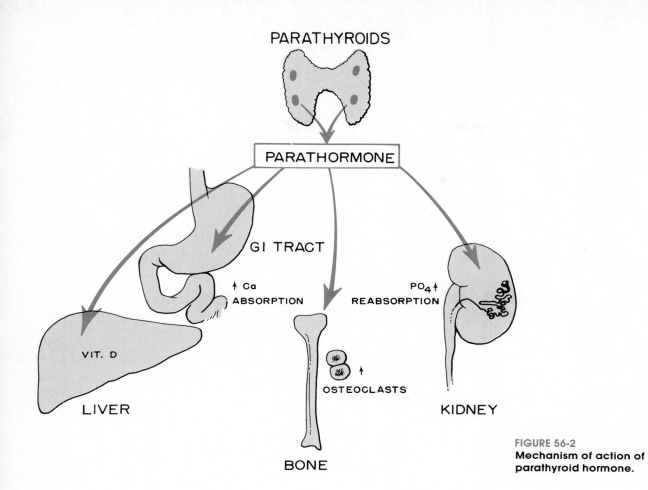

PARATHYROIDS

PARATHORMONE

GI TRACT

↑ Ca ABSORPTION

PO₄↑ REABSORPTION

VIT. D

LIVER

OSTEOCLASTS

BONE

KIDNEY

FIGURE 56-2
Mechanism of action of parathyroid hormone.

FIGURE 56-3
In vivo metabolism of cholecalciferol (vitamin D₃).

CHOLECALCIFEROL (VITAMIN D₃)

25-HYDROXY-CHOLECALCIFEROL

24,25-DIHYDROXYCHOLECALCIFEROL

1,25-DIHYDROXYCHOLECALCIFEROL

LIVER

KIDNEY

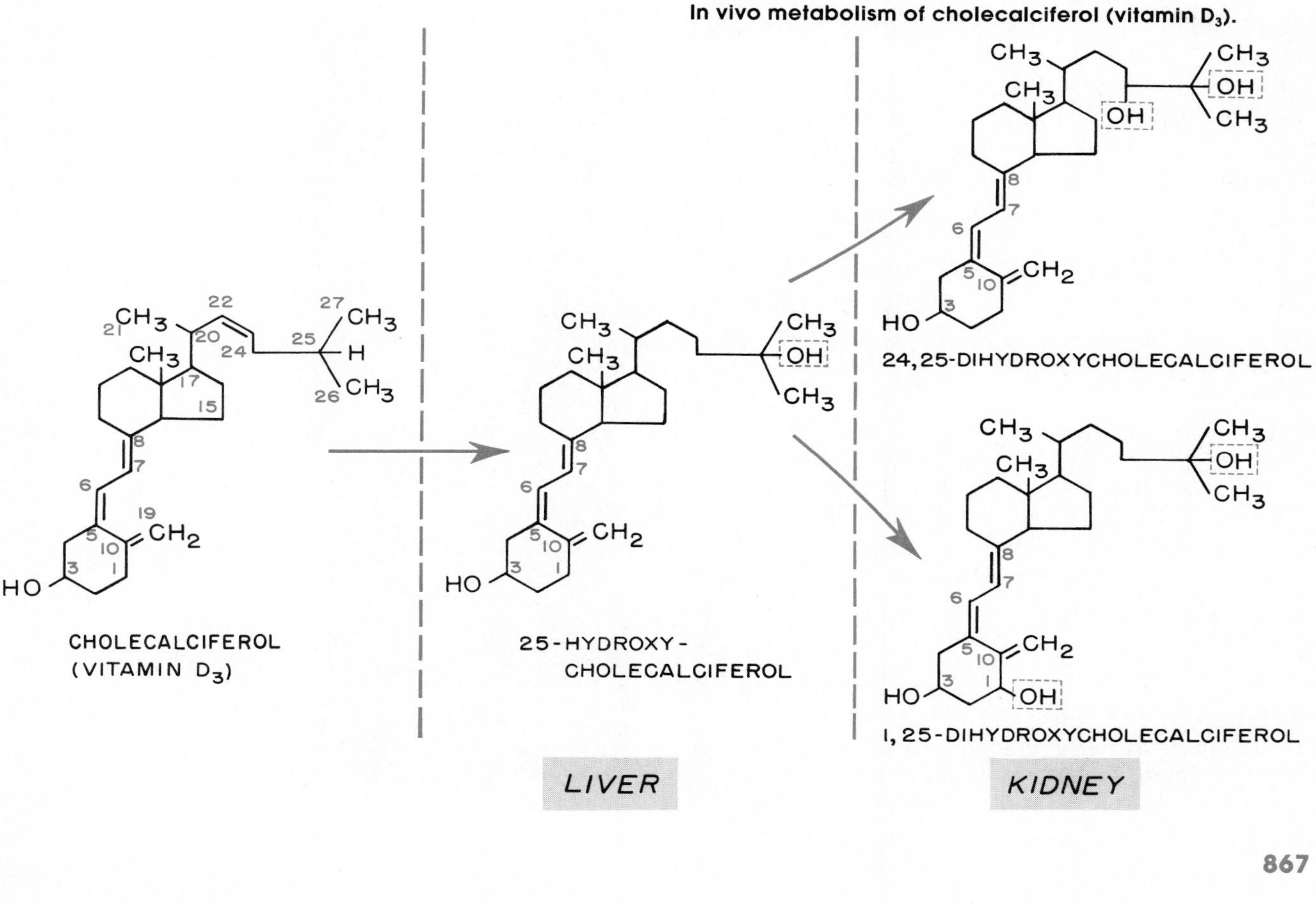

TABLE 56·1

STATE OF CALCIUM IN BLOOD

	Amount, mg/100 ml
Total serum Ca	9.5
Bound to protein	4.0
Not bound to protein	5.5
Ionized	4.5
Complexed (citrate, bicarbonate, phosphate)	1.0

cause. Excessive production of PTH may occur as the result of primary hyperparathyroidism or secretion of a PTH-like peptide by nonparathyroid malignancies. In addition, hypercalcemia may be found in association with tertiary hyperparathyroidism observed in chronic uremia and after dialysis or renal transplantation. Usually, hyperparathyroidism is caused by a benign adenoma of the parathyroid glands. The excessive secretion of PTH by these adenomas is responsible for hypercalcemia, hypophosphatemia, and increased bone reabsorption. Occasionally, hyperparathyroidism may result from hyperplasia of all four parathyroid glands. In this case, all four parathyroids are the source of excessive PTH secretion. Several types of nonparathyroid neoplasms have been found to be associated with hypercalcemia. PTH-like peptides have been identified in some patients with these neoplasms. It is postulated that the neoplasm has acquired the capacity to synthesize and release peptide hormones. Bronchial carcinomas, squamous cell carcinomas, hypernephromas, and carcinoma of the liver are among those neoplasms associated with hypercalcemia.

There are many other types of conditions in which hypercalcemia develops independently of PTH. In fact, PTH is suppressed by the high calcium level. Included among these conditions are vitamin D intoxication, sarcoidosis, acute immobilization, hyperthyroidism, multiple myeloma, and metastatic malignancy with skeletal involvement.

Symptoms and signs of hypercalcemia vary greatly depending on the rapidity of onset and the degree of elevation of serum calcium levels. In mild cases, one may find patients who are completely asymptomatic and whose hypercalcemia is discovered only through routine laboratory investigation. On the other hand, there are severe cases where patients deteriorate rapidly and become dehydrated, confused, and lethargic. Their serum calcium levels are markedly elevated.

Symptoms of hypercalcemia are gastrointestinal, including anorexia, nausea, vomiting, weight loss, and constipation; urinary, including polydipsia, polyuria, and nephrocalcinosis; cardiovascular, including hypertension and electrocardiographic changes; and neuropsychiatric, including lethargy, apathy, myopathy, and electromyographic abnormalities. Patients whose hypercalcemia is secondary to hyperparathyroidism have, in addition to the changes described, skeletal changes caused by the effect of parathyroid hormone on bone. Usually there is increased bone reabsorption, formation of bone cysts, and erosion in the subperiosteal edges of the long bones (see Fig. 56-4). In its fully developed stage, the skeletal manifestations constitute osteitis fibrosa cystica.

The diagnosis of hyperparathyroidism is based on the demonstration of high serum calcium and low serum phosphate levels together with elevated serum PTH levels. When the hypercalcemia is caused by one of the PTH-independent conditions, the hypercalcemia may not be associated with hypophosphatemia, and the serum parathyroid hormone level is usually suppressed.

Treatment

If the condition is caused by hyperparathyroidism, treatment involves the excision of the parathyroid tumor or

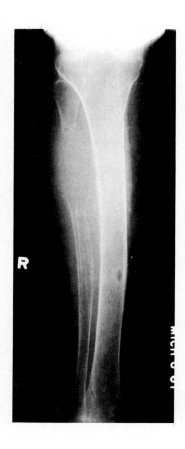

FIGURE 56-4
Lesions of osteitis fibrosa cystica in the tibia and fibula of a patient with hyperparathyroidism.

subtotal removal of all four parathyroid glands. In the PTH-independent types of hypercalcemia, correction depends on the treatment of the underlying disease. Since the underlying disease may be a malignancy which does not respond to therapy, it may be necessary to lower the serum calcium level by other means. These generally include effective hydration and the use of agents that enhance renal calcium excretion or drugs such as calcitonin and mithramycin which inhibit bone reabsorption and therefore decrease the flux of calcium from bone to the extracellular fluid space. Phosphate salts are frequently used for correction of hypercalcemia because phosphate binds calcium and precipitates it out of the bloodstream. A side effect of this treatment may be precipitation of calcium phosphate in the renal parenchyma. Thus, it should not be administered to patients with impaired renal function.

HYPOCALCEMIA

Hypocalcemia is the clinical condition caused by serum calcium levels of less than 9.0 mg/100 ml. It may result from the surgical removal of all four parathyroid glands or may develop as the result of autoimmune destruction of these glands. The parathyroid glands may be removed accidentally in the course of a thyroidectomy. The condition associated with autoimmune destruction of the glands is known as *idiopathic hypoparathyroidism.*

The clinical manifestations of hypocalcemia are tetany, seizures, mental disturbances, and ectodermal lesions. Tetany is characterized by involuntary muscle spasms. It may involve muscles of the upper and lower extremities, causing carpopedal spasms, paresthesias, and occasionally laryngeal stridor. When respiratory muscles are involved, respiratory distress may be a manifestation of hypocalcemia. Usually, the increased neuromuscular excitability can be demonstrated by tapping over the facial nerve anterior to the ear. A unilateral contraction of the facial muscle occurs (Chvostek's sign). It can also be demonstrated by the Trousseau test, which is induction of a carpal spasm by placing a blood pressure cuff on the arm and inflating it above systolic pressure. Occasionally, epileptiform seizures can occur in patients who have an underlying seizure disorder and who subsequently develop hypocalcemia. Patients with hypocalcemia usually complain of a variety of emotional disturbances, including irritability, emotional instability, impairment of memory, and confusion. Prolonged hypocalcemia, as seen in idiopathic hypoparathyroidism, may cause changes in the skin, hair, and nails as well as in the teeth and lenses. The skin may be coarse, dry, and scaly, and alopecia may develop with patchy or absent eyelashes and eyebrows. The nails become thin and brittle with transverse grooves. The teeth may erupt late and appear hypoplastic. Cataracts may develop within a few years of untreated hypocalcemia.

Treatment

Treatment of hypocalcemia is based on the administration of calcium salts and vitamin D or its synthetic metabolites in order to enhance intestinal absorption of calcium. Calcium salts are available as calcium gluconate, calcium lactate, or calcium carbonate. Giving 10 to 15 g calcium gluconate or lactate daily is usually necessary. Vitamin D is given in doses of 50,000 to 150,000 units per day. When patients are treated with the proper combination of calcium and vitamin D, serum calcium levels can be maintained within the normal range.

QUESTIONS

Disorders of calcium metabolism

Directions: Circle the letter preceding each item below that correctly answers the question. More than one answer may be correct.

1. Bodily processes affected by the concentration of calcium ion include:
   a. Contractility of cardiac and skeletal muscle *b.* Permeability of the cell membrane to sodium and potassium *c.* Release of neurotransmitters at synaptic junctions *d.* Excitability of nerve tissue

2. In primary hyperparathyroidism:
   a. Serum levels of PTH are always greater than in persons with hypercalcemia due to vitamin D_3 intoxication *b.* An adenoma of one or more of the parathyroids is often the cause of the hypersecretion *c.* There may be a generalized loss of bone density on x-ray examination

3. PTH-independent causes of hypercalcemia include:
   a. Vitamin D intoxication *b.* Malignant neoplasm with osseous metastasis *c.* Multiple myeloma *d.* Chronic renal failure *e.* Prolonged immobilization

4. Hypocalcemia may be treated by the administration of:

a. Calcitonin   b. Vitamin D   c. Mithramycin
d. Calcium gluconate

5. The most common cause of hypoparathyroidism is:
a. Autoimmune destruction of the parathyroid
glands   b. Damage to the parathyroid glands during thyroid surgery or following removal of the
parathyroid glands for hyperparathyroidism

6. Deficiency of parathyroid hormone results in:
a. Increased renal tubular reabsorption of
phosphate   b. Hypoplasia of developing teeth
c. Decreased density of bones   d. Increased neuromuscular irritability

7. Which hormone increases reabsorption of calcium
from bone?
a. Insulin   b. Thyroxine   c. Parathyroid
d. Calcitonin

*Direction: Complete the following questions by
filling in the blanks with the appropriate responses.*

8. The normal total serum calcium level is_____
to_____ mg/100 ml.

9. The two most important factors affecting calcium
homeostasis are _____ and
_____.

10. The   major   mechanisms   of   calcium   loss
are _____, _____,
and _____.

THE ADRENAL CORTEX— DISORDERS OF HYPERSECRETION

OBJECTIVES

At the completion of this chapter you should be able to:

1. Describe the effects of glucocorticoid excess on the distribution of adipose tissue and on carbohydrate and protein metabolism.

2. Describe the effect of high or low plasma cortisol levels on the feedback control mechanism.

3. Differentiate between a glucocorticoid and a mineralocorticoid.

4. Explain the rationale for altering the basic chemical structure of cortisol in the manufacturing of synthetic steroid analogues.

5. Identify one consequence of glucocorticoid therapy involving large amounts for a long period of time.

6. Describe Cushing's syndrome (include at least three causes, the clinical signs and symptoms, diagnostic tests, and treatment).

7. Differentiate between primary and secondary aldosteronism as to etiology and pathophysiology.

This chapter will focus on two selected clinical entities—Cushing's syndrome and aldosteronism. The first discussion will concentrate on situations in which the plasma concentration of cortisol increases above normal physiological levels and results in Cushing's syndrome. Causes of spontaneously abnormal elevations of plasma cortisol will be considered. The second discussion will focus on another hormone of the adrenal cortex, aldosterone, and the condition known as *aldosteronism*. The chapter will include some aspects of the pharmacology of synthetic corticosteroids and the metabolic side effects which result from their chronic administration.

The adrenal cortex synthesizes and secretes four types of adrenocortical hormones: (1) glucocorticoids, (2) mineralocorticoids, (3) androgens, and (4) estrogens. The physiological glucocorticoid secreted by the human adrenal is cortisol; the physiological mineralocorticoid is aldosterone. There are other compounds, either naturally occurring or synthetic, which may have glucocorticoid or mineralocorticoid activity.

Cushing's syndrome is a clinical condition resulting from the combined metabolic effects of persistently elevated blood levels of glucocorticoids. In order to better understand the clinical manifestations of Cushing's syn-

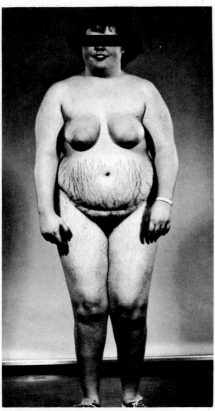

FIGURE 57-1
Abdominal striae in a patient with Cushing's syndrome produced by chronic administration of large amounts of glucocorticoids.

drome, it is useful to begin with a review of the metabolic consequence of glucocorticoid excess.

METABOLIC EFFECTS OF GLUCOCORTICOIDS

Glucocorticoid excess causes alteration in (1) protein and carbohydrate metabolism, (2) distribution of adipose tissue, (3) electrolytes, (4) the immune system, (5) gastric secretion, (6) brain function, and (7) erythropoiesis. In addition, it suppresses inflammation.

Glucocorticoids have catabolic and antianabolic effects on protein, causing a decrease in the ability of protein-forming cells to synthesize protein. As a consequence, there is loss of protein from tissues such as skin, muscles, blood vessels, and bone. Clinically, the skin atrophies and breaks down easily; wounds heal slowly. Rupture of elastic fibers in the skin causes purple stretch marks, or striae (see Fig. 57-1). Muscles also atrophy and become weak. Thinning of blood vessel walls

and weakening of perivascular supporting tissue result in easy bruising (see Fig. 57-2). This condition can be severe enough for petechiae or even large areas of ecchymosis to appear under the cuff when the patient's blood pressure is taken. Bone is also affected. The protein matrix of bone becomes weak, causing a condition known as *osteoporosis*. This may be a serious complication of glucocorticoid excess, since it causes the bone to become brittle and develop pathological fractures. Osteoporosis occurs most frequently in the spine, causing vertebral collapse and resultant back pain and loss of height.

Carbohydrate metabolism is also affected by abnormally high levels of glucocorticoids. Glucocorticoids stimulate gluconeogenesis and interfere with the action of insulin in peripheral cells. As a consequence, patients may develop hyperglycemia. People without diabetes are able to compensate for the effect of glucocorticoids by increasing insulin secretion and subsequently normalizing glucose tolerance. In contrast, patients with diminishing insulin-secreting capacity are unable to compensate, and they develop abnormal glucose tolerance tests, fasting hyperglycemia, and clinical manifestations of diabetes.

Excessive glucocorticoid levels also affect the dis-

FIGURE 57-2
Marked protein catabolism in a patient with Cushing's syndrome. Muscles are markedly atrophic, and there are multiple ecchymoses in the upper and lower extremities.

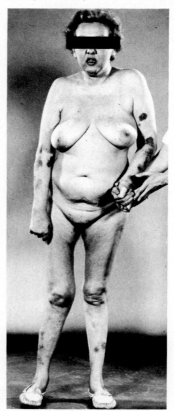

tribution of adipose tissue, which accumulates in the central areas of the body, causing development of truncal obesity, round face (moon facies), supraclavicular fossa fullness, and cervicodorsal hump (buffalo hump) (see Fig. 57-3). The truncal obesity and thinning of the upper and lower extremities as a result of muscle atrophy give patients the classic cushingoid appearance. This appearance is illustrated in Fig. 57-4.

Glucocorticoids have minimal effects on serum electrolytes. However, when given or produced in very large concentrations, they may cause sodium retention and potassium waste, leading to edema, hypokalemia, and metabolic alkalosis.

Glucocorticoids can inhibit the immune response. Immune responses are of two major types: one results in production of humoral antibodies by plasma cells and B lymphocytes following antigenic stimulation; the other depends on sensitized T-lymphocyte–mediated reactions. Glucocorticoids impair humoral antibody production and inhibit proliferation of germinal centers of spleen and lymphoid tissue in the primary response to antigen. Impairment of the immunological response can occur at each of the stages of this response: (1) initial processing of antigens by cells of the monocyte-macrophage system, (2) induction and proliferation of immunocompetent lymphocytes, (3) antibody production, and (4) the inflammatory reaction. Glucocorticoids also suppress delayed hypersensitivity reactions. For example, they may convert the skin test for tuberculosis from positive to negative. In addition, the glucocorticoid-mediated inhibition of cellular immunity is probably important in suppressing transplant rejection.

Gastric secretory activity is increased by glucocor-

FIGURE 57-3
Typical cushingoid facies with roundness of the face, double chin, prominent upper lip, and fullness of the supraclavicular fossae.

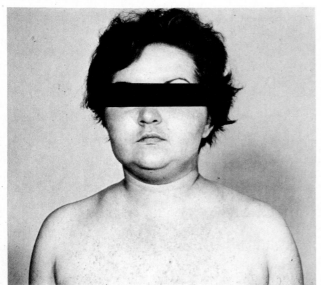

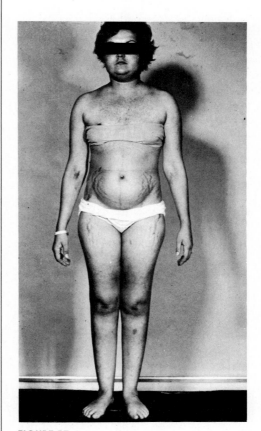

FIGURE 57-4
Patient with Cushing's syndrome with acne over the chest, striae over the abdomen and upper thighs, and relatively thin upper and lower extremities. She also has pretibial edema.

ticoids. Hydrochloric acid and pepsin secretion may be increased in certain individuals taking glucocorticoids. It has also been suggested that mucosal protective factors are altered by steroids and that this may contribute to ulcer formation.

Psychic changes are frequently seen with glucocorticoid excess. They are characterized by emotional lability, euphoria, insomnia, and episodes of transient depression. The neuropsychiatric manifestations of glucocorticoid excess occur in patients with spontaneous Cushing's syndrome and in those receiving pharmacological doses of glucocorticoids. These changes are reversed upon normalization of cortisol levels.

Glucocorticoids cause involution of lymphoid tissue, stimulation of neutrophil release, and enhancement of erythropoiesis.

The most important and clinically useful pharmacological effect of glucocorticoids is their ability to suppress the inflammatory response. In this regard, glucocorticoids can inhibit hyperemia, extravasation of cells, cellular migration, and cellular permeability. They also inhibit the release of vasoactive kinins and suppress phagocytosis. By their effects on mast cells, glucocorticoids inhibit histamine synthesis and suppress the acute anaphylactic reaction based on antibody-mediated hypersensitivity. The anti-inflammatory properties of glucocorticoids have placed them in the foreground of therapeutic agents available for the treatment of a variety of disorders in which suppression of inflammation is desirable. There are clinical conditions in which the immune suppression and anti-inflammatory effect of glucocorticoids may be a disadvantage to the patient. With acute infection, the host may be unable to defend him or herself appropriately while receiving pharmacological doses of glucocorticoids.

Suppression of the hypothalamic-pituitary-adrenal axis

It is well known that the administration of glucocorticoids in doses which surpass the physiological concentrations can significantly suppress the ability of the hypothalamic-pituitary axis to release adrenocorticotropic hormone (ACTH). This is important, since the administration of corticoids on a long-term basis may result in adrenal insufficiency (1) when steroids are withdrawn and (2) in response to stress.

CUSHING'S SYNDROME

Cushing's syndrome may result from long-term administration of pharmacological doses of glucocorticoids (iatrogenic) or from excessive cortisol secretion caused by a disturbance in the hypothalamic-pituitary-adrenal axis (spontaneous).

Iatrogenic Cushing's syndrome is seen in patients with conditions such as rheumatoid arthritis, asthma, lymphoma, and generalized skin disorders who receive synthetic glucocorticoids as anti-inflammatory agents. In spontaneous Cushing's syndrome, adrenocortical hyperfunction develops either as a result of excessive stimulation by ACTH or as a consequence of adrenal pathology leading to abnormal production of cortisol.

Cushing's syndrome can be divided into two types: (1) ACTH-dependent and (2) ACTH-independent (see Fig. 57-5). Among the ACTH-dependent types, adrenocortical hyperfunction may result from abnormal and excessive secretion of ACTH by the pituitary gland. Since this is the type originally described by Harvey Cushing in 1932, it is also designated as Cushing's disease. In 80 percent of these cases there is either a disturbance in corticotropin-releasing hormone (CRH)–ACTH release or an ACTH-secreting pituitary adenoma. In the remaining 20 percent there is histological evidence of pituitary corticotrope hyperplasia. It is not clear if either the microadenomas or the hyperplasia arises from a disturbed release of CRH by the neurohypothalamus. In either case there is excessive secretion of ACTH, loss of normal circadian rhythm of ACTH release, and diminished sensitivity of the feedback control system to levels of circulating cortisol. ACTH may be secreted excessively in patients with ectopic hormone production. These are patients who have neoplasms which have acquired the capacity to synthesize and release peptides resembling ACTH both chemically and physiologically. The excessive amounts of ACTH produced under these circumstances lead to excessive stimulation of cortisol secretion by the adrenal cortex and, secondarily, to suppression of pituitary ACTH release. Thus, the high ACTH levels in such a patient come from the neoplasm and not from the patient's own pituitary gland. A large number of neoplasms can cause the ectopic secretion of ACTH. These

FIGURE 57-5
Classification of Cushing's syndrome.

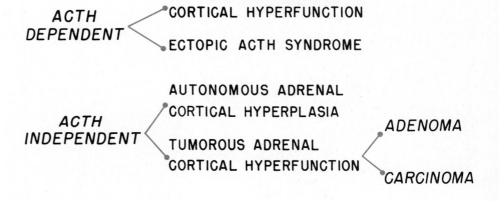

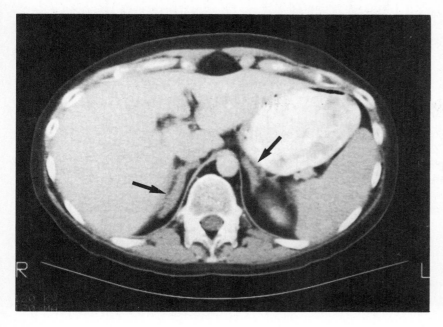

FIGURE 57-6
Computerized axial tomography (CAT) scan of the upper abdomen, demonstrating bilateral adrenal enlargement in a patient with ACTH-dependent Cushing's syndrome.

neoplasms are usually derived from tissues originating in the neuroectodermal layer during embryonic development. Oat-cell carcinoma of the lung bronchial carcinoids, thymomas, and islet-cell tumors of the pancreas are among the most common.

Adrenocortical hyperfunction can occur independently of ACTH control. This happens in conditions where a tumor develops in the adrenal cortex with a capacity to secrete cortisol in an autonomous fashion. Adrenocortical tumors leading to Cushing's syndrome may be benign (adenomas) (see Fig. 57-6) or malignant (carcinomas) (see Fig. 57-7).

The presence of Cushing's syndrome can be determined on the basis of the medical history and the phys-

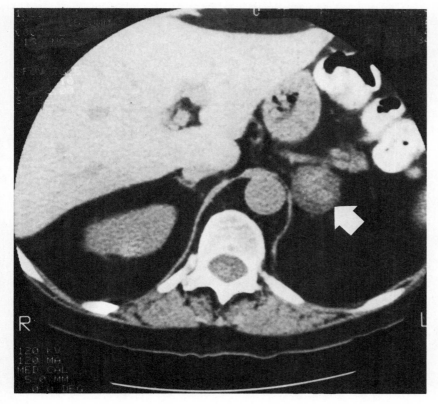

FIGURE 57-7
Computerized axial tomography (CAT) scan of the upper abdomen, demonstrating a left adrenal mass in a patient with Cushing's syndrome secondary to an adrenal cortical adenoma.

ical findings described above. The diagnosis is usually confirmed by the measurement of abnormally high levels of cortisol in plasma and urine. There are specific tests which can be performed to determine the presence or absence of a normal circadian rhythm of cortisol release and a sensitive feedback control mechanism. Absence of circadian rhythm and diminished or absent sensitivity of the feedback control system are characteristic of Cushing's syndrome.

The types of Cushing's syndrome associated with excessive ACTH secretion—pituitary or ectopic—are frequently associated with hyperpigmentation. This hyperpigmentation is caused by the secretion of peptides related to ACTH and by breakdown fragments of ACTH which have melanotropic activity. The pigmentation is recognized in both skin and mucous membranes.

Adrenocortical adenomas may lead to severe Cushing's syndrome, but they usually develop slowly, and symptoms may be present for several years before the diagnosis is finally made (see Fig. 57-6). In contrast, adrenocortical carcinomas develop rapidly and may lead to metastasis and early death (see Fig. 57-7).

Several diagnostic procedures can be used to establish the nature of the underlying pathology in Cushing's syndrome and to help localize a lesion amenable to surgical management.

Physiological testing can help distinguish pituitary from ectopic or primary adrenocortical forms of Cushing's syndrome. In the ectopic and adrenocortical forms of Cushing's syndrome, the abnormal secretion of ACTH and/or cortisol is not likely to be altered by stimulating or suppressive maneuvers which test the presence or absence of a normal negative feedback control mechanism. For example, the administration of metyrapone, a drug that blocks 11-β hydroxylation at the adrenocortical level and thus causes a decrease in plasma cortisol, is unable to stimulate ACTH release in patients with ectopic ACTH syndrome; in contrast, patients with pituitary ACTH-dependent Cushing's syndrome usually respond with an increase in ACTH release. Patients with either ectopic ACTH syndrome or primary adrenocortical disease do not suppress ACTH and/or cortisol levels with high doses of dexamethasone, a feature which is characteristic of most patients with pituitary ACTH-dependent Cushing's syndrome.

Identification of the nature and localization of the lesion responsible for causing Cushing's syndrome is based on the radiographic visualization of pituitary and adrenal lesions and on nuclear scanning of the adrenal glands.

High-resolution computerized axial tomography (CAT) scanning of the pituitary gland can demonstrate areas of decreased density or enhancement consistent with a microadenoma in about 30 percent of these patients. CAT scanning of the adrenal glands usually shows adrenal enlargement in patients with ACTH-dependent Cushing's syndrome and adrenal masses in patients with adrenal adenoma or carcinoma.

Nuclear scanning of the adrenal glands involves the intravenous administration of radioactive cholesterol. Cholesterol labeled with ^{131}I is taken up and concentrated by the adrenal cortex. Images of the adrenal glands can be obtained by scanning techniques within 3 to 7 days after injection of the tracer (see Fig. 57-8). Patterns suggestive of normal adrenal glands, adrenal hyperplasia, or adrenal adenoma or carcinoma can be obtained with adrenal photoscanning.

Treatment of Cushing's syndrome

Treatment of ACTH-dependent Cushing's syndrome differs depending on whether the source of ACTH is pituitary or ectopic. Several approaches to therapy can be used in patients with pituitary hypersecretion of ACTH. If a pituitary tumor is recognized, a transsphenoidal resection of the tumor should be attempted. If there is evidence of pituitary hyperfunction but a tumor is not clearly detected, cobalt irradiation of the pituitary gland can be used instead. This is a treatment modality which is effective, particularly in young people with Cushing's syndrome. Alternatively, cortisol excess can be controlled by a total adrenalectomy and subsequent administration of physiological doses of cortisol or by chemical agents capable of blocking or destroying cortisol-secreting adrenal cortical cells. When the treatment of Cushing's syndrome is successful, remission of the clinical manifestations takes place within 6 to 12 months after institution of therapy (see Fig. 57-9).

When adrenal neoplasms are the cause of cortisol excess, removal of the neoplasms followed by chemotherapy in patients with carcinoma is the preferred mode of treatment.

Treatment of ectopic ACTH syndrome is based on (1) resection of the neoplasm secreting ACTH or (2) adrenalectomy or chemical suppression of adrenal function as prescribed for the patients with the pituitary ACTH-dependent type of Cushing's syndrome.

ALDOSTERONISM

Aldosteronism is a clinical condition resulting from excessive production of aldosterone, the mineralocorticoid steroid hormone of the adrenal cortex. The metabolic effects of aldosterone relate to electrolyte and fluid balance. Aldosterone enhances proximal renal tubule reabsorption of sodium and causes potassium and hydrogen ion excretion. The clinical consequences of aldosterone

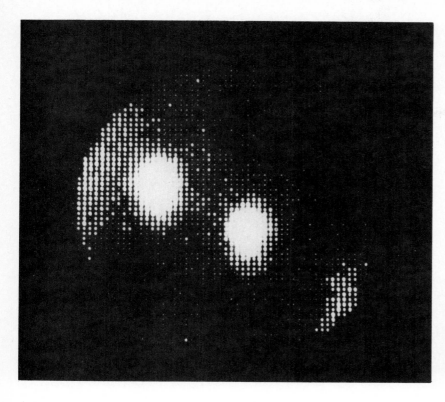

FIGURE 57-8
$^{131}I\ 6\beta$-iodomethyl-19-norcholosterol nuclear scan of the adrenal glands in a patient with ACTH-dependent Cushing's syndrome. There is bilateral increased uptake of radioactivity consistent with adrenal cortical hyperfunction.

excess are sodium and water retention, expansion of the extracellular fluid volume, and hypertension. In addition, there are hypernatremia, hypokalemia, and metabolic alkalosis.

There are two types of aldosteronism: (1) primary and (2) secondary. Aldosteronism is primary when the production of aldosterone occurs as a result of a tumor (see Fig. 57-10), or hyperplasia of the adrenal cortex. The majority of the aldosterone-secreting tumors are benign and of small size—0.5 to 2 cm. Primary aldosteronism represents a form of endocrine hypertension and probably affects 1 to 2 percent of patients with hypertension. Recognition of this condition may lead to the cure of hypertension.

Secondary aldosteronism is present in conditions where there is a decrease in afferent arteriolar pressure in the renal glomerulus, leading to stimulation of the renin-angiotensin system. Angiotensin stimulates aldosterone production. Secondary aldosteronism is seen in congestive heart failure, cirrhosis of the liver, and ne-

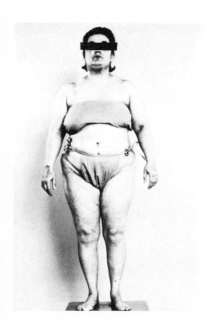
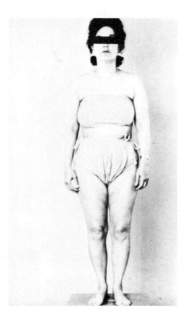

FIGURE 57-9
Response to treatment of Cushing's syndrome with mitotane, an adrenal inhibitor.

877

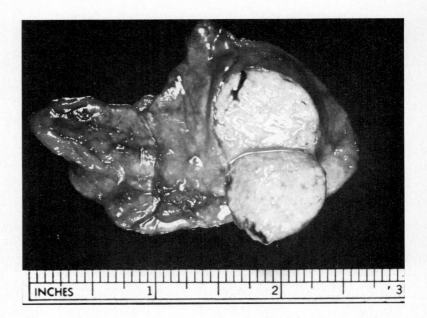

FIGURE 57-10
Aldosterone-secreting adrenocortical adenoma.

phrotic syndrome, conditions in which edema is a prominent clinical feature. Congestive heart failure provides a good example of the way secondary aldosteronism may develop. Patients in congestive heart failure cannot pump blood normally and develop a fall in cardiac output. Perfusion pressure to the afferent arteriole of the renal glomerulus decreases. The fall in pressure is sensed by stretch receptors in the juxtaglomerular apparatus, and renin is secreted in increased amounts. Renin activates angiotensin production, which in turn stimulates aldosterone secretion by an otherwise normal adrenal cortex. The increased production of aldosterone will, in turn, promote sodium and water reabsorption, expansion of the extracellular fluid compartment, and possibly an increase in afferent arteriolar pressure.

Secondary aldosteronism also develops in conditions where there is a partial occlusion of the renal artery, leading to renal vascular hypertension.

The diagnosis of aldosteronism is based on the measurement of increased levels of aldosterone in plasma and urine and measurements of plasma renin. Plasma renin is low in primary aldosteronism, while it is high in secondary aldosteronism.

CAT scanning and nuclear photoscanning can also help detect and localize an adrenal lesion in patients with primary aldosteronism. In addition, samples of adrenal venous blood may be obtained by selective catheterization of the right and left adrenal veins. A significantly higher concentration of aldosterone on the side suspected of harboring a tumor helps confirm the presence of the lesion.

Treatment of primary aldosteronism includes partial adrenalectomy, resection of an aldosterone-secreting adenoma, subtotal or total adrenalectomy in patients with adrenal hyperplasia, and the administration of aldosterone antagonists such as spironolactone.

PHARMACOLOGY AND USE OF SYNTHETIC CORTICOSTEROIDS

Synthetic analogues of cortisol with glucocorticoid and anti-inflammatory activity are frequently employed either topically or systemically in the treatment of many medical conditions. For example, steroids are used topically for the treatment of skin disorders. They are used systemically for treatment of conditions such as rheumatoid arthritis, asthma, and acute allergic reactions.

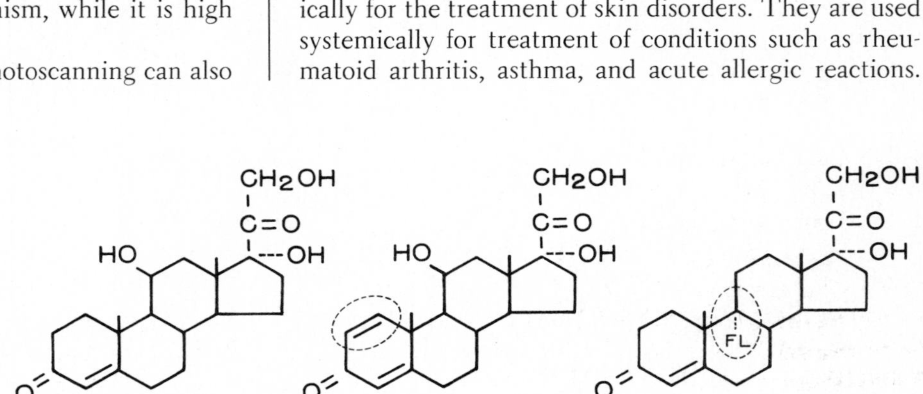

FIGURE 57-11
Changes in the basic chemical structure of cortisol, leading to compounds with different pharmacological characteristics than the parent compound. (A) Cortisol. (B) Prednisolone. (C) 9α-Fluorocortisol.

A B C

Although therapeutically effective, steroids also have side effects. These side effects are related to the metabolic activity and action on various organ systems as described above.

By alteration of the basic chemical structure of cortisol, the naturally occurring glucocorticoid, the pharmacological characteristics of this compound may be altered (see Fig. 57-11). For example, if a double bond is introduced between carbons 1 and 2 in the cortisol molecule, prednisolone is produced, which has, on a milligram-per-milligram basis, less sodium-retaining and more anti-inflammatory activity than the parent compound, cortisol. That is, 1 mg prednisolone is a much more potent anti-inflammatory and immunosuppressive agent than 1 mg cortisol. Another possible structural alteration is the introduction of a fluorine atom in an alpha position on carbon 9 of the steroid nucleus. The resulting compound, 9α-fluorocortisol, has strong sodium-retaining properties similar to aldosterone, a naturally occurring mineralocorticoid. By this substitution a compound with predominantly glucocorticoid activity becomes a mineralocorticoid.

Dozens of synthetic compounds have been created in the manner described above. In most cases, the objective has been the development of steroid compounds with strong anti-inflammatory activity and minimal undesirable metabolic side effects. Although this objective has been reached to some extent, therapy with any of the currently available synthetic corticosteroid preparations, if given long enough and in sufficiently high doses, results in Cushing's syndrome and persistent suppression of endogenous hypothalamic-pituitary-adrenal function. In many instances, steroids are the only effective medication available for treatment of serious systemic diseases. Under those circumstances the development of Cushing's syndrome may be a necessary trade-off in the control of a serious and crippling disease. The undesirable side effects of corticosteriod therapy can be minimized by administering the steroid on an alternate-day schedule instead of giving the corticosteroid preparation daily and in divided doses. One double dose of a preparation with intermediate duration of action is administered every other day in the morning. For example, if a patient needs prednisolone, 20 mg daily, instead of getting it in doses of 5 mg every 6 hours, the patient receives it in doses of 40 mg every other morning.

QUESTIONS

The adrenal cortex—disorders of hypersecretion

Directions: Circle the letter preceding each item below that correctly answers the question. More than one answer may be correct.

1. Glucocorticoids affect the following when present in excess:
   a. Adipose tissue distribution   *b.* The immune system   *c.* Protein metabolism   *d.* Carbohydrate metabolism

2. When synthetic glucocorticoids are administered orally over a long period of time, which of the following events is likely to occur?
   a. The adrenal gland continues to function normally   *b.* The hypothalamic-pituitary axis is suppressed   *c.* CRH and ACTH levels are increased   *d.* Endogenous cortisol secretion is stimulated

3. Abrupt interruption of corticosteroid therapy may result in:
   a. Hyperglycemia   *b.* Severe salt depletion   *c.* Nausea, vomiting, hypotension   *d.* Marked hyperpigmentation

4. Which of the following pathological conditions may cause Cushing's syndrome?
   a. Hypothalamic-pituitary hyperfunction
   b. Adrenal adenoma   *c.* Ectopic hormone production by a neoplasm   *d.* Atrophy of the adrenal glands

5. Which of the following diagnostic tests can be used to determine whether Cushing's syndrome is caused by an adrenal neoplasm or by a primary abnormality of the hypothalamic-pituitary axis?
   a. Adrenal venous angiography   *b.* Adrenal biopsy   *c.* Adrenal photoscanning   *d.* Myelography

6. Mrs. A., 35, presents with the typical signs and symptoms of Cushing's syndrome. All the following signs and symptoms are characteristic of this condition except:
   a. Moonface (full, round face)   *b.* Hypotension
   c. Purple abdominal striae   *d.* Truncal obesity
   e. Osteoporosis

7. Which of the following are characteristic metabolic effects of aldosterone?
   a. Decreased potassium excretion   *b.* Sodium retention   *c.* Regulation of blood glucose
   d. Suppression of ACTH release

8. Primary aldosteronism occurs when the overproduction of aldosterone results from a tumor or enlargement of the:
   a. Pituitary gland   b. Adrenal cortex   c. Adrenal medulla   d. Hypothalamus

9. Which of the following findings are characteristic of primary aldosteronism?
   a. Hypokalemia   b. Hyponatremia   c. Hypertension   d. Nephrotic syndrome

10. The direct effect of stress is an increased secretion of corticotropin by the anterior pituitary. Corticotropin acts on the adrenal cortex to increase secretion, primarily, of:
    a. Glucocorticoids   b. Mineralocorticoids
    c. Epinephrine

11. Cushing's syndrome may develop when which of the following secretes abnormal amounts of the stated hormone?
    a. Adrenal cortex, aldosterone   b. Anterior pituitary, aldosterone   c. Adrenal cortex, adrenocorticotropic hormone   d. Anterior pituitary, adrenocorticotropic hormone

12. In physiological testing for forms of Cushing's syndrome, patients who respond to metyrapone administration with an increase in ACTH release usually have which form of the disease?
    a. Ectopic   b. Tertiary   c. Primary   d. Pituitary

Directions: Answer the following questions on a separate sheet of paper.

13. Explain the statement that glucocorticoids have a catabolic effect on protein metabolism.

14. What effects do abnormally high levels of glucocorticoids have on glucose utilization?

15. The hypothalamic-pituitary axis may be activated under stress. Explain the process by which it occurs.

16. How do the basic chemical structures of 9α-fluorocortisol and prednisolone differ? In relation to pharmacological effects, what is achieved by altering the basic chemical structure of cortisol?

17. List three types of treatment for pituitary ACTH-dependent Cushing's syndrome. What is the purpose of the treatment modalities?

18. What is the preferred treatment for Cushing's syndrome that is secondary to an adrenal tumor?

19. Explain the way secondary aldosteronism develops in response to congestive heart failure.

Directions: Circle T if the statement is true, F if the statement is false. Correct any false statements.

20. T   F   CRH is secreted by the hypothalamus.

21. T   F   CRH stimulates the release of ACTH from the anterior pituitary.

22. T   F   High plasma cortisol levels exert a negative feedback effect on CRH release in the normal state.

23. T   F   CRH directly initiates the secretion of cortisol.

CHAPTER 58

THE ADRENAL CORTEX— DISORDERS OF HYPOSECRETION

OBJECTIVES

At the completion of this chapter you should be able to:

1. Identify several causes of adrenocortical insufficiency.
2. Describe the possible etiologies of primary adrenal insufficiency.
3. Explain why hypoglycemia is often a manifestation of glucocorticoid insufficiency in Addison's disease.
4. State the effect of cortisol insufficiency on the production of melanocyte-stimulating hormone (MSH) and on the response to stress.
5. Identify the fluid and electrolyte disturbances which may result from a deficit in aldosterone production.
6. Define postural hypotension and tachycardia and explain the relationship between these conditions and Addison's disease.
7. Identify the effect of Addison's disease on plasma renin levels.
8. Differentiate between the signs in males and females that result from decreased production of adrenal androgens in Addison's disease.
9. Describe the most comon tests used to diagnose Addison's disease.
10. Describe the treatment of Addison's disease.

Adrenocortical hormone secretion may be insufficient to maintain normal life because of (1) primary disease or insufficiency of the adrenal cortex or (2) deficient secretion of adrenocorticotropic hormone (ACTH). When the cause of adrenocortical insufficiency is a pathological process of the adrenal cortex, the condition is known as Addison's disease. With pituitary ACTH insufficiency there is secondary failure of the adrenal cortex. Patients with Addison's disease have involvement of all zones of the cortex. As a result of this involvement there is deficiency of all the adrenocortical secretions—glucocorticoids, mineralocorticoids, and androgens. Occasionally patients present with partial deficiencies of adrenocortical hormone secretion. This is seen in states of hypoaldosteronism, which involves the zona glomerulosa only and its secretion of aldosterone, or in the adrenogenital syndrome, where an enzyme defect blocks the secretion of a specific steroid hormone.

Addison's disease occurs with an incidence of 4 per 100,000. In the past, tuberculosis was the main cause of Addison's disease. Presently, with better chemotherapy for tuberculosis, this pathological process is the cause of adrenal insufficiency in less than 50 percent of patients with this condition. In more than 50 percent of patients with Addison's disease, destruction of the adrenal cortex occurs as a manifestation of an autoimmune process. Adrenal antibodies are found in high titers in some patients with Addison's disease. These antibodies react with antigens in the adrenocortical tissue and cause an inflammatory reaction which eventually leads to destruction of the adrenal gland. Usually, well over 80 percent of both glands must be destroyed before signs and symptoms of insufficiency develop. Addison's disease may occur concurrently with other endocrine diseases in which autoimmunity plays an etiological role. Among these are Hashimoto's thyroiditis, certain cases of insulin-dependent diabetes mellitus, and hypoparathyroidism. There also appears to be a familial predisposition for autoimmune endocrine disease, which is probably related to abnormal reactivity of the patient's immune system. Less common causes of Addison's disease are the chronic use of anticoagulants, granulomatous diseases, and metastatic neoplasms which involve both adrenal glands.

METABOLIC CONSEQUENCES OF CORTISOL, ALDOSTERONE, AND ANDROGEN DEFICIENCIES

The clinical picture of Addison's disease results from the lack of cortisol, aldosterone, and androgens. Cortisol insufficiency has metabolic consequence in terms of maintenance of blood glucose levels. In the absence of cortisol, gluconeogenesis is diminished, liver glycogen is decreased, and there is increased sensitivity of peripheral tissues to insulin. The combination of these changes in carbohydrate metabolism may cause inability to maintain normal blood glucose levels in the fasting state. Because of the low glycogen storage, patients with adrenal insufficiency are unable to withstand food deprivation for a long period of time. Sensitivity to insulin observed in the presence of cortisol insufficiency may be a problem for insulin-requiring diabetics who also develop Addison's disease. These patients may notice that insulin doses which kept them under control in the past now cause hypoglycemia.

Another consequence of cortisol insufficiency is an increase in ACTH release. This occurs as a result of diminished feedback inhibition of the hypothalamic-pituitary axis. MSH is also suppressed by cortisol. Lack of cortisol is usually associated with an increase in MSH secretion. The clinical consquence of this hormonal response is hyperpigmentation.

Since cortisol is required for a normal stress response, patients with cortisol insufficiency are unable to withstand surgical stress, trauma, infection, etc. Under these circumstances patients may become acutely adrenal-insufficient and develop evidence of vascular collapse.

Aldosterone deficiency is manifested by increased renal sodium loss and enhanced potassium reabsorption. Salt depletion is associated with water and volume depletion. The decrease in circulating plasma volume leads to hypotension. This change is most strikingly evident when the patient changes from the recumbent to the upright position. Patients with Addison's disease may record a normal blood pressure when they are lying down but marked hypotension and tachycardia when they stand up for several minutes. By definition, postural hypotension occurs when systolic and diastolic blood pressures drop by more than 20 mmHg when the patient assumes the upright posture. Postural tachycardia exists when the pulse rate increases by more than 20 beats per minute (bpm) under these circumstances. In both cases, the decrease in blood pressure and the increase in pulse rate should persist for more than 3 minutes after the change in posture. Thus, a person with Addison's disease may have a blood pressure of 120/80 mmHg in the recumbent position but of 60/40 mmHg after assuming the upright posture. Likewise, the pulse may rise from 80 to 140 bpm with a change in posture.

The plasma renin activity is also affected in Addison's disease. The decrease in plasma volume and in arteriolar pressure causes stimulation of renin release and increased production of angiotensin II. The problem in Addison's disease is that since the adrenal cortex is destroyed, angiotensin II is not able to stimulate aldosterone production and bring the serum level back to its initial physiological range. Therefore, high renin levels and low aldosterone secretion are characteristic of aldosterone deficiency.

Androgen deficiency may affect growth of axillary and pubic hair. This effect is masked in the male, where testicular androgens exert the major androgenic metabolic effects. In the female, androgen insufficiency causes loss of axillary and pubic hair and decrease of hair over the extremities.

Pigmentation in Addison's disease

Hyperpigmentation is an important characteristic of primary adrenocortical insufficiency. It is found in the distal portion of the extremities and sun-exposed areas. It is also present in areas which are not normally ex-

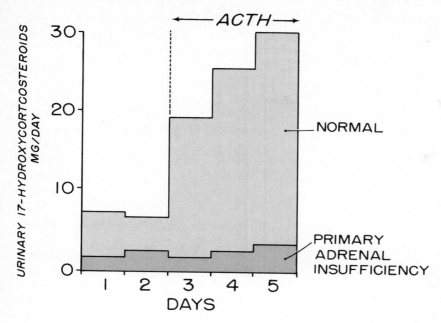

FIGURE 58-1

ACTH stimulation test. Patients with primary adrenocortical insufficiency fail to respond to the administration of ACTH.

posed to the sun. These areas include the nipples, extensor surfaces of the extremities, genitalia, buccal mucosa, tongue, palmar creases, and knuckles. The assessment of pigmentation may be more difficult in a black than in a Caucasian. In blacks the history of color change as ascertained by the patients or their relatives may be the only way of assessing the development of hyperpigmentation. Treatment of Addison's disease reverses the hyperpigmentation.

Diagnosis and treatment

The diagnosis of Addison's disease is based upon the recognition of cortisol, aldosterone, and androgen deficiency. In addition, there are laboratory tests indicative of primary adrenocortical insufficiency. Patients have decreased excretion of the degradation products or metabolites of cortisol, the urinary 17-hydroxycorticoids. Plasma cortisol levels are low, while plasma ACTH levels are found to be elevated. If patients with Addison's disease receive an intravenous infusion with ACTH, there is a lack of rise of plasma cortisol levels in response to ACTH (see Fig. 58-1). Serum electrolytes are abnormal in patients with Addison's disease, who demonstrate hyponatremia, hyperkalemia, and metabolic acidosis. Patients with adrenal insufficiency secondary to ACTH deficiency also present with low levels of cortisol and of its urinary metabolites. However, aldosterone levels are normal and plasma ACTH levels are low. When an intravenous infusion with ACTH is given to these patients, plasma cortisol levels rise, but in subnormal fashion.

Treatment of Addison's disease is based on replacement with cortisol—usually 20 to 30 mg per day in divided doses—and an aldosterone analogue, 9α-fluorocortisol. When both cortisol and 9α-fluorocortisol are employed, patients may return to a normal metabolic state and be able to live a normal life. While in the past patients used to die of Addison's disease, presently patients with this condition, if properly treated, are able to live a normal life and reach normal life expectancy.

QUESTIONS

The adrenal cortex—disorders of hyposecretion

Directions: Circle the letter preceding each item below that correctly answers the question. More than one answer may be correct.

1. Addison's disease occurs when:
   a. There is an increase in levels of aldosterone
   b. Both glucocorticoid and mineralocorticoid deficiencies develop simultaneously   *c.* Serum potassium levels decrease   *d.* There is increased sodium reabsorption by the kidney

2. Autoimmune destruction of the adrenal gland is caused by:
   a. Tuberculosis or other granulomatous diseases
   b. Malignant neoplasm of the lung which metastasizes to the adrenal gland   *c.* Adrenal tissues

becoming antigenic, causing the production of antibodies

3. Factors contributing to hypoglycemia in Addison's disease are:
   a. Decreased gluconeogenesis in the liver
   b. Increased glycogen storage in the liver
   c. Increased sensitivity of the peripheral tissues to insulin   d. Increased insulin secretion by the pancreas

4. Which of the following sequences best explains the postural hypotension and tachycardia associated with Addison's disease?
   a. Aldosterone deficiency → increased sodium and water excretion → hypovolemia → fall in systolic and diastolic blood pressure upon standing → compensatory increase in heart rate to maintain cardiac output   b. Cortisol deficiency → decreased protein synthesis → hypoproteinemia → decreased osmotic pressure → edema → decreased intravascular plasma volume → fall in systolic and diastolic blood pressure upon standing → compensatory increase in heart rate to maintain cardiac output   c. Antidiuretic hormone deficiency → inability of kidney to conserve water → hypovolemia → fall in systolic and diastolic blood pressure upon standing → compensatory increase in heart rate to maintain cardiac output

5. Adrenocortical insufficiency is associated with:
   a. Increased plasma renin activity and decreased plasma aldosterone   b. Decreased plasma renin activity and increased plasma aldosterone   c. Hyperkalemia and hyponatremia   d. Hypokalemia and hypernatremia

6. The pigmentary changes observed in patients with Addison's disease are a result of:
   a. Decreased production of MSH   b. Decreased production of ACTH by the pituitary gland and associated increased production of MSH   c. Decreased production of cortisol, causing an increase in ACTH and MSH secretion   d. Increased production of cortisol by the adrenal cortex, causing increased production of MSH

7. The diagnosis of primary adrenocortical insufficiency can be made with certainty when:
   a. Plasma cortisol levels are low   b. Hyperkalemia, hyponatremia, and hypertension are present   c. Urinary 17-hydroxycorticosteroid levels are less than 2 mg in 24 hours (normal = 2 to 8 per 24 hours) and fail to rise after ACTH infusion   d. Urinary 17-ketosteroid levels are less than 10 mg in 24 hours in an adult male (normal = 10 to 22 mg per 24 hours)

8. Treatment of Addison's disease commonly includes the administration of:
   a. ACTH   b. Cortisol   c. Pitressin   d. 9α-fluorocortisol   e. Pituitary extract

9. Loss of pubic and axillary hair:
   a. May be a manifestation of adrenal androgen insufficiency in females but not in males   b. Commonly occurs in males with Addison's disease   c. Is uncommon in males with Addison's disease, since serum testosterone levels are generally normal

THE PANCREAS—GLUCOSE METABOLISM AND DIABETES MELLITUS

OBJECTIVES

At the completion of this chapter you should be able to:

1. Explain the mechanism which regulates blood glucose levels.
2. Identify a condition leading to fasting hyperglycemia.
3. Identify a condition leading to fasting hypoglycemia.
4. Explain the difference in response to a glucose load exhibited by non-diabetic versus diabetic individuals.
5. Define—in milligrams per 100 ml of plasma—normal blood glucose, hyperglycemia, hypoglycemia, and normal renal threshold for glucose.
6. Explain (in relation to administration, interpretation, sensitivity, and applicability to the diagnosis of diabetes mellitus) the test of glucose tolerance, including fasting plasma glucose, 2-hour postprandial plasma glucose, and oral glucose tolerance.
7. Give a general definition of diabetes mellitus.
8. Describe the types of disturbances presently being postulated as possible causes of diabetes.
9. State the prevalence rate for diabetes in the United States.
10. Differentiate between insulin-dependent and non-insulin-dependent diabetes as to severity, symptoms, and rationale for treatment.
11. List the complications usually associated with diabetes mellitus.
12. State the principles that guide any management program for a diabetic patient.
13. Explain the purpose of the food exchange system.
14. Identify the treatment of a patient with severe insulin deficiency, and describe the rationale for that treatment.
15. Differentiate between the three types of insulin preparations as to their time of action and indications for use.
16. Explain the way exercise influences blood glucose levels in both non-diabetic and diabetic persons.
17. State two examples in each of the two major categories of complications of diabetes mellitus—metabolic and peripheral vascular.

ROLE OF THE PANCREAS IN THE REGULATION OF GLUCOSE METABOLISM

Carbohydrates are important components of the diet. They are chemical substances present in various forms, including simple sugars, or monosaccharides, and complex chemical units, disaccharides and polysaccharides. Following ingestion, carbohydrates are digested to monosaccharides and absorbed, preferentially in the duodenum and proximal jejunum. Following absorption, the blood glucose level rises temporarily and eventually returns to baseline. The physiological regulation of blood glucose levels depends to a large extent on hepatic (1) extraction of glucose, (2) synthesis of glycogen, and (3) glycogenolysis. In addition, peripheral tissues—muscles and adipocytes—utilize glucose for their energy needs. Although quantitatively in lesser magnitude than the liver, these tissues also contribute to the maintenance of normal blood glucose levels.

The hepatic uptake and output of glucose and the utilization of glucose by peripheral tissues depend on the physiological balance of several hormones. These hormones can be classified as those which (1) lower blood glucose or (2) raise blood glucose. Insulin is the blood glucose–lowering hormone. It is produced by the beta cells of the islets of Langerhans of the pancreas. In contrast, several hormones are capable of raising blood glucose levels. These include (1) glucagon secreted by the alpha cells of the islets of Langerhans, (2) epinephrine secreted by the adrenal medulla and other chromaffin tissues, (3) glucocorticoids secreted by the adrenal cortex, and (4) growth hormone secreted by the anterior pituitary gland. Glucagon, epinephrine, glucocorticoids, and growth hormone constitute a counterregulatory mechanism which prevents hypoglycemia under the effect of insulin (see Fig. 59-1).

A normal fasting plasma glucose level (Autoanalyzer technique) is 80 to 115 mg/100 ml. Hyperglycemia is defined as a fasting plasma glucose level greater than 115 mg/100 ml, and hypoglycemia as a level less than 80 mg/100 ml. Glucose is filtered by the renal glomerulus and almost totally reabsorbed by the renal tubule as long as the concentration of glucose in plasma does not exceed 160 to 180 mg/100 ml. When the plasma glucose concentration rises above this level, glucose appears in the urine, a condition called *glycosuria*. Thus, the normal renal threshold for glucose is defined by a plasma glucose concentration of 160 to 180 mg/100 ml.

Tests of carbohydrate tolerance

There are various methods of testing an individual's ability to regulate plasma glucose levels within the normal range. These methods test (1) the fasting plasma glucose and (2) the plasma glucose response to a glucose load.

FIGURE 59-1
Outline of regulation of blood glucose.

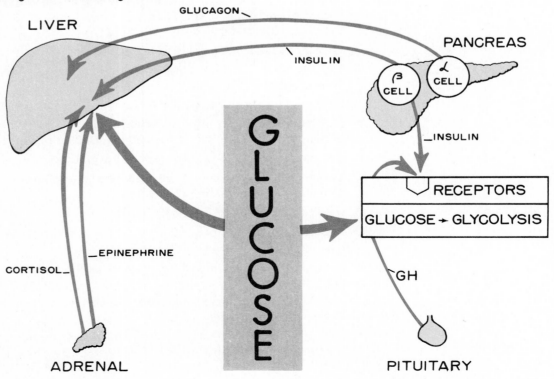

In the fasting state when food is not being absorbed, maintenance of normal fasting glucose levels depends upon a well-integrated interaction among the liver, peripheral tissues, and hormones which lower and raise plasma glucose levels. If an individual is unable to regulate plasma glucose normally, this inability is reflected by either an increase or decrease in fasting plasma glucose. For example, a patient with an insulin-producing tumor which secretes insulin in inappropriately large amounts develops hypoglycemia. On the other hand, a patient with insulin deficiency is unable to maintain glucose levels at a normal range and becomes hyperglycemic. Thus, the measurement of fasting plasma glucose levels can help evaluate the integrity of the mechanism regulating plasma glucose. In the case of diabetes, a condition of relative or absolute insulin deficiency, these levels become abnormal only in the advanced state of the disease. Therefore, their measurement does not provide information about early abnormalities in glucose metabolism.

A more sensitive method for uncovering abnormalities in glucose metabolism is the measurement of plasma glucose following a glucose load. A nondiabetic individual who ingests a glucose load absorbs this glucose and exhibits a temporary rise in plasma glucose levels. Mechanisms for glucose disposal are then brought into action, and the plasma glucose level returns to normal. The mechanism which mediates this reponse is insulin, and the main stimulus to insulin release is glucose. The tests used to make the pertinent measurements after a glucose load are the (1) 2-hour postprandial plasma glucose, and (2) oral glucose tolerance.

The 2-hour postprandial plasma glucose test is a simple *screening test* for the ability of an individual to dispose of a glucose load. The test consists of measuring the patient's plasma glucose level 2 hours following the administration of 75 g glucose orally. If the plasma glucose is less than 140 mg/100 ml 2 hours after the ingestion of the glucose load, one can conclude that the plasma glucose level must have returned to baseline after an initial rise, indicating that the subject has a normal mechanism for glucose disposal. In contrast, if the patient's plasma glucose level is still high after 2 hours, one can conclude that there is a disturbance in the mechanism regulating glucose levels.

If a 2-hour postprandial plasma glucose level is abnormal, an *oral glucose tolerance test* (OGTT) can provide additional and more complete information about the presence of a disturbance in carbohydrate metabolism. For a glucose tolerance test, a patient receives 75 g glucose orally within 5 minutes. Plasma glucose levels are measured fasting and at half-hour intervals for a period of 2 hours after the glucose load. In healthy, ambulatory people with normal glucose tolerance, the fasting plasma glucose is 80 to 115 mg/100 ml. After the ingestion of glucose, the plasma glucose level rises initially but returns to baseline within 2 hours. Normal values for the OGTT have been defined as plasma glucose

less than 200 mg/100 ml at ½, 1, and 1½ hours and less than 140 mg/100 ml at 2 hours (National Diabetes Data Group criteria). Criteria differing slightly from these values have been proposed by other investigators and health organizations.

DIABETES MELLITUS

Diabetes mellitus can be defined as a genetically and clinically heterogeneous group of disorders of metabolism which is manifested ultimately by loss of carbohydrate tolerance. In its fully developed clinical expression, diabetes is characterized by fasting hyperglycemia, atherosclerotic and microangiopathic vascular disease, and neuropathy. The clinical manifestations of hyperglycemia usually precede by many years the clinical recognition of vascular disease. Occasionally, however, there are patients with only mild abnormality of glucose tolerance who suffer the severe clinical consequences of vascular disease.

There is evidence that diabetes mellitus has heterogeneous etiology; that is, different types of lesions may ultimately lead to insulin insufficiency. The following types of disturbances are presently being postulated as possible causes of diabetes:

1. A genetically determined abnormality in beta-cell function or number
2. Environmental factors altering beta-cell function and integrity
3. A defective immune system
4. Abnormality of insulin activity

While there is substantial evidence in favor of some of these proposed etiologies, the role played by others is still hypothetical.

Genetic determinants are thought to be important in most patients with diabetes. In patients with insulin-dependent diabetes mellitus, these genetic determinants are expressed by an associated increased or decreased frequency of certain histocompatibility antigens (HLA) and an abnormal immune response leading to the production of islet-cell autoantibodies. In patients with non-insulin-dependent diabetes mellitus, the disease has a strong familial pattern of occurrence. It frequently affects children, adolescents, and adults of the same family with autosomal-dominant inheritance. The inherited abnormality could affect the beta cell directly and alter its ability to recognize or propagate the secretory stimulus or the complex series of steps involved in the synthesis or release of insulin. More likely, it may increase the susceptibility of affected individuals to the action of environmental factors, including certain viruses or dietary characteristics.

Several *environmental factors* can alter the integrity and function of the beta cell in susceptible individuals. These factors include:

1. Infective agents, such as Coxsackie B and mumps viruses
2. Diet—excessive intake of calories, carbohydrates, refined sugars
3. Obesity
4. Pregnancy

Most of these factors do not, by themselves, cause diabetes but may affect genetically susceptible individuals and precipitate decompensation of beta-cell function.

A *defective immune system* may be the basis for development of diabetes in certain people. It may operate by:

1. Autoimmunity with development of antipancreatic cell antibodies and eventual destruction of insulin-secreting cells
2. Increased susceptibility to beta-cell damage by viral agents

Decreased sensitivity to endogenous insulin can also lead to diabetes. This mechanism occurs in patients with obesity and diabetes. The reason for this impaired sensitivity of tissues to insulin may be a decreased number of insulin receptor sites in the cell membrane of insulin-responsive cells or interference with intracellular glycolysis.

Epidemiology

The prevalence rate of diabetes is high. Estimates are that there are 10 million cases of diabetes in the United States and that 600,000 new cases are diagnosed every year. Diabetes is the third leading cause of death in the United States by disease and the leading cause of blindness, through the development of diabetic retinopathy. Heart attacks occur at least 1½ times as frequently in diabetics as in nondiabetics of a comparable age.

Seventy-five percent of diabetic patients eventually die of vascular disease. Heart attacks, kidney failure, strokes, and gangrene are the major complications. In addition, there is an increased rate of intrauterine neonatal death in infants of diabetic mothers.

The economic impact of diabetes is substantial. The approximate loss is $5 billion a year in medical expenses and lost wages without even including the financial consequence of many of the complications such as blindness and vascular disease.

Classification of diabetes mellitus and glucose intolerance

Several classifications of diabetes mellitus have been proposed, based on the modalities of clinical presentation, age of onset, and natural history of the disease. Table 59-1 describes a classification proposed by the National Diabetes Data Group of the National Institutes of Health, based on contemporary knowledge of the diabetic syndrome and disorders of glucose tolerance. Three clinical classes of disorders of glucose tolerance are described: (1) diabetes mellitus (DM), (2) impaired glucose tolerance (IGT), and (3) gestational diabetes (GDM). Among individuals with diabetes mellitus, three types are recognized: Patients with insulin-dependent diabetes (IDDM), or Type I, are ketosis-prone and have increased or decreased frequency of certain histocompatibility antigens (HLA) on chromosome-6 and islet-cell antibodies. This type has been termed *juvenile-onset type* in the past. However, it can occur at any age. Non-insulin-dependent (NIDDM), or Type II, patients are non-ketosis-prone. Obesity is frequently associated with this type. Secondary diabetes develops in association with other conditions and syndromes, such as underlying pancreatic disease, Cushing's syndrome, and acromegaly. Some patients present with primary insulin-receptor abnormalities such as those seen with acanthosis nigricans and the insulin-resistant syndrome.

In nonpregnant adults, the diagnosis of diabetes mellitus is based on the finding of (1) classic symptoms of diabetes and unequivocal hyperglycemia, (2) fasting plasma glucose equal to or greater than 140 mg/100 ml on more than one occasion, and (3) if the fasting plasma glucose is less than 140 mg/100 ml, glucose levels obtained during an oral glucose tolerance test equal to or greater than 200 mg/100 ml at 2 hours and at least at one other time between times 0 and 2 hours following ingestion of glucose.

The diagnosis of diabetes in children is also based on the finding of classic symptoms of diabetes and a random plasma glucose of greater than 200 mg/100 ml.

Patients with impaired glucose tolerance do not meet the criteria described for diagnosis of diabetes. However, their glucose tolerance tests show abnormal values. These patients are asymptomatic. Biochemically, they exhibit fasting plasma glucose levels of less than 140 mg/100 ml and values during an oral glucose tolerance test equal to or greater than 200 mg/100 ml at ½, 1, or 1½ hours and 140 to 200 mg/100 ml at 2 hours. Some patients with impaired glucose tolerance may

TABLE 59-1

889
DIABETES MELLITUS

CLASSIFICATION OF DIABETES MELLITUS AND OTHER CATEGORIES OF GLUCOSE INTOLERANCE

Clinical classes
1. Diabetes mellitus (DM)
a. Insulin-dependent type (IDDM), Type I
b. Non-insulin-dependent type (NIDDM), Type II
(1) Nonobese NIDDM
(2) Obese NIDDM
c. Secondary diabetes
2. Impaired glucose tolerance (IGT)
3. Gestational diabetes (GDM)

Statistical risk classes
1. Previous abnormality of glucose tolerance (Prev AGT)
2. Potential abnormality of glucose tolerance (Pot AGT)

have underlying conditions which may be responsible for secondary types of diabetes. In other individuals, an IGT may be the expression of an early stage in the development of diabetes. These individuals are not considered to be diabetic but are recognized as being at higher risk than the general population for the development of diabetes. Some of these patients may remain in this class for many years. Many return to normal glucose tolerance spontaneously, but 1 to 5 percent of persons with IGT proceed to overt clinical diabetes per year. Although clinically significant renal and retinal microangiopathic complications of diabetes are absent in patients with IGT, many studies of such groups have shown an increased prevalence of arterial disease, electrocardiographic abnormalities, and cardiac death or increased susceptibility to atherosclerotic disease. Appropriate intervention, including caloric restriction or weight loss in obese persons with IGT, may lead to improvement in glucose tolerance and a possible change in the occurrence of these complications.

Gestational diabetes is the glucose intolerance that has its onset or recognition during pregnancy. Because of the increased secretion of various hormones with metabolic effects on glucose tolerance, pregnancy is a diabetogenic condition. Patients with underlying predisposition for diabetes may show glucose intolerance or clinical manifestations of diabetes with pregnancy. The recommended criteria for the biochemical diagnosis of gestational diabetes are those proposed by O'Sullivan and Mahan. According to these criteria, gestational diabetes is present when two or more of the following values are met or exceeded after a 100-g oral glucose challenge: fasting, 105 mg/100 ml; 1 hour, 190 mg/100 ml; 2 hours, 165 mg/100 ml; and 3 hours, 145 mg/100 ml. Recognition of this type of diabetes is important because these patients are at increased risk for perinatal morbidity and mortality and they have increased frequency of viable fetal loss.

Two statistical risk classes of patients are included

in the classification of diabetes. These are (1) previous abnormality of glucose tolerance (Prev AGT) and (2) potential abnormality of glucose tolerance (Pot AGT). Prev AGT applies only to people who at the time of their examination have a normal glucose tolerance but have previously demonstrated diabetic hyperglycemia or impaired glucose tolerance which appeared spontaneously or in response to an identifiable stimulus. Included in this class are patients with gestational diabetes who have recovered glucose tolerance postpartum and patients with impaired glucose tolerance or NIDDM who have normalized their glucose tolerance following weight reduction.

Persons with Pot AGT include those who have never exhibited abnormal glucose tolerance but who are at substantially increased risk for the development of diabetes. Individuals who are at increased risk for IDDM include persons with islet-cell antibodies; monozygotic twins of IDDM diabetics; siblings of IDDM diabetics, especially with identical HLA haplotypes; and offspring of IDDM diabetics. Individuals who are at an increased risk for NIDDM include monozygotic twins of NIDDM diabetics, first-degree relatives of NIDDM diabetics, mothers of neonates weighing more than 9 lb, obese individuals, and members of racial or ethnic groups with a high incidence of diabetes. Patients with Pot AGT used to be classified as prediabetic. However, this diagnosis can be established only retrospectively once individuals have developed diabetes and, therefore, cannot be used in individuals who may be at risk but who have normal glucose tolerance.

Clinical manifestations of diabetes

The clinical manifestations of diabetes are related to the metabolic consequence of insulin deficiency. Patients with insulin deficiency are unable to maintain normal fasting plasma glucose levels or glucose tolerance following the ingestion of carbohydrate. If the hyperglycemia is severe and exceeds the renal threshold for this substance, glycosuria supervenes. Glycosuria leads to osmotic diuresis, which causes increased urinary output—polyuria—and thirst—polydipsia. Because of the loss of glucose through the urine, patients develop negative caloric balance and weight loss. Increased hunger—polyphagia—may also develop as the result of calorie loss. Patients complain of fatigue and sleepiness.

Patients with IDDM frequently exhibit an explosive onset of symptoms, with polydipsia, polyuria, weight loss, polyphagia, fatigue, and somnolence occurring within a few days or weeks. They may become very ill and develop ketoacidosis, and they may die if treatment is not instituted promptly. They usually require insulin therapy for metabolic control and are generally sensitive to insulin. In contrast, patients with NIDDM may be completely asymptomatic, and the diagnosis made only following a laboratory examination of their blood and performance of tests of glucose tolerance. With more severe degrees of hyperglycemia, these patients may develop polydipsia, polyuria, fatigue, and somnolence. They usually do not develop ketoacidosis. If the hyperglycemia is severe and patients do not respond to diet therapy, insulin therapy may be required in order to normalize glucose levels. These patients usually exhibit diminished peripheral sensitivity to insulin. Their own insulin levels may be diminished, normal, or high but inadequate to maintain normal blood glucose levels. They are also resistant to exogenous insulin. Since many of these patients are obese, it is postulated that high carbohydrate intake, large adipose cells, and impairment in intracellular glucose metabolism are responsible for their decreased sensitivity to insulin.

Principles of management of diabetes

The management of diabetes is based on (1) diet, (2) hypoglycemic agents, and (3) controlled physical activity.

In people without diabetes, an intact capacity to secrete insulin compensates for varying amounts of food intake and exercise. In diabetics who are unable to secrete insulin normally, this ability is lost. While normal individuals adjust to hour-to-hour changes in food intake and exercise by varying their insulin secretion, diabetic patients on insulin are unable to do so unless they concomitantly adjust their insulin dose in order to prevent wide fluctuations in blood glucose levels.

The diet of diabetic patients is aimed at controlling the number of calories and the amount of carbohydrates ingested daily. The recommended number of calories varies depending on the need for maintaining, reducing, or increasing body weight. For example, if the patient is obese, a calorie-restricted diet should be prescribed until weight has dropped into the ideal range for that person. In contrast, young patients with IDDM may lose weight during the state of decompensation. They should receive sufficient calories to help restore their best weight.

Diabetic patients should avoid intake of excessive amounts of carbohydrates in order to prevent excessive postprandial hyperglycemia and glycosuria. Usually, carbohydrates make up 40 percent of the total daily calorie allowance. This carbohydrate allowance must be distributed in such a way that the intake matches the patients' requirements throughout the day. For example, larger amounts are given at times of greater physical activity. A food exchange system has been developed to help patients manage their own diets. Food exchange lists are available which identify food choices on the basis of calorie and carbohydrate values and compare these values among various types of foods.

In general, a diabetic patient is instructed on the food exchange system by a dietician. Alternatively, pa-

TABLE 59-2

INSULIN

Type	Description	Effect on blood glucose (hours after administration)		
		Onset	Peak	Termination
Short acting				
Regular (crystalline zinc)	Clear	Immediate	2–4	6–8
Semilente (SL)*	Cloudy: amorphous insulin Zn suspension, no protamine	1	4–6	12–16
Intermediate acting				
NPH†	Cloudy: crystaline Zn insulin suspension) 50% saturated with protamine	2–3	8–12	18–24
Lente	Cloudy: mixture 30% SL + 70% UL, no protamine	2–3	8–12	18–24
Long acting				
PZI†	Cloudy: excess protamine	6	14–20	24–36
Ultralente (UL)*	Cloudy: crystalline insulin suspension, high Zn content, no protamine	6	16–18	30–36

*Lente insulins (semi and ultra) do not contain protamine and are prepared in sodium acetate buffer. Their time of action depends on their variable Zn content and crystal size.
†Delayed action of NPH and PZI is controlled by their protamine content; they are prepared in sodium phosphate buffer.

TABLE 59-3

ORAL HYPOGLYCEMIC AGENTS

Agent	Action	Half-life	Timing dose	Initial priming (not necessary)	Maintenance dose	Toxicity	Tablet size
Tolbutamide (Orinase)	Stimulates insulin release	4.5–6 h	BID or TID	2–3 g 2–4 days	0.5–2.0 g	Skin GI Hematologic	500 mg
Chlorpropamide (Diabinese)	Stimulates insulin release	36 h	Single	250–500 mg	100–500 mg	Hepatic Hematologic Skin GI	100 mg 250 mg
Acetohexamide (Dymelor)	Stimulates insulin release	4–6 h	Single or divided	250 mg–1.5 g	250 mg–1.5 g	Hepatic Hematologic Skin GI	250 mg 500 mg

tients may receive standardized diets of appropriate calorie value and composition prepared by the American Diabetes Association (ADA diets).

Patients with mild diabetes may be able to maintain normal blood glucose levels by means of a diet alone. Patients with severe insulin insufficiency, however, require a hypoglycemic agent in addition to the diet. The physiological hypoglycemic agent is insulin, which is available only in injectable form. Several insulin preparations are available for treatment of diabetics (see Table 59-2). They are classified as short acting, intermediate acting, or long acting, according to the time required for maximal plasma glucose-lowering effect following their injection. Short-acting insulins produce their maximal effect within 2 to 6 hours after injection and are employed in the treatment of acute diabetic decompensation and in the management of patients with diabetic ketoacidosis. They also may be used to supplement longer-acting insulins. Intermediate-acting insulins have their peak effect within 14 to 20 hours after their administration and are usually used for day-to-day control of the diabetic patient. Long-acting insulin preparations with a peak effect within 18 to 24 hours after their administration are rarely used in the routine management of diabetic patients.

Control of the diabetic patient is usually achieved by the use of intermediate-acting insulin administered either as a single dose before breakfast or as a split dose, with the larger portion being given before breakfast and the smaller before supper. Short-acting insulin is frequently combined with intermediate-acting insulin for physiological regulation of glucose levels during postprandial periods. In any case, it is important to know the kind of insulin preparation a patient receives in order to anticipate maximal effects and possible hypoglycemic reactions.

Other hypoglycemic agents can be administered orally. The most common type is the sulfonylureas. They should be used only in patients with mild diabetes who have some remaining islet-cell function. This excludes patients with insulin-dependent diabetes. Sulfonylureas stimulate beta-cell function and increase secretion of insulin. They also appear to enhance the peripheral action of insulin and are therefore useful in the management of patients with NIDDM who frequently exhibit an impaired response to insulin.

There are potential side effects from the use of oral hypoglycemic drugs (see Table 59-3). In addition, the chronic use of sulfonylureas may be associated with increased incidence of cardiovascular deaths among diabetics.

Physical exercise also influences the control of blood glucose levels in patients with diabetes. Exercise appears to facilitate the transport of glucose into cells. Normally, nondiabetic individuals are able to decrease insulin release during exercise and avoid hypoglycemia. In contrast, patients who receive insulin are unable to exert this control. In these patients, exercise can potentiate the hypoglycemic action of insulin. This is particularly important when a patient engages in physical exercise at the time when the insulin dose has maximally depressed the glucose level. By appropriate timing of their physical exercise, patients may be able to improve the control of their glucose levels. For example, if patients exercise at the time when the blood glucose level is high, they may be able to lower this level with exercise alone. Conversely, if patients need to exercise when the blood glucose level is low, it is important that they receive additional carbohydrate in order to prevent hypoglycemia.

Diabetic patients can lead a relatively normal life if they are well informed about their disease and its management. They learn in time to regulate their insulin dose, administer their own insulin, and plan their diet and exercise in such a way that they minimize hyper- or hypoglycemia. Patients with NIDDM who are obese and asymptomatic, with moderately elevated glucose levels, learn that the treatment of choice is dietary restriction and weight reduction. However, the success rate in weight reduction among these patients is low, and they may eventually require therapy with hypoglycemic agents.

Complications of diabetes mellitus

Complications of diabetes mellitus can be divided into two major categories: (1) acute metabolic complications and (2) long-term vascular complications.

The metabolic complications of diabetes are the consequence of relatively acute changes in plasma glucose concentration. The most serious metabolic complication is diabetic ketoacidosis. With severe insulin insufficiency, patients develop severe hyperglycemia and glycosuria, decreased lipogenesis, increased lipolysis, and increased oxidation of free fatty acids with production of ketone bodies (acetoacetate, hydroxybutyrate, and acetone). The increase in ketones in plasma causes ketosis. The increased production of ketones causes an increased hydrogen ion load and metabolic acidosis. Marked glycosuria and ketonuria also lead to osmotic diuresis and resultant dehydration and loss of electrolytes. Patients may become hypotensive and develop a state of shock. Eventually, owing to decreased cerebral oxygen utilization, patients may go into coma and die. Coma and death from ketoacidosis are a rare occurrence today, because patients and health care personnel are aware of the potential dangers of this complication and treatment of ketoacidosis can be instituted early.

The principles of therapy of diabetic ketoacidosis involve (1) reversal of the metabolic derangement caused by the lack of insulin, (2) restoration of water and electrolyte balance, and (3) treatment of conditions which may have precipitated ketoacidosis. Treatment with short-acting (regular) insulin—administered as a continuous intravenous infusion or as frequent intramuscular injections—and glucose increases glucose utilization, decreases lipolysis and ketone body production, and restores acid-base balance. In addition, patients are treated with intravenous infusions of water, bicarbonate, and electrolytes, especially potassium. Since intercurrent infections can increase insulin requirements in diabetic patients, it is not unusual for infection to precipitate acute diabetic decompensation and ketoacidosis. Thus, treatment with antibiotics may be necessary in the management of patients with this condition.

Another frequent metabolic complication of diabetes is hypoglycemia. This is mainly a complication of insulin therapy. Insulin-dependent diabetics may, at times, receive insulin in amounts larger than needed to maintain normal glucose levels. Hypoglycemia follows. Symptoms of hypoglycemia are caused by epinephrine release (sweating, shakiness, headache, palpitations) and by lack of glucose in the brain (bizarre behavior, dullness of sensorium, and coma). Management of hypoglycemia requires the prompt administration of carbohydrate, either orally or intravenously. Occasionally, glucagon, a glycogenolytic hormone, is administered intramuscularly to raise blood glucose levels.

The long-term vascular complications of diabetes involve small vessels—microangiopathy—and middle- and large-size vessels—macroangiopathy. Microangiopathy is a specific lesion of diabetes which affects capillaries and arterioles of the retina (diabetic retinopathy), renal glomeruli (diabetic nephropathy), peripheral nerves (diabetic neuropathy), and muscles and skin. Histochemically, this thickening is accompanied by in-

FIGURE 59-2

Diabetic retinopathy. Note the hemorrhages, exudates, neovascularization, and dilatation of veins in the fundus of a patient with diabetes mellitus. (Reproduced with permission from the Ophthalmology Department, University Hospital, University of Michigan.)

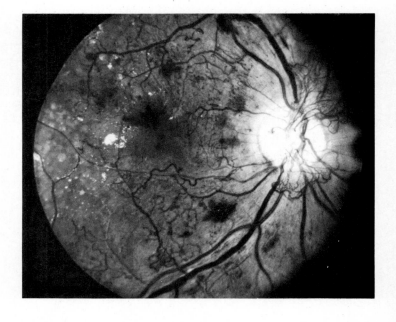

creased accumulation of glycoprotein. In addition, since all the chemical components of the basement membrane can be derived from glucose, there is an increased rate of formation of basement membrane cells with hyperglycemia. These cells do not require insulin for glucose utilization.

Histological evidence of microangiopathy is already apparent in patients with IGT. However, clinical manifestations of vascular disease, retinopathy, or nephropathy usually appear 15 to 20 years after the onset of diabetes.

An early manifestation of retinopathy is the presence of microaneurysms (tiny saccular dilatations) of the retinal arterioles. Subsequently, hemorrhages, neovascularization, and retinal scars may lead to blindness (see Fig. 59-2).

Early manifestations of nephropathy are proteinuria and hypertension. As the loss of functioning nephrons progresses, patients develop renal insufficiency and uremia.

Other frequent complications resulting from insulin insufficiency are neuropathy and cataracts. They result from disturbances in the polyol pathway (glucose → sorbitol → fructose) caused by lack of insulin. In the lens, there is increased accumulation of sorbitol, leading to formation of cataracts and blindness. In nerve tissue, there is an increased accumulation of sorbitol and fructose and a decreased concentration of myoinositol, leading to neuropathy. The biochemical alteration in nerve tissue interferes with metabolic activity of the Schwann cells and causes axonal loss. Motor conduction velocity decreases early in the course of neuropathy. Subsequently, there are pain, paresthesias, decreased vibratory and proprioceptive sensations, and motor impairment with loss of deep tendon reflexes, muscle weakness, and atrophy. Neuropathy may involve peripheral nerves (mono- and polyneuropathy), cranial nerves, or the autonomic nervous system. Involvement of the autonomic nervous system may be accompanied by nocturnal diarrhea, delayed gastric emptying, postural hypotension, and impotence.

Diabetic macroangiopathy has the histopathological characteristics of atherosclerosis. A combination of biochemical disturbances caused by insulin insufficiency probably leads to this type of vascular disease. The disturbances include (1) accumulation of sorbitol in the vascular intima, (2) hyperlipoproteinemia, and (3) abnormality in blood coagulation. Diabetic macroangiopathy eventually leads to vascular occlusion. When it involves peripheral arteries, it may result in peripheral vascular insufficiency with intermittent claudication and gangrene of the extremities. When it involves the aorta and coronary arteries, it may lead to angina and myocardial infarctions.

Diabetes also interferes with pregnancy. Diabetic women are prone to spontaneous abortions, intrauterine fetal death, large fetal size, and premature infants with a high incidence of respiratory distress syndrome and fetal malformations. The outcome of pregnancy in diabetic mothers has improved with tighter diabetic control during pregnancy, early delivery, and advances in the field of neonatology and in the management of complications in the newborn. Frequently, pregnancy's change in the hormonal milieu has a marked influence on insulin requirement and on the level of glucose control. In general, pregnancy causes a progressive increase in insulin requirement, which reaches a peak in the third trimester.

Present clinical and experimental evidence suggests that development of long-term diabetic complications relates to the chronic abnormality in metabolism caused by insufficient insulin secretion. It is possible that diabetic complications could be minimized or prevented if diabetic patients were able to completely normalize glucose metabolism with appropriate insulin therapy at all times. Unfortunately, even with the best possible control, the treatment of diabetes is not effective enough to totally normalize glucose metabolism. Persistent abnormalities in glucose metabolism are likely to lead to the vascular complications which can eventually bring death to diabetic patients.

QUESTIONS

The pancreas—glucose metabolism and diabetes mellitus

Directions: Circle the letter preceding each item below that correctly answers the question. More than one answer may be correct.

1. Glucose is removed from the bloodstream by:
   a. Conversion to glycogen by the liver   b. Peripheral glucose utilization by muscle or adipose tissue

2. Fasting hypoglycemia will usually occur when there is:

   a. Pancreatic islet-cell tumor   b. Cirrhosis of the liver where the patient is unable to synthesize glycogen   c. Excessive production of cortisol   d. Excessive production of growth hormone

3. Which of the following tests is the most sensitive in the diagnosis of diabetes mellitus?
   a. Fasting plasma glucose   b. 2-hour postprandial plasma glucose   c. Standard oral glucose tolerance

4. The purpose of the 2-hour postprandial plasma glucose test is to:
   a. Assess the ability of an individual to dispose of a glucose load   b. Test the insulin-secreting capacity of the islets of Langerhans under stress
   c. Determine insulin requirements   d. Detect gestational diabetes

5. The major defect in diabetes mellitus is a disorder in the secretion of:
   a. Epinephrine   b. Cortisol   c. Insulin
   d. Growth hormone

6. Current theories of the pathogenesis of diabetes mellitus include:
   a. Autoimmune destruction of beta cells
   b. Viral destruction of beta cells   c. Genetically determined defects in insulin release   d. Decreased growth hormone production

7. The prevalence rate of diabetes mellitus is calculated at a *minimum* of how many million cases in the United States?
   a. 1   b. 3   c. 6   d. 10

8. Robert M., a 30-year-old male, is being treated in an outpatient clinic. His history reveals that he has a bilateral family history of diabetes mellitus. His 2-hour postprandial blood glucose test shows levels of 115 mg/100 ml. Robert would most probably be classified as having:
   a. Insulin-dependent diabetes   b. Potential diabetes   c. Non-insulin-dependent diabetes
   d. Impaired glucose tolerance

9. Which of the following are the usual characteristics of a non-insulin-dependent diabetic patient?
   a. Relative insensitivity to insulin   b. Obesity
   c. Very low islet-cell reserve   d. Proneness to diabetic ketoacidosis

10. The individual with insulin-dependent diabetes usually presents with all the following except:
    a. Weight gain   b. Polydipsia   c. Polyuria
    d. Fatigue   e. Polyphagia

11. Jane S., a 10-year-old, is admitted to the hospital and diagnosed as having insulin-dependent diabetes. The medical management that would most likely be prescribed for Jane is:
    a. A fixed amount of carbohydrate, fat, and protein distributed throughout the day plus an oral hypoglycemic agent   b. A fixed amount of calories and carbohydrate, protein, and fat plus insulin therapy   c. Education about diabetes and oral hypoglycemic agents

12. If a diabetic patient is given an excessive dose of lente insulin at 7 A.M., when would one expect to see a hypoglycemic reaction (if such a reaction occurs)?
    a. Within ½ hour   b. 11 A.M.   c. 4 P.M.
    d. Midnight

13. The most common metabolic complication of insulin therapy is:
    a. Hypoglycemia   b. Hyperglycemia   c. Ketoacidosis   d. Diabetic coma

14. Long-term complications of diabetes mellitus include which of the following?
    a. Peripheral vascular insufficiency   b. Diabetic nephropathy   c. Ketoacidosis   d. Retinopathy

Directions: Answer the following questions on a separate sheet of paper.

15. What is the purpose of measuring the fasting blood glucose level?

16. Administration of a glucose load to a nondiabetic individual causes a rise in blood glucose. Which is the mechanism that brings glucose back to baseline levels?

17. What is the purpose of the food exchange system?

Directions: Match the glucose level in col. B with the appropriate term in col. A.

Column A

18. ____ Hypoglycemia

19. ____ Normal plasma glucose

20. ____ Renal threshold for glucose

21. ____ Hyperglycemia

Column B

a. 160 to 180 mg/100 ml
b. 210 mg/100 ml
c. 40 mg/100 ml
d. 80 to 115 mg/100 ml

Directions: Circle T if the statement is true and F if the statement is false. Correct any false statements.

22. T   F   Heart attacks occur at least 2½ times as frequently in diabetics as in nondiabetics of comparable age.

23. T   F   Twenty-five percent of all diabetics eventually die of vascular disease, heart attacks, kidney failure, strokes, or gangrene.

24. T   F   Exercise tends to increase blood sugar by blocking transport of glucose into the tissues.

25. T   F   Obesity is a frequent finding in patients with NIDDM.

CHAPTER

60

DISORDERS OF THE FEMALE REPRODUCTIVE CYCLE

OBJECTIVES

At the completion of this chapter you should be able to:

1. Describe the function of the hypothalamus and the anterior pituitary gland in ovulation.
2. Describe the anatomical structure of an ovarian follicle.
3. State the process by which a follicle initiates the development cycle.
4. Describe the general biochemical process under which estrogens and progesterone are synthesized.
5. Describe the hormonal endometrial changes which follow the fluctuations during the menstrual cycle.
6. Describe menarche in terms of age of onset, sexual maturation events, and critical body weight.
7. State the hormonal and ovarian changes and associated signs and symptoms that occur during climacteric and menopause.
8. Define primary and secondary amenorrhea.
9. Differentiate between primary and secondary amenorrhea which results from hypothalamic-pituitary failure and gonadal disorders according to etiology, chromosomal abnormality, presenting features, and harmful levels.
10. Explain the importance of the clinical investigation and laboratory assessment of the amenorrheic patient.
11. Explain the rationale for the treatment of the amenorrheic patient.
12. Explain the theories that best describe the pathophysiology of women with premenstrual syndrome (PMS).
13. Describe the relationship between physical training and menstrual dysfunction.
14. Identify factors which determine hair growth patterns in men and women.
15. Describe the typical manifestations of hirsutism and virilism in females.
16. Identify and describe the source, metabolism, and excretion of three types of androgens in men and women.

17. Compare the androgenic potency of dehydroepiandrosterone, Δ4-androstenedione, and testosterone.
18. Identify several possible causes of hirsutism in females.
19. Describe the pathogenesis of adrenal cortical hyperplasia and its consequences in congenital deficiency of C_{21}-hydroxylase.
20. Describe clinical differences among various causes of hirsutism.
21. Describe the treatment of androgen excess.

REGULATION OF THE NORMAL MENSTRUAL CYCLE

A normal menstrual cycle is achieved by the coordinated operation of the central nervous system, the pituitary gland, the ovary, and the uterus. The central nervous system, through the hypothalamus, causes the release of gonadotropin-releasing hormone (GnRH). GnRH reaches the anterior pituitary gland by way of the hypothalamic-hypophyseal portal system and causes the release of the two gonadotropins, follicle-stimulating hormone (FSH) and luteinizing hormone (LH).

OVARIAN FUNCTION

At the time of puberty, the ovary contains about 300,000 follicles. Every month, one of these follicles initiates a developmental cycle under stimulation by pituitary gonadotropins. The follicle consists of an ovum and its two surrounding cell layers. The inner layer of granulosa cells synthesizes progesterone, which is secreted into the follicular fluid during the first half of the menstrual cycle and serves as precursor for estrogen synthesis by the surrounding layer of theca interna cells. Estrogen is synthesized in the luteinized cells of the theca interna. The pathway of estrogen biosynthesis proceeds from progesterone and pregnenolone via 17-hydroxylated derivatives to androstenedione, testosterone, and estradiol. A high content of aromatizing enzyme in these cells facilitates the conversion of androgens to estrogens. Once the developing follicle matures, ovulation occurs and the ovum and surrounding cells are extruded. The granulosa layer becomes vascularized and intensely luteinized, forming the yellow corpus luteum, which is active in progesterone secretion and which lasts for 2 weeks until the termination of that particular cycle.

CYCLIC HORMONE CHANGES

A regular, repetitive monthly occurrence of a menstrual cycle depends on a series of cyclic, well-coordinated steps which involves hormone secretion at various levels of this integrated system. These steps have been carefully studied through daily measurements of the levels of FSH and LH in the blood and levels of estradiol and progesterone in the blood and urine. The changes in the levels of these hormones during a menstrual cycle are illustrated in Fig. 60-1.

The earliest hormonal event responsible for initiating a new cycle is a rise in FSH levels at the end of the luteal phase of the previous cycle. FSH stimulates the secretion of estradiol by the granulosa cells and helps in the development of LH receptors in the ovary. Concomitant with the increase in FSH secretion, serum estradiol levels rise. However, this rise in estradiol causes FSH levels to decline. Estradiol levels continue to increase independently of FSH. LH secretion is maintained at its basal level without significant fluctuations. A further rise in estradiol at midcycle triggers, through a positive feedback effect on the pituitary gland, a peak release of LH and FSH. LH rises more than fivefold above its basal level; the FSH peak is of lower magnitude. This peak release of LH and FSH causes the rupture of the developing ovarian follicle and ovulation. The peak lasts for 2 or 3 days, and the levels of LH and FSH quickly fall back to baseline. FSH levels decline until the end of the luteal phase, when they begin to rise again in preparation for the next cycle. At the same time, LH levels show minor fluctuation.

Following ovulation, estradiol levels promptly drop, but they rise again toward the end of the luteal phase. The major feature of the luteal phase is the activity of the corpus luteum and progesterone secretion, starting within 2 or 3 days of the midcycle peak of LH and FSH and progressing for the next 12 to 14 days until

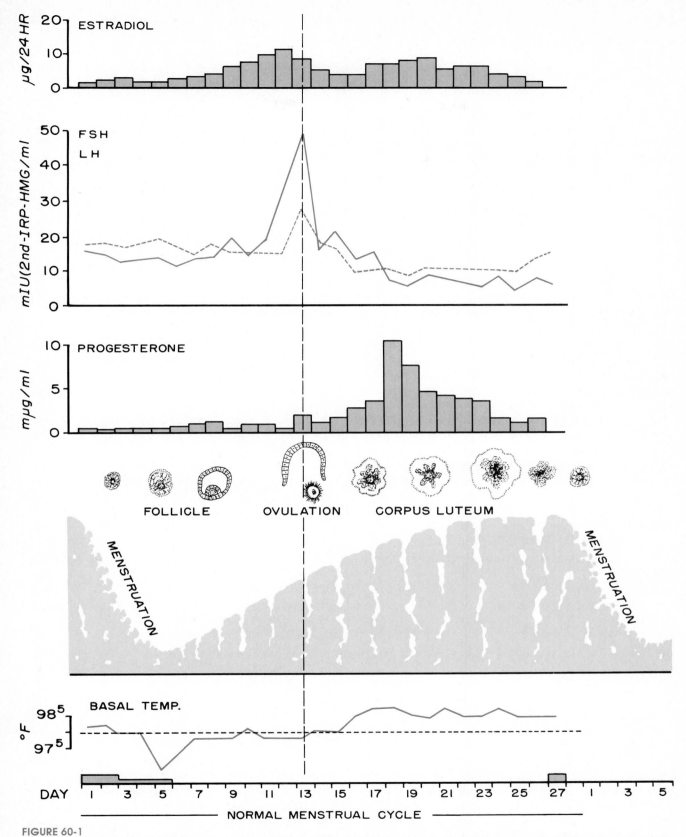

FIGURE 60-1
Change in hormone levels throughout a reproductive cycle in a menstruating normal woman. The horizontal bars on the time scale indicate the occurrence of menses. The interrupted vertical line at midcycle depicts the time of ovulation. Basal body temperature rises during the luteal phase of the cycle, coinciding with the onset of progesterone secretion.

the end of the cycle. At the completion of the cycle, estradiol and progesterone levels fall and menses occurs. The menstrual episode is the culmination of the cyclic changes which occur in the endometrium in coincidence with the changes in estradiol and progesterone secretion.

ENDOMETRIAL CHANGES

At the beginning of the cycle during the follicular phase, the rising levels of estradiol cause endometrial glandular proliferation. During this proliferation phase, the glands and stroma grow at about an equal pace. The glands become longer while maintaining their straight, tubular form. The glandular epithelium is columnar with uniform eosinophilic cytoplasm and central nuclei. The stroma is fairly compact in the basal layer but looser toward the surface. Vessels follow a slightly spiraling course and are of smaller caliber. During the luteal phase, under the influence of progesterone the secretory phase of the endometrium begins. This is characterized by greater and more elaborate convolution of glands and infolding of the glandular epithelium, giving a "sawtooth" appearance. The nuclei of the cells move downward, and the surface of the epithelium acquires a frayed appearance. The stroma becomes edematous. Just preceding menstruation, heavy infiltration with leukocytes occurs and the blood vessels become more and more tightly coiled and dilated. With the drop in estrogen and progesterone levels at the end of the cycle, the superficial layer of the endometrium sheds. The tissue and the blood eliminated in this manner constitute the menstrual flow. Normal menses usually lasts from 3 to 5 days. The cessation of the flow is followed by the development of a new follicular cycle (see Fig. 60-1).

MENARCHE

The onset of menstrual cycles at puberty is called *menarche*. There appears to be a relationship between the onset of the pubertal process and a critical body weight. A minimum body mass seems to be required for the maturation of the hypothalamic-pituitary-ovarian axis. For American girls of European ancestry, the average weight at which menarche occurs is 48 kg. The usual age range for menarche is 11 to 16 years. Menarche is normally preceded by a period of sexual maturation which may span a 2-year period. During this interval, an orderly sequence of events occurs which includes breast development, growth of pubic and axillary hair, and a spurt in somatic linear growth.

During the prepubertal years, the pituitary gonadotropins are at a low level and do not exhibit the cyclic pattern observed in the adult female. Puberty in the female probably begins as a consequence of increased secretion of GnRH by the hypothalamus or increased responsiveness of the pituitary cells to the secretion of hypothalamic GnRH. During early puberty, gonadotropins are released principally during sleep. The peaks of gonadotropin release become more pronounced as puberty advances. This stage of sleep-related gonadotropin release is followed by the normal cyclic release of gonadotropins which characterizes the ovulatory cycle.

CLIMACTERIC AND THE MENOPAUSE

The reproductive phase of life fades out with the gradual decline of ovarian function. This transitional period between the childbearing age and senescence is defined as the *climacteric*. *Menopause*, the cessation of menstruation, is the most important manifestation of the climacteric and usually occurs between ages 47 and 50 years. There are women who may reach menopause at 35 years and others who may continue to menstruate until age 55. Many factors are probably responsible for the age of menopause, but heredity appears to be the most significant.

With the onset of menopause, estradiol levels decrease and the ovary decreases in size and is virtually devoid of follicles. Microscopic examination reveals cortical thinning and a relative thickening of the medulla from increased fibrous connective tissue. Blood vessels at the hilus and medulla become progressively sclerotic. The anatomical involution of the ovary is accompanied by a decrease in its ovulatory and endocrine functions. The decrease in circulating estradiol levels increases by negative feedback pituitary gonadotropin secretion. This increased production of FSH and LH continues for many years after the onset of menopause.

The decline of ovarian function is associated with a variety of symptoms. These symptoms are vasomotor, nervous and psychic, genital and skeletal. The most common symptom is the hot flush, described as a sensation of heat over the body, especially over the face and neck, accompanied by reddening of the skin of these areas. This is often followed by diffuse perspiration and chilliness. These vasomotor disturbances may occur only once or twice a day or as often as every half hour. If they occur at night, they may interfere with the patient's rest. They usually last for a few minutes and are often precipitated by excitement or emotional upset. They are mild to moderate in most women and disappear spontaneously without treatment but may be severe in some women and require therapy. It is estimated that 75 percent of women experience vasomotor flushes in the perimenopausal period or later, and the problem continues for 5 years or more in 20 percent of these women. Physiological concomitants of the hot flush include an acute rise in skin temperature, peripheral vasodilatation, a transient increase in heart rate, fluctuations in the electrocardiographic baseline, and pronounced decrease in skin resistance. The exact cause of this symptom has yet to be determined. The current theory is that decreases in estrogen levels cause instability of the autonomic nervous system, mediated centrally at the hypothalamic level. Of interest is that the hot flush episodes also appear to correlate with the pulsatile pituitary release of luteinizing hormone. However, the exact relationship between the vasomotor symptoms and high gonadotropin levels in menopausal women remains uncertain. For example, an increase in gonadotropins has been observed in menopausal women who have not complained of flushes; the administration of large doses of gonadotropic hormones does not produce vasomotor symptoms; hot flushes are rarely seen in males with elevated gonadotropin levels, and they may be favorably influenced by doses of estrogens too small to inhibit gonadotropin release.

Variable degrees of depression, anxiety, and emotional lability are also associated with the onset of menopause. It is likely that the degree of psychic involvement observed in the climacteric is predetermined largely by the patient's personality characteristics. Some of the psychiatric changes observed during the climacteric may be related to the hormonal changes associated with it. In addition, concern about aging and loss of femininity and reproductive capacity may also have detrimental psychological effects.

Most postmenopausal women experience symptoms referable to atrophy of the urogenital tissues. This is especially evident in the vagina, where the mucosa shrinks and thins to a marked degree and vaginal secretions become scant and less acid. These changes render the vaginal tissues more susceptible to trauma, inflammation, and infection. Atrophic vaginitis, pruritus vulvae, and dyspareunia develop with increasing frequency as the postmenopausal changes progress. Changes in muscle strength and muscle replacement by fibrous connective tissue cause loss of flexibility and easy contractility at the posterior urethra and trigone of the bladder, leading to urgency, incontinence, and frequency. Loss of libido is a common complaint during the climacteric, and the changes in the vaginal mucosa may be associated with discomfort during intercourse.

The incidence of osteoporosis increases for both sexes with age, but in women, loss of bone density accelerates significantly when endogenous estrogen production is reduced by natural or surgical menopause. Because of this complication of aging, 25 percent of white women older than 60 years suffer vertebral compression fractures. The risk of pathological fracture varies with the family history and other poorly defined factors. Fractures of the hip and other bones are even more frequent in elderly women and constitute a major source of morbidity; they are responsible for a mortality rate as high as 15 percent.

Associated with the decrease in estrogen levels, there is an increase in facial or body hair growth. This increase is most likely related to the unopposed effect of circulating androgens and a decrease in androgen binding by sex hormone–binding globulin.

Women in the perimenopausal period should seek medical care and should be encouraged to see a physician at least twice a year. The periodic examination should include a careful physical examination including palpation of the breasts, inspection of the cervix, and a Pap smear for cytologic examination. It should also provide an opportunity for a physician's psychological support, which should be offered to the patient when needed. Although there remain some physicians who oppose treatment for the climacteric woman, most physicians agree that estrogen replacement therapy is beneficial. The use of estrogen therapy in menopausal women poses a small relative risk, but the risk should be balanced against the benefits derived from this type of treatment. The Council on Scientific Affairs of the American Medical Association recommends the following principles in the management of menopause: (1) As with any form of drug therapy, estrogens should be used only for specific indications in the smallest effective doses and for the shortest period that satisfies therapeutic need. (2) Estrogens are effective in the treatment or prevention of vasomotor flushes, atrophic urogenital conditions, and osteoporosis. Recent evidence also supports the protective effect against certain manifestations of arteriosclerotic heart disease. (3) When estrogen is given to menopausal women with intact uteri, cyclic administration is recommended, to avoid continuous stimulation of the endometrium and the possible risk of endometrial carcinoma. A progestin may be added on the last 7 to 10 days of each estrogen cycle, to enhance the spontaneous removal of the proliferated endometrium. (4) Topical estrogen preparations are useful in the treatment of vulvovaginal atrophic symptoms, but the ready absorption through the intact but atrophic epithelial surface requires that cumulative dosage be considered. (5) Any vaginal bleeding in the postmenopausal patient *must* be investigated promptly so that endometrial cancer can be ruled out. (6) At least yearly monitoring of asymptomatic patients treated with estrogens should be performed and may include histological or cytologic sampling. Pelvic and breast examinations and measurements of blood pressure should also be done. (7) Estrogen replacement therapies are specifically contraindicated in those patients with estrogen-dependent neoplasms of the breast or the history of such lesions. (8) As in all therapeutic decisions, the patient should be fully informed of relative risks and benefits before treatment is initiated, and the question of continued need should be reviewed periodically.

In those women where the menopausal symptoms are mild and there is no concern about osteoporosis, the patients may be followed periodically without hormonal therapy and with the use of mild tranquilizing preparations for any psychiatric symptoms attributable to menopause.

PREMENSTRUAL SYNDROME

Definition

Premenstrual syndrome (PMS) is a complex psychoneuroendocrine disorder which results in recurrent temporary disruption of the personal and professional lives of a large number of women throughout their reproductive years. It is not clear to what extent the disorder is primarily a psychological disorder with secondary neuroendocrine manifestations or primarily a neuroendocrine abnormality with secondary psychological consequences. It may start as early as 7 to 10 days before menses and is characterized by a variety of complaints of variable severity. In some women, the symptoms are mild and transient, while in others they are severe and long-lasting. PMS needs to be distinguished from premenstrual exacerbation of other conditions which may be chronically present but are accentuated during the week prior to menstruation.

Clinical presentation

The constellation of symptoms present in PMS appears to be linked to the cyclic activity of the hypothalamic-pituitary-ovarian axis. Symptoms include breast tenderness, lower abdominal bloating, fatigue, emotional lability, and depression. As menses approach, anxiety, restlessness, irritability, and hostility predominate. Although women complain of fullness and swelling, true weight gain and edema are not always clearly demonstrable. As symptoms intensify, some women develop an inability to concentrate, forgetfulness, feelings of impaired judgment, and loss of self confidence. The onset of menses is generally associated with the prompt resolution of psychological symptoms, but the appearance of dysmenorrhea may sometimes prolong the discomfort.

The clinical manifestations of PMS range from mild to severe. However, many women may express reluctance to discuss their symptoms, in particular the psychological ones, with their physicians or gynecologists for fear that these manifestations may be interpreted as expressions of psychoneurosis. It is important for physicians and other health professionals to inquire about premenstrual symptoms when obtaining a detailed menstrual history. Taken in that context, the PMS symptoms are more easily recognized, and the legitimacy of their presence may provide an opportunity for more effective management.

Pathophysiology

Numerous theories have been proposed to explain the pathophysiology of PMS, but none has been conclusively proven. Some of these theories suggest that women with PMS are very sensitive to mild physical changes associated with their menstrual cycle and that they report these changes as very distressing symptoms. In a study in which women were led to believe that their menses would occur at a time other than the actual one, those who thought they were premenstrual reported many more symptoms than those who thought they were intermenstrual. It is also known that placebo medication frequently improves PMS. Other theories propose a neuroendocrine disturbance as the cause of PMS. It was initially thought that, since PMS occurs as the levels of estrogen and progesterone decline prior to menses, the hormonal changes were responsible for the physical and psychological symptoms. Progesterone deficiency was proposed by some investigators as a possible cause of PMS, and this led numerous clinicians to treat PMS with progesterone. However, progesterone levels in women with PMS are not abnormally low, and the doses advocated for the treatment of PMS with progesterone are consistent with its pharmacological rather than physiological action, which through some unknown central effect may explain the apparent amelioration of PMS. It is possible that a change in levels of estrogen and/or progesterone can influence PMS by inciting other neuroendocrine changes or changes in central neurotransmitters capable of affecting brain function.

It has also been postulated that the underlying problem in patients with PMS is fluid retention which, by causing edema at different anatomical levels, causes the varied manifestations of PMS. For example, brain edema could cause depression and irritability; abdominal edema, bloating; etc. However, women who have been closely observed during PMS have not shown definitive weight gain and fluid retention. In the minority of women who show weight gain and edema, other factors, such as excessive ingestion of carbohydrate and salt premenstrually, may lead to this finding. No definitive abnormality has been found in the secretion of mineralocorticoids, with its potential for sodium and water retention, or of vasopressin, with its potential for decreasing free water clearance. Prolactin has been suggested as a possible mediator of sodium and water retention, because it seems to have mineralocorticoid effects in lower animals. Initial reports that prolactin levels were elevated in PMS have not been confirmed in subsequent studies, and the use of pharmacological agents such as bromocriptine that are capable of suppressing prolactin secretion has not been useful in the treatment of PMS. Another theory which requires confirmation is that cyclic changes in endogenous opiate activity occur during the menstrual cycle and that an excessive secretion of opiate peptides may be ultimately responsible for the manifestations of PMS. It has been speculated that estrogen and progesterone acting either alone or in combination can increase central endogenous opiate activity. At the time of maximal exposure to opiates during the luteal phase of the menstrual cycle, depression may result from diminished brain release of norepinephrine or dopamine occasioned by opiate inhibition of biogenic amine systems. Acute withdrawal of opiate inhibition as the menses approach may produce rebound hyperactivity of these neural pathways, resulting in irritability, anxiety, tension, and aggression. Not only opiate hyperactivity may explain the psychological changes observed in PMS, but other manifestations of PMS may also be due to increased levels of endogenous opiates. These include increased appetite and thirst and increased release of vasopressin or prolactin, which may lead to some of the bloating and occasional weight gain that patients manifest, as well as the breast tenderness.

Treatment

The treatments proposed for PMS are as numerous and as varied as the theories of its causes. Numerous therapeutic regimens have been based on anecdotal observations and poorly controlled trials without sufficient consideration for the striking placebo response which is present in this disorder. Since the etiology of PMS remains ill defined, there is no treatment which at present is capable of eliminating all of the symptoms of PMS. The treatment is, therefore, palliative and directed toward the most uncomfortable symptoms expressed by the patient. It is essential to educate both the patient with PMS and her family about the nature of her illness and to reassure them that the symptoms are not all imagined. The patient and her family should allow for modifications of family activities during the period in which the patient is most disabled by her PMS. There is little evidence that oral contraceptive steroids reduce premenstrual symptoms. However, since some women report definite improvement when taking this medication, it seems reasonable to try a low-dose oral contraceptive, particularly in patients who require contraception. Prostaglandin inhibitors such as ibuprofen or naproxen should be used mainly for the treatment of dysmenorrhea and other symptoms such as headache and minor musculoskeletal pains associated with PMS. Diuretic therapy is of some benefit but frequently overprescribed. Potassium-sparing diuretics or spironolactone should be preferred to other, more potent and kaliuretic drugs. Low-carbohydrate diets should be prescribed during the premenstrual period, since these diets are likely to cause diuresis and minimize the feelings of bloating and swelling complained of by the patient. Patients showing marked variations in mood and manic or severe depressive symptoms and those exhibiting psychotic behavior should have the benefit of a complete psychiatric evaluation. Psychotherapy, lithium carbonate, tricyclic antidepressants, and minor tranquilizers have been employed in the treatment of the psychological symptoms associated with PMS; these agents are particularly helpful in patients with predominant psychiatric disorders, but they are relatively ineffective in the treatment of the psychological manifestations of PMS in other types of patients. Both bromocriptine and danazol have proven useful in the treatment of the breast symptoms associated with PMS. Large doses of progesterone and pyridoxine have also been used, with questionable results.

It is possible that, if the role of opiate peptides in the pathogenesis of PMS is confirmed, treatment with long-acting opiate antagonists may be helpful in the treatment of this condition. Similarly, the use of luteinizing hormone–releasing factor (LHRF) agonists and antagonists, which are capable of altering the pituitary ovarian axis, may be of some benefit in the treatment of PMS.

AMENORRHEA

Primary amenorrhea is the failure to begin spontaneous menstruation by the age of 16 years. Secondary amenorrhea is present when a woman who previously had regular cycles has not menstruated for longer than 3 months.

Etiology

Pregnancy is the most common physiological cause of secondary amenorrhea. It should always be ruled out in someone who presents with secondary amenorrhea. In most other instances, secondary amenorrhea is a manifestation of an endocrine disorder. It may, in fact, be the presenting symptom of a number of endocrine syndromes. In patients with hypothalamic or pituitary insufficiency, amenorrhea caused by failure of gonadotropin secretion may precede by several years symptoms of insufficiency of other pituitary tropic hormones.

Uterine malformations or defects should always be ruled out in patients with primary amenorrhea. In the absence of a responsive endometrium, menses do not occur even in the presence of an otherwise intact hypothalamic-pituitary-ovarian axis. Causes of secondary amenorrhea may appear early in the course of pubertal development and may lead to an apparent primary amenorrhea, since menarche fails to develop.

Primary amenorrhea may occur as the result of (1) hypothalamic-pituitary failure or (2) gonadal disorders. Isolated gonadotropin deficiency and panhypopituitarism, either idiopathic or as a result of hypothalamic (craniopharyngioma) or pituitary tumors, may result in insufficient secretion of GnRH or pituitary gonadotropins. Patients with isolated gonadotropin deficiency fail to go through puberty or to exhibit normal menstrual cycles. In the these patients, other indices of hypothalamic-pituitary function are normal. In contrast, patients with panhypopituitarism show, in addition to primary amenorrhea, evidence of growth hormone, thyroid-stimulating hormone (TSH), and adrenocorticotropic hormone (ACTH) insufficiency. They present with dwarfism, hypothyroidism, and secondary adrenal insufficiency.

Gonadal disorders accounting for primary amenorrhea include gonadal dysgenesis (Turner's syndrome) and the syndrome of testicular feminization. In patients with gonadal dysgenesis, the ovaries have been replaced by streaks due to a chromosomal abnormality resulting in the deletion of one of the X chromosomes in all the body cells (46,XO karyotype) or in some of the body cells, including the gonad (46,XO/XX mosaics). Patients with Turner's syndrome present with a characteristic phenotype, including short stature (<5 ft), webbed neck, cubitus valgus, shieldlike chest, and foreshortened fourth metacarpals or metatarsals (Fig. 60-2). Lymphedema is present in the newborn baby with this syndrome. Because of the failure of estrogen production in a subject with an otherwise intact anterior pituitary gland, low estradiol levels are associated with high levels of FSH and LH.

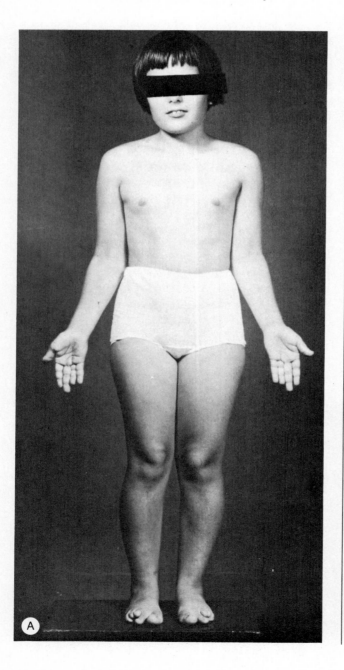

FIGURE 60-2

Appearance of a patient with gonadal dysgenesis (Turner's syndrome). She has a 46,XO/XX mosiac karyotype. To be noted are: (A) the cubitus valgus, broad chest, widely set nipples, and foreshortened fourth and fifth digits in both hands, and (B) the upward growth of nuchal hair.

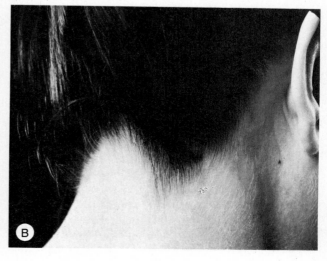

Patients with testicular feminization have a 46,XY karyotype but are phenotypically female. They have functioning testes in the abdomen or in the inguinal canals which secrete normal male levels of testosterone. However, the circulating testosterone is ineffective in causing masculinization of the fetus because of a complete or partial absence of testosterone receptors in the cytoplasm of target cells. Since testosterone is also ineffective at the hypothalamic level, serum LH and FSH levels are elevated. In the complete form of this disorder, the patient has scanty pubic hair and normal breast development. These subjects are usually raised as females and are well adjusted to their gender.

Secondary amenorrhea

Patients with secondary amenorrhea may also suffer from (1) hypothalamic-pituitary disease or (2) a gonadal disorder. Hypothalamic-pituitary disorders causing secondary amenorrhea result from (1) hyperprolactinemia and pituitary tumors, (2) changes in body weight, (3) oral contraceptives, (4) isolated gonadotropin deficiency, and (5) psychic stress.

Prolactin-secreting pituitary adenomas causing galactorrhea-amenorrhea syndrome have been described in Chap. 54. Changes in body weight such as marked weight loss or weight gain can lead to cessation of menstrual periods. In patients with weight loss caused by anorexia nervosa, a regression to the prepubertal pattern of release of gonadotropins has been observed. The loss of the adult pattern of LH secretion appears to be related to a diminished secretion of GnRH by the hypothalamus. All anorectic patients are amenorrheic when their body weight drops below 75 percent of normal. Menstrual cycles return to normal when body weight is regained. The menstrual irregularity and amenorrhea seen in obesity are not well understood. Increased aromatization of androgens to estrogens in adipose tissue may lead to increased levels of estrogens in these patients and interference with the normal hypothalamic feedback control mechanism.

The use of oral contraceptives may lead to secondary amenorrhea. A large number of women in the United States and around the world take oral contraceptives for years at a time. Amenorrhea, after oral contraceptives are stopped, may occur in 1 to 2 percent of patients. In half of these patients, the amenorrhea is due to a specific endocrine disorder, and the withdrawal bleeding induced by the oral contraceptives has simply masked the appearance of amenorrhea. In other patients who present with this type of amenorrhea, a specific cause is not found. They fall into the category of hypothalamic amenorrhea. Gonadotropin levels in these patients are low or normal, but normal cyclic changes do not occur. The disorder is often self-limited, and 80 percent of the patients resume menstruation within 12 months.

Psychic stress is the most common cause of secondary amenorrhea. This occurs in patients who suffer from marked emotional distress as a result of major changes in their life patterns, such as traveling, separation, and environmental changes. During World War II, many nurses who were sent overseas on military duty failed to menstruate until they returned home. Young women who go away to college and leave home for the first time frequently develop amenorrhea which may last for many months. Serum LH, FSH, and estradiol levels in these patients are normal or low as seen in other forms of hypothalamic amenorrhea. As is the case with the post-oral-contraceptive amenorrhea, the problem is often self-limited and menses resume within 6 to 12 months.

In some women, amenorrhea results from gonadotropin deficiency which is not accompanied by failure of secretion of other pituitary-tropic hormones. This isolated gonadotropin deficiency is believed to result from a partial or complete deficiency of hypothalamic GnRH secretion. The disorder may be associated with other congenital defects such as anosmia (as in Kallmann's syndrome), harelip and cleft palate, and color blindness. Pituitary function in these patients is otherwise normal, and gonadotropin secretion may occur in response to repetitive stimulation with exogenous GnRH.

The most common gonadal causes of secondary amenorrhea are polycystic ovarian disease and ovarian failure in women who experience premature menopause. Patients with polycystic ovarian disease (PCOD) present with a history of hirsutism, starting in early teen age, and irregular menses. Hirsutism is frequently progressive over the years, and menses may become increasingly irregular. Amenorrhea may eventually develop. Obesity is a common feature of this disorder. The ovaries are enlarged, with multiple cysts and a thickened and glistening capsule. This constellation of findings is called the *Stein-Leventhal syndrome*. Serum testosterone and dehydroepiandrosterone levels are elevated; estradiol levels are normal or elevated, and serum LH levels are increased, with an abnormal and sustained pattern of release. Stein-Leventhal syndrome results from excessive ovarian androgen secretion. In addition, 20 to 30 percent of these patients have combined ovarian and adrenal androgen overproduction.

Premature menopause may occur in women in the third or fourth decade of life. It has the clinical characteristics of the menopause which occurs physiologically in older women. The cause of premature ovarian failure appears to be autoimmune destruction of the ovaries. This condition is often associated with other types of autoimmune endocrinopathy, including Addison's disease, Hashimoto's thyroiditis, hypoparathyroidism, and pernicious anemia.

Physical training and menstrual dysfunction

Female athletes have an increased incidence of oligomenorrhea and amenorrhea and a later age of menarche compared with the general population. Studies obtained in premenarche-trained athletes have indicated a mean menarcheal age several years older than in postmenarche-trained athletes. In addition, of the premenarche-trained athletes, 61 percent had irregular menstrual cycles and 22 percent were amenorrheic, whereas 60 percent of postmenarche-trained athletes had regular menstrual cycles and none were amenorrheic. Physical training increases the incidence of oligomenorrhea and amenorrhea among both premenarche- and postmenarche-trained athletes. The exact physiological basis for this phenomenon is not known, but it has been suggested that a minimum weight for height, representing a critical lean/fat ratio, is necessary for menarche and for the maintenance of regular ovulatory cycles. Women with anorexia nervosa who lose 10 to 15 percent of their body weight become amenorrheic. Weight gain above the critical level restores normal menses after varying intervals of time. Since human female adipose tissue converts androgen to estrogen, the adipose tissue is a significant extragonadal source of estrogen. Therefore, fatness also affects the pathway of metabolism of estrogen to its most potent or least potent form. The amount of adipose tissue may, therefore, directly affect hormonal regulation of short-term or long-term feedback mechanisms controlling the menstrual cycle and ovulation. Athletes with a very low fat/lean ratio may undergo suppression of the neurohypothalamic-pituitary axis through a decrease in estrogen levels. In addition, these women may also exhibit suppression of gonadotropin release by psychogenic factors related to the stress of competition and intense training.

Clinical investigation of the amenorrheic patient

The clinical investigation of the amenorrheic patient should focus on important historical clues which may lead to the differential diagnosis of the type of amenorrhea present. A history of normal development of secondary sexual characteristics and onset of menarche followed by amenorrhea rules out primary gonadal disorders such as gonadal dysgenesis or testicular feminization syndrome. The presence of hirsutism in an amenorrheic patient should raise the possibility of a vi-rilizing syndrome or polycystic ovarian disease. A history of hot flushes associated with cessation of menses suggests early menopause. The presence of galactorrhea suggests hyperprolactinemia and a prolactin-secreting pituitary adenoma. A recent history of weight loss may easily explain the onset of secondary amenorrhea. The presence of emotional factors may be important for the diagnosis of psychogenic amenorrhea. Symptoms of deficiency of other pituitary tropic hormones suggest amenorrhea associated with panhypopituitarism.

Laboratory assessment of amenorrhea

The first step is to determine whether the hormonal failure is due to a hypothalamic-pituitary problem or to a gonadal disorder. This is assessed by measurement of serum FSH. If the serum FSH is repeatedly elevated, the patient most likely has primary ovarian failure. If the serum FSH is normal or low, the problem most likely lies in the hypothalamus or the pituitary gland. In this case, evaluation of thyroid and adrenal function may determine if the patient has isolated gonadotropin deficiency or panhypopituitarism. In the presence of galactorrhea, a serum prolactin level should be obtained. An x-ray examination of the pituitary fossa and computerized axial tomography of the pituitary gland may help determine if the patient has a pituitary tumor with or without suprasellar extension. In patients in whom the amenorrhea is associated with hirsutism, measurement of urinary 17-ketosteroids and serum testosterone and dehydroepiandrosterone should be carried out. Levels are usually elevated in patients with excessive androgen secretion. More specific tests to determine the source of the excessive secretion of androgens include a pelvic examination, laparoscopy, adrenal scintiscanning, and abdominal CAT scanning. Ultimately, selective catheterization and sampling of blood from the adrenal and gonadal veins may help localize the source of androgen hypersecretion.

Treatment of the amenorrheic patient

Treatment of amenorrhea is often based on the type of underlying pathology causing the problem. Patients with prolactin-secreting pituitary adenomas should be treated with either transsphenoidal resection of the pituitary tumor or suppression of prolactin secretion with bromocriptine. Patients with excessive androgen secretion should receive suppressive therapy with corticosteroids or oral contraceptives. Both of these preparations are capable of suppressing the excessive secretion of androgens, probably by inhibiting gonadotropin release.

Patients with hypothalamic-pituitary or ovarian deficiency should receive replacement therapy with estrogens and progesterone administered in a cyclic fashion. Physiological doses of estrogens are given for the first 21 days of each month, and physiological doses of progesterone from days 15 to 21 of each month. With-drawal uterine bleeding follows within 5 to 7 days after interruption of hormone therapy. Combined treatment with estrogens and progesterone helps maintain secondary sexual characteristics and prevent vaginal and breast atrophy and osteopenia. Therapy can be continued through the expected time of menopause (age 40 to 47).

Patients with primary gonadal disorders remain infertile. However, ovulation can be induced and fertility restored in some women with isolated gonadotropin deficiency, PCOD, post-oral-contraceptive or psychogenic amenorrhea, or amenorrhea following weight loss, after patients have regained weight. Ovulation and fertility can be obtained with clomiphene citrate, a nonsteroidal compound which has both estrogenic and antiestrogenic properties, depending on the site of action. In the hypothalamus, clomiphene blocks estradiol receptors and probably, as the result of increased GnRH secretion, causes secretion of LH and to a lesser extent FSH from the pituitary. The drug may also increase pituitary sensitivity to GnRH, resulting in increased LH output. The drug is given in doses of 50 to 100 mg per day for 5 to 7 days. In responsive patients, ovulation occurs 4 to 8 days and menstruation 14 to 21 days after clomiphene has been stopped. Several courses of treatment may be necessary before ovulation and fertility or normal menstrual cycles are established. An otherwise intact pituitary gland is required for a positive response to therapy.

In patients with hypopituitarism or pituitary tumors, fertility can be restored by treatment with human FSH and human chorionic gonadotropin (HCG), which acts like LH. This therapy is expensive and requires careful control of dosage and estradiol response to avoid multiple pregnancies or the production of ovarian cysts.

SYNDROMES OF ANDROGEN EXCESS

One of the most common problems seen by the endocrinologist among young women is hirsutism. It is the simplest and earliest clinical expression of androgen excess.

It is well documented that there is a complex relationship between the growth of hair in men and women and sex hormones. For example, the growth of beard; hair in the ears, nasal tip, and upper pubic triangle; and coarse hair over the trunk and limbs are dependent upon adult male levels of circulating androgens. The growth of hair at the axilla, lower pubic region, and, in part at least, the limbs is initiated by pubertal events in both sexes and is mediated by weaker adrenal androgens. Androgen-type hair is coarse and dark. Certain

hair growth appears to be independent of sex hormones. This hair is fine and light in color and includes the lanugal hair, the eyebrows, and the eyelashes.

Hirsutism is defined as excessive growth of body hair in the female in a characteristic masculine distribution over the facial, periareolar, abdominal, and sacral areas (see Fig. 60-3). It may be associated with baldness (see Fig. 60-4) or temporal recession of the hairline (see Fig. 60-5). It may be present by itself or be part of a virilizing syndrome, which is the clinical picture observed in girls and women of all ages with signs and symptoms of defeminization and masculinization. The characteristic findings in defeminization include amenorrhea, decrease in libido, atrophy of the breasts, and loss of feminine body contour. Masculinization includes hirsutism, seborrhea, acne, deepening of the voice, increased muscular development, and enlargement of the clitoris (see Fig. 60-6).

True virilism is currently recognized as a rare condition, almost always associated with adrenal or ovarian tumors or with the syndrome of congenital adrenal hyperplasia. In contrast, hirsutism—often without any other signs of virilism but frequently accompanied by

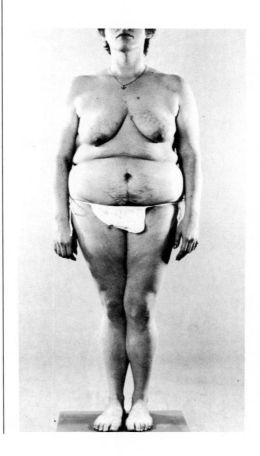

FIGURE 60-3
Hirsutism in the female. Excess of body hair over the breasts, abdomen, and extremities.

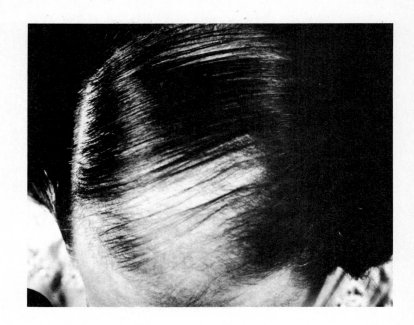

irregular or absent menstrual periods and acne—is a common clinical entity. While it is often thought that simple hirsutism is a mild form of virilism because it has a similar cause, no specific hormonal abnormality or etiological mechanism has been found as the sole cause of

these types of hirsutism. Ethnic and genetic factors play an important role in the development of hair growth patterns. However, there is evidence that androgen excess is present in most cases of hirsutism.

Androgen physiology

Various types of androgens are normally secreted by both men and women. The three major types are (1) dehydroepiandrosterone (DHEA), (2) Δ 4-androstenedione, and (3) testosterone (see Fig. 60-7).

Dehydroepiandrosterone and its metabolites, dehydroepiandrosterone sulfate and androstenediol, are

FIGURE 60-5
Recession of the hairline in a woman with androgen excess. Note the excessive facial hair growth over the upper lip, chin, and sideburn areas.

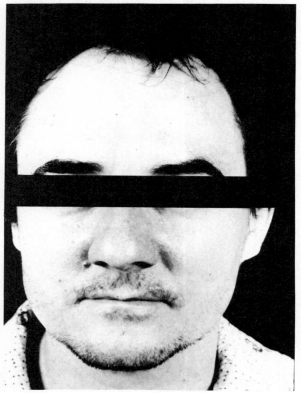

FIGURE 60-6
Clitoral enlargement in a woman with androgen excess.

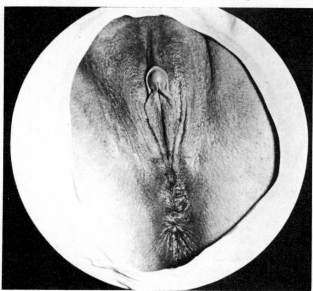

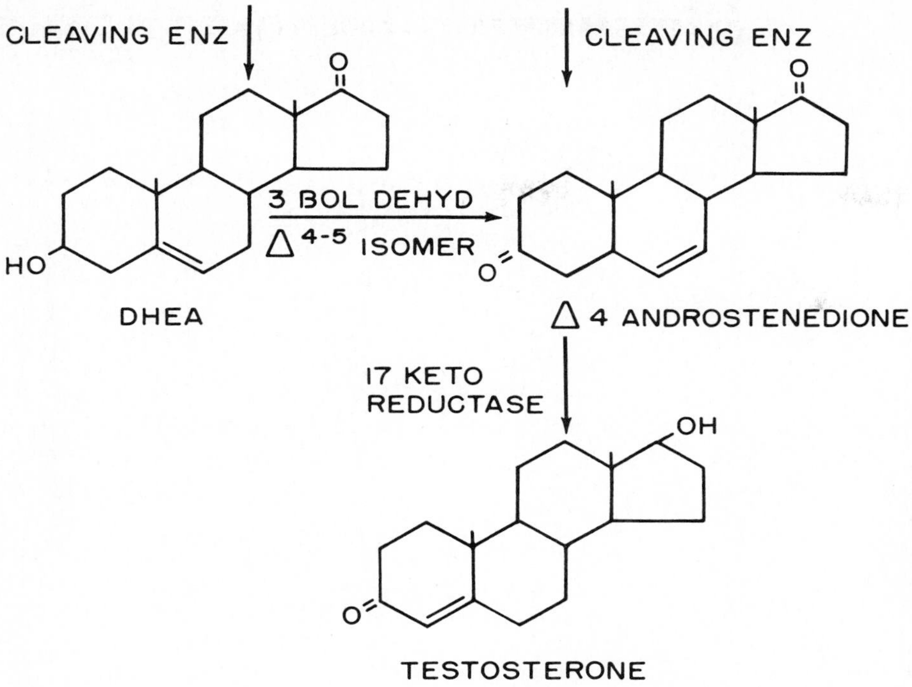

FIGURE 60-7

Three major types of androgens in the female. 17-α-Hydroxypregnenolone is the immediate precursor of DHEA, while 17α-hydroxyprogesterone is the immediate precursors of Δ4-androstenedione. The transformation of the precursor to the androgen hormones is catalyzed by a cleaving enzyme. Δ4-Androstenedione can, in turn, be converted to testosterone by a step catalyzed by 17-ketoreductase.

generally considered to be weak androgens. The adrenal is the main source of this type of androgen, although the ovary also contributes to the level of androstenediol. These androgens can be measured in the urine as 17-ketosteroids, of which dehydroepiandrosterone makes up 60 percent of the total.

Δ 4-Androstenedione is a stronger androgen product than dehydroepiandrosterone but weaker than testosterone, of which it is a precursor. Like dehydroepiandrosterone, Δ 4-androstenedione is also produced by the adrenal cortex and the ovary.

Testosterone is the most potent of the three androgen compounds. There are several sources of testosterone, including the adrenal cortex, the ovary, the testes, and peripheral tissues. Testosterone is metabolized to a potent androgen, dihydrotestosterone (DHT); finally, both testosterone and DHT may be converted to androstenediol in peripheral tissues and excreted as such in the urine.

Testosterone can be produced in several endocrine and peripheral tissues from precursors. It circulates in the plasma partially bound to a carrier protein [sex hormone–binding globulin (SHBG)], and it is removed through metabolic degradation in the liver and other peripheral tissues (see Fig. 60-8). Testosterone levels are therefore a balance between production and metabolic clearance. While a large portion of circulating androgens is bound to SHBG, a small fraction is present in a free state. The biological effects of circulating androgens are related to the levels of free androgens in plasma. Women with hirsutism usually present with abnormalities in testosterone secretion and metabolism. For example, in normal women testosterone is extracted and metabolized almost in its entirety by the liver; in contrast, in virilized women 32 percent of secreted testosterone is extracted and metabolized by extrahepatic peripheral tissues. These tissues are then subject to greater androgenic activity than that found in normal women. Similarly, hirsute women have less testosterone binding, higher free testosterone levels, and more active metabolic clearance rates than women without hirsutism.

Differential diagnosis of androgen excess

Four major categories of conditions are associated with androgen excess: (1) adrenal cortical, (2) ovarian, (3) sim-

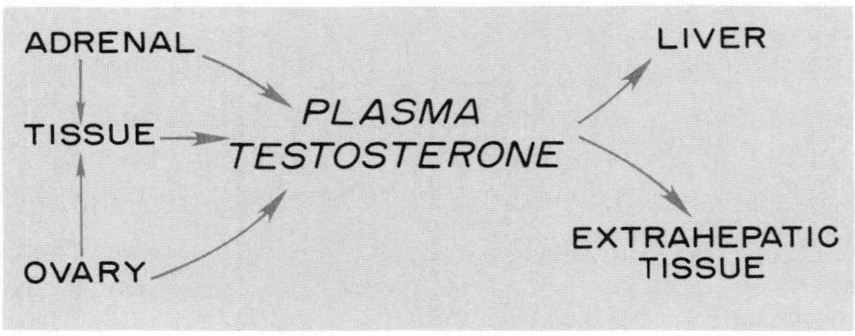

FIGURE 60-8

Metabolism of plasma testosterone. The plasma level of testosterone results from a balance between adrenal, ovarian, and peripheral tissue production of testosterone and clearance by the liver and extrahepatic tissues.

ple or idiopathic hirsutism, and (4) miscellaneous states (see Table 60-1).

Among the adrenal cortical states associated with androgen excess is Cushing's syndrome. In Cushing's syndrome manifestations of androgen excess are superimposed on signs and symptoms of cortisol excess.

Clinically, patients demonstrate coarse, dark hair growth; balding; deepening of the voice; and occasional clitoral enlargement. Biochemically, they demonstrate high urinary 17-ketosteroids and high levels of dehydroepiandrosterone and androstenediol. Androgen excess is found most commonly among the ACTH-dependent type of Cushing's syndrome and in patients with adrenal carcinoma.

There are adrenocortical disorders associated with androgen excess only and with normal secretion of cortisol. Prenatally, such a disorder is found in patients with congenital adrenal hyperplasia. In this condition there is an inborn defect in one of the enzymes involved in cortisol biosynthesis. The most common type is a defect in 21-hydroxylase (see Fig. 60-9). As a consequence of 21-hydroxylase deficiency the adrenal cortex has an impaired capacity to secrete cortisol. The decrease in

cortisol production causes an increase in ACTH secretion in response to the negative feedback activation of pituitary function. ACTH stimulates the adrenal cortex in such a manner that the precursors of cortisol biosynthesis prior to the deficient step are shunted to the biosynthesis of androgens (see Fig. 60–10). When the fetus is exposed to increased androgen production, it undergoes changes in the development of the external genitalia. For example, a female fetus with this defect develops an enlargement of the clitoris and fusion of the labia majora. The genitalia then resemble male external genitalia. At the time of birth this ambiguity in sexual development may create difficulties in sexual identification of the newborn. The syndrome of a masculinized genetic female fetus caused by androgen excess in utero is called *female pseudohermaphroditism* (see Fig. 60-11).

Manifestations of androgen excess of adrenal origin can also develop postnatally and before puberty. Such a condition may be the result of late manifestation of congenital andrenal hyperplasia as described above or of an androgen-secreting adrenal carcinoma. Finally, the clinical picture of androgen excess may develop at puberty or after puberty. It may be part of the syndrome of polycystic ovaries or may be secondary to an adrenal carcinoma.

Several ovarian conditions can cause androgen excess. Tumors of the ovary such as arrhenoblastomas and hilus-cell neoplasms are capable of secreting large amounts of testosterone. Other types of androgens are seen in patients with these tumors, depending on the cell type involved. Manifestations of androgen excess can also be seen in patients with Leydig-cell hyperplasia. These patients usually have high plasma testosterone levels. Occasionally masculinization in association with Leydig-cell hyperplasia and Leydig-cell tumors is seen in patients with gonadal dysgenesis, a sex chromosome abnormality leading to abnormal development of the ovaries.

In polycystic ovary syndrome, hirsutism is frequently associated with infertility, amenorrhea, obesity, and enlarged ovaries. In these patients, testosterone production rates are clearly increased and are responsible for the manifestations of androgen excess. The increased production of androgens in the polycystic ovary syndrome may result from biosynthetic defects in the production of estrogens or from abnormalities in the physiological cyclic release of gonadotropins. Patients with polycystic ovary syndrome frequently present with sustained elevations of serum luteinizing hormone. These changes in gonadotropin secretion may lead to anatomical changes in the ovary and stimulation of ovarian androgen production.

Many women present with hirsutism without any other clinical manifestations of androgen excess. The problem usually begins after puberty and progresses slowly over a period of years. Patients may or may not have menstrual irregularities and may or may not pres-

TABLE 60-1

ANDROGEN EXCESS: DIFFERENTIAL DIAGNOSIS

  I. Androgen excess of adrenal cortical origin
    A. Cortisol excess: Cushing's syndrome
    B. Androgen excess only
        1. Prenatal: congenital adrenal hyperplasia (CAH)
        2. Postnatal: prepubertal
          a Late manifestations of CAH
          b Carcinoma
        3. Pubertal or postpubertal
          a Hyperplasia, with or without polycystic ovaries
          b Carcinoma
 II. Androgen excess of ovarian origin
    A. Neoplasms: arrhenoblastoma, adrenal rest cell neoplasms, hilus cell neoplasms, luteoma
    B. Hilus-cell or Leydig-cell hyperplasia
    C. Polycystic ovary syndrome
III. Simple or idiopathic hirsutism
IV. Miscellaneous causes
    A. Endocrine
        1. Acromegaly
        2. Pregnancy
        3. Hypothyroidism
        4. Menopause
        5. Androgen therapy
        6. Inanition
    B. Nonendocrine
        1. Immobilization
        2. Body cast
        3. Porphyria
        4. Congenital ectodermal dysplasia

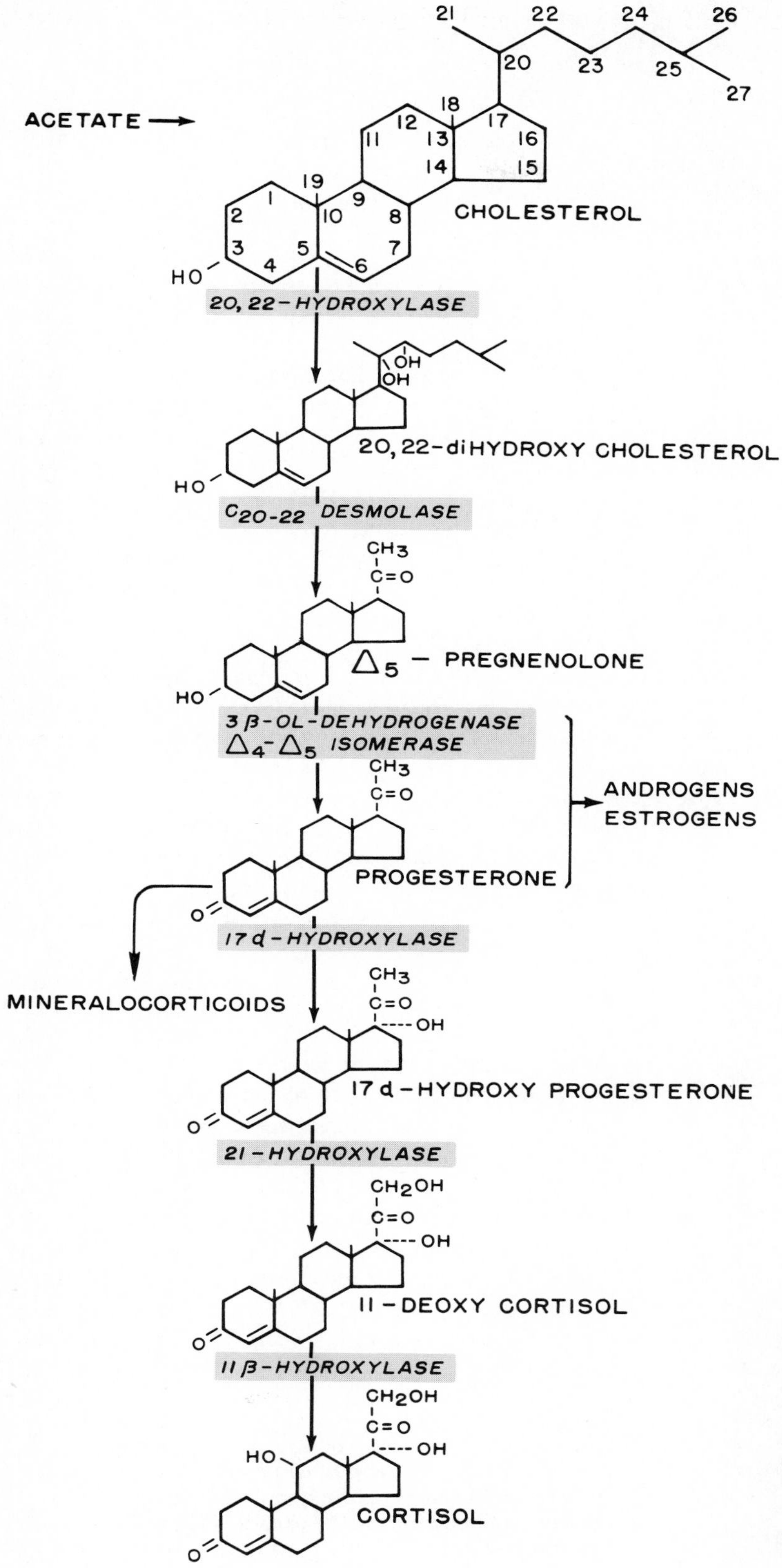

FIGURE 60-9
Pathway of cortisol biosynthesis. Δ5-Pregnenolone and progesterone are also precursors of androgens and estrogens. Progesterone is also a precursor of mineralocorticoids. The biosynthesis of cortisol takes place in the adrenal cortex. Each step is controlled by specific enzymes. A defect in 21-hydroxylase is the cause of the most common type of congenital adrenal hyperplasia.

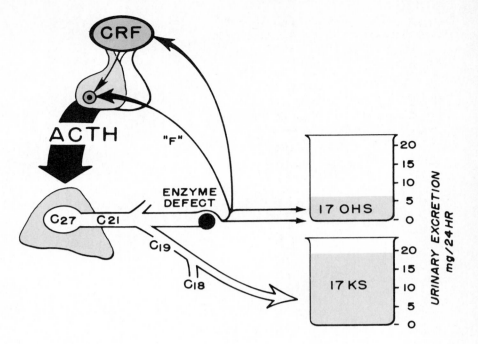

ent with polycystic ovaries. Urinary 17-ketosteroids are frequently slightly or moderately elevated, and testosterone production rates are increased. Free testosterone levels are also elevated. The specific biochemical defect and pathophysiology of this type of androgen excess are not well understood.

There are a number of miscellaneous causes of hirsutism. Some of them are of endocrine origin and include the hirsutism associated with acromegaly, pregnancy, hypothyroidism, menopause, androgen therapy, and inanition. Increased hair growth may occur without hormonal stimulation. It is seen in disorders such as porphyria and congenital ectodermal dysplasia or in areas of the body which have been either immobilized or placed in a body cast.

Clinical and laboratory evaluation of hirsute women

If a patient presents with complaints of excessive hair growth, it is necessary to determine whether the hirsutism is present by itself or accompanied by manifestations of virilization as described above. It is also important to determine whether the symptoms are those of androgen excess alone or are accompanied by symptoms of cortisol excess. A history of recent onset and rapid progression of excessive hair growth frequently suggests a malignancy as the source of excessive androgen production. In that case, one should suspect either an adrenal or ovarian tumor and perform such procedures as a

FIGURE 60-11
Female pseudohermaphroditism in a patient with congenital adrenal hyperplasia due to 21-hyrdoxylase deficiency. This patient had a male phenotype but was genetic female. Note the masculine muscle development and body hair growth. On casual examination the patient appeared to have a developed penis. However, on closer examination this penis was seen to be an enlarged clitoris. The patient also had developed gynecomastia as a result of increased estrogen production accompanying the androgen excess.

pelvic examination, laparoscopy, adrenal venography, and adrenal photoscanning in order to confirm or rule out this diagnosis. In patients with simple idiopathic hirsutism, measurements of androgens in the urine and plasma help confirm the presence of excessive androgen production. If one desires to identify the source of the androgens, suppression tests with glucocorticoids, estrogens, and progestogens as well as ovarian and adrenal vein catheterization for measurement of regional androgen levels may help distinguish between adrenal and ovarian sources.

Treatment

The treatment of states of androgen excess relates to the underlying pathology. If androgen excess is part of Cushing's syndrome, correction of Cushing's syndrome in the manner described in Chap. 57 result in remission of the manifestations of androgen excess. Congenital adrenal hyperplasia can be effectively suppressed by chronic suppressive therapy with glucocorticoid analogues. Patients with adrenal or ovarian tumors should undergo resection of these tumors. Patients with simple or idiopathic hirsutism can be treated by androgen suppression with (1) oral contraceptives, (2) synthetic corticosteroids, (3) spironolactone, or (4) antiandrogens.

QUESTIONS

Disorders of the female reproductive cycle

Directions: Circle the letter preceding each item below that correctly answers the question. More than one answer may be correct.

1. The cyclic events associated with a normal menstrual cycle are regulated by the:
   a. Cerebral cortex and the adrenal gland
   b. Parathyroid glands   c. Hypothalamus and the anterior pituitary gland   d. Cerebellum

2. During the first half of the menstrual cycle estrogen is synthesized in the:
   a. Follicular fluid   b. Luteinized cells in the theca interna   c. Inner layer of granulosa cells
   d. Granulosa cells of the corpus luteum

3. The earliest hormonal event responsible for initiating a new cycle at the end of the luteal phase is a:
   a. Decrease in follicle-stimulating hormone
   b. Increase in serum estradiol levels   c. Increase in luteinizing hormone   d. Increase in follicle-stimulating hormone

4. Which of the following are characteristic signs and symptoms of gonadal dysgenesis (Turner's syndrome):
   a. Short stature (less than 5 ft)   b. Scanty pubic hair   c. Webbed neck   d. Cubitus valgus

5. Testicular feminization is associated with which of the following chromosomal defects?
   a. 46,XO/XX mosaics   b. 46,XO karyotype
   c. 46,XY karyotype

6. The most common cause of secondary amenorrhea is:
   a. Use of oral contraceptives   b. Changes in body weight   c. Psychic stress   d. Pituitary tumors   e. Pregnancy

7. A 25-year-old obese female presents with premature menopause. A pregnancy test is negative. History reveals hirsutism diagnosed at age 13 and irregular menses. Physical examination reveals enlarged ovaries with multiple cysts; serum testosterone and dehydroepiandrosterone levels are elevated, estradiol levels are normal, and serum LH levels are increased. The above data are suggestive of:
   a. Turner's syndrome   b. Panhypopituitarism
   c. Polycystic ovarian disease   d. Primary hypothyroidism

8. In postmenopausal women, the most common signs and symptoms associated with atrophy of the urogenital tissue include:
   a. Decreased vaginal secretions   b. Increased acidity of vaginal secretions   c. Dyspareunia
   d. Atrophic vaginitis

9. A 52-year-old woman with an intact uterus presents with erratic, episodic menstrual bleeding for the past 18 months. Initial treatment includes progestin on the last 7 days of each estrogen cycle. The *primary* rationale for this regime is to:
   a. Reduce vasomotor flushes   b. Prevent osteoporosis   c. Prevent atrophic urogenital conditions   d. Enhance the spontaneous removal of the proliferated endometrium

10. Which of the following theories best describes the pathophysiology of women with premenstrual syndrome:
    a. Progesterone levels are abnormally low and require pharmacological treatment with progesterone   b. Elevated prolactin levels are responsible for the salt and water retention, and bromocriptine has been found to be an effective

treatment   *c.* Evidence suggests that cyclic changes in endogenous opiate activity during the menstrual cycle, along with excessive secretion of opiate peptides, may have a role in the manifestations of PMS   *d.* Premenstrual symptoms may be reduced by a regime of low-dose oral contraceptives, particularly in patients who require contraception

11. A female with hirsutism may present with which of the following signs and symptoms?
    a. Amenorrhea, or irregular menstrual period
    b. Increased breast size   *c.* Hair growth under the chin   *d.* Increased fertility

12. Androstenedione, a steroid precursor of testosterone, is:
    a. Produced in the ovary and adrenal cortex of adult females   *b.* Produced only in the male testes   *c.* A 17-ketosteroid   *d.* Present in higher concentration in the plasma of hirsute and virilized females   *e.* A less potent androgen than dehydroepiandrosterone

13. Congenital adrenal hyperplasia, of the 21-hydroxylase variety, is characterized by:
    a. A masculinized genetic female fetus   *b.* A feminized genetic male fetus   *c.* High ACTH levels   *d.* Low serum cortisol levels   *e.* Increased urinary 17-ketosteroids

14. Which of the following conditions may result in excessive androgen production?
    a. Polycystic ovary syndrome   *b.* Arrhenoblastoma   *c.* Adrenal carcinoma   *d.* Hilus-cell tumor of the ovary

15. Manifestations of virilism include all of the following except:
    a. Acne   *b.* Receding hairline, balding   *c.* Decreased body hair growth   *d.* Clitoral enlargement   *e.* Deepening of voice

Directions: Circle T if the statement is true and F if it is false. Correct any flase statements.

16.   T   F   At puberty, the ovary contains about 100,000 follicles.

17.   T   F   A follicle initiates a development cycle under stimulation by pituitary gonadotropins.

18.   T   F   Following ovulation, estradiol levels immediately rise.

19.   T   F   During the follicular phases of the menstrual cycle endometrial glandular proliferation occurs.

20.   T   F   Secondary amenorrhea is the failure to begin spontaneous menstruation by age 16.

21.   T   F   Climacteric is the transitional period between the childbearing age and senescence.

22.   T   F   A deficiency of 21-hydroxylase causes an increase in cortisol production and decrease in ACTH secretion.

23.   T   F   Prostaglandin inhibitors are used for symptoms associated with PMS, such as weight gain and fluid retention.

24.   T   F   Any vaginal bleeding in the postmenopausal patient must be investigated promptly to rule out endometrial cancer.

25.   T   F   In menopausal women osteoporosis accelerates significantly because of the decrease in endogenous estrogen production.

Directions: Answer the following questions on a separate sheet of paper.

26. What is the apparent relationship between the onset of the pubertal process and a critical body weight?

27. What are the hormonal and ovarian changes which occur during menopause?

28. Explain the rationale for the treatment of the amenorrheic patient.

29. Briefly describe a current theory that reflects on the etiology of hot flushes as a common symptom of menopause.

30. Explain the postulated physiological basis for increased incidence of oligomenorrhea and amenorrhea in female athletes.

REFERENCES FOR PART IX

BAXTER, J. D. and P. H. FORSHAM: "Tissue Effects of Glucocorticoids," *American Journal of Medicine*, **53**(5):573–589, November 1972.

CATT, K. J.: *An ABC of Endocrinology*, Little, Brown, Boston, 1971.

Council on Scientific Affairs: "Estrogen Replacement in

the Menopause", JAMA, **249**(3):359–361, January 21, 1983

EDIS, A. J., L. A. AYALA, and R. H. EGDAHL: *Manual of Endocrine Surgery*, Springer-Verlag, New York, 1984, pp. 66–88.

EZRIN, C., J. L. GOODEN, R. VOLPE, and R. WILSON (eds.): *Systematic Endocrinology*, 2d ed., Harper & Row, Hagerstown, Md., 1979.

FRISCH, R. E., et al.; "Delayed Menarche and Amenorrhea of College Athletes in Relation to Age of Onset of Training," *JAMA*, **246**(14):1559–1563, October 2, 1981.

GANNON, L.: "Evidence for a Psychological Etiology of Menstrual Disorders: A Critical Review," *Psychological Reports*, **48**: 287–294, 1981.

KIRSCHNER, M. A. and C. W. BARDIN: "Androgen Production in Normal and Virilized Women," *Metabolism, Clinical and Experimental*, **21**(1):7, January 1972.

National Diabetes Data Group: "Classification and Diagnosis of Diabetes Mellitus and Other Categories of Glucose Intolerance," *Diabetes*, **28**(12):1039–1057, December 1979.

PETERSDORF, R., et al. (eds.): *Harrison's Principles of Internal Medicine*, 10th ed., McGraw-Hill, New York, 1980, sec. 10, pp. 1657–1849.

RABIN, D. and T. J. McKENNA: *Clinical Endocrinology and Metabolism Principles and Practice, vol. 9: The Science and Practice of Clinical Medicine*, J. M. Dietschy (ed.), Grune & Stratton, New York, 1982.

REID, R. L., and S. S. C. YEN: "Premenstrual Syndrome," *American Journal of Obstetrics and Gynecology*, **139**(1):85–104, January 1, 1981.

RUBLE, D. H.: "Premenstrual Symptoms: A Reinterpretation," *Science*, **197**:291–292, July 6, 1977.

PART X

LARRY S. MATTHEWS

ORTHOPEDICS

Orthopedics is concerned with prevention or corrective treatment of deformities or diseases of the musculoskeletal system, including bones, muscles, joints, ligaments, tendons, and fascia of the body. This part includes a discussion of fractures (definitions, the "four R's" of fractures, and fracture complications) dislocations (types, diagnosis, and treatment), accidental injury and its initial treatment, and osteomyelitis. Also included is a discussion of orthopedic diseases of children and a rationale for the treatment of tumors of the musculoskeletal system.

OBJECTIVES

At the completion of this part you should be able to:

1. Identify the characteristics of fractures and dislocations according to their classification, description, recognition, reduction, retention of reduction, complications, types of dislocations, and treatment.
2. Develop skill in identifying causes, pathogenesis, and treatment of various orthopedic diseases of children.
3. Explain the rationale for the treatment of tumors of the musculoskeletal system.

FRACTURES AND DISLOCATIONS

OBJECTIVES

At the completion of this chapter you should be able to:

1. Explain the primary functions of bone.
2. Describe the composition of bone.
3. Locate and describe the function of the parts of the long bone—diaphysis (shaft), metaphysis, physis, epiphysis, periosteum, and nutrient arteries.
4. Explain why the specific histology of the physis is important in understanding some specific injuries in children.
5. Define a *fracture*.
6. Explain complete vs. incomplete fracture.
7. Differentiate between the types of fractures [transverse, oblique, spiral, segmental, compression, pathologic, stress (fatigue), greenstick, avulsion] in terms of radiologic appearance, location, cause, treatment, and complications.
8. State what a comminuted fracture indicates.
9. Explain the significance of angulation and opposition in the description of long-bone fractures.
10. Differentiate between open and closed fractures in terms of area involved, treatment, and likely complications.
11. Describe the sequential stages or changes that occur in the process of fracture healing.
12. Identify the "four R's" of fractures.
13. Cite at least three considerations for dealing with recognition of fractures.
14. Explain the importance of crepitus.
15. Define *reduction*.
16. Identify the characteristics of both closed and open reductions.
17. Identify the advantages and disadvantages of closed reduction and external immobilization by the various types of retention, and of open reduction and retention by fixation.
18. Identify the medical implications of fracture treatment.
19. Explain the purpose of and general rule for the application of casts.

20. Describe the optimal appearance of a cast and the purpose of careful molding of the soft plaster over bony prominences.

21. List the signs and treatment of neurovascular dysfunction of the exposed portions of the distal limb.

22. State the rationale for the treatment of a limb with a compromised vascular supply.

23. Identify the signs, symptoms, and immediate treatment if a cast has not been properly applied over bony prominences.

24. Describe traction by identifying the contribution that it makes to maintenance of limb length, position control, and observation.

25. State at least two important factors that must be considered when applying or maintaining traction.

26. List at least three advantages traction provides as the definitive early treatment of fractures.

27. Describe the potential complication associated with the use of skin tractions.

28. Identify, for Bryant's skin traction, the location of the fracture, the positioning, and the rationale for age and weight requirements.

29. Describe balanced skeletal traction by identifying the type of fracture it is used with, the position of the skeletal pin and traction bail, and the application and use of a Thomas splint and Pearson attachment.

30. List advantages of using balanced skeletal traction for the treatment of fractures.

31. Describe Russell's traction as to its purpose, the type of fracture associated with it and positioning of the patient.

32. Explain the purpose of the ninety-ninety-ninety traction.

33. Describe the operative procedure referred to as open reduction and internal fixation (ORIF).

34. List the advantages and disadvantages of operative fracture treatment.

35. State the most frequently encountered reasons for using open reduction and internal fixation of fractures.

36. State the rationale for operative fracture treatment in an elderly patient with a hip fracture.

37. Identify the advantages of the telescoping hip nail and other implant devices.

38. Explain the major advantage of a femoral head replacement arthroplasty in an elderly patient.

39. State the rationale for planning for an orderly rehabilitation program from the first day of injury.

40. Differentiate between malunion, delayed union, and nonunion of a fracture, and identify an example of each type.

41. Differentiate between dislocation and subluxation.

42. Describe shoulder dislocation by identifying its appearance, the age group affected, and treatment.

43. Explain the rationale for examining the neurovascular status of the limb at the time of initial evaluation of a shoulder dislocation, prior to any manipulative reduction.

44. Describe the sustained anterior traction method of reduction of a dislocated shoulder.

45. Identify the characteristics of a dislocated hip according to the signs, symptoms, prognosis, and consequences of delayed reduction.

46. Explain the advantages and disadvantages of total hip arthroplasty and total knee replacement in the treatment of severe joint arthritis.

47. State the prime objective of treatment at the scene of a serious accident.

48. Describe external cardiac massage by identifying the purpose, time to begin, and necessary duration of massage.

49. Describe the emergency treatment of any injured person who is cyanotic and in obvious respiratory distress.

50. List the characteristics of arterial bleeding.

51. Describe the sequence of steps used to stop arterial bleeding.

52. Explain the procedure used in the application of a tourniquet and the precautions that must be taken.

53. Explain the rationale for treatment of a seriously injured limb.

54. Differentiate between the emergency treatments when the fracture is located at the midpoint of a long bone, in a lower or upper extremity, or near a joint.

55. Describe the rationale for the procedure used in applying splints.

56. Differentiate between acute and chronic osteomyelitis as to cause, pathogenesis, signs and symptoms, treatment, and prognosis.

57. Explain the importance of early recognition of osteomyelitis, especially in children.

ANATOMY AND HISTOLOGY OF THE LONG BONE

Bones form the supporting and protecting framework of the body's skeletal system. They also provide the attachments of the muscles which move the skeleton. The central cavity of certain bones contains hematopoietic tissue, which forms a variety of blood cells (see Part III). Bone also performs an important role in the regulation of calcium and phosphate (see Part IX). Bone is composed of a supportive rigid connective tissue which consists of an organic matrix referred to as osteoid. Osteoid consists of an abundant matrix of collagen fibers embedded in a cementing gel of protein polysaccharide. Deposited on the collagen fibers is a mineral (hydroxyapatite) which is made up of calcium and phosphate in a specific crystalline array.

Figure 61-1 illustrates the location of the parts of a long bone. The diaphysis, or shaft, is the cylindrical midportion of the bone. It is composed of cortical bone which has great strength. The metaphysis is the flared region near the end of the shaft. This region is largely of trabecular or spongy bone and contains marrow, which is also found in the epiphysis and diaphysis of a bone. The metaphysis also supports the joint and pro-

vides appropriate areas for epiphyseal attachment of tendons and ligaments. The epiphyseal plate is the region of longitudinal growth in children. It disappears at skeletal maturity; the epiphysis directly adjacent to the joint of the long bone fuses to the metaphysis, causing cessation of growth in bone length. The entire bone is covered with a fibrous layer, the periosteum, which contains the proliferating cells that contribute to the transverse growth of a long bone. Most long bones have specific nutrient arteries. The location and patency of these may govern the success of bone healing after fracture.

The specific histology of the epiphyseal plate, or growth plate, is important in understanding some specific injuries in children (see Fig. 61-2). The uppermost layer of cells near the epiphysis is referred to as the area of resting cells. The next layer is the area or zone of proliferation. In this area active cell division is occurring, and this is where the growth of long bones begins. These cells are pushed toward the shaft into the area of hypertrophy, where they swell and become metabolically inactive. These swollen cells are weak. Epiphyseal fracture separations in children commonly occur in this region, with extension of the injury into the area of provisional calcification. In the zone of provisional calcification the cells first begin to become hard and resemble

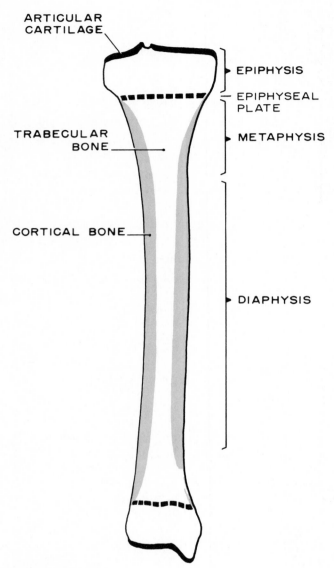

FIGURE 61-1
Anatomy of a long bone.

normal bone. Damage to the proliferating area may cause growth arrest with either retardation of the longitudinal growth of the limb or progressive deformity in case of serious damage to only a portion of the plate.

FRACTURES

Classification of fractures

A *fracture* is a structural discontinuity or break in a bone usually caused by trauma or physical force. The

amount of force, along with other factors, determines whether a fracture is complete or incomplete. Complete fractures result in structural discontinuity of the entire thickness of the bone, whereas incomplete fractures do not extend through the entire thickness of the bone. For effective communication regarding fractures, several important descriptive terms must be introduced.

Angle of break

A *transverse fracture* is one which proceeds directly across the bone. When the broken segments of such a transversely fractured bone are repositioned, or reduced, back to their original location, they are stable and usually easy to control with casts (see Fig. 61-3A). *Oblique fractures* proceed at an angle across the bone. They are unstable and difficult to control (see Fig. 61-3B). *Spiral fractures* are the result of torsion of a limb. They are typical in ski injuries where the toe of the ski becomes lodged in a snowbank and the ski twists around until the bone breaks. Interestingly, this low-energy fracture is associated with little soft-tissue damage, and such fractures tend to heal readily with external immobilization (see Fig. 61-3C).

Multiple fractures in one bone

Segmental fractures are two adjacent fractures which isolate a central segment from its blood supply. These fractures are difficult to treat. Frequently the fracture at one or the other end of the avascular segment fails to heal and may require operative treatment (see Fig. 61-4A). *Comminuted fractures* refer to splintering or disruption in continuity of tissue in which there are more than two fracture fragments.

Impaction fractures

Compression fractures occur when two bones crush (by impaction) a third bone between them, such as a vertebra between two other vertebrae. These fractures of the vertebral bodies are diagnosed by their radiographic appearance. Lateral views of the spine show a decrease in vertical height and a mild angulation at one or a few vertebrae. Although compression fracture patients do not usually require sophisticated treatment, they should be hospitalized for care of the possible serious, indirect complications which may arise. In young people, a compression fracture may be associated with considerable retroperitoneal hemorrhage. As in pelvic fractures, the patient may rapidly develop hypovolemic shock and die if repeated accurate assessments of the pulse, blood pressure, and respiration are not obtained during the first 24 to 48 postinjury hours. Ileus and urinary retention may also result from these injuries (see Fig. 61-4B).

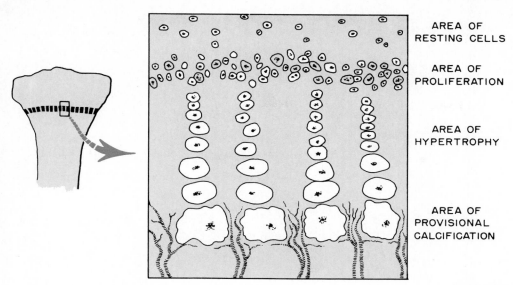

AREA OF
RESTING CELLS

AREA OF
PROLIFERATION

AREA OF
HYPERTROPHY

AREA OF
PROVISIONAL
CALCIFICATION

FIGURE 61-2
Growth of normal bone.

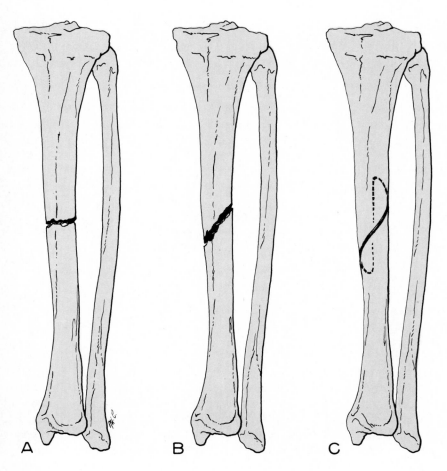

FIGURE 61-3
Classification of fractures. (A)
Transverse. (B) Oblique. (C) Spiral.

A

B

C

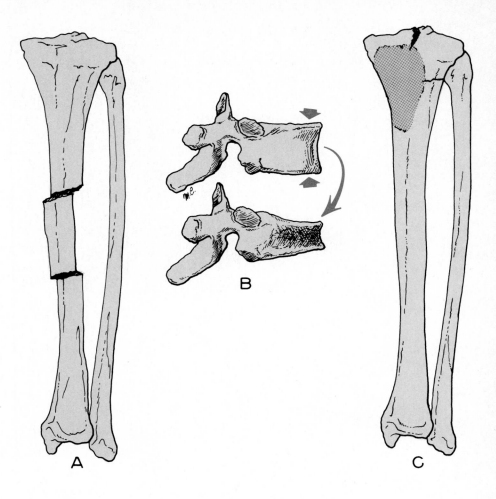

FIGURE 61-4
(A) Segmental. (B) Compression.
(C) Pathologic.

Pathologic fractures

Pathologic fractures occur through regions of bone that have been weakened by a tumor or some other pathologic process. Frequently the adjacent bone shows decreased bone density. The most frequent cause of such fractures is a primary or metastatic tumor (see Fig. 61-4C).

Other stress (fatigue) fractures

Stress, or fatigue, fractures occur in people who have recently increased their activity level—recruits in the army in basic training or people who have recently taken up jogging. With the onset of symptoms, the radiographs may not demonstrate the fracture. However, usually after 2 weeks, linear radiopaque lines later appear perpendicular to the long axis of the bone. Such fractures heal well if the bone is immobilized for a few weeks. However, if they are not diagnosed, the bones can become displaced and cause an increase in morbidity. Thus, any patient with severe extremity pain after a recent increase in activity may have such a lesion and should be protected by the use of crutches or an appropriate cast. After 2 weeks, radiographs should be obtained (see Fig. 61-5A)

Greenstick fractures

Greenstick fractures occur in children and are incomplete fractures. The cortex is partially intact, as is the periosteum. They will heal readily and remodel rapidly back to a normal shape and function (see Fig. 61-5B).

Avulsion fractures

Avulsion fractures separate a fragment of bone at a site of tendon or ligament insertion. Frequently no specific treatment is required. However, if joint instability or another cause of disability is expected to result from such a fracture, the displaced fragment may be operatively excised or replaced in most cases (see Fig. 61-5C).

Joint fractures

Specific note should be made of fractures which involve joints, particularly if the joint geometry is significantly disturbed by displacement of these fragments. Unless adequately treated, this type of injury may lead to a progressive posttraumatic degenerative arthritis of the injured joint (see Fig. 61-6).

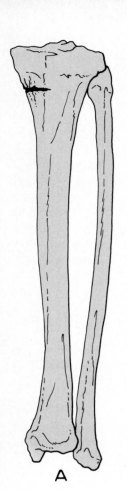

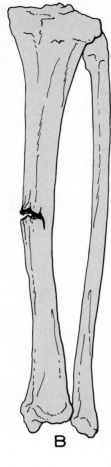

A

B

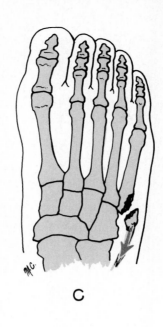

C

FIGURE 61-5
(A) Stress (fatigue). (B) Greenstick. (C) Avulsion.

Description of fractures

Angulation and *opposition* are two terms frequently used in the description of long-bone fractures. The degree and direction of angulation from the normal position of a long bone may indicate the degree of fracture severity and the type of treatment program. Angulation is described by estimating the degrees of deviation of the distal fragment from the normal longitudinal axis, indicating the direction of the apex of the angle (see Fig. 61-7A). Opposition refers to the extent of displacement of the fracture surfaces and is used to describe what proportion of the fractured portion of one fragment touches its mate (see Fig. 61-7B).

Exposure to environment

Closed (simple) and *open (compound)* are terms frequently used in fracture description. A closed, or simple, fracture is one in which the skin is not perforated from without or within, so the fracture site is not exposed to the environment.

Technically, an open, or compound, fracture is one in which the skin on the involved limb has been penetrated. The important concept is whether the contaminated outside environment has come into contact with the fracture site. A fracture fragment may frequently perforate the skin at the time of injury, become contaminated, and then return to near its normal position. Under these conditions operative irrigation, debridement, and administration of intravenous antibiotics may be necessary to prevent osteomyelitis. In general, open

FIGURE 61-6
Fracture of the distal radius with extension into the wrist joint.

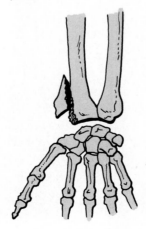

fractures should have operative irrigation and debridement within 6 hours of the time of injury for the best chance of preventing infection.

A typical description of a fracture might then be: "This patient has a midshaft, open, transverse, uncomminuted fracture of the right femur; it is angulated 30°, the apex directed posteriorly. The fragments are separated widely with no opposition. The neurovascular supply to the limb is intact." Such a description would immediately indicate that the limb is apt to survive but that surgery is needed within a short time. The purpose of the surgery is to protect the patient from infection and, if necessary, to reposition the fracture fragments.

Fracture healing

When a bone is fractured, the adjacent soft tissues are damaged, the periosteum is separated from the bone, and considerable bleeding takes place. A blood clot develops in the area. The clot forms granulation tissue, within which the primitive bone-forming (osteogenic) cells differentiate into chondroblasts and osteoblasts. The chondroblasts secrete phosphate, which stimulates deposition of calcium. A thickened band (the callus) forms around the fracture site. The band continues to thicken and expand across the fracture site and converges with the band from the opposite fragment and fuses with it. Fusion of the two fragments, fracture healing, progresses as osteoblasts form trabeculae, which adhere to the bone and extend across the fracture site. This provisional bony union undergoes metaplastic transformation to become stronger and more organized. The bone callus remodels to assume the shape of intact bone as osteoblasts form new bone and osteoclasts remove the damaged and temporary bone (see Fig. 61-8).

FOUR R'S OF FRACTURES

Four basic concepts should be considered for fractures: *recognition, reduction, retention,* and *rehabilitation.* Recognition concerns the diagnosis at the scene of the accident and later in the hospital. Reduction is the repositioning of the fracture fragments as nearly as possible to their normal location. Retention refers to the methods which are applied to hold the fragments while they are healing. A rehabilitation plan should be initiated immediately and concurrently with the fracture treatment.

Recognition

The history of the accident, the severity, the force involved, and the description of the event by the patient determine the likelihood of broken bones and the need for specific examination for fractures. The pain of fractures of long bones is very specific. For example, the patient's leg is severely painful and tender at the fracture site, but other areas such as the knee and ankle may feel nearly normal. Obvious deformities define discontinuities in the skeletal integrity. The association of localized pain and tenderness, deformity, and instability frequently leads to the presumptive diagnosis of fracture at the scene of the injury. *Crepitus* refers to the feeling as if two pieces of rough sandpaper are rubbing together. Although it occurs in other orthopedic conditions, crepitus indicates the presence of a fracture and it is, in fact, the sensation generated by the rubbing of the fracture fragments together. Fracture fragments are usually very sharp. Their relative motion after injury may sever the neurovascular supply to the limb. Therefore, upon recognition of the possibility of fracture of a

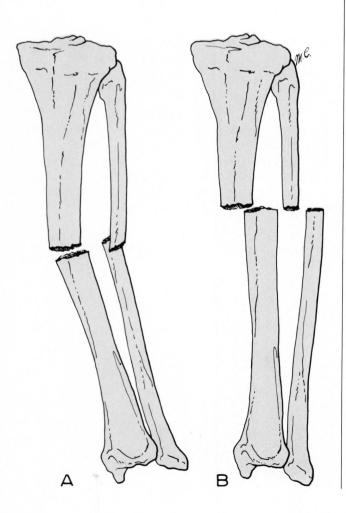

FIGURE 61-7

(A) Angulation. (B) Opposition.

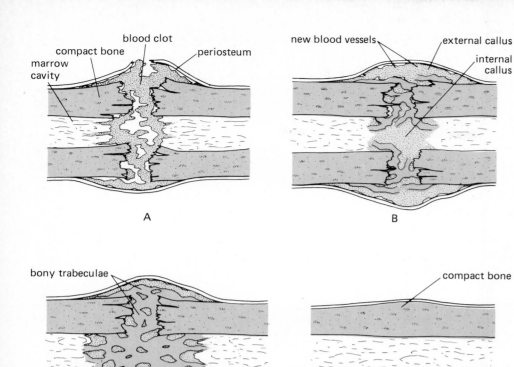

marrow cavity
compact bone
blood clot
periosteum

A

new blood vessels
external callus
internal callus

B

bony trabeculae

C

compact bone

D

FIGURE 61-8

(A) In a fracture usually the periosteum is torn, blood vessels are damaged, and bone fragments are separated. (B) Rapid division of bone- and cartilage-forming cells in the region of the break forms a thickened band that is composed of an internal and external callus. (C) Osteoblasts form trabeculae, which adhere to existing bone and extend across the break. (D) The break is bridged by compact bone, and the contour of the new intact bone is remodeled. (From Luciano, Vander, and Sherman, 1983.)

long bone, the injured limb should be splinted to protect it from further damage.

Obvious soft-tissue damage may also indicate the possibility of a fracture and the need for immediate splinting and further examination. This is especially true for injuries to the cervical spine, where contusions and lacerations of the face and scalp indicate the need for radiographic evaluation, which may demonstrate a cervical spine fracture and/or dislocation and the possible need for surgical stabilization.

Reduction

The act of manipulating broken bone fragments back as nearly as possible to their original location is known as reduction. Closed fractures of long bones are frequently treated by *closed reduction*. This may often be effectively carried out in the emergency room or cast room at the time of the initial evaluation. Intravenous narcotics, sedatives, or local nerve block anesthesia may be used to diminish the patient's pain during the procedure. It is very important that the patient and family recognize the extent of the injury and the need for re-

positioning of the fracture fragments and for immobilization. Since all forms of outpatient analgesia require several minutes for maximum effect, this allows sufficient time for reevaluating the nature of the injury. It is necessary to assess the following factors when planning the patient's treatment program: the social situation, the availability of family support, the likely effect of the injury on the patient's life during the next several months, and the expectations of the patient.

Initial treatment

During the initial treatment, the patient and/or significant others should be instructed regarding the reduction. These instructions include the possibility that reduction will not be successful, the expected consequences of the fracture, and the expected period and nature of disability. It is also very important to outline problems and complications which may possibly be associated with the injury, rather than to have to explain them after their occurrence. For example, after an elbow fracture it is rare for the patient to be able to fully extend and to "lock" the elbow. An early explanation eliminates the necessity of exhaustive excuses for the patient's inability to regain full range of motion several weeks after the incident.

Repositioning

When the patient and the family are aware of the medical implications of the fracture and when analgesia is maximal, a manual effort is generally used to reposition the broken bones. It is more advantageous to use all necessary force on the first attempt, which often rapidly accomplishes a satisfactory reduction, than to be excessively gentle and make multiple skin-damaging attempts. If a closed manual reduction is not successful under outpatient analgesia, it is mandatory that the physician not repeat the effort. Under such circumstances, the patient should be admitted to the hospital, prepared for general anesthesia, and scheduled for a reduction under anesthesia in the operating room. In this situation a fracture table can greatly amplify the force which needs to be used and can frequently ensure control of the fragments until a cast is applied to maintain the reduction.

Retention of reduction

As a general rule, casts applied to maintain a reduction should extend past the joint above and the joint below the fracture. If adjacent joints are positioned at an angle to the central longitudinal axis of the broken bone, angulation and opposition corrections may be maintained, and at the same time rotational displacements may be prevented. A cast should always be smooth, nonlaminated, and in conformity with the geometry of the limb to which it is applied. Careful molding of the soft plaster over bony prominences generally prevents the development of pressure ulcerations and maximizes the ability of the cast to retain the fracture fragment positions.

Postreduction neurovascular supply

Reduction and cast application are frequently completed a few hours after the injury, when the maximum soft-tissue swelling has not occurred. In addition, the act of reduction itself may cause further tissue edema. Consequently, because a cast is an unyielding circumferential dressing, great attention must be paid to the postreduction neurovascular supply to the limb. Therefore, the limb should be elevated, usually by a rope and sling to a fracture frame. The exposed portions of the distal limb should be repeatedly examined for the de-

velopment of pain, pallor, paresthesias, and pulselessness, all of which are signs of neurovascular dysfunction. If there is any indication that the neurovascular supply to the limb is being impaired, the cast should be split from one end to the other. *All* layers should be cut, and the cast should be loosened until the signs and symptoms of neurovascular dysfunction have been reversed. Usually most limbs with fractures are not very painful after reduction and immobilization. All persistent patient complaints during this postreduction period must be taken seriously, and effective steps initiated to relieve the source of discomfort.

An injured limb with a compromised vascular supply may sustain irreversible pathologic changes within 1½ hours; thus an immediate effective response to these signs of danger is mandatory. During the first several hours after injury, repeated administration of narcotic medication is definitely *contraindicated*. For example, if a cast has not been molded or padded sufficiently over bony prominences—the ulnar styloid process, the olecranon, or the medial or lateral malleolus—the patient may develop persistent burning pain at the pressure sites. This is a sign of developing skin and soft-tissue necrosis. Immediate relief from the localized pressure is necessary. This excessive pressure may be relieved by cutting and re-forming the cast; however, on occasion a new, properly fitted and molded cast may be necessary to prevent costly and painful soft-tissue ulceration.

Traction

Another excellent method of maintaining a satisfactory reduction of limb fractures is traction. In general, traction is achieved by weights which are attached by ropes to the patient's limb. The location of pulleys through which the ropes run is adjusted until the direction of pull is in line with the long axis of the fractured bone.

Although longitudinal traction often maintains a satisfactory reduction, usually splints, casts, or slings are used to cradle the limb and assist in holding the fracture fragments in place. As a general rule, skeletal traction with a sterile surgical steel pin drilled through the distal fragment or a more distal bone is preferable to skin traction. When skeletal traction is used, skin necrosis and the neurovascular complications of a circumferential dressing tend to be avoided. Although requiring hospitalization, traction provides many advantages as the definitive method of maintaining a reduction. Most forms of traction ensure dependable limb elevation, which minimizes swelling and promotes soft-tissue healing. The injured extremity may be easily observed for compromised neurovascular circulation. Wound care is facilitated. Appropriate application of traction allows convenient bed care for the patient. The patient may be quite mobile in bed if the longitudinal ropes are appropriately positioned and the splints, casts, or slings used to support the limb are properly balanced. Bedpans can be positioned and removed without discomfort, and bedclothing may be changed without fear of displacement of the fracture fragments.

Some important factors must be considered in applying or maintaining traction. The major rope, which is usually attached to a skeletal pin, should generally pull in line with the normal long axis of a fractured long bone. Both the weight of the limb and the supporting devices should be counterbalanced by weights to ensure stable maintenance of reduction and support of the injured limb during bed care. As much as possible, pulleys and ropes should be located well above and to the side of the patient. Great care should be taken that bony prominences, i.e., the heel, malleoli, and fibular head, are properly padded or otherwise protected. The traction ropes should run freely through the pulleys. The weights should be sufficiently high above the floor with the patient in a normal bed care position so that required routine repositioning does not allow a weight to rest on the floor, thereby removing the necessary tension from the attached rope. Appropriately applied and maintained traction is always comfortable.

Buck's skin traction

The simplest form of traction is Buck's skin traction. This traction method is appropriately used in young people for short periods of time. The most frequent indication for this form of traction is the need to rest the knee joint after trauma prior to possible knee exploration and repair. Utilization of this method of traction ideally begins with application of a thick coating of skin cement, tincture of benzoin, or elastic adherent to the patient's skin below the knee. A rolled tubular stockinette is then applied smoothly over the distal limb below the knee. Adhesive traction strips are applied medially and laterally to the stockinette, and they are, in turn, wrapped smoothly and gently with an elastic bandage. The ends of the traction strips at the ankle are connected to a spreader bar to prevent pressure on the malleoli. A rope which is attached to the center of the spreader bar is then threaded through a pulley at the foot of the bed. Rarely should a weight

greater than 5 lb be applied. Many potential complications are associated with the use of skin traction. The circumferentially wrapped elastic bandage can further compromise the circulation to the foot in a patient with prior vascular disease. Skin allergies to the adhesives may cause a problem. If great care is not taken, pressure ulceration may develop at the malleoli. Excessive traction can avulse the fragile skin of the elderly. In general, this form of traction should not be used to treat elderly patients. Even in the treatment of young adults, skeletal pin traction is preferable if such treatment will be required for more than a few days (see Fig. 61-9).

Bryant's skin traction

Bryant's skin traction is frequently used in the treatment of small children with a femoral fracture or fractures. In this type of traction the patient is positioned with the hips flexed, the knees extended, and the limbs in a vertical position slightly spread apart. Because the periosteum of children's bones is so strong, it is rarely completely separated at the time of fracture; thus this pure longitudinal form of traction almost always accomplishes an adequate reduction and maintenance of fragment position until early healing. Bryant's traction should not be applied to children over the age of 3 years or to children weighing greater than 30 lb. Severe damage to the skin can result from exceeding these limits. In addition, the vascular supply to the feet in older and larger children may be compromised by the considerable hydrostatic effect of vertical limb placement and by the constrictive elastic wraps. Posttraction x-rays often demonstrate bayonette apposition with approximately ½ in of overriding of the bone fragments. This is not only acceptable, but also advantageous, since usually the injured limb of a child grows faster than the normal one for several years following a fracture (see Fig. 61-10).

FIGURE 61-9
Buck's skin traction.

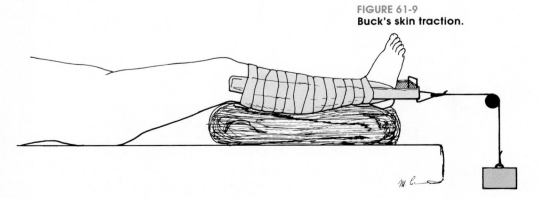

Balanced skeletal traction

Balanced skeletal traction, used primarily for the treatment of femoral shaft fractures in adults, at first glance appears complex. In essence, however, a skeletal pin is positioned transversely through the distal femur or proximal tibia. A traction bail is attached, and the primary traction rope is attached to the bail. The patient's limb is positioned with the hip and knee in approximately 30° of flexion. The primary pulley is adjusted so that the line of tension is coaxial with the longitudinal axis of the fractured femur. Sufficient weight is attached to achieve normal femoral length.

The patient's thigh is supported by a sling or padding attached to the proximal portion of a *Thomas splint*. The distal limb is supported by the Pearson attachment, and the limb itself is suspended by appropriate ropes, pulleys, and weights so that the limb is freely suspended in air. Thus bed care is greatly facilitated. This form of traction is extremely valuable for the treat-

ment of many varieties of femoral fracture. The entire splint may be adducted or abducted to correct angular deformities in the mediolateral plane. Greater or lesser degrees of hip and knee flexion allow lateral corrections. The position and angulation of the Pearson attachment may be adjusted to correct rotational deformities.

Balanced skeletal traction demonstrates many of the major advantages of traction treatment of fractures (see Fig. 61-11). The advantages are elevation, longitudinal coaxial traction on the fractured long bone, easy access to the injured limb for repeated examination of the neurovascular status and for local wound care, and facilitation of nursing care. As is the case with all forms of traction utilizing skeletal pins, the patient should be examined daily for signs of pin tract inflammation or infection, of loosening or sliding of the pin, and of the pin's having been pulled from the bone.

Russell's traction

While balanced skeletal traction may be used for the treatment of most fractures of the femur, better reductions of fractures of the hip may frequently be obtained by using Russell's traction. In this case the thigh is supported by a sling. The longitudinal traction is applied by a pin positioned through the tibia and the fibula transversely above the ankle. The affect of this arrangement is to provide a traction force (derived from the vertical pull of the thigh sling combined with the horizontal pull of the two ropes at the foot) which is in alignment with the injured bone and is of appropriate magnitude. This type of traction is most frequently used to provide comfort for patients with hip fractures during the preoperative evaluation and preparation for surgery.

Although Russell's traction (see Fig. 61-12) may be used as the definitive and final treatment of hip fractures in selected patients, the elderly or debilitated patient with a fractured hip cannot usually tolerate the dangers of long-sustained bed rest, i.e., decubitus ulcers, pneumonia, and thrombophlebitis. The most common problem seen with Russell's traction is that the patient slips toward the foot of the bed, the distal pulleys jam together, and the weight then rests on the floor. Considerable care must be directed toward maintaining the position of the patient in bed; it may be necessary to place blocks under the foot casters of the bed to gain the assistance of gravity.

Ninety-ninety-ninety traction

Ninety-ninety-ninety traction is particularly useful in the treatment of children from the age of 3 years

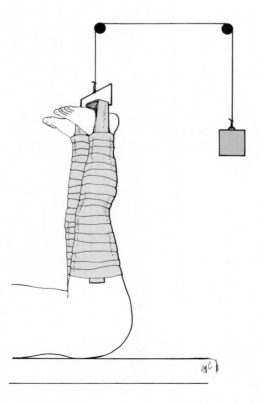

FIGURE 61-10
Bryant's skin traction.

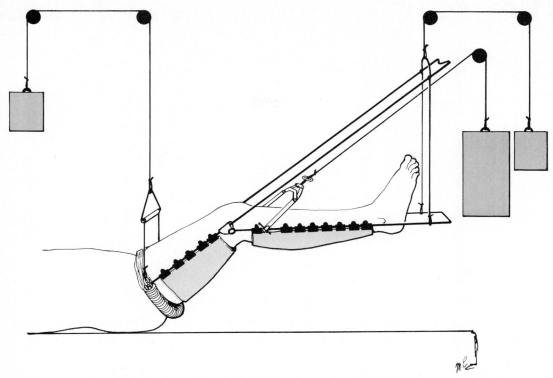

FIGURE 61-11
Balanced skeletal traction.

through young adulthood (see Fig. 61-13). Control of fragments in a femoral shaft fracture is nearly always satisfactory with 90-90-90 traction. The patient has considerable mobility in bed.

Treatment Principles

While only lower-limb traction methods have been described in detail, all the principles apply to the treatment of fractures of the upper limb.

Traction treatment of fractures is generally safe, provides considerable patient comfort and mobility in bed, allows for repeated examination of the injured limb, provides valuable elevation, and does not increase

FIGURE 61-12
Russell's traction.

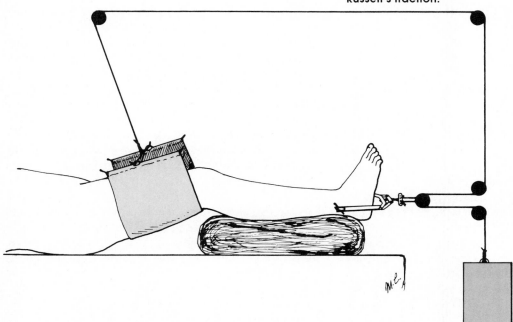

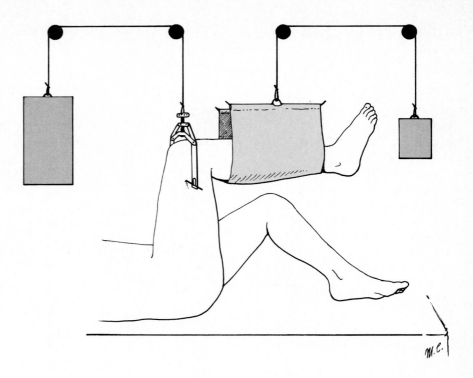

FIGURE 61-13
Ninety-ninety-ninety traction.

the risk of infection. However, traction treatment of fractures should be used with caution with the elderly patient, since it requires continuous hospitalization, which is associated with danger of complications, expense, and inconvenience.

Surgical procedures

Open reduction and internal fixation

At times, the most advantageous fracture treatment method may include surgery. This method of treatment is referred to as open reduction and internal fixation (ORIF). In general, an incision is made at the fracture site and carried along anatomic planes to the fracture. The fracture is observed and studied. Fracture hematoma and nonviable fragments are irrigated from the wound. The fracture is then manually repositioned to a normal position. The fracture fragments, after reduction, are stabilized by the use of appropriate orthopedic devices such as pins, screws, plates, and nails. The advantages of operative fracture treatment include accuracy in repositioning of the fracture fragments, the opportunity for inspection of the adjacent vessels and nerves, the considerable fixation stability that may be achieved, the frequent absence of a need for external casts or appliances after stabilization, a relatively short hospital course in uncomplicated cases, and the potential for maintenance of nearly normal joint function and muscular strength during fracture treatment. However, there are also potential disadvantages. Every anesthesia and operation has a possible risk of complication, even death, from the procedure itself. While closed fractures treated conservatively by casts or traction rarely become infected, operative management greatly increases the chances of infection. The use of a metallic internal stabilization device allows for the possibility of device failure. Surgery itself is additional trauma to the soft tissues, and a previously uninjured structure can accidentally be cut or damaged at operation.

It is extremely difficult to treat the deep infection that may occur. Infection of bone, osteomyelitis, is extremely resistant to antibiotic treatment. The presence of implanted metal devices increases the difficulties of treating the infection. In cases of postoperative infection it is usually necessary to remove the metal device before the infection can be controlled. The decision to use open reduction and internal fixation is of critical importance because of the potential serious complications that can result from this treatment.

An individual with a femoral shaft fracture who is treated by nonoperative methods usually spends 6 weeks in a hospital in traction. When the fracture is partially healed, a cast is applied extending from the toes to the nipple line. This cast is worn until the fracture demonstrates clinical and radiographic evidence of healing stability and cortical remodeling. It is rare that a person can return to work during this period, which may extend for 6 to 12 months. Because employment medical benefits are generally 50 to 60 percent of regular earnings, and remaining immobile at home usually causes the patient additional expenses, a simple closed fracture of the femur treated by closed techniques may be a tragedy for the family.

The nonoperative methods should be compared with treatment by open reduction and internal intramedullary fixation, where, in successful cases, the patient may be discharged from the hospital 3 weeks after the injury. At the time of discharge from the hospital the patient is usually able to ambulate on crutches with partial weight bearing and may frequently return to many types of employment. Self-care, shopping, and virtually any other activities that can be engaged in while using crutches can frequently be managed after the third week. Although this may seem to be the best form of therapy, the omnipresent danger of infection, which occurs in 2 to 6 percent of cases, must always be considered. Deep wound infection following intramedullary fixation of a fractured femur requires long-term antibiotic therapy. It may require removal of the intramedullary rod and other operative procedures, and it may endanger the life of the patient. Obviously the decision as to the most appropriate form of treatment is a major one and requires a major consideration of the patient, health care team, and family.

One of the most frequently encountered reasons for using open reduction and internal fixation of fractures is the inability to obtain an adequate reduction by closed means. This is a frequent occurrence in the treatment of midshaft fractures of the radius and ulna in adults. After three or four failed attempts to achieve a manual reduction, the following conditions occur: the skin becomes red, the soft tissue has sustained further damage, and there is no certainty that the reduction, if it is obtained, can be maintained in a cast for a sufficient period of time. Therefore, a decision for open reduction and internal plate or intramedullary rod fixation of the fractured bones is reasonable and prudent.

In other instances an excellent anatomic reduction is possible, but on repeated radiographic examination the reduction cannot be maintained by cast or traction. A typical example is a Piedmont or Galeazzi fracture of the radius with dissociation of the distal radioulnar joint (see Fig. 61-14). Although these fractures are often easily reduced, the reductions are unstable and may lead to malposition of the fragments a short time later. If this failure to maintain reduction is disregarded and the radius is allowed to heal in this displaced position, the wrist is likely to develop severe arthritis and painful permanent limitation of forearm pronation and supination. Thus, failure of maintenance of adequate reduction by closed means is an excellent reason for open therapy.

Another rationale for surgical treatment of fractures is the need for direct observation and possible repair of vital neurovascular structures.

In open fractures, irrigation, mechanical cleansing of the wound, and debridement of necrotic tissue are essential to prevent postinjury osteomyelitis. Frequently, the contaminated wound can be converted to the equivalent of a clean, aseptic surgical wound. Under these circumstances internal fixation may be a rational treatment choice. If surgical cleansing of an open fracture is required, and adequate irrigation and debridement are accomplished, then internal fixation may be deemed advantageous and utilized immediately, although there is increased risk of infection.

In some cases open reduction and internal fixation may be the optimal form of treatment for the general condition of the patient. For example, elderly patients with hip fractures treated by traction frequently succumb to the complications of bed rest: pressure ulceration, pneumonia, and pulmonary embolism after an extended period of painful hospitalization. Nursing care of these patients is extremely difficult. Adequate bed mobilization is nearly impossible, owing to the fracture pain. The extended period of hospitalization required is expensive, and often the social isolation of the patient displaced from the normal environment leads to an emotional state which may contribute to death. Although the surgical risks and complications of open reduction and internal fixation in this patient population are serious, there is no other method of treatment that results in a rapid recovery to a nearly pain-free, mobile state. Thus, in many cases of fractures in the elderly patient, a surgical procedure is the optimal elective form of treatment.

Recent advances in metallurgy and in the design of implant devices have made open reduction and internal fixation more attractive. The telescoping hip nail (see Fig. 61-15A) has great intrinsic strengths and allows the fracture fragments to settle toward each other as necessary during the healing process. Other devices such as the Holt nail (see Fig. 61-15B) are exceptionally strong.

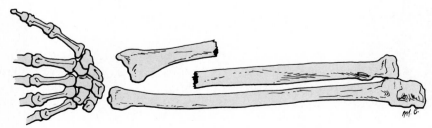

FIGURE 61-14
Galeazzi fracture with disruption of the distal radioulnar joint.

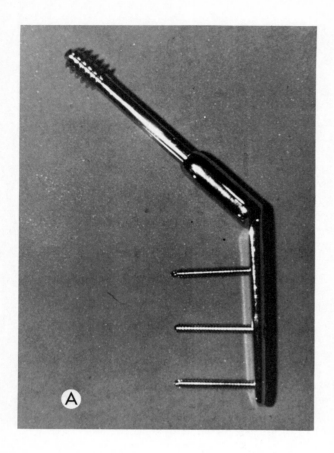

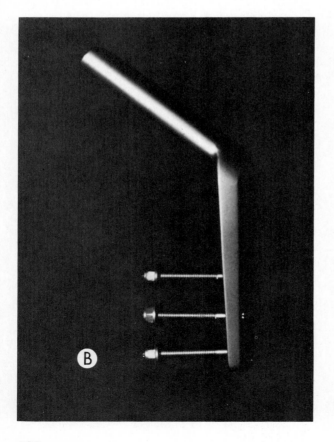

Implanted in a fractured human femur, the Holt nail supports loads in excess of 2000 lb, far more than the loading expected during normal unsupported walking.

Surgical open reduction and internal fixation may allow accurate reduction, increased stability of reduction, examination of neurovascular structures, a decreased need for external immobilization, rapid healing of joints adjacent to the fracture, shorter hospitalization, and a more rapid return to the previous life-style. The risks and potential complications demand a sophisticated analysis of the patient's situation and choice for the most satisfactory overall treatment program.

Replacement of a damaged part

Another surgical method to treat fractures is replacement of the damaged part. Even with the most optimal combinations of device and surgical technique, the complication rates for displaced femoral neck fractures have remained at a high level. Nonunion and aseptic necrosis of the femoral head usually result in a painful, nonfunctional outcome. Since the elderly patient with a displaced femoral neck fracture usually cannot physiologically afford such a complication, femoral head replacement arthroplasty has become a frequently utilized treatment method (see Fig. 61-16). Nonunion of the fracture and aseptic necrosis are impossible with this technique. Full weight bearing may be tolerated soon after the surgery. Yet, this method has its own difficulties. Postoperative dislocation of the femoral head replacement prosthesis is possible. At times, this may be prevented by avoidance of lower-limb flexion, adduction, and internal rotation. Following femoral head replacement, patients should not cross their legs or sit in low chairs until several weeks after their surgery. Migration of the metallic femoral head through the osteoporotic bone into the pelvis has been reported. Finally, after years of satisfactory service, the prosthesis may become painfully loose within the proximal femur, and reoperation may become necessary.

Total hip arthroplasty with stable surgical replacement both of the acetabulum and proximal femur has been infrequently utilized in the past. However, the extraordinary results of this procedure in the treatment of arthritic patients may hasten its use in selected elderly patients with femoral neck fracture. The role of total hip arthroplasty as the primary treatment of femoral neck fractures in the elderly will certainly be investigated and defined in the near future.

FIGURE 61-15
(A) Telescoping hip nail. (B) Holt nail.

Recognition of a fracture, accurate reduction, and maintenance of reduction are the primary treatment modalities, while a fourth major one remains sadly neglected: rehabilitation. The ultimate goal of fracture treatment is to return the patient as rapidly as possible to the preinjury state.

Treatment program

Frequently the effects of the injury and the associated treatment program may unnecessarily result in imperfect or delayed recovery. Since the approximate duration of serious disability may frequently be predicted, it is important to plan for an orderly rehabilitation program from the day of injury. If social assistance is to be required for the family, the appropriate time to initiate procurement procedures is shortly after the injury. It should be anticipated that a patient with severely injured lower extremities will be required to use crutches for an extended time period. Accordingly, exercises to maintain upper-extremity strength and mobility should be initiated as soon as feasible after the injury. Plans for a rational vocational rehabilitation program are best organized during the initial period of hospitalization, when all the concerned individuals can conveniently meet, discuss the problem, and plan for the future. If

special assisting devices will be required upon discharge from the hospital, this is the time to plan for their construction. The nurse, social worker, physical therapist, occupational therapist, vocational rehabilitation representative, and prosthetist-orthotist should develop a comprehensive treatment program during this period, rather than wait until the day of discharge from the hospital to formulate a plan.

Fracture complications

Although most patients with fractures progress toward rapid healing and recovery using standard treatment techniques, there is a significant number who are disabled because of complications of the injury and the treatment program. Therefore, it is appropriate to examine some of the specific complications which relate to fracture treatment and to discuss some of the techniques which may be used to minimize their incidence and severity.

Malunion

Malunion is, as the term implies, a condition in which the fracture has healed in an inappropriate, angulated, or twisted position. A typical example is that of a fractured femur treated by traction and later by cast immobilization where insufficient attention was paid to the rotational alignment of the fracture fragments. The results, discovered upon removal of the final cast, are that the distal limb is either internally or externally rotated and the patient is unable to maintain it in a neutral position. These complications may be avoided by both careful analysis of the reduction and accurate maintenance of reduction during the initial healing period.

Loose casts should be changed as needed. Slippage of fracture fragments following reduction should be detected early by sequential radiographic examination. This condition should be reversed as indicated by repeat reduction and immobilization or perhaps by operative treatment.

Delayed union and nonunion

Delayed union is healing that is continuing to occur but at a rate slower than average. Nonunion of a frac-

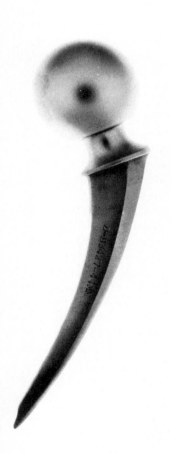

FIGURE 61-16
Femoral head replacement.

ture may be a catastrophic complication for the patient. There are many factors which may predispose a fracture to nonunion, among them inadequate reduction resulting in continued separation of the fracture fragments, inadequate immobilization either by open or closed means, interposition of soft tissues (usually muscle) between the fragments, severe degrees of soft-tissue injury, massive bone loss, infection, and specific anatomic circulatory patterns in which the fracture may damage the blood supply to one or more of the fragments.

If postreduction radiographs demonstrate excessive separation of the fragments, the reduction must be repeated. At times, it is necessary to perform an open reduction to reposition the fracture fragment to an acceptable position. During surgery, a large mass of muscle may be found lying between the fragments. This mass must be displaced to achieve reduction. The quality of maintenance of reduction position and degree of immobilization should be assessed repeatedly throughout the entire treatment program. At times, it may be necessary to apply new casts successively to eliminate excessive fragment mobility when there is a progressive reduction in size of the limb due to a loss of edema fluid and muscle atrophy. Early aggressive treatment of soft-tissue infection may prevent osteomyelitis and its associated nonunion implications.

The overwhelming majority of nonunions of fractures are related to a specific anatomic circulatory situation. The blood supply to a fractured bone may be compromised by the fracture's passing through major arteries to major fragments. Fractures of the carpal scaphoid are particularly prone to nonunion, since they pass through the vascular supply to the proximal fragment (see Fig. 61-17). A similar situation holds for fractures of the femoral neck and fractures of the neck of the talus.

DISLOCATION AND SUBLUXATION

The mating articular cartilage-bearing surfaces of normal joints fit one another with considerable accuracy. Thus for the ball-in-socket hip joint there is little deviation from sphericity of the component parts (see Fig. 61-18). *Subluxation* refers to any deviation from the normal relationship where the articular cartilage is still touching any portion of its mating cartilage. If no portion of its articular cartilage touches the usual mate, the joint is said to be *dislocated*.

Shoulder dislocations are most common in the young and usually result from a traumatic exaggerated abduction, extension, and external rotation position of the upper extermity (see Fig. 61-19). The cocked position for throwing a ball is an example of the position which most frequently, if exaggerated, may cause dislocation. The humeral head is generally displaced anteriorly and inferiorly through a traumatic rent in the shoulder capsule. Characteristically the patient is seen in the emergency room sitting bent over, supporting the injured limb in a flexed position away from the chest or the side. The humeral head may be easily palpated in the anterior axilla. There is a palpable depression beneath the central origin of the deltoid at the acromion. This situation, in addition to the patient's pain and the appropriate history of the incident, is sufficient to indicate the need for roentgenograms for confirmation of the diagnosis. When these films are ordered, it is important to specifically request an axillary view which documents the position of the humeral head with respect to the glenoid cavity and clearly defines the anterior or posterior nature of the dislocation.

During the initial evaluation it is important to examine the neurovascular status of the limb by testing the sensation in the area of the insertion of the deltoid on the humerus. This area is uniquely served by the sensory fibers of the axillary nerve. Local circumscribed anesthesia indicates the likelihood of an axillary nerve injury. Similarly, the ability of the patient to minimally tense the deltoid in a voluntary attempt to initiate abduction also allows an estimate of the function of the axillary nerve. Axillary nerve function is necessary for the shoulder abduction so that the patient is able to functionally position the arm. Since this nerve is fre-

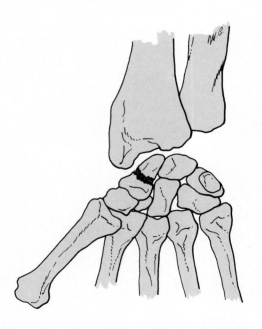

FIGURE 61-17
Fracture of carpal scaphoid.

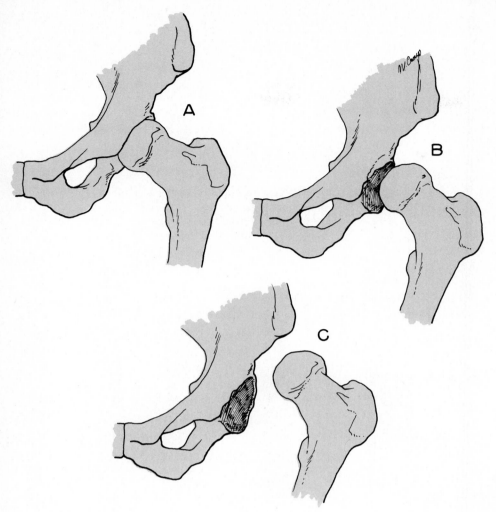

FIGURE 61-18
(A) Normal joint. (B)
Subluxation. (C) Dislocation.

quently injured by the trauma of dislocation, it is imperative that the injury be recognized *prior* to any attempts at replacement of the shoulder or reduction. If this very serious axillary nerve deficit is discovered after manipulation, there is no convincing proof that the attempts to treat the patient did not cause this injury.

Ulnar nerve deficit occurs with nearly the same frequency as axillary nerve injury in shoulder dislocations. Ulnar nerve palsy has a severe effect on hand function, and it is equally imperative that the ability to actively abduct and adduct the four medial digits be initially evaluated. It is absolutely essential that the neurovascular status of the entire extremity be *recorded* prior to any attempt at manipulative reduction, lest the damage be attributed to the medical care.

Circulation, sensation, reflexes, and motor power must be examined repeatedly in all injured limbs, primarily for the patient's benefit and secondarily to ascertain the true relationship of the lesion to the trauma. This examination allows the recognition of any additional dysfunction which may have been caused by attempts at reduction.

FIGURE 61-19
Shoulder dislocation.

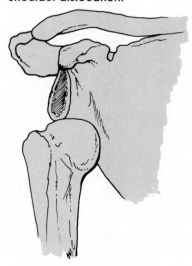

Sustained anterior traction is the safest and most dependable method of reduction of a dislocated shoulder. With this type of traction, the patient is given an analgesic, generally a narcotic, and is in a prone position on an examination table or cart with the affected limb hanging over the side. Slow, gentle, sustained traction toward the floor is applied. In the majority of cases the reduction can be felt as a "clunk." This method of reduction is extremely successful and virtually without complications. A postreduction roentgenogram should demonstrate normal anatomy.

Dislocation of the hip is one of the few orthopedic emergencies. If a dislocated hip is not reduced within 12 or, at the most, 24 hours of the injury, the probability of the patient's developing aseptic necrosis is extremely great. Hip dislocation is recognized usually by gluteal, groin, and thigh pain in association with a rigid position of the limb in adduction, internal rotation, and flexion. With appropriate initial reduction of uncomplicated hip dislocations, the patient is frequently capable of living a normal postinjury life. However, with delay and possible aseptic necrosis, the individual may be crippled for life. Thus, early recognition and early reduction of hip dislocation are the key elements to a satisfactory end result.

In general, early recognition and reduction of all dislocations are essential for a satisfactory end result. The circulation, sensation, reflexes, and motor power examination of the injured limb should be recorded immediately and repeated several times during the care of a patient with a dislocation.

HIP REPLACEMENT

While many forms of arthritis may be well controlled by medical management, at times the progressive destruction of a major joint or joints may prematurely disable an individual. When the pain and disability are so great that the person is unable to independently carry out the basic activities of living, surgical replacement of the diseased joint may be indicated.

Over 10 years ago John Charnley in England developed the first generally successful prosthetic hip joint. His design includes a prosthetic acetabular socket made of ultra-high-molecular-weight polyethylene mated to a prosthetic femoral head of polished metal. Significantly, the friction between the plastic socket and the metal ball is very low during normal activities, and there is little tendency for the prosthetic components to become loosened from the pelvis or femur. In addition,

he discovered that the very firm and lasting fixation of the prosthetic components could be accomplished by the use of self-polymerizing methyl methacrylate cement.

Now, with more than 10 years' experience and after hundreds of thousands of total hip replacements, it is evident that in more than 90 percent of cases the severe disability due to hip arthritis can be virtually eliminated by total hip arthroplasty.

The same technology has also been applied to the knee, ankle, wrist, and shoulder. Because of the lack of knowledge regarding the long-term effects of implanted methyl methacrylate on the body, the possibility that the component will loosen and the danger of infection, these operations have been done primarily on elderly arthritic patients. However, outstanding rehabilitation successes have resulted from these procedures, and there is a continued interest in both the technical developments of the implants and the identification of appropriate patents to maximize the value of total joint replacement.

TOTAL KNEE REPLACEMENT

Total knee replacement as a treatment for patients with very severe knee joint arthritis was introduced by B. Walldius in the 1950s. His prosthesis was essentially a heavy-metal-on-metal hinge joint. With chronic usage, metallic wear debris was generated, causing severe synovitis. This same debris may have been the cause of the serious infection rate associated with the use of this type of prosthesis. In addition, the natural knee has the ability not only to flex and extend, but also to allow internal and external rotation of the tibia relative to the femur; the uniaxis hinge prosthesis did not allow this natural function. As a result the prosthetic fixation stems would twist themselves from their position in the intramedullary canals of the bones.

With the advent of the successful metal-on-polyethylene total hip joint, similar materials and design principles were enlisted for the knee. Presently total knee prostheses consist of femoral components that are similar in shape to the natural lower end of the femur, and tibial components shaped to replace the tibial plateau. Usually the inner surface of the patella is replaced with a polyethylene "button" insert. After appropriate bone sculpting, the components are secured into place with the same methyl methacrylate bone cement that is used with total hip replacement (see Fig. 61-20).

The collateral and usually the posterior cruciate ligaments, as well as the majority of the strong joint capsule, are preserved at surgery. Correction of angular deformity and accomplishment of normal straight knee alignment is essential for satisfactory long-term function.

Considerable improvements in design of total knee prosthesis components and in surgical techniques, including the provision of a patellofemoral replacement, designs to limit excessive stresses on the cement, and metal support of the polyethylene, have resulted in more certain long-term success. The success rate with current total knee replacement is between 80 and 90 percent.

Presently the limiting factor is the durability of the cement. The most reasonable solution to this problem appears to be porous ingrowth fixation. Bone predictably grows into pores in biocompatible materials if they are 100 to 400 μm in diameter. Ingrowth of bone into the porous surface of metal components can provide very stable long-term fixation. Application of this technique will most likely be used in younger patients, for whom great durability is essential.

EMERGENCY TREATMENT OF FRACTURES

Circulation and respiration

At the scene of a serious accident the prime objective is to preserve life and to maximize the potential for rapid and complete rehabilitation of the injured person. Therefore, maintenance of cardiovascular and respira-

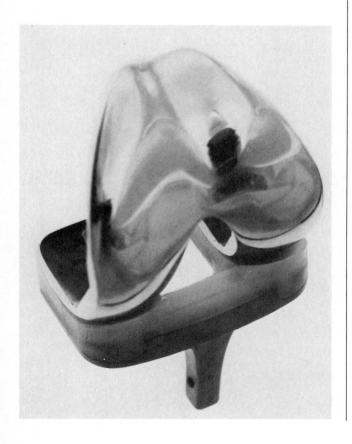

tory functions is of prime importance, rather than the orthopedic concern—immobilization of a fracture site, for instance. Death, defined as irreversible brain damage due to cerebral anoxia, usually begins within 5 minutes after cardiac standstill. The time to begin external massage is *immediately* when pulselessness is discovered. External cardiac massage must be effectively continued until either the individual's heart has resumed unaided function or the patient is under the care of appropriate emergency personnel. Likewise, respiration must be continuous and effective, or death begins in approximately 8 minutes. The most frequent cause of failure of respiration at the scene of an accident is obstruction of the nasopharynx. Debris and clotted blood must be manually removed from the mouth and throat immediately. The prone position allows continuous drainage. When an injured person is cyanotic and in obvious respiratory distress, obstructing material should immediately be removed from the nasopharynx. Success is obvious, with a rapid rush of air and a change in the patient's color. Another maneuver which is frequently successful is to rapidly compress the abdomen from behind. This raises the intrathoracic pressure and may "blow out" debris which is lodged in the trachea. Finally, if all attempts to remove the obstruction fail, a tracheostomy must be done if the injured person is to survive. If obstruction is not the problem, or if it has been successfully eliminated and no respiratory efforts are being made by the injured individual, external respiration should be started and continued until definitive care is available.

Arterial bleeding is red, pulsatile, and voluminous. A transected femoral artery can lead to exsanguination and death in a few minutes. Such bleeding must be stopped. If the application of simple pressure dressing wound does not stop the bleeding, then digital pressure on the major artery proximal to the area of bleeding will usually be temporarily effective. A tourniquet (a belt, rope, tape, or the like) should be tightened circumferentially, proximal to the wound, until the bleeding is controlled. The time of application of a tourniquet must be recorded, since the limb begins to sustain irreversible damage if reparative surgery is not initiated within approximately 1½ hours. The injured individual must be rapidly transported to a hospital where such surgery may be performed.

FIGURE 61-20
Knee prosthesis.

Splinting of limb deformities

Limb deformities and obvious skeletal instability are frequently evident. Motion of sharp fracture fragments can shear and irreparably damage the neurovascular supply to a limb. All seriously injured limbs should be splinted to prevent this unnecessary damage during tansportation of the patient. If the limb fracture is located at the midportion of a long bone, the limb should be gently straightened to a nearly normal position and bound to an appropriate stable object. For the lower extremity, tying the injured limb to the naturally adjacent, uninjured one is frequently convenient. An upper extremity can be supported in a sling or simply bound to the chest. If the deformity is near a joint, e.g., an elbow or knee, no attempt should be made to straighten the limb, since in these locations the nerves and vessels lie close to the bone and further damage may result from attempts at fracture reduction. The limb should be secured in a soft support, such as a pillow, in its deformed state.

The distal pulse should be checked before and after splinting to ensure that the circulation has remained intact. All splints should be extremely well padded to prevent skin ulceration. An ulceration over a bony prominence may cause more disability and require more care than the fracture itself. Open wounds should be bandaged to prevent further contamination. Any clean cloth is satisfactory if sterile bandages are not available. In many cases the time from the incident until final emergency room treatment may determine the outcome, so be sure that an ambulance is called.

OSTEOMYELITIS

Infection of bone tissue is termed *osteomyelitis*, which may be acute or chronic. The acute form is characterized by rapid onset of fever with systemic as well as local manifestations. In children infections of bone commonly develop as a complication of infection from other sites, such as the pharynx (pharyngitis), ear (otitis media), and skin (impetigo). The bacteria (*Staphylococcus aureus*, *Streptococcus*, *Haemophilus influenzae*) travel via the bloodstream to the metaphysis near the growth plates, where the blood flows into sinusoids. With bacterial proliferation and tissue necrosis, the localized area of inflammation is very tender and painful.

It is extremely important that osteomyelitis, especially in children, be diagnosed early so that appropriate antibiotic and surgical treatment can be administered to prevent the local spread of infection and crippling destruction of the entire bone. Any severely ill child with a painful limb should be examined; the anticipated diagnosis is osteomyelitis, not thrombophlebitis, which is extremely rare in children. An incorrect diagnosis in children with osteomyelitis can lead to serious delay in the initiation of appropriate therapy. In adults osteomyelitis may also be initiated by bloodborne bacteria, but more frequently it is the result of tissue contamination at the time of injury or surgery.

Chronic osteomyelitis results from inadequately treated acute osteomyelitis. As mentioned previously, osteomyelitis is extremely resistant to antibiotic therapy. It is theorized that this is partially due to the avascular nature of cortical bone. Appropriate quantities of antibodies may never reach the infected tissue. Bone infections are extremely difficult to eradicate, and even treatment by surgical drainage and debridement with appropriate antibiotic therapy is often insufficient to eliminate the disease.

QUESTIONS

Fractures and dislocations

Directions: Circle the letter preceding each item below that correctly answers the question. More than one answer may be correct.

1. Which of the following are characteristics of bone:
   a. Provides the supporting and protecting framework for the musculoskeletal system *b.* Plays a minor role in the regulation of calcium and phosphate *c.* Composed of supportive, rigid connective tissue referred to as apatite *c.* Is uniform in structure

2. Which of the following fractures is illustrated in the accompanying diagram? (See Fig. 61-21A.)
   a. Segmental *b.* Compression *c.* Greenstick *d.* Transverse

3. Which type of fracture is illustrated in the accompanying diagram? (See Fig. 61-21B.)
   a. Pathologic *b.* Greenstick *c.* Stress (fatigue) *d.* Avulsion

4. Which of the following best describes the periosteum?
   a. It is a region of longitudinal growth in children. *b.* It is a heavy fibrous band attached to the flared end of the long bone. *c.* It is composed mainly of cortical bone. *d.* It contains proliferating cells which contribute to transverse growth of bone.

5. In young children epiphyseal fractures involving the area of provisional calcification most likely will result in:

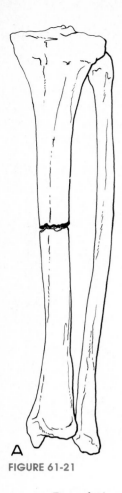
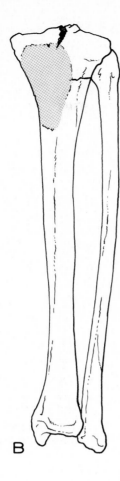

FIGURE 61-21

a. Retardation of longitudinal bone growth
b. Hypertrophy of collagen fibers in the diaphysis
c. Obliterated nerve supply to the diaphysis
d. Progressive deformity of the involved limb

6. Which of the following best describes a complete fracture?
a. The fracture crosses or involves the entire width or thickness of the bone.   b. The fracture contains more than two fragments of bone.
c. There is a structural discontinuity or break in a bone in which the surface opposite the break is intact.   d. A fragment of the bone at the involved area is separated at a tendon site.

7. The *initial* stage in the repair of a fracture is the:
a. Division of osteogenic cells, which causes a callus to form around the fracture site   b. Proliferation of osteoblasts, which form trabeculae   c. Remodeling of the fracture site   d. Formation of a blood clot in the area

8. Opposition refers to the:
a. Degree of severity   b. Degrees of deviation from the normal longitudinal axis and the direction of the apex of the angle   c. Extent of displacement of the fracture surfaces   d. Percentage of the fractured portion of one fragment that touches its mate

9. Which of the following is a definite sign of a fracture?
a. Generalized pain and tenderness   b. Crepitus
c. Abrasions   d. Shock

10. A cast that is applied to maintain a reduction should usually be placed:
a. Past the joint above and the joint below the fracture   b. Over the fractured area only
c. Over the smallest area possible, to prevent pressure and decubitus formation

11. The advantages of operative fracture treatment include:
a. Increased accuracy in repositioning the fracture fragments   b. Opportunity for inspection of adjacent vessels and nerves   c. No need for external casts or appliances after stabilization   d. Potential for maintenance of nearly normal joint function and muscular strength during fracture treatment

12. The most frequent reasons for using open reduction and internal fixation of fractures are:
a. To avoid deep wound infections   b. Inability to obtain an adequate reduction by closed means
c. To avoid complications resulting from prolonged bed rest in elderly patients

13. Mr. W. was diagnosed with a fractured femur and was treated by traction and later cast immobilization. Upon removal of the final cast, the distal limb is either internally or externally rotated and cannot be maintained in a neutral position by the patient. This fracture complication is referred to as:
a. Nonunion   b. Delayed union   c. Malunion
d. Osteomyelitis

14. Bill, a 19-year-old college student, severely injured his knee while playing soccer. At the time of admission his knee is too severely swollen, painful, and tender to make a definitive diagnosis. The most appropriate traction to use for comfort until his condition improves and a diagnosis can be made is:
a. Buck's   b. Balanced skeletal   c. Russell's
d. Bryant's

15. Balanced skeletal traction is frequently used in the treatment of fractures of the:
a. Patella   b. Tibia   c. Femur   d. Humerus

16. The traction shown in the following figure is used in the treatment of femoral fractures in children:
a. Above 5 years of age and weighing over 40 lb
b. Three years of age and weighing 30 lb
c. Three years of age and weighing 40 lb   d. Six years of age and weighing 60 lb

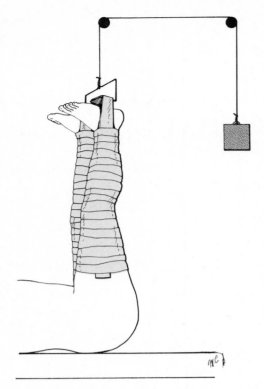

17. Which of the following are possible complications if the age and weight limitations are exceeded in Bryant's traction:

    a. The vascular supply to the feet in older and larger children may be compromised by the hydrostatic effect of vertical limb placement and constrictive elastic wraps.   b. The osmotic pressure of the blood is decreased.   c. Severe damage to the skin can result from exceeding these limits.   d. The heart rate is slower.

18. One complication of operative fracture treatment is osteomyelitis. Which of the following is a characteristic of osteomyelitis:

    a. A benign neoplasm consisting of osteoblastic connective tissue   b. Infection of the bone marrow and adjacent bone and cartilage   c. A sarcoma in bone containing foci of neoplastic cartilage

19. Subluxation:

    a. Occurs when no portion of a cartilaginous surface is in contact with its mating cartilage
    b. Refers to the angle of fracture in the femur
    c. Occurs when parts of articular cartilage are partially separated   d. Is a method of reducing a fractured limb

20. All the following are signs and symptoms indicative of a shoulder dislocation except:

    a. The patient supports the injured limb in a flexed position away from the chest or the side.
    b. The humeral head can be palpated in the anterior axilla.   c. There is localized pain in the area of the injury.   d. There is a definite sensation of crepitus.

21. Before attempting to reduce a dislocated shoulder, one must observe and record which of the following:

    a. The amount and duration of pain the victim is experiencing   b. The presence of tactile sensation within a small designated area over the deltoid muscle   c. Blood pressure and pulse rate   d. Ability of the patient to minimally elevate the injured limb away from the body

22. The important structure that is necessary for shoulder abduction and is most frequently injured as a complication of a shoulder dislocation is the:

    a. Radial nerve   b. Brachial artery   c. Axillary nerve   d. Radial artery

23. Mr. M., 30 years old, was brought to the emergency room after falling down his basement stairs. He is experiencing pain in his left groin and in the gluteal region. His right leg is flexed at the hip, adducted, and internally rotated. Mr. M.'s most likely diagnosis is:

    a. Fractured acetabulum   b. Dislocated hip   c. Fractured femoral head   d. Fractured femur

24. In treating an orthopedic emergency, the primary objective is to:

    a. Reduce the fracture   b. Preserve the life of the injured person   c. Use a sling to cradle the limb and hold it in position   d. Maximize the potential for rapid and complete rehabilitation of the injured person

25. External cardiac massage should be started immediately when there is:

    a. A weak, thready pulse   b. Absence of a pulse   c. Slow, shallow respiration   d. Gurgling sound on inspiration and expiration

26. Which of the following techniques of emergency treatment should be used for an injured person who is cyanotic and in obvious respiratory distress?

    a. Place the person in the supine position to allow for continuous drainage.   b. Manually remove debris and clotted blood from the mouth and throat.   c. From the front position, rapidly compress the chest.   d. If all attempts to remove the obstruction fail, perform a tracheostomy.

27. Which of the following best describes arterial bleeding?

    a. Red, pulsatile, and voluminous   b. Continuously flowing dark red   c. Red and scant

28. At the scene of an accident you have been unable to stop the victim's massive femoral arterial hemorrhaging by applying a series of compress pressure dressings. You decide to apply a tourniquet. Where in relation to the hemorrhaging site should a tourniquet always be applied?

    a. Distal to   b. Proximal to   c. At (the site)

29. The most important precaution, when using a tourniquet, is to note the exact time of application. Al-

though changes are usually reversible up to 2 hours, an extremity is likely to die if a touniquet is left in place longer than how many hours?
a. 4   *b.* 6   *c.* 10   *d.* 12

30. The correct emergency treatment for a limb deformity near a knee joint is to:
a. Tie the injured limb to the adjacent, uninjured one   *b.* Straighten the limb to a near-normal position and bind it to a stable appropriate object   *c.* Not attempt to straighten the limb, because of the close proximity of nerves and blood vessels to the fractured fragments   *d.* Support the limb on a soft support without attempting to straighten it

31. When splinting an injured limb, the following applies:
a. No padding is necessary   *b.* Check the distal pulse before and after the procedure   *c.* Only sterile bandages are to be applied to open wounds   *d.* Ample padding is necessary

32. Label the parts of the long bone—diaphysis, epiphysis, physis, periosteum—in the accompanying diagram.

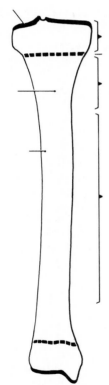

Directions: Match the type of fracture in col. A with its characteristic in col. B. Each letter may be used more than once.

Column A
33. ____ Spiral
34. ____ Oblique
35. ____ Greenstick

Column B
a. Heals rapidly; occurs in children
b. Results from torsion of a limb
c. Occurs in people who have

36. ____ Pathologic
37. ____ Stress (fatigue)
38. ____ Comminuted

recently increased their activity level
d. Is typical in ski injuries
e. Is most frequently caused by primary or metastatic tumors
f. Proceeds at an angle across the bone
g. Contains more than two fragments of bone

Directions: Circle T if the statement is true and F if it is false. Correct any false statements.

39. T   F   A closed fracture is one where the skin on the involved limb has been penetrated.

40. T   F   The most frequently used method of reduction is manual manipulation.

41. T   F   Comminution involves *more* than two fracture fragments.

42. T   F   Closed reduction of a fracture involves detailed and precise surgical approximation of the bone ends.

Directions: Answer the following questions on a separate sheet of paper.

43. Explain the changes that occur in the process of fracture healing.

44. Describe the type of pain, what this usually indicates, and the treatment when a cast has not been molded or padded sufficiently over bony prominences.

45. Why is skeletal traction generally preferable to skin traction?

46. What are the principles used in traction to maintain satisfactory reduction of limb fractures?

47. List the advantages of traction as a method of reduction of a limb.

48. List the advantages of implant devices such as the telescoping hip nail.

49. What is the ultimate goal of fracture treatment, and how is this achieved?

50. What is the ultimate goal of total hip arthroplasty or total knee replacement surgery?

51. List all the signs of neurovascular dysfunction.

52. Why is it important to immediately treat a limb with a compromised neurovascular supply by splitting all layers of the cast from one end to the other?

CHAPTER 62

ORTHOPEDIC DISEASES OF CHILDREN

OBJECTIVES

At the completion of this chapter you should be able to:

1. Explain the special characteristics of children's fractures and their treatment as compared with those in adults.

2. State the rationale for accepting bayonette apposition instead of end-on-end reduction when treating children's fractures.

3. Identify the characteristics of congenital dislocation of the hip according to: causes, pathogenesis, signs and symptoms, diagnostic tests, treatment, and prognosis.

4. Describe talipes equinovarus (clubfoot) by identifying its appearance, age group affected, treatment, and prognosis.

5. Differentiate between Calvé-Legg-Perthes disease and slipped capital femoral epiphysis according to the causes, pathogenesis, age group affected, signs and symptoms, treatment, and prognosis.

6. Identify the causes, age group affected, diagnosis, treatment, and prognosis for scoliosis.

HEALING POTENTIAL OF CHILDREN'S FRACTURES

Children's fractures heal rapidly and well. The active periosteal sleeve around the tubular bones in children is very strong. Since this area is rarely completely ruptured, fracture fragments tend to be maintained in acceptable position after fracture. Children's bones have great potential for corrective remodeling. Thus, a considerable postreduction angular deformity may be accepted with confidence that the mature bone will be straight without evidence of injury. In addition, there is a tendency of the injured limb to grow faster than normal. *Bayonette apposition* is often preferable to an end-on-end reduction, in order to achieve equal adult limb lengths (see Fig. 62-1). While angular deformities do rapidly correct, there is no similar tendency for rotational deformities to spontaneously resolve. Thus it is of utmost importance to maintain a normal rotational position during healing.

Most fractures in children are appropriately treated by closed reduction and external immobilization with

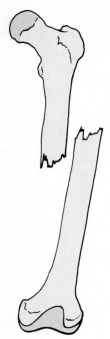

FIGURE 62-1
Bayonette apposition.

casts or traction. Only a few very specific children's fractures are optimally treated surgically. An example is a fracture of the lateral condyle of the humerus which extends into the joint and which may also involve an injury to the epiphyseal growth plate. Failure to accurately reduce the fragment back to its normal anatomic position may lead to a reduction of elbow function and growth arrest of the limb, which may result in gross deformity developing with increasing maturity. Fractures of the head of the radius and of the hip in children also frequently demand surgical treatment. In general, fractures which extend into joints or which pass across or through growth plates require surgery more often than do other fractures.

SPECIFIC DISEASE CONDITIONS

Congenital dislocation of the hip

Congenital dislocation of the hip is a condition in which the femoral head is not positioned normally in the acetabulum at birth (see Fig. 62-2). In addition, there is usually a delay in the maturity, size, and development of both the femoral head and the socket itself. The femoral head is small and frequently located superiorly and laterally out of the acetabulum.

Normal congruous development of the hip requires a normal congruent relation between the femoral head and the acetabulum. Long-term dissociation (separation) leads to inadequate development of the femoral head and acetabulum and results in ultimate *crippling*

of the individual. *All* newborn children should be examined for congenital hip dislocation within a few days of birth. This neonatal examination should specifically test for the ability to manually dislocate and then reduce the abnormal hip. The baby is placed in a supine position with both hips flexed. A gentle pressure is applied at the knees toward the examining table, and the knees and the thighs are manually abducted. At the same time an upward and medial pressure is applied to the proximal thighs. This initial downward knee pressure causes complete dislocation of the affected hip. When the thighs are abducted as described above, the hip can be felt to spontaneously reduce with a "clunk." Then with adduction the hip can be felt to dislocate. The hip instability demonstrated by this provocation test is diagnostic of congential hip disease and is known as a *positive Ortolani's sign* (see Fig. 62-3).

An inability to fully abduct one or both hips is frequently seen in a congenital dislocated hip (see Fig. 62-4). Additional signs include the Addis test, where obvious pathologic shortening of the thigh is noted (see Fig. 62-5). Asymmetric skin folds, extra gluteal folds, or inguinal creases are less definitive signs, but they do identify the need for further careful examination.

The most important radiographic view is an anterior-posterior projection of the pelvis and hips with the hips extended, the thighs together, and the lower limbs in neutral rotation. This position ensures maximal separation of the femoral head and acetabulum. If the fem-

FIGURE 62-2
(A) Congenital dislocation of the hip. (B) Normal hip.

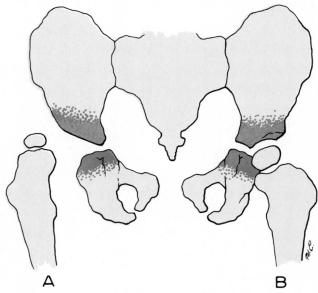

A   B

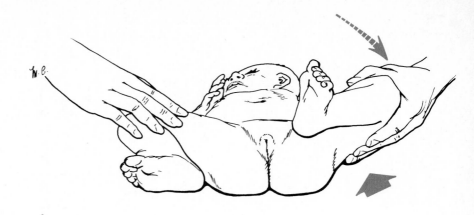

FIGURE 62-3
Ortolani's sign.

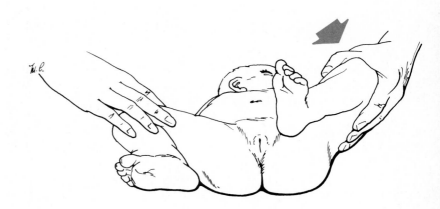

FIGURE 62-4
Limitation of abduction.

oral head does not lie in the lower inner quadrant as defined by Hilgenringer's line (drawn horizontally through the triradiate cartilage connecting the bones of the pelvis) and Perkin's line (drawn vertically downward from the superior lateral margin), congenital dislocation of the hip is the most likely diagnosis (see Fig. 62-6). The femoral head of the affected side is usually smaller than normal. The acetabular angle is greater than normal. However, of greater diagnostic signifi-

cance is absence of the normal cupping depression of the acetabulum.

FIGURE 62-6
X-ray changes in congenital dislocation of the hip.
(Modified from Smith et al., 1968.)

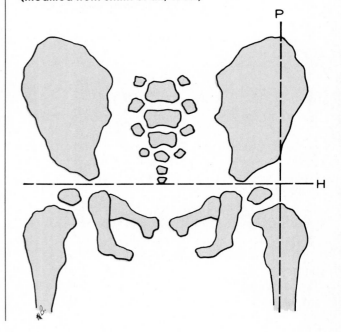

FIGURE 62-5
Addis test.

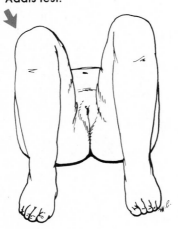

If congenital hip disease is diagnosed in the newborn infant, the appropriate treatment is reduction or relocation of the femoral head within the socket. This reduction must be maintained until the mutual relationship between the ball and the socket have stimulated a normal development and resolution of the disease. Gentle manipulation will generally allow seating of the femoral head in the acetabulum. Immobilization to maintain reduction must not be in an extreme position. Forceful reduction and extreme positions often lead to rapid development of aseptic necrosis of the femoral head, which may be a situation *more disabling* than the congenital hip dislocation itself. Many orthopedists rely on casts applied during anesthesia to maintain the first reduction for a period of a few months and continue the treatment with splints or braces until the radiographs demonstrate symmetric and normal hip development.

While braces may be used from the outset, it is possible for the hip to become dislocated during the infant's diaper changes. When the brace or splint is reapplied, the femoral head may be forced against the pelvic wall in a dislocated position. It is more advantageous to maintain the limb in a reduced position in a carefully applied cast until a relative degree of stability is achieved.

Nearly all patients with congenital dislocation of the hip who are diagnosed in the neonatal period and treated as described above develop hips which function normally throughout their lives. The success of this treatment in the neonatal period emphasizes the need for early diagnosis of *all* cases. If the diagnosis is not made until the child is 1 or 2 years of age, the chances for success are greatly compromised. Although closed reduction and immobilization may be a successful mode of treatment, operative care is often necessary. Many operative procedures have been described for the late treatment of congenital dislocation of the hips; this wide variety of treatment indicates the lack of predictable success for any specific procedure.

Talipes equinovarus

Talipes equinovarus (clubfoot) is another childhood disease which is optimally treated by early diagnosis and conservative management. In this condition the newborn foot is abnormally directed downward and turned in (see Fig. 62-7). It cannot be passively corrected to a normal position. While some spontaneous normalization may occur with time, the optimal immediate treatment to achieve maximal correction is the application of a small, short leg cast in the position of correction. This treatment is repeated on a daily or alternate-day basis. The newborn has an amazing potential for a plastic response to corrective forces which are applied early. Most clubfoot deformities can be corrected in a few weeks, and the correction need be maintained only until the foot is stable in the new, more normal position. With this treatment program the need for operative repositioning is decreased enormously. Prior treatment programs involved manipulation and cast application on an every-other-week basis. This procedure is to be condemned, since it fails to take maximal advantage of the great flexibility and rapid corrective response characteristic of the neonatal period.

Calvé-Legg-Perthes disease

Calvé-Legg-Perthes disease is a condition affecting the hip joint of children, the majority of whom are 5 to 7 years of age. Although frequently classified as an osteochondritis, the cause is unknown. Avascular necrosis of the epiphyseal ossification center results because of loss of cartilage and bone tissue supply. Reabsorption of dead bone and replacement with immature cells occurs in various stages.

Frequently a healthy child begins to complain of groin or knee pain on an intermittent but increasingly frequent basis. The knee is often examined. The negative examination and normal knee roentgenograms delay the important process of hip evaluation. The fact that the pain usually originates in the hip region and radiates directly to the knee tends to delay the diagnosis. Finally, the continued pain and limp eventually lead to an examination of the hip. The hip is painful during a forced range of motion examination. Roentgenograms

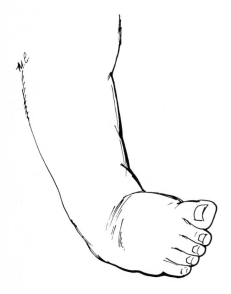

FIGURE 62-7
Talipes equinovarus (clubfoot).

usually demonstrate an increase in the apparent joint space and a slight lateral displacement of the femoral head by the presence of moderately tense effusion. At times, the joint capsule may be seen bulging. The femoral epiphysis appears somewhat flat (see Fig. 62-8B). In this early stage the epiphysis is probably relatively avascular and somewhat soft.

With time, cystic changes appear (see Fig. 62-8C), and frequently the epiphysis appears to fragment (see Fig. 62-8D). After many months revascularization occurs (see Fig. 62-8E), and the epiphysis regains its blood supply and strength.

Historically, treatment has relied on methods which can minimize the deforming forces on the affected epiphysis, such as crutches with a leather sling to support the distal limb and discourage weight bearing, non–weight-bearing crutch walking, or bed rest. After a few weeks, the child usually becomes symptom-free and discontinues the treatment program before reconstitution has progressed, but with unprotected ambulation the femoral head becomes increasingly deformed and a permanent crippling deformity results.

For many years long-limb suspension ischial weight-bearing braces were used to attempt to accomplish the goal of sustained protection of the hip. Frankel recently proved that the voluntary acceleration of the brace and limb during normal gait requires muscular activity about the hip which imposes loads on the involved epiphysis. These loads are at least as great in magnitude and deformation potential as those experienced during normal unprotected gait. This type of brace is therefore ill-advised.

Another, more recent treatment method depends upon the normal spherical anatomy of the uninvolved acetabulum. This concept is that if the capital femoral epiphysis can be positioned and maintained within the spherical acetabulum, it can be protected from significant deformation during the natural course of the disease. Thus, abduction braces and casts have been used to accomplish this goal. Although theoretically correct, the treatment method is cumbersome, and the brace is often discarded before the final safe stage of the disease.

In Scandinavia, bed rest or bed rest with traction (Mose) imposed throughout the course of the disease has been demonstrated to produce the best results, as documented by repeated roentgenograms. However, the required period of inactivity is approximately 18 months. There is considerable disagreement whether the disease has such serious or disabling consequences as to warrant this extreme treatment.

In summary, the essence of treatment would appear to be minimization of muscular and weight forces on the femoral head until reconstitution has occurred. Con-

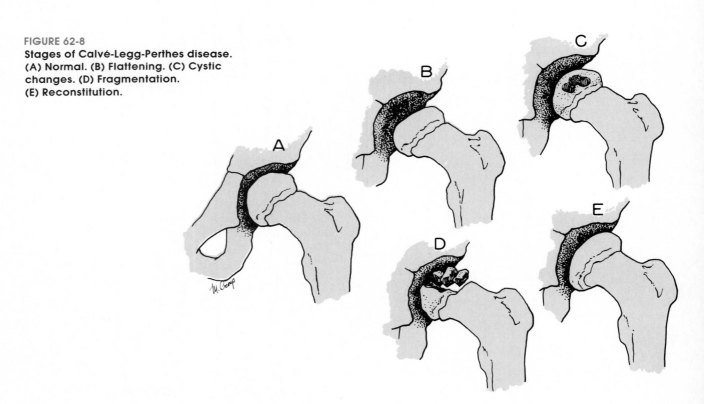

FIGURE 62-8
**Stages of Calvé-Legg-Perthes disease.
(A) Normal. (B) Flattening. (C) Cystic
changes. (D) Fragmentation.
(E) Reconstitution.**

tainment of the soft femoral head in the acetabulum may be of some value. Surgical reshaping or repositioning of the acetabulum to increase the coverage or protection of the femoral head has recently been attempted. Until the end results have been documented, it is too soon to adequately judge this new treatment method.

Slipped capital femoral epiphysis

Slipped capital femoral epiphysis is another fairly common disease of children. These children are usually in their early teens and have no associated disease. They are usually obese and large for their age, but may also be notably thin. The incidence is greater in males.

In this condition the epiphyseal plate of the proximal femur has insufficient shear strength to prevent deformation, and slippage of the femoral epiphysis occurs from its normal position directly on the end of the femoral neck. It may progressively slip medially (varus) and posteriorly relative to the femoral neck (see Fig. 62-9).

These patients also complain of pain on a forced end range of motion examination. When hip flexion is attempted, the limb automatically assumes a position of external rotation. Internal rotation in a flexed position is markedly limited. The knee on the same side feels painful, and again excessive medical interest in the knee may misdirect the diagnosis away from the diseased hip joint. Children, as well as adults, with complaints of knee pain should have an examination of the hips. In this condition an accurate early diagnosis may make a great difference in the patient's subsequent course. If the disease is diagnosed early, when minimal slippage and deformity have occurred, a simple internal pin fix-

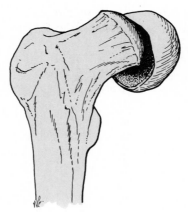

FIGURE 62-9
Slipped capital femoral epiphysis.

ation may stabilize the epiphysis, and nearly normal function frequently may be expected. However, if the individual continues untreated with unrestricted activity, increased deformity and the associated loss of normal range of motion may result. The incidence of aseptic necrosis and resultant crippling hip disease parallels delay in treatment. When a teenager is examined for suspicious knee, groin, or hip pain, an x-ray is indicated. A positive result for slipped capital femoral epiphysis indicates the immediate need for crutches, at least, and possibly for early or immediate hospitalization and treatment (see Fig. 62-10A and B).

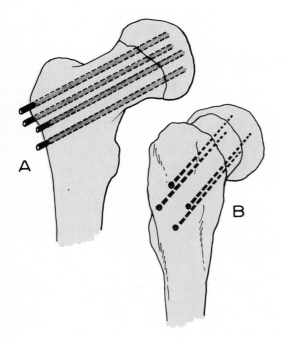

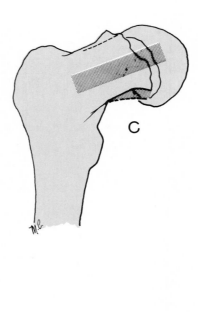

FIGURE 62-10
Surgical treatment for slipped capital femoral epiphysis.

While multiple pin stabilization is frequently satisfactory treatment for mild slips, those with more deformity may require extensive surgery to identify the diseased epiphyseal plate. The growth plate is then wholly or partially removed. An iliac bone graft is impacted across the plate region into the epiphysis. This procedure ensures immediate mechanical stability and early solid union of the epiphysis to the shaft. It is important to note that full unprotected activity is not completely safe until this union has taken place. Since forcible attempts at reduction of the epiphysis to its normal position are strongly related to head necrosis, it is generally best to accept even a moderate degree of deformity and to attempt union in this position. Since the bulge of the lateral proximal femoral neck may restrict abduction and internal rotation, this protrusion is surgically removed during the operation (see Fig. 62-10C).

Scoliosis

Scoliosis means curvature of the spine as observed by an anteroposterior x-ray. Although there are many rec-

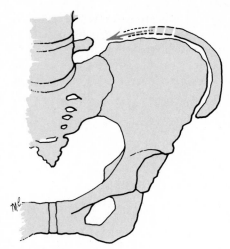

FIGURE 62-12
Risser's sign. (Modified from Keim, 1972.)

ognized causes of scoliosis, the most frequent type is referred to as *idiopathic scoliosis*. A typical example of this condition is an 11- or 12-year-old girl noted to have a protrusion of the right posterior chest with the right scapula appearing high and prominent. Her clothing drapes poorly, and there is an apparent difference in the lengths of the lower limbs. Although initially mildly deforming, with adolescent prematuration rapid growth the curvature may very quickly become much more severe. As the curvature increases, a rotation of the spine develops, and the deformity of the thorax becomes very offensive (see Fig. 62-11).

If an early diagnosis of idiopathic scoliosis is made, the youngster may usually be effectively treated with a Milwaukee brace. This sophisticated device not only tends to hold the spine straight in tension, but, of greater importance, it encourages the patient to use his or her own muscles to maintain the correction. With further growth in the corrected position, progression of the deformity is halted and at times reversed. The brace must be worn 23 hours daily, and a series of breathing, straightening, and strengthening exercises must be carried out. The brace must be worn until there is definite objective evidence of skeletal maturity and cessation of further spinal growth. The iliac apophysis must appear and progress toward the sacrum (Risser's sign), and the vertebral ring apophysis must fuse to the central mass of the vertebral bodies (see Fig. 62-12). A regular menstrual cycle and secondary sex characteristics, i.e., development of axillary and pubic hair and of breasts, should be established before brace treatment may be safely discontinued. Although the deformity documented at diagnosis can rarely be reversed by brace treatment, further progression is usually prevented. After skeletal maturity, a slight progression of the deformity is anticipated, but the patient can be expected to lead a nearly normal life.

FIGURE 62-11
Scoliosis.

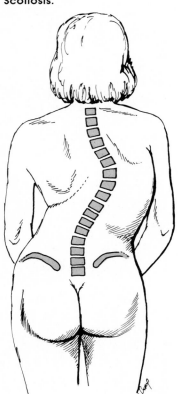

In the case of a late diagnosis or failure of brace treatment, surgical straightening of the spine and spinal fusion in the corrected position may be the best treatment. Special surgical implants such as Harrington rods may be used to straighten the spine at fusion. A skeletal brace traction, the Halo pelvic brace, may be required in severe cases. Spinal fusions are massive operations with a significant complication rate. Therefore, the best expected end result is a stiff spine in a partially cor-

rected position. It is very important that the diagnosis be made early and the Milwaukee brace therapy be initiated before the deformity becomes excessive or the spine too stiff.

QUESTIONS

Orthopedic diseases of children

Directions: Circle the letter preceding each item below that correctly answers the question. More than one answer may be correct.

1. All newborn babies in the nursery should be examined for the presence of the following signs of congenital hip dislocation:
   a. Limitation of abduction in initial flexion
   b. Impaction of the two bone ends   *c.* A positive Ortolani's sign (palpable click on adduction and abduction)   *d.* Limitation of adduction

2. The treatment (early after birth) of a congenital dislocated hip is:
   a. To place the proximal head of the ischium into the acetabulum and hold it until stable in that position   *b.* Open reduction to establish a new acetabulum and to reposition the head of the femur in that   *c.* To place the proximal head of the femur into the acromion process and hold it in a cast until stable   *d.* To relocate the femoral head within the socket and to maintain this reduction in a cast in abduction with the femoral head reduced in position

3. Talipes equinovarus is best treated by:
   a. Use of multiple casts   *b.* Surgical procedures to shorten the calcaneal tendon   *c.* Bryant's traction   *d.* Buck's traction

4. The condition characterized by flattening, cystic changes, breakup, and reconstitution of the femoral head is:
   a. Slipped capital femoral epiphysis   *b.* Calvé-Legg-Perthes disease   *c.* Osteoarthritis of the femoral head   *d.* Osteogenic sarcoma

5. John, an obese, large-in-stature 13-year-old, presents with moderate groin and knee pain in his left leg. While John's hip is flexed, his leg abducts and externally rotates. The most likely diagnosis of John's condition is:
   a. Congenital dislocation of the hip   *b.* Slipped

capital femoral epiphysis   *c.* Calvé-Legg-Perthes disease   *d.* Fracture of the femoral head

6. A 7-year-old boy with a history of knee pain for several days presents with a history of sudden acute hip pain and inability to bear weight. The most likely diagnosis is:
   a. Fracture of the hip   *b.* Congenital hip dislocation   *c.* Slipped capital femoral epiphysis *d.* Calvé-Legg-Perthes disease

7. The most likely treatment is:
   a. Multiple pin stabilization   *b.* Bed rest, with use of a leather sling to support the distal limb   *c.* Aspiration of the hip joint and antibiotic therapy

8. An 11-year-old girl presents with a "curve in the back" which is associated with back pain after exercise and at the end of each day. There is no history of neuromuscular disease. Physical examination reveals a thoracic idiopathic scoliosis. Anterior x-ray views of the pelvis reveal open iliac epiphysis. The most likely treatment is:
   a. Spinal fusion and Harrington rod instrumentation   *b.* Milwaukee brace   *c.* Halo pelvic brace   *d.* Hyperextension and hyperflexion exercises

9. Optimum treatment for idiopathic scoliosis depends primarily upon:
   a. Surgery after the curvature is of significant magnitude and fixed   *b.* Brace treatment for 2 years   *c.* Early examination and diagnosis at a stage of relative skeletal immaturity   *d.* Use of casts prior to surgery

Directions: Answer the following questions on a separate sheet of paper.

10. Explain why children's fractures usually heal rapidly and well.

11. Why is bayonette apposition often preferable in reduction of children's fractures?

TUMORS OF THE MUSCULOSKELETAL SYSTEM

OBJECTIVES

At the completion of this chapter you should be able to:

1. List the signs and symptoms associated with tumors of the musculoskeletal system.
2. Explain the rationale for treatment of a lesion that is benign and self-limiting, as opposed to a lesion that is less certainly benign. State an example of each type of lesion.
3. List the complications that may result in the use of a cannulated needle to obtain a tissue biopsy.
4. State the advantages and disadvantages of performing an open excisional biopsy to obtain a tissue specimen.
5. For osteogenic sarcoma, identify the age group affected, sites of occurrence, appearance, treatment, and prognosis.
6. For osteoma, enchondroma, and chondrosarcoma, identify sites of occurrence, appearance, and treatment.
7. List the clinical signs and symptoms that increase concern for malignant tumor potential.
8. Identify the radiographic appearance and the cause for the "onion-skin" appearance of Ewing's sarcoma.
9. Describe the specific radiologic signs that may be associated with a chondroblastoma, a benign unicameral cyst, a giant-cell tumor, osteogenic sarcoma, Ewing's sarcoma, and osteoid osteoma.
10. State the causes of the major type of bone tumor in adults.

SIGNS, SYMPTOMS, AND DIAGNOSIS

A complete presentation of the diagnosis, characterization, pathophysiology, and treatment of tumors found in

tissue within the musculoskeletal system is beyond the scope of this chapter. Therefore, it is more appropriate to focus the discussion on information pertaining to these lesions as they confront the health care team. The emphasis of this chapter will be on the rationale for an appropriate plan for care.

The patient frequently presents with a painful, enlarging mass. Characteristically the pain is minimal, related to activity, and frequently more intense at night. There is usually no previous history of specific serious trauma. Occasionally the tumor has weakened the bone to such an extent that a pathologic fracture has occurred. The tumor may be discovered by x-ray examination that is done for unrelated reasons. No matter how the patient presents, the immediate concern is whether the mass should be biopsied.

Some tumors or lesions may be directly identified by a consideration of the characteristics of the patient, the family history, the course of the condition, and the radiographic appearance of the lesion. In cases where the condition is definitively diagnosed as benign and self-limiting, e.g., a bone island or degenerative cyst, no further diagnostic studies are needed and no further medical care is usually necessary. In other cases the lesion may be diagnosed as benign with a lesser degree of certainty, e.g., osteochondroma or a unicameral bone cyst. When uncertainty exists about the lesion, it may be reasonable to reexamine the patient at intervals and to repeat the radiographs. The dimension of time and the rate of change used in this treatment regimen may eliminate the need for a surgical procedure. When this method of treatment is used, assessment must be made as to whether the patient and the family are responsible and will return for repeat examinations. If a series of examinations over several months reveals no change in the lesion or in the condition of the patient, follow-up visits may be discontinued. The patient should be instructed to return for a further examination should any changes become evident. Many lesions may not be easily identified and may leave doubts as to return for repeated examinations; a biopsy is necessary for a definitive diagnosis.

In obtaining a sample of tissue from the lesion, use of a cannulated needle is convenient and often successful. However, several problems are associated with this technique. The needle may macerate the tissue and thus destroy its important architecture. There is no certainty as to the exact location sampled, and so the tumor cells may not be included in the examined material. There is also the potential of injury to vascular or vital structures, which may be recognized as a late complication.

Although inconvenient for the patient and usually requiring hospitalization, open excisional biopsy may be the procedure of choice. This procedure is most appropriate for a patient who has a small, circumscribed lesion of uncertain identity. For example, in osteoid osteoma the lesion may be totally removed and positively identified, and the treatment may be completed with an excisional biopsy; or such a biopsy may identify a tumor with considerably greater malignant potential, which may require more extensive definitive treatment.

TYPES OF TUMORS

Giant-cell tumor

A characteristic feature of a giant-cell tumor is the vascular and cellular stroma which is made up of oval-shaped cells containing small, elongated, darkly staining nuclei. The giant cell is a large cell with pink-staining cytoplasm; it contains numerous nuclei, which are vesicular and appear similar to stromal cells. Although this tumor is usually considered to be benign, there are varying degrees of malignancy, depending upon the sarcomatous nature of the stroma. In the malignant types, the tumor becomes anaplastic and has areas of necrosis and hemorrhage.

Giant-cell tumors occur chiefly in young adults. They occur more frequently in women. The common sites are the ends of the long bones, especially at the knee and the lower end of the radius. The most common symptom is pain. Joint motion limitation and weakness may also be seen. This type of tumor usually requires a definitive gross local excision after biopsy identification. Removal of a safe border of normal tissue is in this case necessary. Characteristics of this tumor are that it tends to be locally recurrent (probably 60 percent or greater) and of increasingly malignant character after incomplete excision. With prior biopsy, diagnosis, and gross local removal, an immediate reconstruction of the area may be possible. In the case of a large giant-cell tumor of the distal radius (see Fig. 63-1A) the patient's proximal fibula can be substituted to reconstruct the forearm (see Fig. 63-1B).

Osteoma

Osteomas are benign bone lesions characterized by an abnormal outgrowth of bone. The classic osteoma presents as a slowly growing, painless, hard bump. Radiographically, peripheral osteomas present as radiopaque lesions which extend from the surface of bone; central osteomas are seen as well-delineated sclerotic masses inside the bone. Surgical excision of the osteoma is the preferred treatment when the lesion is symptomatic, enlarging, or causing disability. Removal is also done for diagnostic purposes for large lesions. Excision usually produces curative results.

Chondroblastoma

Chondroblastoma is a rare, usually benign tumor. It occurs most frequently in adolescent males. This tumor is uniquely found in the epiphysis. The most common site of occurrence is the humerus. The most frequent symptom is joint pain arising from cartilaginous tissue. Treat-

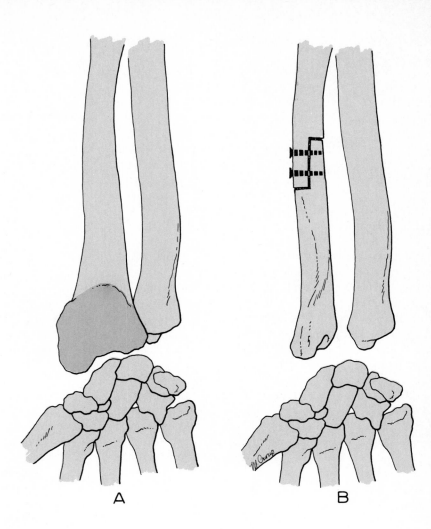

FIGURE 63-1

(A) Giant-cell tumor of the distal radius. (B) Use of a bone transplant to reconstruct the limb after total excision of a giant-cell tumor.

A

B

ment consists of surgical excision. Recurrence is treated with surgical excision, cryosurgery, or radiotherapy.

Enchondroma

Enchondroma, or central chondroma, is a benign tumor of dysplastic cartilage cells occurring in the metaphysis of tubular bones, particularly of the hands and feet. Radiographically, spotty calcification in the circumscribed, enlarged, rarefied lesion is characteristic of this tumor. It is believed to develop during the growth period in children and adolescence. This condition increases the likelihood of pathologic fractures. Surgical curettage and bone grafting are usually the treatment of choice for this lesion.

Osteogenic sarcoma

Osteogenic sarcoma, or osteosarcoma, is a very malignant primary neoplasm of bone. The tumor arises in the metaphysis of the bone. The most common sites are at the ends of the long bones, especially at the knee. The incidence of osteogenic sarcoma is greatest in adoles-

cents and young adults, but it may also affect people, usually over 50 years of age, who have Paget's disease. Severe pain associated with bone destruction and erosion is a usual symptom of this condition.

The gross appearance of osteogenic sarcoma is variable. It may be (1) osteolytic where the bone is destroyed and the soft tissue is invaded by the lesion, or (2) osteoblastic as a result of the formation of new sclerotic bone. Periosteal new bone may be deposited adjacent to the lesion itself, appearing as a triangle on x-rays (see Fig. 63-2). Although this is seen with many malignancies of bone, it is characteristic of osteogenic sarcoma; the tumor itself may produce a somewhat abortive form of bone. The radiographic appearance of such a lesion is referred to as a "sunburst," as depicted in Fig. 63-3.

Some primary tumors such as osteogenic sarcoma may be best treated by amputation or radical ablative surgery. While chemotherapy and immunotherapy appear to have some potential benefits, complete surgical removal of the tumor and all surrounding tissue is usually necessary. Twenty percent of patients with osteosarcoma survive for 5 years. The mean survival rate is 18 months.

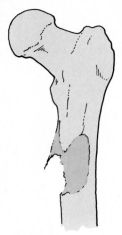

FIGURE 63-2
Osteogenic sarcoma with Codman's triangle.

Chondrosarcoma

Chondrosarcoma is a malignant bone tumor composed of anaplastic chondrocytes which may occur as a central or peripheral bone tumor. It occurs most often in males over 35 years of age. A painless mass of long duration is the most frequent presenting symptom. For example, peripheral lesions are often asymptomatic for long periods of time, presenting with only minor discomfort and palpable enlargement. However, rapid aggressive growth may occur. The pelvis, femur, ribs, shoulder girdle, and craniofacial bones are the most frequent sites of the lesion.

Chondrosarcomas appear as radiolucent areas with stippled and blotchy calcification of radiographs. Radical surgical excision is the treatment preferred; however, cryosurgery, radiotherapy, and chemotherapy may also be used. For large, aggressive, or recurrent lesions, amputation may be an appropriate treatment.

FIGURE 63-3
Radiographic "sunburst" appearance seen in osteogenic sarcoma.

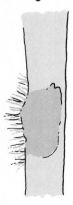

Ewing's sarcoma

Ewing's sarcoma is another very malignant bone tumor. This tumor is most often seen in preteenage children. The common site is the shaft of long bones. The gross appearance is a soft, gray tumor arising into the bone marrow reticulum which erodes bone cortex from within. Under the periosteum, layers of new bone are deposited parallel to the shaft, producing an onion-skin effect (see Fig. 63-4). The typical signs and symptoms are pain, tender swelling, fever (30° to 40°C), and leukocytosis (20,000 to 40,000 leukocytes per cubic millimeter). Treatment consists of radiation therapy, cytotoxic drugs, and surgical removal of the tumor. A poor prognosis is associated with this tumor. Recent reports indicate that new techniques of chemotherapy may significantly increase the survival rate.

FIGURE 63-4
Radiographic "onion skin" appearance seen in Ewing's sarcoma. (Courtesy of Dr. William Martel.)

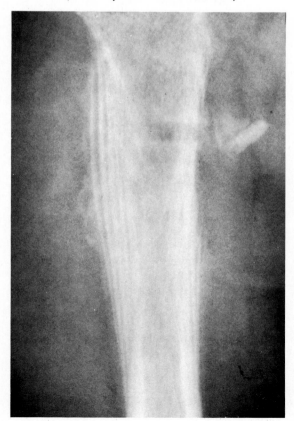

SIGNS AND SYMPTOMS ASSOCIATED WITH MALIGNANT TUMORS

What are the clinical signs and symptoms that may indicate a malignant tumor potential? The rate of increase in the size of mass is important. Benign lesions grow very slowly or not at all, while a very malignant tumor may double in size within a month. Increasing nightly pain and sleeplessness that are associated with weight loss in a presumably healthy individual are important indications. Fatigability in a young person is a very significant sign. A persistent fever and localized temperature increase in the region of the tumor indicate an increase in cellular activity. Finally, a physiologic dysfunction such as obstruction of the ureters, obstruction of a major vessel, or neurologic dysfunction is frequently seen in malignant tumors.

DIAGNOSTIC MEASURES

As a general rule the radiographic appearance of a specific lesion may be very helpful in determining its relative malignancy. For example, a lesion with discrete rounded margins tends to be benign. Such a lesion frequently has a sclerotic margin, indicating that the bone has had the time and ability to respond to the mass. The lack of a definable margin indicates invasion of the tumor into adjacent bone (see Fig. 63-5A). This lesion is growing rapidly and the bone has not had sufficient time or a defense response to react against it. Extension of the lesion through the cortex of the bone is typical of a malignancy. When the tumor penetrates the cortex, the periosteum may be lifted off. The bone may respond by depositing a thin layer of reactive bone, which is then lifted off, and the periosteal reaction begins again. As mentioned previously, this produces an onion-skin effect typical of Ewing's sarcoma (see Fig. 63-5B).

While the previous radiographic signs indicate the degree of malignancy of a lesion, there are other specific x-ray signs that lead to a more definitive diagnosis. For example, a radiolucent lesion located within the epiphysis of a growing bone is apt to be a chondroblastoma (see Fig. 63-6). A sclerotic marginated cystic lesion in the metaphysis of a long bone near an active growth plate is likely to be a benign unicameral bone cyst (see Fig. 63-7). A lucent lesion in an adult in the metaphysis

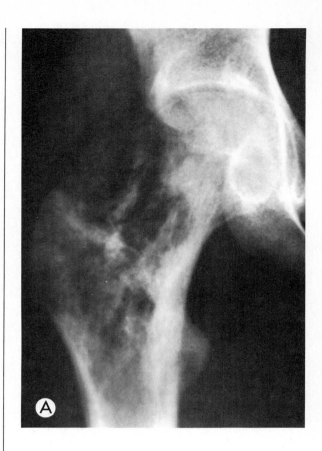

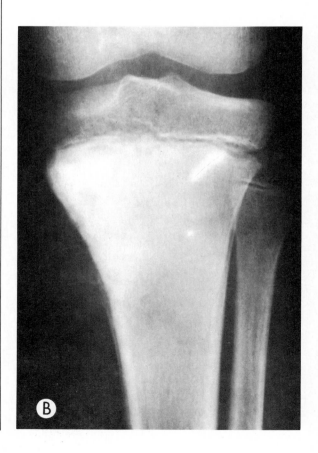

FIGURE 63-5
Radiographic appearance of a malignant tumor. (A) Femur. (B) Tibia. (Courtesy of Dr. William Martel.)

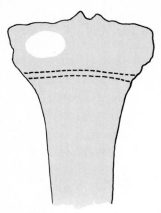

FIGURE 63-6
Chondroblastoma.

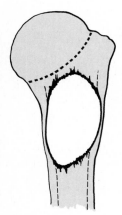

FIGURE 63-7
Unicameral bone cyst.

near the old growth plate is likely to be a giant-cell tumor (see Fig. 63-8).

A large, destructive lesion penetrating the cortex of the metaphysis of a long bone of an adolescent or young adult is very indicative of osteogenic sarcoma. A retic-

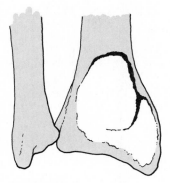

FIGURE 63-8
Radiographic appearance of a giant-cell tumor.

ulated, spotty, and extensive radiolucent cortical lesion in a child is very likely to be Ewing's sarcoma. A "target" or "bull's-eye" lesion, sclerotic bone around a radiolucent area surrounding a central dense nucleus, in an individual with night pain which responds to salicylates is nearly always an osteoid osteoma.

The age of the patient offers significant diagnostic information. For example, children are often affected by unicameral cysts, eosinophilic granuloma, or Ewing's sarcoma, while slightly later chondroblastoma becomes relatively more prevalent. As mentioned previously, adolescents and young adults are usual victims of osteogenic sarcoma, which also affects people in the late middle years who have Paget's disease.

The major type of bone tumor in adults is metastasis from other primary sites such as the lungs, breasts, thyroid, kidneys, and the prostate. Multiple myeloma is the most common primary tumor of bone in adults (see Chap. 17).

QUESTIONS

Tumors of the musculoskeletal system

Directions: Answer the following questions on a separate sheet of paper.

1. What is the rationale for treatment of a lesion that is benign, as opposed to a lesion that is less certainly benign?

2. Cite the complications that occur in the use of a cannulated needle to obtain a tissue biopsy.

3. What are the advantages vs. disadvantages of performing an open excisional biopsy to obtain a tissue specimen?

4. What are the clinical signs and symptoms that indicate a malignant tumor potential?

Directions: Circle T if the statement is true and F if the statement is false. Correct any false statements.

5. T   F   Osteochondroma occurs frequently near joints and has a potential for malignant change.

6. T   F   Pathologic fractures usually do not re-

sult from metastasis of malignant tumor to bone.

7. T F Benign giant-cell bone tumors have a tendency to become aggressive and spread locally if there is incomplete surgical removal and/or unsuccessful radiation therapy.

8. T F The major type of bone tumor found in children results from metastasis from the primary tumor site to bone.

9. T F Chondrosarcoma occurs frequently in males over 35 years of age.

Directions: Circle the letter preceding each item below that correctly answers the question. More than one answer may be correct.

10. Which of the following are characteristic of an osteoma?
    a. Usual presentation as a slowly growing, painless, hard bump *b.* Commonly affects elderly males *c.* An increase in the likelihood of pathologic fractures *d.* Benign bone lesion occurring near the joints in children and adolescents

11. The onion-skin pattern of subperiosteal new bone formation is most likely in which of the following tumors involving long bones?
    a. Ewing's sarcoma *b.* Osteosarcoma
    c. Chondroblastoma *d.* Reticulum cell sarcoma

12. The bone most frequently involved in chondroblastoma is the:
    a. Femur *b.* Humerus *c.* Tibia *d.* Ulna

13. Concerning chondroblastoma, which of the following is *not* true:
    a. The tumor is found in the epiphysis *b.* Severe pain associated with bone destruction is commonly encountered *c.* Occurs most frequently in adolescent males *d.* It is a rare, usually benign tumor

14. The mean survival rate of patients with osteosarcoma is:
    a. Less than 6 months *b.* 6 months to 1 year
    c. 18 months *d.* 3 to 5 years

15. James B., age 16, was admitted to the hospital with an enlarging primary mass in the right distal femur at the knee. Microscopic studies revealed numerous abnormal bone-forming cells with great variation in size and shape. Radiologic studies revealed extension of the tumor into adjacent soft tissue—cortical breakthrough. Which one of the following diagnoses would you suspect?
    a. Ewing's sarcoma *b.* Osteogenic sarcoma
    c. Osteoid osteoma *d.* Giant-cell tumor

REFERENCES FOR PART X

ADAMS, J. C.: *Standard Orthopaedic Operations,* 2d ed., Churchill Livingstone, London, 1980.

APLEY, A. G. and L. SOLOMON: *Apley's System of Orthopaedics and Fractures,* 2d ed., Butterworth, London, 1982.

BLOUT, W.: *Fractures in Children,* Williams & Wilkins, Baltimore, 1955.

BROWN, P.: *Basic Facts in Orthopaedics,* Blakiston, London, 1981.

BRUNNER, L. and D. SUDDARTH: *Textbook of Medical-Surgical Nursing,* 4th ed., Lippincott, Philadelphia, 1980.

COZEN, L.: *An Atlas of Orthopedic Surgery,* Lea & Febiger, Philadelphia, 1966.

DONAHOO, C. and J. DIMON: *Orthopedic Nursing,* Little, Brown, Boston, 1977.

DUTHIE, R. and A. B. FERGUSON: *Mercer's Orthopaedic Surgery,* 7th ed., Williams & Wilkins, Baltimore, 1973.

HILT, N. and S. COGBURN: *Manual of Orthopedics,* Mosby, St. Louis, 1980.

HUVOS, A.: *Bone Tumors, Diagnosis, Treatment, and Prognosis,* Saunders, Philadelphia, 1979.

KEIM, H.: "Scoliosis," *Clinical Symposia* 24:1, 1972.

LANGLEY, L. L., I. R. TELFORD, and J. B. CHRISTENSEN: *Dynamic Anatomy and Physiology,* 5th ed., McGraw-Hill, New York, 1980.

LARSON, C. and M. GOULD: *Orthopedic Nursing,* 6th ed., Mosby, St. Louis, 1978.

LATTES, R.: *Tumors of the Soft Tissue,* Armed Forces Institute of Pathology, Washington, D.C., 1982.

LUCIANO, D., A. VANDER, and J. SHERMAN: *Human Anatomy and Physiology,* McGraw-Hill, New York, 1983.

MACAUSLAND, W. and R. MAYO: *Orthopedics,* Little, Brown, Boston, 1965.

MARCONE, R.: *The Surgery of Tumors of Bone and Cartilage,* Grune & Stratton, New York, 1981.

MERCER, L. R. and F. J. PETID: *Practical Orthopedics,* Year Book, Chicago, 1980.

MUSTARD, W., et al. (eds.): *Pediatric Surgery,* 2d ed., Year Book, Chicago, 1969.

ROCKWOOD, C. and D. GREEN (eds.): *Fractures*, vols. 1–2, Lippincott, Philadelphia, 1975.

RUBIN, P.: *Dynamic Classification of Bone Dysplasia,* Year Book, Chicago, 1964.

SALTER, B.: *Textbook of Disorders and Injuries of the Musculoskeletal System,* Williams & Wilkins, Baltimore, 1970.

SMITH, W., et al.: "Correlation of Postreduction Roentgenograms and Thirty-one Year Follow-up in Congenital Dislocation of the Hip," *Journal of Bone and Joint Surgery,* 50-A(6):1081–1098, 1968.

PART XI

MICHAEL A. CARTER

RHEUMATIC DISORDERS

The diverse group of rheumatic disorders are very common. Twenty percent of the United States population is affected with one or more of these disorders, and over half of all individuals over 65 years of age have some form of arthritis. These figures do not include the millions of Americans who have mild forms of arthritis which have not been reported. Rheumatoid disorders affect women more frequently than men, and no racial group is spared. The costs these disorders exact are enormous when one considers the lost days from work because of pain and limitations in mobility, costs for medications and professional services, and the large amount of monies spent for unproven remedies.

In this part a number of rheumatic disorders are covered, although no attempt is made to cover the more than 100 different disorders. Rheumatic disorders share the common characteristics of inflammation or pain of the muscles, joints, or connective tissues of the body. For the most part, these disorders are long-term illnesses which can involve multiple organ systems. Rheumatic disorders most frequently affect the diarthrodial or freely movable joints of the body. The synovial membranes in these joints are particularly at risk for developing inflammation and pain.

The classification of rheumatic disorders is undergoing constant change as new knowledge of the pathophysiological mechanisms that underlie these disorders becomes available. Also, research in the association of certain rheumatologic disorders to HLA antigens has contributed to the development of new forms of classification. The Nomenclature and Classification Committee of the American Rheumatism Association provides frequent revision and updating of classification as new knowledge about these disorders is obtained.

Rheumatologic disorders become increasingly common with advancing age. Figures reporting the frequency of arthritis may significantly underestimate the true number of people with these disorders. For example, many people may have radiographic evidence of degenerative joint disease but few symptoms. Other persons may have what they consider minor aches, pains, or stiffness that they attribute merely to increasing age. These persons may have never been seen by a health care practitioner for this problem and therefore cannot be reported in frequency figures. Health care practitioners may fail to report these symptoms since they are so ambiguous.

The focus of this part is twofold. First, there is a focus upon the anatomy and physiology of joints and connective tissues, since these are sites commonly affected in rheumatologic disorders. The second focus of this part is upon selected rheumatologic disorders. No attempt has been made to cover all of these disorders; instead, certain ones have been chosen for inclusion because they are common or very disabling.

OBJECTIVES

At the completion of this part you should be able to:

1. Describe the anatomical and pathophysiological alterations seen in the major rheumatologic disorders presented.
2. Describe the basis of therapy for these disorders based upon an understanding of the anatomical and pathophysiological alterations.

CHAPTER 64

ANATOMY AND PHYSIOLOGY OF THE JOINTS

OBJECTIVES

At the completion of this chapter you should be able to:

1. Formulate a definition of rheumatic disorders.

2. State the importance of the joints and surrounding connective tissues in rheumatic disorders.

3. Differentiate between the three types of joints (synarthrodial or fibrous, cartilaginous, diarthrodial) as to location, function, and degree of involvement in rheumatic disorders.

4. Describe the composition of a joint capsule.

5. Identify for normal joint synovial fluid the appearance, amount, white cell count, and function.

6. Differentiate between hyaline cartilage and articular cartilage as to composition and function.

7. Explain the mechanism of lubrication of a joint.

8. Describe the unique characteristics of the blood supply to the joint.

9. Explain why the inflammatory process is especially pronounced in the synovium.

10. Identify for the autonomic and sensory nerves the ligaments, joint capsule, synovium sensitivity factor, and rationale for referred pain.

11. Define *connective tissue*.

12. State the role of temporary cells found in connective tissues (i.e., mast cells, lymphocytes) in the inflammatory and immune reactions that are indicative of rheumatic disorders.

13. Indicate the function of permanent cells in the connective tissue.

14. List the six forms of collagen classified according to their location.

15. Differentiate between collagen and elastin fibers by location, synthesis, process, and results of alterations in synthesis.

16. Define *proteoglycans*.

17. Identify the relationship of proteoglycans in articular cartilage to the inflammatory and immunologic processes.

18. Identify at least four factors that appear to predispose individuals to rheumatic disorders.

19. List the assessment measures applied in the evaluation of joints.
20. Describe the seven kinds of angular movements of a joint.
21. Explain the rationale for the difficulty in evaluating joint pain.
22. Differentiate between the three types of joint swelling as to location, causes, and complications.
23. Describe the mucin clot test.
24. Describe the way selected rheumatic disorders affect synovial fluid.

Rheumatic disorders produce pain and stiffness in some portion of the musculoskeletal system. These disorders primarily affect the joints and the surrounding connective tissues, although other connective tissues throughout the body can be affected. *Arthritis* is the term used when the joint is affected, and *soft tissue rheumatism* refers to inflammation of connective tissue not in a joint.

JOINTS

Joints are areas in the body where two or more bones meet. These bones are held together by various means such as joint capsules, fibrous bands, ligaments, tendons, fasciae, or muscles. There are basically three types of joints. Synarthrodial, or fibrous joints are those in which the bones are held together by fibrous tissues which allow no movement. Fibrous joints include the sutures of the skull, the tibiofibular attachments, and the tooth sockets. These joints are not usually affected by rheumatic disorders.

Cartilaginous joints are those in which the bones are joined by cartilage and are slightly movable. The symphysis pubis and the intervertebral discs are examples of cartilaginous joints.

Diarthrodial or synovial joints are the joints that are freely movable. These are the ones most frequently affected by rheumatic diseases. The bones in diarthrodial joints do not touch but are held together by a variety of connective tissues and surrounded by a joint capsule (see Fig. 64-1).

The joint capsule is made up of a dense fibrous outer covering, an inner layer of highly vascularized connective tissue, and synovium. The synovium forms a sac that lines the entire joint and covers tendons that pass through the joint. The synovium does not extend across to the articular surface of the joint. The syno-vium is folded in such a way as to allow full joint motion. The linings of the bursae throughout the body resemble synovium. The periosteum does not extend into the joint capsule.

The synovium produces a highly viscous liquid that lubricates the joint surfaces. Normal synovial fluid is clear, nonclotting, and either colorless or straw-colored. Relatively small amounts (1 to 3 ml) are found in normal joints. The white cell count of the fluid is normally less than 200 cells per cubic millimeter and is primarily of mononuclear cells. Hyaluronic acid is responsible for the viscosity of synovial fluid and is synthesized by synovial lining cells. The liquid component of the synovial fluid is thought to be a transudate from plasma. Synovial fluid also serves as a source of nutrition for the articular cartilage. Rheumatic disorders can cause a variety of changes in the synovium and the synovial fluid.

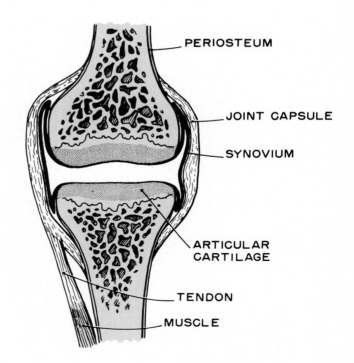

FIGURE 64-1
Normal joint.

Hyaline cartilage covers the load-bearing portions of the bones in diarthrodial joints. This cartilage serves an important role in distributing weight loads. Articular cartilage is made up of very few cells and a large amount of ground substance. This ground substance consists of Type II collagen and proteoglycans that are produced by the cartilage cells. The proteoglycans found in articular cartilage are very hydrophilic, which adds to their ability to resist wear with heavy joint use.

Articular cartilage in the adult does not have any blood supply, lymphatic channels, or nerves. Oxygen and other necessary products for metabolism are carried by the synovial fluid which bathes the cartilage. There can be alterations in collagen and proteoglycan synthesis following injury or with increasing age. Some of the new collagen produced at this time begins to resemble Type I collagen and is much more fibrous. The proteoglycans can lose some of their hydrophilic abilities. These changes mean that the cartilage can lose its ability to resist wear with heavy usage. The variables that cause these changes are not understood at this time.

The joint is lubricated by the synovial fluid and by hydrostatic changes in the interstitial fluid of the cartilage. Pressure on the cartilage causes fluid to move from the cartilage to an area of less pressure. As the joint glides forward, this weeping fluid moves ahead of the load. The fluid moves back into the portions of the cartilage from which the pressure is relieved. The articular cartilage and the bones of the joint are normally held apart during action by the film of fluid. The articular cartilage cannot be worn out by excessive use as long as there is an adequate fluid film present.

The blood supply to the joint is richest in the synovium. The vessels arise from the subchondral bone at the level of the margin of the capsule. The capillary network is particularly thick in the portions of the synovium immediately adjacent to the joint space. This allows products from the plasma to diffuse easily into the joint space. The inflammatory process can be especially pronounced in the synovium, since there is such a rich supply of blood vessels as well as the presence of a large number of mast cells and other cells and chemicals that dynamically interact to stimulate and amplify the inflammatory response.

Autonomic and sensory nerves are widely distributed in the ligaments, joint capsule, and synovium. These nerves account for the sensitivity of these structures to position and movement. Nerve endings in the capsule, ligaments, and adventitia of blood vessels are particularly sensitive to stretching or twisting. Pain that arises from the joint capsule or synovium tends to be diffuse rather than localized. Joints are innervated by peripheral nerves that cross the articulation. This means that pain from one joint may be reported as coming from another. For example, pain arising in the hip can be felt by the person as knee pain.

CONNECTIVE TISSUE

The tissues found in the joints and adjoining areas are primarily connective tissues. Connective tissues are composed of cells and ground substance. The cells found in connective tisusue are of two types. One type includes cells that do not develop in or permanently remain in connective tissue and includes mast cells, plasma cells, lymphocytes, monocytes, and polymorphonuclear leukocytes. These cells play an important role in the inflammatory and immune reactions seen in the rheumatic disorders. The second type of cells found in connective tissue includes those permanently located there—fibroblasts, chondrocytes, and osteoblasts. These cells synthesize the various fibers and proteoglycans of the ground substance and gives each type of connective tissue its unique properties.

The fibers found in the ground substance include collagen and elastin. There are at least six forms of collagen that can be classified by their molecular chain structure, location, and function. Type I collagen is a widely distributed form found in the cornea, conjunctiva, skin, sclera, synovium, bone, and tendon. Type II collagen is found in cartilage and the vitreous. Type III collagen is found in skin, synovium, and blood vessel walls along with Type I. Type IV collagen is present in basement membrane. Type V collagen is found in the placenta and the corneal stroma. Type VI collagen is found in embryonic tissues and in corneal scar tissue.

Collagen can be broken down by the action of collagenases. These proteolytic enzymes cleave the stable molecule in such a way that it becomes unstable at physiological temperatures and is hydrolyzed by other processes. Alterations in the synthesis of cartilage collagen are seen with increasing age and may be a major factor in the development of degenerative joint disease. Increased collagenase activity is seen in immune-mediated forms of rheumatic disorders such as rheumatoid arthritis.

Elastin fibers have a unique cross-linking property that provides important elastic properties. These fibers are found in the ligaments, the walls of the larger blood vessels, and the skin. Elastin is broken down by enzymes called elastases. Elastases may be important in the development of arteriosclerosis and emphysema. There is some evidence that changes in the cardiovascular system because of aging may be a result of increased breakdown of elastin fibers.

Proteoglycan is the other important product found in the ground substance along with the fibers. Proteoglycan is a class of large molecules that are made up of long polysaccharide chains attached to polypeptide cores. Proteoglycans in articular cartilage are responsible for the cushioning properties that are necessary for the joints to withstand large physical forces. The relationship of the proteoglycans to the inflammatory and immunologic processes is complex. Lymphokines can induce connective tissue cells to produce new proteoglycans, inhibit their production, or increase their breakdown. Proteoglycans can become the focus of autoimmunity action in disorders such as rheumatoid arthritis. Increasing age brings changes in porteoglycans in cartilage. They become less able to aggregate with each other and interact with collagen. The major structural and functional changes that are a part of the normal aging process are a result of changes in the biochemistry of the connective tissues and primarily in the fibers and proteoglycans. The rheumatic disorders are characterized by specific biochemical changes in these same components.

THE IMMUNE AND INFLAMMATORY PROCESSES IN RHEUMATIC DISORDERS

Major components of rheumatic disorders are alterations in the immune and inflammatory processes. An in-depth knowledge of the immune system (see Chaps. 4 and 5) is required to understand the changes seen in rheumatic disorders. Additional knowledge of the concept of autoimmunity (see Chap. 12) is required to understand the autoimmune rheumatic disorders of rheumatoid arthritis and systemic lupus erythematosus.

Why some people develop chronic inflammatory disorders is not known. There are several factors that appear to predispose individuals to these disorders. These factors include chronic trauma over years to connective tissue; genetic predispositions, especially those associated with the HLA markers; abnormal connective tissue synthesis; the presence of certain sex hormones; and the compromised repair processes of aging tissue. Substantial basic research currently under way is designed to show the relationships between host responses and environmental phenomena in the development of these disorders. Rheumatic disorders appear to be the result of normal immune and inflammatory processes that somehow are not functioning appropriately. This assumption forms the basis for the interventions used in the treatment.

EVALUATION OF JOINTS

Joints are evaluated by examining their range of motion and the presence of pain and tenderness, swellings, dis-

colorations, and deformities. Various rheumatic disorders differ in the way that they affect the joints, and evaluation of the joints is helpful in making the diagnosis and monitoring responses to therapy.

There are seven kinds of angular movement possible by a joint. These are (1) *flexion*, which decreases the angle between bones, or brings the bones together, (2) *extension*, which increases the angle, or separates the bones, (3) *abduction*, which is movement away from the body, (4) *adduction*, which is movement toward the body, (5) *internal rotation*, which is a turning of the joint toward the center of the body, (6) *external rotation*, which is a turning of the joint away from the center of the body, and (7) *circumduction*, which is a circular motion of the joint (Malasanos, 1981). Rheumatic disorders usually restrict full range of motion, particularly full extension.

Evaluation of joint pain can be particularly difficult, since periarticular pain may be hard to distinguish from pain arising from the joint. The location of the pain and any tenderness should be described as accurately as possible. There is no pain or discomfort with full active use of normal joints.

There are three types of swellings that can occur in or around a joint. The joint can swell because of an increase in synovial fluid production. This will produce an enlarged joint space. An increase in joint space can also follow trauma that causes bleeding into the joint.

The second type of joint swelling is synovial enlargement. Normally the synovial tissues are not palpable in the joint space, but with inflammation they can become quite large and boggy.

The third type of joint swelling is bony enlargement. This occurs particularly in people with degenerative joint disease and is usually along the lateral margins of the joint. These enlargements are permanent, while joint effusions and synovial enlargements are transitory.

Periarticular swellings can occur around the joint. These include ganglia, rheumatoid nodules, tophi, and swelling of the tendon sheaths.

Discolorations of joints are also assessed. The skin over the joint can become red (active inflammation), white (swelling that decreases circulation), or blue (cyanosis). The skin over the joint usually feels warm or hot if the color is red but is normal or cool if the color is white or blue.

The rheumatic disorders can produce characteristic joint deformities as they progress. These deformities are covered in the following chapters for each disorder.

EVALUATION OF SYNOVIAL FLUID

The synovial fluid may be affected differently by each of the rheumatic disorders. Table 64-1 compares normal synovial fluid with the changes seen in some of the more common disorders. The mucin clot test is performed by

TABLE 64·1

SYNOVIAL FLUID

	Normal	Degenerative joint disease	Systemic lupus erythematosus*	Gout†	Rheumatoid arthritis	Reiter's syndrome	Infectious arthritis‡
Color and clarity	Straw-colored; clear	Straw-colored; clear	Straw-colored; clear	Straw-colored or white; cloudy	Straw-colored or light yellow; cloudy	Opaque	Gray, purulent; cloudy
Mucin clot	Good	Usually good	Fair to good	Poor	Poor	Poor	Poor
White cell count (average)	$<200/mm^3$	$1000/mm^3$	$5000/mm^3$	$10,000$–$20,000/mm^3$	$15,000$–$20,000/mm^3$	$20,000/mm^3$	$50,000$–$75,000/mm^3$

*LE cells may be present.
†Uric acid crystals are present.
‡Bacteria can be cultured.

adding acetic acid to the synovial fluid. This forms a precipitate by interaction with hyaluronic acid. The mucin clot has poor results with the more inflammatory fluids because the hyaluronic acid has been broken down by the lysosomal enzymes and therefore is not available to precipitate when treated with acetic acid. The clarity of normal synovial fluid is diminished by an increase in the cells and protein in pathological conditions.

QUESTIONS

Anatomy and physiology of the joints

Directions: Answer the following questions on a separate sheet of paper.

1. Define *rheumatic disorders.*
2. Describe the relationship of the joints and surrounding connective tissue to rheumatic disorders.
3. List the various means by which joints are held together.
4. Explain the process by which a joint is lubricated.
5. List the assessment measures utilized in the evaluation of joints.
6. What are the factors that appear to predispose individuals to rheumatic disorders?

Directions: Circle the letter preceding each item that correctly answers the question below. More than one answer may be correct.

7. Which of the following is an example of a truly movable joint:
   a. Diarthrodial (synovial)   b. Synarthrodial (fibrous)   c. Cartilaginous
8. An example of a synarthrodial (fibrous) joint is:
   a. A skull suture   b. The synovium   c. The symphysis pubis   d. An intervertebral disc

9. The function of ligaments is to:
   a. Attach muscle to bone   b. Cover the surface of bones   c. Hold bones together at joints   d. Cover tendons that pass through joints
10. The load-bearing portions of the bones in diarthrodial joints is covered with:
    a. Synovial fluid   b. Hyaline cartilage   c. Fibrocartilage   d. Fascia
11. Which of the following contains the richest blood supply to the joint?
    a. Articular cartilage   b. Synovium   c. Hyaline cartilage   d. Serous membrane
12. The cells that develop and remain in connective tissue are:
    a. Mast cells   b. Plasma cells   c. Fibroblasts   d. Osteoblasts
13. The type of collagen found in the cornea conjunctiva, skin, sclera, synovium, bone, and tendon is Type:
    a. II   b. I   c. III   d. IV
14. Which of the following is responsible for the synthesis of collagen fibers?
    a. Fibroblasts   b. Proteolytic enzymes   c. Polysaccharides   d. Elastin

15. The function of proteoglycans in articular cartilage is to:
a. Allow full joint motion   b. Distribute weight loads   c. Lubricate the cartilage

16. All of the following depict causes of swellings that can occur in or around a joint *except:*
a. An increase in synovial fluid production
b. Synovial enlargement due to inflammation
c. Bony enlargements along the lateral margins of the joint   d. An increase in production of collagenases

Match the type of angular movement by a joint in col. A with the description in col. B.

Column A

17. ____ Extension
18. ____ Adduction
19. ____ Circumduction
20. ____ Internal rotation
21. ____ Flexion
22. ____ External rotation

Column B

a. Turning of the joint away from the midline of the body
b. Movement away from the midline of the body
c. Turning of the joint toward the midline of the body
d. Circular motion of the joint
e. Decrease in the angle between bones

23. ____ Abduction

f. Movement toward the body
g. Increase in the angle or separation between bones

Directions: Circle T if the statement is true and F if it is false. Correct the false statements.

24. T   F   Pain from the synovium tends to be localized.

25. T   F   Autonomic and sensory nerves in the ligaments, joint capsule and synovium account for the sensitivity of these structures to position and motion.

26. T   F   The mucin clot test is most effective with the more inflammatory fluids.

Directions: Match the conditions in col. A with the synovial fluid white cell counts in col. B.

Column A

27. ____ Normal joint
28. ____ Rheumatoid arthritis
29. ____ Infectious arthritis
30. ____ Systemic lupus erythematosus

Column B

a. 15,000 to 20,000 per cubic millimeter
b. 5000 per cubic millimeter
c. <200 per cubic millimeter
d. 50,000 to 75,000 per cubic millimeter

CHAPTER
65

RHEUMATOID ARTHRITIS

OBJECTIVES

At the completion of this chapter you should be able to:

1. Formulate a definition of rheumatoid arthritis.
2. Identify for rheumatoid arthritis the frequency of occurrence, incidence, and prevalence.
3. Explain the association with the genetic markers, and the hypothesis concerning the causes of rheumatoid arthritis.
4. Describe the destruction of tissues in the joint that occurs in rheumatoid arthritis.
5. Identify and describe the eight clinical features of rheumatoid arthritis.
6. Evaluate the laboratory tests and radiologic features that are used in diagnosing rheumatoid arthritis.
7. List the diagnostic criteria developed by the American Rheumatism Association and explain the three categories of diagnosis for rheumatoid arthritis.
8. Describe two of the systemic organ involvements which may be seen in rheumatoid arthritis.
9. List the overall goals of the therapeutic program for rheumatoid arthritis.
10. Evaluate the therapeutic prescriptions that are designed to meet those goals.
11. List the major components of an educational program for rheumatoid arthritis patients.
12. Discuss the goals for the rest, exercise, and thermotherapy therapeutic programs.
13. Explain the nutritional therapeutic plan.
14. State the purposes of medication therapy.
15. Describe the nonsteroidal anti-inflammatory drugs (NSAIDs) as to class of therapeutic agents and pharmacologic mechanism used in rheumatoid arthritis.
16. List and explain the goals of treatment with disease-modifying anti-rheumatic drugs (DMARDs).
17. Explain the rationale for the utilization of corticosteroid therapy.

Rheumatoid arthritis is a chronic disorder that affects multiple organ systems. This disorder is one of a group of diffuse connective tissue diseases that are immune-mediated and of unknown cause. There is usually progressive joint destruction, although the episodes of joint inflammation may have periods of remission (see Fig. 65-1).

Rheumatoid arthritis affects women about 2½ times more frequently than men. The incidence increases with age, especially in women. The peak incidence is between 40 and 60 years of age. The disease is seen worldwide in all racial groups. About 1 percent of all adults have definite rheumatoid arthritis, and about 750 new cases per million population are reported each year in the United States.

The causes of rheumatoid arthritis are still unknown even though a great deal is known about the pathogenesis. The disorder cannot be shown to have a definite genetic link. There is an association with the genetic markers of HLA-Dw4 and HLA-DR5 in whites. Only an association with HLA-Dw4 has been shown in blacks, Japanese, and Chippewa Indians. A current hypothesis concerning the cause of this disorder is that there are genetic factors that lead to the development of the disorder following some viral illness such as an infection by Epstein-Barr virus.

Destruction of the tissues in the joint occurs in two ways. First, there is a digestive destruction that is brought about by the production of proteases, collagenases, and other hydrolytic enzymes. These enzymes break down the cartilage, ligaments, tendons, and bones in the joints and are released along with oxygen radicals and arachidonic acid metabolites by polymorphonuclear leukocytes in the synovial fluid. The process is thought to be part of an autoimmune response to locally produced antigens.

The second way in which tissue destruction occurs appears to be through action of rheumatoid pannus. This is a vascular granulation tissue that forms from the inflamed synovium and later extends into the joint. Along the edge of the pannus there is destruction of collagen and proteoglycans through the production of enzymes by cells in the pannus.

CLINICAL FEATURES

There are several common clinical features seen in persons with rheumatoid arthritis. These may not all be present at one time in any particular individual, since the disorder is so variable.

1. Constitutional symptoms—these include fatigue, anorexia, weight loss, and fever. At times the fatigue can be disabling.
2. Symmetrical polyarthritis primarily of peripheral joints—this includes the joints of the hands, usually sparing the distal interphalangeal joints. Almost any diarthrodial joint can be affected.
3. Morning stiffness of greater than 1 hour—this may be generalized stiffness but primarily involves the joints. This stiffness is different from the stiffness seen in degenerative joint disease, which usually lasts only a few minutes and always less than an hour.
4. Erosive arthritis is a radiologic characteristic of this

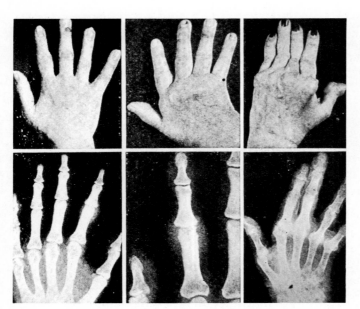

FIGURE 65-1
Early, moderate, and advanced rheumatoid arthritis in the hands. Note the swelling of the second proximal interphalangeal (PIP) joint as part of the early changes. In the moderate stage there is swelling of the metacarpophalangeal (MCP) joints. The advanced stage shows subluxation of the MCP joints.
(Reproduced with permission from Dwight C. Ensign, "Osteoarthritis and Rheumatoid Arthritis," *Modern Medicine*, March 1, 1955, p. 128, copyright 1955 by Harcourt Brace Jovanovich.)

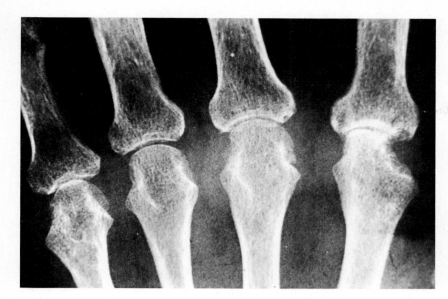

FIGURE 65-2
X-ray of a rheumatoid hand. Note the joint space narrowing, erosion of the second metacarpal head, and early erosion of the third metacarpal head. The cortex of the fourth metacarpal head remains indistinct. Compare this with the nice, well-defined cortex of the fifth metacarpal head. (Reproduced with permission from the Canadian Arthritis and Rheumatism Society, Dr. J. B. Houpt, editor.)

disorder. The chronic inflammatory response results in loss of the marginal aspects of the bones (see Fig. 65-2).

5. Deformity—there is destruction of the supportive structures of the joints as the disease progresses. Ulnar drift or deviation of the fingers, subluxation of the metacarpophalangeal joints, and boutonniere and swan neck deformities (see Fig. 65-3) are some of the common deformities of the hands. There is a protrusion of the metatarsal heads secondary to metatarsal subluxation in the feet. Large joints may also be involved and have a decreased range of motion primarily in extension.

6. Rheumatoid nodules are subcutaneous masses occurring in about one-third of adults with rheumatoid arthritis. The most common site for these is in the olecranon bursa (elbow) or along the extensor surface of the forearm; however, they can occur elsewhere. The presence of these nodules is usually indicative of an active or more severe disease (see Fig. 65-4).

7. Extraarticular manifestations—rheumatoid arthritis may involve organs other than the joints. The heart (pericarditis), lungs (pleuritis), eye, and blood vessels can be damaged. Table 65-1 outlines extraarticular manifestations of this disorder.

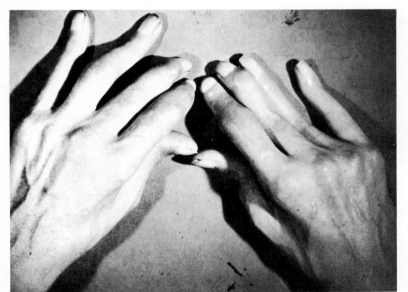

FIGURE 65-3
Rheumatoid hand with boutonniere and swan neck deformities. Polyarthritis of the joints of the hands. Among the advanced deforming changes is the muscle wasting in the anatomical snuffbox (between thumb and forefinger). Boutonniere deformity of the left fourth digit. Swan neck deformity involving the right third and fourth digits. (Reproduced with permission from the Arthritis Division, University Hospital, University of Michigan.)

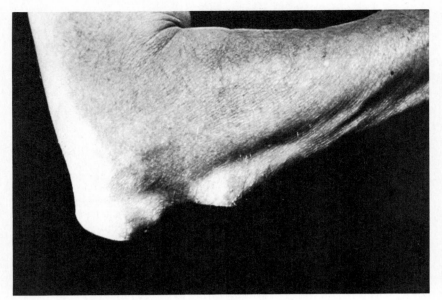

FIGURE 65-4
Rheumatoid nodules in the elbow. Two large subcutaneous nodules are located about the elbow. One is in the olecranon bursa, and the other is on the extensor surface of the forearm. Nodules may be fixed or movable and are usually tender. They occur most commonly at the elbow but may also be found elsewhere, as on the feet, fingers, occiput, heels, and buttocks. Nodules occur in about 20 percent of patients with rheumatoid arthritis, may fluctuate in size, and are usually associated with high titers of rheumatoid factor. (Reproduced with permission from the Arthritis Foundation, New York, copyright 1972.)

TABLE 65-1

EXTRAARTICULAR MANIFESTATIONS OF RHEUMATOID ARTHRITIS

1. Subcutaneous and subperiosteal features (rheumatoid granulomas)
2. Organ involvement:

Heart	Pericarditis: only occasionally symptomatic and only rarely progressing to chronic constricting disease
	Valvular lesions: chiefly aortic due to rheumatoid granulomas (rare)
Lung	Pleurisy: with or without effusion
	Multiple pulmonary (rheumatoid) nodules
	Rheumatoid pneumoconiosis (Caplan's syndrome)
	Progressive interstitial fibrosis: with formation of honeycomb lung
Eye	Scleritis
	Iridocyclitis (in *juvenile* rheumatoid arthritis)
Nervous system	Peripheral neuropathy (associated with vasculitis)
	Peripheral compression syndromes, including carpal tunnel syndrome (median nerve neuropathy), ulnar nerve neuropathy, peroneal palsy, and cervical spine abnormalities

3. Systemic complications:
   Anemia (common)
   Generalized osteoporosis
   Felty's syndrome (in 10% of cases of rheumatoid arthritis)
   Sjögren's syndrome (keratoconjunctivitis sicca)
   Amyloidosis (rare)
4. Features associated with vasculitis:
   Fever
   Digital arteritis (focal ischemic areas in nail fold, nail edge, or digital pulp, gangrene, rare)
   Raynaud's phenomenon
   Skin lesions (rash and gangrene)
   Chronic leg ulcers
   Peripheral neuropathy (mononeuritis multiplex)
   Erosions in mucosa of gastrointestinal tract with hemorrhage
   Necrotizing arteritis involving mesenteric, coronary, renal vessels

Source: Modified from Committee of the American Rheumatism Association, 1973, p. 34.

LABORATORY FINDINGS

Several laboratory tests are used in diagnosing rheumatoid arthritis. Rheumatoid factor is found in the serum of about 85 percent of the people who have rheumatoid arthritis. This autoantibody is an anti–gamma globulin factor, IgM, that reacts against altered IgG. Higher titers, greater than 1:160, are usually associated with rheumatoid nodules, severe disease, vasculitis, and a poor prognosis. Rheumatoid factor is a helpful diagnostic test but is not an exclusive test for rheumatoid arthritis. A positive test can indicate other connective tissue disorders such as systemic lupus erythematosus, progressive systemic sclerosis, and dermatomyositis. In addition about 5 percent of the normal population has a positive test. The incidence of positive rheumatoid factor in the normal population increases with age. As many as 20 percent of people over 60 years of age may have positive factors with low titers.

The erythrocyte sedimentation rate (ESR) is a nonspecific index of inflammation. In rheumatoid arthritis there may be very high values (100 mm per hour or higher). This means that the ESR may be useful for monitoring disease activity.

Rheumatoid arthritis can cause a normocytic normochromic anemia through action on the bone marrow. This anemia does not respond to usual forms of therapy and can make the person very tired. Often there is an iron deficiency anemia as a consequence of drug therapy for the illness. This form of anemia may respond to iron replacement.

Normal synovial fluid is a clear, light-yellow fluid with a white cell count of less than 200 per cubic millimeter. In rheumatoid arthritis the synovial fluid loses its viscosity and the white cell count is increased to 15,000 to 20,000 per cubic millimeter. This makes the fluid turbid. The fluid may clot, but the clot is usually poor and friable.

In the early stages of the illness, there may be no radiologic findings other than soft-tissue swelling. As the joint damage progresses, there may be narrowing of the joint space because of the loss of articular cartilage. Bone erosions at the margin of the joint and decreased bone density occur. These changes are not usually reversible.

DIAGNOSTIC CRITERIA

The diagnosis of rheumatoid arthritis can be a very complex process. In the early stages there may be a few or no positive laboratory tests; the joint changes can be minor; and the symptoms can be transitory. The diagnosis does not rest on any single characteristic but is based on the evaluation of a number of signs and symptoms. The diagnostic criteria developed by the American Rheumatism Association are the ones that are widely used. These are:

1. Morning stiffness
2. Pain on motion, or tenderness in at least one joint
3. Swelling (not bony) in at least one joint
4. Swelling of at least one other joint within a 3-month period
5. Symmetrical joint swelling
6. Subcutaneous nodules
7. X-ray changes typical of rheumatoid arthritis
8. Positive serologic test for rheumatoid factor
9. Poor mucin precipitate from synovial fluid
10. Characteristic histologic change in nodules
11. Characteristic histologic change in synovial tissue

There are three categories of diagnosis for rheumatoid arthritis: probable rheumatoid arthritis means three of the criteria are met; definite rheumatoid arthritis means five of the criteria are met; and classic rheumatoid arthritis means seven criteria are met. These criteria are combined with a set of exclusions to rule out other related illnesses.

TREATMENT

The treatment of rheumatoid arthritis is based upon an understanding of the pathophysiology of the disorder. In addition, attention needs to be directed toward the psychophysiological manifestations and the attendant psychosocial disruptions caused by the chronic, fluctuating course of the problem. Making an accurate diagnosis may take years, but treatment is initiated early.

The overall goals of the therapeutic program are to:

1. Relieve pain and inflammation
2. Maintain joint function and maximum functional capacity of the person
3. Prevent and/or correct joint deformities

There are a number of therapeutic prescriptions designed to achieve these goals: education, rest, exercise and thermotherapy, nutrition, and medication.

The first step of the therapeutic program is to provide an adequate education about the illness to the patient, the family, and those with whom the patient comes into contact. This education includes an understanding of the pathophysiology, causes, and prognosis of the illness, all the components of the management program including the complex drug regime, sources of assistance for coping with the illness, and effective methods of management offered by the health care team. The educational process is a constant one. Assistance is provided by patient clubs, community agencies, and by other people with rheumatoid arthritis and their families.

Rest is important because rheumatoid arthritis usually is accompanied by profound fatigue. While there may be some fatigue each day, there are times in which the person will be better or worse. Stiffness and discomfort may worsen with rest. This means that the person can frequently awaken at night with pain. Methods of decreasing nighttime pain should be prescribed, such as long-acting anti-inflammatory drugs. In addition, the treatment plan should cover activity pacing. The person should be assisted in breaking each day into periods of activity followed by rest. If there is to be a particularly heavy activity, such as a party, then the rest period should be prior to that activity.

Specific exercises are useful in maintenance of joint function. These include active and passive range of motion to all affected joints at least twice a day. Pain medications may be necessary before beginning these exercises. Heat applications to painful and swollen joints may decrease pain. Special temperature-regulated paraffin baths and contrast baths of heat and cold can be used at home.

The exercise and thermotherapy program is best prescribed by a health care provider with special training such as physical therapy or occupational therapy. Overuse of exercise can tear supporting structures of the joint that are already weakened by the illness. Adaptive and assistive equipment may be necessary for the person to perform activities of daily living. Materials are available from the Arthritis Foundation or from one of the many local chapters that show how to use these devices and where to purchase them.

There is no specific nutritional prescription for rheumatoid arthritis. There are a number of unproven claims about various types of dietary interventions. The general principle is that a well-balanced diet is important. The illness may affect the temporomandibular joint, making chewing difficult at times. A number of the medications used to treat the illness can cause stomach discomfort and decrease adequate nutrition. Keeping the body weight in the proper limits is very important. Weight can be easily gained, since activity levels usually are low. This increased weight can place additional stress on hip, knee, and foot joints. Referral to a registered dietitian can be of assistance.

Medication therapy is a very important part of the overall treatment program. Medications are prescribed to reduce pain, to decrease the inflammation of the illness, and to attempt to modify the course of the illness. Different drugs may be used for each of these goals.

Pain is a constant part of rheumatoid arthritis. This means that the use of dependency-causing drugs should be kept to a minimum. Therapeutic measures such as heat and exercise can do a lot to diminish pain. Many nonsteroidal anti-inflammatory drugs have both an analgesic and anti-inflammatory action and are used for both purposes.

The mainstay of drug therapy in rheumatoid arthritis is the use of nonsteroidal anti-inflammatory drugs (NSAIDs). Twenty individual drugs currently compose this class of therapeutic agents, and they can be subdivided into six chemical classes. These are the salicylates, pyrazolones, propionic acids, oxicams, indole/indenes, and anthranilic acids. Although their chemical structures are diverse, the pharmacology is very similar. This class of drugs reduces inflammation by interrupting the cascade of production of inflammatory mediators. Specifically, they act by inhibition of either cyclooxygenase or prostaglandin synthetase. These enzymes are responsible for the conversion of the endogenous systemic fatty acid, arachidonic acid, to prosta-glandins, prostacyclins, thromboxanes, and oxygen radicals. The historical standard drug in this class is aspirin, and all other NSAIDs are considered equally effective to aspirin at appropriate doses of each drug.

Additional drug therapy is indicated when the NSAIDs do not control the rheumatoid arthritis. Disease-modifying antirheumatic drugs (DMARDs) are a group of drugs used for this purpose. These drugs are a diverse group of agents that include antimalarials, gold compounds, immunosuppressive agents, and penicillamine. The goals of treatment with DMARDs are to control the clinical manifestations and to arrest or slow the progression of the illness. The onset of response to DMARDs is often very gradual and can be delayed 3 to 6 months. Maximum response usually occurs after 1 year of therapy. NSAID therapy is continued during this initial latency period in order to control pain and inflammation. NSAID therapy may be necessary even after the full effect of the DMARD therapy, to control pain. Each of the DMARDs acts differently and often through a poorly understood mechanism. The adverse effects vary with the agent being used.

There are at least four indications for the utilization of corticosteroid therapy. Chronic oral therapy is used in those persons with rheumatoid arthritis who do not respond to NSAIDs and DMARDs. The second indication is for the control of symptoms during the waiting period before the onset of action of DMARD therapy. Third, intraarticular injections are indicated for acute exacerbations of synovitis in single joints in which mobility is significantly impaired. The fourth indication is high-dose oral therapy for short periods for severe attacks. The mechanism of action of these agents is twofold through anti-inflammatory and immunosuppressive properties. Inflammation is reduced by blockage of prostaglandin formation, inhibition of leukocyte and monocyte chemotaxis and phagocytosis, stabilization of lysosomal enzymes, and prevention of changes in capillary membranes. Immunosuppression is caused by decreased reticuloendothelial, or monocyte-macrophage, procession of antigens and altered functions of lymphocytes. There are many adverse effects from the use of these drugs, particularly in chronic use. Almost all organ systems are disturbed by their use.

QUESTIONS

Rheumatoid arthritis

Directions: Answer the following questions on a separate sheet of paper.

1. Define *rheumatoid arthritis*.
2. What is the association between the genetic markers HLA-Dw4 and HLA-DR5 and the development of rheumatoid arthritis?
3. Describe the two ways in which destruction of tissues in the joint occurs in rheumatoid arthritis.
4. List the 11 diagnostic criteria developed by the American Rheumatism Association, and explain the three categories of diagnosis for rheumatoid arthritis.

5. What are the overall goals of the therapeutic program for rheumatoid arthritis?

6. Describe the mechanism by which nonsteroidal anti-inflammatory drugs (NSAIDs) reduce inflammation.

7. Cite the four indications for the utilization of corticosteroid therapy in persons with rheumatoid arthritis.

8. What is the mechanism of action of these corticosteroid drugs?

9. Discuss two of the systemic organ involvements which may be seen in rheumatoid arthritis.

Directions: Circle the letter preceding each item below that correctly answers the question. More than one answer may be correct.

10. Rheumatoid arthritis typically affects which of the following segments of the population:
    a. Both sexes equally   *b.* Females more than males(2.5:1)   *c.* Males more than females (2.5:1)

11. The peak incidence of rheumatoid arthritis is between which years of age?
    a. 10, 20   *b.* 40, 60   *c.* 20, 40   *d.* 60, 80

12. The joints most commonly affected by symmetrical polyarthritis are the:
    a. Joints of the hands, including distal interphalangeal joints   *b.* Peripheral joints   *c.* Symphysis pubis   *d.* Intervertebral discs

13. Common clinical features seen in rheumatoid arthritis are:
    a. Skin rash, psoriasis   *b.* Sun sensitivity   *c.* Fatigue, anorexia, weight loss   *d.* Morning stiffness lasting less than 1 hour   *e.* Joint swelling of the hands, including distal interphalangeal joints

14. Which of the following laboratory findings is indicative of rheumatoid arthritis?
    a. Rheumatoid factor in the serum   *b.* An erythrocyte sedimentation rate of less than 100 mm per hour   *c.* Urate crystals in the synovial fluid   *d.* A positive mucin clot test

15. Typical radiologic findings found in rheumatoid arthritis are:
    a. Asymmetrical soft-tissue tophi   *b.* Narrowing of the joint space   *c.* Irregular loss of joint space   *d.* Bony cystic erosion

16. The therapeutic program for rheumatoid arthritis usually includes:
    a. Rest periods and decreased activity during the day   *b.* An educational program covering the pathophysiology, etiology, management (drugs and sources of assistance), and prognosis   *c.* A vigorous exercise program to strengthen structures of the joint   *d.* Specific dietary prescriptions recommending either high-dose B or C vitamins   *e.* Initial prescription of disease-modifying antirheumatic drugs (DMARDs)

Directions: Circle T if the statement is true and F if it is false. Correct the false statements.

17. T   F   Salicylates, pryrazolones, propionic acids, indole/indenes, and anthroanilic acids are classified as nonsteroidal anti-inflammatory drugs.

18. T   F   An association with the genetic marker HLA-DR5 has been shown in blacks and Japanese.

19. T   F   The most common site for rheumatoid nodules is the olecranon bursa.

20. T   F   Rheumatoid factor (RF) is a measure of the IgM antibody, which reacts against the altered IgG and is detected in about 99 percent of patients with rheumatoid arthritis.

CHAPTER
66

SERONEGATIVE SPONDYLOARTHROPATHIES

OBJECTIVES

At the completion of this chapter you should be able to:

1. State the reason that ankylosing spondylitis, psoriatic arthritis, and Reiter's syndrome are called seronegative.

2. Identify the characteristics of ankylosing spondylitis, including the diagnostic criteria, sex differences, and joint involvement.

3. Explain the significance of the laboratory and radiologic findings in ankylosing spondylitis.

4. Describe the aim of the treatment measures and prognosis for ankylosing spondylitis.

5. State the relationship between psoriasis and psoriatic arthritis.

6. Identify for psoriatic arthritis the clinical features and significance of the laboratory and radiologic findings.

7. Discuss the goals of treatment of psoriatic arthritis.

8. Identify for Reiter's syndrome the predisposing factors, triad of symptoms and association with psoriatic arthritis.

9. Describe the clinical features and laboratory and radiologic findings in Reiter's syndrome.

10. State two components of the treatment program for Reiter's syndrome.

Seronegative spondyloarthropathies are a group of related disorders that include ankylosing spondylitis, psoriatic arthritis, and Reiter's syndrome. These disorders are called seronegative because there is a lack of rheumatoid factor in the serum. In addition, there is an association of these disorders with HLA-B27.

ANKYLOSING SPONDYLITIS

Ankylosing spondylitis is a chronic inflammatory disease that can be progressive. The illness usually involves the sacroiliac joints and the spinal articulations. The hips and costovertebral articulations can be affected as the disease progresses. Ankylosing spondylitis was once thought to be a variant of rheumatoid arthritis. This is no longer the case, based upon the criteria of negative rheumatoid factor, the absence of rheumatoid nodules, and the differences in the bone changes in the spine. The 9:1 male-to-female ratio of the illness no longer is believed accurate, now that better criteria for diagnosis have been established. Men tend to have a more progressive spinal disease and are more likely to be diagnosed as having ankylosing spondylitis. This gives a clinical ratio of about three men for each woman with spinal involvement. Ankylosing spondylitis occurs less frequently in Japanese and blacks but more frequently in Pima Indians.

Ankylosing spondylitis affects the cartilaginous and fibrocartilaginous joints of the spine and paravertebral ligaments. Calcification of the joints and articular structures occurs when intervertebral discs become invaded by vascular and fibrous tissue and later become calcified. Calcified soft tissue bridges one vertebra to another. The synovial tissue around the joints involved becomes inflamed. Heart disease can also occur with ankylosing spondylitis.

The causes of ankylosing spondylitis are still unknown. There appears to be a genetic factor involved. Approximately 90 percent of persons diagnosed as having ankylosing spondylitis have a positive HLA-B27 antigen; incidentally, 50 percent of their unaffected relatives are positive for the same antigen (Katz, 1977).

Clinical features

Ankylosing spondylitis has an insidious onset, beginning with feelings of fatigue and intermittent low-back or hip pain. Morning stiffness which is relieved by mild activity may occur. The symptoms can be so mild and unprogressive that many people are never diagnosed. In addition, the symptoms of ankylosing spondylitis can be confused with those of mechanical back problems.

The evaluation indicates a basically healthy person who gives a history of persistent back pain with insidious onset. The person is usually under 40 years of age. The back pain is made better with exercise and worse with rest and has diffuse radiation throughout the lower back and buttock. The physical exam shows no scoliosis, a symmetrical decrease in range of motion, diffuse tenderness, and a negative straight-leg-raising test. The peripheral neurologic system is usually unchanged. As the illness progresses, there is a loss of normal lumbar lordosis, fusion of the dorsal spine into kyphosis, and restriction of thoracic excursion. At the late stages of the illness there is fusion of the spine that can result in hip flexion contractures and the use of flexed knees to maintain an erect position (see Fig. 66-1). Pain is usually diminished after ankylosis is complete, and there is a marked decrease in synovitis.

Laboratory Findings

There are no specific laboratory tests used in diagnosing ankylosing spondylitis. The erythrocyte sedimentation is usually elevated during active phases of the illness. The rheumatoid factor is usually negative. The antigen HLA-B27 is likely to be positive, but this is not specific to ankylosing spondylitis.

Radiologic findings

There are characteristic x-ray changes that occur in ankylosing spondylitis. In the very early stages of the illness, there may be only blurring of sacroiliac joint and diffuse osteoporosis of the spine. As the illness progresses, there is joint erosion, squaring of the vertebrae, and narrowing of the disc spaces. In the last stages of the illness, calcification of the discs and paravertebral ligaments occurs. Vertical bony growths, called syndesmophytes, can be demonstrated bridging the gaps between the vertebrae (see Fig. 66-2). In about 25 percent of the people with ankylosing spondylitis, there is complete fusing of the spine, including the cervical spine.

Treatment

Treatment of ankylosing spondylitis is multifocal and related to the stage of the illness. There is a focused intervention aimed at increasing the understanding of the illness by the person and the family. Changes in the work patterns may be necessary, since bending, lifting, and prolonged static positions are difficult. Medication therapy is aimed at decreasing the synovitis and the resulting pain. Nonsteroidal anti-inflammatory drugs are used for this purpose, particularly those with high prostaglandin-blocking ability and a long half-life. Indomethacin is frequently the drug of choice. Corticosteroids, disease-modifying drugs, and muscle relaxants are of limited value. An active program of physical therapy is often helpful, focused upon breathing exercises, muscle strengthening, maintaining or improving posture, and range of motion exercises. Braces and splints may be used for limited time periods to decrease muscle spasm and pain.

Prognosis

Not all persons with ankylosing spondylitis develop the disabling stages of the illness. About half have a slow, extended course than can last for decades. A number of the remaining persons can be successfully treated with

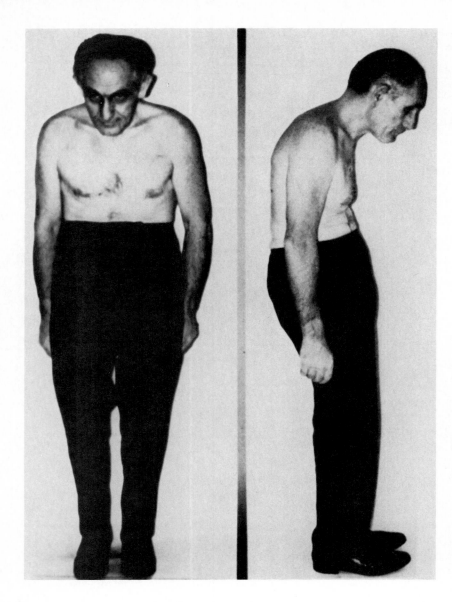

FIGURE 66-1
Ankylosing spondylitis: on the left a frontal view demonstrates the characteristic upward gaze of the eyes when they look straight ahead, necessitated by the flexion deformity of the neck. The lateral view demonstrates forward protrusion of the head, flattening of the anterior chest wall, thoracic kyphosis, protrusion of the abdomen, and flattening of the lumbar lordotic curvature. Slight flexion of the hip is also present due to hip involvement. (Reprinted from the Revised Clinical Slide Collection on the Rheumatic Diseases, copyright 1981. Used by permission of the Arthritis Foundation, New York.)

a focused program of education, drug therapy, and physical therapy. These individuals can develop a fulfilling life-style within the confines of their illness. Less than 5 percent develop fatal manifestations of their illness.

PSORIATIC ARTHRITIS

About 7 percent of people with psoriasis (see Chap. 74) develop inflammatory joint disease. Usually the arthritis occurs after the appearance of the skin lesions, but it can occur before or at the same time as the skin lesions.

Clinical features

Psoriatic arthritis most commonly occurs as an asymmetric inflammation involving only a few peripheral joints at a certain time. The distal joints of the hands and feet are the ones usually affected (see Fig. 66-3), but other joints that can become affected include all joints of the hands, feet, knees, and hips. There is a tendency for the activity of the arthritis to vary with the psoriasis, particularly the nail involvement of psoriasis. Psoriatic arthritis can present itself as a symmetrical arthritis resembling rheumatoid arthritis, as arthritis mutilans in which the entire joint is completely resorbed, or as spondylitis similar to that of ankylosing spondylitis. Psoriatic arthritis generally tends to be much less debilitating than rheumatoid arthritis.

Laboratory and radiologic findings

There are no specific laboratory tests for psoriatic arthritis. The erythrocyte sedimentation rate can be elevated during acute phases of the illness. The antigen HLA-B27 is positive about 20 percent of the time. This increases to a 50 percent positive rate if the person has sacroiliac inflammation with the illness. The presence

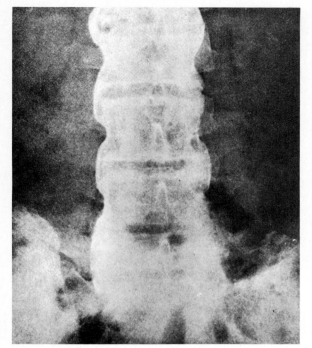

FIGURE 66-2
Ankylosing spondylitis: spine x-ray. Advanced ankylosing spondylitis of the lumbar spine. There is generalized symmetrical osseous bridging between the vertebrae (syndesmophytes). The apophyseal and sacroiliac joints are fused. (Reproduced with permission from J. L. Hollander (ed.), *Arthritis and Allied Conditions, A Textbook of Rheumatology*, 8th ed., Lea & Febiger, Philadelphia, 1972.)

of rheumatoid factor is the same as for the general population.

X-rays in the early stages of the illness are usually normal. A characteristic finding in later stages of the illness is what is called the "pencil-in-cup" sign. There is erosion of the distal end of the proximal phalanx to a

rather sharp point and a concomitant bony overgrowth of the proximal end of the distal phalanx where the tendons insert.

Treatment

The treatment for psoriatic arthritis is appropriate doses of aspirin or other nonsteroidal anti-inflammatory drugs. These measures are combined with treatment of the skin lesions. Corticosteroids are not generally used because such large doses are required and the undesirable adverse effects are beyond acceptable levels. Other drug therapies include gold and immunosuppressive drugs. These drugs are usually reserved for very severe cases that do not respond to other forms of therapy.

The long-term treatment involves a multifocal approach that includes physical therapy, alterations in activities of daily living, and occasionally hospitalization and surgery. The majority of people with psoriatic arthritis, however, do not require extensive medical intervention. They have periods of remission that are frequent and last for several months.

REITER'S SYNDROME

Reiter's syndrome is one of the leading causes of arthritis in young adult males. The syndrome is named for Hans Reiter, who described the clinical picture of nongonoccocal urethritis, arthritis, and conjunctivitis in 1916. This syndrome rarely occurs in women, children, or the elderly. In the United States the syndrome begins suddenly, usually following venereal exposure. In other

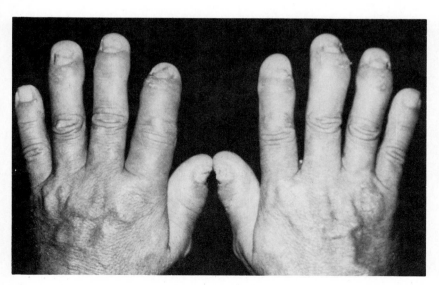

FIGURE 66-3
Psoriatic arthritis: swelling and deformity of distal interphalangeal (DIP) joints are present, together with typical psoriatic involvement of the skin and nails. Several digits, including the left thumb and index finger, are diffusely swollen, suggesting a sausagelike appearance. (Reprinted from the Revised Clinical Slide Collection on the Rheumatic Diseases, copyright 1982. Used by permission of the Arthritis Foundation, New York.)

parts of the world the syndrome follows an infection with *Shigella flexneri*.

Reiter's syndrome is accompanied by a triad of symptoms—urethritis, arthritis, and conjunctivitis. Oral mucocutaneous lesions, keratoderma blennorrhagicum (a characteristic dermatitis; see Fig. 66-4), and balanitis circinata are also seen.

The causes are unknown. There is an association between the antigen HLA-B27 and the development of Reiter's syndrome. Psoriatic arthritis and Reiter's syndrome may be nearly the same disease, since the dermatitis and nail changes are very similar in the two. A history of sexual exposure or dysentery leads to the suspicion that these illnesses are immune responses to some infectious agent.

Clinical features

Constitutional symptoms, weight loss, and fever may occur at the onset of Reiter's syndrome. A purulent or watery urethritis that the person may think is a venereal

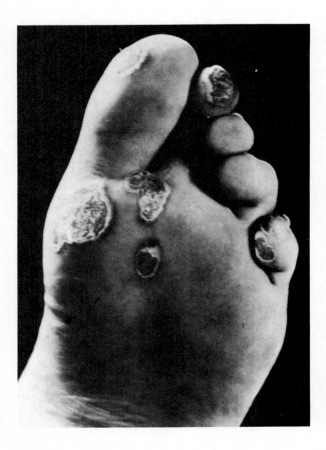

disease is often the factor that precipitates a visit to seek health care.

Articular manifestations most commonly involve the joints of the feet and ankles, the knees, and the sacroiliacs. Heel pain is fairly common. Conjunctivitis can occur with a purulent discharge and photophobia. The oral and penile lesions are usually painless. In a few cases, there are electrocardiographic changes and aortic valve involvement.

The course of the illness is unpredictable. Reiter's syndrome can be acute, subacute, or chronic. The majority of people recover from the first attack in several months, but most have one or two more attacks within 2 years. Thirty percent develop long-term disability or permanent sequelae, including residual joint damage following severe joint involvement and long-term back pain following sacroiliac involvement.

Laboratory and radiologic findings

There are no specific laboratory tests for Reiter's syndrome. Ninety percent of the people with Reiter's syndrome have a positive antigen HLA-B27, but the frequency of positive rheumatoid factor is equal to that in the general population. Synovial fluid is inflammatory, with 15,000 to 20,000 white blood cells per cubic millimeter.

There are x-ray changes that are specific for Reiter's syndrome. These include a tendency for joints of the lower extremities to be involved, isolated osteoporosis, articular erosive changes, periostitis at the insertion of the Achilles tendon, calcaneal spurs, sacroiliac inflammations, and nonmarginal spurs along the vertebral column.

Treatment

The treatment of Reiter's syndrome is primarily symptomatic. Therapeutic doses of nonsteroidal anti-inflammatory drugs are used to relieve the inflammation and pain. The use of corticosteroids systemically or locally is a controversial issue. Antibiotics are not of proven value.

FIGURE 66-4
Reiter's syndrome: keratoderma blennorrhagicum in the foot. Discrete, circinate, scaly, and plaquelike lesions on the foot are due to Reiter's syndrome and resemble secondary syphilis and psoriasis. Note two small lesions in an early phase of keratoderma. (Reproduced with permission from the Arthritis Foundation, New York, copyright 1972.)

Seronegative spondyloarthropathies

Directions: Answer the following questions on a separate sheet of paper.

1. Explain the goals of the treatment measures and the prognosis for ankylosing spondylitis.

2. What is the relationship between psoriasis and psoriatic arthritis?

3. What are the components of the treatment program for Reiter's syndrome?

Directions: Circle the letter preceding each item below that correctly answers the question. More than one answer may be correct.

4. The group of related disorders known as seronegative spondyloarthropathies includes:
   a. Psoriatic arthritis   *b.* Reiter's syndrome
   c. Polyarthritis   *d.* Ankylosing spondylitis

5. Which of the following statements is not true concerning seronegative disorders?
   a. There is a high titer of rheumatoid factor in the serum in 95 percent of the patients   *b.* Rheumatoid factor in serum is usually negative
   c. The antigen HLA-B27 is likely to be positive
   d. There are no specific laboratory tests used in diagnosing these conditions

6. The joints which are most commonly involved in Reiter's syndrome are:
   a. Weight-bearing joints (feet and ankles, knee)
   b. Sacroiliac joints   *c.* Hips and costoverterbal articulations   *d.* Cartilaginous and fibrocartilaginous joints of the spine

7. Ankylosing spondylitis usually involves the:
   a. Distal joints of the hands and feet   *b.* Joints of the ankles   *c.* Sacroiliac joints   *d.* Spinal articulations

8. Which of the following clinical features are seen in the late stages of ankylosing spondylitis?
   a. Erosion of the distal and of the proximal phalanx   *b.* Increase in pain over sacroiliac joints
   c. Hip flexion contractions and flexed knees
   d. Evidence of increase in synovitis

9. Radiologic findings that occur in the early stages of ankylosing spondylitis are:
   a. Blurring of the sacroiliac joint   *b.* Joint erosion and squaring of the vertebrae   *c.* Diffuse osteoporosis of the spine   *d.* Calcification of the discs and paravertebral ligaments

10. The drugs of choice prescribed for ankylosing spondylitis are:
    a. Nonsteroidal anti-inflammatory drugs
    b. Corticosteroids   *c.* Disease-modifying drugs
    d. Muscle relaxants

11. In very severe cases of psoriatic arthritis that are unresponsive to anti-inflammatory drug therapy, the drugs used are:
    a. Corticosteroids   *b.* Gold   *c.* Immunosuppressive agents   *d.* Muscle relaxants

Directions: Circle T if the statement is true and F if it is false. Correct the false statements.

12. T   F.   The psoriasis usually precedes the arthritis in psoriatic arthritis.

13. T   F   Psoriatic arthritis is usually much more destructive to the joints than rheumatoid arthritis.

14. T   F   Reiter's syndrome is characterized by a triad of symptoms—urethritis, arthritis, and conjunctivitis.

15. T   F   The male/female ratio for occurrence of ankylosing spondylitis is 9:1.

CHAPTER

67

POLYMYOSITIS, DERMATOMYOSITIS, AND PROGRESSIVE SYSTEMIC SCLEROSIS (SCLERODERMA)

OBJECTIVES

At the completion of this chapter you should be able to:

1. Contrast polymyositis and dermatomyositis as to muscle and skin involvement, sex predilection, and age groups affected.

2. List the groups in the classification of polymyositis and dermatomyositis developed by Bohan.

3. Describe the clinical course, significance of the signs and symptoms, and related conditions of polymyositis and dermatomyositis.

4. State the significance of the laboratory findings in polymyositis and dermatomyositis.

5. Evaluate the therapeutic program and prognosis for polymyositis and dermatomyositis.

6. Identify for progressive systemic sclerosis (scleroderma) the area of involvement, characteristic fibrotic and degenerative changes, sex ratio, and age groups involved.

7. Describe Raynaud's phenomenon and its relationship to progressive systemic sclerosis.

8. Discuss the importance of the CREST variant in progressive systemic sclerosis.

9. Describe the signs and symptoms associated with progressive systemic sclerosis.

10. State the significance of the laboratory and radiologic findings in progressive systemic sclerosis.

11. Identify the therapeutic measures patients use for progressive systemic sclerosis.

Polymyositis, dermatomyositis, and progressive systemic sclerosis (scleroderma) are diffuse connective tissue disorders. Each of these disorders can have overlapping symptoms in the early stages, and it may be difficult to distinguish one from the other.

POLYMYOSITIS AND DERMATOMYOSITIS

Polymyositis and dermatomyositis are diffuse inflammatory disorders that affect the striated muscle. They cause muscle weakness and atrophy. Dermatomyositis is a variant of polymyositis, with characteristic skin involvement. These disorders can affect a person of any age, but dermatomyositis occurs more often in children or in persons over 40 years of age. Females are affected twice as often as males. Malignancies are associated with these disorders approximately five times more frequently than in the general population. The sex distribution of these diseases is equal in the presence of a tumor. Prognosis is better for children, young adults, and those without a malignancy.

The classification of polymyositis and dermatomyositis has been confusing. The classification by groups developed by Bohan and Peter (1975) is helpful:

1. Primary idiopathic polymyositis
2. Primary idiopathic dermatomyositis
3. Dermatomyositis (or polymyositis) associated with neoplasia
4. Childhood dermatomyositis (or polymyositis) associated with vasculitis
5. Polymyositis or dermatomyositis associated with collagen-vascular disease

Clinical features

The mode of onset and rate of progression of these disorders can be quite varied. Generally, these disorders begin with a gradual weakening of the proximal muscles. The course is further complicated by a high rate of spontaneous remissions and exacerbations. Muscle weakness can be so profound as to suggest severe myasthenia gravis. Other signs and symptoms include weight loss, fever, fatigue, arthralgias, and arthritis involving the small joints of the hands, the wrists, and the knees.

Muscle weakness generally affects the proximal muscles of the lower extremities first. This may result in difficulty in climbing stairs or rising from a sitting position. Upper-extremity involvement of the proximal muscles may prevent the person from hair brushing or from holding the arms elevated for any extended period of time. Neck musculature can also be affected and can prevent the person from raising the head from the pillow. Dysphagia (difficulty swallowing) may result from inflammation of the voluntary muscles of the pharynx.

Hypomotility of the lower esophagus, such as is found in scleroderma, may occur. Pain and tenderness of the affected muscles are directly related to the acuity of the disease process but are experienced by fewer than 25 percent of people with these disorders.

Pulmonary function can be impaired because of the inflamed intercostal muscles. Pulmonary fibrosis or aspiration pneumonitis can develop secondary to these disorders.

Involvement of distal muscles may occur in severe or chronic disease. Long-term complications may include muscle atrophy and contractures. Calcinosis may result from severe muscle inflammation and is seen more frequently in children or adolescents than in adults.

The dermal involvement of dermatomyositis includes the appearance of dark-red patches that are slightly scaly (see Plate 32). These eruptions often appear over the proximal interphalangeal or metacarpophalangeal joints, as well as over the elbows and knees. A butterfly malar rash may appear, as in systemic lupus erythematosus. A dusky erythematous rash on the eyelids is referred to as a heliotrope rash and is considered pathognomonic.

The occurrence of malignancy in conjunction with these disorders is demonstrated at a higher frequency rate than the occurrence of malignancies alone. The lungs, breasts, ovaries, uterus, and prostate are the most common sites for the malignancy. Generally, the myositis presents itself 1 to 2 years prior to the discovery of the malignancy, but it may follow the appearance of malignancy. The successful treatment of the malignancy may also resolve the myositis.

Laboratory findings

The erythrocyte sedimentation rate is often elevated. Rheumatoid factor may also be present. The most helpful laboratory tests for both diagnosis and regulation of therapy are the serum muscle enzymes (creatine phosphokinase, aldolase, and transaminases). These enzymes are released from damaged muscle tissue into the serum. Measurement of the elevated serum enzymes indicates the extent of muscle injury. Electromyography and muscle biopsy are also useful in establishing the correct diagnosis.

Treatment

The first principle of therapy is rest, particularly during the acute and active phase of the disease. Corticosteroids, usually in the range of 40 to 60 mg per day in divided doses, should be promptly instituted. Steroid doses in this range generally suppress the disease activity, although patients with malignancies are often steroid-resistant. In some cases immunosuppressive or cytotoxic agents may be used.

The corticosteroid medications can be reduced as muscle strength improves and muscle enzymes approach normal levels. A reduction of corticosteroid levels that is too rapid may result in a flare of the illness. Some persons may require long-term low-dose steroid therapy. Immunosuppressive medication may be considered if the illness does not respond to steroid therapy.

Occupational and physical therapy are utilized for maintenance of range of motion in joints, for prevention of contractures, and for alterations in activities of daily living. Overstretching of muscles should be avoided, as it can damage them. The person may need assistance with gait retraining, since the pelvic girdle is so frequently involved.

Prognosis

The prognoses of polymyositis and dermatomyositis are usually unpredictable. The best outcome is seen in persons who are in Group 1 or Group 2. Children with dermatomyositis usually have a better course than do adults. Persons with associated malignancies usually do not have a favorable outcome. Persons over the age of 50 usually have the poorest prognosis.

PROGRESSIVE SYSTEMIC SCLEROSIS

Progressive systemic sclerosis is often referred to as scleroderma, since one of the characteristics is fibrosis and degenerative changes in the skin. This is a systemic, generalized disorder of the body's connective tissue. Fibrosis and degenerative changes are also seen in the synovium, digital arteries, and parenchyma and the small arteries of the esophagus, intestine, lungs, heart, kidney, and thyroid gland. The cause of progressive systemic sclerosis is not known, although a number of serologic and cellular immune reaction abnormalities exist, indicating that there is an immunologic mechanism involved.

The disorder is seen worldwide in all races. Women are affected three times as often as men. The disease onset is usually in the third to fifth decades; only rarely does the disorder affect children. The disease occurs with particularly high frequency in coal miners leading to the suggestion that silicosis is a predisposing factor.

Progressive systemic sclerosis is similar to other connective tissue disorders in that there may be remissions and exacerbations with a generally slow progression which allows for a reasonably long life. The disorder may be rapidly progressive, however, and lead to an early death when vital organs are affected and damaged. Renal failure is the leading cause of death for persons with progressive systemic sclerosis.

The changes seen in the skin and other organs are the result of the overproduction of collagen. Why this is so is not known. The changes in the blood vessels are similar. The lesions that develop in the small arteries and arterioles begin as proliferations on the intimal side of the internal elastic membrane. A medial thinning

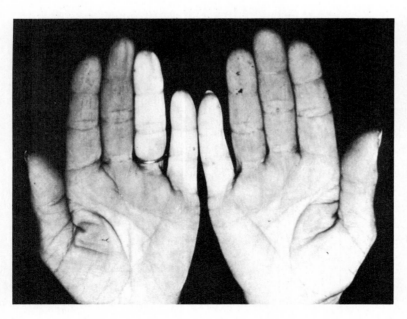

FIGURE 67-1
Scleroderma: Raynaud's phenomenon. The marked pallor of the fourth and fifth digits of the left hand and of the fifth digit of the right hand is characteristic of Raynaud's phenomenon. Vasospastic changes are common in systemic sclerosis. (Reproduced with permission from the Arthritis Foundation, New York, copyright 1972.)

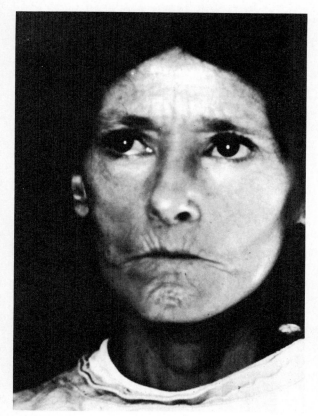

FIGURE 67-2
Scleroderma: skin changes. This young woman demonstrates many features of systemic sclerosis: drawn pursed lips, shiny skin over the cheeks and forehead, and atrophy of muscles of the temple, face, and neck. Such facial changes are known as *Mauskopf* (mousehead). (Reproduced with permission from the Arthritis Foundation, New York, 1972.)

volving the arms, chest, and face. The face becomes very taut (see Fig. 67-2), the oral orifice becomes wrinkled, and the opening of the orifice is restricted. The forehead loses its normal wrinkles. Polyarthralgia, joint stiffness, and polyarthritis are also seen.

One form of progressive systemic sclerosis is the CREST variant. This mnemonic stands for the first letter in calcinosis, Raynaud's phenomenon, esophageal dysmotility, sclerodactyly, and telangiectasia (see Fig. 67-3).

The colon may be affected, which results in diarrhea or constipation, cramping, malabsorption, and, in a few cases, perforation.

Exertional dyspnea is usually the first sign of pulmonary involvement. Pulmonary function studies may show alteration in the gas exchange, that is, decrease in breathing capacity and an increase in the residual air.

FIGURE 67-3
Scleroderma: telangiectasias. Multiple telangiectases are present on the face. They blanch with pressure. Telangiectasia occurs frequently in this disorder, at times leading to confusion in differentiation from hereditary hemorrhagic telangiectasia. (Reproduced with permission from the Arthritis Foundation, New York, 1972.)

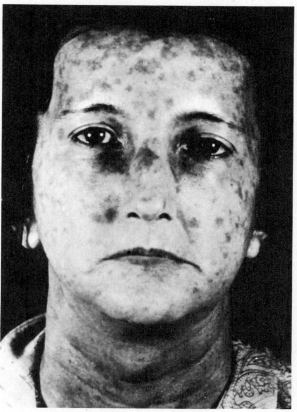

then occurs, and finally the deposit of a connective tissue cuff rich in collagen proceeds. All these changes are thought to be brought on by alterations in B-cell and T-cell activity.

Clinical features

Raynaud's phenomenon (see Fig. 67-1) is the most common manifestation seen in persons with progressive systemic sclerosis. Raynaud's phenomenon is a paroxysmal vasospastic disorder in which there is an abnormal spasm of the arteries of the hand in response to cold temperatures or extreme emotions. This causes the digits to become white (vasospasm), then blue (cyanosis), then red (reactive hyperemia). Other common symptoms are swelling and puffiness of the hands and gradual thickening and tightening of the skin of the fingers and other body parts. The fingers develop a sausagelike appearance. The skin slowly thickens and becomes very taut, shiny, and tightly bound to the underlying subcutaneous tissue. This process progresses proximally, in-

Pericarditis, arrythmias, and/or electrocardiogram changes may occur with cardiac involvement.

Renal involvement manifested as proteinuria, microscopic hematuria, and hypertension may rapidly deteriorate to renal failure. Any vital organ involvement, especially when rapidly deteriorating, indicates a poor prognosis.

Laboratory and x-ray findings

The erythrocyte sedimentation rate may be elevated. A small group of patients may demonstrate rheumatoid factor in their serum. A positive antinuclear antibody

and hypergammaglobulinemia may be demonstrated. Skin biopsies are the most specific way of making the diagnosis but are usually not necessary because of the striking clinical picture.

Radiologic examination may demonstrate subcutaneous calcifications of the digits of the hand (see Fig. 67-4). Esophageal and intestinal abnormalities may also be detected.

Treatment

Persons with progressive systemic sclerosis need to protect themselves from exposing their hands to cold, in order to decrease the frequency of attacks of Raynaud's phenomenon. Grasping a cold glass can initiate an attack. Gloves may be necessary for most of the time. The person should stop the use of all tobacco products, because of the adverse effects of nicotine on the blood ves-

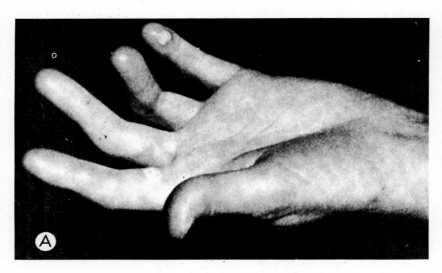

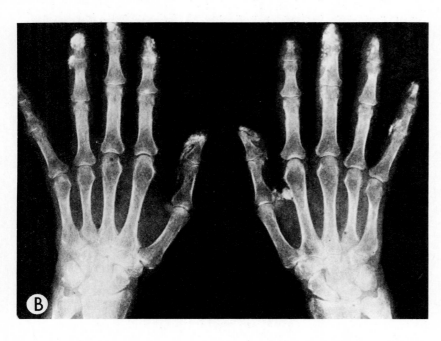

FIGURE 67-4

Scleroderma: subcutaneous calcification. (A) Hand of an adolescent girl with progressive systemic sclerosis. Note the circumscribed lesions of calcinosis in the skin of the volar surface of the proximal portion of the second and the distal portion of the fifth digit. (B) X-ray of the hands of a woman with progressive systemic sclerosis as depicted by the extensive subcutaneous calcinosis in the fingers and near the joint of the right hand. (Reproduced with permission from J. R. Hollander (ed.), *Arthritis and Allied Conditions, A Textbook of Rheumatology,* 8th ed., Lea & Febiger, Philadelphia, 1972.)

sels. Vasodilators are sometimes of benefit in treatment of Raynaud's phenomenon.

Low doses of corticosteroids may relieve joint complaints but are usually not of great benefit for treatment of progressive systemic sclerosis. Nonsteroidal anti-inflammatory agents can be used to decrease discomfort.

Antibiotics have been used with some success in the treatment of small-bowel involvement. The hypomotility of the bowel allows for an overgrowth of microorganisms, and these interfere with absorption. Treatment with antibiotics reduces the overgrowth.

Dimethyl sulfoxide (DMSO) has been used in the treatment of scleroderma with variable results. Immunosuppressive drugs and alkylating agents are sometimes used.

Physical therapy is a very important component of therapy. This modality can decrease or prevent contractures. The characteristic restriction of the opening of the mouth can interfere with the person's ability to eat. Functioning of the mouth can be greatly improved through stretching and muscle strengthening.

QUESTIONS

Polymyositis, dermatomyositis, and progressive systemic sclerosis (scleroderma)

Directions: Answer the questions on a separate sheet of paper.

1. In what sex do polymyositis and dermatomyositis occur more frequently and at what ratio of occurrence?

2. Outline the therapeutic program for polymyositis and dermatomyositis.

3. Describe the skin and other organ changes in progressive systemic sclerosis (scleroderma).

4. Describe a potential problem which may occur in a patient with polymyositis when the intercostal muscles are involved.

5. Identify the therapeutic measures used for patients with progressive systemic sclerosis.

Directions: Circle the letter preceding each item below that correctly answers the question. More than one answer may be correct.

6. Polymyositis and dermatomyositis are diffuse inflammatory disorders affecting:
   a. Smooth muscle   *b.* Striated muscle

7. In polymyositis and dermatomyositis, the incidence of malignancy is approximately how many times greater than in the general population?
   a. 2   *b.* 3   *c.* 5   *d.* 10

8. The most common site for the malignancy is the:
   a. Lungs   *b.* Colon   *c.* Breasts   *d.* Prostate

9. In Bohan and Peter's classification of polymyositis and dermatomyositis, Group 3 is classified as:
   a. Primary idiopathic polymyositis   *b.* Dermatomyositis (or polymyositis) associated with neoplasia   *c.* Childhood dermatomyositis (or polymyositis) associated with vasculitis   *d.* Primary idiopathic dermatomyositis

10. A butterfly malar rash, as seen in systemic lupus erythematosus, may appear in:
    a. Polymyositis   *b.* Dermatomyositis   *c.* Progressive systemic sclerosis

11. In polymyositis and dermatomyositis, muscle weakness generally *initially* affects the:
    a. Facial musculature   *b.* Proximal muscles of the lower extremities   *c.* Voluntary muscles of the pharynx   *d.* Proximal muscles of the upper extremity

12. Which of the following laboratory values are suggestive of polymyositis and dermatomyositis?
    a. Elevated erythrocyte sedimentation rate
    b. Negative rheumatoid factor   *c.* Elevated creatine phosphokinase   *d.* Elevated aldolase, transaminases, and creatine phosphokinase

13. The initial dosage of corticosteroids in polymyositis and dermatomyositis is:
    a. 15 to 20 mg once daily   *b.* 25 to 35 mg once daily   *c.* 40 to 60 mg per day in divided doses

14. The most common manifestations associated with progressive systemic sclerosis is:
    a. Perforation of the colon   *b.* Raynaud's phenomenon   *c.* Pericarditis   *d.* Exertional dyspnea

Directions: Circle T if the statement is true and F if it is false. Correct the false statements.

15. T   F   In dermatomyositis, children usually have a better prognosis than do adults.

16. T   F   Raynaud's phenomenon is a paroxysmal vasospastic disorder where there is an abnormal spasm of the arteries of the hand in response to cold temperature or extreme emotions.

17. T   F   Radiographic studies of progressive systemic sclerosis may demonstrate subcutaneous calcifications of the great toe.

CHAPTER
68

SYSTEMIC LUPUS ERYTHEMATOSUS (SLE)

OBJECTIVES

At the completion of this chapter you should be able to:

1. Define *systemic lupus erythematosus* (SLE).
2. Identify for SLE the sex predilection, age and racial groups involved, characteristic features, and difficulty in diagnosis.
3. Describe the clinical features associated with SLE.
4. Differentiate between rheumatoid arthritis and the polyarthritis of SLE.
5. Explain the antinuclear antibody (anti-DNA) process that occurs in lupus nephritis.
6. List the 11 criteria developed by the American Rheumatism Association for the classification of SLE.
7. Explain the importance of drug-induced SLE.
8. Describe the laboratory tests utilized in diagnosing SLE.
9. Discuss the importance of counseling females of childbearing age regarding SLE.
10. Evaluate the drug therapy program administered in treating SLE.
11. Discuss the rationale in SLE for avoidance of exposure to the sun.

Systemic lupus erythematosus (SLE) is a multisystem, chronic autoimmune disease. The signs and symptoms of this disorder can be very diverse, transitory, and difficult to diagnose. Therefore, exact figures as to the number of people with the disorder are difficult to obtain. SLE affects women about eight times as often as men. The disorder frequently begins in late adolescence or early adulthood. In the United States, black women are affected about three times as often as white women.

The disorder is usually milder and more easily controlled if SLE develops after the age of 60.

SLE was originally described as a skin disorder in the 1800s and given the name lupus because of the characteristic "butterfly rash" across the bridge of the nose and the cheeks that resembles the coloring of a wolf (*lupus* is the Latin word for wolf). *Discoid lupus* is the name now given to the disorder when it is limited to cutaneous involvement.

SLE is one of a group of diffuse connective tissue disorders of unknown etiology. These include SLE, scleroderma, polymyositis, rheumatoid arthritis, and Sjögren's syndrome. These disorders frequently have overlapping symptoms and may be present at the same time making an accurate diagnosis very difficult. SLE can vary from a mild disorder to one that is rapidly fulminating and fatal. The most common situation, however, is one of exacerbations and near remissions that can last for long periods. Early identification and treatment of SLE usually leads to a more favorable prognosis.

CLINICAL FEATURES

The clinical picture of SLE can be very confusing, particularly in the early stages of the disorder. The most common symptom is a symmetrical arthritis or arthralgia that is present 90 percent of the time, often as an initial manifestation. The most frequently affected joints are the proximal joints of the hands, wrists, elbows, shoulders, knees, and ankles. The polyarthritis of SLE differs from that of rheumatoid arthritis in that it is not permanently deforming. Also subcutaneous nodules are rarely seen in SLE.

Constitutional symptoms of fever, fatigue, weakness, and weight loss generally occur early but may recur throughout the course of the disorder. Fatigue and weakness may be secondary to a mild anemia that is caused by SLE.

Skin manifestations include an erythematous rash which may appear on the face (see Fig. 68-1), the neck, the extremities, or the trunk. Exposure to sunlight may aggravate this rash. Alopecia (hair loss) can develop and can sometimes be severe. Hair growth usually returns without major problems. Small ulcerations of the oral or nasopharyngeal mucous membranes can occur.

Pleurisy (chest pain) may occur as a result of the chronic inflammatory process of SLE. SLE can also cause carditis involving the myocardium, endocardium, or pericardium.

Raynaud's phenomenon occurs in about 40 percent of the people with SLE. Some cases may be so severe that gangrene of the digits occurs. Vasculitis may affect all sizes of arteries and veins.

Lupus nephritis occurs as the antinuclear antibody (anti-DNA) attaches to its antigen (deoxyribonucleic acid, or DNA) and is deposited in the renal glomerulus. DNA is not normally antigenic in humans but becomes so in SLE. Complement is fixed to this immune complex, and the inflammatory process begins. Renal inflammation, tissue damage, and scarring may result.

About 65 percent of the people with SLE develop some renal involvement. Only 25 percent, however, develop severe problems. Lupus nephritis is detected by examining the urine for protein, red blood cells, or casts. A kidney biopsy may be necessary for an accurate diagnosis.

SLE may affect the central or peripheral nervous system. Symptoms include behavioral changes (depression, psychosis), convulsions, cranial nerve disorders, and peripheral neuropathies. Central nervous system changes are often associated with severe forms of the disorder and are frequently fatal.

DIAGNOSIS

The American Rheumatism Association has developed revised criteria for the classification of SLE. The presence of four or more of the 11 criteria either serially or simultaneously is considered diagnostic.

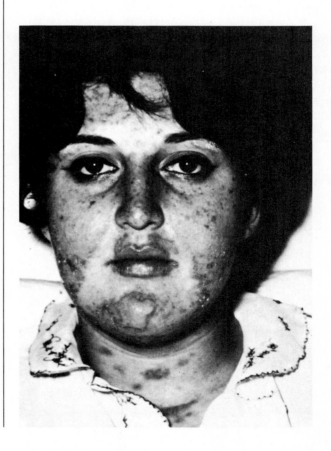

FIGURE 68-1

SLE: rash on the face and neck. Widespread discrete and confluent erythematous lesions are present on the face and neck. Typical peeling is noted on the chin and cheeks. (Reproduced with permission from the Arthritis Foundation, New York, copyright 1972.)

1. Malar rash
2. Discoid rash
3. Photosensitivity
4. Oral ulcers
5. Arthritis—nonerosive, of two or more peripheral joints
6. Serositis—pleuritis or pericarditis
7. Renal disorder—persistent proteinuria with greater than 0.5 g per day, or cellular casts
8. Neurologic disorder—seizures or psychosis
9. Hematologic disorder—hemolytic anemia or leukopenia or lymphopenia or thrombocytopenia
10. Immunologic disorder—positive lupus erythematosus (LE) cells or anti-DNA or anti-Sm or a false positive serologic test for syphilis
11. Antinuclear antibody

DRUG–INDUCED SLE

A number of drugs are able to induce in susceptible people a syndrome that is very similar to SLE. This syndrome includes most of the symptoms of SLE, including positive tests for antinuclear antibodies (ANA), but renal and central nervous system affectations rarely occur. The SLE symptoms begin to disappear within a few weeks following the discontinuation of these drugs. The positive ANA test reverts to negative after several months. Hydralizine and procainamide are two of the more common drugs. A number of other drugs are capable of producing a positive ANA. These drugs include penicillamine, isoniazid, chlorpromazine, and anticonvulsants such as barbiturates, phenytoin, ethosuximide, methsuximide, and primidone. Some drugs can cause an exacerbation of SLE in people who are in a remission. These include sulfonamides, penicillin, and oral contraceptives.

LABORATORY TESTS

Antinuclear antibodies are positive in greater than 95 percent of those with SLE. This test indicates whether there are antibodies capable of destroying the nucleus of one's own body cells. In addition to the presence of ANA, the ANA pattern and the specific antibodies are evaluated. The pattern refers to the appearance of the slide when viewed under ultraviolet light. A differential evaluation of the specific types of ANA is now available and is useful in differentiating SLE from other types of disorders.

A laboratory test that was previously used and may occasionally be used today is the lupus erythematosus factor. The LE cell is formed by damaging some of the person's white cells so that they will release their nucleoprotein. This protein reacts with IgG, and the complex is phagocytosed by the remaining white cells. The resulting cell is easily identified (see Fig. 68-2). This factor can usually be demonstrated at some time in the course of the disorder if enough tests are done. LE cells can be demonstrated in other immune-mediated systemic forms of rheumatic disorders.

The urine is examined for the presence of protein, white blood cells, red blood cells, and casts. These tests are used both to determine the presence of renal complications of SLE and to monitor the progression of the illness.

TREATMENT

The treatment of the person with SLE is multifaceted and includes a variety of measures, including counseling, complex drug therapy, and preventive measures. The most frequent onset period of SLE is during late adolescence and early adulthood for females. As these are the prime reproductive years, a great deal of counseling is needed to assist in making the decision concerning having children. Pregnancy may cause a flare of SLE, which can be dangerous for women with renal damage. Cytotoxic drugs may be necessary in order to control the illness, and these can potentially affect the fetus. Contraception methods cannot usually include birth control pills, since these may aggravate SLE. The intrauterine device can be a problem for women taking systemic corticosteroids, because of the potential for infection.

The drug therapy includes nonsteroidal anti-inflammatory drugs (NSAIDs) and disease-modifying anti-rheumatic drugs (DMARDs), usually antimalarials or immunosuppressive agents, and corticosteroids. The selection of appropriate drug therapy depends upon the specific organs affected by the illness. NSAIDs are used to control the arthritis and arthralgia. Aspirin is used

FIGURE 68-2
SLE: LE cell. A neutrophil within which is contained homogeneous material, the LE body. The nucleus is pushed to one side and flattened around the mass.

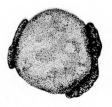

less frequently now because it produces the highest incidence of hepatotoxicity and some people with SLE have hepatic involvement. People with SLE are at a higher risk of the cutaneous, hepatic, and renal adverse effects of NSAIDs and these should be monitored closely.

Antimalarial therapy is sometimes effective if the NSAIDs cannot control the symptoms of SLE. Antimalarials are usually given at initially high doses to achieve a remission. The clearance of skin lesions offers a monitoring parameter to use in dosage adjustment. Immunosuppressive therapy (cyclophosphamide or azathioprine) can be used in an effort to suppress the autoimmune activity of SLE. These drugs are usually prescribed when there is (1) a well-established diagnosis, (2) the presence of severe, life-threatening symptoms, (3) failure of other therapeutic measures, such as a failure to respond to steroids or the need for reduction of steroids because of the adverse effects, and (4) the absence of infection, pregnancy, and neoplasm.

Acute flares of SLE, especially in those with interstitial nephritis, are treated with high-dose oral corticosteroids for short periods. These drugs are then gradually reduced in dosage over the next several weeks. Both SLE and systemic corticosteroids can produce behavioral changes and can be difficult to distinguish.

An important aspect of the prevention of flares of SLE is avoidance of exposure to the sun. Just how the sun causes SLE to flare is not fully understood. One explanation is that DNA exposed to ultraviolet light normally becomes antigenic and this leads to the flares seen after sun exposure. People with SLE should be encouraged to utilize umbrellas, hats, and long-sleeved shirts when out of doors. There may be problems getting teenagers to follow these suggestions. A sunscreen with a protection factor of 15 should be used to block the ultraviolet light exposure. The sunscreen should be reapplied after swimming or heavy exercise. The person should receive a list of drugs that can cause exacerbations, in order to prevent this type of flare.

PROGNOSIS

The prognosis for SLE is variable and depends upon the severity of the symptoms, the organs involved with the disorder, and the length of time remissions may be maintained. There is no cure for SLE, and treatment is focused upon the management of the symptoms. The prognosis is related to how well the symptoms are managed.

QUESTIONS

Systemic lupus erythematosus (SLE)

Directions: Answer the following questions on a separate sheet of paper.

1. Formulate a definition of systemic lupus erythematosus.

2. Contrast the antinuclear antibody test with the LE factor test.

3. Discuss the importance of counseling females of childbearing age regarding SLE.

4. Explain the rationale in SLE for avoidance of exposure to the sun.

5. What is the rationale for the selection of drugs used in the treatment of SLE?

Directions: Circle the letter preceding each item below that correctly answers the question. More than one answer may be correct.

6. In systemic lupus erythematosus, approximately how many times more are females affected than males?
   a. 5 *b.* 7 *c.* 8 *d.* 10

7. The most common *initial* manifestation of SLE is:
   a. Symmetrical arthritis or arthralgia *b.* Subcutaneous nodules *c.* Fatigue and weakness *d.* Weight loss

8. Which of the following laboratory tests will be positive in greater than 95 percent of those with SLE?
   a. Antinuclear antibodies *b.* Increased serum complement levels *c.* Decreased erythrocyte sedimentation rate *d.* Positive rheumatoid factor

9. Which of the following drugs are able to induce a syndrome (symptoms of SLE) that is similar to SLE?
   a. Isoniazid *b.* Procainamide *c.* Hydralazine *d.* Chlorpromazine

10. The serial or simultaneous presence of which of the criteria listed below is considered diagnostic of SLE:
    a. Photosensitivity, a positive ANA test, symmetrical joint swelling, subcutaneous nodules *b.* Malar rash, pain on motion, morning stiffness of less than 30-minute duration, ulcers *c.* Photosensitivity, malar rash, a positive ANA test, hemolytic anemia *d.* Photosensitivity, a positive rheumatoid factor, oral ulcers, pleuritis

Directions: Circle T if the statement is true and F if it is false. Correct the false statements.

11.   T   F   The onset of systemic lupus erythematosus is most frequently seen in late adolescence or early adulthood.

12.   T   F   Cyclophosphamide or azathioprine is prescribed for SLE to control the symptoms and achieve a remission.

13.   T   F   Lupus nephritis is a serious disorder that occurs in over 80 percent of the individuals with SLE.

14.   T   F   DNA is not usually antigenic to humans in SLE.

CHAPTER
69

GOUT

OBJECTIVES

At the completion of this chapter you should be able to:

1. Define *gout*.
2. Contrast the causes of primary and secondary gout.
3. Explain the consequences when crystals of monosodium urate monohydrate form in the joints and surrounding tissues.
4. Identify the sex and age groups affected.
5. Contrast the four stages in the clinical progression of gout in relation to the serum uric acid values, signs and symptoms, gout attacks, and inflammatory reactions.
6. State the rationale for the development of tophi in chronic gout.
7. State the significance of males who develop monarticular arthritis.
8. Explain the response of the joint symptoms to colchicine.
9. Discuss the factors that contribute to the development of gout.
10. State the principles of the treatment of gout.
11. Describe the pharmacologic action of allopurinol and uricosuric agents in the treatment of chronic gout.

Gout is a metabolic disorder that was described in ancient Greece by Hippocrates. Early ideas were that gout was a problem only of the elite social classes and was caused by overindulgence in food, wine, and sex. Many etiologic and therapeutic theories have been proposed over the ages, but today a great deal is known about gout, and there is a very high success rate for treatment.

Gout is a term used for a group of at least nine metabolic disorders that are characterized by an elevation in the serum uric acid concentration (hyperuricemia).

Gout may be primary or secondary. Primary gout is the direct result of the body's overproduction of or decreased excretion of uric acid. Secondary gout occurs when the overproduction or decreased excretion of uric acid is secondary to another disease process or medication.

The problem develops when crystals of monosodium urate monohydrate form in the joints and surrounding tissues. These needlelike crystals are responsible for the acute inflammatory reaction which develops, resulting in the severe pain commonly associated with an acute gouty attack. These crystal deposits can lead to extensive joint and soft-tissue damage if left untreated.

CLINICAL FEATURES

The serum urate level in males normally begins to increase after puberty. The urate level does not increase in females until after menopause, since estrogens increase the renal excretion of uric acid. Following menopause, the serum urate levels of women begin to rise to that of men.

Gout is seldom seen in women. Men account for almost 95 percent of the cases. Gout is seen worldwide in all racial groups. There is a familial prevalence which suggests a genetic basis. A number of factors likely influence the expression of the illness, however, including diet, body weight, and lifestyle.

There are four stages in the clinical progression of gout that is untreated. The first stage is asymptomatic hyperuricemia. The normal value of serum uric acid in adult males is 5.1 ± 1.0 mg/100 ml, and in adult females the value is 4.0 ± 1.0 mg/100 ml. These levels rise to an average of 9 to 10 mg/100 ml in persons with gout. At this stage the person has no symptoms other than an elevated serum uric acid. Only 5 percent of the people with asymptomatic hyperuricemia go on to develop an acute gouty attack.

The second stage is acute gouty arthritis. At this stage there is a sudden onset of exquisitely painful swelling and tenderness usually of the great toe and metatarsophalangeal joint (see Fig. 69-1). The arthritis is monarticular and shows signs of local inflammation. There may be fever and an elevated white cell count. The attack may be precipitated by surgery, trauma,

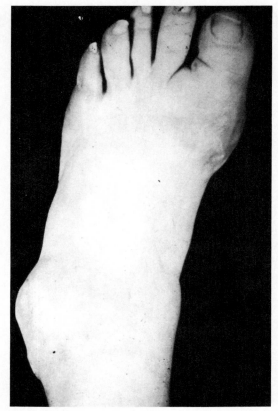

FIGURE 69-1
Gout: great toe. Typical inflammatory response of gout involving the great toe. This is the most common site of acute gout. (Reproduced with permission from the Arthritis Division, University Hospital, University of Michigan.)

drugs, alcohol, or emotional stress. This stage usually leads the person to seek prompt medical attention. Other joints can be affected, including the finger joints, knees, ankles, wrists, and elbows. Acute gouty attacks usually resolve if untreated but may take 10 to 14 days to do so.

The development of the acute attack of gout generally follows a set sequence of events. First there is a

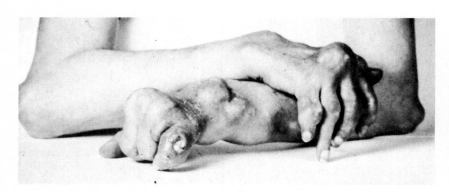

FIGURE 69-2
Gout: tophi on the hands and olecranon bursa. Many tophi are present on the hands. One asymmetrically shaped tophus on the little finger has ulcerated. Tophi are also present in both olecranon bursae; these are common sites for tophi. Swelling of some joints due to synovitis is also present. (Reproduced with permission from the Arthritis Foundation, New York, copyright 1972.)

supersaturation of urate in the plasma and body fluids. This is followed by a deposition into and around the joints. The mechanism of the crystallization of urates out of the serum is not clearly understood. Gout attacks frequently follow local trauma or the rupture of tophi (deposits of sodium urate), which accounts for a rapid increase in local concentrations of uric acid. The body may not be able to appropriately handle this increase, resulting in the precipitation of uric acid out of the serum. Crystallization and deposition of the uric acid then triggers the gout attack. These uric acid crystals trigger a phagocytic response by leukocytes, and as the leukocytes ingest the urate crystals, the responses of other inflammatory mechanisms are triggered. The inflammatory response may be influenced by the site and magnitude of uric acid crystal deposition. The inflammatory reaction may become self-propagating and self-enhancing, owing to the deposition of additional crystals from the serum.

The third stage, which follows the acute gouty attack, is the intercritical stage. There are no symptoms during this period, which may last for months to years. Most people have a repeat gouty attack in less than 1 year if they are untreated.

The fourth stage is the chronic gout stage, in which the urate pool continues to expand over a period of years if treatment is not begun. Chronic inflammation from the presence of urate crystals results in the development of pain, aching, and stiffness as well as large and nodular joint swelling. Acute attacks of gouty arthritis may occur during this stage. Tophi develop in chronic gout because of the relative insolubility of urates (see Fig. 69-2). The onset and the size of tophi may be proportionally related to the level of serum urate. The olecranon bursa, Achilles tendon, extensor surface of the forearm, infrapatellar bursa, and helix of the ear (see Fig. 69-3) are the most common sites for tophi. These tophi may be very difficult to distinguish clinically from rheumatoid nodules. Tophi are rarely seen today and will resolve with appropriate therapy. The kidneys can be damaged by gout, leading to even poorer excretion of uric acid.

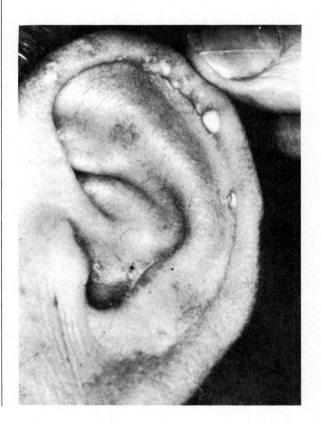

FIGURE 69-3
Gout: tophi on the ear. Small tophi can be seen on the helix of the ear, having a typical whitish appearance as a result of urate deposition. Small cartilaginous nodules are commonly present in the ears of normal individuals and can be mistaken for tophi. A tophus characteristically stands out as a discrete white nodule when pressed by the examiner's fingers; in contrast, the cartilaginous nodule blanches out and blends with the rest of the ear. Transillumination reveals an opaque center in the tophus but not in the cartilaginous nodule. (Reproduced with permission from the Arthritis Foundation, New York, copyright 1972.)

DIAGNOSTIC CRITERIA

Gout should be considered in males who develop monarticular arthritis, particularly of the great toe, that is acute in onset. An elevated serum uric acid is helpful in making the diagnosis but not specific, since a number of drugs can elevate the serum uric acid level. Also, there is a fairly large number of people with asymptomatic hyperuricemia.

Another test used to diagnose gout is the rapid response of the joint symptoms to colchicine. Colchicine is a drug that inhibits phagocytic leukocytes and thereby produces a dramatic and rapid relief of symptoms. Radiologic changes other than soft-tissue swelling are usually not present in the early stages of gout. The demonstration of urate crystals in the synovial fluid of an involved joint is considered diagnostic (see Fig. 69-4).

CONTRIBUTING FACTORS

The factors that contribute to the development of gout depend upon the cause of the hyperuricemia. A diet

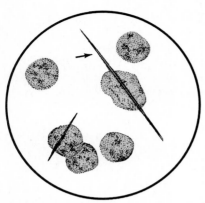

FIGURE 69-4
Gout: uric acid crystal. One uric acid crystal in a white blood cell in synovial fluid.

high in purines can trigger a gouty attack in a person with one of the inborn errors of purine metabolism that cause an overproduction of uric acid. A low-purine diet, however, will not usually lower the serum urate level to any great extent.

The ingestion of alcohol can bring on a gouty attack. Blood lactate levels increase as a by-product of the normal metabolism of alcohol. Lactic acid blocks the renal excretion of uric acid with a concomitant rise in serum levels.

A number of drugs can block the renal excretion of uric acid and lead to a gouty attack. These include aspirin in low doses (less than 1 to 2 g per day), most diuretics, levodopa, diazoxide, nicotinic acid, acetazolamide, and ethambutol.

TREATMENT

The treatment of gout depends upon the stage. Asymptomatic hyperuricemia usually requires no treatment. The acute attack of gouty arthritis is treated by the use of nonsteroidal anti-inflammatory drugs or colchicine. These are given in high doses or in loading doses to reduce the acute inflammation of the joint. The dose is then decreased gradually over the next few days.

The treatment of chronic gout is based upon decreasing the production of uric acid or on increasing the renal excretion of uric acid. The drug allopurinol blocks the formation of uric acid from its precursors (xanthine and hypoxanthine) by inhibiting the enzyme xanthine oxidase. This drug can be given in a convenient once-a-day dose.

Uricosuric agents enhance the excretion of uric acid by blocking renal tubular reabsorption. An adequate kidney function is necessary for uricosuric agents to be effective. The creatine clearance is evaluated to determine kidney function (normal is 115 to 120 ml per minute). Probenecid and sulfinpyrazone are two widely used uricosuric agents. Fluid intake of at least 1500 ml per day is needed to promote the excretion of uric acid while a patient is taking a uricosuric. All aspirin products should be avoided, as they block the uricosuric action of these drugs. Figure 69-5 depicts gout pathophysiology and drug actions.

Strict dietary modifications are not usually necessary in the treatment of gout. The person can be helped to avoid those things that precipitate an attack, but this is usually determined by trial and error for each person. Obviously, products very high in purines may be problematic. These include organ meats such as liver, kidneys, sweetbreads, and brains as well as a number of luncheon meats. Excessive use of alcohol can also precipitate an attack.

FIGURE 69-5
Gout pathophysiology and drug actions. (Reproduced with permission from M. B. Weiner and G. A. Pepper, *Clinical Pharmacology and Therapeutics in Nursing*, 2d ed., McGraw-Hill, New York, 1985, p. 407.)

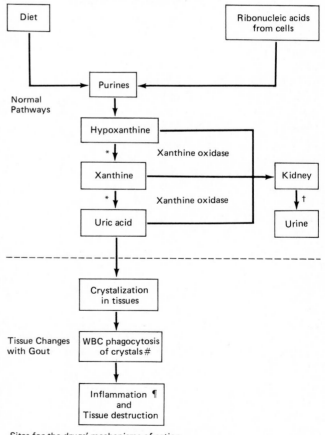

Sites for the drugs' mechanisms of action.

* Allopurinol
† Probenecid and sulfinpyrazone
# Colchicine
¶ NSAIDS

Gout

Directions: Answer the following questions on a separate sheet of paper.

1. Formulate a definition for gout.

2. Differentiate between the causes of primary and secondary gout.

3. Explain the rapid response of the joint systems to the colchicine test used to diagnose gout.

4. Discuss the contributing factors which result in development of gout.

5. State the rationale for the treatment of chronic gout.

Directions: Circle the letter preceding each item below that correctly answers the question. More than one answer may be correct.

6. The pathogenesis of gout is characterized by:
   a. Changes in the composition of articular cartilage which results in loss of compressibility
   b. Formation of crystals of monosodium urate monohydrate in joints and tissue   c. Formation of an antinuclear antibody (anti-DNA) that attaches to its antigen (DNA) whereby complement is fixed to this immune complex and an inflammatory process is caused   d. Changes in the collagen of the cartilage where Type II replaces Type I cartilage, resulting in an alteration of the biomechanics of the cartilage

7. In asymptomatic hyperuricemia, the serum uric acid levels usually average how many mg/100 ml?
   a. 4.0 to 5.0   b. 5.0 to 6.0   c. 8.0 to 9.0   d. 9.0 to 10.0

8. In the first stage of gout, the individual usually experiences:
   a. Painful swelling and tenderness   b. Fever and an elevated white cell count   c. No symptoms
   d. Elevated serum uric acid

9. The most common sites for tophi in chronic gout are the:
   a. Helix of the ear   b. Olecranon bursa   c. Cervical vertebrae   d. Achilles tendon

10. A classical sign of gout that is acute in onset in a 50-year-old male is:
    a. Fusion of the dorsal spine into kyphosis
    b. Monarticular arthritis of the great toe   c. Inflammation of the distal joints of the hands and feet   d. Severe heel pain

11. Tophi develop in chronic gout because of:
    a. Relative instability of urates   b. Chronic inflammation from the presence of calcium crystals
    c. Biochemical changes which occur within a joint
    d. Recent viral illness such as infection by Epstein-Barr virus

12. Which of the following depict the third stage of gout?
    a. Development of tophi   b. Asymptomatic hyperuricemia, which may last for months or years
    c. Pain, stiffness, large nodular swelling   d. A repeat gout attack in an untreated person

13. Treatment of an acute attack of gouty arthritis consists of initially administering high doses or loading loses of:
    a. Allopurinol   b. Nonsteroidal anti-inflammatory drugs   c. Aspirin   d. Colchicine

DEGENERATIVE JOINT DISEASE (OSTEOARTHRITIS)

OBJECTIVES

At the completion of this chapter you should be able to:

1. Define *degenerative joint disease* (DJD).
2. Identify the prevalence, sex predilection, and age groups affected by DJD.
3. Describe the pathogenesis of DJD.
4. Describe the role of genetic and hormonal factors in DJD.
5. List the most commonly involved joints in DJD.
6. Identify at least four variants of DJD.
7. Contrast the joint pain of DJD and rheumatoid arthritis.
8. Describe the characteristic changes that occur in the hands and the spine.
9. Explain the laboratory and radiologic findings.
10. Identify the goals of treatment of DJD.
11. Evaluate the therapeutic measures which may be employed in treatment of DJD.
12. Cite the problems encountered related to lifestyle of individuals with DJD.

Degenerative joint disease (DJD, osteoarthritis, hypertrophic arthritis, osteoarthrosis) is a disorder of movable joints. The disorder is chronic, slowly progressive, and noninflammatory and is characterized by the deterioration and abrasion of articular cartilage and formation of new bone at the articular surface.

DJD is the most common form of arthritis. A little over half of all cases of arthritis are DJD. The disorder is more common in women than in men and is found primarily in people over the age of 45. This disorder was once thought to be a normal consequence of the aging process, since the incidence increases with age. DJD was given the name of "wear and tear" arthritis, based upon the idea that the joint wore out with age. Newer findings of the biochemistry and biomechanics of the joint have shown that the joint does not wear out with age.

DJD develops with changes in the makeup of the

articular cartilage. The proteoglycan content of the ground substance of the cartilage begins to decrease for an unknown reason. The problem may originate in the proteoglycan synthesis mechanism. The articular cartilage then loses its unique compressibility. In addition, there are changes in the collagen of the cartilage. There is a small amount of Type I cartilage that replaces the normal Type II, and there are changes in the collagen fiber diameters and orientation. These changes alter the biomechanics of the cartilage.

The synthesis of proteoglycans and collagen is greatly increased in the joint with DJD. There is a net loss of proteoglycans and collagen over time, since degradation is even more rapid. What initiates this process is still unknown, but a number of factors seem to be related to the development of the disorder. The aging process seems to be related to the development and progression of DJD through changes in the chondrocyte functioning. These are the cells responsible for the formation of the proteoglycans and collagen in the articular cartilage. The aging chondrocytes may lose their ability to function appropriately.

Genetic factors play a role in some forms of DJD. The development of DJD of the distal interphalangeal joints of the hands (Heberden's nodes) is sex influenced and dominant in females. Women develop Heberden's nodes 10 times more frequently than men.

Sex hormones and other hormonal factors seem to be related to the development of DJD. The relationship between estrogens and bone formation and the prevalence of DJD in women both strongly suggest that hormones play an active part in the disease's factors of development and progression.

The joints most commonly affected in DJD are the weight-bearing joints, including the knees, hips, lumbar and cervical spine, shoulders, elbows, and phalangeal joints. A distinguishing feature of DJD is that the proximal and distal phalangeal joints are frequently affected, whereas the metacarpophalangeal joints are usually unaffected. In rheumatoid arthritis, however, the proximal phalangeal joints and the metacarpal joints are affected, while the distal interphalangeal joints are spared.

DJD primarily involves biochemical and biomechanical changes within the joint; it is not an inflammatory disorder. Synovitis frequently accompanies the changes seen in the joint, however, and is a source of the pain and discomfort seen in this illness.

In addition to the common form of DJD there are several variants. Primary generalized DJD is different in that there is an increase in the number and severity of the joints involved. Erosive inflammatory DJD affects primarily the finger joints and is associated with acute inflammatory episodes that lead to deformities and alkylosis. Alkylosing hyperostosis involves ossification of the vertebrae. Secondary DJD develops as a consequence of some other illness such as rheumatoid arthritis or gout.

CLINICAL FEATURES

The most common feature of DJD is an aching pain in the joint, especially with movement or weight bearing. There may be stiffness after resting, but this goes away with motion. Morning stiffness, if present, usually lasts only a few minutes compared with the much longer period of morning stiffness characteristic of rheumatoid arthritis. Muscle spasm or pressure on the nerves in the region of the joint are likely to be the source of pain. Other features of DJD include restriction of range of motion (especially full extension), local tenderness, bony enlargements around the joint, small effusions, and crepitation.

Characteristic changes occur in the hands. Heberden's nodes, or bony enlargements of the distal interphalangeal joints, are frequently seen. Less common are Bouchard's nodes (see Fig. 70-1), which are bony enlargements of the proximal interphalangeal joints.

FIGURE 70-1
Degenerative joint disease. (A) Primary osteoarthritis of the hands with marked proximal interphalangeal involvement (Bouchard's nodes) along with distal interphalangeal joint involvement. (B) X-ray of the same hands. (Reproduced from J. L. Hollander (ed.), *Arthritis and Allied Conditions, A Textbook of Rheumatology*, 8th ed., Lea & Febiger, Philadelphia, 1972.)

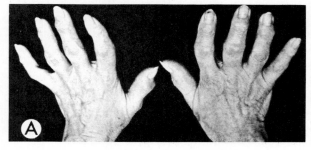

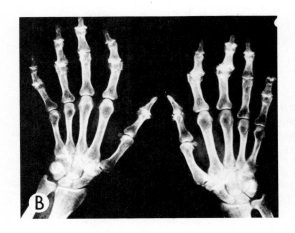

Characteristic changes are also seen in the spine, which becomes painful, stiff, and limited in range of motion. Bony overgrowths or spurs may irritate the nerve roots as they pass through the vertebrae. This results in neuromuscular changes such as the presence of pain, stiffness, and limited range of motion. Some people complain of headaches that are a direct result of DJD of the cervical spine.

LABORATORY FINDINGS

DJD is a local arthritic disorder, so there are no specific blood tests that are used in the diagnosis. Laboratory tests are sometimes used to exclude other forms of arthritis. Rheumatoid factor may be present in the serum of people with DJD, since it normally increases in frequency with aging. The erythrocyte sedimentation rate may be slightly elevated if there is extensive synovitis.

RADIOLOGIC FINDINGS

A common characteristic of DJD seen with x-rays is narrowing of the joint space. This happens because of loss of cartilage. In the knee the joint space may be narrowed in only one compartment. In addition to narrowing, there is an increase in bone density around the joint. Osteophytes (spurs) can be seen at the marginal aspects of the joint (see Fig. 70-2). Cystic changes of various sizes are sometimes seen.

The extent of the change in the joints noted with x-ray may not be related to the presence of symptoms. Radiologic evidence of DJD can be demonstrated in up to 85 percent of the people over 75 years of age, although a much lower percent actually complain of pain and stiffness.

Specialized x-rays may be helpful in evaluating DJD. Weight-bearing x-rays of the knees may give a

FIGURE 70-2

Degenerative joint disease: spine x-ray. This anteroposterior projection of the lumbar spine shows scoliosis and narrowing of the intervertebral spaces on the concave side, where extensive osteophyte formation is present. The osteophytes are not continuous as seen in ankylosing spondylitis. Adjacent bony margins are sclerosed. (Reproduced with permission from the Arthritis Foundation, New York, copyright 1972.)

better picture of the effects of the illness than non-weight bearing views. DJD is not a symmetrical disorder, so views of the contralateral joint can be helpful.

TREATMENT

The treatment of DJD is multifocal and consists of an individualized plan for each person. The goals of treatment are to retard or prevent further damage to the joint and to manage pain and stiffness in order to maintain mobility.

The protection of the joints from additional trauma is important to assist in slowing the progression of the disorder. Evaluation of work patterns and activities of daily living assist in eliminating those activities that increase the load bearing strain to an affected joint. Canes and walkers can significantly decrease the weight load on knees and hips. Reducing weight, if the person is overweight, can greatly decrease the load placed upon knees and hips.

Physical therapy measures are important for relieving pain and preserving muscle strength and range of motion. The use of ice or heat on the involved joints may provide temporary relief of pain. Range of motion exercises may be helpful in maintaining full range of

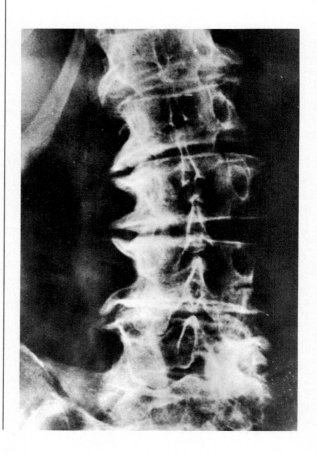

motion of involved joints. Isometric exercises will be helpful for building the muscles that support the joints. Isotonic exercises should not be used with resistance, since this can add additional stresses to the joint.

Drug therapy is designed to control the pain in the joint. An additional function of the drug therapy is to control any synovitis. Over-the-counter analgesic drugs such as acetaminophen, aspirin, and ibuprofen are usually adequate for pain relief. Aspirin and ibuprofen have the added advantage of controlling the synovitis. Other nonsteroidal anti-inflammatory drugs are frequently used for pain and synovitis control. Adverse effects of these drugs are generally more common in elderly; drug therapy should be considered carefully in this case, since so many elderly have DJD.

Disease-modifying antirheumatic drugs are not used in the treatment of DJD, since this is not a systemic disorder. Oral corticosteroids are usually contraindicated in the treatment of DJD. These agents are generally ineffective in improving symptoms, and their toxic potential makes their use risky. Intraarticular injections can provide relief of synovitis. If used too frequently, the agents deplete the normal ground substance of the cartilage and can accelerate the arthritic progression.

Surgical treatment of DJD is designed to remove loose bodies, repair damaged supporting tissues, or replace the entire joint. The introduction of the arthroscope allows a variety of surgical procedures to be performed with much lower morbidity rates than are associated with open surgeries. Particles of cartilage can be removed as efficiently as in other surgical procedures.

Another form of surgery used in DJD is angulation osteotomy. This is used to treat DJD of the knee that affects only one compartment. Pain is relieved in the joint by correcting the varus or valgus deformity and bringing healthy articular cartilage into contact with other healthy articular cartilage.

Total joint replacements for hips and knees have been successful in maintaining near normal function for many people with DJD. DJD is a hypertrophic form of arthritis, which indicates that the bone adjacent to the artificial joint is strong, forming an excellent base for attachment. There are a number of complications that can occur with joint replacement, and these are weighed against the acquired benefits. Long-term evaluation studies of total prostheses for finger and other joints are still underway (see Chap. 61).

Joint fusions may be necessary for the relief of pain in advanced cases of DJD. The cervical spine is an area in which joint fusion can provide dramatic pain relief.

PROGNOSIS

DJD generally progresses very slowly. The major problems encountered are pain upon the use of a joint and increasing instability with weight bearing, particularly in the knee. These problems mean that the person usually must develop a new lifestyle. This new lifestyle often includes altering lifelong patterns of eating and exercise, manipulating complex drug regimes, and utilizing adaptive and assisting devices.

QUESTIONS

Degenerative joint disease (osteoarthritis)

Directions: Answer the following questions on a separate sheet of paper.

1. Define *degenerative joint disease*.
2. Describe the synthesis of proteoglycans and collagen in DJD.
3. Explain why the aging process seems to be related to the development of DJD.
4. Explain the rationale for total joint replacements for hips and knees in DJD.
5. Explain the radiologic findings for DJD.
6. Identify the goals of treatment of DJD.

Directions: Circle the letter preceding each item below that correctly answers the question. More than one answer may be correct.

7. The pathogenesis of degenerative joint disease develops with changes in the:
   a. Articular cartilage   *b.* Articular joints
   c. Collagen of the cartilage, where a small amount of Type I cartilage replaces normal Type II
   d. Collagen fiber diameters and orientation
8. The highest incidence of DJD is found in people between which years of age?
   a. 15, 20   *b.* 25, 34   *c.* 35, 44   *d.* 45, greater

duration   *b.* Aching pain in the joint with working   *c.* Restriction of range of motion *d.* Muscle spasm or pressure on nerves in the region of the joint

9. In DJD, the development of Heberden's nodes in the distal interphalangeal joints of the hands occurs how many times more frequently in which sex?
   a. 5, men   *b.* 10, men   *c.* 5, women   *d.* 10, women

10. The joints most commonly affected in DJD include the:
   a. Lumbar and cervical spine   *b.* Knees   *c.* Distal phalangeal joints   *d.* Metacarpal phalangeal joints

11. Common clinical features of DJD include:
   a. Morning stiffness of less than 30-minute

Directions: Circle T if the statement is true and F if it is false. Correct the false statements.

12. T   F   DJD is considered an inflammatory disease.

13. T   F   Erosive inflammatory DJD is a variant of DJD which involves ossification of the vertebrae.

14. T   F   Oral corticosteroids are used in the treatment of DJD.

15. T   F   Evidence of positive rheumatoid factor is indicative of DJD.

REFERENCES FOR PART XI

CARTER, M. A., et al.: "Immune and Inflammatory Disorders," in M. B. Weiner and G. A. Pepper, *Clinical Pharmacology and Therapeutics in Nursing*, McGraw-Hill, New York, 1985, pp. 389–419.

CHEUNG, H. S., et al.: "In Vitro Biosynthesis in Healing and Normal Rabbit Articular Cartilage," *Journal of Bone and Joint Surgery*, 60A(8): 1076–1081, 1978.

KATZ, W. A. (ed.): *Rheumatic Diseases: Diagnosis and Management*, Lippincott, Philadelphia, 1977.

KELLEY, W., et al.: *Textbook of Rheumatology*, Saunders, Philadelphia, 1981.

MALASANOS, L., et al.: "Musculoskeletal Assessment," *Health Assessment*, 2d ed., Mosby, St. Louis, 1981, pp 443–517.

McCARTY, D. J. (ed.): *Arthritis and Allied Conditions*, 9th ed., Kimpton, London, 1979.

RADIN, E. L.: "Biomechanics of the Knee Joint," *Orthopaedic Clinics of North America*, 4(2): 539–546, 1973.

RADIN, E. L.: "Mechanical Aspects of Osteoarthrosis," *Bulletin of Rheumatic Diseases*, 26: 862–865, 1976.

RAVECHE, E. S., et al.: "Studies of the Effects of Sex Hormones on Autosomal and X-Linked Genetic Control of Induced Spontaneous Antibody Production," *Arthritis and Rheumatism*, 22(11): 1177–1187, 1979.

RIGGS, G. and E. GALL: *Rheumatic Diseases: Rehabilitation and Management*, Butterworth Publishers, Boston, 1984.

RODNAN, G. P., et al. (eds.): *Primer on the Rheumatic Diseases*, 8th ed., Arthritis Foundation, Atlanta, 1983.

ROBINSON, D. R., et al.: "Prostaglandins: Their Regulation in Rheumatoid Arthritis," *Annals of the New York Academy of Science*, 332: 279–294, 1979.

ROTHSCHILD, B. M.: *Rheumatology: A Primary Care Approach*, Yorke Medical Books, New York, 1982.

TRANG, L. E.: "Prostaglandins and Inflammation," *Seminar of Arthritis and Rheumatism*, 9: 153–190, 1980.

PART XII

MAREK A. STAWISKI
JEFFREY P. CALLEN

DERMATOLOGY

Dermatology is concerned with the structure, function, and diseases of the skin. The skin forms a protective barrier around the entire body and has a role in body thermoregulation, glandular secretion, and sensory communication with the external environment. Any structure of the skin has a potential for disease. A skin disorder may be restricted to cutaneous involvement or be indicative of a major systemic disease.

This section includes a review of skin anatomy and physiology. Selected cutaneous diseases, their etiology, pathogenesis, and treatment are also discussed

OBJECTIVES

At the completion of this part you should be able to:

1. Describe the structure and function of the skin.
2. Identify the causes, pathogenesis, and principles of treatment associated with some of the more important dermatological disorders.

CHAPTER 71

THE STRUCTURE AND FUNCTIONS OF THE SKIN

OBJECTIVES

At the completion of this chapter you should be able to:

1. Identify the basic functions of the skin.
2. Differentiate between the three layers of skin—epidermis, dermis, and subcutaneous fat—in terms of location, function, and composition.
3. Name and describe the function of the three distinct layers of the epidermis.
4. Describe the process of skin proliferation.
5. Identify the characteristics of basal cells, keratinocytes, and melanocytes.
6. Differentiate between melanosomes in blacks and Caucasians.
7. Identify the functions of the adnexal structures in the dermis.
8. Differentiate between sweat, sebaceous, and apocrine glands as to location and function.
9. Explain the composition and process of hair and nail formation.
10. Describe the essential elements of a skin examination.
11. Identify at least two systemic diseases that may be detected by skin abnormalities.

DERMATOLOGICAL VOCABULARY

1. Macule—a nonpalpable circumscribed area usually demarcated by a change of color; example: tinea versicolor (Plate 13).
2. Papule—an elevated palpable lesion usually smaller than 5 mm; example: a blue nevus (Plate 22).
3. Nodule, tumor—a palpable lesion usually larger than 5 mm; example: basal cell carcinoma (Plate 17).
4. Plaque—a palpable lesion that has a greater dimension in area than in thickness; example: psoriasis (Plate 8).
5. Vesicle, bulla—a fluid-filled, elevated lesion; example: a vesicle of herpes simplex (Fig. 75-5).

6. Pustule—a lesion that contains pus; example: acne vulgaris (Fig. 72-4).

7. Wheal—a transitory palpable lesion; example: hives (Plate 6).

8. Comedo—a plugged pilosebaceous opening; example: acne vulgaris (Fig. 72-3).

9. Burrow—a linear trail produced by a parasite; example: scabies (Fig. 77-7).

10. Scale—an excessive accumulation of keratin; example: psoriasis (Plate 8).

11. Crust—an excessive accumulation of serum and cellular, bacterial, and squamous debris; example: impetigo (Plate 15).

12. Fissure—a crack in the skin extending to the dermis; example: hand eczema (Plate 5).

13. Lichenification—an area of accentuated skin markings associated with a thickening of the skin caused by scratching and rubbing; example: neurodermatitis (Fig. 73-1).

14. Erosion—a loss of epidermis only; example: impetigo (Plate 15).

15. Ulcer—a loss of epidermis and dermis; example: an ulcer (Plate 18).

16. Excoriations—a linear erosion, frequently self-inducement is implied; example: neurotic excoriation (Fig. 73-2).

17. Atrophy—a loss of epidermal and dermal substance; example: atrophy following treatment with topical steroids.

18. Verrucous—wartlike; example: verruca vulgaris (Fig. 75-1).

19. Telangiectasis—a dilatation of superficial vessels; example: dilated vessels in a basal cell carcinoma (Plate 17).

20. Eczematoid lesion—an eczema-like inflammatory lesion with scale, vesiculation, crust, and weeping; example: poison ivy (Plate 4).

21. Hyperkeratosis—a lesion with excessive scales; example: psoriasis (Plate 8).

22. Circinate lesion— an arcuate lesion; example: urticaria (Plate 6).

23. Annular lesion—a ring-shaped lesion with an active margin and often a clear center; example: ringworm (Fig. 75-12).

24. Nummular lesion—a coin-shaped lesion; example: nummular eczema.

25. Guttate—drop-sized; example: guttate psoriasis (Fig. 74-2).

26. Iris, or target, lesion—two or three concentric circles that form an irislike lesion; example: erythema multiforme (Fig. 73-8).

27. Herpetiform—having groups of vesicles; example: herpes simplex (Fig. 75-5).

28. Morbilliform lesions—a small confluent maculopapular lesion; example: a viral exanthem.

29. Confluent—blending into adjacent lesions; example: tinea versicolor (Plate 13).

30. Zosteriform—having a linear dermatomal distribution; example: herpes zoster (shingles) (Plate 11).

31. Photodistribution—distribution in areas exposed to sunlight; example: sunburn.

32. Koebner's phenomenon—lesions that form in areas of previous trauma of the skin; example: psoriasis.

The skin, which is the largest organ of the human body, envelops the muscles and internal organs. It is an endless network of blood vessels, nerves, and glands, all of which have a potential for disease. Since the number of cutaneous diseases is very extensive, only the most commonly encountered will be discussed. The most common dermatological condition—acne—and new advances in its treatment will be described. Another frequently seen disease is eczema, which can be inherited or caused by allergens. Psoriasis is thought to be the most economically and psychologically ravaging skin disease. Most dermatological hospital admissions are caused by severe exacerbations of psoriasis.

Cutaneous infections with viruses causing warts and herpes simplex have captured the attention of not only the health care community but also the press and public. Fungal infections are responsible for ringworm, athlete's foot, and jock itch. Presentation and treatment of these fungal infections and bacterial skin infections will be included.

Neoplasms of the skin are the most common of the cancers encountered in humans. They range from non-invasive basal cell carcinoma to aggressive and frequently fatal melanomas. Description of diagnostic features and etiology of these tumors should help the reader to diagnose and prevent these malignancies.

Classic venereal diseases such as syphilis and gonorrhea are included. However, the attention of the nation has been captured by presentation and complications of herpes simplex and acquired immune deficiency syndrome (AIDS). Appropriate diagnostic, preventive, and therapeutic aspects of venereal diseases should be familiar to all health personnel. Diagnosis, prevention, and treatment of infestations with scabies and lice can be a considerable challenge to nurses, especially public health and/or school nurses. However, before the various skin diseases are considered, the basic structure and functions of the skin will be summarized.

FUNCTIONS OF SKIN

The skin protects the body from trauma and shields it from bacterial, viral, and fungal infections. Heat loss and conservation are regulated by cutaneous vasodilatation or secretion by the sweat glands. After complete loss of skin, essential body fluids evaporate and electrolytes are lost within hours; an example of this is seen in burn patients. The pleasant or unpleasant odors of the skin serve as social and sexual signs of acceptability or rejection. Epidermal appendages of the skin, such as nails and hair, have their well-established cosmetic values unique to specific cultures. The skin also provides the sensations of touch, pressure, temperature, pain, and pleasure by an intricate network of nerve endings.

SKIN STRUCTURE

Microscopically skin consists of three layers: epidermis, dermis, and subcutaneous fat (see Fig. 71-1). The epidermis, the outermost portion of the skin, is divided into two main layers—a stratum of anucleate cornified cells, (the stratum corneum, or horny layer) and the inner, malpighian layer, from which the surface cornified cells arise by differentiation. The malpighian layer is subdivided into the (1) basal cell layer (or stratum germinativum), (2) stratum spinosum, and (3) stratum granu-

losum. The stratum granulosum lies just below the stratum corneum. Stratum granulosum has an important function in the production of stratum corneum proteins and chemical bonds.

The basal layer consists largely of undifferentiated epidermal cells which undergo constant mitosis, renewing the epidermis. When such a cell undergoes mitosis, one of the daughter cells remains in the basal layer to divide again while the other cell migrates outward toward the stratum spinosum.

The major differentiating cell of the epidermis is the keratinocyte, which produces keratin, a fibrous protein. As keratinocytes leave the malpighian layers and move upward, they undergo changes in shape, orientation, cytoplasmic structure, and composition. This leads to the transformation of viable, actively synthesizing cells into the dead, cornified cells of the stratum corneum, a process termed *keratinization*. Keratinocytes of the basal layer are cylindrical in shape. They become polyhedral in the stratum spinosum, flatter in the granular layer, and lamellar in the stratum corneum. Important changes also occur in their cytoplasmic constituents, the nucleus, and the cell membranes. The keratinocytes synthesize tonofilaments, filamentous proteins. In the stratum germinativum the tonofilaments are arranged in bundles which surround the nucleus of the cell. In the stratum spinosum, synthesis continues

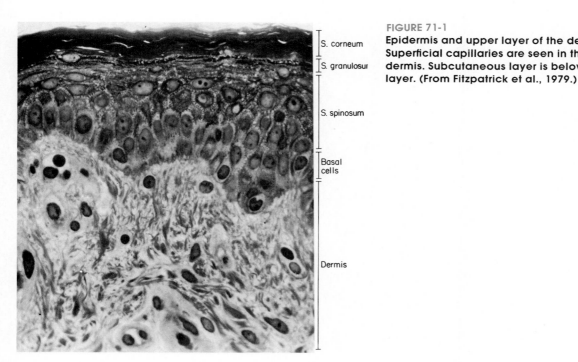

S. corneum

S. granulosur

S. spinosum

Basal cells

Dermis

FIGURE 71-1

Epidermis and upper layer of the dermis. Superficial capillaries are seen in the upper dermis. Subcutaneous layer is below the dermal layer. (From Fitzpatrick et al., 1979.)

and these tonofilament bundles become more compact, forming an interlacing network extending through the cytoplasm. As they move through the stratum granulosum, keratohyalin granules appear within these cells, deposited within and around the tonofilament bundles. In the stratum corneum the granules appear tightly packed. Keratohyalin is not sufficiently defined chemically, and its final role in the keratinization process is not clear. It does appear to contribute to the amorphous, electron-dense matrix of the cornified cells.

As stated above, it appears that during differentiation keratinocytes pass through a synthetic phase in which tonofilaments, keratohyalin, lamellar bodies, and other cell constituents are formed. Finally they enter a transition phase, in which the cytoplasmic components are dissociated and degraded. The remaining cell constituents form a fibrous, amorphous complex surrounded by a reinforced impermeable membrane, the horny cell. This programmed process of epidermal cell migration normally takes about 28 days.

The second major cell of the epidermis is the melanocyte, found in the basal layer. The ratio of basal cells to melanocytes is 10:1. Within the melanocyte, pigment granules called *melanosomes* are synthesized. Melanosomes contain brown biochrome called *melanin*.

The melanosomes are transferred to keratinocytes through long dendritic processes. Each melanocyte is connected through these projections, and about 36 keratinocytes form what is referred to as the epidermal melanin unit (Fig. 71-2). Melanosomes are hydrolyzed at varying rates by enzymes. The amount of melanin within the keratinocyte determines the color of the skin. Melanin protects the skin from harmful effects of the sun. Paradoxically it is the sun's rays which increase the production of melanosomes and melanin. Both blacks and Caucasians have the same number of melanocytes. Black persons have large melanosomes which resist destruction by the hydrolyzing enzymes, while Caucasians have smaller melanosomes which are more readily destroyed.

The dermis is located immediately below the epidermis and is composed of collagen fibers, elastin, and reticulin embedded in a ground substance. The dermal matrix contains blood vessels and nerves, which provide support and nourishment to the growing epidermis. Surrounding the small blood vessels are lymphocytes, histiocytes, mast cells, and leukocytes, which protect the body from infections and foreign body invasion. Specialized collagen fibers anchor the epidermal basal cells into the dermis. The adnexal appendages of the dermis are hair, nails, and eccrine (sweat), sebaceous, and apocrine glands.

Underlying the dermis is the third layer of skin—the subcutaneous fat. This layer provides a cushion for the skin, insulation to maintain body heat, and a store

FIGURE 71-2

The epidermal melanin unit. Relationship of a single melanocyte to multiple epidermal cells is well illustrated. (From Fitzpatrick et al., 1979.)

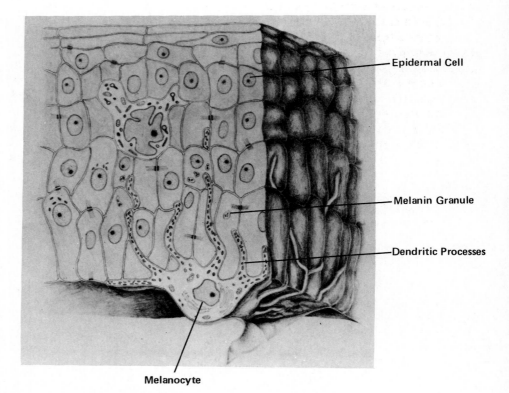

Epidermal Cell

Melanin Granule

Dendritic Processes

Melanocyte

of energy. Cosmetically, subcutaneous fat influences the attractiveness of either sex.

Sweat glands are present almost everywhere on the skin except in the ears and on the lips. These glands produce a hypotonic solution which is clear and watery and has a high content of urea and lactate. Sweat glands aid in maintaining the appropriate body temperature.

Sebaceous glands are lobulated structures which consist of lipid-filled cells. The oily substance referred to as sebum is passed to the central duct and drained to the pilosebaceous ducts of the hair follicles (Fig. 71-3). Sebaceous glands are concentrated over the face, the chest, the back, and the proximal arms. Their activity is hormonally regulated primarily by androgenic hormones.

The apocrine glands are found primarily in the axilla, in the genital skin, around the nipples, and in the perianal area. The apocrine duct empties into the hair follicle above the entrance of the sebaceous duct (Fig. 71-4). The apocrine secretions do not serve any useful function in humans but contribute to the axillary odor when apocrine secretions are decomposed by bacteria. Apocrine glands produce a milky, viscous substance which results from a high content of organic components. They begin their secretory activity at puberty.

Hair is formed from keratin. By a predetermined differentiating process certain epidermal cells form the hair follicle. The hair follicle is supported by dermal matrix and differentiates into the hair (Fig. 71-5). An epithelial canal is formed, through which the hair passes to the surface. Hair is dead keratin just like scale, and it is formed at a predetermined rate. Cystine and methionine, sulfur-containing amino acids, contribute strong covalent bonds, giving strength to hair. On the scalp the rate of the growth of hair is usually 3 mm per day. Each hair follicle goes through a cycle of: growth (anagen hair), intermediate stage (catagen hair), and involution (telogen hair). The anagen stage on the scalp lasts about

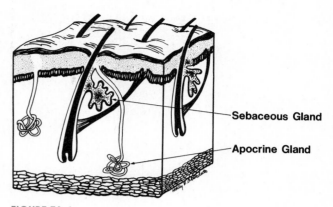

FIGURE 71-4
Apocrine gland empties above the entrance of the sebaceous duct. (From the Biomedical Media Production Unit, University of Michigan Medical Center.)

3 years, while the telogen stage lasts only about 3 months. Once the hair follicle reaches the telogen stage, the hair falls out. Eventually, the hair follicle regenerates into the anagen stage and a new hair is produced. This cycle of activity for hair follicles is independent for each hair follicle. The mosaic pattern prevents occurrence of temporary baldness of the scalp. The process stops when the person becomes permanently bald. Various commercial preparations advertised to strengthen hair are of questionable value. Protein shampoos affect only the dead keratin and not the hair follicle and therefore cannot prevent hair loss.

The nail is a dead keratin plate produced by epidermal cells of nail matrix (Fig. 71-6). The nail matrix is located beneath the proximal portion of the nail plate

FIGURE 71-3
Sebaceous gland which opens into the central duct. (From the Biomedical Media Production Unit, University of Michigan Medical Center.)

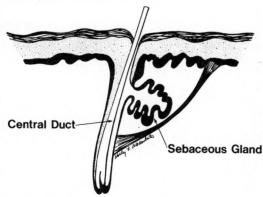

FIGURE 71-5
Hair matrix is supported by a dermal papilla and differentiates into hair. (From the Biomedical Media Production Unit, University of Michigan Medical Center.)

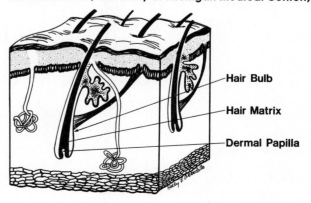

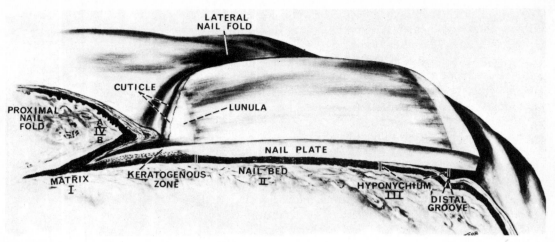

FIGURE 71-6
Diagrammatic drawing of adult normal fingernails. (From Fitzpatrick et al., 1979.)

in the dermis. It is visible as a white area, called the lunula, which is covered by the proximal nail fold and cuticle. Since both nail and hair are dead keratin structures, they have no nerve endings and no blood supply.

SKIN EXAMINATION

Skin should be examined in a well-illuminated room, preferably in natural daylight. A dimly illuminated hospital room is the least desirable place to inspect the skin, and examination there may lead to serious errors in diagnosis. The color of the skin should be recorded. Purplish, cyanotic discoloration of the toes or fingers can provide a useful clue to the presence of internal diseases. Pallor can be a sign of anemia (see Chap. 16). Skin has turgor and elasticity on palpation. Excessive dryness causes this organ to be scaly and wrinkled. This may indicate dehydration or thyroid disease. Skin ridges are visible over the palms and feet and are also present over the entire body surface. They are called dermatoglyphics and form the pattern unique for every individual and species (Fig. 71-7). These dermatoglyphics over the volar aspects of the fingers are used for the process of fingerprinting. They are useful in criminology; however, health care professionals are also interested in the presence of these whorls. Their disappearance over fingertips can be a first sign of vascular insufficiency, as in progressive systemic sclerosis (scleroderma), see Chap. 67.

There is an expected pattern of hair distribution in both males and females. In many men, and some women, temporal and occipital scalp thinning becomes evident with advancing age. However, a sudden hair loss over the scalp or even the entire body must be investigated for possible thyroid abnormalities (see Chap. 55). The lack of hair over distal extremities can be the first sign of vascular insufficiency, whereas abnormal hair growth over the face, especially in females, should be investigated for a hormone-producing tumor.

Nails can be damaged and thinned in many diseases such as psoriasis, fungal infections, and thyroid abnormalities. Excessive sweat production can be a sign of anxiety or an underlying internal illness.

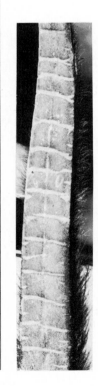

FIGURE 71-7
Underside of the spider monkey with characteristic dermatoglyphics. (From Fitzpatrick et al., 1979.)

The structure and functions of the skin

Directions: Circle the letter preceding each item below that correctly answers the question. More than one answer may be correct.

1. Which of the following are functions of the skin?
   a. Regulating heat loss and conservation   *b.* Protecting against trauma and infection   *c.* Replacing utilized corticosteroids   *d.* Providing tactile sensations

2. The epidermis contains the:
   a. Stratum spinosum   *b.* Basal layer
   c. Keratinocytes   *d.* Hair roots   *e.* Collagen fibers

3. The dermis is composed of:
   a. Stratum germinativum   *b.* Melanocytes
   c. Blood vessels and nerves   *d.* Elastin and reticulin

4. Which of the following skin conditions is most likely to have the greatest economic and psychological impact:
   a. Herpes simplex   *b.* Psoriasis   *c.* Basal cell carcinoma   *d.* Scabies

Directions: Answer the following questions on a separate sheet of paper.

5. Explain the process by which skin proliferates by identifying the layer of the skin that produces new cells and the direction of movement of the new cells.

6. List the functions of two of the adnexal structures in the dermis—sweat glands and sebaceous glands.

7. Describe the essential elements of a skin examination.

8. What is the function of the subcutaneous fat layer of the skin?

Directions: Circle T if the statement is true and F if it is false. Correct the false statements.

9. T   F   Abnormal hair loss in the scalp should be investigated for possible thyroid abnormalities.

10. T   F   The absence of whorls over the fingertips may be indicative of vascular insufficiency, as in scleroderma.

11. T   F   The stratum granulosum layer contains the partially keratinized epidermal cells.

12. T   F   Hair is composed of particular living keratinocytes which are bonded together with sulfur bonds into longitudinal strands.

13. T   F   Nails are composed of keratin produced by epidermal cells.

14. T   F   Melanosomes are hydrolyzed by enzymes.

15. T   F   Racial differences in pigmentation are due to differences in number of melanocytes.

16. Label the three layers of the skin—epidermis, dermis, and subcutaneous fat—on the following diagram (Fig. 71-8).

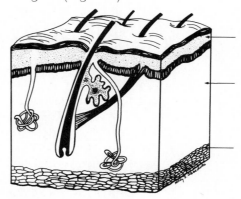

FIGURE 71-8

CHAPTER 72

ACNE AND RELATED CONDITIONS

OBJECTIVES

At the completion of this chapter you should be able to:

1. Identify for acne the probable causes, age of occurrence, and distribution.
2. Describe the steps that occur in the formation of acne lesions (comedones, papules, pustules, cysts).
3. Discuss two variants of acne.
4. Explain the goal of acne therapy.
5. Describe the mechanism of action in topical acne therapy.
6. Discuss the systemic antibiotics used in the treatment of acne as to rationales for use, mechanisms, contraindications for use, side effects, and laboratory analyses.
7. Differentiate acne rosacea from acne vulgaris in terms of age of occurrence, predisposing factors, presenting signs, and treatments.

ACNE VULGARIS

Acne is a chronic inflammatory process of sebaceous glands. It generally occurs among most adolescents and young adults and spontaneously resolves around 20 to 30 years of age. However, many middle-aged adults experience acne eruptions. Acne is usually associated with a high rate of sebum secretion. Androgens are known stimulants of sebum secretion, and estrogen reduces sebum production. A sudden onset of severe acne associated with hirsutism and/or menstrual abnormalities may be indicative of an endocrine disorder in a female patient. Acne which presents in women in their 20s,

30s, and 40s is frequently caused by comedo-producing oil-based cosmetics and moisturizers. Mechanical factors, which include rubbing, friction pressure, and stretching of the skin rich in sebaceous glands, can trigger acne. Among the more common mechanical causes are football helmets, surgical tape, shirt collars, and wrestling.

Medications can also precipitate the onset of acne. Chronic oral corticosteroids used for treatment of other conditions (e.g., systemic lupus erythematosus, renal transplants) can trigger superficial pustules over the face, chest, and back. Contraceptive birth control pills usually are helpful in acne treatment, because of their estrogen content. However, in some women, contraceptives can exacerbate the disease. Other drugs known to aggravate or precipitate acne are bromides, iodides, diphenylhydantoin, lithium, and isonicotinic acid hydrazide. Workers employed in industry can be exposed to chlorinated hydrocarbons which are acnegenic.

Management of acne patients requires a careful history to rule out acnegenic factors and more serious endocrine abnormalities. It should be noted that in most acne patients there is a family history of acne.

The distribution of acne corresponds to the areas of sebaceous glands and occurs over the face, neck, chest, back, and shoulders (Fig. 72-1). The earliest lesion to appear in the skin is the *comedo. White comedones*, or closed comedones, are more likely to progress to inflammatory papules and pustules of acne. *Black comedones*, or open comedones or blackheads, have a dark, horny material plugging up dilated pilosebaceous ducts. These comedones obstruct the flow of sebum to the surface. The sebum, bacteria (*Propionibacterium acnes*), and fatty acids are thought to be responsible for the development of inflammation around the pilosebaceous ducts and sebaceous glands. This inflammation leads to formation of erythematous papules, inflammatory pustules, and inflammatory cysts (Fig. 72-2). The pustules and cysts, in time, drain and heal. Deeper papules and cysts

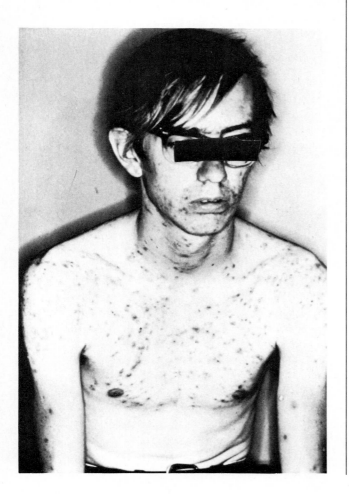

can leave permanent scars, while mild acne resolves without scarring. The tendency to scar varies among individuals and is greater when the person attempts to empty the lesions.

Acne is classified as comedonal (black and white comedones) (Fig. 72-3), papulopustular (papules and pustules) (Fig. 72-4), or cystic (Plate 1). Comedonal and papulopustular acne are given numerical grades. Grade I acne has less than 10 comedones, papules, or pustules on one side of the face (Fig. 72-3); Grade II, 10 to 20 comedones, papules, or pustules; Grade III, 25 to 50; Grade IV, greater than 50 (Plate 1).

Variants of acne

Several variants of acne should be recognized. Acne excoriate occurs in individuals who obsessively manipulate the acne lesions; doing this can cause a great deal of scarring. Acne conglobata is the most severe cystic acne, having deep cysts, multiple comedones, and marked scarring. It can be associated with malaise and fever, and it may even require hospitalization (Fig. 72-4 and Plate 1). Acne keloidalis presents with multiple scars and keloids in the areas where acne lesions were present (Fig. 72-5).

Treatment of acne

The goal of acne therapy is to decrease the inflammatory process of pilosebaceous glands until spontaneous remission occurs. Treatment of acne and related conditions improves the patient's cosmetic appearance and self-image, and it prevents scars related to acne.

Acne treatment includes halting the use of all exacerbating factors such as oil-based makeup and moisturizing creams. Dietary restrictions are usually not required or effective. However, it is reasonable to omit certain foods such as colas, chocolate, milk products, and iodides if a patient reports flare-ups of acne after ingestion of these.

Cleaning and scrubbing of the face with soap removes the surface oil and dislodges some comedones. The affected areas should be washed twice daily. Soaps such as Lava, Dial, Pernox, Fostex, Neutrogena, and Desquam-X Wash are recommended. An abrasive sponge such as a Buf-Puf is useful in dislodging super-

FIGURE 72-1
Characteristic distribution of acne pustules over the face, chest, and shoulders.

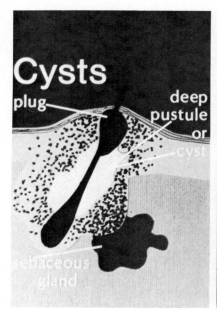

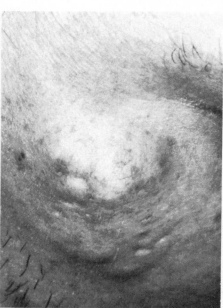

FIGURE 72-2
Inflammation around the pilosebaceous duct and sebaceous glands which leads to formation of papules, pustules, and cysts.

FIGURE 72-4
Severe scarring can follow obsessive manipulation of acne papules and pustules.

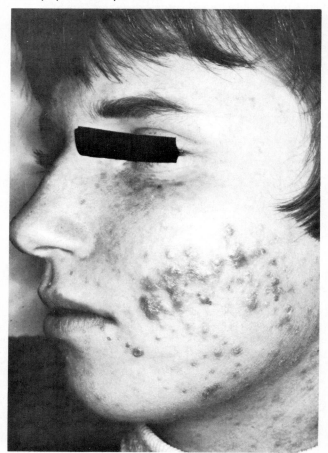

FIGURE 72-3
Multiple comedones in a superficial comedonal acne.

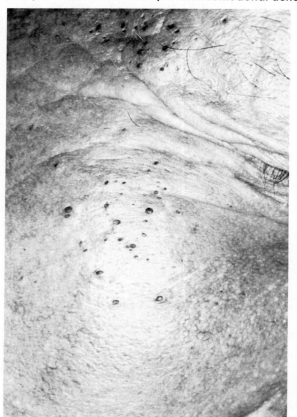

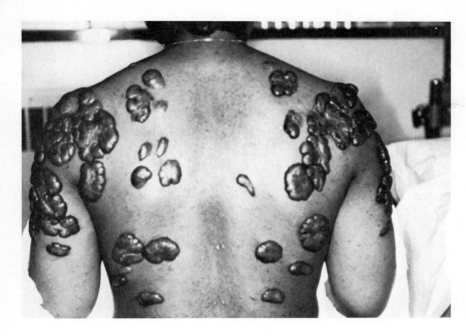

FIGURE 72-5
Keloids can complicate a course of acne vulgaris.

ficial comedones. A keratolytic agent such a benzoyl peroxide at a concentration of 5 to 10% is used daily. Precipitated sulfur (1 to 2%) is useful in drying pustules, especially of acne rosacea. Vitamin A acid [Retin-A] cream (0.05%) and gel (0.01%) is useful because of its keratolytic effect on the superficial comedones. However, Retin-A derivatives can enhance irritability of the skin from exposure to the wind, sun, or cold weather. Topical tetracycline (Topicycline), topical clindamycin (1% Cleocin-T), topical erythromycin (Staticin, Ery-Derm, A/T/S), and topical meclocycline (Meclan) are used in the treatment of superficial acne papules and pustules.

Systemic antibiotics remain the principal mode of therapy of deep pustular, deep papular, and cystic acne. Patients are usually treated with tetracycline, erythromycin, or minocycline. For superficial pustular acne the dose of tetracycline is between 250 and 500 mg daily. For severe deep papulopustular or cystic acne, 1000 mg of tetracycline daily is administered. Long-term tetracycline therapy has been shown to be safe. Children under age 12 are not treated with tetracycline, since permanent staining of the teeth can occur. Tetracycline is not given to pregnant women, because there may be enamel hypoplasia and permanent discoloration of the teeth in newborns. Some patients may develp photosensitivity, nausea, and/or candidiasis while receiving tetracycline. Erythromycin is less effective in treatment of acne. Minocycline at a dose of 50 to 100 mg daily is very effective but usually too expensive for chronic use. The pharmacological action of tetracycline on acne is not completely understood. The antibiotic decreases the population of *Propionibacterium* in the pilosebaceous gland. This bacterium produces lipases which hydrolyze sebum to fatty acids. Tetracycline also inhibits these lipases. Fatty acids may be responsible for inflammation of the pilosebaceous duct.

Outpatient therapy for acne includes acne surgery, which consists of removal of comedones and opening and drainage of pustules. Self-manipulation of acne lesions usually results in more scar formation and should be discouraged. The benefit of ultraviolet light is minimal, and home sunlamps are not recommended. Cryotherapy has been very effective in the treatment of superficial pustules and cysts.

A new oral drug, isotretinoin (Accutane), has been released by the Food and Drug Administration for treatment of severe antibiotic-resistant cystic-conglobate acne. A single (4-month) course at the dose of 1 mg/kg per day results in remission of the disease in about 80 to 90 percent of patients. In many of these patients remission appears to be permanent, even after a 3-year follow-up.

The exact mechanism of isotretinoin is unknown. Chemically it is related to vitamin A. In contrast to vitamin A, isotretinoin is not stored in the liver but is rapidly excreted; the half-life of oral isotretinoin is approximately 10 to 20 hours. Consequently, the drug has fewer side effects than vitamin A. Isotretinoin inhibits sebaceous gland function, and this presumably is its mechanism of action in acne.

Since isotretinoin is a known teratogen, the drug *must not be used in females who are pregnant or who intend to become pregnant* while undergoing therapy or soon after completion of therapy. Before isotretinoin is administered to women of childbearing age, a pregnancy test should be performed, and an effective mode of contraception should be used for 2 months before therapy, throughout the therapy, and for 2 months following discontinuation of therapy.

1013

Cheilitis, xerosis, conjunctivitis, and drying of nasal mucosa with nosebleeds are the most common side effects, which are reversible upon discontinuation of the medication. Other side effects include myalgias, transient arthralgias, and thinning of scalp hair. Very rare but serious side effects include increased intercranial pressure with papilledema, nausea, vomiting, headaches, and visual disturbances. Since the drug ingestion has been associated with inflammatory bowel diseases, it should not be used in patients with inflammatory bowel diseases. If signs of increased intracranial pressure or severe diarrhea develop, isotretinoin must be stopped immediately. Transient elevation of triglycerides has been observed in 25 percent of the patients. Furthermore, elevation of uric acid and liver enzymes and very minor depression of red cell counts and white cell counts have been reported. Patients on isotretinoin should have blood lipid determinations, white cell counts, red cell counts, and levels of platelets, alkaline phosphatase, serum glutamic-oxaloacetic and pyruvic transaminases (SGOT and SGPT), and lactic acid dehydrogenase (LDH) obtained before therapy and at intervals throughout the therapy.

There is much optimism regarding the potential role of isotretinoin in the treatment of severe acne. Its use should be restricted to short-term, low-dose therapy of patients with antibiotic-resistant cystic acne. Patients who are obese, diabetic, or alcoholic or have high triglycerides and women planning families in the near future *should not* be treated with this medication. Furthermore, only physicians who are experienced or trained in its use should prescribe this drug.

Dermabrasion is used to smooth and plane the scars and pits that develop as a result of acne. However, as a surgical procedure which often requires hospitalization, it is reserved for more severe cases of scarring. Patients with broad-based scars respond better than those patients with deep, pitted lesions. The procedure involves the use of a high-speed brush to plane the skin to various levels. Improvement occurs in about 50 percent of patients. Scarring, hyperpigmentation, and hypopigmentation are the main complications of the procedure. Only the most skilled dermatologist or plastic surgeon should perform this procedure on very carefully screened patients.

Recently, bovine collagen (Zyderm) has been used for the purpose of improvement of superficial acne scars. After skin testing with bovine collagen, the preparation is injected into the dermis. In spite of enthusiastic reports by many dermatologists, many others remain skeptical about the long-term efficacy of this product.

RELATED CONDITIONS

Acne rosacea is a separate disease entity which usually occurs in persons between the ages of 40 and 60. It presents with pronounced erythema and superficial pustules and papules over the central portion of the face. A large multilobulated rhinophyma is rare but can result from this acne as the sebaceous glands become larger (Fig. 72-6 and Plate 2).

Blepharitis can complicate acne rosacea. The predisposing factors of acne rosacea are not known, but there is frequently a family history of acne rosacea and of ruddy complexion. Acne rosacea patients have an increased number of sebaceous glands over the face associated with erythema and multiple small telangiectasias. The acne rosacea patient should avoid foods and liquids

FIGURE 72-6
Large rhinophyma of the nose in acne rosacea. The skin is erythematous, and multiple pustules are present.

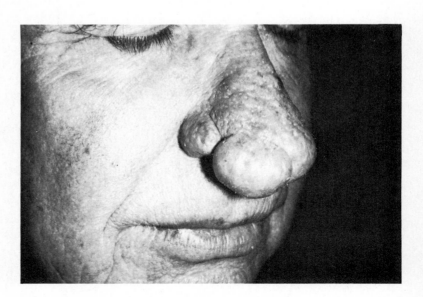

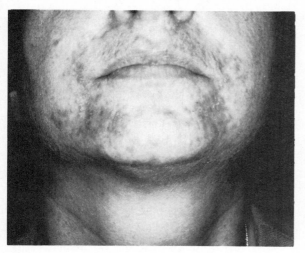

FIGURE 72-7
Erythema, papules, and scaliness in perioral distribution is characteristic of perioral dermatitis.

that are hot in temperature. Alcohol ingestion can contribute to facial erythema. The main therapeutic modality is oral tetracycline. It is usually started at doses of 500 to 1000 mg daily. As the pustules and papules decrease in number, tetracycline is gradually tapered. Topically, 1% hydrocortisone cream with or without 1 to 2% precipitated sulfur can help in treatment of erythema and superficial pustules. Acne rosacea is a chronic disease which may have to be treated for a prolonged period of time. Dermabrasion of large rhinophyma is occasionally recommended.

Young women in their 20s and 30s can develop superficial pustules, papules, and erythematous, greasy, scaly patches in perioral distribution (Fig. 72-7). This disorder is called perioral dermatitis, or perioral acne,

FIGURE 72-8
Multiple papules and pustules in perifollicular distribution over the neck of a patient with pseudofolliculitis barbae.

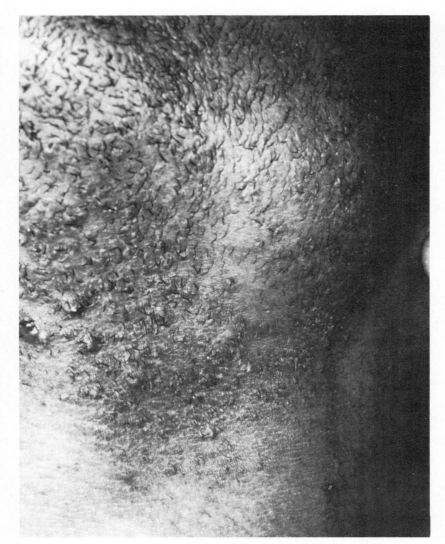

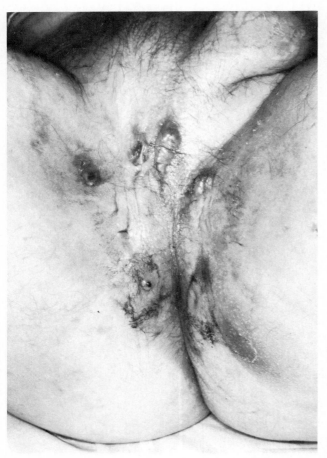

FIGURE 72-9
Painful nodules, cysts, and sinus tracts in hidradenitis suppurativa of the groin.

lips. These patients frequently report a previous use of strong fluorinated steroid creams on the face. However, the cause of this condition is unknown. In therapy of this condition, all strong topical steroid creams should be stopped. A 1% hydrocortisone cream helps erythema and prevents exacerbation of this acne when stronger topical steroids are stopped. Oral tetracycline, 250 to 500 mg daily, is usually effective. The antibiotic is gradually tapered over a few months. Frequently, resolution of perioral acne occurs within 4 months.

Pseudofolliculitis barbae occurs predominantly in bearded areas of black males. Curved, stiff beard hairs, when shaved close to the skin surface, reenter the skin and cause foreign body granulomas. The patients develop perifollicular inflammatory papules and pustules (Fig. 72-8). Patients frequently form scars and keloids secondary to these foreign body granulomas. The disease starts at the time when individuals begin shaving. The most practical way to treat this condition is to grow a beard. Since this is not always acceptable, as in the armed forces and some places of employment, other remedies are utilized. Depilatories (Magic Shave, for example) are helpful but can cause severe irritation of the skin. Using a toothbrush to comb and remove the ingrown hairs from the skin is helpful.

A chronic inflammation of the apocrine glands results in hidradenitis suppurativa. Painful nodules, cysts, and sinus tracts form in the axillae, the groin, the perianal area, and the breasts where the apocrine glands are present (Fig. 72-9). Frequently, there is a history of cystic acne in the family and patients have cystic acne over the face, chest, and back. However, the etiology of hidradenitis suppurativa is unknown. Cysts are frequently sterile or grow a common epidermal contaminant, *Staphylococcus epidermidis*. The inflammatory process of apocrine glands may be secondary to bacteria or their breakdown products. In treatment of this condition, drainage of the cysts is helpful. Systemic tetracycline or erythromycin is useful in management of inflamed, painful cysts. In chronic, refractory cases of hidradenitis suppurativa surgical resection of the affected area is sometimes indicated.

and is the most frequent acne seen in adult women. Perioral acne spares the skin immediately adjacent to the

QUESTIONS

Acne and related conditions

Directions: Answer the following questions on a separate sheet of paper.

1. Define *acne*.
2. What age groups have the highest incidence rates of acne?
3. Describe the formation of acne lesions.
4. Explain the purpose of each of the following treatments for acne:
   a. Proper cleansing of the skin with a good soap
   b. Antibiotic therapy (identify two examples of a commonly used antibiotic)   c. Dermabrasion
5. Discuss at least two predisposing factors contributing to the development of acne.

Directions: Circle the letter preceding each item below that correctly answers the question. More than one answer may be correct.

1017

QUESTIONS

6. Isotretinoin can be administered to which of the following patients:
   a. Women with severe, cystic acne who stopped birth control pills 3 months before the flare-up of acne   *b.* Patients with Grade III acne which is inflammatory and scarring but which has not been treated with systemic antibiotics   *c.* Females with severe cystic acne who are allergic to tetracycline and use adequate contraception   *d.* Patients with severe, cystic acne who have normal triglyceride levels and borderline serum chloride levels who did not respond to oral antibotics.

7. Acne is classified as to the number of comedones, papules, or pustules; how many comedones, papules, or pustules on one side of the face depicts Grade III acne?
   a. 5   *b.* 10 to 15   *c.* 15 to 20   *d.* 25 to 50

8. Acne rosacea occurs most frequently in which of the following age groups:
   a. Infants   *b.* Children under 15   *c.* Young adults (20 to 30 years)   *d.* Middle-aged adults (40 to 60 years)   *e.* Older adults (70 to 80 years)

9. The most severe cystic acne, consisting of deep cysts, multiple comedones, and scarring, is which of the following variants:
   a. Acne rosacea   *b.* Acne conglobata   *c.* Acne excoriate   *d.* Acne keloidalis

ECZEMA AND VASCULAR DISORDERS

OBJECTIVES

At the completion of this chapter you should be able to:

1. Differentiate between the clinical presentations of acute and chronic eczema.
2. Identify for atopic eczema the causes, populations affected, areas involved, characteristic lesions, and treatments.
3. List five causes of allergic contact eczema.
4. Identify the most common sites of neurodermatitis, seborrheic dermatitis, and stasis eczema.
5. Describe the characteristics of urticaria (hives) and cutaneous vasculitis.
6. Differentiate between erythema multiforme and erythema nodosum as to the types of skin lesions, areas involved, complications, and treatments.

ECZEMA

Eczema encompasses all types of red, blistering, weeping, scaly, thickened, itchy skin lesions. Acute eczema presents with vesicles, bullae, erythema, weeping, and crusting. Chronic eczema has thickened, scaly, pruritic patches and plaques. Examples of eczema include (1) atopic eczema, characterized by weeping, crusted, dry, scaly, pruritic patches on the faces of infants and in the larger folds of skin found in the antecubital and popliteal fossae in adolescents and adults, (2) allergic contact eczema, characterized by pruritic vesicles, erythema, and patches in areas where patients have touched allergens such as poison ivy, poison sumac, cosmetics, rubber, and cement, among many others, (3) hand eczema characterized by erythematous, scaly, fissured patches over the hands, (4) neurodermatitis, characterized by excoriated patches and lines secondary to compulsive scratching of the skin, (5) seborrheic dermatitis, characterized by yellow-red-brown, greasy, scaly patches over the scalp and face, and (6) stasis eczema, characterized by stasis edema hyperpigmentation and scaliness of the lower legs.

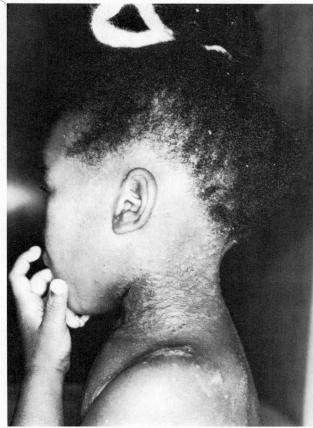

FIGURE 73-1
Lichenified, thickened, scaly skin over the neck area in childhood atopic eczema.

Atopic eczema

Atopic eczema, or atopic dermatitis, is a hereditary chronic skin disease which can appear at any age (see Chap. 9). There is often a family history of this eczema and associated allergic rhinitis and/or extrinsic asthma. Some children outgrow the cutaneous eczema only to develop hay fever or extrinsic asthma in later years. Infantile atopic eczema frequently presents with weeping, eroded, erythematous patches in the diaper area and on the cheeks and scalp (Plate 3). Since the eruptions are pruritic, the infants are irritable. Secondary infections with bacteria are common. In most of the infants eczema disappears spontaneously. In some infants it can progress into childhood or adult forms. Pruritus is the universal complaint of all these patients.

In children or adults, the areas of involvement include the popliteal spaces, the antecubital fossae, the neck areas, and other flexural surfaces (Fig. 73-1). In adults, eczematous skin changes can become generalized over the entire body. Spontaneous remission of adulthood eczema is uncommon. Patients present with erythematous, excoriated, thickened skin over the face, trunk, and extremities (Fig. 73-2). Changes in the weather and irritation from wool clothing, soap, and water frequently exacerbate the disease. Upper respiratory infections and bacterial skin infections can also aggravate the skin condition. These patients should not be vaccinated against smallpox, as disseminated vaccinia can develop. Exposure to herpes virus can result in disseminated herpetic infection of the skin.

The causes of atopic eczema are unknown. Hereditary factors definitely play a role. Irritation of the skin with wool, water, harsh soaps, climate changes, stress, and infection frequently results in clinical exacerbations. Many of the patients have abnormal levels of serum IgE. The number of thymus-derived lymphocytes is decreased in some patients. Some investigators have postulated an abnormality in the receptors responsible for production of cyclic adenosine monophosphate (AMP) nucleotides. How these abnormalities produce an extremely pruritic, eczematous skin is not understood.

Therapy of the disease focuses on prevention and

FIGURE 73-2
Thickened skin with multiple excoriated papules of chronic eczema.

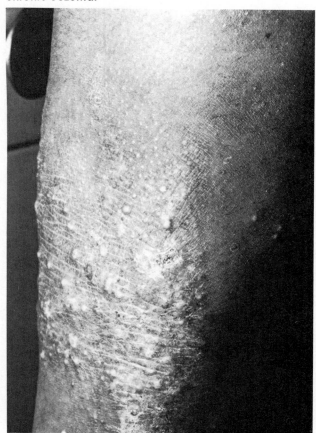

treatment. All possible exacerbating factors must be avoided or eliminated. Superfatted soaps, mineral oil, and lubricating creams are recommended. In infants, dietary restrictions may be helpful (avoidance of orange juice, and cow's milk), but they are not useful with older children and adults. A humidifier may be installed in the house. Antibiotics are used to treat secondary bacterial infections. Pruritus is controlled with antihistaminics such as diphenhydramine (Benadryl), hydroxyzine (Atarax), or cyproheptadine (Periactin). The dosages of these medications are increased to levels that relieve pruritus or produce drowsiness, whichever comes first. Topical corticosteroids in the weakest possible strength are used for children. Topical 1% hydrocortisone is usually prescribed for infants, while 0.025% triamcinolone in a lubricating cream is given to adults.

Hyposensitization immunotherapy may exacerbate, benefit, or have no effect on atopic eczema. It is, therefore, not indicated in this form of eczema.

Contact eczema

Contact eczema is very common and occurs in localized areas where an allergen comes into contact with the skin. The skin reaction to the oil of poison ivy, *Rhus* dermatitis, is best known. Linear areas of vesiculation, weeping, and erythema occur in the places where the skin has touched the poison ivy, poison sumac, or poison oak plant (Fig. 73-3 and Plate 4). The oil can be carried in many ways—on a pet's fur, on clothing, on shoes, or on fingernails. Once the oil is washed off, the dermatitis does not spread. *Rhus* dermatitis is not transmitted from person to person through the blister fluid.

A frequent cause of contact eczema is nickel. This metal is found in virtually all jewelry, metal eyeglass frames, and coins. A patient sensitive to nickel presents with crusted, well-defined patches of eczema at the site of exposure (i.e., the neck, ears, wrists, or abdomen). Patients allergic to potassium dichromate develop eczema when exposed to it or to cement or leather shoes. Shoes can also contain rubber, which is a frequent cause of shoe contact eczema. The medications neomycin and benzocaine and the preservative ethylenediamine are common causes of allergic eczema. In photodermatitis, topical agents (e.g., halogenated salicylamides in soaps) or oral medication (e.g., tetracycline) in combination with sunlight cause erythema, edema, and occasionally

vesiculation. Photodermatitis usually occurs on sun-exposed areas of the face, neck, and forearms.

Contact eczema is mediated through a cellular Type IV delayed hypersensitivity (see Chap. 12). After primary exposure, a second contact with the allergen is required to produce eczema. This type of eczema can be reproduced by patch-testing the patient in whom the allergy is suspected. A careful history is required for selection of appropriate allergens to be tested. Patch testing is usually done over the back of the patient after the eczema is under control.

In therapy, the removal of offending allergens is necessary. Patients must learn how to identify *Rhus* plants. Cosmetics, jewelry, and other objects that contain the allergen responsible for eczema should be avoided. Topical care of acute allergic eczema includes soaks and corticosteroid creams and gels. Frequently, severe allergic eczema, such as poison ivy, is treated with systemic steroids. A short treatment with systemic prednisone at the initial dose of 40 to 60 mg per day is tapered over 7 to 14 days.

Hand eczema

Hand eczema most often occurs in persons who must wash their hands frequently or who are under stress.

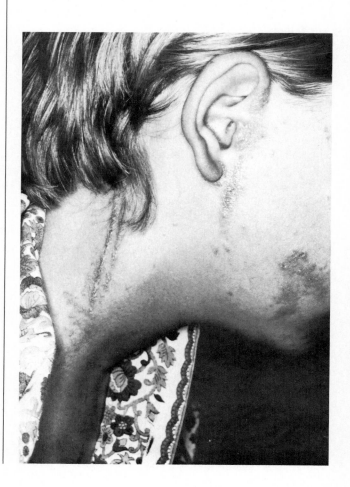

FIGURE 73-3
Grouped and linear vesicular eruptions are characteristic of poison ivy dermatitis.

Small vesicles appear on the lateral aspects of fingers, toes, and feet. Pruritus accompanies the appearance of vesicles. The small blisters develop into scaly, eczematous patches over the palms and soles (Plate 5). Hand eczema is exacerbated by water, detergents, and stress. It can be a chronic problem which is extremely difficult to control. When hand eczema is exacerbated by exposure to an industrial chemical, patch testing is required to rule out allergic eczema.

Hand eczema is sometimes prevented through avoiding harsh soaps and wearing protective gloves. Oral antihistamines and strong fluorinated topical corticosteroids (Lidex, Halog) are used to suppress this kind of eczema. Occasionally, a short course of a systemic corticosteroid is required, such as prednisone at a dosage of 30 to 40 mg initially, tapered daily over 6 to 8 days. Secondary bacterial infections are treated with appropriate systemic antibiotics.

Neurodermatitis

Neurodermatitis is caused by compulsive scratching of pruritic skin. It can be localized to the neck, scrotum, or anywhere on the body. Linear, thickened, dry patches of eczema result from persistent scratching (Fig. 73-4).

Generalized neurodermatitis frequently occurs during the cold, dry winter months in older patients who have dry, pruritic skin. Compulsive scratching can result in factitious ulcers (Fig. 73-5). These self-induced ulcers have odd angles and square borders, which should alert the examiner to this diagnosis. However, diffuse pruritus and scratching can also be caused by scabies, atopic eczema, systemic lymphoma, hypothyroidism, diabetes mellitus, cirrhosis, and severe uremia. These conditions must be carefully ruled out before the diagnosis of neurodermatitis is made.

Treatment of this condition consists of lubrication

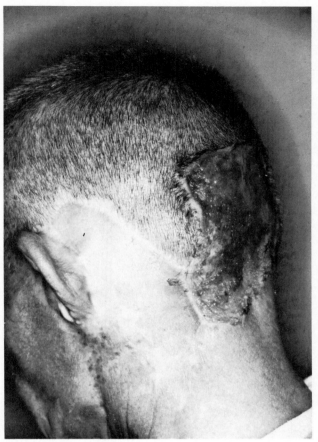

FIGURE 73-5
Compulsive scratching can result in factitious ulcers associated with hair loss.

and application of topical corticosteroids to the skin. Systemic antihistaminics are useful in control of pruritus. Psychotherapy may be required in treating severe neurodermatitis, especially if the face is affected.

Seborrheic dermatitis

Seborrheic dermatitis commonly involves the scalp, the eyebrows, the nasolabial folds, the ears, and the anterior chest. Erythematous, scaly patches appear intermittently. The condition may begin any time from infancy to old age. It may be slightly pruritic. The cause is unknown, but genetic factors seem to play an important part.

Therapy of scalp seborrheic dermatitis includes shampoos which contain selenium sulfide (Selsun), tar (Tegrin, Sebutone), and salicylic acid (Sebulex). Topical corticosteroid sprays or solutions are useful. Weak topical corticosteroids (1% hydrocortisone) combined with

FIGURE 73-4
Persistent scratching causes a localized patch of thickened, excoriated skin. (From Fitzpatrick et al., 1979.)

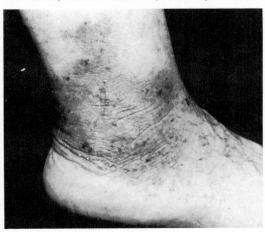

precipitated sulfur (0.5 to 1%) are used to treat seborrheic dermatitis of the face and the chest.

Stasis eczema

Stasis eczema is localized to the areas of venous stasis and edema on the lower legs. Crusted, scaly, weeping, erythematous patches appear (Fig. 73-6). The eruptions are pruritic and can lead to secondary excoriations, erosions, and ulcers.

Therapy requires removal of edema fluid and improvement of circulation. The legs are elevated; wraps and Jobst stockings are frequently recommended. Eczema is treated with weak or intermediate strength topical corticosteroids (1% hydrocortisone, 0.025% triamcinolone). Ulcers are soaked, cleansed, and debrided.

VASCULAR DISORDERS

Urticaria

Urticaria (hives) is the most common cutaneous reaction in which edema and erythema result (Fig. 73-7 and Plate 6) (see Chap. 11). Within a few hours after onset, lesions disappear. Pruritus frequently accompanies urticaria. Sometimes angioedema, resulting in swelling of the lips, tongue, eyelids, and larynx, can accompany cutaneous urticaria. Laryngeal angioedema is a medical emergency. Acute urticaria is frequently caused by the ingestion of a food (shellfish, nuts, food additives, food preservatives, or food dyes). Virtually every drug can cause acute urticaria, the most common being aspirin, laxatives, and antibiotics.

Chronic urticaria is usually idiopathic but may be caused by food preservatives, collagen vascular diseases, medications, or infections. Occasionally, cold temperatures, sun, exercise, stress, or alcohol can trigger urticaria. Urticaria results from release of histamines, serotonins, bradykinins, and other mediators. These mediators result in vasodilatation and edema in the dermis and subcutaneous layers. Since so many mediators of inflammation are involved in formation of urticaria lesions, treatment can be difficult. Equally difficult can be the search for an underlying cause. Patients with chronic urticaria are evaluated by a complete history, physical examination, and blood tests, including tests for differential leukocyte count, sedimentation rate, and antinuclear factor. Blood tests should also include liver tests such as those for serum glutamic-oxaloacetic and pyruvic transaminases (SGOT and SGPT), lactic acid dehydrogenase (LDH), alkaline phosphatase, and bilirubin. Search for the infectious agent includes examination of stool for ova and parasites, chest x-rays, sinus x-rays, and a dental checkup. Skin tests are of little merit in evaluation of urticaria.

In therapy, all precipitating factors (medications, dyes, foods) should be eliminated. Urticaria is treated symptomatically. Acute urticaria with angioedema is treated with subcutaneous epinephrine. Less severe urticaria is treated with oral antihistamines such as diphenhydramine, hydroxyzine, and cyproheptadine. These medications can cause severe drowsiness and sleepiness; patients should be advised about this potentially dangerous side effect. A diet which avoids artificial preservatives and dyes is prescribed for many patients.

Erythema multiforme

Erythema multiforme presents with macules, papules, and vesicles. The characteristic lesion has the central "target" discoloration or necrosis (Fig. 73-8). The lesions are symmetrical and frequently involve the palms of the hands. Erythema multiforme is usually asymptomatic but can be painful and pruritic.

When the mucous membranes of the lips, mouth, genitalia, and conjunctiva are involved, erythema multiforme is called *Stevens-Johnson syndrome* (Fig. 73-9). These patients are toxic and febrile. Corneal scarring

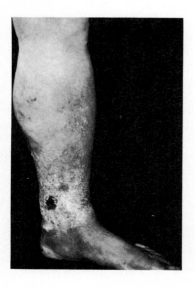

FIGURE 73-6

Stasis dermatitis localized to the area of chronic venous insufficiency. Secondary ulceration is seen over the region of the malleolus medialis. (From Fitzpatrick et al., 1979.)

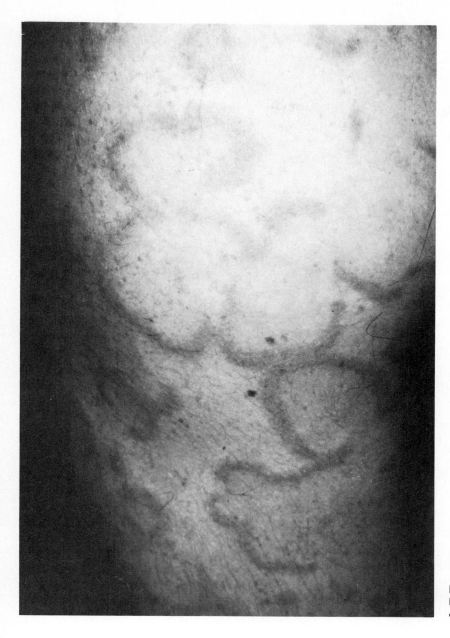

FIGURE 73-7
Edema, erythema, and pruritus are the clinical features of urticarial welts.

can result. Death occurs in about 10 percent of the cases. The causes of erythema multiforme include drugs (sulfa, penicillin, barbiturates) and infections (particularly herpes simplex). However, in over 50 percent of cases the cause is idiopathic. Severe erythema multiforme, or Stevens-Johnson syndrome, is treated with systemic corticosteroids.

Erythema nodosum

Erythema nodosum presents with painful, erythematous nodules usually localized to the anterior aspect of the legs. Fever, arthritis, and arthralgia accompany the eruptions. In only about 20 to 30 percent of the cases can specific causes be determined. These include streptococcal infections, sarcoidosis, pregnancy, drug ingestion, and inflammatory bowel disease. Patients are usually treated with bed rest, aspirin, and occasionally oral corticosteroids.

Cutaneous vasculitis

In cutaneous vasculitis, persistent urticarial lesions, hemorrhagic macules, papules, ulcers, and purpura are observed (Plate 7). The lesions are usually found over the distal extremities. Cutaneous vasculitis can be as-

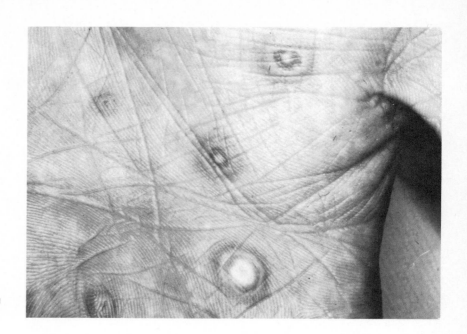

FIGURE 73-8
Targetlike lesions are seen in erythema multiforme.

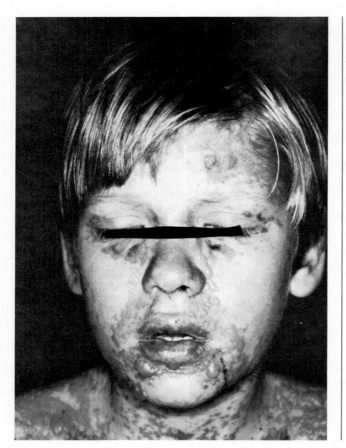

sociated with systemic vasculitis of the kidney, gastrointestinal tract, and other organs. Therefore, a patient can present with fever, arthralgia, gastrointestinal bleeding, or hematuria. The causes of vasculitis include drugs, infections (particularly *Streptococcus*), collagen vascular diseases (rheumatoid arthritis, systemic lupus erythematosus), and hepatitis type B virus. In most patients, the cause is idiopathic. Patients with clinical lesions of cutaneous vasculitis require skin biopsy to confirm this diagnosis. Once the diagnosis is established, patients are evaluated for systemic involvement by urinalysis, evaluation of creatinine clearance, and tests for the presence of cryoglobulins, antinuclear factor, rheumatoid factor, and hepatitis B antigen. Therapy is based on the severity of cutaneous involvement and on systemic involvement. Usually systemic corticosteroids help in resolution of the process.

FIGURE 73-9
Erosions of the lips and conjunctiva associated with fever in this boy with Stevens-Johnson syndrome.

QUESTIONS

Eczema and vascular disorders

Directions: Answer the following questions on a separate sheet of paper.

1. Describe the characteristic lesions of acute and chronic eczema.

2. List five of the causes of allergic contact eczema.

3. What are the most frequent causes and treatments of hand eczema?

4. Describe neurotic excoriations (neurodermatitis).

5. List at least three drugs that are most often implicated in acute urticaria.

Directions: Circle the letter preceding each item below that correctly answers the question. More than one answer may be correct.

6. Bill, a 15-year-old, presents with erythematous, excoriated, scaly, thickened skin over antecubital and popliteal fossae. His past history reveals erythematous pruritic eruptions during childhood. It reveals no known allergies. The most likely condition is:
   a. Contact eczema   *b.* Atopic eczema   *c.* Neurodermatitis   *d.* Stasis eczema   *e.* Urticaria

7. Which of the following are typical of the skin lesions of seborrheic dermatitis?
   a. Localization to the area of the lower legs
   b. Involvement of the scalp, eyebrows, and ears
   c. Crusted, scaling, weeping patches over the arms   *d.* Lesions which are frequently erythematous, scaly patches.

Directions: Circle T if the statement is true and F if it is false. Correct the false statements.

8. T   F   Urticaria is a common cutaneous reaction in which edema, erythema, and pruritus are usually present.

9. T   F   Skin tests are very useful in establishing the causative agent(s) in urticaria.

10. T   F   A skin biopsy is frequently necessary to confirm the diagnosis in cutaneous vasculitis.

CHAPTER 74

PSORIASIS AND PITYRIASIS ROSEA

OBJECTIVES

At the completion of this chapter you should be able to:

1. Describe the areas involved in and the classic lesions of psoriasis.
2. Explain the pathogenesis of psoriasis.
3. Describe pustular psoriasis as to causes, lesions, and complications.
4. State the rationale of the various treatment modalities used in psoriasis.
5. Identify for pityriasis rosea the lesions, areas involved, causes, and treatments.

Disorders of the skin characterized by the presence of plaques, patches, and scales are called *papulosquamous* diseases. These include psoriasis and pityriasis rosea.

PSORIASIS

Psoriasis is reported in 2 to 5 million Americans. Psoriasis appears as thick, erythematous plaques and papules covered by a silvery white scale. The plaques are usually located over the knees, elbows, and scalp (Fig. 74-1 and Plate 8). However, the skin eruptions can affect any part of the body, with the exception of the mucous membranes. The nails frequently appear thickened, with yellowish discoloration, multiple pits, and separation from the nail bed. Arthritis can also accompany this skin disease and classically involves the distal interphalangeal joints. In these patients, the rheumatoid factor is not present. Arthritis does not always correlate with

severity of the psoriasis. Psoriasis is usually not pruritic; however, some patients report severe pruritus, especially associated with the development of new papules.

Psoriasis is a chronic disease which can occur at any age. Fluctuations mark the natural course of this condition. For example, sunlight, relaxation, and the summer season are usually beneficial to psoriasis patients. An upper respiratory tract infection can trigger an acute exacerbation of psoriasis, as evidenced by eruptions of multiple small papules over the trunk (Fig. 74-2). Generalized psoriasis, as characterized by multiple pustules with inflammatory plaques, is called *pustular psoriasis*. This condition can be accompanied by chills, high fever, and electrolyte imbalances. Pustular psoriasis is a medical emergency which can be fatal.

Psoriasis is an inherited disease, although the mode of inheritance is not well understood. A family history of psoriasis is found in 66 percent of psoriasis patients. Histocompatibility antigens HLA-B13 and HLA-B17

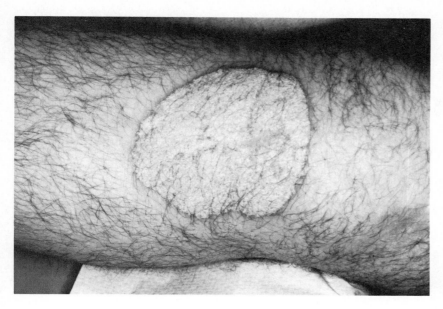

FIGURE 74-1
Thick psoriatic plaques with white silvery scale as seen in the psoriatic patient.

are increased fourfold in psoriatics. Environmental factors also play a significant role in the disease. Trauma to the skin can produce new lesions of psoriasis, especially in the area where the skin is punctured, scraped, or cut.

Histopathologic examination of a psoriatic skin biopsy reveals thickened epidermis and stratum corneum and dilated upper dermal blood vessels. The number of basal cells undergoing mitosis is markedly increased. These fast-dividing cells move rapidly to the surface of the thickened epidermis. This rapid proliferation and migration of epidermal cells results in thick epidermis covered by a thick keratin (silvery scale). Abnormal levels of cyclic nucleotides, especially of cyclic adenosine monophosphate (AMP) and cyclic guanosine monophosphate (GMP) may be partially responsible for this

rapid mitosis rate of epidermal cells. Prostaglandins and polyamines are also abnormal in the disease. The exact role of each of these abnormalities in influencing the formation of a psoriatic plaque is not clearly understood.

Treatment

Therapy of chronic psoriasis requires knowledge of various treatment modalities, patience, and an experienced physician. The treatment must be flexible, and alternative therapy must be administered if the patient fails to respond to the original program of treatment. Localized disease is treated with topical corticosteroids over the face and intertriginous areas, and in children weak steroids such as 1% hydrocortisone are used. Over the trunk, extremities, and scalp, intermediate strength ste-

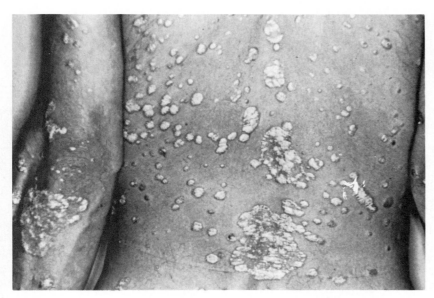

FIGURE 74-2
Multiple small psoriatic papules can erupt following an upper respiratory infection. This form of psoriasis is termed guttate psoriasis.

roids such as triamcinolone or fluocinolone are recommended. The strong steroids—fluocinonide, halcinonide, and betamethasone—are reserved for resistant plaques. A tar preparation in cream or shampoo is frequently used. A bath oil with tar (Balnetar) is also helpful. All these medications result in decreased cell proliferation, which makes the epidermis thinner and results in disappearance of plaques and scales of psoriasis.

Severe generalized psoriasis requires hospitalization for intensive topical steroid, tar, and ultraviolet light therapy. Unfortunately, relapses of psoriasis often occur 3 to 6 months after hospitalization. The newest modality of treatment combines the use of psoralen, an oral photosensitizing medication, with long ultraviolet light (so-called PUVA). This treatment is not indicated in patients with a previous history of x-ray radiation, skin cancer, or cataracts. The skin carcinogenic potential of this therapy is still unknown. An oral antineoplastic medication, methotrexate, may be useful in treating patients with severe plaque-type psoriasis, pustular psoriasis, and/or debilitating arthritis. However, this oral agent may cause irreversible cirrhosis of the liver and/or bone marrow suppression. The most effective and safe treatment of severe psoriasis may be tar and then ultraviolet light, which is administered to patients on an outpatient basis in what are referred to as day-care psoriasis centers.

PITYRIASIS ROSEA

In contrast to psoriasis, pityriasis rosea is an acute, self-limited eruption seen in young adults and adolescents. Pityriasis rosea begins with an oval, scaly lesion called the "herald patch." Within a week, multiple, pale-red, oval patches with a fine scale around the periphery appear over the neck, trunk, and proximal extremities (Figs. 74-3 and 74-4 and Plate 9). Pruritus is usually not severe. Lesions of pityriasis rosea usually do not occur on the face, palms, and soles, in contrast to secondary syphilis. The cutaneous eruptions, which can be accompanied by malaise and fever, persist for 4 to 8 weeks and

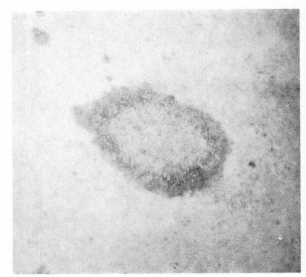

FIGURE 74-3
Oval-shaped, scaly lesion of pityriasis rosea—a so-called herald patch with typical peripheral scale.

rarely recur. The cause of this common disease is unknown; however, viral agents have been implicated.

Obtaining an adequate history is necessary to rule out drug eruptions and viral exanthems. Syphilis can mimic pityriasis rosea, so serology is required (see Chap. 77). Treatment for pruritus consists of oral antihistamine agents and topical corticosteroids.

FIGURE 74-4
Oval-shaped papules and patches in pityriasis rosea showing the dermatome-type pattern. (From Fitzpatrick et al., 1979.)

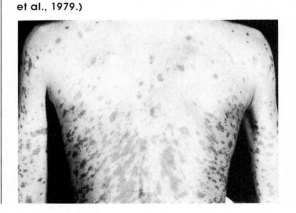

QUESTIONS

Psoriasis and pityriasis rosea

Directions: Answer the following questions on a separate sheet of paper.

1. Explain the pathogenesis of psoriasis.

2. What is the latest treatment modality used in psoriasis? What are contraindications for its use?

3. Describe the skin, cell, and blood vessel findings ev-

ident in a histopathologic examination of a psoriatic
skin biopsy.

*Directions: Circle the letter preceding each item
below that correctly answers the question. More
than one answer may be correct.*

4. An oval, scaly lesion termed the herald patch is
characteristic of which of the following?
a. Psoriasis   *b.* Pityriasis rosea   *c.* Neurodermatitis   *d.* Atopic eczema

5. Psoriasis can be treated with the use of psoralen and
long ultraviolet light (PUVA) therapy. This treatment is contraindicated in patients who:
a. Are heavy cigarette smokers (more than 2
packs per day)   *b.* Have a previous history of x-
ray radiation   *c.* Have been treated with topical
steroids   *d.* Have a history of skin cancer

6. Treatment of pruritus associated with pityriasis
rosea is:
a. Benzoyl peroxide   *b.* Topical corticosteroids
c. Tar preparation in cream   *d.* Oral antihistamine agents

7. The incidence of psoriasis is reported in how many
million Americans?
a. More than 1   *b.* 2 to 3   *c.* 2 to 5   *d.* 8 to 10

CUTANEOUS INFECTIONS

OBJECTIVES

At the completion of this chapter you should be able to:

1. Identify verrucae vulgaris (warts) by identifying their causes, pathogenesis, and treatments.

2. Describe the appearance and course of molluscum contagiosum.

3. Identify for herpes simplex, chickenpox (varicella), and herpes zoster the causes, pathogenesis, signs and symptoms, age groups affected, treatments, complications, and prognoses.

4. Contrast herpes simplex Type I and Type II as to areas affected and modes of transmission.

5. Differentiate rubeola, rubella, and infectious mononucleosis as to causes, signs and symptoms, and complications.

6. Identify the characteristics of tinea capitis, corporis, versicolor, cruris and pedis, and onychomycosis according to causes, pathogenesis, lesions, areas involved, and treatments.

7. Describe the causes and characteristic clinical symptoms and treatments of candidiasis infections.

8. Describe the etiologic agent and characteristic lesion of impetigo.

9. Describe erysipelas and superficial folliculitis in terms of causes and lesions.

WARTS

Verrucae vulgaris, or warts, are caused by the DNA papovavirus. The virus replicates in the epidermal cells and is transmitted from person to person. Warts are also contagious to the patient's self by autoinoculation. The virus is contagious to those people who lack the virus-specific immunity in the skin. The immunity to warts is not well understood. Verrucae appear as rough, warty nodules over the trunk, legs, hands, or arms (Fig. 75-1). Flat warts are more prevalent on the face. Plantar warts grow into the thick stratum corneum of the foot and have small black dots within, which represent infarcted capillaries. In the groin area verrucae are called *condylomata acuminata*. They appear as verrucous, moist nodules which may occur in large numbers (Fig. 75-2). The warts resolve spontaneously when immunity against the virus develops. However, the immune re-

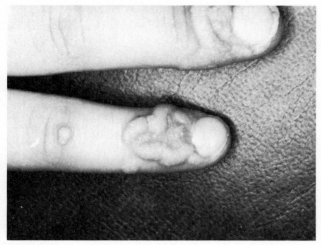

FIGURE 75-1
Rough nodules of verrucae vulgaris over the fingers.

sponse can be delayed for many years. Small numbers of verrucae are usually removed by cryosurgery or curettage combined with electrodesiccation. Large num-

bers of those which occur in children are removed with preparations of salicylic acid, lactic acid, or glacial acetic acid. Cantharidin solution and salicylic acid preparations are preferred for plantar warts. Podophyllin is usually applied to condylomata acuminata. Treatment of warts is often difficult and prolonged and can be painful.

MOLLUSCUM CONTAGIOSUM

Molluscum contagiosum is a dome-shaped, smooth, umbilicated nodule (Fig. 75-3). It is caused by a DNA virus of the pox family. It is transmitted from person to person. The virus is contagious to people who lack immunity to this specific virus. The lesions are most common in children and occur on the head and trunk. In young adults they usually appear in the groin area. The preferred modes of treatment are cantharidin solution in

FIGURE 75-2
Moist, verrucous nodules of condyloma acuminatum in the groin area.

FIGURE 75-3
Smooth, umbilicated, dome-shaped nodules of molluscum contagiosum over the face of a child.

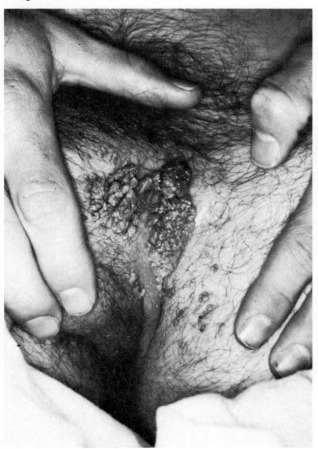

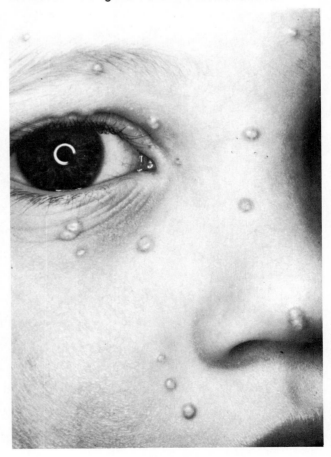

children and gentle curettage or liquid nitrogen cryo-surgery in adults.

HERPES SIMPLEX

Herpes simplex is caused by a DNA virus. An infectious DNA particle enters the nucleus of the cell and uses the reproductive machinery of the cell for its own replication. The number of patients with genital herpes increased from 29,000 in 1966 to 261,000 in 1979. Probably 20 million persons have or have had the infection today. Herpes labialis of the lip is even more common. There are two types of herpes—Type I and Type II. Type I usually affects the lips, mouth, nose, and cheeks. This form of herpes is acquired from close contact with an infected family member or friend in a nonsexual manner. It is transmitted by kissing, touching, and the use of common towels. Type II herpes simplex virus usually infects the genital areas. It frequently follows a sexual encounter, but not necessarily. It is estimated that up to 20 percent of sexually active persons, or 20 million persons, in the United States have or have had herpes Type II.

Multiple, grouped, painful vesicles appear following primary exposure of the patient to the virus. Primary infections occur anywhere on a person's skin, though they usually occur around the mouth and nose, causing gingivostomatitis; around the eyes, causing con-junctivitis; the fingers, causing herpetic whitlow; and the buttocks and genitals, causing vulvovaginitis. Primary infections cause intense skin edema, extensive vesiculation, and exquisite pain (Fig. 75-4). Nurses frequently develop extremely painful edematous vesicles on their fingers. This so-called herpetic whitlow follows exposure to a patient with herpetic infection. This primary infection lasts for up to 4 weeks, and the nurse should not work around surgical, debilitated, or immunosuppressed patients during this period of time. During the primary infection, the virus ascends via peripheral nerves to dorsal root ganglia, where it is present in the dormant stage. Some patients are subject to recurrent reactivations of the latent virus. *Most patients do not* experience recurrent infections. Recurrent infections are usually less painful and frequently localized to the lips and genitals. Recurrences can be triggered by fever, sunlight, or trauma. Grouped vesicles (Fig. 75-5) become pustules within a few days and usually resolve spontaneously within 2 weeks.

Herpes progenitalis has been the most prominent sexually transmitted disease in the United States during the past 10 years. Recurrent herpes progenitalis causes painful vesicles and ulcers. The recurrent herpetic infection can follow primary infection within weeks, months, or years. Since the initial herpetic infection can be very mild, a patient may not realize that she or he has had the primary infection. Years later, when a recurrent infection appears, mistaken accusations of infidelity by a partner can arise. In humans, only 14 percent of patients with Type I herpes acquire recurrent herpes, whereas 60 percent of herpes Type II infections become recurrent. Ninety-eight percent of recurrent genital herpes are caused by Type II virus. Many factors affect

FIGURE 75-4
Multiple vesicles, edema, erythema in a primary herpetic infection causing conjunctivitis.

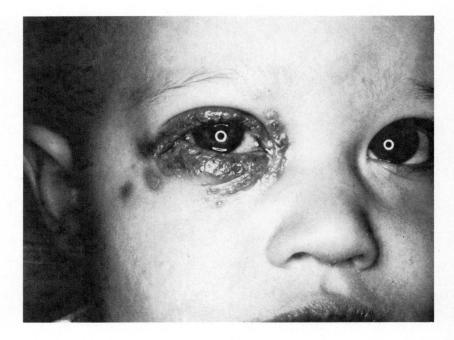

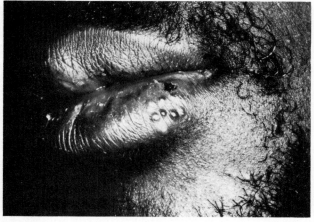

FIGURE 75-5
Grouped, localized, painful vesicles of recurrent herpes simplex of the lips.

recurrence. It can be triggered by fever, sunlight, ovulation, and physical trauma.

Herpes infection has serious implications if the infection occurs in the eye, around the cervix, in newborns, or in immunosuppressed individuals. The herpes infection of the eye may lead to herpetic keratitis. Scarring of the cornea, and even corneal perforation, can result. A pregnant woman with active genital herpes at the time of delivery can transmit the virus to the baby as it passes through the birth canal. Severe encephalitis in a newborn, complicated by death or mental retardation, can result. Cesarean section is indicated in women who have genital herpes at the time of delivery. Similarly, if the mother or a person working in the nursery has active vesicles of herpes on the lips or the hands,

the baby can become infected. The infection with herpes Type I can result in the same severe condition as Type II herpes infection. Herpes infection in seriously ill or immunosuppressed patients can result in chronic, nonhealing ulcers (Plate 10), dissemination, and encephalitis. Women who have had genital herpes have 5 to 8 times greater risk of cervical cancer. Frequent Pap smears can detect this cancer.

The diagnosis of herpes is ususally made on the basis of history and clinical appearance. The diagnosis can be confirmed by a herpetic culture, which is positive in about 80 percent of the patients with herpes. The Tzanck test is positive in 50 to 80 percent of patients with herpes. In this test, the material from the vesicle is placed on a glass slide and stained with 1% toluidine blue. Large multinucleated giant cells can be seen in a patient with herpes simplex (Fig. 75-6). The Tzanck test takes only a few minutes to perform and is much cheaper than a herpes culture.

There is no adequate treatment for cutaneous herpes infections. No vaccine has been developed to prevent these infections from recurring. Recurrent episodes of herpes of the lips can sometimes be prevented by use of opaque sunscreens or avoidance of excessive sun exposure. Sexual spread of genital herpes is frequently aborted by use of rubber condoms when vesicles are present and for 7 days afterward. Sexual abstinence when vesicles are present is an alternative method of prevention. Furthermore, towels, underclo-

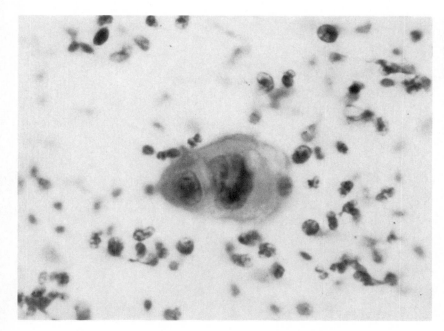

FIGURE 75-6
Giant cells seen in vesicles of a patient with herpes simplex. The cells are surrounded by neutrophils. Slide is stained with 1% toluidine blue.

thing, and swimming suits should not be shared. One promising drug is acyclovir (Zovirax). This drug, administered in intravenous fluids and as an ointment, is effective in treatment of cutaneous herpes infection in immunosuppressed patients. Acyclovir ointment does not prevent recurrence or shorten the duration of the herpetic eruption in otherwise healthy individuals. Acyclovir ointment decreases the duration of viral shedding in patients with primary herpes. Oral acyclovir is now available in the United States. Usually, patients with recurrent herpes are treated symptomatically, using soaks, topical antibiotics, and pain medications.

CHICKENPOX (VARICELLA) AND HERPES ZOSTER

The virus which causes varicella is a DNA virus. When the disease is active, it is highly contagious. The incubation period is 14 to 21 days. The infection usually occurs in school-aged children but occasionally affects young adults. Varicella is characterized by malaise and fever, followed by the eruption of multiple small erythematous macules, papules, and vesicles.

The vesicles become purulent and crusted and heal spontaneously, usually within 1 week. Characteristically, multiple stages of the lesions are present. The lesions initially appear on the trunk and face and spread peripherally to the extremities. Adults can develop varicella pneumonitis or encephalitis. In immunosuppressed children, complications from varicella infection include pneumonitis and encephalitis, both of which can be fatal.

Herpes zoster is caused by the same herpes virus as varicella, or chickenpox. Following the primary varicella infection, the virus apparently persists in the dorsal root ganglia. Herpes zoster, or shingles, usually occurs in elderly patients. The dormant varicella virus is activated, and inflammatory vesicles appear unilaterally along a single dermatome. The adjacent skin is edematous and hemorrhagic (Fig. 75-7 and Plate 11). This condition is usually preceded or accompanied by intense pain and/or burning. Even though any nerve can be involved, the thoracic, lumbar, and cranial nerves are most often affected. Herpes zoster persists for about 3 weeks. The pain whch may follow an attack of herpes zoster is referred to as postherpetic neuralgia and frequently may persist for a period of several months or, rarely, many years. Postherpetic neuralgia is more common in elderly patients. Dissemination of herpes zoster to the entire body surface, lungs, and brain can be fatal. This dissemination is usually seen in patients with lymphoma or leukemia. Thus, any patient who develops disseminated herpes zoster should be evaluated for a possible underlying malignancy.

Treatment of localized herpes zoster is symptomatic with soaks and pain medication. If the ophthalmic branch of the trigeminal nerve is affected, an ophthalmologist should also be consulted because corneal perforations may result from the infection. Early administration of systemic corticosteroids may be helpful in the prevention of postherpetic neuralgia.

FIGURE 75-7
Inflammatory vesicles appear along a single dermatome on edematous and hemorrhagic skin in herpes zoster.

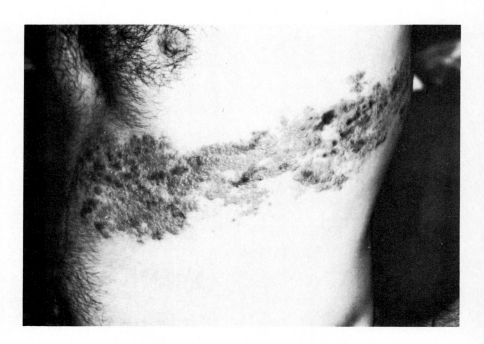

Rubeola, or measles, is caused by an RNA myxovirus. About 2 weeks after exposure, the patient develops fever, cough, headache, and conjunctivitis. The exanthem appears on the face, trunk, and proximal extremities. It consists of brightly erythematous, confluent macules. Over the buccal mucosa or the upper palate, mottled bright spots called *Koplik's spots* appear. These eruptions last 5 to 10 days. Treatment of this infection is symptomatic. Administration of the rubeola vaccine has substantially decreased the incidence of the disease.

Rubella, or German measles, is also caused by an RNA myxovirus. The disease occurs 2 to 3 weeks after exposure and is associated with malaise and a mild fever. Pale-red macules appear over the face and within a day spread to the trunk. The exanthem fades within a few days. Painful postauricular and suboccipital enlarged lymph nodes are usually present. The diagnosis is confirmed by rising antibody titers. If the infection occurs in the first trimester of pregnancy, congenital defects (cataracts, mental retardation, heart defects, deafness) are common. Therapy is symptomatic; vaccination of school-aged children and women in childbearing age with low rubella titers is advisable.

Erythema infectiosum, also called fifth disease, is a viral disease usually seen in children. Pale, reticulated macules appear over the cheeks and extremities, sometimes accompanied by a low-grade fever, malaise, and pruritus of skin eruptions. The infection persists for 1 to 2 weeks, and no treatment is necessary.

Infectious mononucleosis is caused by an Epstein-Barr virus. The infection presents with malaise, fever, exudative pharyngitis, postauricular adenopathy, and hepatosplenomegaly. The cutaneous eruptions occur over the trunk as erythematous macules. Patients with mononucleosis who receive ampicillin invariably develop erythematous, confluent, hemorrhagic macules, and therefore, this therapy is contraindicated (Fig. 75-8).

An interesting infection caused by a Coxsackie A16 virus is *hand-foot-and-mouth disease.* Multiple oval-shaped vesicles surrounded by erythema appear on the palms, fingers, soles, and mucous membranes of the mouth. The infection subsides within a week.

FUNGAL SKIN INFECTIONS

Superficial fungal infections can involve the skin, hair, and nails. Fungal infections of the scalp and the skin are known as *ringworm infections.*

FIGURE 75-8
Confluent, bright, erythematous macules following administration of ampicillin to a patient with infectious mononucleosis.

Most fungal infections in humans are caused by three genera of fungi: *Microsporum, Trichophyton,* and *Epidermophyton.* The fungi are transmitted from human to human (anthropophilic), from animal to human (zoophilic), or from soil to human (geophilic). A suspected fungal infection can be confirmed by microscopic examination of skin scrapings in a solution of potassium hydroxide (Fig. 75-9). Multiple hyphae can be found on microscopic examination of the skin scrapings of a patient with a fungus infection.

A fungal culture is done to identify the fungus responsible for the infection, to confirm a diagnosis, and to suggest a mode of transmission (Fig. 75-10).

Tinea capitis, or fungal infection of the scalp, is usually caused by *Trichophyton tonsurans* or *Microsporum canis. T. tonsurans* is transmitted by child-to-child contact and results in oval patches of hair loss. Individual hairs are broken at various lengths, and the scalp surface is scaly (Fig. 75-11). *M. canis* is usually transmitted from young kittens to children and causes inflammatory, purulent patches of hair loss. The patch

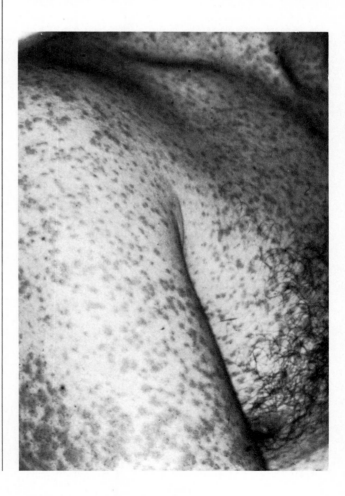

is frequently crusted with multiple pustules and can result in permanent alopecia. Every patch of hair loss associated with scaly, crusted scalp should be suspected for a possible fungal infection. To confirm the diagnosis of tinea capitis, hairs are plucked, examined under a microscope after potassium hydroxide treatment, and cultured.

Tinea corporis is a fungal infection of the skin over the face, trunk, and extremities. Frequently, peripheral scale associated with erythema and pustules appears with a ringlike shape (Fig. 75-12). This infection can be contracted from animals from *M. canis* or *Trichophyton mentagrophytes* and from humans from *Trichophyton rubrum.* The diagnosis is confirmed by potassium hydroxide examination and fungal culture.

Tinea cruris is a fungal infection of the groin. The infection is more frequent in males and is associated with severe pruritus and annular or arclike lesions with peripheral erythema and scale which frequently extend to the thighs. The scrotum is usually not involved. A common term for this infection is jock itch (Plate 12).

Tinea pedis and *tinea manuum,* fungal infections of the feet and hands, are probably the most common fungal infections. *T. rubrum* causes scaly, erythematous patches on the soles and palms. Both feet and only one hand are frequently involved. *T. mentagrophytes* cause inflammatory, crusty, pustular eruptions on the feet. Tinea pedis, manuum, and cruris are confirmed by microscopic examination of potassium hydroxide–treated skin scrapings and fungal cultures.

Tinea versicolor is caused by *Malassezia furfur.* Sharply marginated, scaly, white or brownish patches appear over the trunk, neck, and extremities (Fig. 75-13 and Plate 13). The infection is more apparent in the summer. Microscopic examination of potassium hydroxide–treated scale confirm the diagnosis. Multiple short hyphae and spores are present.

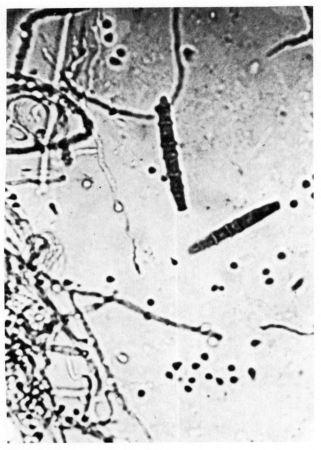

FIGURE 75-9
Multiple hyphae and spores can be seen on microscopic examination of skin scrapings from a patient with superficial fungal infection of the skin.

FIGURE 75-10
Trichophyton rubrum, the most common cause of superficial fungal skin infection, as seen on fungal culture grown at room temperature.

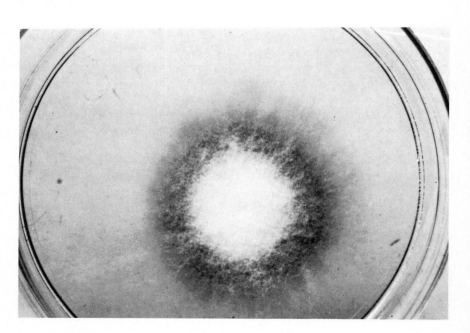

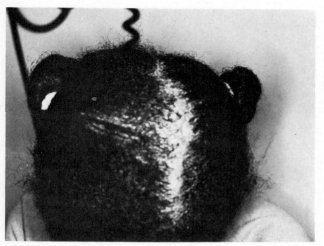

FIGURE 75-11
Verrucous, superficial nodule of seborrheic keratosis, which appears to be glued to the surface.

Fungal infection of the nails, *onychomycosis*, presents with dystrophic nails. There is subungual hyperkeratosis and separation of the nail plate from the nail bed (Fig. 75-14). The diagnosis is confirmed by fungal cultures and potassium hydroxide examination. This common fungal infection is extremely resistant to fungal therapy and frequently recurs when treatment is discontinued.

Treatment

The usual treatment of tinea pedis, tinea cruris, and tinea corporis is with topical antifungal agents, which include miconazole (Micatin), clotrimazole (Lotrimin), and haloprogin (Halotex). These agents are used twice daily, generally for a period of 1 month. Patients are also instructed in proper foot hygiene and told to wear loose-fitting cotton underwear and nonocclusive shoes. For prevention of infections, the useful agents available include undecylenic acid (Desenex) and tolnaftate (Tinactin). These over-the-counter agents are usually ineffective in the *treatment* of fungal infections. Resistant infections of the feet and pruritic infections of the groin can also be treated with oral griseofulvin, an effective, oral antifungal agent. Oral griseofulvin is also used for infections of the scalp and severe infections of the nails. The treatment is continued until the organisms are eradicated. Tinea capitis usually requires 4 to 6 weeks of 250 to 500 mg of griseofulvin daily; tinea corporis, 2 to 4 weeks; tinea pedis, 4 to 8 weeks; and tinea unguium, 6 to 12 months. It is important to note that this drug is phototoxic and interferes with the activity of such medications as warfarin and barbiturates. Ketoconazole is an oral agent approved for the treatment of serious *systemic not cutaneous* fungal infections. Serious liver disorders can complicate the therapy with ketoconazole. Tinea versicolor is treated with selenium sulfide (Selsun), which is applied twice to the affected areas for at least 60 minutes. However, pigmentary changes may persist for several months.

CANDIDIASIS

Candidiasis is caused by *Candida albicans*, a type of yeast infection. The organism is normally present in the gastrointestinal tract, but it can cause an opportunistic infection (see Chap. 6). Persons who are obese, have diabetes mellitus, or are on broad-spectrum antibiotics

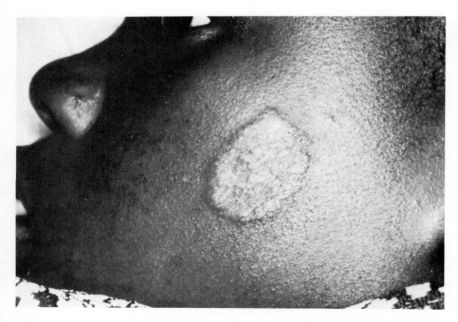

FIGURE 75-12
Tinea corporis of the face, with peripheral scale and ringlike shape.

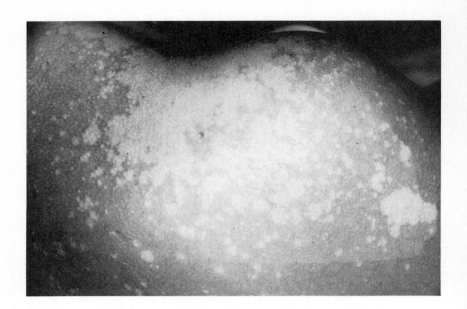

FIGURE 75-13
Sharply marginated, scaly hypopigmented patches of tinea versicolor are usually seen over the back.

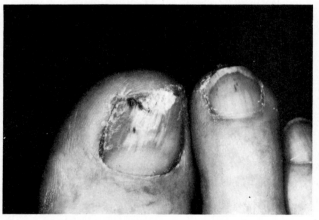

FIGURE 75-14
Subungual hyperkeratosis and discoloration of the nail plate seen in onychomycosis.

(tetracycline) or corticosteroids can develop the infection. In the groin and intertriginous areas, candidiasis presents with erythema, whitish pseudomembrane, and peripheral papules and pustules (Fig. 75-15 and Plate 14). The infection frequently occurs in infants and obese patients. *Candida* infection of the paronychial area causes swelling, erythema, and pus formation. *Candida* of the mouth, or *thrush*, presents with a white coating of the tongue and occasional macerated, fissured patches in the corners of the mouth. Systemic candidiasis in debilitated leukemia or cancer patients can be fatal when complicated by candidal meningitis, endocarditis, or septicemia. Diagnosis of *Candida* infection is confirmed by a microscopic examination of a potassium hydroxide–treated skin scraping and culture.

Treatment consists of removing predisposing fac-

FIGURE 75-15
Plaque of candidiasis in the axilla with a whitish pseudomembrane and peripheral papules.

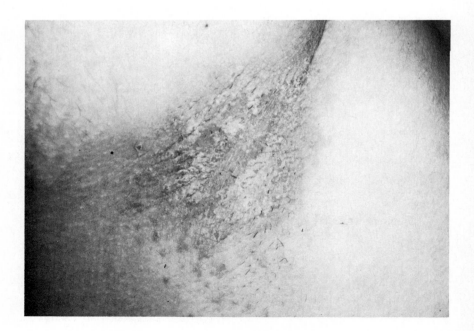

tors. *Candida* infection is treated with oral or topical nystatin, topical miconazole, topical clotrimazole, or amphotericin cream. These medications are also used for vaginal candidiasis. Systemic infection is treated by intravenous amphotericin B. A new oral medication, ketoconazole (Nizoral), is effective in treatment of systemic candidiasis and chronic mucocutaneous candidiasis. Several cases of severe hepatic toxicity have been reported with use of this medication.

CUTANEOUS BACTERIAL INFECTIONS

Impetigo is the most common bacterial infection of the skin. It is caused by streptococci and staphylococci. The infection is transferred by human-to-human contact, usually among children. Hot, humid temperatures and poor hygiene predispose one to this infection. Patients with eczema occasionally develop impetigo secondary to excoriations of pruritic skin lesions. Impetigo begins as a purulent vesicle. As the lesion spreads, it becomes eroded and a golden crust develops on the surface (Fig. 75-16 and Plate 15). The infection usually starts on the face and extremities but can spread to any surface of the body.

Treatment should include instructions in proper hygienic techniques in order to control spread of the infection. Topical antibiotics (polymixin, neomycin, bacitracin) and antiseptics (Betadine) are used. Oral penicillin or erythromycin therapy is indicated when large or multiple lesions are present. This can prevent the incidence of poststreptococcal glomerular nephritis, especially in children. Impetigo usually heals without scar formation.

Erysipelas is a serious, toxic, streptococcal infection of the skin. The lesions are brightly erythematous,

sharply marginated, and tender and have indurated areas (Plate 16). They frequently occur over the face or the extremities. The patient has high fever and malaise, and is toxic. Regional lymph nodes are enlarged. Complications such as endocarditis and septicemia can result. Patients with erysipelas are usually hospitalized and treated with intravenous penicillin. Occasionally, a prolonged treatment is required to eradicate the infection and prevent secondary lymphedema in the affected areas.

Erythrasma casues erythematous, dry, scaly patches in the intertriginous areas. It is caused by *Corynebacterium minutissimum*. The infection is most often seen in obese individuals and can be confirmed by a characteristic coral-red fluorescence under a Wood's light examination. Erythrasma is usually treated with topical antibiotics, but systemic tetracycline and erythromycin are also effective.

Trichomycosis axillaris is an infection of the axillary and, rarely, pubic hair. Yellow, red or black concretions form on the hair (Fig. 75-17). The infection is asymptomatic and not contagious. The patients report an abnormal coloring of sweat, and there may be an axillary odor. *Corynebacterium* species isolated from these infections can be treated by topical application of antibiotics or by shaving of the hair from the affected areas.

Superficial folliculitis is caused by staphylococci. The disease presents with small pustules surrounded by erythema. The scalp and extremities are the usual sites. Poor hygiene practices, maceration, and excoriations

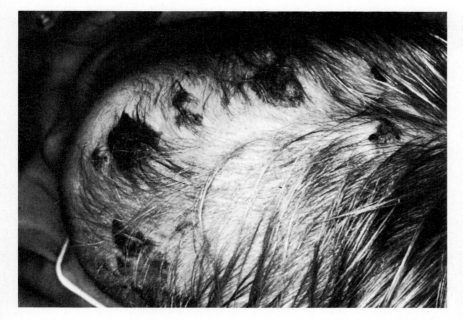

FIGURE 75-16
Crusted, eroded patches of impetigo on the scalp.

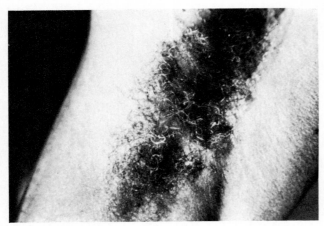

FIGURE 75-17
Trichomycosis axillaris with yellow concretions on the hair.

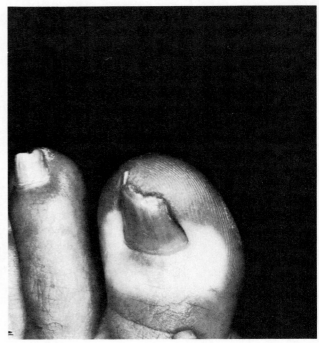

FIGURE 75-18
Swollen, painful toe secondary to bacterial paronychia. The whitish area contains purulent material.

are the predisposing factors of this infection. Treatment is with antibacterial soaps (pHisohex) and, occasionally, systemic antibiotics. Recurrent chronic folliculitis can be difficult to eradicate and may require systemic antibiotics after appropriate bacterial cultures, and sensitivities are obtained.

Deep staphylococcal infections are responsible for furuncles (boils) and carbuncles (multiple confluent furuncles). Deep-seated, erythematous, tender nodules occur over the buttocks, neck, and axillae. The nodules become fluctuant in a few days and discharge a purulent necrotic material. Furuncles can be very painful when located in the nasal area, axillae, or ears. Boils are treated with surgical draining, hot wet dressings, and appropriate systemic antibiotics. The antibiotics are se-

lected after aerobic and anaerobic cultures and sensitivity studies are performed.

Infection of the nail fold with staphylococci and streptococci can lead to a painful infection called *paronychia*. The infection can follow a hangnail and is common among people whose hands are frequently immersed in water. The nail folds are erythematous, swollen, and painful in this infection (Fig. 75-18). Since paronychia can be also caused by *Candida*, fungal cultures are required to confirm the disease. Bacterial paronychia is treated with systemic antibiotics, and localized pus is drained. The patient is instructed to avoid prolonged exposure to water.

QUESTIONS

Cutaneous infections

Directions: Circle the letter preceding each item below that correctly answers the question. More than one answer may be correct.

1. The etiology of verrucae (warts) and herpes simplex is similar. The causative agent is:
   a. Candida albicans *b.* DNA virus *c.* RNA virus *d.* Bacteria

2. Untreated warts over the finger area:
   a. Persist indefinitely *b.* Invade the dermis
   c. Disappear spontaneously in 2 to 5 years
   d. Are not infectious

3. Mr. A., 40 years of age, presented with a series of many small, painful vesicles appearing on an edematous, hemorrhagic area of the skin on his trunk. These inflammatory vesicles appeared unilaterally along a single dermatome, starting at its origin on the back and continuing to his middle. His history revealed chickenpox as a child. You would suspect which of the following?
   a. Herpes simplex *b.* Herpes zoster *c.* Molluscum contagiosum *d.* Rubeola

4. Herpes zoster is usually self-limiting and lasts:

a. 3 to 4 days   *b.* 3 to 4 weeks   *c.* 1 to 2 months
d. 3 to 4 months

5. A highly effective vaccine is used to control which of the following?
a. Herpes simplex   *b.* Rubella   *c.* Verrucae
d. Infectious mononucleosis

6. The usual mode of transmission of Type II herpes simplex is by:
a. Use of common towels   *b.* Kissing, touching
c. Sexual encounters   *d.* Contaminated drinking water

7. The recurrence rate of herpes Type I infections is approximately what percent?
a. 10   *b.* 14   *c.* 50   *d.* 80

8. The percentage (or number) of sexually active individuals who have had Type II herpes simplex is estimated to be:
a. 5 (5 million)   *b.* 10 (10 million)   *c.* 30 (20 million)   *d.* 50 (50 million)

Directions: Circle T if the statement is true and F if it is false. Correct the false statements.

9.   T   F   Tinea versicolor is characterized by erythematous, scaly, edematous eruption, with satellite lesions on the periphery, which occur in the groin.

10.   T   F   Candidiasis can be treated with nystatin.

11.   T   F   *Candida albicans* is a type of yeast that causes skin infections.

12.   T   F   Erysipelas is a serious, toxic, streptococcal infection of the skin.

13.   T   F   Impetigo is a viral infection.

Directions: Answer the following questions on a separate sheet of paper.

14. List the most common sites of occurrence following primary exposure to the herpes simplex virus.

15. Describe the two tests used to attempt to confirm the diagnosis of herpes simplex.

16. What are the therapeutic measures that can be used in an attempt to prevent recurrent infections of cutaneous herpes infections?

17. Describe the serious complications associated with:
a. Herpes simplex infection of the eye
b. Herpes infection of the female genital area

18. Describe the lesion characteristic of impetigo.

19. Contrast impetigo and erysipelas as to etiologic agent and pathogenesis.

20. State the predisposing factors associated with superficial folliculitis.

TUMORS OF THE SKIN

OBJECTIVES

At the completion of this chapter you should be able to:

1. List the characteristics of malignant tumors of the skin (basal cell carcinoma, squamous cell carcinoma, melanoma).

2. Identify the causes and treatments of basal cell carcinoma and squamous cell carcinoma.

3. Describe nevi by identifying their appearance and treatment.

4. Explain the rationale for the treatment of a giant congenital nevus.

5. Describe the appearance of malignant melanoma.

6. Differentiate between superficial spreading and nodular melanomas as to occurrence and prognosis.

7. Describe the causes and treatment of melanoma.

8. Describe the characteristics of nevus flammeus, strawberry angioma, spider angioma, cherry angioma, and pyogenic granuloma.

9. Identify for dermatofibromas, acrochordons, and keloids the characteristic lesions and treatments.

10. Describe seborrheic keratosis, actinic keratosis, and keratoacanthoma as to their appearances, and treatments.

Cutaneous tumors can derive from various cell types in the skin (e.g., epidermal cells, and melanocytes). These tumors can be benign or malignant and either localized in the epidermis or invasive to the dermis and subcutaneous tissue.

MALIGNANT SKIN TUMORS

Basal cell carcinoma

Basal cell carcinoma is the most common malignant tumor of the skin. It arises from the epidermal cells **1042**

along the basal layer of the epidermis. The incidence of basal cell carcinoma is directly proportional to the age of the patient and inversely proportional to the amount of melanin pigment in the epidermis. There is also a direct correlation between this condition and the total lifetime exposure to sunlight. About 80 percent of basal cell cancers occur on the sun-exposed areas of the face, head, and neck. Fortunately, the tumor rarely metastasizes. However, a patient with a single basal cell cancer is likely to develop future skin cancers and must be followed indefinitely on an annual basis.

The carcinogenic sun rays are found in the solar

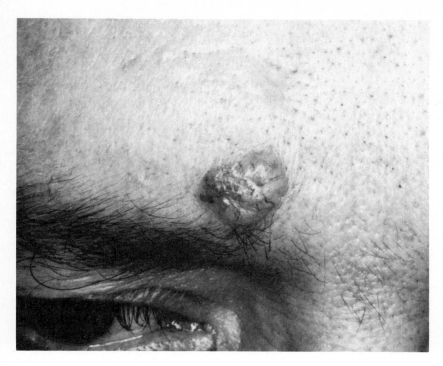

FIGURE 76-1
A smooth, pearly nodule of early basal cell carcinoma.

FIGURE 76-2
Ulcerated tumor with elevated smooth borders in a patient with advanced basal cell carcinoma.

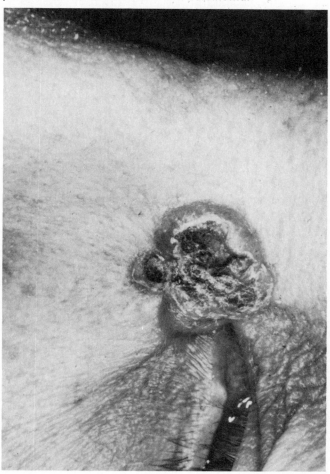

spectrum primarily between 280 and 320 nm. This spectrum is primarily responsible for burning and tanning of the skin exposed to the sun. Sunscreens, sun blocks, and avoidance of excessive sunlight exposure are recommended for patients with a family history of skin cancer, and for fair-skinned individuals who have a tendency to sunburn easily. Also, patients with a history of basal cell carcinoma should use sunscreens or protective clothing to avoid carcinogenic sun rays. Sunscreens most commonly used contain para-aminobenzoic acid, which absorbs the carcinogenic rays.

Other causes of basal cell carcinoma include previous x-ray therapy of other skin disorders, contact with arsenic, and rare genetic disorders (xeroderma pigmentosum and nevoid basal cell carcinoma syndrome). The use of suntanning booths also damages the epidermis and is considered to be carcinogenic.

The tumor is characterized by an erythematous, smooth, pearly nodule (Fig. 76-1). The borders are frequently elevated and have telangiectatic vessels on the surface. Central ulceration and bleeding are frequently observed (Fig. 76-2 and Plate 17). The tumor bleeds frequently, invades the dermis, and destroys normal tissue.

Basal cell carcinoma should be treated promptly. Treatments include curettage with electrodesiccation, scalpel surgery, irradiation, chemosurgery, and cryosurgery. A small basal cell cancer under 2 cm in diameter is usually treated with scalpel excision or electrodesiccation and curettage after biopsy is obtained to confirm the diagnosis. The cure rate is about 95 percent. Roentgen therapy may be used in patients over 60 to 70 years who have very large tumors around the eyelids, earlobes, or lips. Chemosurgery is useful in the treatment of large, infiltrating, and recurrent cancers, especially around the ears, the nasolabial folds, and the eyes. In chemosurgery, the microscopic excision of the tumor is accomplished by removing layer by layer with a scalpel; frozen sections are prepared, and a map of the tumor is constructed, then the undersurface of each removed frozen section is examined for evidence of basal cell cancer. This is the most tedious, effective, and expensive technique which has a cure rate of over 97 percent. Cryosurgery utilizes liquid nitrogen, and the cure rate is similar to that for electrodessication and curettage.

Squamous cell carcinoma

Squamous cell carcinoma is a malignant neoplasm of keratinocytes. It arises from more differentiated cells of epidermis (keratinocytes), while basal cell carcinoma arises from basal cells. Frequently, the tumor is seen in older, fair-skinned individuals. Commonly, it arises on sun-damaged skin with multiple actinic keratoses present. Sunlight is the main etiologic factor causing squamous cell carcinoma of the skin. As in basal cell carcinoma, sunlight in the ultraviolet light (UV) spectrum between 280 and 320 nm (UV-B spectrum) is responsible. However, recent cooperative studies on the use of long ultraviolet light, between 320 and 400 nm (UV-A spectrum), combined with oral psoralens in treatment of psoriasis have demonstrated that prolonged, chronic exposure to UV-A with psoralens can also produce squamous cell carcinoma.

Fair-skinned persons of Celtic origin who are chronically exposed to the sunlight (farmers, sailors) have a very high incidence of squamous cell carcinomas. Both basal cell carcinomas and squamous cell carcinomas are much more common in sunbelt areas of this country than in midwest or northeast areas. The incidence of skin squamous cell carcinoma and basal cell carcinoma in blacks is extremely low.

Other causes of squamous cell carcinoma include ingestion of arsenic, x-ray irradiation, burns, scars, and genetic susceptibility. Patients who were treated for acne or hemangiomas with x-ray therapy many years ago can develop basal cell cancers and squamous cell cancers. Those individuals who 30 to 40 years ago were treated with arsenic for psoriasis or asthma, ingested arsenic in their drinking water, or inhaled it in smelting plants have a tendency to develop squamous cell carcinomas. A few rare genetic diseases (albinism and xeroderma pigmentosum) also predispose individuals to these cancers. Excessive use of suntanning booths will likely lead to an increased incidence of squamous cell carcinoma in future years.

Squamous cell carcinomas which arise in sun-damaged skin generally do not metastasize and rarely cause death. Squamous cell cancers rising on sun-unexposed areas (lips, buttocks, groin), after ingestion of arsenic, or on an old scar have the greatest risk of metastasis. Squamous cell carcinoma which occurs on sun-unexposed areas can be a cutaneous marker of internal malignancy. Once it is diagnosed, a thorough history and physical examination are required.

A variant of squamous cell carcinoma is localized to the epidermis and is called Bowen's disease. Bowen's disease is usually caused by chronic sun exposure. It can also be caused by ingestion of arsenic. Some sources feel that there is an increased incidence of internal malignancies with this tumor. Patients with Bowen's disease should undergo a workup which includes a complete history and physical examination if this cancer occurs on sun-unexposed areas.

Squamous cell carcinoma presents with an ulcerated, scaly, thickened nodule or tumor which bleeds occasionally (Fig. 76-3 and Plate 18). The nodules usually arise on sun-damaged skin of the face, scalp, ears, neck,

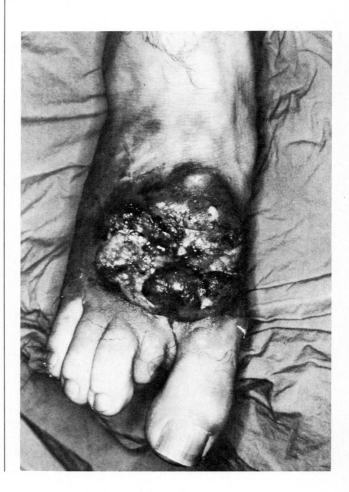

FIGURE 76-3
Verrucous, ulcerated tumor of squamous cell carcinoma following x-ray therapy to the foot.

hands, or forearms. Frequently, they are surrounded by multiple actinic keratoses, many of which, if left untreated, would degenerate into squamous cell cancers. Bowen's disease presents as an erythematous plaque with undulating borders, scaliness, and frequently central erosion. It can be indistinguishable from eczema or psoriasis (Fig. 76-4 and Plate 19). A lesion of psoriasis or eczema which is unresponsive to appropriate therapy should, therefore, be biopsied.

The treatment of squamous cell carcinoma and its variant, Bowen's disease, is primarily surgical excision. Radiation therapy, cryosurgery, and chemosurgery have been utilized and have cure rates of 95 to 98 percent. Skin tumors less than 2 cm can be treated utilizing electrodesiccation and curettage, with a cure rate of 94 percent. Bowen's disease is best treated with surgical excision, but radiation therapy, cryotherapy, chemosurgery, and electrodesiccation with curettage have been successfully used. The lymph nodes are not removed if they are clinically negative, but they should be carefully palpated during the surgical procedure. Metastatic lesions of squamous cell carcinoma do not respond well to chemotherapy. As with basal cell carcinoma patients, those with squamous cell carcinomas must be followed indefinitely, since there is a high risk for development of new squamous cell carcinomas. The lymph nodes are palpated during these follow-up visits. Of these patients, 20 to 50 percent with one squamous cell carcinoma eventually develop another squamous cell carcinoma or basal cell carcinoma.

Melanoma

Malignant melanoma comprises only 3 percent of all primary cutaneous malignancies but is responsible for over two-thirds of the deaths secondary to skin cancers. Furthermore, the incidence of melanoma is increasing. Early diagnosis and surgical treatment is the only way to ensure long-term survival and even cure. Unless recognized and treated early, melanomas invade deeper layers of the dermis and the subcutaneous tissues and metastasize to distant sites. Most melanomas occur in the 40- to 70-year age group, but there has been an increase in the number of cases among the ages of 20 to 40 years. One of the explanations for this increased incidence is a greater sun exposure secondary to recreation and attire changes. Further evidence for the role of ultraviolet light in causing melanomas is the increased frequency of this tumor in sunbelt states. The mode of inheritance of melanomas is undetermined, and only a small percentage of melanoma patients (about 2 percent) have a family history of melanoma. However, all family members should be examined for atypical nevi by an experienced dermatologist. Atypical nevi in individuals with a family history of melanomas should be removed, since they can degenerate to malignant mel-

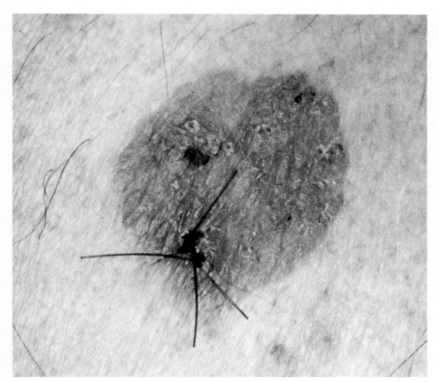

FIGURE 76-4
Undulating borders and central erosion of plaque in Bowen's disease.

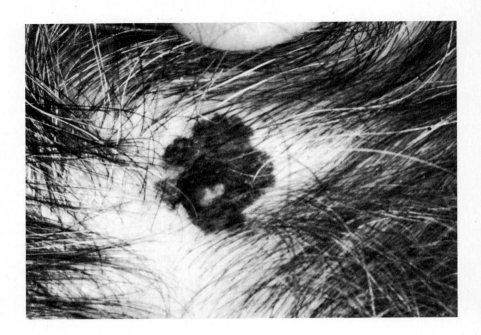

FIGURE 76-5
Irregular borders, uneven pigmentation, and ulceration in a superficial, spreading malignant melanoma.

anomas. Large congenital nevi give rise to malignant melanomas in 2 to 13 percent of patients, and these should be surgically excised.

Diagnosis is based on the change in shape, color, and configuration of a pigmented lesion. Irregular pigmentation with shades of blue, purple, red, and brown should alert the examiner. The borders of this tumor are irregular, and the surface is frequently ulcerated (Fig. 76-5). Satellite lesions and diffusion of pigment into the surrounding skin are also observed (Fig. 76-6 and Plate 20).

The superficial spreading melanoma is the most common type (60 to 80 percent) and has the best prognosis. It presents as a flat growth with bizarre colors and configuration (Fig. 76-7). The nodular melanoma is less common (20 percent) and presents as a tumor (Fig. 76-

FIGURE 76-7
Bizarre colors and irregular borders in a superficial, spreading, malignant melanoma.

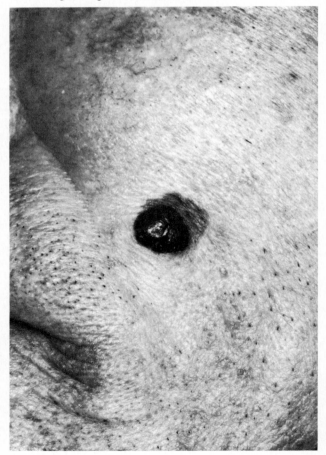

FIGURE 76-6
Nodule with diffusion of pigment in nodular malignant melanoma.

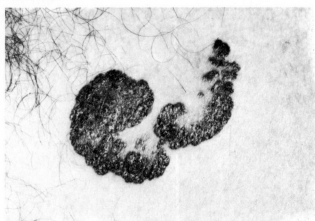

6). This variant has the worst prognosis. The lentigo maligna melanoma occurs on a preexisting, irregularly pigmented, brown patch (lentigo maligna) (Plate 21). This tumor is even less common (5 to 10 percent) and, if detected early, has a good prognosis.

The prognosis for patients with malignant melanoma is not as poor as once thought. The great majority of patients survive for 5 years or more, and many are cured. Early diagnosis and surgical treatment are responsible for these improved statistics. Several factors determine survival of melanoma patients. Patients with superficial spreading melanoma have the best prognosis, followed by lentigo maligna melanoma; nodular melanoma has the worst prognosis. Lesions located over the posterior scalp, back, and posterior arms have a worse prognosis. Clinical ulceration of the tumor carries a poor prognosis. Histological levels of primary malignant melanoma invasion of the dermis, as defined by Clark, determine prognosis: the best survival rates are seen with Level I and II melanomas, confined to the epidermis and upper dermis; intermediate survival rates are seen with Levels III and IV, extending to the lower dermis; and the worst rates are seen with Level V, invading the subcutaneous tissue. Breslow was able to correlate vertical tumor thickness with prognosis of malignant melanomas: melanomas less than 0.76 mm in thickness do not metastasize if removed locally, melanomas greater than 1.5 mm in thickness are likely to develop metastasis, and tumors between 0.76 and 1.5 mm are less likely to metastasize.

The treatment of malignant melanoma is primarily surgical. There is a controversy over whether Level I and II melanomas should be widely excised. Many authorities feel that a narrow excision with 1- to 2-cm margins is adequate. Level III melanomas are excised with a wide margin (5 to 10 cm). Level IV and V melanomas should receive a wide excision and elective regional lymph node dissection, if feasible. Patients with disseminated melanomas receive chemotherapy using 5-imidazole-4- carboxamide and immunotherapy with bacillus Calmette-Guérin (BCG) administration. Unfortunately, *disseminated* melanoma has a 1-year mortality as high as 83 percent. The most effective treatment of melanoma remains early detection and aggressive surgical removal.

BENIGN SKIN TUMORS

Nevi, or moles, are the most common tumors derived from the melanocyte. The melanin pigment produces uniform brown, dark brown, light brown, or blue color in flat or elevated nevi (Fig. 76-8 and Plate 22). Flat nevi do not infiltrate the dermis and can occur anywhere on the body. Nevi are rarely excised unless they become irritated, bleed, grow rapidly, or change in appearance.

The compound nevus is an elevated nodule, usually brown in color. It is elevated because melanocytes are found in the dermis. It is also composed of melanocytes in the epidermis and can occur anywhere on the body. Surgical excision is not necessary unless it is irritated by clothing or is cosmetically unattractive (Fig. 76-9).

Large nevi present at birth are called giant congenital nevi (Fig. 76-10). Since melanomas can arise in giant congenital nevi, they should be excised by surgical removal down to the layer of subcutaneous fat. Regrowth of the nevus will occur if this is not done. The skin should be replaced with grafts if necessary.

Seborrheic keratosis

Seborrheic keratosis appears as a verrucous, brown growth which appears to be glued to the surface of the epidermis (Fig. 76-11). The cause of this benign tumor is unknown. The tumor cells are derived from small basal cells which are localized in the epidermis. Older patients develop multiple seborrheic keratoses usually over the trunk, face, and upper extremities. Treatment is not necessary except for cosmetic and/or diagnostic reasons.

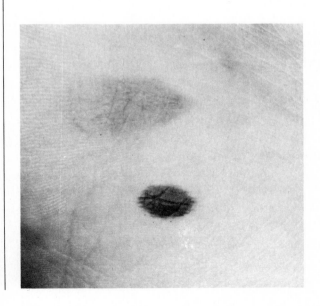

FIGURE 76-8
Dark-brown, flat macules with uniform pigment; no skin ulceration; and no history of recent change are typical of benign junctional nevi.

Actinic keratosis

Actinic keratosis usually occurs on the sun-exposed areas of the face, neck, scalp, and extremities. It appears as an erythematous, scaly, rough suface lesion (Plate 23). The lesion is caused by chronic exposure to sun, particularly in older patients. This premalignant growth can develop into squamous cell carcinoma and should be treated. Treatment measures include electrodesiccation with curettage or cryosurgery. Patients are warned about future exposure to the sun and instructed in the use of sunscreens. The sunscreens which block UV-B light with protection factor 8 or 15 are recommended (PreSun, Eclipse). Also effective in the treatment of actinic keratosis is 1 to 5% topical 5-fluorouracil applied daily for 30 days.

Keratoacanthoma

Keratoacanthoma is a dome-shaped tumor with a central keratotic crater or ulceration (Fig. 76-12). The tumor grows rapidly over a period of a few months and usually occurs in elderly persons. The tumor is benign and may undergo spontaneous involution. Since the tumor can resemble squamous cell carcinoma, it should be excised and examined by a histopathologist.

Dermatofibroma, acrochordon, keloid

Three common benign tumors are dermatofibromas, acrochordons (skin tags), and keloids. Dermatofibroma is a brown nodule usually found on the legs, the trunk, or the arms. On palpation it has a hard buttonlike consistency. The tumor is excised only for cosmetic or diagnostic reasons, since it is benign. Skin tags (acrochordons) are frequent over the neck, axilla, and groin of middle-aged and elderly persons (Fig. 76-13). Acrochor-

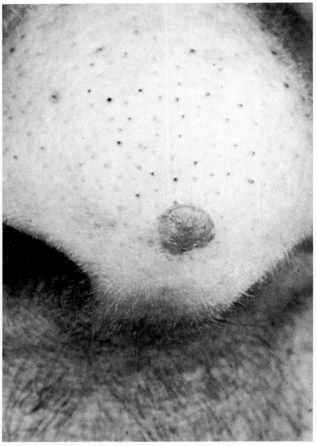

FIGURE 76-9
Brownish, elevated papule with uniform color and no history of recent change is typical of benign compound nevus.

FIGURE 76-10
Giant pigmented nevus present at birth has an increased incidence of progression to a melanoma.

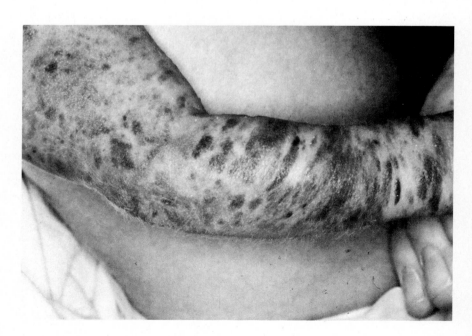

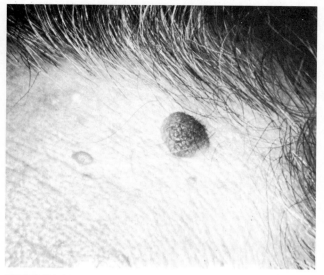

FIGURE 76-11
Verrucous, superficial nodule of seborrheic keratosis, which appears to be glued to the surface.

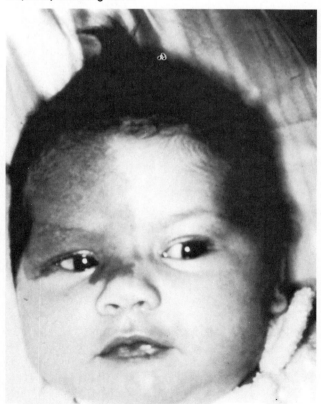

FIGURE 76-13
Pedunculated, filiform lesions of acrochordons over the neck.

FIGURE 76-12
Rapidly growing dome-shaped tumor with central keratotic crater is a benign keratoacanthoma.

FIGURE 76-14
Proliferation of capillaries causes a pink skin discoloration known as nevus flammeus or capillary hemangioma.

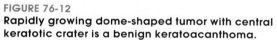

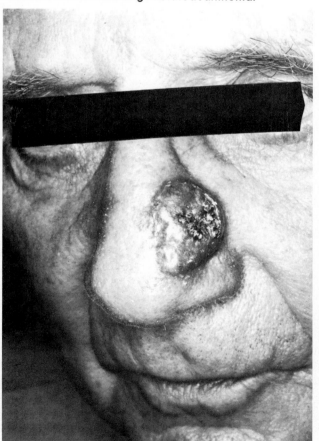

dons are more common in obese patients and in pregnant women. They are excised if associated with pain and for cosmetic reasons. Keloids are caused by an abnormal scar formation following even a minor injury (Fig. 72-5). They are more common in blacks, and the tendency to form them is genetic. Surgical excision of keloids may be attempted for cosmetic reasons. Excision of keloids in combination with injection of corticosteroids into the lesions is frequently an effective treatment.

Benign tumors of blood vessels

Among the numerous tumors of blood vessels of the skin, the most commonly encountered are nevus flammeus, strawberry angioma, cherry angioma, spider angioma, and pyogenic granuloma.

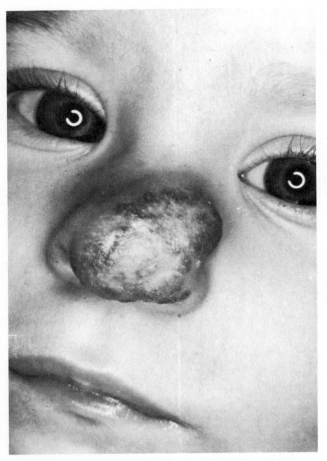

FIGURE 76-15
Strawberry angioma presents with an elevated, erythematous tumor, shown here over the nose.

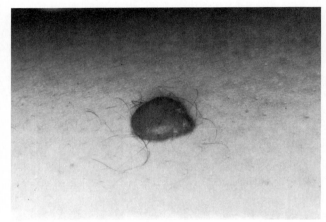

FIGURE 76-16
Elevated, erythematous papule of cherry angioma.

FIGURE 76-17
Pedunculated, red, moist nodule of pyogenic granuloma of the finger.

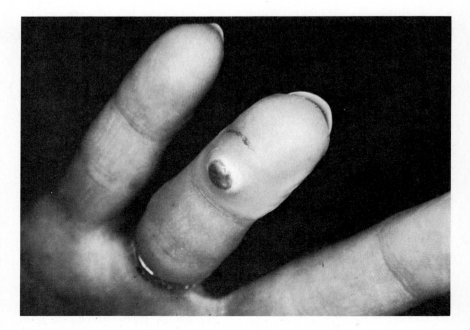

Proliferation of mature capillaries can produce a pink discoloration of the skin on newborns that is called nevus flammeus (Fig. 76-14). When the capillaries follow a branch of the trigeminal nerve, the condition can be associated with angioma of the ipsilateral eye and the central nervous system (*Sturge-Weber syndrome*). This can lead to glaucoma and contralateral seizures. Nevus flammeus can fade or persist indefinitely. If the lesion persists, a cover-up makeup (Covermark) is recommended.

Strawberry angioma arises after birth and involutes spontaneously by age 5 in 90 to 95 percent of cases. Proliferating capillaries in the dermis cause an elevated bluish-red nodule (Fig. 76-15 and Plate 24) usually on the head or upper trunk, but it can occur anywhere on the body's surface. Since most of these tumors involute spontaneously, no treatment is usually required.

Cherry angiomas are red, slightly elevated papules over the trunk and extremities of middle-aged and el-

derly persons (Fig. 76-16). They are asymptomatic and benign, and treatment is not necessary.

Spider angiomas appear in women at the times of pregnancy, in alcoholics, and also in children. A central arteriole feeds multiple small branches of this tumor. Multiple spider angiomas can be associated with liver disease such as cirrhosis. Most spider angiomas in children and pregnant women resolve spontaneously. Persistent spider angiomas can be electrodesiccated.

Pyogenic granuloma is caused by an abnormal proliferation of granulation tissue. The tumor occurs after trauma to the site. Red or purple pedunculated, moist nodules appear (Fig. 76-17). This benign tumor bleeds occasionally and is treated by surgical removal.

QUESTIONS

Tumors of the skin

Directions: Answer the following questions on a separate sheet of paper.

1. Describe the characteristic appearance of the lesion, cause, prognosis, and treatment of malignant melanoma.

2. What are the causes and common sites of occurrence of basal cell carcinoma?

3. Discuss the preventive measures recommended for patients with a family history of skin cancer and for fair-skinned individuals.

4. What is the usual treatment of basal cell carcinoma?

5. Describe the causes, pathogenesis, type of lesion, and treatment of squamous cell carcinoma.

Directions: Circle the letter preceding each item below that correctly answers the question. More than one answer may be correct.

6. Carcinogenic sun rays in the solar spectrum occur primarily in what nm range (UV-B spectrum)?
   a. 50, 100 *b.* 100, 150 *c.* 175, 200 *d.* 280, 320

7. Cutaneous tumors are derived from which of the following skin cell types?
   a. Fibroblasts *b.* Melanocytes *c.* Epidermal cells

8. The classic presentation of squamous cell carcinoma of the skin is:
   a. Irregular pigmentation with shades of blue and purple *b.* Ulcerated, hyperkeratotic nodules

with evidence of dermal invasion on palpation
   c. A smooth, pearly appearance with multiple telangiectasis

9. The natural history of untreated basal cell carcinoma is characterized by:
   a. Involvement of regional lymphatics *b.* An ulcerated tumor *c.* Gradual local enlargement
   d. Metastasis

10. A benign, verrucous, flat lesion commonly found in elderly people, which resembles dried mud hardened on the skin is:
    a. Melanoma *b.* Urticaria *c.* Seborrheic keratosis *d.* Psoriasis

11. Mr. M., a 47-year-old male, a construction worker, presents with several lesions on his forearm. Examination reveals erythematous ulcerated plaques with undulating borders. A biopsy is negative for psoriasis and eczema. The most likely condition is:
    a. Melanoma *b.* Basal cell carcinoma *c.* Seborrheic keratosis *d.* Bowen's disease

Directions: Match the type of tumor in col. A with the appropriate characteristic in col. B.

Column A	Column B
12. ____ Flat nevi	*a.* Elevated, nodular, usually
13. ____ Compound nevi	brown in color, composed of melanocytes in the epidermis and dermis
14. ____ Giant congenital nevi	*b.* Caused by abnormal scar formation following injury
15. ____ Keloids	

16. _____ Straw-
       berry angiomas

c. Sharply marginated, caused
   by proliferation of melanocytes, characterized by uniform pigment, flat in appearance

d. Arising after birth and invo-
   luting spontaneously in 90 to
   95 percent of cases

e. Treated by surgical removal
   of nevi to the subcutaneous
   layer and replacement with
   skin grafts (regrowth of nevi
   will occur if this is not done)

f. Does not infiltrate the dermis

CHAPTER 77

VENEREAL DISEASES AND INFESTATIONS

OBJECTIVES

At the completion of this chapter you should be able to:

1. Describe the incidence, causes, diagnosis, and incubation period of syphilis.
2. Differentiate between secondary syphilis and pityriasis rosea.
3. Explain the course of untreated syphilis.
4. Identify the organ systems which can be affected by tertiary syphilis and the signs and symptoms that result.
5. Explain the measures used to treat syphilis.
6. Describe the causes, signs and symptoms, and treatment of gonorrhea.
7. Identify for scabies and pediculosis pubis the causes, signs and symptoms, and treatments.
8. List the characteristics of bites for fleas, chiggers, bedbugs, and ticks.
9. Identify for autoimmune deficiency syndrome (AIDS) the incidence, probable causes, signs and symptoms, complications, and treatments.

SYPHILIS

There has been an increase in the number of reported cases of primary and secondary syphilis each year since 1977. In 1982, reported cases increased 7.5 percent over the number which had been reported the previous year (Centers for Disease Control, 1983). This increase has led to an intensified interest in diagnosis and treatment of this disease.

Primary syphilis

The causative agent of syphilis, *Treponema pallidum*, is transmitted only by direct contact with an infectious lesion. After an incubation period of 10 to 90 days a painless ulcer, a primary lesion called a chancre, develops at the site of contact (Fig. 77-1 and Plate 25). On palpation, this chancre is painless and indurated. It heals spontaneously after 3 to 12 weeks. Dark-field micros-

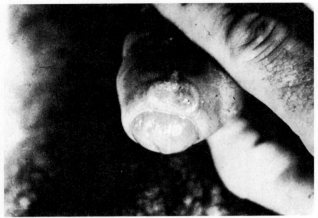

FIGURE 77-1
Painless, hard ulcer of primary syphilitic chancre on the penis.

copy is the most important diagnostic test and must be done by an experienced examiner. The Venereal Disease Research Laboratory (VDRL) serologic test is positive in only 50 percent of cases when a chancre initially appears, whereas the fluorescent treponemal-antibody absorption (FTA-ABS) test is positive in 90 percent of cases. In the diagnosis of primary syphilis, the chancre must be differentiated from herpes progenitalis, chancroid, granuloma inguinale, and drug eruptions. A characteristic indurated ulcer and positive dark-field examination along with a positive FTA-ABS test confirm the diagnosis of syphilis.

Secondary syphilis

Approximately 6 weeks to 6 months following exposure, untreated primary syphilis patients develop cutaneous manifestations of secondary syphilis. The lesions consist of brownish papules and macules with a slight scale which classically occur over the palms and soles (Fig. 77-2). Generalized eruptions over the trunk can resemble pityriasis rosea. Moist, flat, wartlike condylomata lata can appear over the genitalia. *All* lesions of secondary syphilis are contagious. Alopecia and lymphadenopathy frequently accompany the cutaneous lesions. The diagnosis is established on the basis of VDRL and FTA-ABS tests, which are almost always positive.

Latent syphilis

If not treated, the lesions of secondary syphilis heal in 4 to 12 weeks, and the patient enters the latent stage of syphilis. During the first 4 years, the only evidence of active syphilis is positive FTA-ABS or VDRL serology, or positive cerebrospinal fluid serology.

Tertiary syphilis

Tertiary syphilis occurs in about 30 percent of cases of untreated syphilis. The other patients have no symptoms but positive FTA-ABS serology; over half have positive VDRL serology or positive cerebrospinal fluid serology. Benign cutaneous lesions called gummata are destructive ulcers and tumors of the skin, bone, or liver which occur in 17 percent of untreated syphilitic patients (Fig. 77-3). Approximately 10 percent of these patients develop the most serious complication of syphilis, which is cardiovascular disease with associated thoracic aneurysms. This development is usually fatal. Another 10 percent develop neurosyphilis, which can cause strokes, personality changes, paresis, ataxia, areflexia, and paresthesia.

Congenital syphilis

Congenital syphilis is acquired by the fetus in utero. *Treponema pallidum* can cross the placenta from the

FIGURE 77-2
Brownish macules over the palms in secondary syphilis.

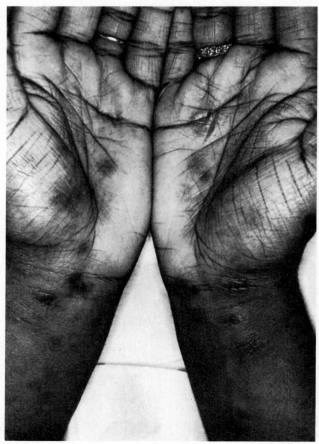

PLATES

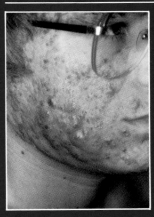

1. Acne grade IV, conglobata. Cysts and scars.

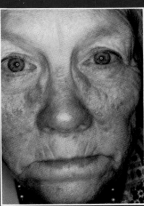

2. Acne rosacea. Central facial erythema and pustules.

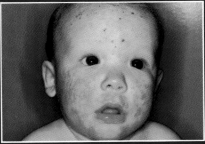

3. Infantile eczema. Weeping, erythematous patches.

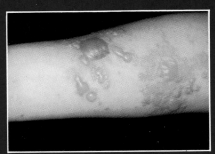

4. Poison ivy. Vesicles in linear and grouped configuration.

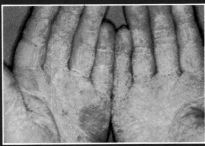

5. Hand eczema. Scaliness, fissures.

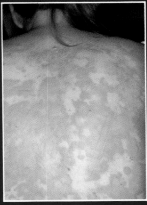

6. Urticaria. Annular and arciform wheals.

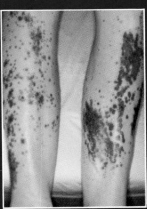

7. Vasculitis. Hemorrhagic, necrotic patches and papules.

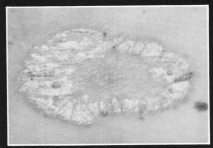

8. Psoriasis. Sharply marginated plaque with thick white scale.

PLATES

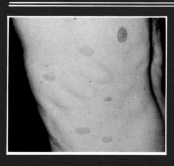

9. Pityriasis rosea. Oval shaped patches on the trunk. [From T.B. Fitzpatrick et al. (eds.), *Dermatology in General Medicine*, 2d ed., McGraw-Hill, New York, 1979.]

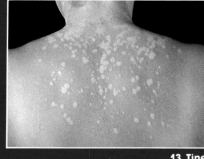

13. Tinea versicolor. Whitish, scaly, confluent macules. [From T.B. Fitzpatrick et al. (eds.), *Dermatology in General Medicine*, 2d ed., McGraw-Hill, New York, 1979.]

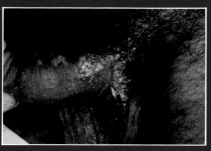

10. Chronic **herpes simplex** in an acquired immune deficiency syndrome (AIDS) patient. Chronic ulceration 3 months in duration with positive herpetic culture.

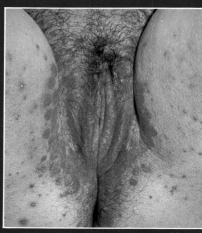

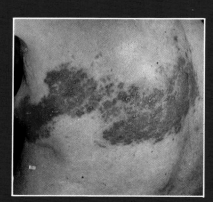

11. Herpes zoster. Linear vesicles on erythematous base along one dermatome. [From T.B. Fitzpatrick et al. (eds.), *Dermatology in General Medicine,* 2d ed., McGraw-Hill, New York, 1979.]

14. Intertriginous candidiasis. Sharply marginated, scaly plaque and satellite pustules. [From T.B. Fitzpatrick et al. (eds.), *Dermatology in General Medicine*, 2d ed., McGraw-Hill, New York, 1979.]

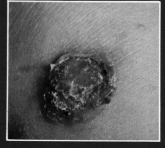

15. Impetigo. Crusts, erosion, moist patch. [From T.B. Fitzpatrick et al. (eds.), *Dermatology in General Medicine,* 2d ed., McGraw-Hill, New York, 1979.]

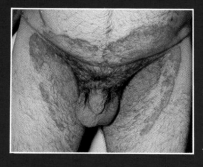

12. Tinea cruris. Peripheral extension of sharply marginated plaques. [From T.B. Fitzpatrick et al. (eds.), *Dermatology in General Medicine,* 2d ed., McGraw-Hill, New York, 1979.]

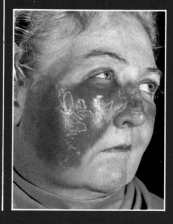

16. Facial erysipelas. Bright red, sharply marginated, painful, hot lesion. [From T.B. Fitzpatrick et al. (eds.), *Dermatology in General Medicine,* 2d ed., McGraw-Hill, New York, 1979.]

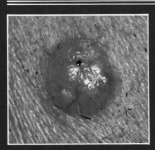

17. Basal cell carcinoma. Early nodule with pearly appearance and peripheral telangiectatic vessels. [From T.B. Fitzpatrick et al. (eds.), *Dermatology in General Medicine*, 2d ed., McGraw-Hill, New York, 1979.]

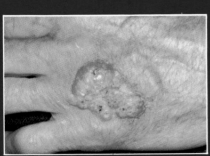

18. Early squamous cell carcinoma. Erythematous, infiltrating, ulcerated tumor on sun-exposed area.

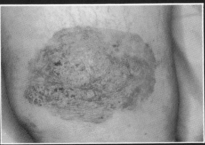

19. Bowen's disease. Erythematous, irregular in configuration, scaly patch on sun-exposed area.

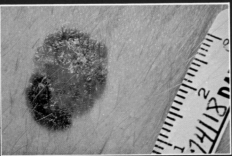

20. Superficial spreading melanoma. Variegated colors, infiltration of surrounding skin with diffusion of pigment. [From T.B. Fitzpatrick et al. (eds.), *Dermatology in General Medicine*, 2d ed., McGraw-Hill, New York, 1979.]

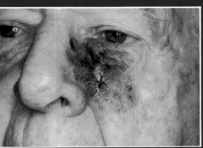

21. Lentigo maligna melanoma. Brown, black patch with central black nodule of melanoma arising.

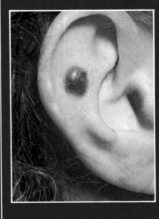

22. Blue nevus. Blue, uniform color of a benign nevus. [From T.B. Fitzpatrick et al. (eds.), *Dermatology in General Medicine*, 2d ed., McGraw-Hill, New York, 1979.]

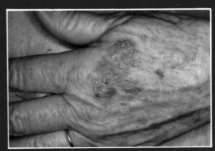

23. Actinic keratosis. Erythematous, scaly, firm on papulation plaque.

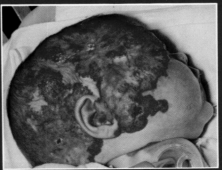

24. Extensive capillary ("strawberry") hemangioma. [From T.B. Fitzpatrick et al. (eds.), *Dermatology in General Medicine*, 2d ed., McGraw-Hill, New York, 1979.]

PLATES

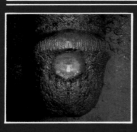

25. Primary syphilis. Painless ulcerated papule. [From T.B. Fitzpatrick et al. (eds.), *Dermatology in General Medicine*, 2d ed., McGraw-Hill, New York, 1979.]

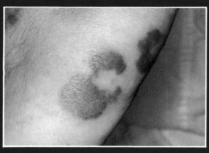

26. Kaposi sarcoma. Hemorrhagic, violaceous tumor of the dermis.

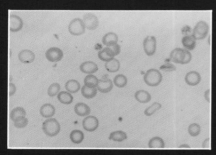

27. Hypochromic, microcytic red cells characteristic of **iron deficiency anemia.** Poikilocytosis is seen. 1000x. (Courtesy of Dr. Koichi Maeda, Henry Ford Hospital, Detroit, Mich.)

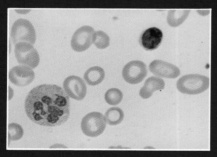

28. Peripheral blood findings seen in **megaloblastic anemia.** A hypersegmented neutrophil and macroovalocytic red cells are evident. (Courtesy of Dr. Sheikh M. Saeed, Div. Head Hematopathology, Henry Ford Hospital, Detroit, Mich.)

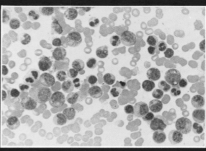

29. Bone marrow characteristic of **chronic granulocytic leukemia.** Marrow is hypercellular with an increase in the granulocytic line. 500x. (Courtesy of Dr. Koichi Maeda, Henry Ford Hospital, Detroit, Mich.)

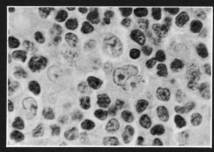

30. Reed-Sternberg cell—giant binucleated cell in the center typically seen in **Hodgkin's disease.** Small mature lymphocytes are seen in the background. To the left of the Reed-Sternberg cell is an eosinophil containing red-orange cytoplasmic granules. (Courtesy of Dr. Koichi Maeda, Henry Ford Hospital, Detroit, Mich.)

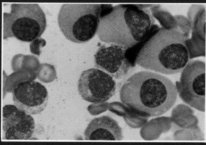

31. Bone marrow aspirate depicting cells seen in **multiple myeloma.** (Courtesy of Dr. Sheikh M. Saeed, Div. Head Hematopathology, Henry Ford Hospital, Detroit, Mich.)

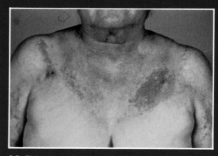

32. This woman has **acute onset dermatomyositis.** An erythematous eruption is prominent in a mantle distribution of light-exposed areas. Talengiectiasia are present. Marked inflammatory changes have caused a breakdown in the skin in several areas. (Reprinted from the Revised Clinical Slide Collection on the Rheumatic Diseases copyright 1981. Used by permission of the Arthritis Foundation.)

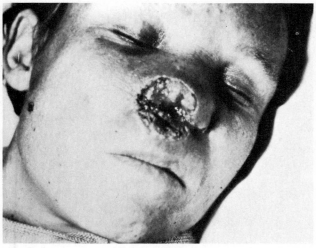

FIGURE 77-3
Cutaneous gumma presenting as an ulcer over the nose.

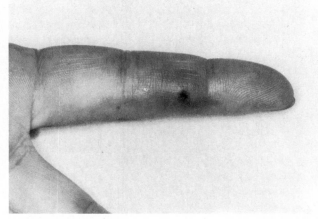

FIGURE 77-4
Necrotic pustules over the palms are characteristic of disseminated gonorrhea.

mother to the fetus after the eighteenth week of pregnancy. Infection of the fetus, which occurs in the second trimester, results in late congenital syphilis. Newborns fail to thrive and develop mulberry molars (extra cusps), saber shins, interstitial keratitis, neural deafness, frontal bossing, and saddlenose. If infection occurs in the last trimester, the infant is born with a hemorrhagic nasal discharge known as snuffles and hepatosplenomegaly, fever, and lymphadenopathy. Many of these infants die within weeks after birth. A positive FTA-ABS immunoglobulin M antibody test establishes the diagnosis, since the IgM antibody cannot cross the placenta.

Treatment

Penicillin is the most effective therapy for primary, secondary, latent, tertiary, and congenital syphilis. Primary, secondary, and early latent stages are treated with a single injection of 2.4 million U of benzathine penicillin G. Treatment of tertiary syphilis requires a large amount of penicillin—7.2 to 9.6 million U divided into four weekly doses. Congenital syphilis is also treated with benzathine penicillin, 50,000 U per kilogram of body weight. Tetracycline and erythromycin are used in the treatment of patients allergic to penicillin. Treatment of syphilis must be followed by serial VDRL tests every 3 months for 1 year to confirm the cure. Patients treated with penicillin therapy must be informed that the unpleasant symptoms of Jarisch-Herxheimer reaction may occur. This reaction is likely due to a rapid release of antigenic material after spirochetes are killed by penicillin. The reaction intensifies skin lesions and causes fever and malaise within 12 hours of treatment; it subsides after 24 hours. All patients must be observed for at least 30 minutes following a penicillin injection, to watch for possible systemic anaphylactic reactions.

GONORRHEA

Approximately 2 million people in the United States have gonorrhea, and the disease is increasing in prevalence. Gonorrhea is caused by the bacterium *Neisseria gonorrhoeae*. Symptoms of the disease, when they occur, consist in males of a painful discharge from the urethra, accompanied by painful urination (dysuria) which occurs 3 to 10 days after contact. In women, cervical discharge can be frequently asymptomatic. Local spread of the gonococcus can cause pelvic inflammatory disease. Pharyngeal and rectal gonorrhea have increased in frequency. Untreated gonorrhea can progress to disseminated, septic gonococcal septicemia, in which scattered hemorrhagic, necrotic pustules can be observed on the skin (Fig. 77-4). The lesions have a predilection to occur over the joints, fingers, and palms. Arthralgia, fever, arthritis, and tenosynovitis accompany the cutaneous lesions. Disseminated gonorrhea is much more common in women, since many women have asymptomatic cervical gonorrhea.

Unlike syphilis, there is no serologic test to confirm the diagnosis of gonorrhea. The diagnosis is confirmed by smear and culture of the purulent urethral or cervical material. Since the disease can be asymptomatic, there are many carriers of this disease who spread it for years by sexual contact. In the case of disseminated systemic gonorrhea, cultures must be obtained from the cervix, urethra, pharynx, rectum, and blood.

Treatment

Treatment of localized urethral or cervical gonorrhea is intramuscular procaine penicillin at a dose of 4.8 million U with 1 g of oral probenecid. The gonococcus organism is sometimes resistant to penicillin. Intravenous penicillin is sometimes required in disseminated gonorrhea. Recently, oral ampicillin in combination with probenecid has been effective in disseminated gonorrhea. Tetracycline, spectinomycin, ampicillin, and erythromycin are other antibiotics effective in gonorrhea.

Cultures for gonorrhea should be repeated 2 and 4 weeks following treatment. Every patient with gonorrhea should be evaluated for presence of syphilis with a serologic VDRL test. Other sexual contacts of both syphilis and gonorrhea patients should be located and treated. The use of rubber prophylactics during intercourse is a reasonably effective way to avoid contracting cervical gonorrhea.

Among other venereal diseases transmitted through sexual intercourse are chancroid, lymphogranuloma venereum, warts (condyloma acuminatum) (Fig. 77-5), and herpes progenitalis (Fig. 77-6).

ACQUIRED IMMUNE DEFICIENCY SYNDROME (AIDS)

Acquired immune deficiency syndrome is a clinical diagnosis. Patients with this syndrome have opportunistic infections and/or cancer. Although anyone can contact AIDS, 73 percent of U.S. cases occur in homosexual or bisexual men (4 among every 3000 homosexuals). AIDS is also seen in past or present intravenous drug abusers (17 percent), hemophiliacs (1 among every 1000 hemophiliacs), Haitians, sexual partners of persons at increased risk (1 percent), and infants born to parents at increased risk.

It is transmitted following heterosexual or homosexual intercourse or through blood. There have been no documented cases of AIDS transmission to medical personnel, family, or household members caring for AIDS patients. A cause of AIDS is a T-lymphotropic virus, Type III (HTV-III) with an incubation period varying between 6 months and 5 years. Patients with AIDS develop diarrhea; lymphadenopathy; fever; fatigue; opportunistic infections of the lungs, usually secondary to *Pneumocystis carinii*; and disseminated cytomegalovirus infections. Immunological abnormalities can be detected by simple office procedures which test for persistent lymphopenia and skin allergy to mumps and *Candida* antigens.

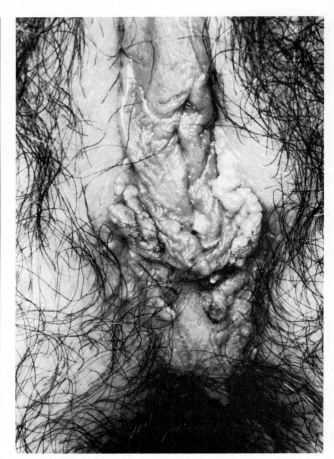

FIGURE 77-5
Verrucous, moist nodules of condyloma acuminatum of the vulva.

Localized symptoms of AIDS are frequently cutaneous. A neoplasm called Kaposi's sarcoma presents with purplish, hemorrhagic patches, plaques, and nodules (Plate 26). Anogenital herpes appears with persistent, chronic ulcerations over the penis, vulva, or buttocks (Plate 10). Mouth soreness and dysplagia are caused by candidiasis.

FIGURE 77-6
Grouped, painful vesicles in herpes progenitalis.

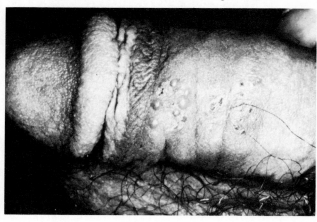

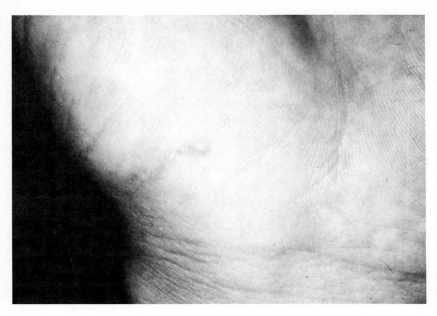

FIGURE 77-7
Linear, pruritic papules of scabies on the wrist with a typical linear burrow.

Mortality related to AIDS is 100 percent within 2 to 3 years, usually secondary to disseminated cytomegalovirus infection. The prognosis in milder cases of AIDS seems much better. There is no effective treatment, but two experimental drugs (interleukin-2 and gamma interferon) have been used. The major steps to prevent spread of AIDS are sexual precautions, a policy of not sharing blood-contaminated objects, and careful screening of blood donors. Reasonable isolation precautions should be followed by hospital workers who take care of AIDS patients.

INFECTIONS AND BITES

Bites are not generally included with venereal diseases. However, some mites can be transmitted through sexual contact. These include scabies and pediculosis pubis. Other bites described in this chapter include those from pediculosis capitis, fleas, chiggers, bedbugs, and ticks.

Scabies is a common infestation caused by the mite *Sarcoptes scabiei*. It is transmitted by close human contact. The infection is especially common among chil-

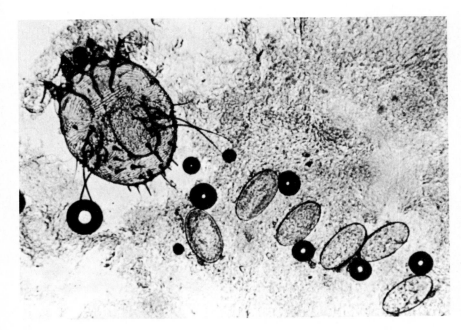

FIGURE 77-8
Microscopic examination of scraped scabies reveals a mite and multiple eggs.

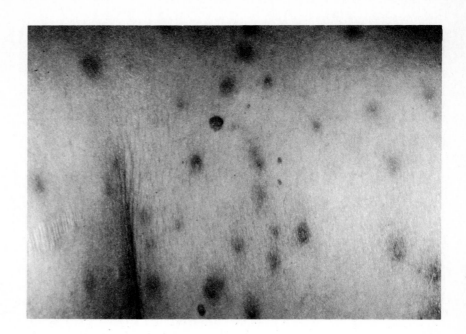

FIGURE 77-9
Multiple pubic lice located in the suprapubic area.

dren and sexually active adults. Pruritus is the chief complaint of these patients. Excoriated linear papules and vesicles are classically found between the fingers and over the elbows, wrists, breasts, and genitalia (Fig. 77-7). Scabies must be suspected if one or more family members develop nocturnal pruritus. The diagnosis is confirmed by microscopic demonstration of the female mite and/or hatching larvae from a skin scraping (Fig. 77-8). Occasionally, the microscopic examination is negative for scabies. Treatment consists of application of gamma benzene hexachloride (Kwell) for two 24-hour periods. Children under 5 years of age are treated for a limited time with crotamiton (Eurax). Secondary irritant eczema can complicate the treatment and result in persistence of pruritus. All family members must be treated prophylactically overnight with gamma benzene hexachloride or crotamiton, even if they present no evidence of scabietic lesions or pruritus.

Pediculosis pubis (pubic crabs) is a frequent infection of the pubic hair and skin. The infection is transmitted by human contact. Lice and nits, which attach to the pubic hair and can be seen with the naked eye, cause intense pruritus (Fig. 77-9). *Pediculosis capitis* (head lice) is caused by lice which are transmitted from person to person and which often cause epidemics, particularly in schools. Pruritus usually is the only complaint. Kwell shampoo is the treatment of choice for both types of louse infestations. Patients are instructed to apply the shampoo two times. Nits may also be removed with a fine-toothed comb soaked in vinegar.

Flea bites are caused by animal fleas which live on pets and furniture, carpeting, etc. A flea bites a person and then leaves the skin; the usual result is a group of erythematous papules with central puncta, which are localized to the lower extremities (Fig. 77-10). Only some family members may react with pruritus and clinical le-

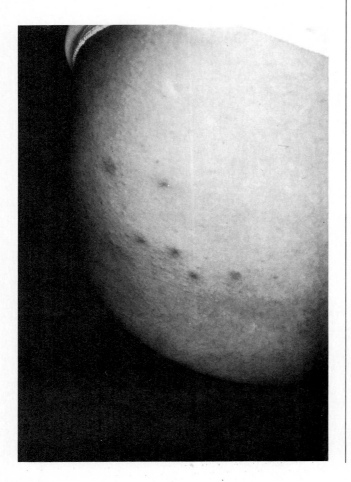

FIGURE 77-10
Grouped erythematous papules secondary to flea bites over the knee area.

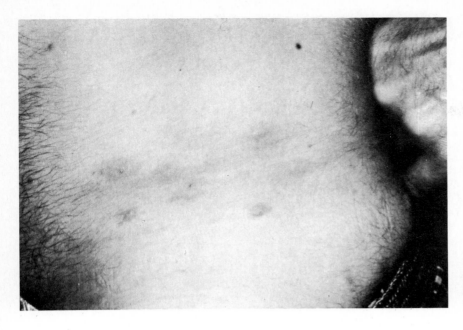

FIGURE 77-11
Erythematous, urticarial papules secondary to chigger bites over the trunk.

sions, even though all members are bitten. Household furniture (e.g., carpeting) and pets must be fumigated. Bites are treated symptomatically with topical steroids and oral antihistaminics.

Chiggers bite from July through September. The bites usually occur in lines under tight-fitting clothing. Multiple pruritic, erythematous papules or vesicles with central puncta are observed (Fig. 77-11). Symptomatic relief from these bites with antipruritics and topical corticosteroids is usually helpful.

Bedbugs live in wood surfaces near beds or in bed-

ding. Bites occur during the night and characteristically appear as grouped vesicles and erythematous papules. Extermination of the bedbugs is required, and clinical lesions are treated symptomatically.

Ticks live in forests, grass, and on animals. Once attached to the skin, the tick will engorge itself with blood and remain attached. It can be removed by use of forceps. Ticks can transmit viral encephalitis and Rocky Mountain spotted fever. When visiting certain areas, people should be warned about the possibility of developing Rocky Mountain spotted fever.

QUESTIONS

Venereal diseases and infestations

Directions: Answer the following questions on a separate sheet of paper.

1. What is the causative organism in syphilis?

2. What is the usual course of the infectious process of syphilis without treatment?

3. Describe the treatments for primary, secondary, early latent, and tertiary syphilis.

4. When the diagnosis of gonorrhea is confirmed by culture, what is the usual treatment?

5. Identify for autoimmune deficiency syndrome the probable causes, modes of transmission, signs and symptoms, and treatments.

Directions: Circle the letter preceding each item below that correctly answers the question. More than one answer may be correct.

6. Which of the following should always be included in a differential diagnosis of syphilis?
   a. Tinea versicolor   *b.* Pityriasis rosea   *c.* Acne   *d.* Seborrheic keratosis

7. One sign of primary syphilis which develops at the site of the infection about 3 weeks following initial contact is:
   a. Skin rash   *b.* Painless chancre   *c.* Painful ulcers   *d.* Pruritus

8. The principal test to positively confirm early primary syphilis is the:
   a. Fluorescent treponemal-antibody absorption (FTA-ABS) test   *b.* Dark-field examination   *c.* VDRL test   *d.* KOH preparation

9. Which of the following statements are true of secondary syphilis?
   a. It develops several months to many years later

b. One hundred percent of those affected develop skin eruption and positive serology   *c.* Untreated, it almost always leads to cardiovascular syphilis

10. Which of the following are some signs and symptoms of tertiary syphilis?
    a. Gummata on the skin, bones, or liver
    b. Ataxia (loss of coordination and reflexes) and dementia (as a result of central nervous system involvement)   *c.* Aortic aneurysms (as a result of cardiovascular involvement)   *d.* Malignant tumors (as a result of gastrointestinal involvement)

11. Gonorrhea infections are increasing because:

a. The majority of women with the disease are asymptomatic   *b.* The incubation period for the causative organism is only 3 to 10 days   *c.* Males can be asymptomatic carriers of the disease
d. The gonococcus organism is usually resistant to penicillin

Directions: Circle T if the statement is true and F if it is false. Correct the false statements.

12.   T   F   A common cause of nocturnal pruritus around the pubic area is scabies.

13.   T   F   Treatment with gamma benzene hexachloride destroys pubic lice.

14.   T   F   Pediculosis capitis is transmitted from person to person and may result in epidemics, particularly in schools.

REFERENCES FOR PART XII

ARNDT, K. A.: *Manual of Dermatological Therapeutics,* 3d ed., Little, Brown, Boston, 1983.

BREATHNACH, A. S. and K. WOLFF: "Structure and Development of Skin," in T. B. Fitzpatrick et al. (eds.), *Dermatology in General Medicine,* 2d ed., McGraw-Hill, New York, 1979, pp. 41–84.

CALLEN, J. P.: *Cutaneous Aspects of Internal Disease,* Year Book, Chicago, 1981.

———: "Squamous Cell Carcinoma of the Skin," *Primary Care,* 5(2):299–311, 1978.

———, M. A. STAWISKI, and J. J. VORRHEES: *Manual of Dermatology,* Year Book, Chicago, 1980.

Centers for Disease Control: "Annual Summary 1982: Reported Morbidity and Mortality in the United States," *Morbidity, Mortality Weekly Report,* 31(54):77–82, 1983.

CHANDA, J. J.: "Primary Cutaneous Malignant Melanoma," *Primary Care,* 5(2):325–337, 1978.

——— and J. P. CALLEN: "Erythema Multiforme and the Stevens-Johnson Syndrome," *Southern Medical Journal,* 71(1):566–570, 1978.

DEMIS, D. J., R. L. DOBSON, and J. I. McGUIRE: *Clinical Dermatology,* Harper & Row, Hagerstown, Md., 1972.

DOMONKOS, A. N.: *Andrews' Diseases of the Skin: Clinical Dermatology,* 7th ed., Saunders, Philadelphia, 1982.

FISHER, A. A.: *Contact Dermatitis,* 2d ed., Lea & Febiger, Philadelphia, 1973.

FITZPATRICK, T. B., et al. (eds.): *Dermatology in General Medicine,* 2d ed., McGraw-Hill, New York, 1979.

KLIGMAN, A. M. and G. PLEWIG: "Classification of Acne," *Cutis,* 17(3):520–522, 1976.

LEWIS, G. M. and C. E. WHEELER: *Practical Dermatology,* 3d ed., Saunders, Philadelphia, 1971.

MAIZE, J. C.: "Atopic Dermatitis," *International Journal of Dermatology,* 15(8):555–556, 1976.

MELANBY, K.: *Scabies,* 2d ed., Classey, Hampton, England, 1943.

MONROE, E. W. and H. E. JONES: "Urticaria," *Archives of Dermatology,* 113(1):80–90, 1977.

MOSCHELLA, S. L., D. M. PILLSBURG, and H. J. HURLEY (eds.): *Dermatology,* Saunders, Philadelphia, 1975.

NAHMIAS, H. J.: "Herpes Simplex Virus Infection. Present Status of Diagnosis and Management," *Southern Medical Journal,* 68(10):1191–1194, 1975.

NASEMANN, J., W. SAUERBERY, and W. BURGDORF: *Fundamentals of Dermatology,* Springer-Verlag, New York, 1983.

ROOK, A., D. S. WILKINSON, and F. J. G. EBLING (eds.): *Textbook of Dermatology,* Blackwell, Oxford, 1979.

SHELLEY, W. B.: *Consultations in Dermatology with Walter B. Shelley,* vols. 1–2, Saunders, Philadelphia, 1973.

SOTER, N. A.: "Clinical Presentations and Mechanisms of Necrotizing Angitis of the Skin," *Journal of Investigative Dermatology,* 67(1):354–359, 1977.

———, D. S. WILKINSON, and T. B. FITZPATRICK: "Clinical Dermatology," pt. 1, *New England Journal of Medicine,* 289(4):189–195, 1973.

———, ———, and ———: "Clinical Dermatology," pt. 2, *New England Journal of Medicine,* 289(5):242–249, 1973.

———, ———, and ———: "Clinical Dermatology," pt. 3, *New England Journal of Medicine*, **289**(6):296–302, 1973.

STAWISKI, M. A.: "Basal Cell Carcinoma," *Primary Care*, **5**(2):283–297, 1978.

———: "Gonorrhea," *Michigan Medical Center Journal* **40**:72–73, 1974.

——— and H. V. DUBIN: "Diagnosis and Treatment of Syphilis," *Michigan Medical Center Journal*, **40**:67–71, 1974.

ANSWERS

CHAPTER 1

General concepts of disease—health versus disease

1. *Pathology* is the science or study of disease. It includes study of the pathogenesis of disease and the structural and functional alterations which result from disease. Pathology is literally abnormal biology, the study of sick or disordered life. *Pathophysiology* is a science that emphasizes disease of living organisms. It is concerned with the disruption of normal physiology; with the alterations, derangements, and mechanisms involved in disruption and how they are manifested as signs, symptoms and as physical and laboratory findings. Pathophysiology provides the basic link between the sciences of anatomy, physiology, and chemistry and their application to clinical practice.

2. *Anatomic pathology* is the study of the morphology of cells, organs, and tissues in disease. Clinical pathology refers to the application of laboratory techniques to the study of disease. Examples of anatomic pathology include surgical pathology, exfoliative cytology, autopsy pathology. Examples of clinical pathology include clinical chemistry, microbiology, hematology, immunology, and immunohematology.

3. *Etiology* refers to the causal agent(s) of disease. *Pathogenesis* is the way disease unfolds, the mechanism of development.

4. The concept of *normalcy* is a complex one and difficult to define succinctly. Selecting any parameter which might be applied to an individual or group, the concept of *normal* involves some average value for that parameter. For example, average values for height and weight are derived from observations on many individuals. Implicitly a certain amount of variation from the average is accepted as being per-

missible or normal. The usual concept of normalcy involves both an average value and some range of variation either above or below that value.

5. *b*
6. *a*
7. *c*
8. *d*

CHAPTER 2

Heredity, environment, and disease; interaction of heredity and environment

1. (a) DNA may instruct a cell to produce a specific chemical product. (b) Other kinds of DNA can instruct cells to develop certain kinds of structures. (c) Portions of the DNA thus determine the limits of the individual's stature, facial features, etc. (d) DNA molecules can instruct the cell to make exact duplicates of themselves when the cell is about to divide.

2. Cellular DNA is arranged in twin strands forming a double helix—the base sequence in one strand complements that of the other. As DNA replicates, the sequence of bases in one strand automatically determines that of the other; the base-paired strands of the double helix separate, and each one is a template for the synthesis of a new complementary strand. Just before a cell divides its DNA content is doubled, so that identical genetic information is passed to each daughter cell.

3. A chromosomal abnormality develops when one or more chromosomes break and the broken ends stick inappropriately to other chromosomes, forming a fused, abnormal chromosome. Another type of abnormality involves failure of separation of the two chromosomes of a given pair during the meiotic re-

duction division which normally leads to 23 chromosomes. A germ cell would be formed with a pair of chromosomes in a particular location instead of a single one, which would result in 24 instead of 23 chromosomes.

4. The prevention of genetic disorders requires the identification of couples who are capable of producing defective genotypes. The task of human genetics is also one of identifying subjects at unusual risk on a genetic basis and minimizing that risk by some environmental manipulation. The genetic counselor must render as accurate a diagnosis as possible. When parental genotypes are determined, the genetic prognosis is usually presented in terms of probability that a given couple will produce an affected offspring. The counselor must make certain that the couple understands the meaning of these absolute figures and the variability in clinical expression. The counselor must possess the ability to explain to the parents, humanely but understandably, the nature and prognosis of the disease and its impact on affected individuals, the mode of treatment available, and the means of preventing the occurrence of the disease.

5. *a, d*

6. *a, c*

7. *a, c, d*

8. *a, d*

9. *c*

10. *b*

11. *b, d*

12. *b, c*

13. *c*

14. *a, c, d*

15. *c*

16. False; these abnormalities cannot be identified by microscopic examination, since the karyotype of the affected individual is normal.

17. True

18. True

19. True

20. False; *transcription* refers to the transfer of genetic information from DNA to messenger RNA.

CHAPTER 3

Cellular injury and death

1. *d*

2. *b*

3. *d*

4. *e*

5. *b*

6. *c*

7. *b*

8. *a*

9. *d*

10. *a*

11. *d*

12. Biochemical, functional, anatomic

13. Dystrophic, metastatic, stone formation

14. Rigor mortis

15. *d*

16. *c*

17. *b*

18. *e*

19. *a*

CHAPTER 4

Response of the body to injury—inflammation and repair

1. *d*

2. *c*

3. *a, b, c*

4. *a, c, e*

5. *b, d*

6. *a, c*

7. *a, b, c*

8. *a, c*

9. *b*

10. *a, c, d*

11. *a, d*

12. *b, c*

13. *c, d*

14. *c*

15. *d*

16. *e*

17. *d*

18. *a*

19. *a, b, d*

20. *a, c*

21. All are correct.

22. *b, c, e*

23. All are correct.
24. *b, d, e*
25. *a, c*
26. *a, b, c*
27. *b, d, e*
28. All are correct.
29. *a, b, c*
30. True
31. False; the host is capable of forming and liberating endogenous substances with a chemotactic effect.
32. True
33. True
34. True
35. True
36. False; it is called a *macrophage.*
37. True
38. True
39. True
40. True
41. False; they are formed by fusion of macrophages.
42. False; this is characteristic of chronic inflammation. Subacute inflammation involves only *early* repair.
43. False; it is caused by abnormal production or remodeling of collagen in the healing wound.
44. True
45. True
46. *b*
47. *e*
48. *a*
49. *d*
50. *c*
51. Abscess
52. Ulcer
53. Empyema
54. Sinus
55. Fistula
56. -itis
57. Margination
58. Emigration
59. Resolution
60. Repair
61. Lymphadenitis
62. *a, b, e, d, c*

CHAPTER 5

Response of the body to immunologic challenge

1. The offending foreign material is neutralized, destroyed, or eliminated from the host more rapidly than would otherwise occur, i.e., in the absence of immunity.

2. Antigens are of relatively high molecular weight. Most antigens are proteins, but polysaccharides, polypeptides, or nucleic acids of large sizes may also function antigenically. Antigens may be chemically pure proteins, or they may be incorporated in complex form as part of the structure of a bacterium, a virus, or a living tissue. In provoking an immunologic response, only certain active portions of the molecule (determinant groups) are essential to the specificity of the reaction. Certain molecules too small to behave as antigens by themselves are able to join chemically with larger molecules within the host, creating molecules which may behave as antigens.

3. (a) Humoral immunity, in which immunoglobulin antibodies are formed, or (b) cellular immunity, in which a population of specifically sensitized lymphocytes is developed; the result in either case is enhanced elimination of the antigen.

4. (a) Self-recognition—these reactions will be mounted only against materials which are sensed as being foreign and will not ordinarily be mounted against constituents of the host's own body. (b) Memory—immunologic reactions proceed more rapidly with repeated introduction of the antigen. (c) Specificity—antibodies whose formation is elicited by a particular antigen react uniquely with that antigen.

5. Some stimulated lymphocytes are capable of secreting lymphokines. Other types of lymphocytes modulate their structure, acquire the cytoplasmic "machinery" of protein synthesis, and produce immunoglobulin antibody. Other lymphocytes undergo "blast formation," that is, they become dividing lymphoblasts, giving rise to expanding numbers of cells having the same properties.

6. When the antigen enters the body, phagocytosis of the antigen by macrophages occurs. The macrophages present the antigen to the B lymphocytes, which have surface receptors to which the antigen binds. The stimulated B lymphocytes differentiate into plasma cells and secrete an antibody which is specific for the original antigen: In the case of most antigens a population of T lymphocytes function as helper cells, influencing B lymphocyte activities. Thus the induction of antibody response generally involves the collaboration of B cells, T cells, and macrophages.

7. Compare your answer with Table 5-1.

8. False; they are filled with blood.

9. True

10. False; the spleen is a major locus of antibody production.

11. False; it is active, not passive, immunization that is described.

12. True

13. False; this is an antibody-mediated, not a cell-mediated, response.

14. True

15. c

16. a

17. e

18. c

19. d

20. a, c

21. d

22. c

23. c

24. d

25. b

26. b

27. d

28. d, e

29. c

30. c

31. b, c

32. a, b

33. a

34. b

35. a

36. a

37. a

38. a

39. b

CHAPTER 6

Response of the body to infectious agents

1. Infection can be said to be present if some microbial agent has been able to adhere to the body surface or to colonize and invade the tissues of the host and then grow and multiply. The presence of infection, however, only indicates the relation of the parasite to the host and does not necessarily indicate disease. Infectious disease is usually manifested by clinical illness. Infection may be totally asymptomatic.

2. *Skin* (especially if traumatized): Ordinarily the mulilayered epithelium, dry keratin layer, and shedding of cells provide a mechanical barrier to infection. The chemical properties of sweat and sebaceous secretions have a mild bactericidal effect, and the normal flora provides a biological barrier.

   Mouth, pharynx, gastrointestinal tract: The entire alimentary canal is lined with mucous membrane, which, along with the protective layer of mucous, provides a mechanical barrier to invasion by microbes. The flow of saliva washes away many microbes mechanically. Rapid peristalsis in the stomach and especially in the small intestine provides another mechanical barrier. The high acidity of the stomach provides an excellent chemical barrier. Finally, the normal flora of the mouth, throat, and especially the large intestine provides a biological barrier to microbial proliferation and invasion. The gastrointestinal mucus contains antibodies which provides immunologic defense.

   Respiratory tract: A mechanical barrier is provided by a layer of mucus covering the surface and the constant action of the cilia, which move the secretions toward the exterior of the body. Antibody is present in respiratory secretions, and motile macrophages in the alveoli engulf and destroy microbes.

   Urinary tract: Defense is provided by the multilayered epithelium and the flushing action of urine flow.

   Eyes: The flow of tears is a defense; antibody also is present in tears.

   The defenses of the body surfaces against microbial invasion are mechanical, chemical, biological (normal flora of each surface area), and immunologic.

3. The microorganisms may spread locally along fascial planes or tubular structures such as a bronchus or ureter. The organisms may be passively carried by the fluid currents of the body. They may spread via lymphatics, ultimately to infect lymph nodes, or may be transferred to another location by a phagocyte if it does not kill the ingested organism. The next step is systemic spread of the microorganisms via the circulating blood. Organisms may even enter blood vessels directly in the local area of initial invasion.

4. If an infectious agent is not contained locally by the inflammatory response or the regional lymph nodes, the microorganisms may enter the systemic blood (bacteremia) and possibly disseminate throughout the body. The phagocytic cells of the monocyte-

macrophage system, chiefly in the liver and spleen, cleanse the blood of the microorganisms.

5. An infectious disease is produced in a debilitated host by an organism ordinarily harmless to a healthy individual with intact defenses.

6. *(a)* Antimicrobial therapy, which would suppress part of the normal flora and allow a normal resident organism to overgrow or might cause the treated person to become very susceptible to an exogenous invader. *(b)* Adrenocorticosteroids, which would be affecting inflammatory and immunologic mechanisms, might allow overgrowth of bacteria which would ordinarily be held in check. *(c)* Radiation therapy and cancer chemotherapy, which might depress the bone marrow and lymphoid tissue, possibly resulting in severe infection. *(d)* Immunosuppressive therapy (used to prevent rejection of a transplanted organ) causes a depression of immune defenses against microbes. *(e)* Unavoidable situations in hospitalized patients—anesthesia, shock, burns, which lower many defenses. *(f)* Primary disease conditions—for example, virus infection of upper respiratory tract, which may be followed by bacterial pneumonia. *(g)* Environmental factors—overcrowding, famine, weather, etc.

7. Bacterial flora modifies the surface on which it grows and by competitive or direct inhibition prevents others potentially more pathogenic microorganisms from establishing residence.

8. Some pathogenic organisms may damage tissue by immunologic means, producing cellular hypersensitivity (tuberculosis), or may produce circulating antigen-antibody complexes (poststreptococcal glomerulonephritis). Others may produce exotoxins or endotoxins. Viruses act as intracellular parasites, altering cellular metabolism and synthetic activity.

9. *d*
10. *c*
11. *b, d*
12. *c*
13. *b*
14. *a*
15. *d*
16. *b*
17. *a*
18. *c*

CHAPTER 7

Disturbances of circulation

1. In active congestion more blood than usual is actively flowing into the area. This increase in local blood flow is accomplished by dilatation of arterioles, which behave as valves governing the flow into the local microcirculation. In passive congestion there is some impairment of drainage of blood from the area. Anything which compresses the venules and veins draining a tissue or otherwise hinders flow may produce passive congestion.

2. When the heart fails in its pumping action, impaired venous drainage results. For example, if the left side of the heart fails in its pumping action, the flow of blood returning to the heart from the lung will be impaired. The blood will be dammed back into the lung, producing passive congestion of the pulmonary vasculature.

3. If the passive congestion is short-lived, there are no effects on the involved tissue. However, in chronic passive congestion there may be permanent effects on the tissue, because in a passively congested area, if the change in blood flow is severe enough, there is an element of tissue hypoxia which may lead to shrinkage or loss of cells of the involved tissue. Also, in many areas there is evidence of local breakdown of red blood cells, which results in the deposition of certain pigments within the tissues. Fibrosis may also ensue.

4. Edema is an accumulation of excess fluid between the cells of the body or within the various body cavities or, according to some, within cells.

5. *c*
6. *c*
7. *a, d*
8. *c*
9. *a, c*
10. *a, b, c*
11. *c*
12. *a, c*
13. *b*

14. The commonest cause of hemorrhage is loss of integrity of vascular walls, permitting the escape of blood. This is most often due to external trauma, as with injuries accompanied by bruising.

15. *(a)* Blood platelet system. With a small hole in the blood vessel, the blood platelets may aggregate over the hole and simply plug it up. *(b)* Blood clotting system. A fibrin clot is formed by the activation of a series of clotting factors in the blood.

16. The local effects of hemorrhage are related to the presence of extravasated blood in the tissues and

can range from trivial to lethal. The most trivial local effect is perhaps a bruise, which may be of only cosmetic importance, whereas a small volume of hemorrhage in a vital area of the brain can produce death. Systemic effects depend on two factors: (a) rate of loss and (b) volume of blood extravasated. If blood loss is rapid, the patient may actually die or may go into a state of hemorrhagic shock. With survival and the passage of time, the patient may develop blood-loss anemia.

17. (a) Thrombosis may result in obstruction of an artery or vein, with possible ischemia or congestion, respectively. (b) It provides a source of possible emboli.

18. (a) Thrombus in an artery, (b) narrowing of an atherosclerotic artery, (c) embolus in an artery, (d) tumor pressing on a vessel.

19. (a) Functional disturbance (pain, such as angina), (b) atrophy of ischemic tissue, (c) infarction of ischemic tissue.

20. c

21. a

22. a

23. c

24. a, c

25. a, b

26. d

27. b

28. a

29. b

30. False; Mönckeberg's sclerosis is not clinically significant; the lining of the involved vessel is not roughened nor is the lumen narrowed.

31. True

32. True

33. False; atherosclerosis is a multifactorial disease.

34. True

35. True

36. False; *infarct* is used to denote tissue necrosis *due to* a circulatory abnormality.

CHAPTER 8

Disturbances of growth, cellular proliferation, and differentiation

1. c

2. d

3. f

4. e

5. a

6. g

7. b

8. b, c

9. b

10. a

11. b

12. b

13. a, c

14. c

15. d

16. c

17. d

18. b, d

19. True

20. False; the current state of knowledge about the existence of immunologic defenses against the neoplasm does not permit the routine widespread use of immunotherapeutic measures.

21. False; this tumor is sometimes referred to as *scirrhous.*

22. True

23. False; this neoplasm is classified as a leiomyosarcoma.

24. False; this smear may be made of any of a variety of body fluids such as gastric aspirates or sputum specimens as well as uterine cervical scrapings.

25. Some causes of atrophy are ischemia, advancing age related to decreasing hormone production (e.g., breast tissue), and disuse (e.g., leg in a cast).

26. The ability to invade normal tissue and the ability to form metastases.

27. Via lymphatic channels; via direct "transplantation," as across serosal cavities (or, in fact, into incisions via surgical instruments); via the bloodstream.

28. Neoplasms can produce a variety of local-mechanical symptoms by impinging upon normal structures, producing obstruction of passages, destroying vital functions, etc. They may ulcerate, may become secondarily infected, or may give rise to hemorrhages. Neoplasms may have endocrine function and produce signs and symptoms on that basis. Advanced malignant growths may produce a state of cachexia.

29. The most important criterion is the distinction between benign and malignant biological behavior.

That is, if a neoplasm has invaded neighboring non-neoplastic tissue or has produced metastases, it is malignant. When neither invasion nor metastasis is evident, a neoplasm can still be classified as malignant if its *potential* for malignant behavior can be predicted on the basis of its microscopic appearance alone; it is known from experience that untreated neoplasms of certain types will invade and metastasize. Also included is the cell type of origin of the neoplasm and the organ of origin of the neoplasm.

30. This concept is not completely understood at the present time. It is thought that the behavior of cancer cells is "antisocial" with regard to normal cells of the body. Malignant cells disobey the usual territorial rules and grow in inappropriate locations. Evidence is beginning to accumulate which indicates that the important abnormalities of cancer cells seem to lie within the cell membrane. On the cell membrane homeostatic signals are received from other cells and from other points in the body and are transmitted to the interior of the cell. Abnormalities in this membrane may result in abnormal reception of control signals or abnormal responses to them. Evidence also indicates that events at the cell membrane are important in controlling cellular proliferation. The antigenic structure of cell membranes is important with regard to the immunologic interactions of the cell with its surroundings.

31. (a) A classic notion is that of somatic mutation, which suggests that the basic carcinogenic event involves a chemical change in the DNA of a cell, that is, a mutation. This type of mutation would involve a nongerm cell, or somatic cell. This theory of mutation would explain the fact that once a cell is transformed into a neoplastic cell, its characteristics breed true, giving rise to an expanding clone of cells with similar properties, determined by the mutated DNA. (b) Another explanation for the expression of malignant behavior is the "addition" of genetic information to the cell by viral infection, with the "new" genetic information being expressed as abnormal cellular behavior. (c) Finally, there is some evidence that malignancy may be a matter of abnormal differentiation, i.e., abnormal and inappropriate expression of genetic information always present in each cell of the body but usually kept repressed except, for instance, in embryonic life.

32. In most instances of human neoplasia the causes are as yet unknown. However, circumstantial and experimental evidence seems to indicate that the environment is the source of most tumorigenic agents. Many chemical substances in the environment are carcinogenic. This is evident from animal experimentation, from the incidence of certain tumors in industrial workers, and from the devastating incidence of lung cancer in cigarette smokers. The role of viruses of various types in tumorigenesis has been elucidated in many species of animals. Genetic factors do seem to be important in neoplasia. Generally there is inheritance not of an overall susceptibility to cancer of various kinds but of an increased likelihood of developing one particular type of tumor or another.

33. The means used include the confirmation of the neoplasm's presence by physical examination and by radiographic, ultrasonographic, and/or endoscopic means. A final step in determining the diagnosis of neoplasm involves morphologic examination based on microscopic features of the tissue. Decisions about treatment are related to the clinical stage of the cancer. The concept of staging is based on the fact that a given type of cancer is likely to manifest a certain progression. Several different modalities of cancer treatment exist, including extirpation of the cancerous tissue surgically, radiotherapy, application of ionizing radiation to the neoplasm, chemotherapy (based on the differential sensitivity of proliferating cancer cells and normal cells to a variety of cytotoxic chemical agents), and immunotherapy. The approach is not limited to the use of a single treatment modality but is based on the needs of the individual patient with a particular neoplasm at a given clinical stage.

CHAPTER 9

Familiar allergic disorders; anaphylaxis and the atopic diseases

1. Hypersensitivity denotes the immunologic capacity, acquired through contact with a specific, chemically characterizable agent, to hyperreact to that agent. The cellular events that follow exposure and establish a capacity for responses of hypersensitivity are termed *sensitization*.

2. Angioedema reflects a localized inflammatory increase in vascular permeability without frank injury to small veins and capillaries, usually reversible within a short period; whereas lymphedema results from abnormal pressures (due to an obstruction to flow upstream) which promote passage to fluid out into tissues.

3. Evidence suggests that clinical anaphylaxis in both animals and humans involves a sudden multifocal reaction of allergen with mast-cell-bound, specific IgE followed by widespread tissue response to the

mediator substances (e.g., histamine, SRS-A, leukotrienes) released.

4. This seems to reflect differences among species in both the distribution of mast cells and relative responsiveness of tissues to mediator substances.

5. This generally requires the injection of potent allergens, although certain gastrointestinal and respiratory parasites also elicit prominent IgE responses. Many persons also make specific IgE responses to mucosal contact and innocuous materials, including foods, pollens, and animal emanations (danders). In addition, individual capacities to overproduce IgE and to respond immunologically to specific antigens also seem to be involved.

6. Efforts to reduce allergen (and irritant) exposure; suppressive medications to mitigate symptom severity nonspecifically; and specific hyposensitization to reduce responsiveness to unavoidable challenge.

7. c
8. d
9. a, c
10. d
11. a, b, d
12. a
13. c
14. b
15. c
16. a, b, c
17. d
18. b, c, d
19. b
20. b
21. d
22. d
23. a
24. a
25. c
26. b
27. a, b, d
28. True
29. True
30. False; strongly positive reactions indicate only the immunologic "apparatus" for response and provide no assurance that symptoms arise from exposure to the allergens in question.
31. False; aqueous extracts are used, and testing by pricking through the skin is *usually* done first; negative reactors are considered for intracutaneous (IC)

tests. However, where IC tests are done exclusively, very dilute materials must be used.

32. True

CHAPTER 10

Bronchial asthma—allergic and otherwise

1. A clinically defined condition marked by recurrent, discrete episodes of reversible bronchial narrowing, separated by periods in which ventilation approaches normal. These events occur in asthma-prone subjects by a variety of stimuli; this denotes a state of bronchial hyperactivity. Asthma is an abnormal pattern of response rather than a discrete disease.

2. Bronchial narrowing produces an increased resistance to airflow, which underlies an inability to achieve normal rates of flow during respiration (especially expiration). This results in uneven lung aeration and a loss of the normal spatial matching of ventilation and pulmonary blood flow. These defects may produce no symptoms or merely a sense of tracheal irritation; alternatively, respiratory distress may be intolerable.

3. Although atopy is implicated in many instances of bronchial asthma, in a substantial number of asthmatic persons, no allergic factors are demonstrated even after exhaustive study. These persons are often said to have "intrinsic" asthma, although their problem is more properly idiopathic. In addition, many allergic (atopic) asthmatic persons also respond adversely to nonallergic factors.

4. Asthmatic airways behave as if their beta-adrenergic innervation were incompetent, and, at least functionally, partial beta blockage seems to exist. Without adequate bronchodilator tone, bronchoconstrictor influences, known to be mediated normally by parasympathetic (cholinergic) and alpha-adrenergic pathways, would tend to predominate. In clinical practice, the bronchial lability of asthmatic patients may be confirmed by demonstrating their brisk airway obstructive responses to extremely *low* concentrations of inhaled histamine and methacholine.

5. Since invading organisms frequently destroy ciliated epithelium and localize agents of inflammation in labile bronchi, their adverse effect on asthma is predictable. In addition, animal studies have suggested that microbial substances may further weaken beta-adrenergic activity.

6. Slowly released oral theophylline preparations allow successful dosing twice (or even once) daily. In general, these preparations also require lower 24-hour drug totals to maintain stable serum levels than more rapidly absorbed formulations. "Long-acting" theophylline preparations have improved patient compliance and promise to become a standard form of therapy.

7. The effectiveness of these agents is thought to reflect *direct* stimulation of an enzyme, adenyl cyclase, which promotes the synthesis of cyclic AMP. Cyclic AMP–induced effects (i.e., relaxation of bronchial smooth muscle and inhibition of mediator release from mast cells and basophils) are promoted both by beta-adrenergic agents and by theophylline, and additive effects of these two groups of drugs often result.

8. When atopic factors are evident, efforts to reduce exposure and immunotherapy for selected inhalant allergens have established merit. Avoidance of irritants—especially tobacco smoke—as well as prompt treatment of unresolved bacterial respiratory infections are of major benefit to asthmatic persons. Perfumes, aerosol cleaners and cosmetics, solvents, and paint fumes also pose avoidable potential risks that must be appreciated. Cold air is a bronchoconstrictor that may be mitigated by wearing a scarf or gauze mask over the nose and mouth. Adding moisture to dry indoor air may be desirable. Programs of regular medication also can effectively reduce bronchial lability and thereby raise the threshold for obstructive airway responses.

9. *d, e*

10. *b*

11. *b, d, e*

12. *b*

13. *e*

14. *c*

15. *b*

16. *a, b, c, d*

17. *a, b, c*

18. *b*

19. *a*

20. *a*

21. False; EIA is most commonly evident in children and characteristically appears in subjects who are symptom-free before beginning exertion.

22. False; other conditions, such as the impaction of a foreign body or growth of a localized tumor in the bronchi, as well as pulmonary emphysema, may lead to diffuse wheezing simulating asthma.

23. True

24. True

25. *b, d*

26. *a, c*

27. *e*

CHAPTER 11

Atopic dermatitis—urticaria

1. (*a*) Ingestants such as egg, fish, shellfish, and nuts, including peanuts; (*b*) drugs and drug metabolites which are capable of stable bonding to proteins (e.g., penicillins) or which are themselves complete antigens; (*c*) many drugs also appear to cause urticaria, though not typical anaphylaxis, by mechanisms exclusive of IgE (e.g., aspirin).

2. Since bouts of hives generally are self-limited and vary in duration as well as severity, the value of treatment measures for affected individuals often is difficult to discern. Epinephrine has demonstrated effectiveness in speeding resolution. Agents such as diphenhydramine and hydroxyzine also are acknowledged to have value in this condition. Adrenal corticosteroids have been beneficial in severe acute hives. Hydroxyzine often is the single most valuable agent in *chronic* urticaria.

3. Hives (urticaria) probably affect at least 25 percent of the population at some time.

4. Treatment modalities for urticaria are difficult to evaluate, because bouts of hives tend to be self-limiting and vary in duration as well as severity.

5. *a*

6. *b*

7. *a, b, d*

8. *a, d*

9. *b*

10. *c*

11. *a, b, c*

12. *c*

13. *d*

14. *a*

15. *b, d*

16. *a*

17. *c, d*

18. *b, d*

19. False; these factors probably act by direct contact with an abraded epidermis but are rarely implicated.

20. True

21. False; these drugs should be reserved for their anti-inflammatory properties, with bland lubricants used to soften and moisten the skin.

22. True

23. False; tars are rarely used today to reduce licheni-fication and cracking. Urea-containing ointments are more cosmetically acceptable agents to promote healing and restoration of skin texture, and topical corticosteroids are quite helpful for this purpose.

24. False; organic solvents that defat normal skin must be avoided.

25. True

26. False; the resemblance of urticarial wheal to IgE-mediated skin reactions has promoted this false inference.

27. True

28. True

CHAPTER 12

Autoimmune and immune complex–induced diseases

1. The appearance of autoantibodies (antibodies reactive with autologous tissue components) denotes a failure of diverse safeguards which normally prevent immune responses to host tissues (autoimmunity). The responsible factors are rarely demonstrable. These autoantibodies have potential for causing tissue damage and are implicated in various illnesses. In addition, they may serve as diagnostic markers of conditions such as lupus erythematosus.

2. In certain instances the inciting antigens are normally sequestered and may remain "foreign" even to mature tissue. These responses could arise following subtle injury incident to microbial invasion. The possibility that infecting bacteria and viruses may produce limited changes in host tissue components rendering them "foreign" to immune surveillance has been proposed. Antibodies (or sensitized lymphocytes) resulting from this process might have specificities broad enough to permit reaction with native as well as modified tissue determinants. Autoimmune phenomena could arise if an invading organism and host tissues shared an antigen or closely similar antigenic groups as a result of parallel evolution. Mutant ("forbidden") clones of lymphoid cells programmed to recognize normal host components as "foreign" could be involved, as well. Such cells might be antigen-specific or non-specific T_4 (helper/promoter lymphocytes) that foster the immune responses of both T and B lymphocytes. Alternatively, a *decline* of suppressor (T_8^+)

lymphocytes that normally inhibit these responses might be implicated.

3. Circulating antibodies, reactive with glomerular and alveolar basement membranes, are usually present and, along with complement components, form linear deposits at these sites in vivo. The associated tissue damage is thought to reflect complement-mediated cytotoxicity and local effects of recruited neutrophils.

4. Chills, fever, and low back pain occasionally preceded by urticaria or flushing, uneasiness, and mild air hunger. When cell lysis is massive, the resulting debris may trigger widespread intravascular clotting with depletion of coagulation factors and bleeding from wounds and venipuncture sites.

5. All the following measures *must* be used to prevent or mitigate hemolytic transfusion reactions:
   a. The source and proper recipient of blood products must be identified.
   b. There must be continual surveillance of persons receiving blood—especially those whose mobility or awareness is impaired.
   c. Any serious suggestive evidence of an incipient reaction should prompt discontinuance of the questioned unit, maintenance of intravenous access, and careful clinical observation.
   d. A carefully drawn venous sample from the recipient should be checked for serum hemoglobin, a sign of intravascular red cell breakdown, and the compatibility of donor and recipient reconfirmed.
   e. *All* materials used for transfusion should be saved to facilitate serological and microbiological testing.
   f. Special precautions to monitor urine output are essential, and examination of serial centrifuged specimens for hemoglobin may be instructive, since clearance of serum hemoglobin is rapid.
   g. Maintenance of adequate hydration and urine flow are important considerations in all survivors, and osmotic diuresis with cautiously administered IV mannitol may help in achieving this goal.
   h. Safe fluid therapy demands precise and regular evaluation of cardiopulmonary and renal function. Measures to combat shock, pulmonary edema, acute renal failure, and/or defibrination with bleeding may be required.

6. (a) Recipients of leukoagglutinins have developed fever, cough, shortness of breath, and lung shadows

on chest x-ray; several days have been required for full resolution. Persons deficient in IgA also may suffer severe reactions from transfused IgA in plasma as a result of antibodies formed to this immunoglobulin. These episodes often resemble anaphylaxis, with dyspnea, flushing, abdominal cramps and diarrhea, fever, and chills. *(b)* The latter reactions may be averted by using IgA-deficient donors or thoroughly washed red blood cells.

7. False; platelets and red blood cells are attacked predominantly.
8. True
9. True
10. True
11. False; viral invasion may damage $T_8{}^+$ suppressor cells that normally repress T and B cell responses to "self" components.
12. *a, d*
13. *c*
14. *c*
15. *c*
16. *b*
17. *c*
18. *a, c*
19. *e*
20. *a, c*
21. *b, c*
22. *c, d*
23. *a, d*
24. *d*
25. *b*
26. *a, d*

CHAPTER 13

Adverse reactions to drugs and related substances

1. *a, c, d*
2. *a, c*
3. *c*
4. *a, b*
5. *b*
6. *c, d*
7. *a, b*
8. False; since this response to injected antigens is to

be expected in most persons, it is not confined to the atopic population.

9. True
10. True
11. *a, c*
12. *b, c, d*
13. *e*
14. *b, d*
15. *c*
16. Initially complexes of host IgG or IgM and drug (or drug protein conjugate) become attached to one or more blood cell types. Complement components are localized to the cell surface, and their interaction results in discrete membrane lesions, the formed elements being injured as "innocent bystanders" rather than direct participants. Following fixation of complement factors, the immune complexes often dissociate from affected membranes.

17. *(a)* Syncope, hypotension, cardiac rhythm disturbances, and, at times, convulsions. *(b)* These reactions are probably a direct toxic effect of the large doses required for local infiltration.

18. a. An effective approach to the prevention of adverse drug reactions requires knowledge of the potential complications of medication and a willingness to consider adverse drug reactions as a possible cause of *any* unexpected clinical event.

    b. Since untoward responses usually are repetitive, no drug should be given without first assessing the individual's past experience with that agent. The clinical data base requires no less than a comprehensive assessment of past drug reactivity. Health care personnel must also be prepared to accept, at face value, reports of past problems arising from medication until these have been disproved conclusively.

    c. Close surveillance can reveal the earliest stigmata of drug reactions, facilitating prompt withdrawal of the offender and, often, abbreviating morbidity. Once recognized, adverse reactivity must be clearly indicated in the clinical record and, if possible, the sensitivity identified for the patient or responsible family members. Documentation is aided if the patient carries a card, bracelet, or medallion indicating medication(s) to be avoided. Exhaustive instruction is necessary where a risk of reaction from related agents exists or when the offender has many readily available, poorly identified sources.

CHAPTER 14

Approaches to immune deficiency states

1. *d*
2. *c, d*

3. *c*

4. *a, b, c*

5. True

6. False; selective deficit of IgA.

7. True

8. False; T cell defects are generally more evident.

9. False; relatively complete absence of T cell function occurs selectively when the thymus fails to develop.

10 True

11. (a) Determination of naturally occurring (IgM) antibodies to ABO blood group substances absent from the subject's red cells. Normal persons consistently demonstrate such isohemagglutins by the age of 1 year. (b) Schick testing of persons previously immunized with diphtheria toxoid. If adequate levels of (IgG) specific antibody have been produced, tissue breakdown at the site of toxin injection is prevented. (c) Determination of antibody titers before and after nonviable immunizing materials such as tetanus toxoid and typhoid vaccine.

12. Intradermal injections are performed with 0.1-ml portions of substances which elicit DTH and to which a previous sensitizing exposure may be assumed; commonly used materials include PPD (of the tubercle bacillus), streptokinase and streptodornase, enzymes of beta-hemolytic streptococci, etc. Test sites are observed and palpated after 48 hours, and an indurated area with a diameter of 10 mm or larger generally is regarded as a positive reaction. Using a battery of such materials, at least one positive test should be evident in the vast majority of normal persons (excluding infants). For nonreactors, a more stringent test of cellular competence is provided by attempting contact sensitization with dinitrochlorobenzene (DNCB), although this test is now usually deferred in favor of determinations of T cell subsets.

13. (a) Response of lymphocytes in short-term tissue culture to antigens and nonspecific agents that stimulate cell division and associated nucleic acid synthesis. An increase in the incorporation of thymidine tagged with tritium is observed normally in response to these agents. (b) Peripheral aggregation of sheep red blood cells around human peripheral (T) lymphocytes when the two are mixed and incubated. Normally, over 60 percent of lymphocytes demonstrated rosetting, although a teleological basis for the sheep cell receptor is unknown. (c) Assays of lymphokines produced in response to appropriate antigens added to lymphocyte preparations. To date, most studies have focused on the macrophage-inhibiting factor (MIF), and defects at several stages prior to its release have been described.

CHAPTER 15

The composition of the blood and the monocyte-macrophage system

1. A science which deals with blood and the blood-forming tissues. It is the study of blood, its nature, function, and disease.

2. Red blood cells (erythrocytes, red corpuscles, or RBCs); white blood cells (leukocytes, white corpuscles, or WBCs); platelets (or thrombocytes).

3. Since red blood cells, white blood cells, and platelets have a finite life span, a constant optimum production is necessary to maintain levels required to meet tissue needs. In adults, this production, which is called *hematopoiesis* (formation and maturation of blood cells), takes place in the bone marrow of the skull, vertebrae, pelvis, sternum, ribs, and proximal epiphyses of the long bones. However, during periods of increased demand (e.g., hemorrhage or cell destruction), production may resume in all the bones, as is normal in children. All normal cells are thought to derive from a single pluripotential *stem cell*. The stem cell can differentiate into lymphoid and hematopoietic stem cells which become progenitor cells. Progenitor cells differentiate along a single pathway. Through a series of divisions and maturational changes, these cells become specific mature cells in the circulating blood.

4. A complete history or profile (i.e., past and current illnesses, drug exposure, bleeding tendencies, nutritional habits, family history), physical assessment, and selective diagnostic studies. These studies attempt to quantitate the various constituents of blood and bone marrow.

5. *c*

6. *c*

7. *d*

8. *b*

9. *b*

10. *a, b, d*

11. *c*

12. *d*

13. *a*

14. *g*

15. *b*

16. *e*

17. *i*

18. *c*

19. *j*
20. *h*
21. *f*
22. False; men, 4.7–6.1; women, 4.2–5.2
23. True
24. True
25. False; 4000–10,000
26. False; 150,000–400,000
27. True

CHAPTER 16

The red blood cell

1. The major component of the red blood cell is the protein hemoglobin, which transports O_2 and CO_2 and maintains the normal pH through a series of intercellular buffers. The Hb molecule consists of two pairs of polypeptide chains (globin) and four heme groups, each one containing an atom of ferrous iron. This configuration allows the most expedient exchange of gases.

2. It is postulated that red blood cell production is stimulated by a glycoprotein, erythropoietin, believed to originate in the kidney. It is theorized that erythropoietin production is influenced by tissue hypoxia due to such factors as changes in atmospheric O_2, decreased O_2 content of arterial blood, and decreased hemoglobin concentration. The stem cells committed to erythrocyte production appear to be the targets of erythropoietin and initiate proliferation and maturation of red blood cells.

3. *Anemia* is a reduction below the normal level in the number of red blood cells, the quantity of hemoglobin, and the volume of packed red blood cells (hematocrit) per 100 ml of blood.

4. Pallor (nail beds, palms, mucous membranes of the mouth and conjunctivae), tachycardia, shortness of breath, dyspnea, headache, dizziness, faintness, tinnitus.

5. *(a)* Increased red blood cell loss: direct loss from the circulation through bleeding. Bleeding from trauma or ulcers, polyps in the colon, malignant growth, hemorrhoids, menstruation. *(b)* Destruction of red blood cells in the circulation (hemolysis). Hemoglobinopathies (inherited abnormal hemoglobin): sickle cell disease, impaired globin synthesis, thalassemia; red cell membrane defects: hereditary spherocytosis; enzyme deficiencies: glucose 6-phosphate dehydrogenase (G6PD) deficiency.

6. *(a)* Normocytic, normochromic anemia: red blood cells are of normal size and shape, contain the normal amount of hemoglobin (MCV and MCHC are normal or low-normal). Examples are acute blood loss, hemolysis, renal disease, and metastatic infiltrative diseases of the bone marrow. *(b)* Macrocytic, normochromic anemia: red blood cells are larger than normal but are normochromic because the hemoglobin concentration is normal (MCV is increased, MCHC is normal). Examples are deficiency states of vitamin B_{12} and/or folic acid; cancer chemotherapy. *(c)* Microcytic, hypochromic anemia: *microcytic* means small, *hypochromic* means containing less than the normal amount of hemoglobin (MCV and MCHC are decreased). Examples are iron-deficiency anemia, chronic blood loss, and thalassemia.

7. *(a)* Treatment necessitates identification of the cause of the anemia. *(b)* If possible, resolve the underlying cause. *(c)* Start specific treatment only if indicated.

8. Excess *(poly-)* of all the cell lines *(-cythemia)*, but generally used for conditions in which the red cell mass exceeds normal.

9. It may be classified as primary or secondary. *(a)* Primary polycythemia: in polycythemia the pluripotential stem cell is abnormal. There are marked erythrocytosis, leukocytosis, and thrombocytosis. *(b)* Secondary polycythemia: secondary to underlying medical problems such as cardiopulmonary diseases which decrease arterial O_2 saturation, stimulating erythropoiesis, and renal tumors, which increase erythropoietin production.

10. Compare your drawing with Fig. 16-1.

11. Compare your illustration with Fig. 16-6.

12. Normocytic, normochromic

13. Aplastic anemia

14. *c*

15. *a*

16. *c*

17. *b, c*

18. *a*

19. *a, c*

20. *b*

21. *a*

22. *b*

23. *c, d, e, f*

24. *c*

25. *a, d*

26. True

27. True

28. False; 1:600

The white blood cell

1. *d, e*
2. *g, i*
3. *h*
4. *a, e*
5. *c*
6. *b*
7. *f*
8. Granulocytopoietin, or cell-stimulating factor (CSF), is responsible for leukocyte cell differentiation. It is thought that CSF acts directly upon stem cell colony-forming units in the bone marrow, committing them to differentiation to the neutrophil and monocyte lines.
9. Familial leukemia is rare, but there appears to be a higher incidence of leukemia in siblings of affected children, with the incidence increasing to 20 percent in monozygotic (identical) twins. Persons with chromosomal abnormalities seem to have a 20-fold increase in the incidence of acute leukemia.

    Chemicals are being implicated with increased frequency, especially the alkylating agents. There is a likelihood of increased incidence of leukemia in patients treated with both radiation and chemotherapy.
10. A lymphoproliferative disorder associated with plasma cells. This is a malignant disorder that arises in the bone marrow and involves primarily bone.
11. Younger patients: nontender, rubbery-feeling enlarged lymph node in the low cervical or supraclavicular area or a nonproductive cough secondary to hilar adenopathy. Older patients: unexplained fever and/or night sweats; weight loss exceeding 10 percent of body weight.
12. True
13. False; plasma cells do not normally circulate and are found in small numbers in the bone marrow.
14. False; *neutropenia* refers to a decrease in the absolute neutrophil count.
15. True
16. False; 70 percent of the non-Hodgkin's lymphomas are of B cell origin.
17. False; these cells are called *basophils.*
18. Leukemia
19. FAB
20. Reed-Sternberg cells
21. Leukopenia
22. Chronic granulocytic leukemia
23. Neutrophils (neutrophilia), eosinophils (eosinophilia), basophils (basophilia)

24. *b, d*
25. *a, b, d*
26. *d*
27. *c*
28. All are correct.
29. *b*
30. *a, c*
31. *b*
32. All are correct.
33. *a*
34. *i*
35. *b, g*
36. *a, d, g, j*
37. *g, h, j*
38. *f*
39. *c, g*
40. *e*

CHAPTER 18

Coagulation

1. Platelets are derived from a noncommitted pluripotential stem cell, which on demand and in the presence of thrombopoietin differentiates into the committed stem cell pool to form the megakaryoblast. This cell, through a maturation sequence, becomes a megakaryocyte. The cell cytoplasm eventually breaks up into individual platelets.
2. Vasoconstriction is an immediate response to the injury, followed by adhesion of platelets to collagen in the vessel wall exposed by the injury. ADP is released by the platelets, causing them to aggregate. Minute amounts of thrombin stimulate platelet aggregation. Platelet factor III also accelerates plasma clotting. In this way a platelet plug forms. Platelets also play a role in the formation of fibrin and in clot retraction.
3. Factors V and X
4. It is thought that once the platelet level reaches a certain peak level, spontaneous aggregates of platelets occur. In the large vessels this has little effect, but the platelets plug the tiny capillaries. In the process the capillary wall is damaged and there is bleeding into the tissues. Examples of primary thrombocytosis are polycythemia vera and chronic granulocytic leukemia. Examples of secondary thrombocytosis are those occurring temporarily

after stress or exercise with storage pool release from the spleen, or accompanying increased bone marrow demand states (hemorrhage or hemolytic anemia).

5. Treatment is aimed at replacement of the deficient plasma coagulation factors. Teaching patients and their families safety measures and home infusion of factor concentrates at the earliest signs of bleeding has improved the quality of life.

6. *Disseminated intravascular coagulation* refers to a multifaceted complex syndrome in which a normally homeostatic and physiologic system of maintaining fluidity of blood becomes a pathologic system leading to diffuse fibrin thrombi occluding the microvasculature of the body. This syndrome is initiated by the introduction of a procoagulant material or activity into the circulating blood.

7. False; platelets function to maintain capillary integrity and to initiate and retract clots.

8. False; administration of factor VIII.

9. False; factor III (tissue thromboplastin) and factor IV (calcium ion) are the exceptions.

10. True

11. True

12. False; factor VIII is not synthesized by the liver.

13. True

14. False; the partial thromboplastin time (PTT) measures the intrinsic and common pathway.

15. *a*
16. *c*
17. *b*
18. *d*
19. *e*
20. *a*
21. *d*
22. *b*
23. *b, d*
24. *a*
25. *d*
26. *b*
27. *a*
28. *d*
29. *b, d*

CHAPTER 19

The esophagus

1. Transportation of ingested material from the pharynx to the stomach.

2. Lower esophageal closure strength has not developed fully in the infant. In adults, regurgitation reflects both lower esophageal sphincter incompetence and failure of the upper esophageal sphincter to serve as a regurgitation barrier.

3. Varicose veins of the esophagus (enlarged, tortuous veins). Esophageal varices develop in cases of hepatic cirrhosis and portal hypertension because of the communication between the portal and esophageal veins, providing a bypass of the liver to the vena cava. Esophageal varices may rupture, causing a fatal hemorrhage, because they are unable to withstand the high-pressure flow.

4. An *esophagomyotomy* is an operation on the lower esophagus to enlarge the opening into the stomach. A *pyloroplasty* is an operation to repair the pylorus, especially to enlarge the gastric outlet. These procedures are often used to treat achalasia and are often combined, because incompetence of the LES and reflux esophagitis may follow the myotomy. Enlarging the gastric outlet helps to prevent gastric reflux into the esophagus.

5. Avoid hot, cold, or spicy foods; eat bland foods.
   Eat slowly and chew food well before swallowing.
   Sleep with head of bed elevated.
   Take antacids.
   Avoid eating just before going to bed.
   Avoid tight clothes.
   Lose weight, if overweight.
   Avoid stooping, bending.
   Avoid straining to have a bowel movement (stool softeners may be necessary).
   Eat in a quiet, relaxed environment.
   Avoid alcohol and tobacco.

6. Check your drawing with Fig. 19-5. The most important mechanism preventing reflux is the zone of high pressure between the esophagus and stomach (physiologic lower esophageal sphincter). The acute gastroesophageal angle produces a flap-valve effect. The phrenoesophageal ligament produces a pinchcock-valve effect.

7. Chronic reflux esophagitis causes esophageal inflammation, ulcer formation, bleeding, and eventually scarring and stricture.

8. Because these patients often aspirate esophageal or gastric contents into the lungs, especially during sleep

9. The symptom of pyrosis, or heartburn, is poorly correlated with the presence or absence of esophagitis. Some patients with heartburn do not have evidence of esophagitis, and some patients with esophagitis due to reflux may not have symptoms until the condition is advanced. The acid perfusion test is the best method of identifying esophagitis.

10. *d*

11. *c*

12. *b*

13. *c*

14. *a*

15. *b*

16. *a*

17. *a, c*

18. *a*

19. *a*

20. *a*

21. *a, c, d*

22. *b*

23. *b*

24. *d*

25. *c*

26. *a, c*

27. *a*

28. *b*

29. *b, c*

30. *c*

31. *e*

32. *d*

33. *a*

34. *b*

35. *b*

36. *c, e*

37. *a, d*

38. True

39. True

40. False

41. True

42. False

43. True

44. True

CHAPTER 20

Stomach and duodenum

1. Refer to Fig. 20-1.

2. The outer layer of the stomach consists of peritoneum which is reflected off the lesser curvature as the lesser omentum and off the greater curvature as the greater omentum.

3. Mucosal folds which allow for expansion of the stomach.

4. Pepsinogen is converted to pepsin in the presence of a low pH. Pepsin digests proteins.

5. The extrinsic nerve supply of the stomach is entirely from the automatic nervous system. Parasympathetic fibers travel via the vagus nerve and control gastric motor and secretory activity. Sympathetic fibers travel via the greater splanchnic nerves. Sympathetic stimulation inhibits gastric secretion and motility, which is opposite to the effect of vagal stimulation. Auerbach's and Meissner's nerve plexuses are involved in local reflexes and help to coordinate peristalsis. These plexuses constitute the intrinsic gastric innervation.

6. Celiac artery comes off the aorta; right and left gastric arteries and gastroepiploic supply most of the stomach.

7. Because posterior wall duodenal ulcers frequently erode into the gastroduodenal and pancreaticoduodenal arteries located just behind the duodenum.

8. Reservoir function, mixing function, and emptying function.

9. Approximately 1 to 2 liters; there is a receptive relaxation of the smooth muscle as food and liquids are ingested.

10. Intrinsic factor combines with vitamin B_{12} and is necessary for its absorption in the ileum. Vitamin B_{12} is necessary for the normal maturation of red blood cells.

11. There is a basic intrinsic rhythm to the peristaltic activity of the stomach which is modified by nervous and hormonal factors. Gastrin stimulates gastric motility as does parasympathetic stimulation, while sympathetic stimulation inhibits motility. Gastric emptying is also controlled by nervous and hormonal factors which are elicited by distention of the duodenum and the physical and chemical state of the chyme as it enters the duodenum.

12. The gastric mucus forms a protective coat for the gastric mucosa against mechanical and chemical injury (Hollander). The mucus in the columnar epithelial cells and the tight junctions between the epithelial cells prevent back diffusion of hydrogen ion (Davenport). Aspirin, alcohol, and bile salts are the

most common substances causing disruption of the gastric mucosal barrier. The result is increased back diffusion of H^+, mucosal injury, and ulceration due to the action of gastric acid and pepsin.

The duodenum is protected by secretion of a highly alkaline, viscid mucus which neutralizes the acid chyme from the stomach. It is produced by Brunner's glands in the duodenum.

13. Increases closure strength of the lower esophageal sphincter, thus preventing gastric reflux into the esophagus during gastric mixing; increases pyloric sphincter tone, thus preventing gastric emptying until mixing is completed; stimulates the secretion of acid and pepsin in the stomach so that protein digestion may begin; promotes receptive relaxation of the stomach so that filling can occur without an increase in intragastric pressure; stimulates gastric and intestinal motility so that mixing and propulsion of chyme is promoted; stimulates secretion of insulin, bile, and pancreatic juice.

14. Superficial inflammation of the gastric mucosa. If you have ever had "food poisoning" or "intestinal flu" with nausea, vomiting, or diarrhea, you no doubt have had acute superficial gastritis.

15. Cephalic phase—sight, smell, or thought of food is mediated through parasympathetic fibers of the vagus nerve, which stimulates gastric acid secretion.
Gastric phase—antral distention is the prime stimulus to release of the hormone gastrin, which stimulates gastric acid secretion.
Intestinal phase—of little importance in stimulating gastric acid secretion; influence is mainly inhibitory.

16. *d*

17. *a, b, c, d*

18. *a, c, d*

19. *a, b, e*

20. *b*

21. *a, c, d*

22. *c*

23. *a*

24. *c, d*

25. *c*

26. *d*

27. *a, c, d*

28. *c*

29. *a, c*

30. *d*

31. *b*

32. *a, b, d, e*

33. *e*

34. *a*

35. *c*

36. *b*

37. *a, d*

38. *a, b, e, f*

39. False; pepsinogen

40. True

41. True

42. True

CHAPTER 21

Small intestine

1. Cytotoxic drugs interfere with the metabolism of all rapidly proliferating cells (cancer and leukemic cells). Since hair cells and the epithelial cells of the gastrointestinal mucosa are the most rapidly proliferating cells in the body, they are especially vulnerable to the effects of these drugs. Cell division is inhibited, resulting in atrophy of both the villi and the crypts of Lieberkühn, and sometimes there is ulceration and bleeding of the mucosa.

2. Bile salts act as detergents solubilizing fatty acids, glycerides, and fat-soluble vitamins by the formation of micelles. These substances are thus held in solution until absorption takes place.

3. *Maldigestion* means that digestion of a particular nutrient failed to take place somewhere in the step-wise process of food breakdown into the simplest products which can be absorbed. Maldigestion could be caused by general lack of a secretion containing enzymes (pancreatic insufficiency) or lack of a specific enzyme (lactase insufficiency). Other causes of maldigestion are lack of mechanical breakdown of food particles, so that digestive enzymes cannot reach all the food substances, or a transit time through the intestine which is too rapid to allow time for hydrolysis by enzymes. Of course, maldigestion always results in malabsorption, since nutrients cannot be absorbed until they have been hydrolized into the simplest substances.
Malabsorption refers to lack of transport of a substance across the intestinal mucosa.

4. The stool is pale, large in volume, greasy, frothy, and tends to float. It tends to stick to the side of the toilet and is difficult to flush away.

5. The lesion is granulomatous and similar to the lesion of tuberculosis except that cavitation does not

occur. Since the tubercular lesion represents a hypersensitivity reaction (cellular immune mechanism), medical scientists have looked for an infectious agent and autoantibodies but have not been successful in identifying either.

6. Valvulae conniventes, villi, and microvilli

7. *(a)* Inadequate digestion due to rapid emptying of stomach and poor mixing; *(b)* insufficient stimulation of CCK release (which stimulates pancreatic secretion) due to bypass of duodenum in Billroth II gastrectomy; *(c)* deconjugation of bile salts by abnormal bacterial proliferation in blind loop after Billroth II; *(d)* loss of reservoir function, resulting in dumping of stomach contents into small bowel, with rapid transit time

8. When the small bowel is obstructed either mechanically or functionally, it loses its absorptive and forward propulsive capacity, so that gastrointestinal secretions pool within the lumen. The resulting ischemia of the intestinal wall from the distention further compromises the absorptive and motile function of the bowel, so that a vicious cycle of degeneration develops. The pooling of fluids in the gut depletes the ECF volume, resulting in hypovolemic shock. Bacterial proliferation occurs in the pooled fluids, and increased permeability of the ischemic mucosa allows absorption of bacteria and their toxins into the circulation, causing septicemia and toxemia.

9. Superior mesenteric

10. Pyloric; ileocecal

11. Mesentery

12. Greater omentum; infection

13. Ligament of Treitz

14. Valvulae conniventes

15. Villi

16. Crypts of Lieberkühn

17. Lacteal

18. Umbilicus; iliac; appendix

19. *d, f*

20. *c, g*

21. *a, h*

22. *b, e*

23. *b*

24. *d*

25. *c*

26. *b*

27. *c*

28. *d*

29. *a*

30. *c*

31. *b*

32. *d, e*

33. *f*

34. *g*

35. *c, h*

36. *a, f*

37. *b*

38. *d*

39. *g, e*

40. *b*

41. *c*

42. *a*

43. *c*

44. *d*

45. *b*

46. *a, b, d*

47. *b*

48. *c*

49. *c*

50. *d*

51. *a, b, c, d*

52. *c*

53. *a, b, c, d, e*

54. *c*

55. *c, d, e*

56. *a, b, d*

57. *a, b, c, d*

58. True

59. False

60. True

61. True

62. True

CHAPTER 22

Large intestine

1. Check your drawing with Fig. 22-1.

2. The absorption of water and elimination of the wastes of digestion.

3. The large intestine is more than twice as long as the small intestine. It has a diameter more than twice that of the small intestine. The external anal sphincter is under voluntary control, while the

sphincters at each end of the small intestine are under autonomic control. The large intestine has no villi, its longitudinal muscle layer is incomplete throughout most of its length, and the mucosa contains more goblet cells than that of the small intestine. These structural differences between the small and large intestine are in keeping with their primary functions. The villi, large volume of secretions, and active motility pattern of the small intestine serve well its primary function of digestion and absorption. In contrast, the large intestine is much less motile, and although one of its main functions is absorption of water, it only absorbs about ⅓ the amount absorbed by the small intestine. The decreased motility allows more time for absorption, since its ability to absorb is lessened by its lack of villi. One of the functions of the large intestine is to act as a reservoir until elimination can take place. The increased number of goblet cells and increased mucus secretion are important, since the feces are semisolid in the large intestine and lubrication is more necessary for propulsion of the fecal mass.

4. *Haustral churning* refers to back-and-forth pendular movements especially prominent in the transverse colon, caused by annular contractions of short segments of the bowel, especially the circular muscles. These movements allow time for the absorption of water. *Mass peristalsis* is a contraction involving a long segment of the large intestine which serves to propel a large amount of fecal material forward. Feces are frequently moved into the rectum by mass peristalsis and the defecation reflex is initiated.

5. Hemorrhoids, constipation, cancer of the rectum, anorectal abscesses, fissures, and fistulas.

6. Palpation of the abdomen: presence of mass, tenderness.

   Rectal digital examination: palpation of tumors, hemorrhoids.

   Proctosigmoidoscopic examination: direct visualization of tumors, internal hemorrhoids, ulcerated or hyperemic mucosa; biopsy or cell washings may also be obtained for histologic study (lower 25 cm of bowel observed).

   Colonoscopy: direct visualization of entire large bowel with same information obtained as above.

   Barium enema x-ray: neoplasms, strictures, diverticula, and polyps may all be visualized.

   Stool examination: blood, parasites, shape, size, etc. may give clues to many disorders of the GI tract.

7. Only a small percentage of the patients with diverticulitis require surgery. Surgery is indicated when there is severe and extensive disease or complications such as perforation. During an attack of acute diverticulitis, the medical treatment usually consists of bed rest, liquid diet, stool softeners, and antibiotics.

8. Ulcerative colitis of more than 10 years' duration; certain types of colonic polyps; eating a diet low in fiber and high in refined carbohydrates.

9. Burkitt proposed that slow transit with low fiber diets permits bacterial action on bile acids or other normal bowel constituents to produce carcinogens, which then act on the colonic mucosa.

10. Since the superior hemorrhoidal vein is connected to the portal system, increased portal pressure may cause backflow into these veins and hemorrhoids.

11. A *fissure in ano* is a persistent crack in the perianal skin. A *fistula in ano* is an abnormal granulation-lined tract connecting two epithelial surfaces—in this region running between the anal canal and the skin of the perianal area. It is the consequence of anorectal abscess which has been inadequately treated. Any of these conditions may be a complication of hemorrhoids. Crohn's disease of the colon is especially likely to be associated with anorectal fistulas.

12. *a*

13. *a*

14. *e*

15. *a*

16. *a, b, c, d*

17. *a, b, c*

18. *e*

19. *e*

20. *c*

21. *b*

22. *a, c, d, e*

23. *e*

24. *a*

25. *b, c, d*

26. *c*

27. *e*

28. *a, c, e*

29. *d*

30. *a, b, c, e*

31. *b*

32. All of these

33. *b, d, e*

34. *b*

35. *c*

36. *a*

37. *d*

38. *b*

39. *a, c, d*

40. *a, b, d, e*

41. *a, b, c*

42. *a*

43. Diverticulosis; diverticulitis

44. Pedunculated; juvenile; villous; familial polyposis

45. Annular; polypoid

46. Direct extension to adjacent structure, metastasis via lymph nodes, metastasis via bloodstream

47. Superior; middle; inside; inferior

48. Bleeding, thrombosis, strangulation

49. *d*

50. *a*

51. *c*

52. *a*

53. *a*

54. *b*

55. *b*

56. *b*

57. *b*

58. *a*

59. *c*

60. *a*

61. *a*-2; *b*-1; *c*-3

62. True

63. False; it is under voluntary control.

64. False; only a few severe or complicated cases

65. False; vitamin K and some of B group

66. True

67. True

68. False; they are inside both sphincters.

69. True

70. False; 35 percent

71. True

72. True

73. True

74. True

CHAPTER 23

Liver, biliary tract, and pancreas

1. Blood circulation through the liver is unusual because a mixture of portal venous blood and arterial blood flows through the liver sinusoids. The portal blood contains many nutrients absorbed from the intestines which are metabolized in the liver.

2. The gallbladder is a pear-shaped hollow muscular bag having a capacity of about 45 ml. Its primary function is to concentrate hepatic bile which is transported to the gallbladder via the cystic duct. Bile is stored in the gallbladder and released as needed for digestion of fats in the intestine. Cholecystokinin-pancreozymin stimulates the gallbladder to contract and release bile.

   The pancreas is about 6 in long and 1½ in wide and resembles a bunch of grapes. The main pancreatic duct runs through the entire length of the organ and opens into the duodenum. An accessory pancreatic duct (duct of Santorini) may also open into the duodenum at a different point. The pancreas has an exocrine secretion, pancreatic juice from the acini, and endocrine secretions, glucagon and insulin, produced by the alpha and beta cells in the islands of Langerhans. The release of pancreatic juice is controlled by CCK and secretin.

3. Formation and excretion of bile; carbohydrate metabolism, including synthesis, storage, and release of glucose to maintain proper blood level; protein metabolism, including synthesis of most proteins, urea formation, and storage of amino acids; fat metabolism, including cholesterol synthesis and fat storage; storage of many vitamins and minerals; metabolism of steroid hormones; detoxification of both endogenous and exogenous substances potentially harmful; acts as flood chamber and filter.

   The liver is called an organ of defense because of its large concentration of phagocytic Kupffer cells lining the sinusoids. These cells are actually part of the monocyte-macrophage (reticuloendothelial) defense system.

   The liver detoxifies drugs and other potentially harmful chemicals by oxidation, reduction, hydrolysis, or conjugation so that they become physiologically inactive. Conjugation with glucuronic acid, for example, makes the substance water-soluble so that it may be excreted in the urine.

   The liver is capable of holding a liter or more of blood and holds a strategic position between the intestinal and general circulation. It can serve as a reservoir (flood chamber) when blood backs up, as in right ventricular failure. Sudden release of the blood from this reservoir could cause circulatory overload and pulmonary congestion.

   The liver is the central chemical laboratory for

the metabolism of carbohydrates, fats, and proteins, and this role alone makes the liver essential for life. It plays a major role in the regulation of blood glucose, serum lipids, serum proteins, and coagulation factors.

4. Excess production of bilirubin exceeding the processing ability of the liver; impaired uptake of unconjugated bilirubin; impaired conjugation; and impaired excretion of bilirubin.

5. *Kernicterus* is the deposition of bilirubin in lipid-rich brain, especially the basal ganglia, causing damage to the cells by its toxic action. Kernicterus occurs when there are high levels of unconjugated bilirubin (lipid-soluble) in the blood.

6. The jaundice is physiologic, because the immaturity of the liver leads to relative deficiency of the glucuronyl transferase, which conjugates free bilirubin with glucuronic acid. The acceptor proteins may also be inadequate, so that uptake by the hepatocyte is also deficient.

7. No, it is useful only in helping to prevent hepatitis in exposed individuals, especially hepatitis A.

8. Community: Safe and inspected water supply and sewage disposal; inspection of all wells and septic tanks; restaurant inspection; inspection of public swimming pools and beaches for safety of water.
   Home: Good general sanitary habits—hand washing, separate drinking glasses and eating utensils, adequate dish washing and sterilization.
   Clinical unit: Use of disposable syringes, needles, catheters; screening of blood for hepatitis B antigen; careful disposal of urine and feces from infected patients; hand washing; avoidance of needle puncture; isolation of infected patients in a private room with separate bathroom facilities, disposable dishes, and gowns and gloves worn by those attending patient.

9. About 90 percent removal or destruction of the liver is compatible with life. Complete removal results in death in about 10 hours.

10. Triangular, 1500, right upper, kidney, gallbladder, stomach, pancreas; falciform; Glisson

11. Bile, hepatic; hepatic; cystic, bile; pancreatic, Oddi

12. Hepatic, portal, hepatic, vena cava; portal, hepatic; spleen, esophageal, rectal

13. Lobule, sinusoids, Kupffer; canaliculi

14. *b*

15. *d*

16. *a, b, c, d*

17. *d.* Bile is catabolized in the intestine.

18. *a, b, c, d, e*

19. *c*

20. *c*

21. *c*

22. *a*

23. *c*

24. *c*

25. *d*

26. *a*

27. *a, b, d*

28. *d*

29. *b*

30. *d*

31. *d*

32. *a*

33. *d*

34. *a, c, d, e*

35. *c, b, a, b, a, b, d, b, a, b, a*

36. *d, b, c, i, a, g, e, f, h*

37. *Alcoholic hepatitis* is a lesion characterized by hepatocellular necrosis and infiltration with inflammatory cells. It is associated with alcohol ingestion and is believed to be the critical lesion in the development of Laennec's cirrhosis.

38. Because cirrhosis is generally silent until far advanced, when major signs and symptoms appear. Early symptoms are vague and nonspecific, so patients do not seek medical help.

39. *Portal hypertension* is a sustained elevation of the portal venous pressure above the normal 6 to 12 cm water. The primary mechanism causing portal hypertension is increased resistance to blood flow through the liver. This could occur in cirrhosis, congestive heart failure (backup of blood from right atrium), and hepatic vein thrombosis. Increased inflow through the splanchnic arteries in cirrhosis also contributes to portal hypertension.

40. Compression of varices by esophageal and gastric balloons (Sengstaken-Blakemore tube); vasopressin infusion. It is important to remove the blood from the gastrointestinal tract, because large amounts of ammonia may be produced from the action of gut bacteria on the blood protein. The ammonia may reach the systemic circulation, causing hepatic encephalopathy by interfering with cerebral metabolism. Recurrent bleeding from esophageal varices may be prevented by reducing the pressure and blood flow through the varices by creating a surgical shunt between the portal and systemic circulation. Flow through the esophageal veins is reduced,

but ammonia and other protein metabolites may pass directly into the systemic circulation, causing hepatic encephalopathy.

41. *Hepatic encephalopathy* is a form of cerebral intoxication caused by ammonia and/or other protein metabolites. It is manifested clinically by a neuropsychiatric syndrome characterized by mental clouding and neuromuscular dysfunction progressing to coma.

    It occurs when more ammonia is presented to the liver than the failing cells can synthesize into urea or when the ammonia bypasses the liver through shunts and enters the systemic circulation.

    It is important to detect hepatic encephalopathy during the early stages, because prompt treatment may be successful in reversing the process. The mortality is high if it progresses to an advanced stage.

42. *Asterixis* is a peripheral manifestation of impaired cerebral metabolism characterized by a peculiar flapping tremor of the wrists and metacarpophalangeal joints. It is tested by having the patient extend both arms out with fingers spread.

43. *Constructional apraxia* is the inability to construct simple diagrams or to write legibly in the absence of paralysis or motor weakness. Deterioration in the ability to perform purposeful, skilled construction or to write reflects the progress of the encephalopathy, and a serial record can be kept in the patient's records.

44. Stage I: Slowness of mentation and affect, untidiness, slurred speech, personality change, inappropriate behavior, disordered sleep rhythm

    Stage II: Accentuation of stage I, inappropriate behavior, lethargy, asterixis, muscle tremor

    Stage III: Sleeps most of time but can be aroused; marked confusion, may be abusive and violent; abnormal EEG pattern

    Stave IV: Comatose, positive Babinski, hyperactive reflexes, abnormal EEG, hepatic fetor sometimes detected

45. In acute cholecystitis the patient has a sudden onset of severe pain in the right upper quadrant which may last for several hours. It is often associated with the passage of a gallstone through the cystic or common bile duct. There may be tenderness over the gallbladder. Chronic cholecystitis is characterized by symptoms which are much milder. There may be episodes of mild pain in the right upper quadrant and a long history of dyspepsia, flatulence, heartburn, and fat intolerance.

46. Because the liver acts as a filter, with about one-third of the cardiac output traversing it each minute. Malignant cells transported from the intestines, stomach, or pancreas through the portal vein are readily trapped in the liver capillary bed.

47. a, b, c, d
48. c
49. d
50. a
51. d
52. a, c, d
53. a, c
54. b
55. a, b, d
56. c
57. d
58. e
59. d
60. c
61. b
62. c, d
63. d
64. b
65. c
66. a, b, c, d, e
67. a
68. d
69. a, b, d
70. a, b, c
71. False; it is within the peritoneal cavity.
72. True
73. True
74. False; more common in females; history of alcoholism more common in males
75. True
76. True
77. False; pure bilirubin stones
78. False; a pseudocyst forms outside the pancreas, often within lesser omental sac.
79. False; they are uncommon in the United States and are usually diagnosed late, when they are beyond hope; early symptoms are insidious.
80. True
81. True
82. True
83. False; it is a cholecystectomy.
84. f, c, a, b, e, d

CHAPTER 24

Anatomy of the cardiovascular system

1. Venae cavae → right atrium → pulmonary artery → lung capillaries → pulmonary veins → left atrium → left ventricle → aorta → systemic arteries → arterioles → capillaries → venules → systemic veins.

2. The AV node delays the wave of electrical excitation to allow time for ventricular filling during atrial contraction prior to ventricular contraction. It also prevents an excessive number of electrical impulses from reaching the ventricles.

3. The thickness of the right ventricle is only one-third that of the left ventricle. These differences in muscular size reflect their respective pumping functions in the circulatory system. The right ventricle pumps blood through the low-pressure, low-resistance pulmonary circuit. The workload of the left ventricle is much greater than that of the right, since it must generate pressure about five times as high in order to overcome the high resistance of the systemic circulation.

4. To support the atrioventricular valves during ventricular contraction and prevent leaflet eversion into the atria.

5. Three; aortic valve; sinuses of Valsalva; to protect the coronary orifices from occlusion by the aortic valve cusps during ventricular ejection.

6. The visceral and parietal pericardium. This small space contains a small amount of lubricating fluid which functions as protection against friction.

7. Lymph is propelled by muscle compression of the lymph vessels. Flow is aided by lymphatic peristalsis.

8. Sympathetic stimulation of the alpha receptors causes vasoconstriction, while stimulation of beta receptors causes vasodilation. This vasodilatory effect is produced by $beta_2$ receptors. In contrast, the $beta_1$ receptors produce cardiac effects of increased heart rate, force of contraction, and velocity of AV conduction. The $beta_2$ receptors produce vasodilatation.

9. *d*
10. *c*
11. *c*
12. *b*
13. *b*
14. *c*
15. *d*
16. *c*
17. *d*
18. *b*
19. *a, b, c*
20. *a, c, d*
21. *e*
22. *c, d*
23. *a, b*
24. *c, e, f, a, d, b*
25. *c*
26. *a*
27. *e*
28. *d*
29. *b*
30. *f*
31. Automaticity; excitability; conductivity; rhythmicity
32. Valves
33. Collateral
34. Right coronary; left anterior descending
35. 60 to 100; 40 to 60; 20 to 30

CHAPTER 25

Physiology of the cardiovascular system

1. Systole and diastole represent the *mechanical* activity of the heart. Systole is the period when the heart muscle contracts; diastole indicates the resting period of the heart when the muscles relax. The terms *systole* and *diastole* are commonly used in referring to ventricular activity. The ECG represents a body surface recording of the summated *electrical* activity of *all* the myocardial cells. An action potential is an intracellular recording of the electrical activity of a *single* cell. Electrical activity stimulates mechanical activity.

2. Starling's law of the heart states that, within limits, the force of contraction is a function of the length of muscle fibers, i.e., their end-diastolic length. Thus the horizontal axis of the ventricular function curve represents the stretching of the myocardium. It can be seen that as the degree of stretch and EDV increases, the stroke volume (SV), or ventricular performance, increases (vertical axis). However, where the curve flattens, there is no increase in performance as EDV increases. Then, with further EDV increases, dyspnea and finally pulmonary edema develop. The position of the ventricular function curve represents the degree of contractility. When the curve is shifted to the left (increased

contractility due to influence of norepinephrine or Ca^{2+}), there is greater increase in ventricular performance or SV at a given EDV or degree of muscle fiber length (the curve is steeper). A shift of the curve to the right represents myocardial depression and decreased contractility, so that there is a smaller increase in SV for increments in stretch or EDV. The ejection fraction, SV/EDV, is a good index of contractility. Thus the steeper the curve, the greater the contractility. It can be seen from these relationships that contractility has a greater influence on ventricular performance than the Starling mechanism (increasing EDV to increase performance).

3. Poiseuille's law, stated in terms of the circulation, says that the volume of blood circulated per minute is directly related to the systemic blood pressure gradient and inversely related to the resistance ($F = \Delta P/R$). The systemic blood pressure gradient is calculated by subtracting pressures at the arterial and venous end of the circulation (i.e., mean arterial pressure — central venous pressure).

4. SV = EDV − ESV = 100 ml − 30 ml = 70 ml (this is in the normal range). CI = CO ÷ body surface area = 4.5 liters per minute ÷ 1.5 m² = 3.0 (this is also in the normal range). EF = SV/EDV = 70/100 = 0.70 (the ejection fraction should be 2/3, or 0.67, so it is normal).

5. *a*

6. *c*

7. *a, b, c, d*

8. *c*

9. *a, c*

10. *a*

11. *a*

12. *a, b, c*

13. *a, c*

14. *b*

15. *b*

16. *b*

17. *a*

18. All of these

19. *d*

20. *c*

21. *a*

22. *e*

23. *b*

24. *f*

25. *a, h, d, f, g, c, i, b, e*

26. Absolute refractory; relative refractory

27. Negatively; potassium; sodium

28. Open; closed

29. Closed; open

30. AV node

31. *c*

32. *b*

33. *d*

34. *b*

35. *c*

36. *a, d*

37. *f*

38. *e*

CHAPTER 26

Diagnostic procedures in cardiovascular disease

1. Class III

2. The left carotid may be partially occluded, possibly because of an atherosclerotic plague. Her mean arterial pressure is about 126 mmHg. MAP = diastolic BP + pulse pressure/3 = 100 + 78/3 = 126.

3. The hepatojugular test is performed by manually applying pressure over the right upper quadrant of the abdomen for 30 to 60 seconds and simultaneously observing the jugular veins. A rise in the level of the venous pressure head in the neck veins indicates a positive test. A positive test signifies that the right heart was not able to accept the increased venous return (main source, venous reservoir in the liver which is being compressed) which could result from right ventricular failure.

4. The hexaxial reference system is a representation of all the limb leads of the electrocardiogram. It is formed by moving the bipolar limb leads centrally so that these lines intersect. The position of the heart may be pictured at the center of this electrical reference system. When the unipolar limb leads are added to the reference system, the hexaxial reference system is produced. Using this reference system, the summation vector, or electrical axis, for the P, QRS, and T waves can be derived. An analysis of deviations of the electrical axis from the various leads assists in diagnosing conditions such as conduction abnormalities and chamber enlargement.

5. Pressures in the various cardiac chambers and great vessels may be recorded and the waveforms of the pressure tracings analyzed to detect valvular ste-

nosis and regurgitation. The injection of radiopaque material into the various cardiac chambers allows visualization of chamber size and wall movement so that deviations from normal may be detected. Cardiac output may also be determined. Sampling of oxygen content in the right and left sides of the heart allows detection of right-to-left shunts, as from a ruptured septum. Selective coronary artery angiography allows detection of lesions in these vessels.

6. Indications for coronary arteriography: (1) to determine the feasibility of coronary bypass surgery; (2) to evaluate atypical angina; (3) to evaluate the results of coronary revascularization surgery. Characteristics of a bypassable coronary artery lesion: the lesion must be located proximally and must have more than 75 percent obstruction of the lumen, and there must be a patent artery distal to the lesion which can be anastomosed to the bypass graft.

7. *d*

8. *c*

9. *a, c*

10. *b*

11. *d*

12. *d*

13. *b*

14. *b*

15. *d*

16. All of these

17. *d*

18. *a*

19. *b, c*

20. *c*

21. *c*

22. *c*

23. *c*

24. *b*

25. *b*

26. *a*

27. *b*

28. *d*

29. *b*

30. *c*

31. *a*

32. *d*

33. *a*

34. *c*

35. *d*

36. *c*

37. *b*

38. *c*

39. *c*

40. *d*

41. *b*

42. *f*

43. *a*

44. *e*

45. *c*

46. *b*

47. *a*

48. *a*

49. *d*

50. *c*

51. *c*

52. *c*

53. *d*

54. *b*

55. *a*

56. *b*

57. *c*

58. *a*

59. *b*

60. *c*

61. *a*

62. *b*

63. *d*

64. *e*

65. *b*

66. *c*

67. *a*

68. *f*

69. *f*

70. *a*

71. *b*

72. *e*

73. *c*

74. *g*

75. *h*

76. *d*

77. False; it is on top of the foot.

78. True
79. False; the CVP increases during inspiration.
80. True
81. False; it is normal.
82. True
83. False; they are caused by turbulent blood flow through the partially occluded artery during the recording of blood pressure in an extremity.
84. True
85. Regurgitation
86. Five; aortic stenosis
87. Turbulent

CHAPTER 27

Coronary atherosclerotic disease

1. Oxygen demand is greater for the left ventricle than for the right because of its greater workload and larger muscle mass. Oxygen supply is more restricted because little coronary perfusion of the left ventricle occurs during systole. The firm compression of blood vessels by the thick muscular wall limits perfusion during systole. On the other hand, the thinner-walled right ventricle continues to have some perfusion during systole.

2. Atherosclerotic lesions tend to occur in the epicardial proximal segments of the right and left coronary arteries and at points of abrupt curvature, as where the left coronary artery branches into the left anterior descending.

3. Size and location of the infarct; function of the uninvolved myocardium; collateral circulation; cardiovascular compensatory mechanisms.

4. It is a reflex parasympathetic response resulting from pain or stimulation of parasympathetic ganglia in the myocardium. The effect is to slow the heart rate and reduce the blood pressure and cardiac output. Thus the response has an adverse effect in myocardial infarction, since sympathetic support of the compromised circulation is needed.

5. Severe, prolonged chest pain; elevated serum cardiac enzymes; ECG changes in leads overlying the area of necrosis (deep Q waves, ST segment elevation, and inverted T waves).

6. Since cardiac output is a function of heart rate and stroke volume, a slow heart rate can reduce the total volume ejected in a given time by lowering the frequency of ejection. A rapid rate reduces ventricular filling time, so that less blood is ejected per beat. Tachycardia also reduces the length of diastole, so that perfusion time of the myocardium is limited. Thus oxygen supply is reduced at the same time that demand is increased because of the increased cardiac work.

7. Heart rate, force of contraction, and arterial pressure (a determinant of wall tension).

8. Because the diseased coronary blood vessels have a limited ability to dilate and thus increase perfusion and oxygen delivery to the myocardium. Total coronary perfusion is not increased by nitroglycerin, although there is some improvement of flow to ischemic areas by dilatation of collaterals.

9. To allow healing of the infarcted tissue, decrease the incidence of complications, and salvage the ischemic zone surrounding the infarct.

10. In congestive heart failure, digitalis, diuretics, and restriction of fluid and salt intake are utilized to improve cardiac function and prevent the development of pulmonary edema.

    The first priority in the treatment of severe pulmonary edema is to reduce the increased intravascular volume and pressure in the pulmonary vessels and thus reduce transudation of fluid. This may be achieved quickly by the use of rotating tourniquets, phlebotomy, and elevation of the trunk with the legs dependent. Additional treatment includes the use of morphine, which causes peripheral dilatation and helps to pool blood in the extremities. Aminophylline relieves bronchospasm and increases the contractility of the heart. Oxygen therapy helps to correct the hypoxemia, and positive pressure breathing may reduce transudation by opposing the increased pulmonary hydrostatic pressure.

    Cardiogenic shock is treated with vasopressor drugs (and sometimes vasodilators) and sometimes circulatory assistance devices to reduce the cardiac workload. Sodium bicarbonate is utilized to correct acidosis.

11. The patient needs individualized guidance and teaching to achieve maximum functional ability. Both psychological and physical variables are involved.

12. *b*
13. *b*
14. *c*
15. All of these
16. *c*
17. *b*
18. *b*
19. *b*

20. *a*

21. *a*

22. *b*

23. *c*

24. *d*

25. *c*

26. All of these

27. *a, b, d, e*

28. *c*

29. *c*

30. *b*

31. *d*

32. *e*

33. All of these

34. *d*

35. *c*

36. *d*

37. *a, d, e*

38. *d*

39. All of these

40. *b*

41. *c*

42. *a*

43. *b*

44. *a*

45. *b*

46. *True*

47. True

48. False; this is a complication of saphenous vein bypass graft.

49. False; it increases muscle mass and oxygen demand.

50. False; they are a protective response to sinus node failure.

51. Ischemia

52. Increases

53. *b, d, a, c*

54. *a*

55. *b*

56. *b*

57. *a*

58. *b*

59. *a*

60. *a*

61. *a*

62. *b*

63. *b*

64. *c*

65. *d*

66. *a*

67. *d*

68. *a*

69. *c*

70. *b*

71. *c*

72. *a*

73. *b*

74. *e*

75. *d*

76. *b*

77. *c*

78. *a, c, d*

79. *c*

80. *b*

81. *d*

82. *d*

83. *c*

84. *b*

CHAPTER 28

Valvular heart disease

1. Recurrent attacks of rheumatic fever—most common cause

   Subacute bacterial endocarditis—most infections occur in patients with rheumatic or congenital heart deformities.

   Papillary muscle dysfunction or rupture—may be a complication of myocardial infarction

   Congenital malformations

   Inborn defects of connective tissue

2. It is regurgitation secondary to chamber enlargement. As a result of ventricular chamber enlargement, the papillary muscles and chordae tendineae are unable to anchor the valve leaflets securely. The valvular annulus may also enlarge.

3. Prophylactic antibiotics are necessary in order to reduce the risk of bacterial endocarditis in susceptible patients, including those with a history of rheumatic carditis and those with cardiac deformities. Even minor procedures such as dental work

and catheterization may cause a transient bacteremia and the implantation of organisms on the endocardial surface.

4. Pulmonary congestion—diuretics to decrease blood volume; digitalis to increase heart contractility

Atrial fibrillation—antiarrhythmic drugs
Systemic emboli—anticoagulant drugs

5. Splitting of fused valvular commissures by the surgical introduction of an instrument to dilate them by blunt pressure

6. The Jones criteria consist of a list of major and minor manifestations used to help establish a diagnosis of rheumatic fever. If there is evidence that the subject has had a preceding streptococcal infection (positive throat culture, ASO titer) and also has two major manifestations or one major and two minor manifestations, then a diagnosis of rheumatic fever is made. Major manifestations include carditis, polyarthritis, erythema marginatum, and subcutaneous nodules. Minor manifestations are fever, arthralgia, previous rheumatic fever or rheumatic heart disease, and elevated ESR or CRP.

7. *a*

8. *c, b, d, a*

9. *a*

10. *c*

11. *d*

12. *b*

13. *c*

14. *c*

15. *b*

16. *b*

17. *b*

18. *c*

19. All of these

20. *b*

21. *c*

22. *d*

23. *c*

24. *a*

25. *b*

26. *c*

27. *e*

28. *c*

29. *a*

30. All of these

31. *c*

32. *b*

33. *b*

34. *c* or *d*

35. *c*

36. *c*

37. *b, d*

38. *c*

39. *c*

40. *b*

41. *a, c*

42. *c*

43. *a, c, e*

44. *b, d, f*

45. *b*

46. All of these

47. *a, c, e*

CHAPTER 29

Cardiac mechanical dysfunction and circulatory support

1. *c*

2. *a*

3. *b*

4. *d*

5. *b, d*

6. *a*

7. *b*

8. *b, g*

9. *b*

10. *a, c, d, f*

11. *c*

12. *c*

13. *b*

14. *b*

15. *a*

16. *d*

17. *b, c, e*

18. *f*

19. *c*

20. *b*

21. *b*

22. *d*

23. *a, c*

24. *d*

25. *b*

26. *a, d*

27. Circulatory; pump

28. LAP; pulmonary venous; pulmonary edema

29. Heart failure

30. 40

31. Patient; reservoir

32. Venae cavae; oxygenator; aorta; femoral artery

33. 3, 5, 1, 7, 2, 4, 6

34. *b, e, f*

35. *a, c, d*

36. *b*

37. *e*

38. *f*

39. *a*

40. *c*

41. *d*

42. *c*

43. *a*

44. *b*

45. *a*

46. *c*

47. *b*

48. *a*

CHAPTER 30

Vascular diseases

1. *a*-4, *b*-3, *c*-6, *d*-2, *e*-5, *f*-8, *g*-1, *h*-7

2. *Varicose veins* are dilated, tortuous veins generally seen in the lower extremities. Pathogenic factors include inflammatory destruction of valves, weak vein walls, and increased venous pressure (as in pregnancy), all causing varying degrees of valvular incompetence and regurgitation. The two major complications of varicosities are thrombosis and venous ulcer, both resulting from venous stasis. A varicosity differs from an aneurysm in that the vessel is affected throughout a significant segment of its length, whereas an aneurysm generally involves a short segment of a blood vessel.

3. Deep vein thrombosis is more serious because of the potential complication of pulmonary embolus.

The superficial veins may become distended as a result of impaired deep venous drainage.

4. Early ambulation, leg exercises, oral anticoagulants, external intermittent compression, elastic stockings, and elevation of the lower extremities to promote deep venous drainage are all methods of preventing deep venous thrombosis.

5. An *aneurysm* is a localized dilatation of the arterial wall, resulting from degeneration and weakening of the medial layer of the artery. Aneurysms are frequently asymptomatic. The first sign of disease may be a serious, potentially life-threatening complication such as rupture, acute thrombosis, or embolization.

6. The deposition of the products of red blood cell destruction such as hemosiderin, caused by venous stasis with subsequent capillary destruction, results in the brownish skin discoloration seen in patients with chronic venous insufficiency.

7. Stasis of blood flow, endothelial injury, and hypercoagulability.

8. *a*

9. *b*

10. *c*

11. *d*

12. *d*

13. *c*

14. *b, c*

15. *d*

16. *b, c, d*; generally temperature not elevated to this extent; Homan's sign unreliable

17. *a, d, e*

18. *b*

19. *b*

20. Thrombophlebitis; phlebothrombosis

21. Thromboangiitis obliterans

22. *d*

23. *a*

24. *b*

25. *c*

26. *b*

27. *a*

28. *c*

29. *d*

30. *c*

31. *a*

32. *b*

33. *d*

34. *c*

35. *b*

36. *a*

37. False; it is called *embolectomy*.

38. False; they should be slightly dependent.

39. True

40. False; it is called an *embolus*.

CHAPTER 31

Normal respiratory function

1. Infections, malignant diseases, and chronic bronchitis and emphysema

2. *Respiration* is the combined activity of the various mechanisms which supply oxygen to the body cells and remove carbon dioxide.

3. The blanket of mucus serves to trap dust and bacteria, which are then moved by ciliary action to the pharynx, where they are swallowed or expectorated. Inspired air is also humidified and warmed by the mucus blanket and underlying vascular network.

4. The right mainstem bronchus is larger and runs a more vertical course from the trachea than the left.

5. The lung would collapse (atelectasis).

6. The lung has a dual blood supply—the bronchial and the pulmonary circulation. (Did you remember to include the bronchial circulation?) The pulmonary circulation is a low-pressure, low resistance system (the mean pulmonary artery pressure, at 15 mmHg, is only about one-sixth that of the systemic circulation, at about 90 mmHg).

7. Yes, there is a net pressure of 10 mmHg in the direction of the alveolus

8. Larnyx or glottis

9. Surfactant; surface tension

10. Ventilation; respiratory bellows; diaphragm

11. Hering-Breuer

12. Pons and medulla

13. *c*

14. *c*

15. *c*

16. *e*

17. *a*

18. *b*

19. *e*

20. *d*

21. *c*

22. *c*

23. a-6, b-3, c-1, d-5, e-7, f-8, g-9, h-4, i-10, j-2, k-12, l-11

24. a-4, b-5, c-2, d-1, e-7, f-6, g-3

25. Because of dilution with water vapor and other gases in the anatomic dead space

26. The volume of anatomic dead space is equal to 1 ml per pound of body weight; if you weighh 120 lb, your anatomic dead space is about 120 ml.

27. Diffusion; the driving force is the pressure gradient between the partial pressure of the gas in the alveolus and in the pulmonary capillary.

28. No; perfusion increases going from the apex to the base of the lungs because of the effect of gravity in the low-pressure, low-resistance pulmonary circulation. The overall ventilation/perfusion ratio is 0.8, which is less than unity.

29. $V/Q = 3$ liters per minute $\div$ 6 liters per minute $= 0.5$. This value would represent wasted perfusion and would be present in a shunt-producing disease.

30. More oxygen could be transported to the tissues in physical solution, which might make the critical difference in cases where there is very little hemoglobin available to transport oxygen to the tissue cells.

31. No; an increased concentration of oxygen in the inspired air will be wasted, because the blood is already 97 to 98 percent saturated when it leaves the lungs and the oxygen content is normal. An examination of the oxyhemoglobin dissociation curve (flat upper portion) shows that little if any advantage could be gained.

32. The S shape of the oxyhemoglobin dissociation curve indicates that under normal environmental conditions large changes of the P_{O_2} of the inspired air cause only small changes in oxyhemoglobin saturation. Even at a P_{O_2} of 50 mmHg in the alveoli, hemoglobin is 80 to 85 percent saturated with oxygen, which is sufficient to meet tissue demands for oxygen under most conditions.

33. The Bohr effect is the slight shift to the right of the oxyhemoglobin dissociation curve caused by the increase in acidity due to the effect of carbon dioxide being released from the tissues. The rightward shift in the curve causes oxygen to be more easily released from its association with hemoglobin and thus facilitates tissue uptake of oxygen.

34. Although alveolar oxygen tension may be increased slightly by hyperventilation, this does not significantly increase the oxygen content of the arterial blood, because of the sigmoid shape of the oxygen dissociation curve and because blood leaving nor-

mally ventilated alveoli is already almost fully saturated with oxygen. The carbon dioxide dissociation curve, however, is linear in shape, indicating that the CO_2 content of the blood is directly related to the alveola P_{CO_2}. When CO_2 is "washed out" of the lungs during hyperventilation, the carbon dioxide content of the blood is likewise reduced.

35. If diffusion were impaired enough to affect CO_2 transport, the patient would be dead. Carbon dioxide diffuses more readily than oxygen at the same pressure gradient. Even a minute pressure gradient (less than 1 mmHg) is enough to ensure elimination of all the CO_2 produced at rest.

36. No; knowledge of the blood gases does not give information about how well the tissues are being perfused, how much oxygen is being delivered to the tissues, and the P_{O_2} in the tissue cells. One must have data on hemoglobin concentration and adequacy of cardiac function and make other clinical observations to assess the adequacy of respiratory function. All data must be correlated, and the final judgment is a clinical one.

37. All the following are examples of altered mechanisms or conditions which may interfere with normal respiration: (1) low P_{O_2} of inspired air—high altitudes; (2) depression of respiratory center—barbiturate overdose; (3) alveolar hypoventilation due to inadequate bellows function—obesity, deformed chest cage, weak respiratory muscles; (4) impaired diffusion of gases at the alveolar-capillary membrane—pulmonary edema or fibrosis; (5) ventilation/perfusion imbalance—pneumonia or pulmonary embolism; (6) impaired transport of blood gases by systemic circulation—anemia, carbon monoxide poisoning, inadequate cardiac output or shunting by tissues as in shock; (7) impairment of gas diffusion at tissue level—edema.

38. Stage 1 is ventilation—flow of air into and out of the lungs effected by the respiratory bellows.
Stage 2 is transportation—includes the diffusion of gases between the alveolus and the pulmonary blood and between the tissue cells and the systemic blood. Transportation also includes the distribution of the pulmonary and systemic blood and the distribution of air in the lungs.
Stage 3 is cell respiration—oxidation of cell metabolites with the production of energy, water, and carbon dioxide.

39. Normal inspiration is principally caused by contraction of the diaphragm and the muscles elevating the rib cage (sternocleidomastoids, serrati, scalene,

scapular elevators). There is increased activity in these muscles during forceful inspiration. Expiration involves the relaxation of these muscles and is largely passive. The internal intercostal and abdominal muscles are more active during forced expiration.

40. 201 ml/minute (12 g/100 ml $\times$ 1.34 ml/g $\times$ 5000 ml/minute $\times$ 0.25)

41. Mixed venous blood containing reduced hemoglobin from the bronchial circulation is mixed with oxygenated pulmonary blood leaving the lungs, thus accounting for the slight reduction in hemoglobin saturation.

42. Decreases; increases (alkalosis); shifts to the left so that hemoglobin is reluctant to release oxygen to the tissues.

43. 42 mmHg [(247 − 47) × 0.21]; no, a P_{O_2} of 42 would barely be able to supply tissue oxygen requirements at rest. The climber might be expected to pass out unless he uses cylinder oxygen supply.

44. *a*

45. *a, b, c*

46. *b*

47. Increase, decrease, less, into

48. Ascends, decreasing

49. Increase, more, out of

50. Normal, low, low

51. Decrease, increase, alkalosis

52. Right, decreased

CHAPTER 32

Diagnostic procedures in respiratory disease

1. Routine chest film, fluoroscopy, bronchography, angiography, lung scans, and tomograph, including CT scan

2. (a) Status of the thoracic cage, including the ribs, pleura, contour of the diaphragm and of the upper airway as it enters the chest; (b) the size, contour, and position of the mediastinum and hilus of the lung, including the heart, aorta, lymph nodes, and root of the bronchial tree; (c) the texture and degree of aeration of the lung parenchyma; (d) the size, shape, number, and location of pulmonary lesions, including cavitation, fibrous markings, and zones of consolidation.

3. *c*

4. *c*

5. *a*

6. *b*

7. *h*

8. *d*

9. *e*

10. *i*

11. *f*

12. *g*

13. *d*

14. *e*

15. *a, f, g*

16. *c*

17. *b*

18. *f*

19. The chief value of ventilatory function tests is that quantitative data are provided to assess the degree of pulmonary disability, follow the progress of the disability, and assess response to treatment. Ventilatory function test data are not in general specifically diagnostic, although patterns of disordered pulmonary function may be discerned. Blood gas measurements, like ventilatory function tests, provide quantitative data to assess the degree of respiratory insufficiency and are particularly helpful in guiding oxygen therapy, but these data do not provide all the information necessary to assess total respiratory function.

20. Alveolar ventilation takes into account the amount of air wasted in ventilating the dead space.

21. Measurements of the change in volume at different degrees of lung inflation and the change in alveolar or intrapleural pressure measured by means of an esophageal balloon are made simultaneously. Compliance is then calculated by the following formula:

$$\text{Compliance} = \frac{\triangle \text{ volume}}{\triangle \text{ pressure}}$$

22. Causes of decreased lung compliance include pulmonary fibrosis, pulmonary edema, pneumonia, and deficiency of surfactant. Causes of decreased thoracic cage compliance include obesity, abdominal distention, and skeletal deformities of the chest cage.

23. The emphysema patient whose main problem is increased airways resistance due to premature collapse of the airways during expiration adopts a slow, deep pattern of respiration to minimize the work of breathing. Airflow is less turbulent with slow, deep respirations.

24. The chief problem for a patient with very stiff lungs is an increase in the elastic resistance. The work of breathing is minimized by a rapid, shallow pattern of respiration.

25. The radial artery is usually chosen for the arterial puncture because of its easy access. The wrist is extended (positioned over a rolled towel) and the artery is stabilized with two fingers of one hand while the arterial puncture is made with the other hand, using a heparinized syringe. Air is displaced from the blood specimen. Finally, the specimen is placed on ice and taken to the blood gas laboratory.

26. Hyperventilation can occur as a result of anxiety, brain injury, and pneumonia. It may also be secondary to metabolic acidosis occurring as a compensation. Causes of hypoventilation include narcotic or barbiturate overdose and increased physiologic dead space. It may also occur as a compensation for metabolic alkalosis.

27. Hypoxemia is caused by ventilation-perfusion imbalance, alveolar hypoventilation, impaired diffusion, and intrapulmonary anatomic shunts. Hypoxemia caused by intrapulmonary anatomic shunting is not corrected by oxygen administration, because the blood bypasses the pulmonary unit.

28. False; the reason is incorrect. In this case, less effective ventilation results because the total amount of air wasted as dead-space ventilation is greater.

29. True

30. False; $VA = (200 - 120) \times 30 = 2.4$ liters per minute

31. True

32. True

33. True

34. True

35. *a*

36. *b*

37. *c*

38. *c*

39. *b*

40. *d*

41. *a, b*

42. *a, c*

43. *f*

44. *c*

45. *d*

46. *e*

47. *b*

48. *a*

49. *h*

50. *g*

51. Check your answer by referring to Table 32-5.

52. *d*

53. *e*

CHAPTER 33

Cardinal signs and symptoms of respiratory disease

1. *c*
2. *f*
3. *g*
4. *b*
5. *a*
6. *e*
7. *d*
8. True
9. False; a Pa_{O_2} of less than 85 mmHg may or may not be associated with hypoxia. One can be fairly certain, however, that there is associated hypoxia if the Pa_{O_2} is persistently below 50 mmHg.
10. False; the detection of cyanosis is difficult, the cause is highly variable, and it may be absent in the presence of severe hypoxia or present when there is no hypoxia.
11. True
12. False; anemic persons (e.g., Hb = 7 g per 100 ml) may never develop cyanosis even though they have severe hypoxia, because it would be difficult to have 5 g out of 7 g per 100 ml reduced hemoglobin at any one time. Even patients with normal hemoglobin concentration, cyanosis generally is an advanced sign of respiratory insufficiency.
13. True
14. True
15. False; alveolar hyperventilation is the cause of hypocapnia.
16. True
17. *Digital clubbing* refers to a loss of the base angle of the nail so that this angle is greater than the normal 160°; bulbous changes in the digital tips are also indicative of clubbing. Loss of the base angle is the earliest sign of digital clubbing, while the bulbous change is a late sign. Digital clubbing is important to detect, because it is frequently associated with pulmonary disease (especially bronchogenic carcinoma), cardiovascular disease, and gastrointestinal disease.
18. Inspection of the buccal mucosa, especially under the tongue, is the most reliable method of detecting central cyanosis in both black and white patients. The lighting must be good, preferably daylight.

CHAPTER 34

Obstructive patterns of respiratory disease

1. An increased resistance to airflow
2. All three diseases may exist in the pure form, although it is more common for patients to manifest aspects of all these diseases. It is especially common for patients to have features of chronic bronchitis and emphysema at the same time. This overlap and difficulty in separating the diseases are the reason for the label COPD.
3. An asthmatic attack is characterized by orthopnea (having to sit up to breathe), dyspnea, fear of suffocation, prolonged wheezing expirations, and later, cough and sputum production. Treatment consists of bronchodilator drugs and oxygen if the blood gases are abnormal. Corticosteroid drugs are used occasionally for severe attacks. Long-term therapy consists in desensitization and avoidance of known allergens. *Status asthmaticus* is a prolonged, severe attack of asthma which may cause ventilatory insufficiency so severe that death results.
4.

Feature	CLE	PLE
Sex prevalence	More common in males	Equal sex distribution
Etiology	Associated with smoking	Possible genetic factor
Pathologic anatomy	Respiratory bronchioles primarily affected	Entire acinus affected
Part of lung affected	Uneven distribution; upper lobes may be more severely affected	Uniform in distribution; basal lung more severely affected
Type of associated COPD	Chronic bronchitis	Primary emphysema; chronic bronchitis; aging

5. Measures to relieve obstruction of the small airways; cessation of smoking; avoidance of air pollutants; prompt treatment of infection; cautious oxygen administration

6. Excessive production of mucus, chronic cough; 3 months per year and 2 consecutive years

7. Abnormal enlargement of the alveoli and alveolar ducts and destruction of the alveolar walls

8. Blebs; ruptured alveoli

9. Bullae; check valve obstruction of the bronchiole

10. In asthma there is hypersensitivity of the tracheobronchial tree to various stimuli, manifested by periodic, reversible airway narrowing due to bronchospasm.

11. Chronic inflammation causes weakening of the bronchial walls so that they become dilated. The dilated areas may be cylindrical or saccular in shape. The dilated areas serve as a reservoir for the collection of sputum. The stagnant sputum collection, in turn, may lead to chronic reinfection, so that there is progressive destruction and persistence of the process. Precipitating factors include whooping cough, measles, pneumonia, aspiration of a foreign body, and bronchial obstruction due to a tumor.

12. Chronic loose cough, expectoration of a large amount (up to 200 ml per day) of foul-smelling sputum, malnutrition, digital clubbing, cor pulmonale, and right ventricular failure.

13. Daily bronchial hygiene with postural drainage, antibiotics

14. Removal of the obstructing bronchial secretions

15. *b, a, c*

16. *a, c, d*

17. *b, d*

18. *c*

19. *b*

20. *a, b, c*

21. *d*

22. True

23. True

24. False; cystic fibrosis is more common in whites.

25. True

26. True

27. True

28. False; the prognosis is poor and few patients live beyond adolescence.

29. *a*

30. *b*

31. *a*

32. *b*

33. *a*

34. *b*

35. *b*

36. *b*

37. *a*

38. *b*

39. *b, e*

40. *a, c*

41. *d, e*

CHAPTER 35

Restrictive patterns of respiratory disease

1. *f*

2. *e*

3. *a*

4. *b*

5. *d*

6. *c*

7. True

8. False; pectus excavatum is a congenital deformity in which the lower end of the sternum is attached to the thoracic spine by fibromuscular bands, giving the lower end of the anterior chest a "caved-in" appearance.

9. True

10. False; the deformity is symmetrical.

11. *c*

12. *a*

13. *d*

14. *b*

15. Alveolar hypoventilation and an inability to maintain normal blood gas tensions

16. Traumatic—penetrating wound to the chest (knife or gunshot wound)
Therapeutic—induced pneumothorax, which was a common treatment for tuberculosis until about 1960
Spontaneous—rupture of blebs and bullae in emphysema, pneumonia, neoplasm

17. Airtight seal is placed over the wound immediately.

18. Air gains access to the pleural cavity through the defect.

19. A large pneumothorax (more than 20 percent lung collapse) is treated by closed (water sealed) chest tube drainage. A large pleural effusion may be re-

moved by thoracentesis. If a pleural effusion is an exudate it is treated by closed chest tube drainage to prevent fibrothorax.

20. Pleural effusion

21. Pulmonary venous pressure

22. An exudate

23. A transudate

24. (1) Invasion by bacteria, viruses, fungi, malignant cells—infection and destruction of lung tissue; (2) inhalation of irritating dusts—inflammation and pulmonary fibrosis; (3) inhalation of irritating gases—inflammation and pulmonary fibrosis; (4) damage to the alveolar capillary endothelium—edema; (5) deficiency of pulmonary surfactant—atelectasis

25.

	Absorption atelectasis	Compression atelectasis
Common cause	Intrinsic obstruction of airway by mucus plug	Extrinsic pressure on lung from pleural effusion, hemothorax, pyothroax, or pneumothorax
Mechanism	Obstruction prevents air from entering alveoli distal to the obstruction, Air in alveoli is gradually absorbed into bloodstream, and alveoli collapse	External pressure due to the fluid or air causes compression collapse of the alveoli

26. These small pores (between the alveoli) provide a path for collateral ventilation between alveoli and whole segments of the lung in case the normal airway is obstructed. Deep inspiration is effective in opening up the pores and providing ventilation to adjacent obstructed alveoli. Collapse due to absorption of gases into the bloodstream is thus prevented. (Once collapse occurs, reexpansion is much more difficult.) During expiration the pores close and pressure builds up aiding in the expulsion of the mucus plug.

27. Engorgement (4 to 12 hours)—serous exudate from leaking blood vessels pours into alveoli
Red hepatization (next 48 hours)—lung red and granular in appearance (RBCs PMNs and fibrin fill alveoli)
Gray hepatization (3 to 8 days)—lung has grayish appearance (leukocytes and fibrin consolidate in alveoli)
Resolution (7 to 11 days)—lysis and resorption of exudate by macrophages and restoration of tissue to normal

28. Administration of antibiotic effective against the specific infecting organism, oxygen therapy for hypoxemia, and treatment of complications

29. Size of dust particles—those 1 to 5 μm can easily reach alveoli.
Concentration and length of exposure—high concentration and long exposure generally needed to produce adverse affects.
Nature of the dusts—some organic dusts produce an allergic alveolitis; the chemical nature of inorganic dusts is important; some are harmless and inert, while others harm macrophages by which they are phagocytized and form fibrotic nodules.

30. Histoplasmosis, coccidioidomycosis, and blastomycosis

31. Decreased lung compliance; interference with the gas diffusion pathway

32. Restrictive lung disease

33. Interstitial

34. Parenchyma; lung abscess, empyema; poor

35. True

36. True

37. False; the prognosis is generally good.

38. False; erythromycin is effective against mycoplasmal pneumonia. Antibiotics are not effective against viral infections.

39. True

40. False; this statement describes hypostatic pneumonia.

41. True

42. True

43. c

44. a

45. b

46. c, g, j

47. d, h, i

48. a, f

49. b, e

50. c, f, h, i

51. a, b, g

52. d, e

53. c, h

54. *c*
55. *f, g*
56. *d*
57. *a, e*
58. *b*
59. *h*
60. *b, c, d, e*
61. *b, e, f*
62. *a*
63. *a, c, e, g*
64. *d*
65. *a*
66. *b*
67. *e*
68. *c*
69. *d*
70. *b*
71. *c*

CHAPTER 36

Cardiovascular disease and the lung

1. Local injury to the vascular wall; stasis of blood flow; hypercoaguability

2. Chronic obstructive pulmonary disease

3. Increased hydrostatic pressure within the pulmonary capillaries, decrease in the colloid osmotic pressure (as in nephritis), damage to the capillary wall (as when noxious gases are inhaled), left ventricular heart failure

4. It is the name given to attacks of dyspnea caused by pulmonary edema at night. The increased hydrostatic pressure in the lungs is due to the horizontal position in patients with chronic passive congestion of the lungs resulting from left ventricular failure.

5. It is the condition in which hypertrophy and dilatation of the right ventricle develop from disease affecting the structure and function of the lung. (Congenital and left heart disease are not included.)

6. When the left ventricle fails while the right ventricle continues to pump blood, the pulmonary hydrostatic pressure rises until pulmonary edema results. Yes.

7. Prevent the recurrence of pulmonary embolism; relieve symptoms resulting from the embolism; surgically remove a massive embolus

8. To improve the underlying pulmonary disorder and correct the hypoxemia

9. Two mechanisms leading to increased pulmonary vascular resistance are (1) anatomic alterations in the pulmonary blood vessels leading to a reduction of the pulmonary vascular bed and (2) pulmonary functional disorders caused by alveolar hypoventilation or $\dot{V}/\dot{Q}$ imbalances which cause hypoxemia, hypercapnia, and acidosis (blood gas abnormalities); the blood gas abnormalities then cause pulmonary arteriolar vasoconstriction.

10. *a, b, c; d* is associated with a massive pulmonary embolism; *e* is associated with infarction, an uncommon event with pulmonary embolism.

11. *c*
12. *a, b, d*
13. *c*
14. *b, c, d, e*
15. *c*
16. *a, c*
17. *c*
18. *a*
19. *a, b, c, d*
20. Congestive heart failure is first in importance and the postoperative bedridden condition is second.
21. True
22. True
23. True
24. False
25. Embolism
26. 5
27. Pulmonary hypertension

CHAPTER 37

Respiratory failure

1. Respiratory insufficiency refers to an impairment of the normal ability to oxygenate arterial blood and eliminate carbon dioxide, so that there is an inability to maintain normal arterial blood gas levels under conditions of increased demand such as increased activity or exercise.

2. Chronic obstructive pulmonary disease

3. Hypoxemia without hypercapnia (hypoxemic respiratory failure, or oxygenation failure); hypoxemia with hypercapnia (hypercapnic respiratory failure, or ventilatory failure)

4. High concentrations of oxygen will reduce the hypoxic drive for breathing (which patients with this

condition depend on and may aggravate hypoventilation and carbon dioxide retention).

5. Pa_{O_2} about 40 mmHg; Pa_{CO_2} 60 to 70 mmHg

6. Liquefy and remove secretions by adequate hydration and administration of expectorants, aerosols; supervise patient's coughing; use suctioning, percussion, vibration, postural drainage; treat respiratory infection with the appropriate antibiotic

7. Ensure that hypoxemia, acidosis, and hypercapnia do not reach hazardous levels

8. Retained respiratory tract secretions, infection, and bronchospasm, which are all related. For example, bronchospasm can be a response to inflammation and infection or to the inhalation of irritants such as smoke or allergens. Injudicious administration of sedatives or narcotics or inhalation of high oxygen concentration are important iatrogenic factors. Refer to Table 37-2 for a list of other common factors.

9. A $\dot{V}/\dot{Q}$ mismatch means that some regions of the lung have high $\dot{V}/\dot{Q}$ ratios while others have low $\dot{V}/\dot{Q}$ ratios. The high $\dot{V}/\dot{Q}$ gas-exchanging units compensate for the units with a low $\dot{V}/\dot{Q}$ in the case of CO_2 because of linear relationship between CO_2 content and Pa_{CO_2}; consequently the Pa_{CO_2} does not rise. The Pa_{CO_2} is a function of overall alveolar ventilation and CO_2 production. In the case of the Pa_{O_2}, the high $\dot{V}/\dot{Q}$ units cannot compensate for the low $\dot{V}/\dot{Q}$ units, because O_2 content increases little even when there is a large increase in ventilation (flat part of Hb O_2 dissociation curve). Thus the Pa_{O_2} is greatly affected by regional $\dot{V}/\dot{Q}$ imbalance, but the Pa_{CO_2} is not.

10. $P_{A_{O_2}} = P_{I_{O_2}} - (Pa_{CO_2}/R)$
$P_{I_{O_2}} = F_{I_{O_2}} \times (P_B - P_{H_2O})$
$P_{I_{O_2}} = 0.21 (760 - 47) = 149.7$ mmHg (breathing air)
$P_{I_{O_2}} = 0.50 (760 - 47) = 356.5$ mmHg (breathing 50% O_2)
$P_{A_{O_2}} = 149.7 - (80/0.8) = 49.7$ mmHg (predicted breathing air)
$P_{A_{O_2}} = 356.5 - (80/0.8) = 256.5$ mmHg (predicted breathing 50% O_2)
$P_{(A-a)O_2} = 49.7 - 50 =$ essentially 0 (breathing air)
$P_{(A-a)O_2} = 256.5 - 246 = 10.2$ mmHg (breathing 50% O_2)

The hypoxemia is caused by pure hypoventilation, since his A–a gradient breathing air is essentially zero (normal = <20, allowing for some measurement error). The depression of the Pa_{O_2} is accounted for by the increase in Pa_{CO_2} in the situation when he is breathing air and when he is breathing 50% O_2. Note that his hypoxemia was corrected by O_2 therapy but that his Pa_{CO_2} was not. This is because overall alveolar ventilation is reduced because of depression of the respiratory center by the narcotic. He may eventually need to be mechanically ventilated.

11. $P_{A_{O_2}} = 0.21 (747 - 47) - (55/0.8) = 78.25$ mmHg (predicted on admission)
$P_{(A-a)O_2} = 78.25 - 35 = 43.25$ mmHg (on admission)
$P_{A_{O_2}} = 0.24 (747 - 47) - (40/0.8) = 111.75$ (predicted 2 days later)
$P_{(A-a)O_2} = 111.75 - 50 = 61.75$ mmHg (2 days later)

Since A–a gradient breathing air on admission is > 20, he probably has $\dot{V}/\dot{Q}$ imbalance in addition to hypoventilation. Two days later, on 24% oxygen, his condition appears to be deteriorating (even though his Pa_{O_2} has increased) since the A–a gradient has increased. He is not hypoventilating since Pa_{CO_2} is now normal, but his $\dot{V}/\dot{Q}$ imbalance has probably become worse.

12. False; the point when respiratory insufficiency has progressed to failure is hard to detect in these patients, since they have adapted somewhat to the abnormal blood gas tensions.

13. False; it is highly unreliable. (If you missed this question, go back and read the section on cyanosis in Chap. 33.)

14. True

15. True

16. False; hyperventilation causes this.

17. True

18. True

19. True

20. False. The Pa_{O_2} should fall about 12 mmHg for every 10 mmHg rise in the Pa_{CO_2}. Since the Pa_{O_2} rose by 30 mmHg above the value (70 − 40 = 30), the Pa_{O_2} should be expected to fall by 36 mmHg to a value of 59 mmHg (95 − 36 = 59). Since the Pa_{O_2} is 45 mmHg, the patient probably has some $\dot{V}/\dot{Q}$ imbalance or shunting. (You could have used the alveolar gas equation to solve this problem if you had been given data on the barometric pressure, patient's temperature, and $F_{I_{O_2}}$. The rule of thumb approach has been used here on the assumption that the patient is breathing air.

21. False. *Hypoventilation* and *hyperventilation* refer to CO_2 homeostasis and can be assessed *only* by the measurement of the Pa_{CO_2}. CO_2 homeostasis is related to both CO_2 production and alveolar ventila-

tion. One can infer that CO_2 production is increased when the work of breathing is increased (because of airway obstruction or thoracic wall or lung restriction) or when the patient's temperature is increased. On the other hand, CO_2 elimination depends on alveolar ventilation, which in turn is determined by tidal volume, dead space, and breathing frequency. The balance between the CO_2 production and elimination processes cannot be determined accurately by clinical observation.

22. True. An FVC <15 ml per kilogram of ideal body weight indicates a serious reduction of ventilatory reserve. A normal FVC for a 70-kg man is about 4550 to 5250 ml (70 × 65 to 75). See Table 37-4.

23. True. Predicted PA_{O_2} = 1.0 (747 − 47) − (24/0.8) = 670 mmHg P(A − a)O_2 = 670 − 80 = 590 mmHg

24. False. Life cannot be sustained with a 50% shunt except by breathing 100% oxygen, which in itself is toxic to the lung when given for prolonged periods.

25. True. Occurs with breathing of more than 50% O_2 for longer than 48 hours.

26. False. It causes increased cerebral blood flow (CBF) and increased intracranial pressure (ICP).

27. True

28. True. Incr. Pa_{CO_2} → incr. CBF → incr. ICP → papilledema and headache

29. False. Directly related to CO_2 production and inversely related to alveolar ventilation. See formula.

30. True. Both hypoxemia and hypercapnia are generally present in terminal respiratory failure.

31. *d*

32. *b, c*

33. *a*

34. *b, c*

35. *a, b, c, d*

36. All of these

37. *a, b*

38. *e*

39. *d*

40. *b, d*

41. All of these

42. *d*

43. *b, d*

44. *b, c*

45. *b, c*

46. All of these; cardiac output is increased at first but decreases later as myocardial tissue hypoxia becomes severe.

47. $c \rightarrow d \rightarrow a \rightarrow e \rightarrow b \rightarrow g \rightarrow f$. Actually, *d* could occur during sleep, but here it is considered as indicating an exacerbation of the chronic bronchitis. Both *a* and *d* cause a further rise in the Pa_{CO_2} beyond the patient's chronic level.

48. *d*

49. *c*

50. *a, b, c*

51. *a, b, d, e*

52. All of these

53. All of these

54. *a, c, d*

55. *a, b, c*

56. All of these

57. *d; e* will shut off respiratory drive.

58. *c, d, e, g*

59. *a, b, f*

60. *f*

61. *a*

62. *c*

63. *e*

64. *b*

65. *d*

CHAPTER 38

Pulmonary malignant neoplasms

1. The carcinoid syndrome is a symptom complex characterized by attacks of anxiety, tremulousness, hypotension, flushing, dyspnea, and cyanosis due to bronchoconstriction. It is caused by the elaboration of serotonin and other biologically active substances secreted by a carcinoid type of bronchial adenoma.

2. Cough, chest pain, sputum expectoration, mild dyspnea, digital clubbing, and hemoptysis are common, but symptoms may be minimal. Diagnosis on the basis of symptoms is difficult, since the onset may be insidious and the symptoms are not specific. Lung cancer may imitate a number of other lung disorders.

3. Radiology—"coin lesion" on x-ray
Bronchoscopy—direct visualization of tumor and biopsy identification of malignant cells
Cytology—examination of sputum, bronchial washings, or pleural fluid for malignant cells

4. *b, c, h, j*
5. *d, h, j, m, n, o*
6. *e, i, k, l*
7. *a, f, g, i, k, l*
8. True
9. False; there is a positive relationship. The greater the number of cigarettes smoked, the greater the risk.
10. False; it is asbestos.
11. False; secondary metastases are more common.
12. True
13. True
14. *a, c*
15. *c*
16. *a, c,* and *d*
17. *c*

CHAPTER 39

Pulmonary Tuberculosis

1. The factors are (1) completed diagnostic procedures; (2) evidence of tuberculosis infection (i.e., positive tuberculin test); (3) abnormal chest x-ray (not stable, i.e., worsening or improving) and/or clinical evidence of disease; and (4) decision to give a full course of therapy with two or more antituberculosis drugs.

2. These risks are (1) risk of acquiring the infection and (2) risk of developing clinical disease after the infection has occurred. The risk of acquiring the infection and of developing the disease is dependent on infection in the population, crowding, socially disadvantaged populations, and inadequacy of medical care.

3. Both rifampin and isoniazid are bacteriocidal for both extra- and intracellular bacilli. Isoniazid is superior to rifampin in producing an early bactericidal effect on actively metabolizing bacteria, while rifampin is superior for sterilizing lesions which contain dormant bacilli that show only rare and short bursts of metabolic activity. These drugs are effective both for immediate reduction in the large extracellular population of bacilli and for ultimate eradication of the smaller intracellular population.

4. When treatment appears to be failing, the therapy should be changed to an entirely new regimen of at least two new drugs, and care should be taken to ensure that the patient takes the medication regularly.

5. Vaccination with BCG usually leads to the development of tuberculin sensitivity. The degree of sensitivity is highly variable, depending on the strain used in the population vaccinated. Vaccination against tuberculosis in the United States has had only token acceptance. Most authorities agree that the risk of tuberculosis among nonreactors is too small to justify using BCG vaccine.

6. The primary public health measures for prevention and control of tuberculosis in the United States are early detection of cases and sources of infection. Preventive therapy with antimicrobial drugs is an effective tool in the control of the disease.

7. *b, c*
8. *c*
9. *a*
10. *c*
11. *c*
12. *d*
13. *b*
14. *b*
15. *d*
16. *d*
17. *c*
18. *b, c, d*
19. *c*
20. *a, d*
21. True
22. False; the risk of hepatitis is low in persons under 20 years of age and reaches a peak among persons over 50 years of age.
23. True
24. False; both INH and RIF (with or without other drugs) are usually prescribed.
25. False; the classification system is based on the broad host-parasite relationship described by exposure, history, infection, and disease.
26. True
27. *c, d, e*
28. *a, d, j*
29. *c, d, j*
30. *g*
31. *f*
32. *h, i, j*
33. *d, b*

1. 1, Left kidney; 2, right kidney; 3, ureter; 4, bladder; 5, urethra; 6, urinary meatus

2. 1, Eleventh rib; 2, twelfth rib; 3, transversus abdominis muscle; 4, psoas major muscle

3. 1, Fibrous capsule; 2, cortex; 3, medulla; 4, column of Bertin; 5, papilla; 6, pyramid; 7, minor calyx; 8, major calyx; 9, renal pelvis; 10, ureter

4. 1, Proximal convoluted tubule; 2, glomerular capillary tuft; 3, Bowman's capsule; 4, efferent arteriole; 5, juxtaglomerular cells; 7, afferent arteriole; 7, macula densa; 8, loop of Henle; 9, distal convoluted tubule; 10, collecting duct

5. Check your drawing with Fig. 40-1. The hilus of each kidney should be at about the level of the second lumbar vertebra. The superior pole of the left kidney is at about the level of the lower border of the eleventh rib, while the right is at about the level of the twelfth rib.

6. (a) Bowman's capsule; (b) proximal convoluted tubule; (c) distal convoluted tubule; (d) collecting ducts; (e) papillary ducts of Bellini; (f) minor calyces; (g) major calyces; (h) renal pelvis; (i) ureter; (j) bladder

7. (a) Abdominal aorta; (b) renal artery; (c) interlobar arteries; (d) arcuate arteries; (e) interlobular arterioles; (f) afferent arterioles; (g) glomerular capillaries; (h) efferent arterioles; (i) peritubular capillaries; (j) interlobular veins; (k) arcuate veins; (l) interlobar veins; (m) renal vein; (n) inferior vena cava

8. More than 25 percent of the population has more than one renal artery supplying a kidney, which may cause technical difficulties for the surgeon. Some difficulties presented by aberrant blood vessels may be insurmountable.

9. A decrease in the hydrostatic pressure of the blood flowing through the afferent arteriole sensed by the JG cells or an increase in sodium concentration in the distal tubule filtrate sensed by the macula densa cells causes the release of renin from the JG cells. This results in the conversion of angiotensinogen to angiotensin I and finally to the active form, angiotensin II. Angiotensin II increases arterial blood pressure by causing peripheral vasoconstriction and stimulates the secretion of aldosterone. Increased aldosterone levels cause increased sodium reabsorption in the distal tubule. More water is then reabsorbed, resulting in an increase in plasma volume. Both vasoconstriction and increased plasma volume help to elevate blood pressure. An increase in the blood pressure in the afferent arteriole has the op-

posite effect. A decrease in the Na^+ concentration of the distal tubule, however, does not affect renin output.

10. A severe blunt impact over the back, flank, or even the abdomen can cause trauma to the kidney. This situation is common in traffic accidents. The most common trauma in such cases results from the kidney being pushed against a transverse process or being punctured by a fractured twelfth rib. The resulting injury can vary from a simple bruise to a shattering of the renal parenchyma. Complete transection of a kidney by the twelfth rib is not uncommon in severe cases.

11. d
12. f
13. b
14. e
15. c
16. a
17. d
18. a
19. c
20. b
21. d
22. c
23. c
24. a
25. e

26. It is called *ultrafiltration* because the glomerular filtrate has the same composition as plasma with the absence of proteins—almost everything is filtered through and at a high flow rate.

27. The differences in pressure between the glomerulus and Bowman's capsule tend to force fluid into the capsule. Net filtration pressure = intracapillary hydrostatic pressure − colloid osmotic pressure of the blood − intracapsular hydrostatic pressure.

28. The GFR is the rate of appearance of glomerular filtrate from filtration of the blood at the glomerulus. The average GFR in men is 125 ml per minute and in women, 110 ml per minute.

29. To measure the GFR a substance must be used which is freely filtered by the glomerulus but is neither secreted nor reabsorbed along the tubules. A substance which was cleared by both filtration and secretion along the tubule would cause the appar-

ent GFR to be higher than the true GFR. A substance which was both filtered and reabsorbed would cause the apparent GFR to be lower than the true GFR.

30. $\text{GFR} = \dfrac{UV}{P} = \dfrac{(500 \text{ mg}/100 \text{ ml})(2 \text{ ml}/\text{min})}{25 \text{ mg}/100 \text{ ml}}$
    $= 40 \text{ ml}/\text{min}$

A GFR of 40 ml per minute indicates that this patient has moderately severe impairment of renal function. The calculated value is normally corrected for body surface area by means of a normogram. The standard body surface area is 1.73 m² (the body surface area of an average man). The final result is then reported in milliliters per minute/1.73 m².

31. Regulation of water and acid-base balance. Water is reabsorbed in the presence of ADH. Acid-base balance is regulated by regeneration of bicarbonate and hydrogen-ion excretion in combination with phosphates and ammonia.

32. The lungs control the excretion of carbon dioxide, and the kidneys control the reabsorption of bicarbonate, both important components of the bicarbonate–carbonic acid buffer system in the blood. The ratio of these two components is important in maintaining a normal blood pH. This subject may be explored in greater detail in many fine texts dealing with fluid and electrolyte homeostasis.

33. H^+ is excreted in the urine by combining with HPO_4^{2-} to form $H_2PO_4^-$ and by combining with NH_3 to form NH_4^+.

34. (a) Maintain water balance to keep plasma osmolality at 285 mOsm, (b) maintain electrolyte balance, (c) maintain acid-base balance, (d) excrete nitrogenous end products of protein metabolism, (e) produce renin for regulation of blood pressure, (f) produce erythropoietin important in RBC formation, (g) activate vitamin D, (h) degrade insulin, (i) produce prostaglandins.

35. (a) Vapor pressure is lowered, (b) boiling point is elevated, (c) freezing point is lowered, (d) osmotic pressure is increased. Osmotic pressure refers to the external pressure which would have to be applied to a solution with a greater number of particles to prevent water from diffusing across a semipermeable membrane from a solution with a lesser number of particles. It is a measure of water concentration, and there are no real physical pressures present in the solutions—the pressure is that used to charac-

terize the system. Adding particles to water lowers its chemical potential (molar free energy), and water always flows from an area of higher potential (more dilute) to an area of lower potential (more concentrated). The attainment of equilibrium by the application of pressure to the more concentrated solution is due to the fact that its chemical potential is raised so that it is equal to the water in the more dilute solution on the other side of the membrane. The application of pressure prevents an increase in volume in the more concentrated solution due to water diffusion.

36. The osmometer is an apparatus for measuring the freezing point of a solution. The freezing point depression below that of pure water can then be used to accurately calculate the osmotic concentration of the solution, since it depends only on the number of particles in solution. The urinometer actually measures the density or specific gravity of a solution and does not measure true concentration, which depends on the number of particles in solution. Therefore the osmometer is more accurate in estimating the concentration of a solution.

37. $\text{Osmolality} = \dfrac{\Delta T}{K_f} = \dfrac{-0.53}{-1.86} \times 1000 = 285 \text{ mOsm}$

The result is multiplied by 1000 to convert to milliosmols.

38. Check your drawing with Fig. 40-15. Cortical glomeruli should be located high in the cortex, with relatively short loops of Henle which extend slightly into the medullary area. Juxtamedullary glomeruli should be located deep in the cortex next to the medulla, and the loops of Henle should be relatively long, extending deep into the medulla.

39. The vasa recta are medullary blood vessels which form hairpin loops beside the juxtaglomerular loop of Henle. They help maintain the concentration gradient of the medullary interstitial fluid.

40. The purpose of the countercurrent mechanism is the conservation of water (or the concentration of urine) by the kidney. The two basic processes involved are the loop of Henle acting as a countercurrent multiplier of concentration to build up the concentration gradient in the medulla and the vasa recta acting as a countercurrent exchanger to prevent washing out the hyperosmolality built up by the loop of Henle.

41. *d*

42. *a*

43. *b*

44. *c*

45. *c*

46. *d*

47. *c*

48. *d*

49. *d*

50. *b.* It is hyperosmotic even during diuresis.

51. *d.* Increase in medullary blood flow washes out medullary hypertonicity.

52. *b, c*

53. *a, d.* Reabsorption in the proximal tubule is obligatory.

54. *b.* Maximum concentration is about 1400 mOsm; plasma concentration is 285 mOsm.

55. *a*

56. *b*

57. *a*

58. *c*

59. *b*

60. *d.* Hypoosmotic during diuresis because of Na⁺ reabsorption, and water cannot passively follow; isosmotic when water is reabsorbed with Na⁺ during antidiuresis.

61. *a, b,* or *c*

62. *c*

63. *b*

64. All except *f, l*

65. *e, g*

66. *c, d*

67. *i, j, p*

68. *i*

69. *h, j, n.* Actually ammonia is also a nitrogenous substance synthesized from amino acids, especially glutamine, and secreted along the tubule.

70. *a, b*

71. *b, o*

72. *m*

73. *k*

74. *a*

75. *b*

76. *c*

77. *c*

78. *c*

79. *a*

CHAPTER 41

Diagnostic procedures in renal disease

1. A normal healthy adult may excrete up to 150 mg of protein in the urine per day. The amounts in excess of 150 mg per day are considered pathologic and occur most frequently in renal disease, particularly glomerulonephritis. Patients with the nephrotic syndrome excrete more than 3.5 g of protein per day and may excrete as much as 20 to 30 g.

2. The direct cause of proteinuria is always an increase in glomerular permeability.

3. When urine stands for a period of time, urea breaks down to ammonia and the urine becomes more alkaline.

4. Uric acid is derived principally from the catabolism of nucleoproteins in the cells. Cytotoxic drugs cause increased degradation of the rapidly proliferating cells, and thus uric acid production is increased. Two-thirds of the uric acid is normally excreted by the kidneys. The uric acid may crystallize and obstruct the tubules under conditions of acid urine.

5. (*a*) Infection with urea-splitting organisms producing alkaline urine; (*b*) hypercalciuria due to prolonged immobilization; (*c*) urinary stasis due to low fluid intake. All three of these conditions are often present in patients with chronic illness who are confined to bed, thus favoring the formation of urinary calculi, which form in alkaline urine. Calcium salts are mobilized from bone, and precipitation is favored by highly concentrated, alkaline urine.

6. High fluid intake

7. (*a*) Check the accuracy of the urinometer using distilled water; (*b*) gently mix urine to ensure a uniform solution; (*c*) avoid errors of surface tensions; (*d*) read the calibrated units from top to bottom at eye level; and (*e*) correct for temperature.

8. Creatinine is a nitrogenous end product of muscle metabolism. The normal plasma level is 0.7 to 1.5 mg per 100 ml. The plasma level is constant in the healthy person and depends on muscle mass.

9. A substance which is filtered by the glomerulus and is neither secreted nor reabsorbed by the tubules is required for a true measurement of GFR. Creatinine is secreted by the tubules, and there is an error inherent in the laboratory method of measuring the plasma level. These two large errors nearly cancel each other out so that creatinine clearance approximately equals GFR.

10. GFR decreases with increasing age. After age 30 it decreases at the rate of about 1 ml per minute each year.

11. The PAH excretion test is the most accurate test of effective renal plasma flow.

12. The plasma creatinine level, because its production rate in the body is constant. It depends on muscle mass, which changes very little. Urea production varies with dietary protein intake and catabolism of body protein. *Azotemia* means that there is an increase in nitrogenous substances in the blood. This occurs when the kidneys are not able to excrete these substances as rapidly as they are produced.

13. (a) The correct interpretation of a "trace" reading must take into account the concentration of the urine specimen and the time of day it is collected. A trace reading in an early morning concentrated specimen is probably within normal limits. If the urine is collected later in the day and is dilute, a trace response might indicate excessive proteinuria. (b) Contamination by vaginal secretions in the female (contain protein).

14. Albumin; Tamm-Horsfall

15. 6

16. *a*; alkaline

17. *b, c; nocturnal acid*

18. 285

19. 1.001, 1.040; to maintain the osmolality of the ECF at a constant value.

20. 28 percent; this is the minimum for normal renal function; average excretion is 35 percent.

21. 1.025, 1.003

22. Urine acidification or ammonium chloride; 5.3

23. Sodium conservation; *a*

24. *c*

25. *c*

26. *a, c*

27. *c*: $C_{cr} = \dfrac{U_{cr}V}{P_{cr}} = \dfrac{50 \text{ mg/100 ml} \times 1 \text{ ml/min}}{2 \text{ mg/100 ml}}$
$= 25 \text{ ml/min}$

   It is necessary to convert the 24-hour urine volume to milliliters per minute to calculate the problem: 1400 ml per 24 hours × 24 hours per 1440 minutes = 1 ml per minute.

28. *b*; decrease is at the rate of 1 ml per minute a year after the age of 30. A decrease of 60 ml per minute is expected in this 90-year-old man, which is about a 50 percent decrease from the normal GFR in the young, healthy male.

29. Red blood cells, white blood cells, casts, bacteria

30. A bacterial count of 10^5 (100,000) organisms per milliliter of urine is considered significant and is an indication of urinary tract infection (more than three or four WBCs per high-power field during microscopic examination of the urine sediment suggests significant bacteriuria and indicates that a bacterial count should be done). However, the urine must not have been contaminated by bacteria from other sources, as from the container or from the genitalia. Therefore the genitalia must be cleansed with soap and water before voiding into the sterile specimen bottle, and care must be taken to avoid contamination of the urine by the labia or vaginal secretions in the female ("sterile-voided"). Catheterization gives greater insurance that the specimen is "sterile." The urine must be examined immediately or a preservative should be added and the specimen refrigerated to avoid bacterial growth.

31. An IVP is accomplished by injecting into a vein x-ray contrast medium, which is then excreted by the kidneys, while in the retrograde pyelogram a catheter is passed up a ureter and contrast medium is injected directly into the renal pelvis.

   The purpose of an IVP is to visualize the cortex, calyces, renal pelvis, ureters, and bladder. The adequacy of filling of the calyces and renal pelvis may also be determined. The purpose of the retrograde pyelogram is to obtain better visualization when the IVP is not clear and to investigate a nonfunctioning kidney.

32. (a) Hypertension—may be due to renal artery stenosis or other obstruction; (b) possible neoplasm—blood vessels of tumor can be visualized; (c) transplant—to visualize the precise vascular supply prior to surgery; (d) to visualize the blood supply to the cortex—may have patchy appearance indicating ischemia.

33. The GFR is probably low and the dye will not be excreted well; the pyelogram will be difficult to visualize.

34. The entry site should be checked periodically for signs of hematoma or inflammation. Vital signs are checked every 15 minutes until stable and then every 4 hours for 24 hours. Peripheral pulses (in the leg when the femoral artery is used as the entry site) should be checked for diminished strength at the same time intervals as above in order to detect occlusion of blood flow due to thrombus or embolus formation. Color and skin temperature are other signs which should be observed to detect occlusion.

35. The patient should lie prone with a sandbag under the abdomen for 30 minutes after a renal biopsy. Firm pressure with 4 × 4 sponges is applied over the biopsy site for 10 minutes, followed by application of a pressure dressing. The patient should be kept in bed and as quiet as possible for 24 hours.

Vital signs are checked and the abdomen observed for swelling during this period. The urine should also be observed for gross and occult blood.

36. Microscopic; bacteriologic; radiology; biopsy
37. Tamm-Horsfall; distal
38. Cylindruria, protein
39. Culture and sensitivity
40. Clubbing (also may be seen in some other forms of chronic renal disease)
41. *b*
42. *a*
43. *c*
44. *a*. Death occurs in only 0.17 percent of the cases.
45. *c*
46. *d*
47. *a*
48. *b*
49. *b*
50. *c*
51. *d*
52. *a*

CHAPTER 42

Chronic renal failure

1. The time period of development of the disease condition; chronic renal failure is a progressive, slow process over a period of years, whereas acute renal failure develops over a few days to weeks. In both cases the kidneys lose their ability to keep the internal environment of the body normal.

2. (*a*) Chronic glomerulonephritis with primary glomerular involvement; (*b*) chronic pyelonephritis with primary involvement of renal tubules and interstitium; (*c*) polycystic disease with primary involvement of renal tubules; (*d*) hypertensive nephrosclerosis with primary involvement of renal vasculature.

3. Stage I, decreased renal reserve—up to 75 percent of nephron mass destroyed. Stage II, renal insufficiency—75 to 90 percent nephron mass destroyed. Stage III, uremia or end-stage renal failure—90 percent or more of the nephron mass destroyed.

4. First stage—BUN and plasma creatinine levels both normal; second stage—BUN and plasma creatinine levels rising just above normal, unstable; third stage—BUN and plasma creatinine levels both rising sharply with each decrement of GFR.

5. The creatinine clearance progresses toward zero as nephrons are progressively destroyed by the renal disease process (creatinine clearance rate gives a fairly good estimate of the true GFR in the middle range but is much less accurate at either high or low filtration rates).

6. *Polyuria* means an increase in the volume of urine, whereas *oliguria* is just the opposite—urine output is decreased below the normal range. (Do not confuse polyuria and frequency, a common mistake made by students. *Frequency* means an increase in the number of voidings, but there is not necessarily an increase in the volume. With moderate polyuria, there is not necessarily an increase in frequency.) *Nocturia* means that a person has to get up more than once to void during normal sleeping hours or output is 700 ml or more during the night.

7. Polyuria and nocturia occur because of the solute diuresis and inability to concentrate the urine. Both symptoms occur early in the course of progressive renal failure and are compensatory. When most of the nephrons are destroyed, the patient becomes oliguric because total net filtration rate is low (because there are few nephrons), even though the GFR for each individual intact nephron may be high (decompensation stage). Primary lesions of the medulla may interfere with the chloride pump, the countercurrent mechanism, and tubular secretion and reabsorption, while lesions of the glomerulus may prevent glomerular filtration from occurring or cause the loss of protein and formed elements into the urine.

8. An increased solute load may be induced in a normal person by ingestion of a very high protein diet or by giving mannitol intravenously. The usual solute load of the kidneys is thus extended many times. Each normal nephron is undergoing an osmotic diuresis which results in an obligatory loss of water. The kidney loses its flexibility to either concentrate or dilute the urine from the plasma osmolality of 285 mOsm under the stress of water deprivation or overload. Identical principles are involved in progressive renal failure, and both conditions are explained by the intact nephron hypothesis.

9. The remaining intact nephrons compensate by hypertrophying. Filtration rate, solute load, and tubular reabsorption per nephron are all increased, and glomerular-tubular balance is maintained until most of the renal nephrons are destroyed.

10. The renal disease may not be diagnosed until it is far advanced, when functional and morphological characteristics may be similar for a number of chronic renal diseases.

11. Bacteriuria (10^5 bacteria per milliliter of urine) means that there is an infection in the urinary tract, whether symptomatic or asymptomatic, so that there is an increased risk of developing an acute, symptomatic pyelonephritis or perhaps an asymptomatic chronic pyelonephritis.

12. The patient may have a persistent or recurrent asymptomatic bacteriuria, indicating urinary tract infection which is perhaps in the kidney or, if located in the lower urinary tract, can ascend to the kidney.

13. Symptoms may be mild and not revealed by the patient, or the patient may be entirely asymptomatic until end-stage renal disease and thus may not seek help.

14. Arguments for a bacterial etiology of chronic pyelonephritis: (1) at least half the patients have a history of urinary tract infections, including acute pyelonephritis, while the remainder of patients may have had subclinical infections; (2) the hypertonic medulla is especially susceptible to infection, since bacteria can thrive there in the form of protoplasts which can be converted to active bacteria from time to time, causing recurrent or chronic infection; (3) bacteria and leukocyte casts may be discharged into the urine only periodically and consequently may be difficult to detect.

Arguments against a bacterial etiology of chronic pyelonephritis: (1) many patients have no recallable history of urinary tract infection; (2) sex incidence of chronic pyelonephritis is about equal, although the female/male ratio or urinary tract infection and acute pyelonephritis is about 10:1; (3) urinary tract infection is a frequent complication of other renal disease; (4) lesions similar to chronic pyelonephritis are caused by nonbacterial factors such as phenacetin.

15. Acute pyelonephritis: the kidney is swollen, with multiple abscesses on the surface and within the parenchyma; hydronephrosis and blunting of the calyces may be present. Chronic pyelonephritis: the kidney is contracted, has a coarsely granular surface with U-shaped depressions and irregular outline and with scarring and distortion of the pelvis and calyces.

16. *b*

17. *c, d*

18. *d*

19. *b, c*

20. *a*

21. *a, b.* Poor blood supply is probably not important, since most infecting bacteria are not anaerobic; and high glucose content is not normally present.

22. *c*

23. *e*

24. *a*, because it is a result of bacterial infection of the urinary tract which then infects the kidney. Public efforts are needed to detect urinary tract infections (significant bacteriuria) in the population, especially those at high risk. Those infections detected then need to be treated and adequately followed. There is also a need for public health education with respect to prevention measures and information on the signs and symptoms or urinary tract infection or renal disease. Chronic glomerulonephritis might be reduced a small amount by prompt treatment of all streptococcal infections. However, 90 percent of chronic glomerulonephritis has an insidious onset and is not associated with streptococcal infections and cannot be cured. Health education or mass screening programs to ensure early detection of renal disease might be helpful so that conservative medical management could begin and thus prolong renal function.

25. True

26. False; it may be intermittent and so easily missed.

27. True

28. PMNs; tubules; lymphocytes; plasma

29. (*a*) Atrophied tubule containing cast; (*b*) normal tubule; (*c*) area of interstitial fibrosis; (*d*) hypertrophied tubule with atrophy of epithelial cells; (*e*) inflammatory cells (PMNs)

30. The term *glomerulonephritis* was originally used to describe a primary renal disease which involved an inflammatory lesion of the glomerulus and whose chief manifestations were hematuria and proteinuria. This term was also applied to many renal diseases which were poorly understood. Today the term is often used to describe any inflammatory lesion of the glomerulus, even if secondary to a systemic disease.

31. Confusion exists because of the many emerging categories based on histologic findings which do not always correlate with the clinical features of glomerulonephritis. Glomerulonephritis is much more complex than originally believed, and the exact cause is unknown in most cases.

32. Acute glomerulonephritis: In the classic poststreptococcal GN, about 90 percent of children have a complete recovery, but the prognosis is not so good for adults. About 10 percent develop CGN. Acute GN can occur following bacterial endocarditis and during the course of many other renal diseases.

Subacute or rapidly progressive glomerulonephritis: Rapid progression to end-stage renal failure within 2 years; 4 percent of the cases follow APSGN, but in most cases the cause is unknown.

Chronic glomerulonephritis: Slowly progressing GN leading to end-stage renal failure over a period varying from 2 to 40 years; 90 percent of the cases have an insidious onset or the precipitating cause is unknown.

33. Classic case of acute poststreptococcal GN: most prevalent in children aged 3 to 7 years; common nephrotogenic organism is group A β-hemolytic streptococcus, Types 12 and 4 most common; follows streptococcal sore throat or skin infection in about 10 days; common signs and symptoms are anorexia, fatigue, fever, headache, nausea and vomiting, hypertension, edema (especially of face), hematuria; major physiologic disturbances are glomerular damage resulting in hematuria, albuminuria, and urinary casts; decreased GFR from glomerular damage resulting in oliguria, azotemia, salt and water retention. Salt and water retention contributes to both the edema and the development of hypertension. Vasospasm may also play a role in the development of hypertension. Usual treatment is penicillin to eradicate any streptococcal infection, salt restriction, antihypertensive drugs.

34. The *nephrotic syndrome* is a clinical condition characterized by the loss of large amounts of protein in the urine (more than 3.5 g per day), hyperlipidemia, hypoalbuminemia, and edema. Massive edema is common when there is massive loss of protein (rate of loss greater than rate of production by the liver). The resulting hypoalbuminemia reduces the colloid osmotic pressure in the blood vessels, so that fluid tends to move from the intravascular to the interstitial spaces. The edema is further aggravated by the resulting hypovolemia, which causes a decrease in the renal blood flow and GFR and an increase in aldosterone and salt and water retention. More than 75 percent of the cases are associated with the various types of primary glomerulonephritis. About 50 percent of patients with chronic GN have the nephrotic syndrome at some time during the course of the disease. Other diseases commonly associated with the nephrotic syndrome are SLE, diabetes mellitus, and amyloidosis. Principles of treatment include corticosteroid and immunosuppressive drugs directed against the primary disease when appropriate; high protein, salt-restricted diet; diuretics; and protection against infection.

35. Early diagnosis of renal artery obstruction is important because surgical correction of hypertension may be possible. If the condition is left uncorrected, the affected kidney will undergo ischemic atrophy and the contralateral kidney will develop nephro-

sclerosis from the systemic hypertension which is mediated through the renin-angiotensin system of the originally affected kidney.

36. (a) High renal blood flow, (b) hyperosmotic interstitium, (c) excretory route for most drugs and chemicals.

37. c

38. b

39. a

40. b, c, g

41. a, d, e, f, h

42. c, d

43. b, e

44. a, e

45. b, f

46. b, g

47. b, d, i, j

48. b, c, d, i

49. a, b

50. b, h

51. d

52. e

53. c

54. d

55. c

56. b

57. a

58. a

59. c

60. b

61. c

62. d

63. b, c

64. c; Aspirin is believed to potentiate the effect of phenacetin by making the medulla more vulnerable.

65. False; not if the contralateral kidney has developed nephrosclerosis. The ischemic kidney may have better function than the contralateral kidney, so the latter should be removed.

66. False; about two-thirds or more.

67. True

68. True

69. False; the loss of protein is usually not sufficient to cause hypoproteinemia.

70. False; it is often very small, with a granular surface due to ischemia.

71. True

72. True

73. False; it signifies a highly advanced state of destruction; prognosis is very poor.

74. True

75. True

CHAPTER 43

The uremic syndrome

1. The *uremic syndrome* refers to a symptom complex that results from or is associated with retention of nitrogenous metabolites related to renal failure.

2. The first group of symptoms relates to deranged regulatory and excretory functions (i.e., fluid and electrolyte disturbances, acid-base imbalances). The second group of symptoms refers to cardiovascular, neuromuscular, gastrointestinal, and other system abnormalities. The middle molecular hypothesis postulates that molecules of intermediate size present in uremia (guanidines, indican, phenols, amines, etc.) may act as toxins and may be responsible, in part for the multifaribus systemic manifestation of the uremic syndrome. The theory also implies that a treatment method allowing effective removal of middle molecules will reduce the symptoms of the uremic syndrome.

3. Because the total number of nephrons is decreased, not because of a tubular transport problem.

4. H^+ is probably being buffered by calcium carbonate from the bones. No doubt this process contributes to the dissolution of bone, though it is not as important as the increased parathormone levels.

5. Because of the increased solute load of each intact nephron. The osmotic diuresis results in obligatory salt losses.

6. Milk of magnesia and magnesium citrate

7. A fixed urine specific gravity of 1.010 means that the patient has severe renal failure with no ability to either concentrate or dilute the urine. Consequently there is little ability to regulate the fluid balance in the body, and fluid intake must be carefully prescribed.

8. When the GFR falls to about 5 ml per minute in terminal renal failure, both males and females lose their libido and are generally sterile. The male is generally impotent, and the female ceases to menstruate.

9. Poor nutrition, overhydration, indwelling catheters and cannulas, immunosuppressive drugs.

10. White-skinned person—waxy yellow (bronze) cast to the skin; brown-skinned person—yellowish brown coloration; black-skinned person—ashen-gray with yellow tones. All these skin color changes are due to the anemia and retention of urochrome pigments in the uremic patient. Skin color changes in the dark-skinned persons are due to a loss of the red undertones which give the dark skin a "look-alive" appearance. Yellow tones are more evident in the conjunctiva and on the palms and soles.

11. GI bleeding → hypotension → decreased renal
    perfusion → ↓ GFR
    → digestion of blood protein → ↑ BUN
    Vomiting → dehydration → hypovolemia
    → ↓ renal perfusion → ↓
    GFR
    Diarrhea → loss of HCO_3^- → aggravation of acidosis

12. You might expect the patient to complain of tiring easily, of not being able to work long without resting and of being unable to sleep at night or being lethargic during the day. You might observe that the patient's affect seemed flat and there was difficulty in following a complex train of thought. Muscular weakness and muscular twitching might be complaints. The untreated patient in terminal renal failure will eventually become confused and comatose and may have convulsions, especially if severely hypertensive.

13. Stage I: nerve conduction test reveals decreased velocity of nerve conduction. Patient may complain of needing to walk or move the legs (restless leg syndrome). Stage II: sensory nerve changes. Patient complains of burning sensation on the soles of the feet and of feet numbness or prickling sensation moving up legs in stockinglike fashion; may have parethesias of the hands. Stage III: motor nerve involvement. Loss of motor function usually is first observed as foot drop and may progress to paraplegia.

14. Check your illustration with the hand x-ray in Fig. 43-2. The radial aspect of the bone is eroded and has a jagged appearance.

15. See Fig. 43-3 if you have forgotten this sequence of events. Bone disorders associated with secondary hyperparathyroidism might include "honeycombing" demineralization of the bone, especially nota-

ble on skull x-ray, and subperiosteal bone resorption, giving the phalanges a ragged border. Pathological fractures of the long bones and ribs may result. Calcium slats may be deposited in the soft tissues of the body, around joints, in the arteries, and in the eyes.

16. This patient has a calcium-phosphate cross product of $8 \times 10 = 80$, which exceeds the solubility product of calcium and phosphate by a large margin. Soft tissue deposition of calcium phosphate would certainly be expected.

17. Check your illustration with Fig. 43-4. Irritation from the calcium salts deposited in the eye may cause conjunctivitis, called "uremic red eye" from its appearance.

18. *b*

19. *c*

20. *a*

21. *c*

22. *b*

23. *a*

24. *c*

25. *b, c, d*

26. *c*

27. *a, b, c, d*

28. *a, b, c, e*

29. *a, c*

30. *d*

31. True

32. False; if you missed this question, review the description in this chapter.

33. True

34. False; it has no effect on the GFR.

35. True

36. False; certain amino acids are elevated while others are depressed.

37. False; uremic patients are often hyperglycemic.

38. True

39. True

40. Urea, ammonia, infection

41. (*a*) Osteitis fibrosa; (*b*) osteomalacia (rickets); (*c*) osteosclerosis

42. *c*

43. *a, d*

44. *b, e*

45. *b*

46. *f*

47. *d*

48. *e*

49. *c*

50. *a*

CHAPTER 44

The treatment of chronic renal·failure

1. When the patient becomes azotemic. Four causes of sudden deterioration of renal function include (1) ECF volume depletion; (2) urinary tract obstruction; (3) infection, especially of urinary tract; and (4) severe or malignant hypertension. The principles of conservative measure are based on regulating individual solute and fluids in order to achieve as normal an internal milieu as possible in view of the kidney's decreased ability to adapt to a variable intake. Phosphate-binding medications should be given early in the course of chronic renal failure.

2. Dialysis, renal transplantation, or death in terminal renal failure.

3. Some nephrologists restrict protein to 40 g when the GFR is 10 ml per minute; 25 to 30 g with a GFR of 5 ml per minute; and 20 g with a GFR of 3 ml per minute or less. Another approach is to give 0.25 g/kg per day of unrestricted quality protein plus a supplement of essential amino acids. Allowance is much more liberal after dialysis is begun. Protein foods must be restricted somewhat to avoid a high intake of potassium, phosphate, and acid production. Care is taken to provide an adequate carbohydrate intake in order to provide calories and prevent catabolism of body protein. It is usually necessary to restrict dietary potassium even after the patient is undergoing dialysis regularly. Sodium intake must be adjusted carefully to avoid fluid overload or a negative sodium balance, which might lead to dehydration and deterioration of renal function.

4. About 500 ml + 500 ml = 1000 ml

5. Chronic intermittent dialysis and renal transplantation. Dialysis may be used for long-term maintenance of the end-stage renal failure patient. Even if the patient chooses renal transplantation as the mode of therapy, dialysis will undoubtedly play a role in treatment. Dialysis can be used to restore and maintain an optimal physical state in the uremic patient before the transplanted kidney is available and as a backup treatment modality

should the transplanted kidney fail. The patient who has chosen maintenance home or satellite-center dialysis may also opt for a transplant at a later date.

6. *Dialysis* is the process by which water and small molecular-weight solutes pass through a semipermeable membrane from one fluid compartment to another and achieve equilibrium.

7. An artificial shunt is a device for diverting arterial blood to a vein so that the pressure and flow are great enough to allow hemodialysis and provide for easy blood access. With an external shunt or cannula system, an external silicone rubber tubing directs or shunts blood from artery to vein. An internal shunt can be created by anastomosing an artery to a nearby vein (AV fistula) or using a graft of bovine carotid artery.

8. *a, b, d, i*

9. *g*

10. *e, k*

11. *h*

12. *f*

13. *j*

14. *c*

15. *c, d;* unfortunately, erythropoietin is not commercially available, although this would be the ideal way to treat the anemia.

16. *a*

17. *b*

18. *b, c, d;* a BUN of 60 mg per 100 ml is not in itself an indication for dialysis.

19. *c*

20. *c*

21. *c*

22. *a;* not entirely true—some albumin does pass through the pores in the semipermeable membrane. The amount of albumin lost from the blood is generally insignificant during hemodialysis but is quite substantial during peritoneal dialysis.

23. *b*

24. *d*

25. *b;* the purpose is to provide a blood-flow rate high enough for hemodialysis. The enlarged vein allows large-bore needles to be easily inserted.

26. *b*

27. *a, b, c*

28. *c, d*

29. *b*

30. *a, b*

31. *b*

32. *c*

33. *a, d, e*

34. *d*

35. *c*

36. *d*

37. *a*

38. *b*

39. *a*

40. *d*

41. *c*

42. True

43. True

44. False; most recipients go through an acute rejection episode during the first few weeks after transplantation, requiring dialysis because of renal insufficiency. This occurs even when the kidney eventually functions well.

45. False; the only exception might be an identical twin donor who is genetically identical with the recipient. There are undoubtedly other minor and major antigens yet undiscovered which are not matched and which play a role in the immunological response.

46. True

47. True

48. (1) Rapid serologic testing for HLA-DR antigens is highly predictive of success rate. Thus when a cadaver becomes available there is sufficient time to find the best match with the aid of a national computer bank of potential recipients. If the cadaver graft success rate improves sufficiently, it may be possible to solicit nonrelated living donors. (2) Pretransplant blood transfusions greatly improve kidney graft success rate. Patients who become sensitized to certain antigens in the donor population are not given a transplant from donors with those antigens. (3) Cyclosporin A has greatly increased cadaver graft survival.

49. Hemofiltration; CAPD; oral sorbents. All are supposedly more successful in removing middle molecules.

CHAPTER 45

Acute renal failure

1. Because the fumes of CCl_4 (and other organic solvents) inhaled and the ingested ethyl alcohol react

chemically in the body to produce a potent nephro-toxin, which may produce acute tubular necrosis.

2. Nephrotoxic injury and renal ischemia

3. Acute renal failure is superimposed on chronic renal insufficiency due to intrinsic renal disease. Precipitating causes include nausea, vomiting, and infections.

4. Two basic types of lesion are involved in ATN, though in some cases they may be mixed. The less serious lesion results in necrosis of the tubular epithelium only. This lesion commonly results from mild doses of CCl_4 or $HgCl_2$. When only epithelial damage takes place, complete healing of the lesion commonly occurs in 3 to 4 weeks. In the second type of lesion there is necrosis of the epithelium and also the basement membrane. This is commonly associated with severe renal ischemia. The prognosis of this type of lesion depends on the extent of the damage. When the basement membrane is disrupted, epithelial regeneration occurs in a haphazard manner, frequently leading to obstruction of the nephron at the site of necrosis.

5. *Acute cortical necrosis* means that the entire nephron is infarcted. It is commonly associated with pregnancy complications such as postpartum hemorrhage, premature separation of the placenta, eclampsia, and septic abortion. The prognosis is generally poor. If the patient survives the acute phase of illness, calcification and permanent renal damage often occur in the area of cortical necrosis. Glycol (antifreeze) poisoning may also cause this lesion.

6. Infection

7. This classification stresses the identification of extrarenal causes (prerenal, postrenal) and the prevention of progression to intrinsic acute renal failure. The categories provide a systematic diagnostic approach, since the diagnosis of ARF is made on the basis of exclusion of extrarenal (immediately reversible) causes.

8. Bladder outlet obstruction: benign or malignant prostatic hypertrophy; cancer of cervix or rectum. Bilateral ureteral obstruction: cellular debris from necrotizing papillitis in a person with diabetes mellitus; obstruction of the ureter by a calculus in a patient with one functioning kidney; trauma or accidental ligation during extensive pelvic surgery. Intrarenal obstruction: uric acid cyrstallization in the renal collecting ducts in a leukemic patient receiving chemotherapy; obstruction of the renal tubules with Bence-Jones protein in a patient with multiple myeloma (see also Chap. 17). Inadequate hydration and hypovolemia are important predisposing factors in both cited examples of renal tubule obstruction.

9. Penicillin: methacillin; aminoglycosides: neomycin, gentamycin, kanamycin, tobramycin. Chronic renal insufficiency and advanced age (>60 years) are characteristics of patients at high risk for drug-induced ARF.

10. All the theories concerning the pathogenesis of ARF attempt to explain the severe reduction in the GFR. Suggested mechanisms include:
Mechanical obstruction of the renal tubule lumina by necrotic tubular cells which have sloughed off; cellular swelling may also collapse the tubules, blocking them off.
Backleak of filtrate into the peritubular circulation through damaged tubular cells.
Impermeability or reduction in surface area of the glomerular filtration membrane.
Intrarenal vascular dysfunction, with redistribution of blood from cortex to medulla maintained by the release of renin from the juxtaglomerular cells, activation of angiotensin II, and consequent vasoconstriction of the afferent arterioles. Inhibition of prostaglandin synthesis may also play a role in the intrarenal vascular dysfunction.
Stimulation of renin-angiotensin, with consequent vasoconstriction of the afferent arterioles through the tubuloglomerular feedback mechanism. The renin-angiotensin system is activated by the macula densa cells in the distal tubule, which respond to the increased sodium concentration in the tubular fluid. Sodium reabsorption is diminshed because of proximal tubular damage, hence more is present in the distal tubular fluid.

11. Fractional excretion of sodium (FE_{Na}). It is actually the ratio of the renal clearance of sodium to that of creatinine ($C_{Na}/C_{cr} \times 100\%$). Formula for calculation:

$$FE_{Na} = \frac{U_{Na} \times P_{cr}}{P_{Na} \times U_{cr}} \times 100\%$$

The laboratory should be done before a diuretic is given, and only fresh urine should be used. Intermittent urinary tract obstruction and preexisting chronic renal insufficiency cause problems in interpretation. These factors are hazards in the use of renal indices to differentiate prerenal azotemia from ATN. Since the laboratory tests are simple, they should be repeated several times.

12. Mannitol and furosemide

13. *c*

14. *b*

15. *a, b, d, f*

16. *e*

17. *b, c, d*

18. *a, b, c, d, e,*

19. *d* (associated with severe renal infection)

20. *d*

21. *c*

22. *b*

23. *a*

24. True; azotemia characterizes both oliguric and nonoliguric ARF.

25. False; the opposite happens, causing cortical ischemia and shunting renal blood to normally relatively ischemic medulla.

26. True; a nephrotoxic chemical is produced by reaction with ethyl alcohol.

27. False; myoglobin is released from the muscle and excreted in the urine and may induce ARF.

28. False; obstructive uropathy is suggested.

29. True; urea, being a small molecule, back-diffuses because the sluggish movement of filtrate through the tubules gives it more exposure time for this to occur, while creatinine is not reabsorbed because it is a larger molecule. The fever, bleeding, and trauma often associated with prerenal azotemia also produce a catabolic state further increasing the BUN.

30. *b*

31. *c*

32. *a*

33. *a*

34. *a*

35. *a*

36. *b*

CHAPTER 46

The nervous system

1. True

2. True

3. False; toward the cell body

4. False; nerves do not exist in the CNS. Cranial nerves are part of the PNS, although their nuclei are located in the CNS.

5. False; most of them are, but they also exist in ganglia outside the CNS.

6. True

7. False; oligodendroglia perform this function in the CNS; Schwann cells do not exist in the CNS.

8. True

9. True

10. False; it forms the craniosacral outflow.

11. True

12. True

13. True

14. True

15. True

16. False; they are bipolar.

17. False; this is the definition of a Golgi type I neuron.

18. False; transmission of impulses between neurons can occur only at synapses, and the transmission is unidirectional from presynaptic terminal to postsynaptic membrane (called the *law of Bell-Magendie*).

19. True; proteins are transported from the cell body down the axon by axoplasmic flow.

20. True

21. True

22. False; it covers nerve fibers only in the PNS.

23. True

24. False; they are properly called *fiber tracts* or *nerve fiber tracts* to distinguish them from nerves which exist in the PNS.

25. False; lower level of L1

26. *e*

27. *a, c*

28. *a*

29. *c, d*

30. *d*

31. *b*

32. *c*

33. *d*

34. *c*

35. *d*

36. *d*

37. *c*

38. *a*

39. *b, c*

40. *e*

41. *d*

42. *b*

43. *a*
44. *b*
45. *a, b, c, d*
46. *a, b, e*
47. *c, d*
48. *d*
49. *c*
50. *a, b, d*
51. *a, c, d*
52. *b*
53. *a, b, c, d*
54. *a, b, c, e*
55. *a, b, c, d*
56. *c*
57. *a, b, c*
58. *b*
59. *a, b*
60. *c*
61. *c*
62. *c*
63. *a*
64. *d*
65. *a, c, d*
66. *b*
67. *c, d, e*
68. *a, b, d*
69. *b*
70. *b*
71. *b*
72. All of these
73. *a, b, c, d*
74. *a, c, d*
75. *a, b, c*
76. *b, c*
77. *b, c*
78. *a*
79. *b, c, d*
80. *a, c, d*
81. *c*
82. *b*
83. *d*
84. *a, b, c*
85. *b*
86. *c*
87. *a, b*

88. *d*
89. *e*
90. *a*
91. *c*
92. *b*
93. *c, d, e*
94. *a, b, f*
95. *a, b, c, d*
96. *b*
97. Anatomic components of the extrapyramidal system (although difficult to define anatomically) probably include the basal ganglia and their connections to the cerebral cortex, cerebellum, reticular formation, and certain thalamic nuclei. The substantia nigra, red nucleus, and subthalamic nucleus in the brainstem are also considered part of the extrapyramidal system. The main function of this system is to provide coarse control of voluntary muscular movement.

Caudate nucleus		Corpus striatum (some
Lenticular nucleus	{ Putamen, Globus pallidus }	authors include part of adjacent internal capsule)
Amygdaloid nucleus		
Claustrum		
Red nucleus		
Substantia nigra		Structures closely associated with basal ganglia
Subthalamic nucleus (corpus Luysii)		

The basal ganglia function in some way to prevent oscillation and afterdischarge in· motor systems, probably by direct action on the midbrain centers and in part as inhibitory feedback to the motor cortex. They are also involved in the control of stretch reflexes and in the generation of mannerisms and automatic activity.

CHAPTER 47

The neurologic examination: evaluation of the neurologic patient

1. Neurologic illness is usually well defined, and a clear history will provide clues that will assist in an accurate assessment of the patient's condition.

2. Examination of the motor system (i.e., testing the gait, voluntary muscle strength, muscle tone)

Sensory examination (i.e., pain, temperature, vibration sense, examination of the reflexes)
Coordination of arms and legs
Examination of mental status and speech
Examination of cranial nerves
Examination of the reflex status

3. False; the parietal cortex

4. True

5. False; the left hemisphere is dominant.

6. True

7. *e*

8. *h*

9. *d*

10. *g*

11. *a*

12. *f*

13. *b*

14. *c*

15. *b, d*

16. *c*

17. *b*

18. *c*

19. *c*

20. *b*

21. *a*

22. *b*

23. *c*

24. *b*

25. *d*

26. *i*

27. *f*

28. *g*

29. *j*

30. *b*

31. *e*

32. *h*

33. *a*

34. *b*

35. *c*

36. *a*

37. *d*

38. (*a*) Superficial tactile sense; (*b*) proprioceptive (motion or position) sense; (*c*) vibratory sense; (*d*) cortical sensory function

39. *b*

40. *a, c*

41. *a*

42. True

43. False; these are signs of upper motor neuron involvement.

44. True

45. Romberg

46. L5 to S1

CHAPTER 48

Cerebrovascular disease and headache

1. *b*

2. *b*

3. *c*

4. *b, d*

5. The internal carotid enters the skull through the carotid canal, where it gives rise to the ophthalmic artery. It then divides into the anterior and middle cerebral arteries. The anterior cerebral artery supplies the medial surface of the cerebrum and anastomoses with the anterior communicating artery. The middle cerebral artery supplies the lateral surfaces of the cerebral cortex. This branch joins, via the posterior communicating artery, the posterior cerebral branch of the basilar artery. The cerebral arteries and their communicating branches to the basilar artery form the circle of Willis. The basilar artery supplies the cerebellum and the brainstem. It terminates in two posterior cerebral arteries, which supply the inferior surfaces of the temporal and occipital lobes. They communicate with the middle cerebral artery via the posterior communicating artery to complete the circle of Willis.

6. Extrinsic factors: (*a*) Systemic blood pressure: If the BP drops below 60 mmHg, the autoregulatory mechanism of the brain becomes less effective. If the BP continues to drop until CBF is decreased to 30 ml per 100 g of tissue per minute, signs of cerebral ischemia will appear. (*b*) Cardiovascular function: If cardiac output is decreased by more than one-third, there is likely to be a fall in CBF. (*c*) Blood viscosity: CBF may increase by as much as 30 percent with anemia; in polycythemia it may decrease by 50 percent.
Intrinsic factors: (*a*) Cerebral autoregulatory mechanism is related to cerebral perfusion pressure (difference between the cerebral artery and veins).

When systemic BP decreases, there is a compensatory increase in cerebral vascular pressure, whereas when BP increases, the opposite occurs. (b) Cerebral blood vessels: These vessels are considered the most important factor relating to cerebrovascular resistance. A myogenic response suggests that parenchymal tissue of arterioles releases a vasodilatory metabolite in response to their oxygen needs and thereby exerts control on arterial smooth-muscle tone. (c) Intracranial pressure (ICP): An increase in the ICP will increase cerebrovascular resistance. However, CBF does not decrease until ICP has increased to 450 mm water.

7. 200,000; 2 million

8. (a) Transient ischemic attacks (TIAs): Focal neurologic deficits that develop suddenly and disappear within a few minutes to hours. (b) Progressive (stroke in evolution): Evolution of stroke is gradual though acute. (c) Completed stroke: Deficits are maximal at onset, with little improvement.

9. c, d, b, a

10. a, b, c, d

11. e

12. True

13. True

14. False; cerebral tissue necrosis is not associated with TIA.

15. True

16. a

17. d

18. a

19. b

20. d

21. c

22. c

23. c

24. a, b, c

25. c

26. b

27. b

28. a, b, c

29. These factors are (a) stabilization of vital signs—maintaining a patent airway and blood pressure control on an individualized basis, (b) detection and correction of cardiac arrhythmias, (c) bladder care, (d) proper positioning stressed immediately (frequent turning, ROM).

30. (a) Vasodilators have increased CBF experimentally but have not proved beneficial in human strokes. It should be noted that the use of vasodilators may exert an adverse effect on CBF by lowering systemic BP and thereby decreasing intracerebral anastomotic flow. (b) Platelet antiaggregants such as aspirin may be given for prophylaxis against platelet aggregation and subsequent clotting in persons at risk of a stroke. The long-term effectiveness of the therapy needs further evaluation.

31. The primary goal of surgical intervention is improvement of the cerebral blood flow.

32. (a) A revascularization technique by which a superficial temporal artery is anastomosed to a superficial cortical artery or a segment of the saphenous vein is anastomosed to the subclavian artery and the proximal end of the internal carotid. (b) A carotid endarterectomy in which the neck of the carotid artery is exposed. The vessel is incised at the site of stenosis, and the clot and plaque material are removed.

33. To prevent recurrent hemorrhage.

34. (a) Decrease in salt intake—especially with the elderly, and extreme care to maintain blood pressure during surgical procedures; (b) avoidance of oversedation and prolonged bed rest; (c) increased activity; (d) weight control, especially with obese patients; (e) cessation of cigarette smoking.

35. c

36. e

37. a, b, c, e

38. b, c, e

39. a, b, e

40. a, d, e

41. a, b, c, d, e

42. False; this is a description of classic migraine.

43. True, presumably because it is caused by persistent leakage of CSF through the needle site.

44. True

45. True

46. True

47. True

48. Anterior (frontal, temporal, and parietal areas), trigeminal (Vth cranial)

49. Posterior or occipital and neck; upper cervical

50. b, c, e, g, i, j. Migraine is also sometimes precipitated by wine and other alcoholic beverages or foods such as chocolate or cheese. All these foods

contain phenylethylamine. Migraine patients are deficient in monoamine oxidase, responsible for degrading phenylethylamine.

51. *a, c, h, j*

52. *d, f, a, k*

53. Questions need to be asked concerning the onset, frequency, duration, location, and precipitating and relieving factors; whether there are prodromal symptoms or associated symptoms such as dizziness, nausea, vomiting, or blurred vision; type of pain and whether it is incapacitating; whether other members of the family have a headache problem; and whether there has been head injury in the past. Medical conditions must be considered in relation to the headache pattern.

CHAPTER 49

Epilepsy

1. *Epilepsy* is a paroxysmal disorder of the nervous system characterized by recurrent attacks of loss or alteration of consciousness with or without motor convulsive phenomena. This is usually caused by excessive, uncontrolled local discharges of a group of cerebral neurons, ususally in the cortex.

2. The incidence is estimated to be about 0.5 percent or slightly higher. The incidence in the offspring of epileptic persons is higher than that in the general population.

3. Head injury, hypoglycemia, vitamin B_6 deficiency, alcohol withdrawal, encephalitis, brain tumors.

4. Midbrain, thalamus, cerebral cortex

5. Current theory postulates epileptic neurons that have lower thresholds for firing abnormal discharges. A deafferented neuron has been identified in some focal lesions. These neurons are hypersensitive and in a chronic state of depolarization. The cytoplasmic membranes exhibit increased permeability, making them susceptible to activation by various factors (hypoxia, hyperthermia) and circumstances (repeated sensory stimuli).

6. Metabolic needs are increased during convulsions; the electrical discharges of motor nerve cells may be increased to 1000 per second. Cerebral blood flow is increased, and there is some increase in respiration and glycolysis. Acetylcholine appears in the CSF during and following seizures. Glutamic acid may be depleted during seizure activity.

7. *Status epilepticus* refers to a state in which there is a succession (two or more) of generalized seizures with no recovery of consciousness between them.

8. *a, b, c, d*

9. *a, b*

10. *c*

11. *d*

12. *b, d*

13. *a, c, d*

14. *b*

15. *c*

16. *a*

17. *e*

18. *f*

19. *d*

CHAPTER 50

Degenerative and other disorders of the nervous system

1. Basal ganglia; slow degeneration of nerve cells; below the cortex (subcortical)

2. Extrapyramidal motor nerve tract; it regulates semiautomatic movements, such as coordination of hand movements and swallowing.

3. *Parkinson's syndrome* is a chronic disorder of the central nervous system characterized by a specific group of symptoms which get progressively worse until the patient is unable to perform the activities of daily living and becomes bedridden. Parkinson's syndrome may be idiopathic, postencephalitic, or drug-induced (the last a type of pseudo-parkinsonism)

4. A byproduct of catacholamine metabolism is hydrogen peroxide. Its removal is accomplished by two enzymes (peroxidase and catalase) found in the substantia nigra. In parkinsonism patients, the level of these enzymes is significantly reduced, causing a buildup of hydrogen peroxide. The hydrogen peroxide causes destruction of the cells of the substantia nigra and loss of the enzyme (tyrosine hydroxylase) which is responsible for the production of dopamine. Thus the neurotransmitter dopamine is reduced in amount, causing the clinical picture of parkinsonism.

5. (a) Resting tremor—fine or coarse rhythmic alternating contraction of opposing muscle groups, occurring at rest in disease of the basal ganglia and decreasing with voluntary motion; (b) choreiform movement—rapid, irregular, jerky, purposeless contractions of random muscle groups followed by

prompt relaxation; (c) athetoid movement—continuous slow, writhing movements that may be tonic avoiding or grasping reactions; (d) dystonia—slow, powerful movements, like bending a lead pipe; (e) hemiballism—flailing, intense violent movements involving one side of the body.

6. Phenothiazine, *Rauwolfia* agents

7. Hyperactive glabellar reflex; resting tremor (pill-rolling); expressionless face; festinating gait; micrographia; monotone voice; plastic or cogwheel rigidity

8. Acute disseminated encephalomyelitis, in which patchy areas of demyelinization occur in the brain and spinal cord. Preventive measures include regular vaccination for measles in children and avoidance of routine smallpox vaccination. The newer, killed-duck-embryo rabies vaccine should be used when it is necessary to give rabies vaccinations.

9. There are widespread patches of myelin destruction and gliosis in the central nervous system. If the patient reported a temporary blurring of vision in one eye or blindness or an episode of weakness or tingling in an extremity, this would be grounds for suspicion.

10. The major theories are (1) slow viruses, (2) autoimmune process, and (3) aluminum toxicity.

11. *b, c, e*

12. *c*

13. *a*

14. *a, c*

15. *c*

16. *b*

17. *b*

18. *d*

19. *c*

20. *c*

21. *c*

22. *d*

23. *c*

24. *d*

25. *c*

26. All are correct.

27. *a, c*

28. *e*

29. *e*

30. True

31. False; also have been noted in lead encephalopathy and Down's syndrome.

32. True

33. True

34. False; ALS has been tentatively linked to aluminum toxicity.

35. True

36. False; thiamine is the therapy of choice.

37. True

38. False; it is a very serious condition.

39. False; it does not provide complete protection against invasion by viruses.

40. True

41. True

CHAPTER 51

Central nervous system injury

1. Normal intracranial pressure (ICP) is about 4 to 15 mmHg. The basic cause of increased ICP is an expanding mass within the rigid, bony cranium which allows very little room for expansion (about 5 cm³) before pressure starts to increase. Normally the cranial contents consist of tissue, blood, and cerebrospinal fluid (CSF). An increase in ICP can be caused by increased tissue (as from a growing tumor), blood (hematoma secondary to rupture of a blood vessel), blockage of the flow of CSF and its accumulation, and cerebral edema (commonly associated with cerebral trauma). Increased ICP is dangerous because it causes cerebral ischemia, hypoxia, compression of the cortex and herniation of the brainstem through the foramen magnum. This compression causes cessation of function of the vital regulatory centers within the brainstem and death.

2. Compression of cortex: hemiparesis is due to compression of motor cortex; seizures may be due to local cortical disruption; mental dysfunction occurs because cortex is concerned with higher thought processes.

   Displacement of brainstem down into foramen magnum, causing its compression: reticular formation in brainstem is concerned with level of consciousness; systolic blood pressure increases so that it will be higher than ICP and cerebral circulation will be maintained; this also causes decerebrate rigidity from removal of normal influence of higher centers on muscle tone.

   Compression of the oculomotor nerve by herniated uncus causes ipsilateral dilated pupil.

3. (a) Local tissue damage due to direct force (penetration of compression by missiles or bone fragments or damage due to displacement of cranial contents in rapid acceleration or deceleration). (b) Cerebral ischemia due to lack of autoregulation secondary to increasing intracranial pressure.

4. Forceful thrusting of the brain contents against the inner surface of the skull on the side opposite the impact. The areas most likely to be damaged in a decelerating automobile accident are the anterior portion of the frontal and temporal lobes and the upper section of the midbrain.

5. The most common sites are those at which a relatively mobile portion of the vertebral column meets a relatively fixed segment. These sites occur between the lower cervical and upper thoracic spine, between the lower thoracic and upper lumbar spine, and between the lower lumbar spine and the sacrum.

6. Stabilize the spinal column to prevent contusion, laceration, and further damage to the spinal cord from bony fragments and foreign bodies.

7. Epidural hematomas usually result from a tear in the middle meningeal artery. The bleeding occurs between the dura mater and the skull, usually in the temporal area. The development of clinical symptoms and the course are rapid and proceed to completion within a few hours, since the bleeding is arterial. On the other hand, subdural hematomas usually result from the tearing of veins which pass from the surface of the brain to one of the major dural sinuses. Blood escapes between the dura and the arachnoid. Since bleeding is under venous low pressure, the accumulation of blood may be much more prolonged and the clinical course much more protracted.

8. *a*

9. All of these

10. *d*

11. *b, c*

12. *c*; treatment *b* might cause herniation of the uncus.

13. *b*

14. *a, b, c*

15. *b, d*

16. *c*

17. *a*

18. *c*; loss of vibration sense because of destruction of dorsal (uncrossed ascending) columns and increased touch threshold because of destruction of ventral spinothalamic tract (crossed ascending axons)

19. *c, d*

20. *c, e*

21. *a, d*

22. *b*

23. False; it is between the dura and skull.

24. False; this causes quadriplegia.

25. True

26. True

27. True

28. False; surgical decompression is controversial; all agree that is should be done if there is progressive neurologic deficit.

29. True

30. True

31. Nucleus pulposus

32. Annulus fibrosus

33. Annulus; posterior longitudinal

34. *b*

35. *e*

36. *d*

37. *b*; relapses may occur, but the patient may be symptom-free for years

CHAPTER 52

Central nervous system tumors

1. It is difficult because the symptoms are very diverse and depend on the location and size of the growth. However, the symptoms tend to progress. The most common general symptoms are headache, vomiting, and papilledema, all a result of increased intracranial pressure from the expanding mass.

2. *b*

3. *d*

4. *a*

5. *c*

6. *e*

7. *d*

8. *b*

9. *a*

10. *c*

11. *g*

12. *f*

13. *c*

14. *d*

15. *b*
16. *a*
17. *e*
18. *c*
19. *f*
20. *d*
21. *e*
22. *a*
23. *b*
24. *d*
25. *c*
26. *d*
27. *a*
28. *a, c, e*
29. *a*
30. *b*
31. *d*
32. *b*
33. *c*
34. True
35. True
36. False; microglia function as phagocytes.
37. True
38. True
39. False; most commonly in thoracic region
40. False; this is amaurosis fugax. Papilledema involves engorgement and swelling of the optic disc.
41. *a*
42. *b*
43. *c*
44. *d*
45. *c*
46. *b*

CHAPTER 53

Principles of endocrine and metabolic control mechanisms

1. (*a*) Response to stress injury; (*b*) growth and development; (*c*) reproduction; (*d*) maintenance of ionic homeostasis; (*e*) control of energy metabolism

2. One mechanism by which hormones work on cells is the adenyl cyclase system. In this case the polypeptide hormones interact with a specific membrane receptor. As a result of this interaction, adenylate cyclase is activated and ATP is converted to cyclic AMP. Cyclic AMP binds to the regulatory subunit of a protein kinase, liberating a catalytic subunit of the enzyme. This in turn initiates the phosphorylation of certain enzymes that either activate or inactivate the biologic potency of these enzymes.

A second mechanism by which hormones work on target cells is exemplified by steroid hormones, which work directly inside the cell by entering the cell across the cell membrane and binding to cytosol receptor proteins. The steroid receptor complex then is translocated to the nucleus of the cell, where it binds specifically to its locus on the chromatin, activating RNA polymerase with ultimate synthesis of one or several specific messenger RNAs. These products travel from the nucleus to the ribosome, where they direct the synthesis of proteins. By changing messenger RNA, steroids can modify the way protein is synthesized.

3.

Type of hormone	Location of production	Examples
Proteins (polypeptides, glycoproteins)	Posterior pituitary gland	Pitressin
	Beta cells of islets of Langerhans	Insulin
	Thyroid gland	Thyroxine
	Parathyroid gland	Parathyroid hormone
	Anterior pituitary	Tropic hormones
Steroids (lipids)	Adrenal cortex	Cortisol
	Gonads	Estrogen Progesterone

4. A decrease in the pressure of the blood flowing through the afferent arteriole of the renal glomerulus is sensed by JG cells, causing release of renin. This results in the following sequence of events:

Renin → Renin Substrate
↓
Angiotensin I
↓
Angiotensin II
└──────→ Adrenal cortex
↓
Aldosterone

5. The hypothalamus possesses a variety of nuclei which are made up of neurons having a secretory function. These neurons manufacture proteins, called *releasing hormones*, which are secreted

through axons into blood vessels. The hypothalamus receives fibers from other areas of the brain which influence hypothalamic neuronal function.

6. This anatomic mechanism permits the movement of neurostimuli from the hypothalmus to the pituitary gland; this is the mechanism by which the CNS influences the pituitary gland.

7. Any neurostimuli reaching the CR center cause release of CRH into the portal system. CRH causes release of ACTH by cells in the anterior pituitary gland. ACTH stimulates the adrenal cortex to produce cortisol, which affects the rate and amount of CRH-ACTH secreted by the hypothalamic pituitary axis.

8. ACTH production typically exhibits a cyclic pattern throughout the 24-hour period. The levels usually go up early in the day, go down later in the day, and go up again during the night, to reach a peak level by the next morning.

9. The two postulated mechanisms for endocrine disorders are (1) disturbances in which the hormone concentrations are primarily disturbed and (2) disturbances in which the receptors are primarily defective. Most endocrine disorders can be understood conceptually in terms of the metabolic action of the hormone(s) involved.

10. If a disease arises from excessive production of a hormone, the problem may be treated surgically by removing the gland or part of the gland that produces the hormone. This is followed by replacement with normal amounts of the hormone. If a disease is caused by hormone deficit, the treatment is replacement of the hormones which are not being produced.

11. Hyperthyroidism
12. Hypothalamic-hypophyseal portal system
13. Thyroid-stimulating hormone (TSH)
14. True
15. False; they are specific.

CHAPTER 54

Disorders of the pituitary gland

1. b
2. a
3. a
4. c

5. d
6. e
7. g
8. a
9. c
10. b
11. h
12. f
13. a, b, c, d
14. c, d
15. a, c, d
16. c
17. b, c, e
18. e
19. b
20. b, c
21. a, b, c, d
22. a, d
23. a, b, c, d
24. True
25. False; human growth hormone is the only one effective in humans and is used in experimental study for the treatment of hypopituitary dwarfism.
26. True
27. False; radiographic examination of the pituitary gland is mandatory in patients with suspected pituitary disease, since pituitary tumors are a common cause of these disorders.
28. True

CHAPTER 55

Diseases of the thyroid gland

1. a
2. a
3. c
4. b, c
5. a, b, c
6. b
7. b, c
8. a, b
9. a
10. a, b
11. True
12. False; a lesion in the thyroid gland.
13. True
14. True

15. True

16. True

17. The thyroid gland located below the cricoid carti-lage in the neck is made up of nodules of tiny fol-licles. These follicles are lined by cuboidal epithe-lium, and their lumen is filled with colloid. The follicular epithelial cells initiate the synthesis of thyroid hormones and activate their release into the circulation. The thyroid hormones produced by the follicles are thyroxine and triiodothyronine.

18. The process of biosynthesis of thyroid hormones is as follows: (a) Trapping of iodine by the thyroid fol-licular cells. The thyroid takes up and concentrates large amounts of iodine from the circulating iodide pool. (b) Oxidation of iodide to iodine. The thyroid plasma gradient is 20-30:1 at a wide range of plasma inorganic iodide concentrations. Iodide is catalyzed by an iodide peroxidase enzyme and converted to iodine. (c) Organification of iodine into monoiodo-tyrosine. Iodine is incorporated into a tyrosine mol-ecule, which occurs at the cell-colloid interphase. (d) Coupling of iodinated precursors. The resulting compounds, monoiodotyrosine and diiodotyrosine are coupled as follows: two molecules of diiodoty-rosine make thyroxine (T_4), and one molecule of diiodotyrosine and one molecule of monoiodotyro-sine make triiodothyronine (T_3). (e) Storage. The coupling of these compounds and the storage of the resulting hormones take place within thyroglobu-lin. (f) Hormone release for storage. This release oc-curs by incorporation of colloid droplets into the follicular cells by a process called *pinocytosis*. Thy-roglobulin is hydrolyzed, and the hormones are re-leased into the circulation.

19. 4 to 11; 80 to 160

20. Graves' disease; toxic nodular goiter

CHAPTER 56

Disorders of calcium metabolism

1. a, b, c, d

2. a, b, c

3. a, b, c, e

4. b, d

5. b

6. a, b, d

7. c

8. 9 to 10.5

9. Active form of vitamin D_3; parathormone

10. Gastrointestinal losses, deposition of calcium into the bone mineral, and urinary clearance of calcium

CHAPTER 57

The adrenal cortex—disorders of hypersecretion

1. a, b, c, d

2. b

3. c

4. a, b, c

5. a, c

6. b

7. b

8. b

9. a, c

10. a

11. d

12. d

13. The catabolic effect of glucocorticoid excess causes a decrease in the ability of protein-forming cells to synthesize protein from amino acids.

14. Interferes with the action of insulin in the periph-eral cells, which results in the impairment of the ability of the receptor cells to metabolize glucose.

15. Stress causes the CNS to activate the corticotropin-releasing center, causing CRH and ACTH to be re-leased. Increased ACTH leads to an increase in cor-tisol release. The important concept is that stress causes an increased secretion of cortisol by the adrenal gland.

16. 9α-Fluorocortisol has a fluorine group in the 9α-po-sition of the cortisol molecule. Prednisolone has a double bond between carbons 1 and 2 of this mol-ecule. The metabolic effects of these compounds are different from those of the parent compound. For example, prednisolone, compared with cortisol, has less sodium-retaining activity and more anti-in-flammatory activity per milligram. 9α-Fluorocorti-sol has much greater sodium-retaining activity than cortisol.

17. Pituitary irradiation, removal of a pituitary tumor, and adrenalectomy. The excess cortisol is elimi-nated if the procedure is successful.

18. Surgical removal of the neoplasm

19. In congestive heart failure, patients are unable to pump blood normally and cardiac output decreases. The renal afferent arteriole experiences a change in perfusion pressure, causing increased production of renin, which activates synthesis of angiotensin.

This stimulates aldosterone production, causing resorption of Na and water and volume expansion.

20. True
21. True
22. True
23. False; CRF directly initiates the secretion of ACTH.

CHAPTER 58

The adrenal cortex—disorders of hyposecretion

1. *b*
2. *c*
3. *a, c*
4. *a*
5. *a, c*
6. *c*
7. *c*
8. *b, d*
9. *c*

CHAPTER 59

The pancreas—glucose metabolism and diabetes mellitus

1. *a, b*
2. *a, b*
3. *c*
4. *a*
5. *c*
6. *a, b, c*
7. *d*
8. *b*
9. *a, b*
10. *a*
11. *b*
12. *c*
13. *a*
14. *a, b, c, d*
15. Fasting plasma glucose is measured in order to check the function of the regulating mechanisms which control carbohydrate metabolism. This mea-

surement can help evaluate the integrity of the mechanism regulating plasma glucose. In general, these levels become abnormal only in the advanced state of a disease. Therefore, it does not provide information about early abnormalities in glucose metabolism.

16. Insulin. In people without diabetes, a rise in blood glucose stimulates release of insulin which triggers disposal of excess glucose.
17. This system assists diabetics in managing their own diets. The food exchange lists help patients identify food alternatives.
18. *c*
19. *d*
20. *a*
21. *b*
22. True
23. False; 75 percent of diabetic patients eventually die of vascular disease. Heart attacks, kidney failure, strokes, and gangrene are the major complications.
24. False; exercise appears to facilitate the transport of glucose into cells.
25. True

CHAPTER 60

Disorders of the reproductive cycle

1. *c*
2. *c*
3. *d*
4. *a, c, d*
5. *b*
6. *e*
7. *c*
8. *a, c, d*
9. *d*
10. *c, d*
11. *a, c*
12. *a, c, d*
13. All are correct.
14. All are correct.
15. *c*
16. False; 300,000
17. True
18. False; estradiol levels promptly drop.
19. True
20. False; primary, not secondary, amenorrhea
21. True

22. False; a 21-hydroxylase deficiency causes a decrease in cortisol and an increase in ACTH secretion.

23. False; prostaglandin inhibitors should be used mainly for treatment of dysmenorrhea and other symptoms such as headaches and minor muscular skeletal pains associated with PMS.

24. True

25. True

26. There appears to be a relation between the onset of the pubertal process and a critical body weight. A minimum body mass seems to be required for maturation of the hypothalamic-pituitary-ovarian axis. For American girls of European ancestry, the average weight at which menarche occurs is 48 kg.

27. During menopause estradiol levels decrease and the ovary decreases in size and is virtually devoid of follicles. The decrease in circulating estradiol levels increases, by negative feedback, pituitary gonadotropin secretion.

28. Treatment of amenorrhea is often based on the type of underlying disorder causing the problem. For example, patients with prolactin-secreting pituitary adenomas should be treated with either transphenoidal resection of the pituitary tumor or suppression of prolactin secretion with bromocriptine. Patients with hypothalamic-pituitary or ovarian deficiency should receive replacement therapy with estrogens and progesterone administered cyclically.

29. A decrease in estrogen levels causes instability of the autonomic nervous system, mediated centrally at the hypothalamic level. Hot flush episodes also appear to correlate with pulsatile pituitary release of LH. However, the exact relation between the vasomotor symptoms and high gonadotropin levels in menopausal women remains uncertain.

30. The exact physiologic basis for increased incidence of oligomenorrhea and amenorrhea in female athletes is unknown, but it has been postulated that a minimum weight for height, representing a critical lean/fat ratio, is necessary for menarche and for the maintenance of regular ovulatory cycles. Athletes with a very low fat/lean ratio may undergo a suppression of the neurohypothalamic-pituitary axis through a decrease in estrogen levels. These women may also have suppression of gonadotropin release by psychogenic factors related to the stress of competition and intense training.

CHAPTER 61

Fractures and dislocations

1. *a*

2. *d*

3. *a*

4. *d*

5. *d*

6. *a*

7. *d*

8. *c, d*

9. *b*

10. *a*

11. *a, b, d*

12. *b, c*

13. *c*

14. *a*

15. *c*

16. *b*

17. *a, c*

18. *b*

19. *c*

20. *d*

21. *b, d*

22. *c*

23. *b*

24. *b, d*

25. *b*

26. *b, d*

27. *a*

28. *b*

29. *b*

30. *c, d*

31. *b, d*

32. Refer to Fig. 61-1.

33. *b, d*

34. *f*

35. *a*

36. *b*

37. *c*

38. *g*

39. False; penetration of the skin occurs in open fractures.

40. True

41. True

42. False; in many cases closed reduction is the process

of manipulating fragments of broken bone back to their original location without surgical incision.

43. When a fracture occurs, the periosteum is generally torn, blood vessels are damaged, and bone fragments are separated. A blood clot forms, and granulation tissue develops within which osteogenic cells differentiate into chondroblasts and osteoblasts. A band (callus) forms around a fragment at the fracture site and continues to thicken and expand, converging with the band from the opposite fragment and fusing with it. Fusion of the two fragments and fracture healing progress as osteoblasts form trabeculae which adhere to the bone and extend across the fracture site. The bony callus remodels to assume the shape of intact bone, as osteoblasts form new bone and osteoclasts remove the damaged and temporary bone.

44. Persistent burning pain at the pressure sites indicates developing skin and soft-tissue necrosis; pressure may be relieved by cutting and reforming the cast.

45. Skin necrosis and neurovascular complications of circumferential dressing are avoided when skeletal traction is used.

46. Weights are attached by ropes to the patient's limb. The location of pulleys through which the ropes run is adjusted until the direction of pull is in line with the long axis of the fractured bone.

47. Traction (a) provides for limb elevation (reduces swelling) in a dependable way, (b) promotes soft-tissue healing, (c) provides for easy observation for neurovascular dysfunction; and (d) allows convenient bed care for the patient.

48. Implant devices have great intrinsic strength and allow the fracture fragments to settle toward each other as necessary during the healing process.

49. The goal is to return the patient as rapidly as possible to the preinjury state. The approximate duration of serious disability is often predictable, and therefore it is important to plan for rehabilitation from the day of the injury.

50. The progressive destruction of a major joint or joints may prematurely disable a person. When the pain and disability are so great that the person is uable to independently carry out the activities of daily living, surgical replacement of the diseased joint may be indicated.

51. Pain, pallor, pulselessness, anesthesias

52. The limb may sustain irreversible pathologic changes within 1½ hours.

CHAPTER 62

Orthopedic diseases of children

1. *a, c*
2. *d*
3. *a*
4. *b*
5. *b*
6. *d*
7. *b*
8. *b*
9. *c*
10. In children, the periosteal sleeve around the tubular bones is strong and active, allowing for rapid healing.
11. Childrens' limbs grow quickly; bayonette apposition is often used to achieve equal length by adulthood.

CHAPTER 63

Tumors of the musculoskeletal system

1. When a lesion is definitely diagnosed as benign and self-limiting, no further diagnostic studies are generally needed. However, when a lesion is diagnosed as benign with a lesser degree of certainty, the patient should be reexamined at regular intervals with repeat radiographs. If over a period of several months there is no change in the lesion or in the condition of the patient, follow-up visits may be discontinued. The patient must be instructed to return for further examination should any changes occur. It is important to assess whether the patient and the family are responsbile and will follow through with the repeated examination.

2. (a) The cannulated needle may macerate the skin and destroy its architecture; (b) the exact location of the lesion is uncertain, so the sample material may not include tumor cells; and (c) potential injury to vascular or vital structures may result.

3. The disadvantages are that it may be inconvenient for the patient, as hospitalization is usually required. The advantages are that the procedure is most appropriate for a patient who has a small, circumscribed lesion of uncertain identity.

4. The clinical signs and symptoms that may indicate a malignant tumor potential are (a) rate of increase in the size of the mass (a benign lesion may grow very slowly or not at all, while a malignant tumor may double in size within a month); (b) increasing nocturnal pain and sleeplessness associated with weight loss in a healthy person; (c) fatigability in a young person; (d) persistent fever and localized

temperature in the region of the tumor; and (e) physiologic dysfunction (obstruction of the ureters, obstruction of a major vessel, or neurologic dysfunction).

5. True
6. False; pathologic fractures are generally the result of metastasis of malignant tumor to bone.
7. True
8. False; metastasis from a primary site to bone is frequently found in adults, not children.
9. True
10. *a, d*
11. *a*
12. *b*
13. *a*
14. *c*
15. *b*

CHAPTER 64

Anatomy and physiology of the joints

1. Rheumatic disorders share the common characteristics of inflammation or pain of the muscles, joints, or connective tissues. These disorders are generally long-term illnesses which involve multiple organ systems.

2. The importance of the relationship between the joint and the surrounding connective tissues is that these are the sites commonly affected in rheumatic disorders.

3. *Joints* refer to areas in the body where two or more bones meet. These bones are held together by various means, such as a joint capsule, fibrous bands, ligaments, tendons, and so on. For example, synarthrodial, or fibrous, joints are those in which the bones are held together by fibrous tissues which allow no movement.

4. The joint capsule is made up of a dense fibrous outer covering, an inner layer of highly vascularized connective tissue, and synovium. The synovium produces a highly viscous liquid that lubricates the joint surfaces. The joint is lubricated by synovial fluid and by hydrostatic changes in the interstitial fluid of the cartilage. Pressure on the cartilage causes fluid to move from the cartilage to an area of less pressure. As the joint glides forward, this weeping fluid moves ahead of the load. The fluid moves back into the portions of the cartilage from which the pressure is relieved. The articular cartilage and the bones of the joint are normally held apart during action by the film of fluid. The articular cartilage cannot be worn out by excessive use as long as an adequate film is present.

5. Joints are evaluated by examining their range of motion and the presence of pain and tenderness, swelling, discolorations, and deformities. Since various rheumatic disorders differ in the way they affect the joints, the evaluation of the joints is essential to making a diagnosis and monitoring responses to therapy.

6. The factors that appear to predispose persons to rheumatic disorders include chronic trauma to connective tissue over years, genetic predispositions (especially those associated with the HLA markers), abnormal connective tissue synthesis, the presence of certain sex hormones, and aging tissue with compromised repair processes.

7. *a*
8. *a*
9. *c*
10. *b*
11. *b*
12. *c, d*
13. *b*
14. *a*
15. *b*
16. *d*
17. *g*
18. *f*
19. *d*
20. *c*
21. *e*
22. *a*
23. *b*
24. False; it is often difficult to distinguish periarticular pain from pain arising from a joint.
25. True
26. False; the mucin clot test is less effective with the more inflammatory fluids, because the acetic acid added to the synovial fluid forms a precipitate by interaction with hyaluronic acid. The hyaluronic acid has been broken down by the lysosomal enzymes and is not available to precipitate when treated with acetic acid.
27. *c*
28. *a*
29. *d*
30. *b*

CHAPTER 65

Rheumatoid arthritis

1. *Rheumatoid arthritis* is a chronic disorder that affects multiple organ systems and is one of a group of diffuse connective tissue diseases that are immune-mediated and of unknown etiology. There is usually progressive joint destruction, although the episodes of joint inflammation may alternate with periods of remission.

2. The association of the genetic markers HLA-Dw4 and -DR5 in whites with the development of rheumatoid arthritis.

3. Destruction of the tissues in the joints occurs in the following ways: (a) There is digestive destruction caused by the production of proteases, collagenases, and other hydrolytic enzymes. These enzymes break down the cartilage, ligaments, tendons, and bones in the joints and are released along with oxygen radicals and arachidonic acid metabolites by PMNs in the synovial fluid. (b) Destruction of tissue appears to take place through the action of rheumatoid pannus. Along the edge of the pannus there is destruction of collagen and proteoglycans through the production of enzymes of cells in the pannus.

4. The diagnostic criteria developed by the American Rheumatism Association are (a) morning stiffness, (b) pain on motion or tenderness in at least one joint, (c) swelling (not bony) in at least one joint, (d) swelling of at least one other joint within a 3-month period, (e) symmetrical joint swelling, (f) subcutaneous nodules, (g) x-ray changes typical of rheumatoid arthritis, (h) positive serologic test for rheumatoid factor, (i) poor mucin precipitate from synovial fluid, (j) characteristic histologic change in nodule, and (k) characteristic histologic change in synovial tissue.

5. The overall goals of the therapeutic program for rheumatoid arthritis are to relieve pain and inflammation, maintain joint function and the patient's maximum functional capacity, and prevent and/or correct joint deformities.

6. NSAIDS reduce inflammation by interrupting the cascade of production of inflammatory mediators. They act by inhibition of either cyclooxygenase or prostaglandin synthetase. These enzymes are responsible for the conversion of the endogenous systemic fatty acid arachidonic acid to prostaglandins, prostacyclins, thromboxanes, and oxygen radicals.

7. The indications for corticosteroid therapy are as follows: (a) Chronic oral therapy is used in those persons with rheumatoid arthritis who do not respond to NSAIDs and DMARDs. (b) It is used for control of symptoms while awaiting the onset of action by DMARD therapy. (c) Intraarticular injections are indicated for acute exacerbations of synovitis in single joints where mobility is significantly impaired. (d) High dose oral therapy is used for short periods for a severe attack.

8. Corticosteroid agents act through their anti-inflammatory and immunosuppressive properties. Inflammation is reduced by blockage of prostaglandin formation, inhibition of leukocyte and monocyte chemotaxis and phagocytosis, stabilization of lysosomal enzymes, and prevention of changes in capillary membranes. Immunosuppression results from the decreased reticuloendothelial production of antigens and the altered function of lymphocytes.

9. Rheumatoid arthritis may involve the heart (pericarditis), lungs (pleuritis), eye, and blood vessels. Refer to Table 65-1.

10. *b*

11. *b*

12. *b*

13. *c*

14. *d*

15. *b, d*

16. *a, b*

17. True

18. False; only an association with HLA-Dw4 has been shown in blacks and in Japanese.

19. True

20. False; rheumatoid factor is detected in about 85 percent of patients with rheumatoid arthritis.

CHAPTER 66

Seronegative spondyloarthopathies

1. The goals of the treatment of anklosing spondylitis are multifocal and relate to the stage of the illness. There is a focused intervention aimed at increasing the understanding of the illness by the patient and the family. Changes in work patterns may be necessary, since bending, lifting, and prolonged static positions will be difficult. Medication is aimed at decreasing the synovitis and pain. An active exercise program is often focused upon breathing exercises, muscle strengthening, and reducing limitations in range of motion.

2. About 7 percent of people with psoriasis develop inflammatory joint disease (psoriatic arthritis). Usu-

ally the arthritis occurs after the appearance of the skin lesions, but it can occur before or at the same time as the skin lesions.

3. The treatment of Reiter's syndrome is primarily symptomatic. Therapeutic doses of nonsteroidal anti-inflammatory drugs are used to relieve the inflammation and pain. Antibiotics are not of proven value.

4. *a, b, d*

5. *b, c, d*

6. *a, b*

7. *c, d*

8. *b, c, d*

9. *a, c*

10. *a*

11. *b, c*

12. True

13. False; psoriatic arthritis generally tends to be much less debilitating than rheumatoid arthritis.

14. True

15. True

CHAPTER 67

Polymyositis, dermatomyositis, and progressive systemic sclerosis (scleroderma)

1. Polymyositis and dermatomyositis affect females twice as often as males.

2. The therapeutic program for polymyositis and dermatomysitis includes rest, particularly during the acute and active phase. Corticosteroids (40 to 60 mg per day) should be promptly instituted. The corticosteriods can be reduced as muscle strength improves and muscle enzymes approach normal levels. Immunosuppressive medication may be considered if the illness does not respond to steroid therapy. Occupational and physical therapy are instituted for maintenance of range of motion in joints, for prevention of contractures, and for adaptation to alterations in activities of daily living.

3. Scleroderma affects the body's connective tissue. It is characterized by fibrosis and degenerative changes in the skin. Fibrosis and degenerative changes are also seen in the synovium, digital arteries, and parenchyma and small arteries of the esophagus, intestine, lungs, heart, kidney, and thyroid gland.

4. Pulmonary function can be impaired because of the inflamed intercostal muscles (exertional dyspnea).

5. Persons with progressive systemic sclerosis will need to protect themselves from exposure of their

hands to cold in order to decrease the frequency of attacks of Raynaud's phenomenon. Low doses of corticosteroids may relieve joint complaints but are usually not of great benefit for treatment of PSS. Nonsteroidal anti-inflammatory agents can be used to increase comfort. Antibiotics have been used with some success in the treatment of small-bowel involvement. Physical therapy is important and can decrease or prevent contractures.

6. *b*

7. *c*

8. *a, c, d*

9. *b*

10. *b*

11. *b*

12. *a, c, d*

13. *c*

14. *b*

15. True

16. True

17. False; radiographic studies of PSS may demonstrate subcutaneous calcifications of the digits of the hand.

CHAPTER 68

Systemic lupus erythematosus (SLE)

1. *Systemic lupus erythematosus (SLE)* is a multisystem, chronic, autoimmune disease. The signs and symptoms of this disorder can be diverse and transitory.

2. The antinuclear antibody (ANA) test indicates whether there are antibodies capable of destroying the nucleus of the subject's own body cells. In addition to the presence of ANA, the ANA pattern and the specific antibodies are evaluated. The LE factor test may occasionally be used today to identify the lupus erythematosus factor. The LE cell is formed by damage to some of a person's white cells, causing release of their nucleoprotein, which reacts with IgG; this complex is phagocytosed by the remaining white cells. The resulting cell is easily identified.

3. The onset of SLE occurs most frequently during late adolescence and early adulthood in females. Counseling is needed to assist those affected regarding the decision about having children. Pregnancy may cause a flare-up of SLE which can be danger-

ous for women with renal damage. Cytotoxic drugs may be necessary in order to control the illness, and these can affect the fetus. Contraceptives, which include birth control pills cannot be prescribed, since they may aggravate SLE.

4. Just how the sun causes SLE to flare up is not fully understood. One explanation is that DNA exposed to ultraviolet light normally becomes antigenic, and this leads to the flares seen after sun exposure.

5. The selection of appropriate drug therapy depends upon the specific organs affected by the illness. NSAIDs are used to control the arthritis and arthralgia. Aspirin is used less frequently, because it produces the highest incidence of hepatotoxicity, and some people with SLE have hepatic involvement.

6. *c*

7. *a*

8. *a*

9. *b, c*

10. *c*

11. True

12. False; cyclophosphamide or azathioprine can be used in an effort to suppress the autoimmune activity of SLE.

13. False; lupus nephritis occurs in over 65 percent of those with SLE.

14. False; DNA is antigenic to humans in SLE.

CHAPTER 69

Gout

1. *Gout* is a term used for a group of at least nine metabolic disorders that are characterized by an elevation in the serum uric acid concentration (hyperuricemia).

2. Primary gout is the direct result of the body's overproduction or decreased excretion of uric acid. Secondary gout occurs when the overproduction or decreased excretion of uric acid is secondary to another disease process or to medication.

3. Colchicine is a drug that inhibits phagocytic leukocytes and produces a dramatic and rapid relief of the symptoms of gout.

4. The factors that contribute to the development of gout are dependent upon the cause of the hyperuricemia. For example, a diet high in purines can

trigger a gouty attack in a person with one of the inborn errors of purine metabolism. The ingestion of alcohol can produce a gouty attack because blood lactate levels increase as a by-product of the normal metabolism of alcohol. Lactic acid blocks the renal excretion of uric acid, with a concomitant rise in serum levels.

5. The treatment of chronic gout is based upon decreasing the production of uric acid or increasing the renal excretion of uric acid.

6. *b*

7. *d*

8. *c*

9. *a, b, d*

10. *b*

11. *a*

12. *b*

13. *b,d*

CHAPTER 70

Degenerative joint disease (osteoarthritis)

1. *Degenerative joint disease* (DJD, osteoarthritis, hypertrophic arthritis, osteoarthrosis) is a disorder of the movable joints. The disorder is chronic, slowly progressive, and noninflammatory and is characterized by the deterioration and abrasion of articular cartilage and the formation of new bone at the articular surface.

2. The synthesis of proteoglycans and collagen in the joint is greatly increased in DJD. There is a net loss or proteoglycans and collagen over time, since degradation is even more rapid.

3. The aging process seems to be related to the development and progression of DJD through changes in chondrocyte functioning. Chondrocytes are the cells responsible for the formation of the proteoglycans and collagen in the articular cartilage. The aging chrondrocytes may lose their ability to function appropriately.

4. Total joint replacements for hips and knees have been successful in maintaining near normal function for many people with DJD. DJD is a hypertrophic from of arthritis, that is, the bone adjacent to the joint is strong, forming an excellent base for attachment of the artificial joint. A number of complications can occur with joint replacement, and these must be weighed against the benefits.

5. Narrowing of the joint space is commonly seen in DJD because of loss of cartilage. Radiologic findings also reveal an increase in bone density around the joint. Cystic changes of various sizes are sometimes

seen. Osteophytes (spurs) can be seen at the marginal aspects of the joint.

6. The goals of the treatment of DJD are retardation or prevention of further damage to the joint and management of pain and stiffness in order to maintain mobility.

7. *a, c, d*

8. *d*

9. *d*

10. *c*

11. *a, b, c*

12. False; DJD is a noninflammatory disease.

13. False; erosive inflammatory DJD affects primarily the finger joints.

14. False; oral corticosteroids are contraindicated in the treatment of DJD.

15. False; no specific blood tests are used in the diagnosis of DJD.

CHAPTER 71

The structure and functions of the skin

1. *a, b, d*

2. *a, b, c*

3. *c, d*

4. *b*

5. The basal layer consists largely of undifferentiated cells which undergo constant mitoses, renewing the epidermis. One of the daughter cells migrates outward toward the stratum spinosum. These undifferentiated basal-layer cells are precursors of keratinocytes. Keratinocytes migrate upward through the stratum granulosum to the stratum corneum to form a fibrous-amorphous complex surrounded by a reinforced impermeable membrane, the horny cell.

6. Eccrine glands produce a hypotonic solution and allow excess heat to be eliminated from the body, which aids in maintaining appropriate temperature. Sebaceous glands produce sebum, which lubricates the epidermis.

7. (a) Skin should be examined in a well-illuminated room, preferably in natural daylight. (b) Color should be recorded (e.g., purplish, cyanotic discoloration, pallor). (c) Skin characteristics such as turgor and elasticity on palpation should be noted. (d) Hair distribution and condition of nails should be recorded.

8. The subcutaneous layer provides a cushion for the skin, insulation to maintain body heat, and a store of energy.

9. True

10. True

11. True

12. False; hair is composed of dead keratin, not living keratinocytes.

13. True

14. True

15. False; blacks have large melanosomes which resist destruction by the hydrolyzing enzymes; whites have smaller melanosomes which are easily destroyed.

16. Refer to Fig. 71-8.

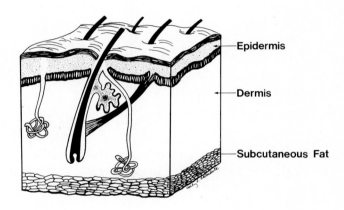

CHAPTER 72

Acne and related conditions

1. *Acne* is a chronic inflammatory process of the sebaceous glands.

2. Acne generally occurs among adolescents and young adults and spontaneously resolves around 20 to 30 years of age.

3. The earliest lesion is the comedo. White comedones are likely to progress to the inflammatory papules and pustules of acne. Black comedones obstruct the flow of sebum to the surface. The sebum, bacteria, and fatty acids are thought to be responsible for the development of inflammation around the pilosebaceous ducts and sebaceous glands. This inflammation leads to the formation of papules, inflammatory pustules, and cysts. The cysts open in time, drain, and heal. Deeper papules and cysts can leave permanent scars, while mild acne resolves without scarring.

4. (a) To remove the surface oil and to dislodge some comedones. (b) Tetracycline. This antibiotic elim-

inates *Propionibacterium acnes* in the sebaceous gland. Tetracycline has an inhibitory effect on the enzyme lipase, thus preventing breakdown of fat into fatty acids. (*c*) Dermabrasion is used to smooth and plane the scars and pits that develop as a result of acne.

5. (*a*) Frequently a family history of acne, especially cystic acne, can be obtained. (*b*) Topically oil-base makeup, external oils, and moisturizing creams can exacerbate acne. (*c*) Systemic corticosteroids, iodides, and/or Dilantin can also aggravate the condition.

6. *c*

7. *d*

8. *e*

9. *b*

CHAPTER 73

Eczema; vascular disorders

1. The characteristic lesions of eczema are pruritic, erythematous, crusty, weepy, and scaly eruptions. Acute eczema presents with many vesicles and bullae and with erythema, weeping, and crusting, whereas chronic eczema presents with thickened (lichenified), scaly, pruritic patches and plaques.

2. (*a*) Skin reaction to the oil of poison ivy, (*b*) nickel sensitivity, (*c*) allergic reaction to potassium and dichromate, (*d*) allergic reaction to shoes which contain rubber, (*e*) allergic reaction to medications such as neomycin or benzocaine

3. Dyshidrotic hand eczema occurs in persons who must wash their hands frequently or are under stress. It is exacerbated by water, detergents, and stress.

4. Generalized neurodermatitis is caused by compulsive scratching of pruritic skin. It may be localized to the neck or scrotum or may occur anywhere on the body.

5. Virtually all drugs can cause acute urticaria, but the most common are aspirin, laxatives, and antibiotics.

6. *b*

7. *b*

8. True

9. False, skin tests are of no use in the evaluation of urticaria.

10. True

CHAPTER 74

Psoriasis and pityriasis rosea

1. Psoriasis is an inherited disease. A family history of psoriasis is found in 66 percent of psoriasis patients. The histocompatibility (HLA) antigens HLA-B13 and HLA-B17 are increased fourfold in persons with psoriasis. Environmental factors play a significant role in the disease.

2. The latest treatment combines the use of psoralen, an oral photosensitizing medication, with long ultraviolet light (PUVA). This treatment is contraindicated in patients with a history of x-ray treatment, skin cancer, or cataracts.

3. A psoriatic skin biopsy reveals thickened epidermis and stratum corneum and dilated upper dermal blood vessels. The number of basal cells undergoing mitosis is increased. These fast-dividing cells move rapidly to the suface of thickened epidermis. This rapid proliferation and migration of epidermal cells results in thick epidermis covered by a thick keratin (silvery scale). Abnormal levels of cyclic nucleotides, especially cyclic AMP and GMP may be partially responsible for this rapid mitosis of epidermal cells. Prostaglandins and polyamines are also possibly abnormal in the disease. The role of these abnormalities in influencing the formation of a psoriatic plaque is not clearly understood.

4. *b*

5. *b, c*

6. *d*

7. *c*

CHAPTER 75

Cutaneous infections

1. *b*

2. *c*

3. *b*

4. *b*

5. *b*

6. *c*

7. *b*

8. *c*

9. False; the description refers to infection with *Candida albicans*. Tinea versicolor produces sharply marginated, scaly white or brownish patches over the trunk, neck, and extremities.

10. True

11. True

12. True

13. False; impetigo is the most common bacterial infection of the skin.

14. Type 1 herpes simplex usually affects the lips, mouth, nose, and cheeks. Type II herpes usually infects the genital areas.

15. The diagnosis of herpes can be confirmed by a positive herpetic culture in about 80 percent of cases. Another test is the Tzank test, which is positive in 50 to 80 percent of patients with herpes. In this test the material from the vesicle is placed on a glass slide and stained with 1 percent toluidine blue. Large multinucleated giant cells can be seen in patients with herpes. This test can be performed in a few minutes; it is cheaper than a herpetic culture.

16. At present there is no vaccine to prevent herpes infections from recurring. Recurrent episodes of herpes of the lips can sometimes be prevented by use of opaque sunscreens or avoidance of exposure to sun. Sexual spread of genital herpes is frequently aborted by use of rubber condoms when vesicles are present and for 7 days afterward. Sexual abstinence when vesicles are present is an alternative method of prevention. Towels, underclothing, and swimming suits should not be shared.

17. (a) A primary herpes simplex infection can cause severe conjunctivitis. (b) The relationship of herpes progenitalis to cancer is highly controversial.

18. Impetigo first appears as a purulent lesion. As the lesion spreads, it becomes eroded, and a golden crust develops on the surface.

19. Impetigo is caused by streptococci and staphylococci. The infection is transferred by human-to-human contact, usually among children. Heat, humidity, and poor hygiene predispose to this infection. Erysipelas, on the other hand, is a serious toxic infection of the skin. The patient has a high fever, malaise, and is toxic.

10. Poor hygiene and excoriations.

CHAPTER 76

Tumors of the skin

1. (a) Characteristic of malignant melanoma is an irregular pigmented lesion with shades of blue, purple, red, and brown. The borders of the tumor are irregular, and the surface is frequently ulcerated. Satellite lesions and diffusion of pigment into the surrounding skin are also observed. (b) The etiology of melanoma is not understood. Exposure to sunlight is an important factor. Approximately 2 percent of all melanomas are familial. (c) Prognosis is determined by the depth of invasion, thickness of the tumor, area of the body surface, clinical variant of melanoma, and presence of lymphatic involve-

ment at the time of diagnosis. (d) Melanoma is treated surgically. A wide cutaneous resection with or without the regional node resection is usually performed. Disseminated melanoma is treated with chemotherapy or immunotherapy.

2. Basal cell carcinoma can be derived from multiple cell types in the skin. This tumor rarely metastasizes. The most common sites of occurrence are on the sun-exposed areas of the face, head, and neck.

3. The preventive measures for patients with a history of skin cancer and for fair skinned individuals are sunscreens, sunblocks, and avoidance of excess sunlight.

4. Treatment includes curettage with electrodesiccation, scalpel surgery, irradiation, or cryosurgery.

5. Squamous cell carcinoma is a tumor which also can be derived from multiple cell types in the skin. This tumor develops in older, fair-skinned persons. The tumor usually presents as an ulcerated, hyperkeratotic nodule with evidence of dermal invasion on palpation. Squamous cell carcinoma of the skin arising in sun-exposed areas rarely mestastasizes. This cancer is treated with scalpel surgery, electrodesiccation with curettage, or irradiation.

6. c

7. All are correct.

8. b

9. b

10. c

11. d

12. f

13. a

14. e

15. b

16. d

CHAPTER 77

Venereal diseases and infestations

1. The causative organism is *Treponema pallidum.*

2. A painless chancre develops at the site of direct contact after a period of 10 to 90 days. It heals spontaneously after 3 to 12 weeks. In primary syphilis the VDRL test is positive in only 50 percent of cases, whereas the FTA-ABS test is positive in 90 percent of cases. In approximately 6 weeks to 6 months, brownish papules and macules with a

slight scale appear. These eruptions classically occur over the palms and soles. Moist, flat, wartlike condylomata lata can appear over the genitalia. In secondary syphilis the VDRL and FTA-ABS tests are almost always positive. The lesions of secondary syphilis heal in 4 to 12 weeks, and the patient enters the latent stage. During the first 4 years about 25 percent of these patients have recurrences of the secondary syphilis lesions. Tertiary syphilis occurs in about 30 percent of untreated cases. Complications such as gummas occur in 17 percent of untreated cases, cardiovascular complications in 10 percent, and neurosyphilis in 10 percent.

3. Primary, secondary, and latent stages are treated with a single injection of 2.4 million units of benzathine penicillin G; the tertiary stage is treated with 7.2 to 9.6 million units divided in four weekly doses.

4. Treatment of localized urethral or cervical gonorrhea is IM procaine penicillin—4.8 million units with 1 g of oral probenecid. Recently oral ampicillin in combination with probenecid has been effective in disseminated gonorrhea. Tetracycline, spectinomycin, ampicillin, and erythromycin are other antibiotics effective in the treatment of gonorrhea.

5. Acquired immune deficiency syndrome (AIDS) is a clinical diagnosis. Patients with AIDS have opportunistic infections and/or cancer. AIDS is seen in homosexual or bisexual men (73 percent of U.S. cases), past or present intravenous drug abusers (17 percent), hemophiliac persons, Haitians, sexual partners of persons at increased risk, and infants born to parents at increased risk. AIDS is transmitted through heterosexual or homosexual intercourse or through blood. A cause of AIDS is a T-lymphotropic virus, Type III, (HTV-III) with an incubation period varying from 6 months to 5 years. Patients develop diarrhea, lymphadenopathy, fever, fatigue, opportunistic infections of the lungs usually from *pneumocystis carinii*, and disseminated cytomegalovirus infections. Localized symptoms are frequently cutaneous. A neoplasm called *Kaposi's sarcoma* presents with purplish hemorrhagic patches, plaques, and nodules. Anogenital herpes appears with persistent chronic ulcerations over the penis, vulva, or buttocks. There is no effective treatment, but two experimental drugs (interleukin-2 and gamma interferon) have been used. The major steps to prevent spread of AIDS are sexual precautions, not sharing blood-contaminated objects, and careful screening of blood donors.

6. *b*
7. *b*
8. *b*
9. *a, b*
10. *a, b, c*
11. *a, b, c*
12. True
13. True
14. True

INDEX